CLINICAL MANIFESTATIONS AND ASSESSMENT OF RESPIRATORY DISEASE

CLINICAL MANIFESTATIONS AND ASSESSMENT OF RESPIRATORY DISEASE

Seventh Edition

Terry Des Jardins, MEd, RRT

Professor Emeritus
Former Director
Department of Respiratory Care
Parkland College
Champaign, Illinois
Faculty/Staff Member
University of Illinois College of Medicine at Urbana-Champaign, Illinois

George G. Burton, MD, FACP, FCCP, FAARC

Associate Dean for Medical Affairs
Kettering College
Kettering, Ohio
Clinical Professor of Medicine and Anesthesiology
Wright State University School of Medicine
Dayton, Ohio

Medical Illustrations by

Timothy H. Phelps, MS, FAMI, CMI

Associate Professor
Johns Hopkins University School of Medicine
Baltimore, Maryland

ELSEVIER

ELSEVIER

3251 Riverport Lane
St. Louis, Missouri 63043

Executive Content Strategist: Sonya Seigafuse
Content Development Manager: Billie Sharp
Content Development Specialist: Charlene Ketchum
Publishing Services Manager: Julie Eddy
Senior Project Manager: Celeste Clingan
Design Direction: Renée Duenow

Printed in Canada

Last digit is the print number: 9 8 7 6 5 4 3 2

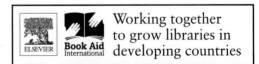

To

Thomas J. DeKornfeld, MD

and

In Memory of Glen N. Gee, RRT

and

Robert (Bob) L. Wilkins, PhD, RRT

Thought Leaders, Innovators, Master Teachers
in the Field of Respiratory Care

Terry Des Jardins, MEd, RRT
George G. Burton, MD

There is a manpower shortage of health-care providers who care for the critically ill. This is one of the most pressing issues affecting the future of our aging population and American medicine … it has been generally acknowledged…that the shortages in nursing, respiratory care practitioners, and pharmacists have already reached crisis levels…a severe shortage of (pulmonary/critical care physicians) can be expected in the very near future.[1]

> *"Respiratory therapists are important for patient outcomes* and their roles might even be expanded beyond traditional boundaries. *More research is needed to define the ICU multidisciplinary staffing that matches patient needs and optimizes patient outcomes."*[2]

Shortfalls in the pulmonary and critical care physician workforce are estimated to be at least 38% and 22%, respectively, by 2020. Advanced Practice Registered Nurses (APRNs) and Physician Assistants (PAs) are now so entrenched in the medical services, they are allowed to act as primary care providers (PCPs), managing everything from diabetes mellitus to heart failure. However, at the time of this writing, the respiratory care profession is in the process of developing a worker with credentials and practice privileges similar to the APRN and PA, who will be designated as an Advanced Practice Respiratory Therapist (APRT). In the final analysis, respiratory therapists (RTs) are the only ancillary medical professionals with comprehensive training in all aspects of pulmonary medicine, including education and management of patients with chronic lung disease.[3,4]

These issues will drive the growth of the respiratory care profession into the twenty-first century: an aging population with complex health-care issues, ever more complex and expensive respiratory care technologies, and concern to find the most cost-effective way to face these challenges. It will become increasing clear to respiratory therapy professionals at all levels that pathophysiology drives intelligent therapy, in a very dynamic fashion! What an exciting time for the profession!

---

[1]Irwin RS, Marcus L, Lever A: The Critical Care Professional Societies address the critical care crisis in the United States, *Chest* 125:1512-1513, 2004.

[2]Kelly MA, Angus D, Chalfin DB, et al: The Critical Care Crisis in the United States, *Chest* 125: 1514-1517, 2004.

[3]Fuhrman TM, Aranson R: Point: Should Medicare allow Respiratory Therapists to Independently Practice and Bill for Educational Activities Related to COPD? Yes. *Chest* 145(2):210-213, 2014.

[4]Barnes TA et al: Transitioning the Respiratory Therapy Workforce from 2015 and Beyond. *Resp Care* 56(5):681-690, 2011.

Preface

The use of **therapist-driven protocols** (**TDPs**)—now often called simply **respiratory protocols** is an integral part of respiratory health services. TDPs provide the much-needed flexibility to respiratory care practitioners and increases the quality of health care. This is because the respiratory therapy can be modified easily and efficiently according to the needs of the patient.

Essential cornerstones to the success of a TDP program are (1) the quality of the respiratory therapist's assessment skills at the bedside and (2) the ability to transfer objective clinical data into a treatment plan that follows agreed-upon guidelines. This textbook is designed to provide the student with the fundamental knowledge and understanding necessary to assess and treat patients with respiratory diseases in order to meet these objectives.

Part I of the textbook, entitled *Assessment of Respiratory Disease*, contains three sections:

Section I, entitled *Clinical Data Obtained at the Patient's Bedside*, consists of two chapters. Chapter 1 describes the knowledge and skills involved in the patient interview. Chapter 2 provides the knowledge and skills needed for the physical examination. This chapter also presents a more in-depth discussion of the pathophysiologic basis for the clinical manifestations associated with respiratory diseases.

Section II, entitled *Clinical Data Obtained from Laboratory Tests and Special Procedures*, is composed of Chapters 3 through 8. Collectively, these chapters provide the reader with the essential knowledge and understanding base for the assessment of pulmonary function studies, arterial blood gases, oxygenation, the cardiovascular system (including hemodynamic monitoring), the radiologic examination of the chest, and important laboratory tests and procedures.

Section III, entitled *The Therapist-Driven Protocol Program— The Essentials*, consists of Chapters 9, 10, and 11.

Chapter 9, entitled *The Therapist-Driven Protocol Program and the Role of the Respiratory Care Practitioner,* provides the reader with the essential knowledge base and step-by-step process needed to assess and implement protocols in the clinical setting. The student is provided with the basic knowledge and helpful tools to (1) gather clinical data systematically, (2) formulate an assessment (i.e., the cause and severity of the patient's condition), (3) select an appropriate and cost-effective treatment plan, and (4) document these essential steps clearly and precisely. At the end of each respiratory disorder chapter, one or more representative case studies demonstrate appropriate TDP assessment and treatment strategies.

Chapter 9 is a cornerstone chapter to the fundamentals necessary for good assessment and critical-thinking skills. The case studies presented at the end of each respiratory disorder chapter often directs the reader back to chapter 9. Note: In the electronic version, there will be a special icon highlighting the protocols featured in this chapter instead of the red bar.

Chapter 10, entitled *Respiratory Failure and Mechanical Ventilation Protocols*, is a new chapter to the 7th edition of this textbook. This chapter describes how respiratory failure can be classified as either (1) hypoxemic (type I) respiratory failure, (2) hypercapnic (type II) respiratory failure, or (3) a combination of both. These categories reflect the pathophysiologic basis of respiratory failure. In addition, this chapter provides the components of mechanical ventilation protocols—including the standard criteria for mechanical ventilation, the clinical indicators for both hypercapnic and hypoxemic respiratory failure, ventilatory support strategies for noninvasive and invasive mechanical ventilation, a mechanical ventilator management protocol, and a mechanical ventilation weaning protocol.

Chapter 11, entitled *Recording Skills: The Basis for Data Collection, Organization, Assessment Skills* provides the basic foundation needed to collect and record respiratory assessments and treatment plans.

Parts II through **XII** (Chapters 12 through 44) provide the reader with essential information regarding common respiratory diseases. Each chapter adheres to the following format: a description of the anatomic alterations of the lungs, etiology of the disease process, an overview of the cardiopulmonary clinical manifestations associated with the disorder, management of the respiratory disorder, one or more case studies, and a brief set of self-assessment questions.

Anatomic Alterations of the Lungs

Each respiratory disease chapter begins with a detailed, colored illustration showing the major anatomic alterations of the lungs associated with the disorder. Although a serious effort has been made to illustrate each disorder accurately at the beginning of each chapter, artistic license ("cartooning") has been taken to emphasize certain anatomic points and pathologic processes. The material that follows this section in each respiratory disorder chapter discusses the disease in terms of the following:

(1) The common pathophysiologic mechanisms activated throughout the respiratory system as a result of the anatomic alterations

(2) The clinical manifestations that develop as a result of the pathophysiologic mechanisms, and

(3) The basic respiratory therapy modalities used to improve the anatomic alterations and pathophysiologic mechanisms caused by the disease.

When the anatomic alterations and pathophysiologic mechanisms caused by the disorder are improved, the clinical manifestations also should improve.

Etiology

A discussion of the etiology of the disease follows the presentation of anatomic alterations of the lungs. Various causes, predisposing conditions, and common co-morbidities are described.

Overview of the Cardiopulmonary Clinical Manifestations Associated With the Disorder

This section comprises the central theme of the text. The reader is provided with the clinical manifestations commonly associated with the disease under discussion. In essence, the student is given a general "overview" of the signs and symptoms commonly demonstrated by the patient. By having a working knowledge—and, therefore, a predetermined expectation—of the clinical manifestations associated with a specific respiratory disorder, the respiratory therapist is in a better position to:

(1) Gather clinical data relevant to the patient's respiratory status,

(2) Formulate an objective—and measurable—respiratory assessment, and

(3) Develop an effective and safe treatment plan that is based on a valid assessment.

If the appropriate data are not gathered and assessed correctly, the ability to treat the patient effectively is lost. As mentioned earlier, the case studies presented at the end of each respiratory disorder chapter frequently refer the reader back to chapter 9 for a broader discussion of the signs and symptoms commonly associated with the disease under discussion—the "clinical scenario." When a particular clinical manifestation is unique to the respiratory disorder, however, a discussion of the pathophysiologic mechanisms responsible for the signs and symptoms is presented in the respective chapter.

Because of the dynamic nature of many respiratory disorders, the reader should note the following regarding this section:

- Because the severity of the disease is influenced by a number of factors (e.g., the extent of the disease, age, the general health of the patient), the clinical manifestations may vary considerably from one patient to another. In fact, they may vary in the same patient from one *time* to another. Therefore the practitioner should understand that the patient may demonstrate *all* the clinical manifestations presented or just a *few*.

  In addition, many of the clinical manifestations associated with a respiratory disorder may never appear in some patients (e.g., digital clubbing, cor pulmonale, increased hemoglobin level). As a general rule, however, the prototypical patient usually demonstrates most of the manifestations presented during the advanced stages of the disease.

- For a variety of practical reasons, some of the clinical manifestations presented in each chapter may not actually be measured (or measurable) in the clinical setting (e.g., age, mental status, severity of the disorder). They are nevertheless conceptually important and therefore are presented here through extrapolation. For example, the newborn with severe infant respiratory distress syndrome, who obviously has a restrictive lung disorder as a result of the anatomic alterations associated with the disease, cannot actually perform the maneuvers necessary for a pulmonary function study.

- It should be noted that the clinical manifestations presented in each chapter are based only on the *one respiratory disorder under discussion*. In the clinical setting, the patient often has a combination of respiratory problems (e.g., emphysema compromised by pneumonia) and may have manifestations related to each of the pulmonary disorders.

This section does not attempt to present the "absolute" pathophysiologic bases for the development of a particular clinical manifestation. Because of the dynamic nature of many respiratory diseases, the precise cause of some of the manifestations presented by the patient is not always clear. In most cases, however, the primary pathophysiologic mechanisms responsible for the various signs and symptoms are known and understood and are described herein.

Management or Treatment of the Disease

Each chapter provides a general overview of the more common therapeutic modalities (treatment protocols) used to offset the anatomic alterations and pathophysiologic mechanisms activated by a particular disorder.

Although several respiratory therapy modalities may be safe and effective in treating a respiratory disorder, the respiratory therapist must have a clear conception of the following:

1. How the therapies work to offset the anatomic alterations of the lungs caused by the disease

2. How the correction of the anatomic alterations of the lungs work to offset the pathophysiologic mechanisms

3. How the correction of the pathophysiologic mechanisms works to offset the clinical manifestations demonstrated by the patient

Without this understanding, the practitioner merely goes through the motions of performing therapeutic tasks with no anticipated or measurable outcomes.*

---

*The reader should understand that this book is not a respiratory pharmacology text. Its emphasis is on the appropriate modalities to be used rather than specific pharmacological agents.

Case Study

The case study at the end of each respiratory disease chapter provides the reader with a realistic example of (1) the manner in which the patient may arrive in the hospital with the disorder under discussion, (2) the various clinical manifestations commonly associated with the disease, (3) the way the clinical manifestations can be gathered, organized, and documented, (4) the way an assessment of the patient's respiratory status is formulated from the clinical manifestations, and (5) the way a comprehensive treatment plan is developed from the assessment.

In essence, the case study provides the reader with a good example of the way in which the respiratory care practitioner would gather clinical data, make an assessment, and treat a patient with the disorder under discussion. In addition, many of the case studies presented in the text describe a respiratory therapist assessing and treating the patient several times—demonstrating the importance of serial assessment and the way therapy is often up-regulated or down-regulated on a moment-to-moment basis in the clinical setting.

References

A list of literature references for each chapter is provided on the Evolve site. The student is encouraged to review these selected references, especially the "state-of-the-art" references regarding the respiratory disorders discussed throughout the textbook.

Self-Assessment Questions

Each disease chapter concludes with a set of self-assessment questions. At the end of self-assessment section, the student is provided the following message:

> *To access additional student assessment questions for application of text material to real-life scenarios, the student may go to the*

following Student Resource web site: http://evolve.elsevier.com/DesJardins/respiratory

Glossary and Appendices

Finally, a glossary and appendices are provided at the end of the text. The appendices include the following:

- A table of symbols and abbreviations commonly used in respiratory physiology
- Medications commonly used in the treatment of cardiopulmonary disorders, including the following:
  - Aerosolized bronchodilators
  - Mucolytic agents
  - Aersolized anti-inflammatory agents
  - Xanthine bronchodilators
  - Expectorants
  - Antibiotic agents
  - Positive inotropic agents
  - Diuretics
- The ideal alveolar gas equation
- Physiologic dead space calculation
- Units of measurement
- Poiseuille's law
- $PCO_2/HCO_3^-/pH$ nomogram
- Calculated hemodynamic measurements
- DuBois body surface area chart
- Cardiopulmonary profile

Approach

In writing this textbook, we have tried to present a realistic balance between the often esoteric language of pathophysiology and the simple, straight-to-the-point approach generally preferred by busy students.

Terry Des Jardins, MEd, RRT
George G. Burton, MD

Acknowledgments

Several people have provided important contributions to the development of the seventh edition of this textbook. First, for their exceptional input, suggestions, and guidance regarding all the Newborn and Early Childhood Respiratory Disorders, a very special thank you goes out to Dr. Robert J. Fink, Director of Pulmonary Medicine, and Sue Ciarlariello, Director of Respiratory Care/Transport/Sleep Center, at Dayton Children's Hospital, Dayton, Ohio. In addition, the folks at Dayton Children's Hospital helped to secure a number of outstanding items for this new edition—including numerous x-rays, clinical pictures, clinical charts and forms, and—importantly—the Newborn/Pediatric Protocols, which now appear in Chapter 32. The addition of these new protocols will, undoubtedly, enhance the respiratory therapist's ability to understand and better develop effective and safe respiratory treatment plans.

For his important suggestions and guidance in the development of our new Congenital Heart Diseases, Chapter 40, we wish to extend a sincere thank you to James Sills. For his outstanding artistic skills, we are thankful to Timothy H. Phelps, Associate Professor, Johns Hopkins University School of Medicine, Baltimore, Maryland, for his work on the new colored illustrations in our new Respiratory Failure and Mechanical Ventilation Protocols chapter (Chapter 10) and our Congenital Heart Disease chapter (Chapter 40). Tim's artistic skills to capture and visually illustrate the various complex subjects described in the textbook have truly enhanced the readability of this textbook. For example, the reader will now be able to easily visualize and understand the anatomic changes that occur in the following heart disorders: Patent Ductus Ateriosus, Atrial Septal Defect, Ventricular Septal Defect, Tetralogy of Fallot, and Transposition of the Great Arteries. In addition, we wish to extend a special thank you to Jeanne Robertson for the more than 30 new black and white and colored illustrations found throughout this new edition.

For their very thorough edits, reviews, and helpful suggestions regarding the depth, breadth, and accuracy of the content presented in this textbook, we thank Suellen Carmody-Menzer, Norma Driscoll, Lindsay Fox, Mary Marcia Fuller, Jill Sand, James R. Sills, and Richard Wettstein. In addition, a special thank you goes out to Robert Kacmarek for his review and edits for the common ventilatory management strategies used to treat specific disorders (good starting points) that we present in Chapter 10.

For their work in the development of the new student and instructor test banks, we are thankful to Trudy Watson, BS, RRT, AE-C, FAARC and Gayle Carr. Great job! Finally, we are very grateful to the team at Elsevier: Content Coordinator, Billie Sharp; Content Development Specialist, Charlene Ketchum; and Senior Project Manager Celeste Clingan. Their work and helpful coordination during the long development of this textbook, and supplemental student and instructor website packages associated with this book, has been most appreciated.

Terry Des Jardins, MEd, RRT
George G. Burton, MD

Contents

PART II

Obstructive Lung Disease, *169*

PART III

Infectious Pulmonary Diseases, *251*

Introduction

The Assessment Process— An Overview

Assessment is (1) the process of collecting clinical information about the patient's health status, (2) the evaluation of the data and identification of the specific problems, concerns, and needs of the patient, and (3) the development of a treatment plan that can be managed by the health-care provider. The clinical information gathered may consist of subjective and objective data (signs and symptoms) about the patient, the results of diagnostic tests and procedures, the patient's response to therapy, and the patient's general health practices.

The first step in the assessment process is **THINKING**—even before the actual collection of clinical data begins. In other words, the practitioner must first "think" about why the patient has entered the health-care facility and about what clinical data will likely need to be collected. Merely obtaining answers to a specific list of questions does not serve the assessment process well. For example, while en route to evaluate a patient who is said to be having an asthmatic episode, the health-care practitioner might mentally consider the following: What are the likely signs and symptoms that can be observed at the bedside during a moderate or severe asthmatic attack? What are the usual emotional responses? What are the anatomic alterations associated with an asthma episode that would be responsible for the signs and symptoms observed? Table 1 presents a broader overview of what the practitioner might think about before assessing a patient said to be having an asthmatic episode.

To collect data wisely, health-care providers must have well-developed skills in observing and listening. In addition, the practitioner must apply his or her mental skills of translation, reason, intuition, and validation to render the clinical data meaningful. Clinically, the collection of data is more useful when the evaluation process is organized into common problem areas, or categories. As the practitioner gathers information in each problem category, a clustering of related data about the patient will be generated. This framework for collecting clinical information enhances the practitioner's ability to establish priorities of care. Furthermore, any time the health-care provider interacts with the patient, for any reason, an assessment of the patient's problems, needs, and concerns should be made. To efficiently and correctly gather data, the health-care provider must make decisions about what type of assessment is needed, how to obtain the data, the framework and focus of the assessment, and what additional data may be needed before a complete treatment plan can be developed.

Purpose of Assessment

Relative to the purpose, an assessment may involve asking just two or three specific questions or it may involve an in-depth conversation with the patient. An assessment may involve a comprehensive focus (head-to-toe assessment) or a specific or narrow focus. The purpose of the assessment may include any of the following:

- To obtain a baseline databank about the patient's physical and mental status
- To supplement, verify, or refute any previous data
- To identify actual and potential problems
- To obtain data that will help the practitioner establish an assessment and treatment plan
- To focus on specific problems
- To determine immediate needs and to establish priorities
- To determine the cause (etiology) of the problem
- To determine any related or contributing factors; e.g., comorbidities
- To identify patient strengths as a basis for changing behavior
- To identify the risk for complications
- To recognize complications

Types of Assessment

There are four major types of assessment: initial, focused, emergency, and ongoing.

The *initial assessment* is conducted at the first encounter with the patient. In the hospitalized patient, the initial assessment is typically performed by the admitting nurse and is more comprehensive than subsequent assessments. It starts with the reasons that prompted the patient to seek care and it entails a holistic overview of the patient's health-care needs. The general objective of the initial assessment is to rule out as well as to identify (rule in) specific problems. The initial assessment most commonly occurs when the patient has sought medical services for a specific problem or desires a general health status examination. The goals of the initial assessment include prevention, maintenance, restoration, or rehabilitation. In general, the thoroughness of the initial assessment is directly related to the length of expected care. Discharge planning should begin at the time of the initial assessment!

The *focused assessment* consists of a detailed examination of the specific problem areas, or patient complaints. The focused assessment looks at clinical data in detail, considers possible causes, looks at possible contributing factors, and examines the patient's personal characteristics that will help—or hinder—the problem. The focused assessment also is used when the patient describes or manifests a new problem. Common patient complaints include pain, shortness of breath, dizziness, and fatigue. The practitioner must be

TABLE 1 Examples of What Might Be Considered Before Evaluating a Patient Having an Asthmatic Episode

Questions and/or Considerations	Likely Responses
What are the likely initial observations?	Shortness of breath, use of accessory muscles to breathe, intercostal retractions, pursed-lip breathing; cyanosis, barrel chest
What might be the patient's emotional response to his or her asthma?	Anxiety, concerned, frightened
What are the anatomic alterations of the lungs associated with asthma?	Bronchospasm; excessive, thick, white, & tenacious bronchial secretions; air trapping; mucus plugging
What are the known causes of asthma?	**Extrinsic factors:** pollen, grass, house dust, animal dander **Intrinsic factors:** infection, cold air, exercise, emotional stress
What are the expected vital signs?	Increased respiratory rate, heart rate, and blood pressure
What are the expected chest assessment findings?	Breath sounds: diminished, wheezing, crackles Percussion: hyperresonant
What are the expected pulmonary function study findings?	Decreased: $PEFR$, FEF_T, FEV_T/FVC Increased: RV, FRC
What are the expected acute arterial blood gas findings?	**Early stage:** Increased pH, decreased $PaCO_2$, decreased HCO_3^- (slightly), decreased PaO_2, decreased SaO_2 and SpO_2 **Late (severe) stage:** Decreased but normal pH, Increased $PaCO_2$, Increased HCO_3^- (slightly), decreased PaO_2, decreased SaO_2 and SpO_2
What are the expected chest radiograph findings?	Translucent lung fields; hyperinflated alveoli; depressed diaphragm
What are the usual respiratory treatments?	Bronchodilator therapy, bronchial hygiene therapy; oxygen therapy
What complications can occur?	Poor response to oxygen & bronchodilator therapy Acute ventilatory failure Severe hypoxia Mechanical ventilation

prepared to evaluate the severity of such problems, assess the possible cause, and determine the appropriate plan of action.

The *emergency assessment* identifies—or rules out—any life-threatening problems or problems that require immediate interventions. When the patient's medical condition is life threatening or when time is of the essence, the emergency assessment will include only key data needed for dealing with the immediate problem. Additional information can be gathered after the patient's condition has stabilized. The emergency assessment always follows the basic "ABCs" of cardiopulmonary resuscitation (i.e., the securing of the patient's *a*irway, *b*reathing, and *c*irculation).

The *ongoing assessment* consists of the data collection that occurs during each contact with the patient throughout the patient's hospital stay. Depending on the patient's condition, ongoing assessments may take place hourly, daily, weekly, or monthly. In fact, for the critically ill patient, assessments often take place continuously via electronic monitoring equipment. Ongoing assessments also take place while a patient is receiving anesthesia, as well as afterward until the effects of the anesthesia have worn off.

Respiratory therapist routinely make decisions about the frequency, depth, and breadth of the assessment requirements of the patient. To make these decisions effectively, the practitioner must anticipate the potential for a patient's condition to change, the speed at which it could change, and the clinical data that would justify a change. For example, when a patient experiencing an asthmatic episode inhales the aerosol of a selected bronchodilator, assessment decisions are based on the expected onset of drug action, expected therapeutic effects of the medication, and potential adverse effects that may develop.

Types of Data

Clinical information that is provided by the patient, and that cannot be observed directly, is called *subjective data*. When a patient's subjective data describe characteristics of a particular disorder or dysfunction, they are known as *symptoms*. For example, shortness of breath (dyspnea), pain, dizziness, nausea, and ringing in the ears are symptoms because they cannot be quantitated directly. The patient must communicate to the health-care provider what symptoms he or she is experiencing and rate them as to severity. The patient is the only source of information about subjective findings.

Characteristics about the patient that can be observed directly by the practitioner are called *objective data*. When a patient's objective data describe characteristics of a particular disorder or dysfunction, they are known as *signs*. For example, swelling of the legs (pedal edema) is a sign of congestive heart failure. Objective data can be obtained through the practitioner's sense of sight, hearing, taste, touch, and smell. Objective information can be measured (or quantified), and it can be replicated from one practitioner to another—a concept called *interrater reliability*. For example, the respiratory therapist can measure the patient's pulse, respiratory rate, blood pressure, inspiratory effort, and arterial blood gases. Because objective data are factual, they have a high degree of certainty.

Sources of Data

Sources of clinical information include the patient, the patient's significant others, other members of the health-care team, the patient's past history, and results of a variety of clinical tests and procedures. The practitioner must confirm that each data source is appropriate, reliable, and valid for the patient's assessment. *Appropriate* means the source is suitable for the specific purpose, patient, or event. *Reliable* means that the practitioner can trust the data to be accurate and honestly reported. *Valid* means that the clinical data can be verified or confirmed.

The Assessment Process—Role of the Respiratory Therapist

When the lungs are affected by disease or trauma, they are anatomically altered to some degree, depending on the severity of the process. In general, the anatomic alterations caused by an injury or disease process can be classified as resulting in an obstructive lung disorder, a restrictive lung disorder, or a combination of both. Common anatomic alterations associated with obstructive and restrictive lung disorders are illustrated in Figure 1. Common respiratory diseases and their general classifications are listed in Table 2.

When the normal anatomy of the lungs is altered, certain pathophysiologic mechanisms throughout the cardiopulmonary system are activated. These pathophysiologic mechanisms, in turn, produce a variety of clinical manifestations specific to the illness. Such clinical manifestations can be readily—and objectively—identified in the clinical setting (e.g., increased heart rate, depressed diaphragm, or an increased functional residual capacity). Because differing chains of events happen as a result of anatomic alterations of the lungs, treatment selection is most appropriately directed at the basic causes of the clinical manifestations—that is, the anatomic alterations of the lungs. For example, a bronchodilator is used to offset the bronchospasm associated with an asthmatic episode.

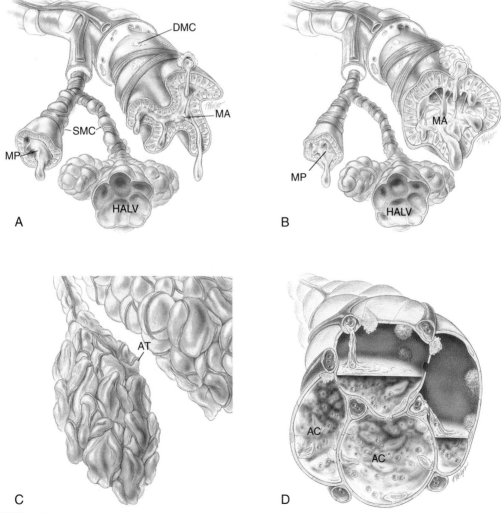

FIGURE 1 *Common anatomic alterations of the lungs in obstructive lung disorders.* **A,** Bronchial smooth muscle constriction accompanied by air trapping (as seen in asthma). **B,** Tracheobronchial inflammation accompanied by mucous accumulation, partial airway obstruction, and air trapping (as seen in bronchitis).
Common anatomic alterations of the lungs in restrictive lung disorders. **C,** Alveolar collapse or atelectasis (as seen in post-operative patients). **D,** Alveolar consolidation (as seen in pneumonia). *AC,* Alveolar consolidation; *AT,* atelectasis; *DMC,* degranulation of mast cell; *HALV,* hyperinflated alveoli; *MA,* mucus accumulation; *MP,* mucous plug; *SMC,* smooth muscle constriction.

TABLE 2 General Classification of Respiratory Diseases

Respiratory Disease	Classification		
	Obstructive	Restrictive	Combination
Chronic obstructive pulmonary disease (chronic bronchitis & emphysema)	X		
Asthma	X		
Bronchiectasis			X
Cystic fibrosis			X
Pneumonia		X	
Lung abscess		X	
Tuberculosis		X	
Fungal disease of the lungs		X	
Pulmonary edema		X	
Flail chest		X	
Pneumothorax		X	
Kyphoscoliosis		X	
Chronic interstitial lung disease			X
Cancer of the lungs		X	
Acute respiratory distress syndrome		X	
Meconium aspiration syndrome			X
Transient tachypnea of the newborn			X
Respiratory distress syndrome		X	
Pulmonary air leak syndrome			X
Respiratory syncytial virus			X
Bronchopulmonary dysplasia			X
Diaphragmatic hernia		X	
Near drowning	X		
Postoperative atelectsis		X	

The Knowledge Base

A strong knowledge base of the following four factors is essential to good respiratory care assessment and therapy selection skills:

1. Anatomic alterations of the lungs caused by common respiratory disorders
2. Major pathophysiologic mechanisms activated throughout the respiratory system as a result of the anatomic alterations
3. Common clinical manifestations that develop
4. Treatment modalities used to correct the anatomic alterations and pathophysiologic mechanisms caused by the disorder

Specific Components of the Assessment Process

The respiratory therapist with good assessment and treatment selection skills must also be competent in performing the actual assessment process, which has the following components:

1. The quick and systematic collection of the important clinical manifestations demonstrated by the patient
2. The formulation of an accurate assessment of the clinical data—that is, identification of the cause and severity of the data abnormalities
3. The selection of the optimal treatment modalities
4. A quick, clear, and precise documentation of this process

Without this basic knowledge and understanding, the respiratory therapist merely goes through the motions of performing assigned therapeutic tasks with no short-or-long-term anticipated outcomes that can be measured. In such an environment, the practitioner works in an unchallenging, task-oriented—rather than a goal-oriented—manner.

Goal-orientated—patient-oriented—respiratory care became the standard of practice in the early 1990s by analyzing the work performance of other health-care disciplines. For example, physical therapists have long been greatly empowered by virtue of the more generic physician's orders under which they work, whereas the respiratory therapists customarily received detailed and specific orders. For example, physical therapists are instructed to "improve back range of motion" or "strengthen quadriceps muscle groups," rather than to "provide warm fomentations to the lower back" or "initiate quadriceps setting exercises with 10-pound ankle weights, four times a day, for 10 minutes." In addition and, importantly, the physical therapist has long been permitted to start, up-regulate, down-regulate, or discontinue the therapy on the basis of the patient's current needs and capabilities—not on the basis of a 2-hour-, 2-day-, or 2-week-old physician assessment. *Goal achievement*, not task completion, is the way the success of physical therapy is routinely measured.

In the current "sicker in, quicker out" cost-conscious environment, a change has come to respiratory care. Under fixed reimbursement programs, shorter lengths of stay have required hospital administrators and medical staff to examine allocation of health-care resources. Recent data suggest that fully one-third of all hospitalized patients receive respiratory care services; therefore such services have come under close scrutiny. Studies using available peer-reviewed clinical practice guidelines have identified tremendous overuse (and, less frequently, underuse) of therapy modalities, and from this misallocation, the now firmly entrenched "therapist-driven protocol" (TDP) approach has emerged as the gold standard of respiratory care practice. Observing that the patient (and more accurately, the pulmonary pathophysiology!) should set the pace, some centers have called these protocols "patient-driven protocols," but the appellation of TDP or just "respiratory therapy protocols" has more strongly caught on. Clinical practice guidelines (CPGs), such as those developed by the American Association of Respiratory Care (AARC) and organizations such as the American Thoracic Society (ATS) and the American College of Chest Physicians (ACCP), are routinely used as the basis for TDPs in respiratory care.

The American College of Chest Physicians defines respiratory care protocols as follows:

> *"Patient care plans which are initiated and implemented by credentialed respiratory care workers. These plans are designed and developed with input from physicians, and are approved for use by the medical staff and the governing body of the hospitals in which they are used. They share in common extreme reliance on assessment and evaluation skills. Protocols are by their nature dynamic and flexible, allowing up- or down-regulation of intensity of respiratory services. Protocols allow the respiratory care practitioner authority to evaluate the patient, [to] initiate care, to adjust, discontinue, or restart respiratory care procedures on a shift- by-shift or hour-to-hour basis once the protocol is ordered by the physician. They must contain clear strategies for various therapeutic interventions, while avoiding any misconception that they infringe on the practice of medicine."*

Numerous studies have now shown beyond a shadow of a doubt that when respiratory care protocol guidelines are followed appropriately, the outcomes of respiratory care services improve. This improvement is noted in both clinical and economic ways (e.g., shorter ventilator weaning time in postoperative coronary artery bypass graft [CABG] patients). Under this paradigm, respiratory care that is inappropriately ordered is either withheld or modified (whichever is appropriate), and patients who *need* respiratory care services (but are not receiving them) should now be able to receive care. (Chapters 9 and 10 discuss structure and implementations of a good TDP program in detail.)

The notion that today's respiratory therapist "might" practice in the TDP setting has passed. Respiratory therapist who find that they are working in an archaic clinical setting—where protocols are not in daily use—should critically re-examine their employment options and career goals! To practice in today's health-care environment without the cognitive (thinking) skills used in the protocol-rich environment is no longer acceptable—*and, importantly, can have serious, negative legal consequences*!

Experience, however, indicates that at least *some* respiratory therapists are not entirely comfortable with the new role and responsibility the TDP paradigm has thrust on them. These workers have difficulty separating the contents of *their* "little black bag" of diagnostic and therapeutic modalities from the one traditionally carried and used by the physician. The choice to be a "protocol safe and ready therapist," however, is no longer elective. The profession of respiratory care has changed and moved on. The Clinical Simulation Examination portion of the National Board for Respiratory Care (NBRC) Advanced Practitioner Examination reflects the actual, no longer just "simulated," bedside practice of respiratory care.

Similar to their physical therapist colleagues, today's respiratory therapists are now routinely asked to participate actively in the appropriate allocation of respiratory care services. Modern respiratory therapists must possess the basic knowledge, skills, and personal attributes to collect and assess clinical data and treat their patients effectively. Under the TDP paradigm, specific clinical indicators (clinical manifestations) for a particular respiratory care procedure must first be identified. In other words, a specific treatment plan is only started, up-regulated, down-regulated, or discontinued on the basis of the following:
1. The presence and collection of specific clinical indicators, and
2. An assessment made from the clinical data (i.e., the cause of the clinical data) that justifies the therapy order or change.

In addition, after a particular treatment has been administered to the patient, all treatment outcomes must be measured and documented. Clearly, the success or failure of protocol work depends on accurate and timely patient assessment.

In view of these considerations, today's respiratory therapist *must* have competent bedside pulmonary assessment skills. Fundamental to this process is the ability to systematically gather clinical data, make an assessment, and develop an appropriate, safe, and effective action plan. Typically, once a treatment regimen has been implemented, the patient's progress is monitored on an ongoing assessment basis. In other words, clinical data are, again, collected, evaluated, and acted on based on the patient's response and progress toward a pre-defined goal.

To be fully competent in the assessment and treatment of respiratory disorders, the respiratory therapist must first have a strong academic foundation in the areas presented in Part I of this textbook. Part I is divided into three sections:
  I. Clinical Data Obtained at the Patient's Bedside
 II. Clinical Data Obtained from Laboratory Tests and Special Procedures
III. The Therapist-Driven Protocol Program—The Essentials

These three sections provide the reader with the essential knowledge base to assess and treat the patient with respiratory disease. The respiratory therapist must master the material in these sections to work efficiently and safely in a good TDP program.

1

The Patient Interview

Chapter Objectives

After reading this chapter, you will be able to:
- Describe the major items found on a patient history form.
- Explain the primary tasks performed during the patient interview.
- Describe the internal factors the practitioner brings to the interview.
- Discuss the external factors that provide a good physical setting for the interview.
- Describe the cultural, religious, and spiritual issues in the patient interview.
- Differentiate between open-ended questions and closed or direct questions.
- Describe the nine types of verbal responses.
- Describe the nonproductive verbal messages that should be avoided during the patient interview.
- List the positive and negative nonverbal messages associated with the patient interview.
- Describe how to close the interview.

Key Terms

Clarification
Closed or Direct Questions
Confrontation
Empathy
Explanation

External Factors
Facilitation
Internal Factors
Interpretation
Nonproductive Verbal Messages
Nonverbal Skills
Open-Ended Questions
Reflection
Silence
Summary

Chapter Outline

Patient History
Patient Interview
  Internal Factors
  External Factors
  Cultural Sensitivity and Religious and Spirituality
    Considerations
Techniques of Communication
  Open-Ended Questions
  Closed or Direct Questions
  Responses—Assisting the Narrative
  Nonproductive Verbal Messages
  Nonverbal Techniques of Communication
Closing the Interview
Self-Assessment Questions

Patient History

A complete patient assessment starts and ends with the patient interview. The purpose of the patient history is to gather pertinent subjective and objective data, which in turn can be used to develop a more complete picture of the patient's past and present health. In most nonacute clinical settings the patient is asked to fill out a printed history form or checklist. The patient should be allowed ample time to recall important dates, health-related landmarks, and family history. The patient interview is then used to validate what the patient has written and collect additional data on the patient's health status and lifestyle. Although history forms vary, most contain the following:

- Biographic data (age, gender, occupation)
- The patient's chief complaint or reason for seeking care, including the onset, duration, and characteristics of the signs and symptoms
- Present health or history of present illness
- Past health, including childhood illnesses, accidents or injuries, serious or chronic illnesses, hospitalizations, operations, obstetric history, immunizations, last examination date, allergies, current medications, and history of smoking or other habits

- The patient's family history
- Review of each body system, including skin, head, eyes, ears, and nose, mouth and throat, respiratory system, cardiovascular system, gastrointestinal system, urinary system, genital system, and endocrine system
- Functional assessment (activities of daily living), including activity and exercise, work performance, sleep and rest, nutrition, interpersonal relationships, and coping and stress management strategies

Patient Interview

The interview is a meeting between the respiratory care practitioner and the patient. It allows the collection of subjective data about the patient's feelings regarding the condition. During a successful interview, the practitioner performs the following tasks:

1. Gathers complete and accurate data about the patient's impressions about his or her health, including a description and chronology of any symptoms
2. Establishes rapport and trust so the patient feels accepted and comfortable in sharing all relevant information
3. Develops and shows an understanding about the patient's health state, which in turn enhances the patient's participation in identifying problems

Interview skills are an art form that takes time—and experience—to develop. The most important components of a successful interview are communication and understanding. Understanding the various signals of communication is the most difficult part. An inability to convey the meaning of messages will lead to miscommunication between the practitioner and the patient.

Communication cannot be assumed just because two people have the ability to speak and listen. Communication is about behaviors—conscious and unconscious, verbal and nonverbal. All these behaviors convey meaning. The following paragraphs describe important factors that enhance the sending and receiving of information during communication.

Internal Factors

Internal factors encompass what the practitioner brings to the interview—a genuine concern for others, **empathy**, understanding, and the ability to listen. A genuine liking of other people is essential in developing a strong rapport with the patient. It requires a generally optimistic view of people, a positive view of their strengths, and an acceptance of their weaknesses. This affection generates an atmosphere of warmth and caring. The patient must feel accepted unconditionally.

Empathy is the art of viewing the world from the patient's point of view while remaining separate from it. Empathy entails recognition and acceptance of the patient's feelings without criticism. It is sometimes described as feeling with the patient rather than feeling like the patient. To have empathy the practitioner needs to listen. Listening is not a passive process. Listening is active and demanding. It requires the practitioner's complete attention. If the examiner is preoccupied with personal needs or concerns, he or she will invariably miss something important. Active listening is a

cornerstone to understanding. Nearly everything the patient says or does is relevant.

During the interview the examiner should observe the patient's body language and note the patient's facial expressions, eye movement (e.g., avoiding eye contact, looking into space, diverting gaze), pain grimaces, restlessness, and sighing. The examiner should listen to the way things are said. For example, is the tone of the patient's voice normal? Does the patient's voice quiver? Are there pitch breaks in the patient's voice? Does the patient say only a few words and then take a breath? Such behaviors are often in opposition to what the patient is verbalizing, and further investigation may be indicated.

External Factors

External factors, such as a good physical setting, enhance the interviewing process. Regardless of the interview setting (the patient's bedside, an office in the hospital or clinic, or the patient's home), efforts should be made to (1) ensure privacy, (2) prevent interruptions, and (3) secure a comfortable physical environment (e.g., comfortable room temperature, sufficient lighting, absence of noise). It should also be noted that the interviewer's use of the *electronic health record* (EHR), also called *electronic medical record* [EMR]) and its associated hardware can also be threatening and may, in some cases, be a potential hazard to good patient communication—especially when combined with the anxiety that is often generated by simply being in the hospital and interacting with the various professional staff members about health issues, test results, and medical procedures—this form of anxiety is often referred to as the "white coat syndrome." In this situation, the patient can be intimidated to the point of "shutting down" and failing to ask questions or to learn from the interview. In addition, the interviewer's focus is often shifted from the patient to the EHR and this can cause them to miss important verbal and nonverbal messages. This situation also has the potential to cause the patient to feel like they are not important.

It should be noted that many respiratory care interviews must be performed in a much more hurried atmosphere than that described in this chapter—that is, relaxed and at the bedside of hospitalized patients. On many occasions, time is of the essence. Indeed, in some instances—such as in a "code" situation or emergency room visit—*no* interview may take place at all! Nevertheless, the thoughtful examiner should take away from this chapter this conclusion: In any clinical setting, the patient should feel that their concerns are being heard—and, when things seem rushed, it should be understood that it is only because the urgency of the situation, *at that moment*, demands it! Even in these situations, however, the good interviewer should be able to modify and adapt their questions to a given clinical situation and patient ability. For example, if the patient is unable to speak, the respiratory therapist can simply phrase their questions so that they can be answered (or signed) with a yes or no.

Cultural Sensitivity and Religious and Spirituality Considerations

Culture, religion, and spirituality strongly influence the way in which people think and behave—and, because of this have a definite and profound impact on the health-care system. For example, in some cultures, the oldest male is the decision maker for the rest of the family—including the making of health-care decisions. In other cultures, elderly patients may be especially upset when an illness or hospitalization interrupts their religious practice. Failure to recognize cultural sensitivities can result in stereotyping, discrimination, racism, and prejudice. Future health-care practitioners are now routinely trained in these considerations in "diversity" classes.

Culture can be defined as the values, beliefs, and practices shared by the majority in a group of people. Culture includes language, religious, or spiritual practices, foods, social habits, music, and art accepted and expected by a cultural group. Although the terms *religion* and *spirituality* are often used interchangeably, they are different. **Religion** refers to a formalized system of belief and worship (e.g., Catholicism, Protestantism, Hinduism, Buddhism, etc.). **Spirituality** entails the spirit, or soul, and is an element of religion. It is intangible and may include a belief in a higher power, creative force, or divine being, or a belief in spirits of departed people and the supernatural.

In the current health-care system, all practitioners must work to develop **cultural awareness**, **cultural sensitivity**, and **cultural competence** to deliver effective care. *Cultural awareness* involves the knowledge of the patient's history and ancestry and an understanding of the patient's beliefs, artistic expressions, diets, celebrations, and rituals. *Cultural sensitivity* refers to refraining from using offensive language, respecting accepted and expected ways in which to communicate, and not speaking disrespectfully of a person's cultural beliefs. *Cultural competence* refers to knowing the health-care practitioner's own values, attitudes, beliefs, and prejudices while, at the same time, keeping an open mind and trying to view the world through the perspective of culturally diverse groups of people.

All health-care practitioners should continue to learn all they can about other cultures. When in doubt, the health-care practitioners should simply ask the patient's preferences, rather than trying to guess or stereotyping the patient based on previous experiences with other cultures. Although mastery of the subject of diversity will forever be a life-long learning process, the following cultural aspects are always a good place to start and should routinely be considered when caring for patients from different cultures:

- What is the patient's preferred method of communication?
- What is the appropriate form of address within the patient's culture?
- Are there potential language barriers (verbal and nonverbal)?
- Is an interpreter needed?
- Is the setting appropriate for the interview? Too private? Too public?
- What roles for women, men, and children are generally accepted within the patient's culture?
- Should a person of the same sex/religious persuasion as the patient be present at the interview?
- Are there religious and/or spiritual beliefs that need to be respected?
- Is direct eye contact considered polite or rude?

- What amount of space between the examiner and the patient is considered appropriate when communicating?
- What are the hidden meanings of nonverbal gestures such as head nodding, smiling, and hand gestures? Are these acceptable or not?
- When, where, and by whom is touch acceptable?
- Who is/are the primary decision makers within the culture and family?
- What are the appropriate manners and dress attire of a person considered a "professional"?

Techniques of Communication

During the interview the patient should be addressed by his or her surname, and the examiner should introduce himself or herself and state the purpose for being there. The following introduction serves as an example: "Good morning, Mr. Jones. I'm Phil Smith, and I'm a Respiratory Therapist. I want to ask you some questions about your breathing so that we can plan your respiratory care here in the hospital."

Verbal techniques of communication used by the examiner to facilitate the interview may include the skillful use of **open-ended questions, closed or direct questions,** and responses.

Open-Ended Questions

An open-ended question asks the patient to provide narrative information. The examiner identifies the topic to be discussed but only in general terms. This technique is commonly used (1) to begin the interview, (2) to introduce a new section of questions, or (3) to gather further information whenever the patient introduces a new topic. The following are examples of open-ended questions:

"What brings you to the hospital today?"
"Tell me why you have come to the hospital today."
"Can you describe what your breathing has been like today?"
"You said that you have been short of breath. Tell me more about that."

The open-ended question is unbiased; it allows the patient freedom to answer in any way. This type of question encourages the patient to respond at greater length and give a spontaneous account of the condition. As the patient answers, the examiner should stop and listen. Patients often answer in short phrases or sentences and then pause, waiting for some kind of direction from the examiner. What the examiner does next is often the key to the direction of the interview. If the examiner presents new questions on other topics, much of the initial story may be lost. Ideally, the examiner should first respond by saying such things as "Tell me about it" and "Anything else?" The patient will usually add important information to the story when encouraged to expand with more details.

Closed or Direct Questions

A closed or direct question asks the patient for specific information. This type of question elicits a short one- or two-word answer, a yes or no, or a forced choice. The closed question is commonly used after the patient's narrative to fill in any details the patient may have left out. Closed questions are also used to obtain specific facts, such as "Have you ever had this chest pain before?" Closed or direct questions speed up the interview and are often useful in emergency situations when the patient is unable to speak in complete sentences. The use of only open-ended questions is unwieldy and takes an unrealistic amount of time, causing undue stress in the patient. Box 1-1 compares closed and open-ended questions.

Responses—Assisting the Narrative

As the patient answers the open-ended questions, the examiner's role is to encourage free expression but not to let the patient digress. The examiner's responses work to clarify the story. There are nine types of verbal responses. In the first five responses the patient leads; in the last four responses the examiner leads.

The first five responses require the examiner's reactions to the facts or feelings the patient has communicated. The examiner's response focuses on the patient's frame of reference; the examiner's frame of reference is not relevant. For the last four responses the examiner's reaction is not required. The frame of reference shifts from the patient's perspective to the examiner's perspective. These responses include the examiner's thoughts or feelings. The examiner should use these responses only when the situation calls for them. If these responses are used too often, the interview becomes focused more on the examiner than on the patient. The nine responses are described in the following sections.

Facilitation

Facilitation encourages patients to say more, to continue with the story. Examples of facilitating responses include the following: "Mm hmm," "Go on," "Continue," "Uh-huh." This type of response shows patients that the examiner is interested in what they are saying and will listen further. Nonverbal cues, such as maintaining eye contact and shifting forward in the seat, also encourage the patient to continue talking.

Silence

Silent attentiveness is effective after an open-ended question. **Silence** communicates that the patient has time to think and organize what he or she wishes to say without interruption by the examiner.

Reflection

Reflection is used to echo the patient's words. The examiner repeats a part of what the patient has just said to clarify or stimulate further communication. Reflection helps the patient focus on specific areas and continues in his or her own way. The following is a good example:

> PATIENT: "I'm here because of my breathing. It's blocked."
> EXAMINER: "It's blocked?"
> PATIENT: "Yes, every time I try to exhale, something blocks my breath and prevents me from getting all my air out."

Reflection can also be used to express the emotions implicit in the patient's words. The examiner focuses on these emotions and encourages the patient to elaborate:

> PATIENT: "I have three little ones at home. I'm so worried they're not getting the care they need."
> EXAMINER: "You feel worried and anxious about your children."

The examiner acts as a mirror reflecting the patient's words and feelings. This technique helps the patient elaborate on the problem and, importantly, further helps the examiner to ensure that they correctly understand what the patient is attempting to communicate.

Empathy

Empathy is defined as the identification of oneself with another and the resulting capacity to feel or experience sensations, emotions, or thoughts similar to those being experienced by another person. It is often characterized as the ability to "put oneself into another's shoes." A physical symptom, condition, or disease frequently has accompanying emotions. Patients often have trouble expressing these feelings. An empathic response recognizes these feelings and allows expression of them:

> PATIENT: "This is just great! I used to work out every day, and now I don't have enough breath to walk up the stairs!"
> EXAMINER: "It must be hard—you used to exercise every day, and now you can't do a fraction of what you used to do."

The examiner's response does not cut off further communication, which would occur by giving false reassurance (e.g., "Oh, you'll be back on your feet in no time"). Also, it does not deny the patient's feelings nor does it suggest that the patient's feelings are unjustified. An empathic response recognizes the patient's feelings, accepts them, and allows the patient to express them without embarrassment. It strengthens rapport.

Clarification

Clarification is used when the patient's choice of words is ambiguous or confusing:

> "Tell me what you mean by bad air."

Clarification is also used to summarize and simplify the patient's words. When simplifying the patient's words, the examiner should ask whether the paraphrase is accurate. The examiner is asking for agreement, and this allows the patient to confirm or deny the examiner's understanding.

Confrontation

In using **confrontation,** the examiner notes a certain action, feeling, or statement made by the patient and focuses the patient's attention on it:

"You said it doesn't hurt when you cough, but when you cough you grimace."

Alternatively, the examiner may focus on the patient's affect:
"You look depressed today."
"You sound angry."

Interpretation

Interpretation links events and data, makes associations, and implies causes. It provides the basis for inference or conclusion:
"It seems that every time you have a serious asthma attack, you have had some kind of stress in your life."

The examiner runs the risk of making an incorrect inference. However, even if the patient corrects the inference, the patient's response often serves to prompt further discussion of the topic.

Explanation

Explanation provides the patient with factual and objective information:
"It is very common for your heart rate to increase a bit after a bronchodilator treatment."

Summary

The **summary** is the final overview of the examiner's understanding of the patient's statements. It condenses the facts and presents an outline of the way the examiner perceives the patient's respiratory status. It is a type of validation in that the patient can agree or disagree with the examiner's summary. Both the examiner and the patient should participate in the summary. The summary signals that the interview is about to end.

Nonproductive Verbal Messages

In addition to the verbal techniques commonly used to enhance the interview, the examiner must refrain from making **nonproductive verbal messages.** These defeating messages restrict the patient's response. They act as barriers to obtaining data and establishing rapport.

Providing Assurance or Reassurance

Providing assurance or reassurance gives the examiner the false sense of having provided comfort. In fact, this type of response probably does more to relieve the examiner's anxiety than that of the patient.
PATIENT: "I'm so worried about the mass the doctor found on my chest x-ray. I hope it doesn't turn out to be cancer! What happens to your lung?"
EXAMINER: "Now, don't worry. I'm sure you will be all right. You have a very good doctor."

The examiner's response trivializes the patient's concern and effectively halts further communication about the topic. Instead, the examiner might have responded in a more empathic way:
"You are really worried about that mass on your x-ray, aren't you? It must be very hard to wait for the lab results."

This response acknowledges the patient's feelings and concerns and, more important, keeps the door open for further communication.

Giving Advice

A key step in professional growth is to know when to give advice and when to refrain from it. Patients will often seek the examiner's professional advice and opinion on a specific topic:
"What types of things should I avoid to keep my asthma under control?"

This is a straightforward request for information that the examiner has and the patient needs. The examiner should respond directly, and the answer should be based on knowledge and experience. The examiner should refrain from dispensing advice that is based on a hunch or feeling. For example, consider the patient who has just seen the doctor:
"Dr. Johnson has just told me I may need an operation to remove the mass they found in my lungs. I just don't know. What would you do?"

If the examiner answers, the accountability for the decision shifts from the patient to the examiner. The examiner is not the patient. The patient must work this problem out. In fact, the patient probably does not really want to know what the examiner would do. In this case, the patient is worried about what he or she might have to do. A better response is reflection:
EXAMINER: "Have an operation?"
PATIENT: "Yes, and I've never been put to sleep before. What do they do if you don't wake up?"

Now the examiner knows the patient's real concern and can work to help the patient deal with it. For the patient to accept advice, it must be meaningful and appropriate. For example, in planning pulmonary rehabilitation for a male patient with severe emphysema, the respiratory therapist advises him to undertake a moderate walking program. The patient may treat the therapist's advice in one of two ways—either follow it or not. Indeed, the patient may choose to ignore it, feeling that it is not appropriate for him (e.g., he feels he gets plenty of exercise at work anyway).

By way of contrast, if the patient follows the therapist's advice, three outcomes are possible: The patient's condition stays the same, improves, or worsens. If the walking strengthens the patient, the condition improves. However, if the patient was not part of the decision-making process to initiate a walking program, the psychologic reward is limited, promoting further dependency. If the walking program does not improve his condition or compromises it, the advice did not work. Because the advice was not the patient's, he can avoid any responsibility for the failure:
"See, I did what you advised me to do, and it didn't help. In fact, I feel worse! Why did you tell me to do this anyway?"

Although giving advice might be faster, the examiner should take the time to involve the patient in the problem-solving process. A patient who is an active player in the decision-making process is more likely to learn and modify behavior.

Using Authority

The examiner should avoid responses that promote dependency and inferiority:
"Now, your doctor and therapist know best."

Although the examiner and the patient cannot have equality in terms of professional skills and experience, both are equally worthy human beings and owe each other respect.

Using Avoidance Language

When talking about potentially frightening topics, people often use euphemisms (e.g., "passed on" rather than "died") to avoid reality or hide their true feelings. Although the use of euphemisms may appear to make a topic less frightening, it does not make the topic or the fear go away. In fact, not talking about a frightening subject suppresses the patient's feelings and often makes the patient more fearful. The use of direct and clear language is the best way to deal with potentially uncomfortable topics.

Distancing

Distancing is the use of impersonal conversation that places space between a frightening topic and the speaker. For example, a patient with a lung mass may say, "A friend of mine has a tumor on her lung. She is afraid that she may need an operation" or "There is a tumor in the left lung." By using "the" rather than "my," the patient can deny any association with the tumor. Occasionally, health-care workers also use distancing to soften reality. As a general rule, this technique does not work because it communicates to the patient that the health-care practitioner is also afraid of the topic. The use of frank, specific terms usually helps defuse anxiety rather than causing it.

Professional Jargon

What a health-care worker calls a myocardial infarction, a patient calls a heart attack. The use of professional jargon can sound exclusionary and paternalistic to the patient. Health-care practitioners should always try to adjust their vocabulary to the patient's understanding without sounding condescending. Even if patients use medical terms, the examiner cannot assume that they fully understand the meaning. For example, patients often think the term *hypertension* means that they are very tense and therefore take their medication only when they are feeling stressed, not when they feel relaxed.

Asking Leading or Biased Questions

Asking a patient "You don't smoke anymore, do you?" implies that one answer is better than another. The patient is forced either to answer in a way corresponding to the examiner's values or to feel guilty when admitting the other answer. When responding to this type of question, the patient risks the examiner's disapproval and possible alienation, which are undesirable responses from the patient's point of view.

Talking Too Much

Some examiners feel that helpfulness is directly related to verbal productivity. If they have spent the session talking, they leave feeling that they have met the patient's needs. In fact, the opposite is true. The patient needs time to talk. As a general rule, the examiner should listen more than talk.

Interrupting and Anticipating

While patients are speaking, the examiner should refrain from interrupting them, even when the examiner believes that she or he knows what is about to be said. Interruptions do not facilitate the interview. Rather, they communicate to the patient that the examiner is impatient or bored with the interview. Another trap is thinking about the next question while the patient is answering the last one, or anticipating the answer. Examiners who are overly preoccupied with their role as interviewer are not really listening to the patient. As a general rule, the examiner should allow a second or so of silence between the patient's statement and the next question.

Using "Why" Questions

The examiner should be careful in presenting "why" questions. The use of "why" questions often implies blame; it puts the patient on the defensive:

"Why did you wait so long before calling your doctor?"

"Why didn't you take your asthma medication with you?" The only possible answer to a "why" question is "because…," and this places the patient in an uncomfortable position. To avoid this trap, the examiner might say, "I noticed you didn't call your doctor right away when you were having trouble breathing. I'd like to find out what was happening during this time."

Nonverbal Techniques of Communication

Nonverbal techniques of communication include physical appearance, posture, gestures, facial expression, eye contact, voice, and touch. Nonverbal messages are important in establishing rapport and conveying feelings. Nonverbal messages may either support or contradict verbal messages—and, thus, generate a positive or negative influence on the interview process. Therefore, an awareness of the nonverbal messages that may be conveyed by either the patient or the examiner during the interview process is important.

Box 1-2 provides an overview of nonverbal messages that may occur during an interview.

Physical Appearance

The examiner's general personal appearance, grooming, and choice of clothing send a message to the patient. Professional dress codes vary among hospitals and clinical settings. Depending on the setting, a professional uniform can project a message that ranges from comfortable or casual to formal or distant. Regardless of one's personal choice in clothing and general appearance, the aim should be to convey a competent and professional image.

Posture

An open position is one in which a communicator extends the large muscle groups (i.e., arms and legs are not crossed). An open position shows relaxation, physical comfort, and a willingness to share information. A closed position, with arms and legs crossed, sends a defensive and anxious message. The examiner should be aware of any posture changes. For example, if the patient suddenly shifts from a relaxed to a

BOX 1-2 Nonverbal Messages of the Interview

Positive	Negative
Professional appearance	Nonprofessional appearance
Sitting next to patient	Sitting behind a desk and/or computer screen
Close proximity to patient	Far away from patient
Turned toward patient	Turned away from patient
Relaxed, open posture	Tense, closed posture
Leaning toward patient	Slouched away from patient
Facilitating gestures	Nonfacilitating gestures
• Nodding of head	• Looking at watch
Positive facial expressions	Negative facial expressions
• Appropriate smiling	• Frowning
• Interest	• Yawning
Good eye contact	Poor eye contact
Moderate tone of voice	Strident, high-pitched voice
Moderate rate of speech	Speech too fast or too slow
Appropriate touch	Overly frequent or inappropriate touch

tense position, it suggests discomfort with the topic. In addition, the examiner should try to sit comfortably next to the patient during the interview. Sitting too far away or standing over the patient often sends a negative nonverbal message.

Gestures

Gestures send nonverbal messages. For example, pointing a finger may show anger or blame. Nodding of the head or an open hand with the palms turned upward can show acceptance, attention, or agreement. Wringing the hands suggests worry and anxiety. The patient often describes a crushing chest pain by holding a fist in front of the sternum. When a patient has a sharp, localized pain, one finger is commonly used to point to the exact spot.

Facial Expression

An individual's face can convey a wide range of emotions and conditions. For example, facial expressions can reflect alertness, relaxation, anxiety, anger, suspicion, and pain. The examiner should work to convey an attentive, sincere, and interested expression. Patient rapport will deteriorate if the examiner exhibits facial expressions that suggest boredom, distraction, disgust, criticism, and disbelief.

Eye Contact

Lack of eye contact suggests that a person may be insecure, intimidated, shy, withdrawn, confused, bored, apathetic, or depressed. The examiner should work to maintain good eye contact but not stare the patient down with a fixed, penetrating look. Generally, an easy gaze toward the patient's eyes

with occasional glances away works well. The examiner, however, should be aware that this approach may not work when interviewing a patient from a culture in which direct eye contact is generally avoided. For example, Asian, Native American, Indochinese, Arab, and some Appalachian people may consider direct eye contact impolite or aggressive, and they may avert their own eyes during the interview.

Voice

Nonverbal messages are reflected through the tone of voice, intensity and rate of speech, pitch, and long pauses. These messages often convey more meaning than the spoken word. For example, a patient's voice may show sarcasm, anxiety, sympathy, or hostility. An anxious patient frequently talks in a loud and fast voice. A soft voice may reflect shyness and fear. A patient with hearing impairment generally speaks in a loud voice. Long pauses may have important meanings. For instance, when a patient pauses for a long time before answering an easy and straightforward question, the honesty of the answer may be questionable. Slow speech with long and frequent pauses, combined with a weak and monotonous voice, suggests depression.

Touch

The meaning of touch is often misinterpreted; it can be influenced by an individual's age, gender, cultural background, past experiences, and the present setting. As a general rule, the examiner should not touch patients during interviews unless he or she knows the patient well and is sure that the gesture will be interpreted correctly. When appropriate, touch (such as a touch of the hand or arm) can be effective in conveying empathy.

To summarize, extensive nonverbal messages, communicated by both the examiner and patient, may be conveyed during the interview. Therefore, the examiner must be aware of the patient's various nonverbal messages while working to communicate nonverbal messages that are productive and enhancing to the examiner-patient relationship.

Closing the Interview

The interview should end gracefully. If the session has an abrupt or awkward closing, the patient may be left with a negative impression. This final moment may destroy any rapport gained during the interview. To ease into the closing, the examiner might ask the patient one of the following questions:

"Is there anything else that you would like to talk about?"

"Do you have any questions that you would like to ask me?"

"Are there any other problems that we have not discussed?"

These types of questions give the patient an opportunity for self-expression. The examiner may choose to summarize or repeat what was learned during the interview. This serves as a final statement of the examiner's and the patient's assessment of the situation. Finally, the examiner should thank the patient for the time and cooperation provided during the interview.

SELF-ASSESSMENT QUESTIONS

ⓔ See Evolve Resources for answers. To access additional student assessment questions visit **http://evolve.elsevier.com/DesJardins/respiratory**.

1. During the patient interview, the practitioner states: "You are worried about your child." This type of statement is an example of which of the following technique:
   a. Reflection
   b. An open-ended question
   c. Confrontation
   d. Facilitation

2. **Which of the following is a closed or direct question?**
   a. Can you tell me why you appear depressed and angry today?
   b. Have you had this pain before?
   c. Tell how you first noticed the problem?
   d. Why did you wait so long before calling your doctor?

3. **Which of the following is considered a negative nonverbal message of the interview?**
   a. Nodding of head
   b. Sitting behind a desk
   c. Moderate tone of voice
   d. Sitting next to the patient

4. Which of the following is/are likely to be found on a complete patient history form?
   1. The patient's family history
   2. Activities of daily living
   3. The patient's chief complaint
   4. Review of each body system
      a. 2 and 3 only
      b. 1 and 4 only
      c. 2, 3, and 4 only
      d. 1, 2, 3, and 4

5. Which one of the following is considered a "facilitation" response?
   a. "You feel anxious about your children."
   b. "It must be hard to not be able to do that now."
   c. "Mm hmmm, go on."
   d. "Tell me what you mean by bad air."

The Physical Examination and Its Basis in Physiology

Chapter Objectives

After reading this chapter, you will be able to:

- Describe the major components of a patient's vital signs.
- Describe the four major components (inspection, palpation, percussion, and auscultation) associated with the systematic examination of the chest and lungs.
- Discuss in more detail the common clinical manifestations observed during inspection, including normal ventilatory pattern and the common pathophysiologic mechanisms that affect the ventilatory pattern.
- Describe the function of the accessory muscles of inspiration.
- Describe the function of the accessory muscles of expiration.
- Discuss the effects of pursed-lip breathing.
- Describe the pathophysiologic basis for substernal and intercostal retractions.
- Explain nasal flaring.
- Discuss splinting and decreased chest expansion caused by pleuritic and nonpleuritic chest pain.
- List abnormal chest shape and configurations.
- List abnormal extremity findings.
- Describe normal and abnormal sputum production.

Key Terms

Abnormal Ventilatory Patterns
Accessory Muscles of Expiration
Accessory Muscles of Inspiration
Adventitious (Abnormal) Breath Sounds
Afebrile
Airway Resistance
Anterior Axillary Line
Aortic and Carotid Sinus Baroreceptor Reflexes
Apnea
Auscultation
Biot's Respiration
Blood Pressure (BP)
Body Temperature (T°)
Bradycardia
Bradypnea
Bronchial
Bronchial Breath Sounds
Bronchovesicular
Cardiac Diastole
Cardiac Output (CO)
Cardiac Systole
Central Chemoreceptors
Central Cyanosis
Chest Excursion
Cheyne-Stokes Respiration

Constant Fever
Core Temperature
Crackles
Crepitus
Deflation Reflex
Diaphragm
Diaphragmatic Excursion
Diastole
Diastolic Blood Pressure
Digital Clubbing
Diminished Breath Sounds
Distended Neck Veins
Diurnal Variations
Dull Percussion Note
External Oblique Muscles
Febrile
Hemoptysis
Hering-Breuer Reflex
Horizontal Fissure
Hyperpyrexia
Hyperresonant note
Hypertension
Hyperthermia
Hyperventilation
Hypotension
Hypoventilation
Inspection
Inspiratory-to-Expiratory Ratio (I : E Ratio)
Intermittent Fever
Internal Oblique Muscles
Irritant Reflex
Juxtapulmonary-Capillary Receptors (J Receptors) Reflex
Kussmaul's Respiration
Lung and Chest Topography
Lung Compliance
Midaxillary Line
Midclavicular Line
Midscapular Line
Midsternal Line
Mild Hypoxemia
Moderate Hypoxemia
Nasal Flaring
Normal Breath Sounds
Oblique Fissure
Palpation
Pectoralis Major Muscles
Pedal (Dorsalis Pedis) Pulse
Percussion
Peripheral Chemoreceptors
Peripheral Edema
Pitting Edema

Chapter Outline

Vital Signs

The four major vital signs—**body temperature (T°), pulse (P), respiratory rate (R), and blood pressure (BP)**—are excellent bedside clinical indicators of the patient's physiologic and psychologic health. In many patient care settings, the oxygen saturation as measured by **pulse oximetry (SpO$_2$)** is considered to be the fifth vital sign. Table 2-1 shows the normal values that have been established for various age groups.

During the initial measurement of a patient's vital signs, the values are compared with these normal values. After several vital signs have been documented, they can be used as a baseline for subsequent measurements. Isolated vital sign measurements are not as valuable as a series of measurements. By evaluating a series of values, the practitioner can identify important vital sign trends for the patient. The identification of vital sign trends that deviate from the patient's normal measurements is often more important than an isolated measurement.

Although the skills involved in obtaining the vital signs are easy to learn, interpretation and clinical application require knowledge, problem-solving skills, critical thinking, and experience. Even though vital sign measurements are part of routine bedside care, they provide vital information and should always be considered as an important part of the assessment process. The frequency with which vital signs should be assessed depends on the individual needs of each patient.

Body Temperature

Body temperature is routinely measured to assess for signs of inflammation or infection. Even though the body's skin temperature varies widely in response to environmental conditions and physical activity, the temperature inside the body, the **core temperature,** remains relatively constant—about 37°C (98.6°F), with a daily variation of ±0.5°C (1°F to 2°F). Under normal circumstances, the body is able to maintain this constant temperature through various physiologic compensatory mechanisms, such as the autonomic nervous system

TABLE 2-1 Average Range of Values for Vital Signs According to Age Group

Age Group	Core Temperature (° F)	Pulse (bpm)	Respirations (breaths/min)	Blood Pressure (mm Hg) Systolic	Diastolic
Newborn	96–99.5	100–180	30–60	60–90	20–60
Infant (1 mo–1 yr)	99.4–99.7	80–160	30–60	75–100	50–70
Toddler (1–3 yr)	99.4–99.7	80–130	25–40	80–110	55–80
Preschooler (3–6 yr)	98.6–99	80–120	20–35	80–110	50–80
Child (6–12 yr)	98.6	65–100	20–30	100–110	60–70
Adolescent (12–18 yr)	97–99	60–90	12–20	110–120	60–65
Adult	97–99	60–100	12–20	110–140	60–90
Older adult (>70 yr)	95–99	60–100	12–20	120–140	70–90

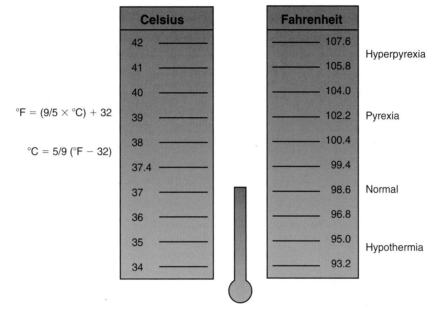

$$°F = (9/5 \times °C) + 32$$

$$°C = 5/9 (°F - 32)$$

FIGURE 2-1 Range of normal body temperature and alterations in body temperature on the Celsius and Fahrenheit scales. See conversion formulas for Fahrenheit and Celsius scales on the left side of the figure.

and special receptors located in the skin, abdomen, and spinal cord.

In response to temperature changes, the receptors sense and send information through the nervous system to the hypothalamus. The hypothalamus, in turn, processes the information and activates the appropriate response. For example, an increase in body temperature causes the blood vessels near the skin surface to dilate—a process called **vasodilation.** Vasodilation, in turn, allows more warmed blood to flow near the skin surface, thereby enhancing heat loss. In contrast, a decrease in body temperature causes **vasoconstriction,** which works to keep warmed blood closer to the center of the body—thus working to maintain the core temperature.

At normal body temperature, the metabolic functions of all body cells are optimal. When the body temperature increases or decreases significantly from the normal range, the metabolic rate and therefore the demands on the cardiopulmonary system also change. For example, during a fever the metabolic rate increases. This action leads to an increase in oxygen consumption and an increase in carbon dioxide production at the cellular level. According to estimates, for every 1°C increase in body temperature, the patient's oxygen

consumption increases about 10%. As the metabolic rate increases, the cardiopulmonary system must work harder to meet the additional cellular demands. Hypothermia reduces the metabolic rate and cardiopulmonary demand.

As shown in Figure 2-1, the normal body temperature is positioned within a relatively narrow range. A patient who has a temperature within the normal range is said to be **afebrile.** A body temperature above the normal range is called **pyrexia** or **hyperthermia.** When the body temperature rises above the normal range, the patient is said to have a *fever* or to be **febrile.** An exceptionally high temperature, such as 41°C (105.8°F), is called **hyperpyrexia.**

The four common types of fevers are **intermittent fever, remittent fever, relapsing fever,** and **constant fever.** An intermittent fever is said to exist when the patient's body temperature alternates at regular intervals between periods of fever and periods of normal or below-normal temperatures. In other words, the patient's temperature undergoes peaks and valleys, with the valleys representing normal or below-normal temperatures. During a remittent fever, the patient has marked peaks and valleys (more than 2°C or 3.6°F) over a 24-hour period, all of which are above normal—that is, the body temperature does not return to normal between the spikes. A relapsing fever is said to exist when short febrile periods of a few days are interspersed with 1 or 2 days of normal temperature. A continuous fever is present when the patient's body temperature remains above normal with minimal or no fluctuation.

Hypothermia is the term used to describe a core temperature below normal range. Hypothermia may occur as a result of (1) excessive heat loss, (2) inadequate heat production to counteract heat loss, and (3) impaired hypothalamic thermoregulation. Box 2-1 lists the clinical signs of hypothermia.

Hypothermia may be caused accidentally or may be induced. Accidental hypothermia is commonly seen in the patient who (1) has had an excessive exposure to a cold environment; (2) has been immersed in a cold liquid environment for a prolonged time; or (3) has inadequate clothing, shelter, or heat. It should be noted that geriatric patients generally display a lower temperature than younger adults. In addition, a reduced metabolic rate may compound hypothermia in older patients. Older patients often take sedatives, which further depress the metabolic rate. Box 2-2 lists common therapeutic interventions for patients with hypothermia.

Induced hypothermia refers to the intentional lowering of a patient's body temperature to reduce the oxygen demand of the tissue cells. Induced hypothermia may involve only a portion of the body or the whole body. Induced hypothermia is often indicated before certain surgeries, such as heart or brain surgery, or after return of spontaneous circulation after a cardiac arrest.

BOX 2-1 Clinical Signs of Hypothermia

- Below normal body temperature
- Decreased pulse and respiratory rate
- Severe shivering (initially)
- Patient indicating coldness or presence of chills
- Pale or bluish cool, waxy skin
- Hypotension
- Decreased urinary output
- Lack of muscle coordination
- Disorientation
- Drowsiness or unresponsiveness
- Coma

BOX 2-2 Common Therapeutic Interventions for Hypothermia

- Remove wet clothing
- Provide dry clothing
- Place patient in a warm environment (slowly increase room temperature)
- Cover patient with warm blankets or electric heating blanket
- Apply warming pads (increase temperature slowly)
- Keep patient's limbs close to body
- Cover patient's head with a cap or towel
- Supply warm oral or intravenous fluids

Factors Affecting Body Temperature

Table 2-2 lists several factors that affect body temperature. Knowing these factors can help the practitioner to better assess the significance of expected or normal variations in a patient's body temperature.

Body Temperature Measurement

The measurement of body temperature establishes an essential baseline for clinical comparison as a disease progresses or as therapies are administered. To ensure the reliability of a temperature reading, the practitioner must (1) select the correct measuring equipment, (2) choose the most appropriate site, and (3) use the correct technique or procedure. The four most commonly used sites are the mouth, rectum, ear (tympanic external auditory canal), and axilla. Any of these sites is satisfactory when the proper technique is used.

Additional measurement sites include the esophagus and pulmonary artery. Temperatures measured at these sites, and in the rectum and at the tympanic membrane, are considered core temperatures. The skin, typically that of the forehead or abdomen, may also be used for general temperature purposes. However, practitioners must remember that although skin temperature–sensitive strips or disposable paper thermometers may be satisfactory for general temperature measurements, the patient's precise temperature should always be confirmed—when indicated—with a glass or tympanic thermometer.

Because body temperature is usually measured orally, the practitioner must be aware of certain external factors that can lead to false oral temperature measurements. For example, drinking hot or cold liquids can cause small changes in oral temperature measurements. The most significant temperature changes have been reported after a patient drinks ice water. Drinking ice water may lower the patient's actual temperature by 0.2°F to 1.6°F. Before taking an oral temperature, the practitioner should wait 15 minutes after a patient has ingested ice water. Oral temperature may increase in the patient receiving heated oxygen aerosol therapy and decrease in the patient receiving a cool mist aerosol. Table 2-3 lists the body temperature sites, their advantages and disadvantages, and the equipment used.

Pulse

A pulse is generated through the vascular system with each ventricular contraction of the heart **(systole).** Thus, a pulse is a rhythmic arterial blood pressure throb created by the pumping action of the ventricular muscle. Between contractions, the ventricle rests **(diastole)** and the pulsation disappears. The pulse can be assessed at any location where an artery lies close to the skin surface and can be palpated against a firm underlying structure, such as muscle or bone. Nine common pulse sites are the temporal, carotid, apical, brachial, radial, femoral, popliteal, **pedal (dorsalis pedis),** and posterior tibial area (Figure 2-2).

In clinical settings the pulse is usually assessed by **palpation.** Initially the practitioner uses the first, second, or third finger and applies light pressure to any one of the pulse sites (e.g., carotid or radial artery) to detect a pulse with a strong

TABLE 2-2 Factors Affecting Body Temperature

Age	Temperature varies with age. For example, the temperature of the newborn infant is unstable because of immature thermoregulatory mechanisms. However, it is not uncommon for the elderly person to have a body temperature below 36.4° C (97.6° F). The normal temperature decreases with age.
Environment	Normally, variations in environmental temperature do not affect the core temperature. However, exposure to extreme hot or cold temperatures can alter body temperature. If an individual's core temperature falls to 25° C (77° F), death may occur. Conversely, in conditions of extreme humidity (>80%) and temperatures (>50° C or >122° F) death may occur.
Time of day	Body temperature normally varies throughout the day, a phenomenon called **Diurnal Variation**. Typically, an individual's temperature is lowest around 3:00 AM and highest between 5:00 PM and 7:00 PM. Approximately 95% of patients have their highest temperature around 6:00 PM. Body temperature often fluctuates by as much as 2° C (1.8° F) between early morning and late afternoon.
Exercise	Body temperature increases with exercise because exercise increases heat production as the body breaks down carbohydrates and fats to provide energy. During strenuous exercise, the body temperature can increase to as high as 40° C (104° F).
Stress	Physical or emotional stress may increase body temperature because stress can stimulate the sympathetic nervous system, causing the epinephrine and norepinephrine levels to increase. When this occurs, the metabolic rate increases, causing increased heat production. Stress and anxiety may cause a patient's temperature to increase without an underlying disease.
Hormones	Women normally have greater fluctuations in temperature than do men. The female hormone progesterone, which is secreted during ovulation, causes the temperature to increase 0.3° C to 0.6° C (0.5° F to 1° F). After menopause, women have the same mean temperature norms as men.

TABLE 2-3 Body Temperature Measurements: Sites, Normal Values, Advantages and Disadvantages, and Equipment Used

Site and Temperature	Advantages and Disadvantages	Equipment
Oral (most common) Average 37° C or 98.6° F	Advantages: Convenient. Easy access and patient comfort. Disadvantages: Affected by hot or cold liquids. Contraindicated in patients who cannot follow directions to keep mouth closed, who are mouth breathing, or who might bite down and break the thermometer. Smoking, drinking, and eating can slightly alter the oral temperature. About 1° F lower than rectal temperature.	Glass mercury thermometer, electronic thermometers
Rectal Average 0.7° C or 0.4° F higher than oral	Advantages: Very reliable. Considered most accurate. Disadvantages: Contraindicated in patients with diarrhea, patients who have undergone rectal surgery, or patients who have diseases of the rectum. General Comment: Used less often now that tympanic thermometers are available.	Glass mercury thermometer
Ear (tympanic) Reflects core temperature. Also calibrated to oral or rectal scales	Advantages: Convenient, readily accessible, fast, safe, and noninvasive. Does not require contact with any mucous membrane. Infection control is less of a concern. With the advent of the tympanic membrane thermometer, the ear is now a site where a temperature can be easily and safely measured. Reflects the core body temperature because it measures the tympanic membrane blood supply—the same vascular system that supplies the hypothalamus. Smoking, drinking, and eating do not affect tympanic temperature measurements. Allows rapid temperature measurements in the very young, confused, or unconscious patient. Disadvantages: No remarkable disadvantages, assuming site is available.	Tympanic thermometer
Axillary Average 0.6° C or 1° F lower than oral	Advantages: Safe and noninvasive. Recommended for infants and children, this is the route of choice in patients whose temperature cannot be measured at other sites. Disadvantages: Considered the least accurate and least reliable site because a number of factors can adversely affect the measurement. For example, if the patient has recently been given a bath, the temperature may reflect the temperature of the bath water. Similarly, friction applied to dry the patient's skin may influence the temperature.	Glass mercury thermometer

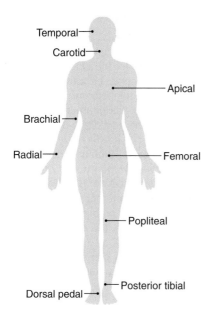

FIGURE 2-2 The nine common pulse measurement sites.

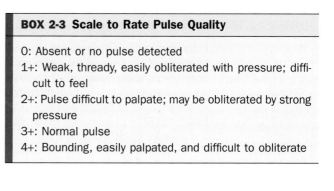

pulsation. After locating the pulse, the practitioner may apply a more forceful palpation to count the rate, determine the cardiac rhythm, and evaluate the quality of pulsation. The practitioner then counts the number of pulsations for 15, 30, or 60 seconds and then multiplies appropriately to determine the pulse rate per minute. Shorter time intervals may be used for patients with normal rates or regular cardiac rhythms.

In patients with irregular, abnormally slow, or fast cardiac rhythms, the pulse rates should be counted for 1 minute. To prevent overestimation for any time interval, the practitioner should count the first pulsation as zero and not count pulses at or after the completion of a selected time interval. Counting even one extra pulsation during a 15-second interval leads to an overestimation of the pulse rate by 4. *The characteristics of the pulse are described in terms of rate, rhythm, and strength.*

Rate

The normal pulse rate (or heart rate) varies with age. For example, in the newborn the normal pulse rate range is 100 to 180 beats per minute (bpm). In the toddler the normal range is 80 to 130 bpm. The normal range for the child is 65 to 100 bpm, and the normal adult range is 60 to 100 bpm (Table 2-1).

A heart rate lower than 60 bpm is called **bradycardia.** Bradycardia may be seen in patients with hypothermia and in physically fit athletes. The pulse may also be lower than expected when the patient is at rest or asleep or as a result of head injury, drugs such as beta-blockers (e.g., propanolol), vomiting, or advanced age. A pulse rate greater than 100 bpm in adults is called **tachycardia.** Tachycardia may occur as a result of hypoxemia, anemia, fever, anxiety, emotional stress, fear, hemorrhage, hypotension, dehydration, shock, and exercise. Tachycardia is also a common side effect in patients receiving certain medications, such as sympathomimetic agents (e.g., adrenaline or dobutamine).

Rhythm

Normally the ventricular contraction is under the control of the sinus node in the atrium, which generates a normal rate and regular rhythm. Certain conditions and chemical disturbances, such as inadequate blood flow and oxygen supply to the heart or an electrolyte imbalance, can cause the heart to beat irregularly. In children and young adults, it is not uncommon for the heart rate to increase during inspiration and decrease during exhalation. This is called **sinus arrhythmia.**

Strength

The quality of the pulse reflects the strength of left ventricular contraction and the volume of blood flowing to the peripheral tissues. A normal left ventricular contraction combined with an adequate blood volume will generate a strong, throbbing pulse. A weak ventricular contraction combined with an inadequate blood volume will result in a weak, thready pulse. An increased heart rate combined with a large blood volume will generate a full, bounding pulse.

Several conditions may alter the strength of a patient's pulse. For example, heart failure can cause the strength of the pulse to vary every other beat while the rhythm remains regular. This condition is called **pulsus alternans.** The practitioner may detect a pulse that decreases markedly in strength during inspiration and increases back to normal during exhalation, a condition called **pulsus paradoxus** that is common among patients experiencing a severe asthmatic episode. This phenomenon can also be observed when blood pressure is measured.

Finally, the stimulation of the sympathetic nervous system increases the force of ventricular contraction, increasing the volume of blood ejected from the heart and creating a stronger pulse. Stimulation of the parasympathetic nervous system decreases the force of the ventricular contraction, thus leading to a decreased volume of blood ejected from the heart and a weaker pulse. Clinically, the strength of the pulse may be recorded on a scale of 0 to 4+ (Box 2-3).

For peripheral pulses that are difficult to detect by palpation, an **ultrasonic Doppler** device may also be used. A transmitter attached to the Doppler is placed over the artery to be assessed. The transmitter amplifies and transmits the pulse sounds to an earpiece or to a speaker attached to the Doppler device. During normal sinus rhythm, the heart rate can also be obtained through **auscultation** by placing a stethoscope over the apex of the heart.

Respiration

The **diaphragm** is the primary muscle of respiration. Inspiration is an active process whereby the diaphragm contracts and causes the intrathoracic pressure to decrease. This action, in turn, causes the pressure in the airways to fall below the atmospheric pressure and air flows in. At the end of inspiration, the diaphragm relaxes and the natural lung elasticity (recoil) causes the pressure in the lung to increase. This action, in turn, causes air to flow out of the lung. Under normal circumstances, expiration is a passive process.

The normal respiratory rate varies with age. For example, in the newborn the normal respiratory rate varies between 30 and 60 breaths per minute. In the toddler the normal range is 25 to 40 breaths per minute. The normal range for the preschool child is 20 to 25 breaths per minute, and the normal adult range is 12 to 20 breaths per minute (Table 2-1).

Ideally the respiratory rate should be counted when the patient is not aware. One good method is to count the respiratory rate immediately after taking the pulse, while leaving the fingers over the patient's artery. As respirations are being counted, the practitioner should observe for variations in the pattern of breathing. For example, an increased breathing rate is called **tachypnea.** Tachypnea is commonly seen in patients with fever, metabolic acidosis, hypoxemia, pain, or anxiety. A respiratory rate below the normal range is called **bradypnea.** Bradypnea may occur with hypothermia, head injuries, and drug overdose. Table 2-4 provides an overview of common normal and **abnormal breathing patterns**.

Blood Pressure

The arterial blood pressure is the force exerted by the circulating volume of blood on the walls of the arteries. The pressure peaks when the ventricles of the heart contract and eject blood into the aorta and pulmonary arteries. The blood pressure measured during ventricular contraction **(cardiac systole)** is the **systolic blood pressure.** During ventricular relaxation **(cardiac diastole),** blood pressure is generated by the elastic recoil of the arteries and arterioles. This pressure is called the **diastolic blood pressure**.

The normal blood pressure in the aorta and large arteries varies with age. For example, in the newborn the normal systolic blood pressure range is 60 to 90 mm Hg. In the toddler the normal range is 80 to 110 mm Hg. The normal range for the child is 100 to 110 mm Hg, and the normal adult range is 110 to 140 mm Hg (see Table 2-1 for both normal systolic and diastolic blood pressures according to age). The numeric difference between the systolic and diastolic blood pressure is the **pulse pressure.** For example, a systolic pressure of 120 mm Hg and a diastolic pressure of 80 mm Hg equal a pulse pressure of 40 mm Hg.

Blood pressure is a function of (1) the blood flow generated by ventricular contraction and (2) the resistance to blood flow caused by the vascular system. Thus, blood pressure (BP) equals flow ($\dot{V}$) multiplied by resistance (R): BP = $\dot{V}$ × R.

Blood Flow

Blood flow is equal to cardiac output. Cardiac output is equal to the product of (1) the volume of blood ejected from the ventricles during each heartbeat **(stroke volume)** multiplied by (2) the heart rate. Thus, a stroke volume (SV) of 75 mL and a heart rate (HR) of 70 bpm produce a **cardiac output (CO)** of 5250 mL/min, or 5.25 L/min (CO = SV × HR). The average cardiac output in the resting adult is about 5 L/min.

A number of conditions can alter stroke volume and therefore blood flow. For instance, a decreased stroke volume may develop as a result of poor cardiac pumping (e.g., ventricular failure) or as a result of a decreased blood volume (e.g., during severe hemorrhage). Bradycardia may also reduce cardiac output and blood flow. Conversely, an increased heart rate or blood volume will likely increase cardiac output and blood flow. In addition, an increased heart rate in response to a decreased blood volume (or stroke volume) may also occur as a compensatory mechanism to maintain normal cardiac output and blood flow.

Resistance

The friction between the components of the blood ejected from the ventricles and the walls of the arteries results in a natural resistance to blood flow. Friction between the blood components and the vessel walls is inversely related to the dimensions of the vessel lumen (size). Thus, as the vessel lumen narrows (or constricts), resistance increases. As the vessel lumen widens (or relaxes), the resistance decreases. The autonomic nervous system monitors and regulates the vascular tone.

Table 2-5 presents factors that affect the blood pressure.

Abnormalities

Hypertension. *Hypertension* is the condition in which an individual's blood pressure is chronically above normal range. Whereas blood pressure normally increases with aging, hypertension is considered a dangerous disease and is associated with an increased risk of morbidity and mortality. According to the Joint National Committee on Detection, Evaluation, and Treatment of High Blood Pressure, the physician may make the diagnosis of hypertension in the adult when an average of two or more diastolic readings on at least two different visits is 90 mm Hg or higher or when the average of two or more systolic readings on at least two visits is consistently higher than 140 mm Hg.

An elevated blood pressure of unknown cause is called *primary hypertension.* An elevated blood pressure of a known cause is called *secondary hypertension.* Factors associated with hypertension include arterial disease (usually on the basis of arteriosclerosis), obesity, a high serum sodium level, pregnancy, obstructive sleep apnea, and a family history of high blood pressure. The incidence of hypertension is higher in men than in women and is twice as common in blacks as in whites. People with mild or moderate hypertension may be asymptomatic or may experience suboccipital headaches (especially on rising), tinnitus, light-headedness, easy fatigability, and cardiac palpitations. With sustained hypertension, the arterial walls become thickened, inelastic, and resistant to blood flow. This process in turn causes the left ventricle to distend and hypertrophy. Hypertension may lead to congestive heart failure.

TABLE 2-4 Common Normal and Abnormal Breathing Patterns

Pattern	Graphic Overview	Description
Eupnea	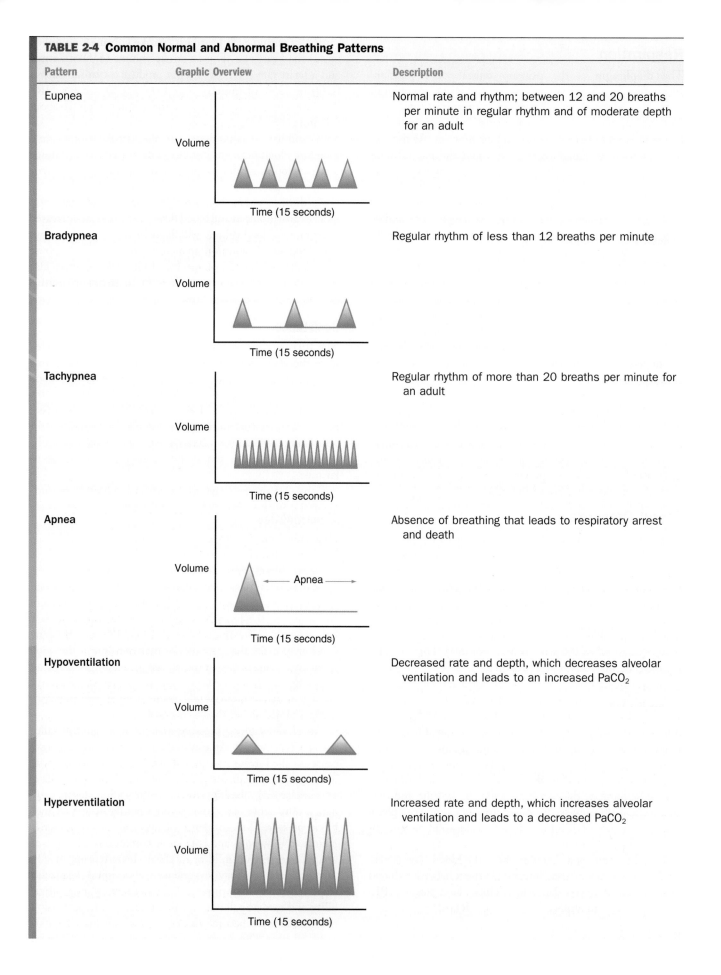	Normal rate and rhythm; between 12 and 20 breaths per minute in regular rhythm and of moderate depth for an adult
Bradypnea		Regular rhythm of less than 12 breaths per minute
Tachypnea		Regular rhythm of more than 20 breaths per minute for an adult
Apnea		Absence of breathing that leads to respiratory arrest and death
Hypoventilation		Decreased rate and depth, which decreases alveolar ventilation and leads to an increased $PaCO_2$
Hyperventilation		Increased rate and depth, which increases alveolar ventilation and leads to a decreased $PaCO_2$

TABLE 2-4 Common Normal and Abnormal Breathing Patterns—cont'd

Pattern	Graphic Overview	Description
Cheyne-Stokes respiration		Respirations that progressively become faster and deeper, followed by respirations that progressively become slower and shallower and ending with a period of apnea
Kussmaul's respiration		Increased rate and depth of breathing. Usually associated with diabetic ketoacidosis as a compensatory mechanism to eliminate carbon dioxide, by buffering the metabolic acidosis
Biot's respiration		Fast, deep respirations with (abrupt, irregular) pauses

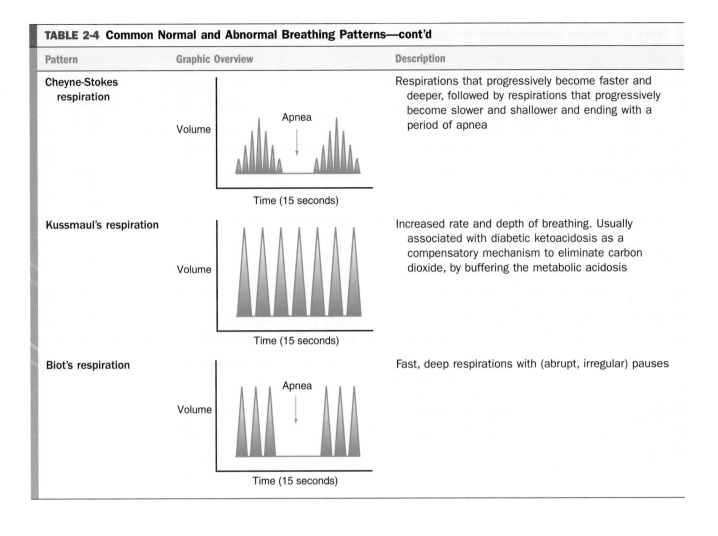

Hypotension. *Hypotension* is said to be present when the patient's blood pressure falls below 90/60 mm Hg. It is an abnormal condition in which the blood pressure is not adequate for normal perfusion and oxygenation of vital organs. Hypotension is associated with peripheral vasodilation, decreased vascular resistance, hypovolemia, and left ventricular failure. Hypotension can also be caused by analgesics such as meperidine hydrochloride (Demerol) and morphine sulfate, severe burns, prolonged diarrhea, and vomiting. Signs and symptoms include pallor, skin mottling, clamminess, blurred vision, confusion, dizziness, syncope, chest pain, increased heart rate, and decreased urine output. Hypotension is life threatening.

Orthostatic hypotension, also called *postural hypotension,* occurs when blood pressure quickly drops as the individual rises to an upright position or stands. Orthostatic hypotension develops when the peripheral blood vessels—especially in central body organs and legs—are unable to constrict or respond appropriately to changes in body position. Orthostatic hypotension is associated with decreased blood volume, anemia, dehydration, prolonged bed rest, and antihypertensive medications. The assessment of orthostatic hypotension is made by obtaining pulse and blood pressure readings when the patient is in the supine, sitting, and standing positions.

Pulsus Paradoxus

Pulsus paradoxus is defined as a systolic blood pressure that is more than 10 mm Hg lower on inspiration than on expiration. This exaggerated waxing and waning of arterial blood pressure can be detected with a sphygmomanometer or, in severe cases, by palpating the pulse at the wrist or neck. Commonly associated with severe asthmatic episodes, pulsus paradoxus is believed to be caused by the major intrapleural pressure swings that occur during inspiration and expiration. The reason for this phenomenon is described in the following sections.

Decreased blood pressure during inspiration. During inspiration the asthmatic patient frequently relies on use of the **accessory muscles of inspiration.** The accessory muscles help produce an extremely negative intrapleural pressure, which in turn enhances intrapulmonary gas flow. The increased negative intrapleural pressure, however, also causes blood vessels in the lungs to dilate, creating pooled blood. Consequently, the volume of blood returning to the left ventricle decreases, causing a reduction in cardiac output and arterial blood pressure during inspiration.

Increased blood pressure during expiration. During expiration, the patient often activates the **accessory muscles of expiration** in an effort to overcome the increased airway resistance (R_{aw}). The increased power produced by

TABLE 2-5 Factors Affecting Blood Pressure

Age	Blood pressure gradually increases throughout childhood and correlates with height, weight, and age. In the adult, blood pressure tends to gradually increase with age.
Exercise	Vigorous exercise increases cardiac output and thus blood pressure.
Autonomic nervous system	Increased sympathetic nervous system activity causes an increased heart rate, an increased cardiac contractility, changes in vascular smooth muscle tone to enhance blood flow to vital organs and skeletal muscles, and an increased blood volume. Collectively, these actions cause increased blood pressure.
Stress	Stress stimulates the sympathetic nervous system and thus can increase blood pressure.
Circulating blood volume	A decreased circulating blood volume, either from blood or fluid loss, causes blood pressure to decrease. Common causes of fluid loss include abnormal, unreplaced fluid losses, such as in diarrhea or diaphoresis, and overenthusiastic use of diuretics. Inadequate oral fluid intake can also result in a fluid volume deficit. Excess fluid, such as in congestive heart failure, can cause blood pressure to increase.
Medications	Any medication that affects one or more of the previous conditions may cause blood pressure changes. For example, diuretics reduce blood volume; cardiac pharmaceuticals may increase or decrease heart rate and contractility; pain medications may reduce sympathetic nervous system stimulation; and specific antihypertension agents may also exert their effects.
Normal fluctuations	Under normal circumstances, blood pressure varies from moment to moment in response to a variety of stimuli. For example, an increased environmental temperature causes blood vessels near the skin surface to dilate, causing blood pressure to decrease. In addition, normal respirations alter blood pressure. Blood pressure increases during expiration and decreases during inspiration. Blood pressure fluctuations caused by inspiration and expiration may be significant during a severe asthmatic episode.
Race	Black males over 35 years of age often have elevated blood pressure.
Obesity	Blood pressure is often higher in overweight and obese individuals.
Diurnal (daily diurnal variations)	Blood pressure is usually lowest early in the morning, when the metabolic rate is lowest.

these muscles generates a greater positive intrapleural pressure. Although increased positive intrapleural pressure helps offset R_{aw}, it also works to narrow or squeeze the blood vessels of the lung. This increased pressure on the pulmonary blood vessels enhances left ventricular filling and results in increased cardiac output and arterial blood pressure during expiration.

Oxygen Saturation

Oxygen saturation, often considered the fifth vital sign, is used to establish an immediate baseline SpO_2 value. It is an excellent monitor by which to assess the patient's response to respiratory care interventions. In the adult, normal SpO_2 values range from 95% to 99%. SpO_2 values of 91% to 94% indicate **mild hypoxemia.** Mild hypoxemia warrants additional evaluation by the respiratory practitioner but does not usually require supplemental oxygen. SpO_2 readings of 86% to 90% indicate **moderate hypoxemia.** These patients often require supplemental oxygen. SpO_2 values of 85% or lower indicate **severe hypoxemia** and warrant immediate medical intervention, including the administration of oxygen, ventilatory support, or both. Table 2-6 presents the relationship of SpO_2 to PaO_2 for the adult and newborn. Table 2-7 provides an overview of the signs and symptoms of inadequate oxygenation.[1]

TABLE 2-6 SpO_2 and PaO_2 Relationships for the Adult and Newborn

	Adult		Newborn	
Oxygen Status	SpO_2	PaO_2 (mm Hg)	SpO_2	PaO_2 (mm Hg)
Normal	95%–99%	75–100	91%–96%	60–80
Mild hypoxemia	90%–95%	60–75	88%–90%	55–60
Moderate hypoxemia	85%–90%	50–60	85%–89%	50–58
Severe hypoxemia	<85%	<50	<85%	<50

Note: The SpO_2 will be lower than predicted when the following are present: low pH, high $PaCO_2$, and high temperature.

Systematic Examination of the Chest and Lungs

The physical examination of the chest and lungs should be performed in a systematic and orderly fashion. The most common sequence is as follows:

- **Inspection**
- **Palpation**
- **Percussion**
- **Auscultation**

Before the practitioner can adequately inspect, palpate, percuss, and auscultate the chest and lungs, however, he

---

[1]For a more in-depth discussion on oxygenation, see Chapter 5, Oxygenation Assessments.

or she must have a good working knowledge of the topographic landmarks of the lung and chest. Various anatomic landmarks and imaginary vertical lines drawn on the chest are used to identify and document the location of specific abnormalities.

Lung and Chest Topography

Thoracic Cage Landmarks

Anteriorly, the first rib is attached to the manubrium just beneath the clavicle. After the first rib is identified, the rest of the ribs can easily be located and numbered. The sixth rib and its cartilage are attached to the sternum just above the xiphoid process (Figure 2-3).

Posteriorly, the spinous processes of the vertebrae are useful landmarks. For example, when the patient's head is extended forward and down, two prominent spinous processes can usually be seen at the base of the neck. The top one is the spinous process of the seventh cervical vertebra (C-7); the bottom one is the spinous process of the thoracic vertebra (T-1). When only one spinous process can be seen, it is usually C-7 (Figure 2-3).

Imaginary Lines

Various imaginary vertical lines are used to locate abnormalities on chest examination (Figure 2-4). The vertical **midsternal line,** which is located in the middle of the sternum, equally divides the anterior chest into left and right hemithoraces. The **midclavicular lines,** which start at the middle of either the right or left clavicle, run parallel to the sternum, traditionally down through the male nipple.

On the lateral portion of the chest, three imaginary vertical lines are used. The **anterior axillary line** originates at the anterior axillary fold and runs down along the anterolateral aspect of the chest, the **midaxillary line** divides the lateral chest into two equal halves, and the **posterior axillary line** runs parallel to the midaxillary line along the posterolateral wall of the thorax.

Posteriorly, the **vertebral line** (also called the *midspinal line*) runs along the spinous processes of the vertebrae. The **midscapular line** runs through the middle of either the right or the left scapula parallel to the vertebral line.

Lung Borders and Fissures

Anteriorly, the apex of the lung extends about 2 to 4 cm above the medial third of the clavicle. Under normal conditions the lungs extend down to about the level of the sixth rib. Posteriorly, the superior portion of the lung extends to about the level of T-1 and down to about the level of T-10 (Figure 2-5).

The right lung is separated into the upper, middle, and lower lobes by the **horizontal fissure** and the **oblique fissure.** The horizontal fissure runs anteriorly from the fourth rib at

TABLE 2-7 Signs and Symptoms of Inadequate Oxygenation	
Central Nervous System	
Apprehension	Early
Restlessness or irritability	Early
Confusion or lethargy	Early or late
Combativeness	Late
Coma	Late
Respiratory	
Tachypnea	Early
Dyspnea on exertion	Early
Dyspnea at rest	Late
Use of accessory muscles	Late
Intercostal retractions	Late
Takes a breath between each word or sentence	Late
Cardiovascular	
Tachycardia	Early
Mild hypertension	Early
Arrhythmias	Early or late
Hypotension	Late
Cyanosis	Late
Skin is cool or clammy	Late
Other	
Diaphoresis	Early or late
Decreased urinary output	Early or late
General fatigue	Early or late

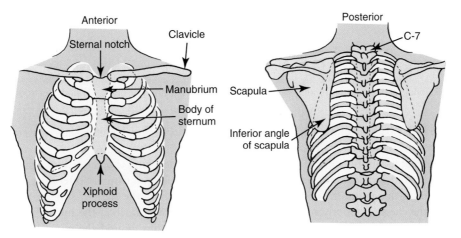

FIGURE 2-3 Anatomic landmarks of the chest.

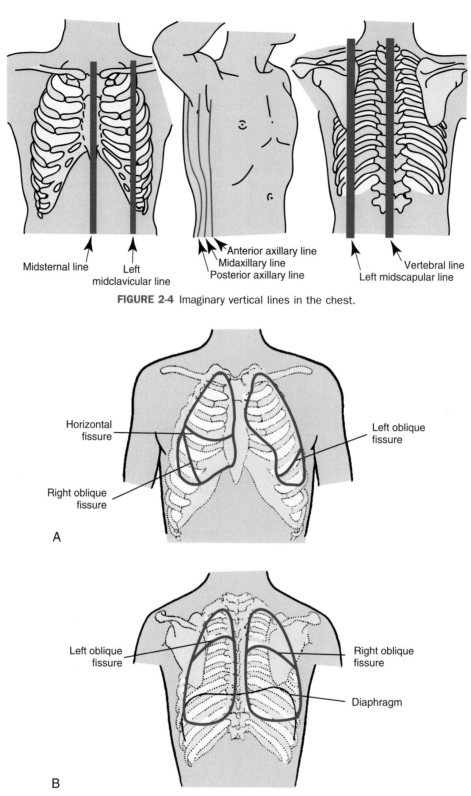

FIGURE 2-4 Imaginary vertical lines in the chest.

Midsternal line

Left midclavicular line

Anterior axillary line
Midaxillary line
Posterior axillary line

Vertebral line
Left midscapular line

Horizontal fissure

Left oblique fissure

Right oblique fissure

A

Left oblique fissure

Right oblique fissure

Diaphragm

B

FIGURE 2-5 Topographic location of lung fissures projected on the anterior chest (A) and posterior chest (B).

the sternal border to the fifth rib at the midaxillary line. The horizontal fissure separates the right anterior upper lobe from the middle lobe. The oblique fissure runs laterally from the sixth or seventh rib and the midclavicular line to the fifth rib at the midaxillary line. From this point, the oblique fissure continues to run around the chest posteriorly and upward to about the level of T-3. Anteriorly, the oblique fissure divides the lower lobe from the lower border of the middle lobe.

Posteriorly, the oblique fissure separates the upper lobe from the lower lobe.

The left lung is separated into the upper and lower lobes by the oblique fissure. Anteriorly, the oblique fissure runs laterally from the sixth or seventh rib and the midclavicular line to the fifth rib at the midaxillary line. The fissure continues to run around the chest posteriorly and upward to about the level of T-3.

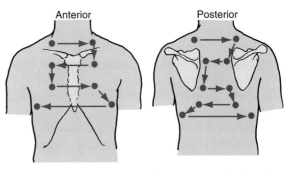

FIGURE 2-6 Path of palpation for vocal or tactile fremitus.

BOX 2-4 Common Clinical Manifestations Observed During Inspection

- Abnormal ventilatory pattern findings
- Use of accessory muscles of inspiration
- Use of accessory muscles of expiration
- Pursed-lip breathing
- Substernal or intercostal retractions
- Nasal flaring
- Splinting or decreased chest expansion caused by chest pain
- Abnormal chest shape and configuration
- Abnormal extremity findings:
  - Altered skin color
  - Digital clubbing
  - Pedal edema
  - Distended neck veins
- Cough (note characteristics)

Inspection

The inspection of the patient is an ongoing observational process that begins with the history and continues throughout the patient interview, taking of vital signs, and physical examination. The inspection consists of a series of observations to gather clinical manifestations—signs and symptoms—that are directly or indirectly related to the patient's respiratory status.

Common Clinical Manifestations Observed During Inspection

Box 2-4 lists common clinical manifestations observed during the inspection of the patient with a pathologic respiratory condition. For example, during a systematic visual inspection, the respiratory practitioner might note the patient's ventilatory pattern. Is the patient using accessory muscles of inspiration? Is the patient engaging in pursed-lip breathing? Are substernal or intercostal retractions occurring during inspiration? Does the patient appear to be splinting or to have decreased chest expansion because of chest pain? Are the shape and configuration of the chest normal? Do the patient's skin, lips, fingers, or toenails appear cyanotic? Does the patient have digital clubbing, pedal edema, or distended neck veins? Is the patient coughing? How strong is the patient's cough? What are the characteristics of the patient's sputum? A more **in-depth discussion of common clinical manifestations observed during inspection** can be found later in this chapter (see page 25).

Palpation

Palpation is the process of touching the patient's chest to evaluate the symmetry of chest expansion, the position of the trachea, skin temperature, muscle tone, areas of tenderness, lumps, depressions, and **tactile and vocal fremitus.** When palpating the chest, the clinician may use the heel or ulnar side of the hand, the palms, or the fingertips. As shown in Figure 2-6, both the anterior and posterior chest should be palpated from side to side in an orderly fashion, from the apices of the chest down.

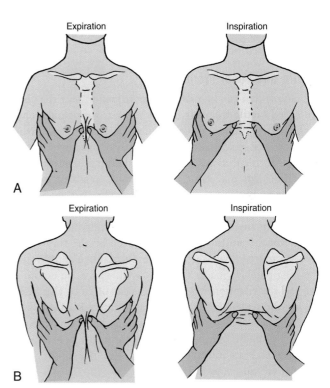

FIGURE 2-7 Assessment of chest excursion. A, Anterior. B, Posterior. Note that the thumbs move apart on inspiration as the volume of the thorax increases.

To evaluate the position of the trachea, the examiner places an index finger over the sternal notch and gently moves it from side to side. The trachea should be in the midline directly above the sternal notch. A number of abnormal pulmonary conditions can cause the trachea to deviate from its normal position. For example, a tension pneumothorax, pleural effusion, or tumor mass may push the trachea to the unaffected side, whereas atelectasis and pulmonary fibrosis pull the trachea to the affected side.

Chest Excursion

The symmetry of chest expansion is evaluated by lightly placing each hand over the patient's posterolateral chest so that the thumbs meet at the midline at about the T-8 to T-10 level. The patient is instructed to exhale slowly and completely and then to inhale deeply. As the patient is inhaling, the examiner evaluates the distance that each thumb moves from the midline. Normally, each thumb tip moves equally about 3 to 5 cm from the midline (Figure 2-7).

The examiner next faces the patient and lightly places each hand on the patient's anterolateral chest so that the thumbs meet at the midline along the costal margins near the xiphoid process. The patient is again instructed to exhale slowly and completely and then to inhale deeply. As the patient is inhaling, the examiner observes the distance each thumb moves from the midline.

A number of pulmonary disorders can alter the patient's **chest excursion.** For example, a bilaterally decreased chest expansion may be caused by both obstructive and restrictive lung disorders. An unequal chest expansion may occur when one or more of the following develop in or around one lung only: alveolar consolidation (e.g., pneumonia), lobar atelectasis, pneumothorax, large pleural effusions, or chest trauma (e.g., fractured ribs).

Tactile and Vocal Fremitus

Vibrations that can be perceived by palpation over the chest are called **tactile fremitus** (also known as **rhonchial fremitus**). This condition is commonly caused by gas flowing through thick secretions that are partially obstructing the large airways. Tactile fremitus is often noted during inhalation and exhalation and may clear after a strong cough. It is often associated with coarse, low-pitched crackles that are audible without a stethoscope. Vibrations that can be perceived by palpation or auscultation over the chest during phonation are called **vocal fremitus.** Sounds produced by the vocal cords are transmitted down the tracheobronchial tree and through the lung parenchyma to the chest wall, where the examiner can feel the vibration. Vocal fremitus can often be elicited by having the patient repeat the phrase "ninety-nine" or "blue moon." These are resonant phrases that produce strong vibrations. Normally, fremitus is most prominent between the scapulae and around the sternum, sites where the large bronchi are closest to the chest wall.

Tactile and vocal fremitus decrease when anything obstructs the transmission of vibration. Such conditions include chronic obstructive pulmonary disease, tumors or thickening of the pleural cavity, pleural effusion, pneumothorax, and a muscular or obese chest wall. Tactile and vocal fremitus increase in patients with alveolar consolidation, atelectasis, pulmonary edema, lung tumors, pulmonary fibrosis, and thin chest walls.

Crepitus (also called **subcutaneous emphysema**) is a coarse, crackling sensation that may be palpable over the skin surface. It occurs when air escapes from the thorax and enters the subcutaneous tissue. It may occur after a tracheostomy and mechanical ventilation, open thoracic injury, or thoracic surgery.

Percussion

Percussion over the chest wall is performed to determine the size, borders, and consistency of air, liquid, or solid material in the underlying lung. When percussing the chest, the examiner firmly places the distal portion of the middle finger of the nondominant hand between the ribs over the surface of the chest area to be examined. No other portion of the hand should touch the patient's chest. With the end of the middle finger of the dominant hand, the examiner quickly

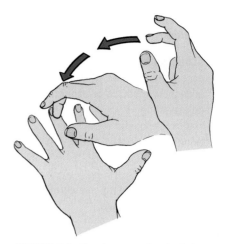

FIGURE 2-8 Chest percussion technique.

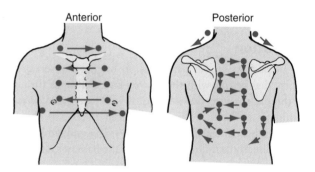

Anterior | Posterior

FIGURE 2-9 Path of systematic percussion to include all important areas.

strikes the distal joint of the finger positioned on the chest wall and then quickly withdraws the tapping finger (Figure 2-8). The examiner should perform the chest percussion in an orderly fashion from top to bottom, comparing the sounds generated on both sides of the chest, both anteriorly and posteriorly (Figure 2-9).

In the normal lung the sound created by percussion is transmitted throughout the air-filled lung and is typically described as loud, low in pitch, and long in duration. The sounds elicited by the examiner vibrate freely throughout the large surface area of the lungs and create a sound similar to that elicited by knocking on a watermelon (Figure 2-10).

Resonance may be muffled somewhat in the individual with a heavily muscular chest wall and in the obese person. When percussing the anterior chest, the examiner should take care not to confuse the normal borders of cardiac dullness with pulmonary pathology. In addition, the upper border of liver dullness is normally located in the right fifth intercostal space and midclavicular line. Over the left side of the chest, tympany is produced over the gastric space. When percussing the posterior chest, the examiner should avoid the damping effect of the scapulae.

Abnormal Percussion Notes

A **dull percussion note** is heard when the chest is percussed over areas of pleural thickening, pleural effusion, atelectasis, and consolidation. When these conditions exist, the sounds

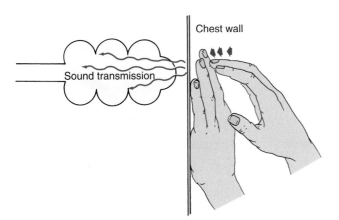

FIGURE 2-10 Chest percussion of a normal lung.

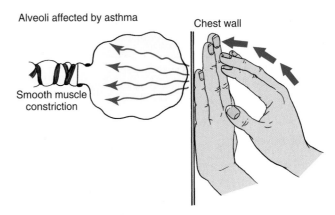

FIGURE 2-12 Percussion becomes more hyperresonant with alveolar hyperinflation.

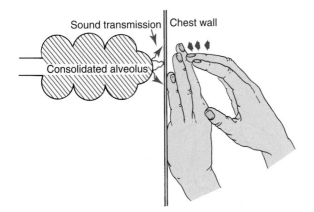

FIGURE 2-11 A short, dull, or flat percussion note is typically produced over areas of alveolar consolidation.

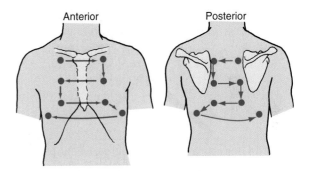

FIGURE 2-13 Path of systematic auscultation to include all important areas. Note the exact similarity of this pathway to Figure 2-6.

produced by the examiner do not freely vibrate throughout the lungs. A dull percussion note is described as flat or soft, high in pitch, and short in duration, similar to the sound produced by knocking on a full barrel (Figure 2-11).

When the chest is percussed over areas of trapped gas, a **hyperresonant note** is heard. These sounds are described as very loud, low in pitch, and long in duration, similar to the sound produced by knocking on an empty barrel (Figure 2-12). A hyperresonant note is commonly elicited in the patient with chronic obstructive pulmonary disease or pneumothorax.

Diaphragmatic Excursion

The relative position and range of motion of the hemidiaphragms can also be determined by percussion. Clinically, this evaluation is called the *determination of* **diaphragmatic excursion.** To assess the patient's diaphragmatic excursion, the examiner first maps out the lower lung borders by percussing the posterior chest from the apex down and identifying the point at which the percussion note definitely changes from a resonant to flat sound. This procedure is performed at maximal inspiration and again at maximal expiration. Under normal conditions the diaphragmatic excursion should be equal bilaterally and should measure about 4 to 8 cm in the adult.

When severe alveolar hyperinflation is present (e.g., severe emphysema, asthma), the diaphragm is low and flat in

position and has minimal excursion. Lobar collapse of one lung may pull the diaphragm up on the affected side and reduce excursion. The diaphragm may be elevated and immobile in neuromuscular diseases that affect it.

Auscultation

Auscultation of the chest provides information about the heart, blood vessels, and air flowing in and out of the tracheobronchial tree and alveoli. A stethoscope is used to evaluate the frequency, intensity, duration, and quality of the sounds. During auscultation the patient should ideally be in the upright position and instructed to breathe slowly and deeply through the mouth. The anterior and posterior chest should be auscultated in an orderly fashion from the apex to base while the right side of the chest is compared with the left (Figure 2-13). When examining the posterior chest, the examiner should ask the patient to rotate the shoulders forward so that a greater surface area of the lungs can be auscultated. Lung sounds are classified as either (1) normal breath sounds or (2) abnormal lung sounds (also called **adventitious lung sounds**).

Normal Breath Sounds

Three different **normal breath sounds** can be auscultated over the normal chest. They are called **bronchial, bronchovesicular,** and **vesicular breath sounds**. Important characteristics of breath sounds include the pitch (vibration

TABLE 2-8 Normal Breath Sounds

Breath Sound	Location	Pitch	Intensity	Sound Diagram*
Bronchial	Over trachea	High	Loud	
Bronchovesicular	Upper portion of anterior sternum, between scapulae	Moderate	Moderate	
Vesicular	Peripheral lung regions	High	Soft	

*For the sound diagram above, the blue upward arrow represents *inhalation*. The red downward arrow symbolizes *exhalation*. The length of the arrow signifies *duration*. The thickness of the arrow denotes in*tensity* or *loudness*. The angle between the blue inhalation arrow and the horizontal line symbolizes *pitch* (i.e., fast or slow vibration frequency).

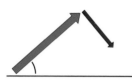

FIGURE 2-14 The normal vesicular breath sound. The blue upward *arrow* represents inhalation. The red downward arrow symbolizes *exhalation*. The length of the arrow signifies *duration*. The thickness of the arrow denotes *intensity* or *loudness*. The angle between the blue inhalation arrow and the horizontal line symbolizes *pitch* (i.e., fast or slow vibration frequency).

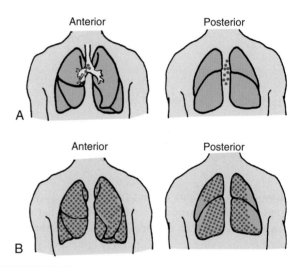

FIGURE 2-15 The location at which bronchovesicular breath sounds (A) and vesicular breath sounds (B) are normally auscultated.

frequency), amplitude or intensity (loudness), and the duration of inspiratory sounds compared with expiration. Figure 2-14 presents a sound diagram that illustrates the audio characteristics of the normal vesicular breath sound. Table 2-8 provides an overview of the normal breath sounds as regards to their location, pitch, intensity, and sound diagram.

Bronchial Breath Sounds. **Bronchial breath sounds** are normally auscultated directly over the trachea and are caused by the turbulent flow of gas through the upper airway. Bronchial breath sounds have a harsh, hollow, or tubular quality. They are loud, high in pitch, and about equal in duration in length of inspiration and expiration. A slight pause occurs between these two components. These sounds are also called *tracheal, tracheobronchial,* and *tubular breath sounds.*

Bronchovesicular Breath Sounds. **Bronchovesicular breath sounds** are auscultated directly over the main stem bronchi. They are softer and lower in pitch and intensity than bronchial breath sounds and do not have a pause between the inspiratory and expiratory phase. These sounds are reduced in pitch and intensity as a result of the filtering of sound that occurs as gas moves between the large airways and alveoli. Anteriorly, bronchovesicular breath sounds can be heard directly over the mainstem bronchi between the first and second ribs. Posteriorly, they are heard between the scapulae near the spinal column between the first and sixth ribs, especially on the right side (Figure 2-15, *A*).

Vesicular Breath Sounds. **Vesicular breath sounds** are the normal sounds of gas rustling or swishing through the small bronchioles and the alveoli. Under normal conditions, vesicular breath sounds are auscultated over most lung fields, both anteriorly and posteriorly (Figure 2-15, *B*). They are primarily heard during inspiration. As the gas molecules enter the alveoli, they are able to spread out over a large surface area and, as a result of this action, create less gas turbulence. Vesicular breath sounds also are heard during the initial third of exhalation as gas leaves the alveoli and bronchioles and moves into the large airways (Figure 2-16).

Abnormal Lung Sounds

Abnormal lung sounds (ALS) are atypical, or uncharacteristic, lung sounds that are not *normally* heard over a specific

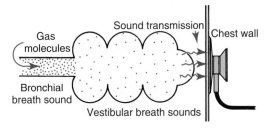

FIGURE 2-16 Auscultation of vesicular breath sounds over a normal lung unit.

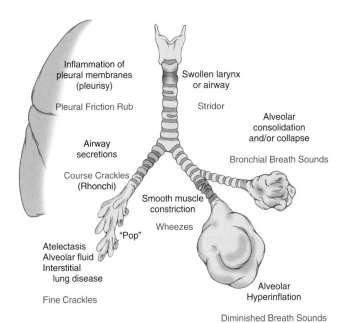

FIGURE 2-17 General location and source of abnormal lung sounds.

area of the thorax. To describe the *pitch* of an ALS, the experts recommend the use of such words as high, moderate, or low—for example, high-pitched wheezes were auscultated. For *the intensity* or *loudness* of the ALS, words such as faint, soft, mild, moderate, or loud should be used—for example, loud bronchial breath sounds were auscultated. The part of the respiratory cycle the ALS occurs should be recorded—for example, **crackles** were heard during inspiration, expiration, or both. In addition, include mention of when the ALS occurs during inspiration—for example, late-inspiratory crackles. Also, document the magnitude of the ALS—for example, small, scant, or profuse crackles. Always record the precise location over the chest the ALS is auscultated—for example, expiratory wheezes were noted over the right lower anterior lobe.

Although the experts have debated for many years the value of some of the terms and adjectives used to describe ALS, they have agreed—for the most part—that several terms or phrases are either ambiguous or very subjective and, therefore, should not be used for clinical reports, charting, and/or electronic documentation. *Terms, adjectives, and phrases not recommended at present are wet, dry, rales, rhonchi, crepitations, sonorous rales, musical rales, and sibilant rales.*

Currently, the recommended terms, adjectives, and phrases for ALS are the following: **fine crackles, medium crackles or coarse crackles, wheezes, bronchial breath sounds, stridor, pleural friction rub, diminished breath sound,** and **whispering pectoriloquy.** Figure 2-17 illustrates the general location and cause for these ALS. Table 2-9 provides an overview and description of the common ALS.

Table 2-10 summarizes the common assessment abnormalities found during inspection, palpation, percussion, and auscultation.

In-Depth Discussion of Common Clinical Manifestations Observed During Inspection

Normal Ventilatory Pattern

An individual's **normal breathing pattern** is composed of a **tidal volume (V_T)**, a **ventilatory rate,** and **an inspiratory-to-expiratory ratio (I:E ratio).** In normal adults, the V_T is about 500 mL (7 to 9 mL/kg), the ventilatory rate is about 15 (with a range of 12 to 18) breaths per minute, and the I:E ratio is about 1:2. In patients with respiratory disorders, however, an abnormal ventilatory pattern is often present (see Table 2-4 for common abnormal ventilatory patterns).

Abnormal Ventilatory Patterns

Although the precise cause of an **abnormal ventilatory pattern** may not always be known, it is frequently related to (1) the anatomic alterations of the lungs associated with a specific disorder and (2) the pathophysiologic mechanisms that develop because of the anatomic alterations. Therefore, to evaluate and assess the various abnormal ventilatory patterns (rate and volume relationships) seen in the clinical setting, the following pathophysiologic mechanisms that can alter the ventilatory pattern must first be understood:

- Lung compliance
- Airway resistance
- Peripheral chemoreceptors
- Central chemoreceptors
- Pulmonary reflexes:
  - Hering-Breuer reflex
  - Deflation reflex
  - Irritant reflex
  - Juxtapulmonary-capillary receptors (J receptors) reflex
  - Reflexes from the aortic and carotid sinus baroreceptors
- Pain, anxiety, and fever

Common Pathophysiologic Mechanisms That Affect the Ventilatory Pattern

Lung Compliance and Its Effect on the Ventilatory Pattern

The ease with which the elastic forces of the lungs accept a volume of inspired air is known as **lung compliance (C_L).** C_L is measured in terms of unit volume change per unit pressure change. Mathematically, it is written as liters per centimeter of water pressure (L/cm H_2O). In other words, compliance determines how much air in liters the lungs will accommodate for each centimeter of water pressure change in distending pressure.

TABLE 2-9 Abnormal Lung Sounds

Abnormal Lung Sound	Sound Diagram*

Crackles

Crackles (previously called *rales*) can be categorized as *fine*, *medium*, and *coarse crackles*.

Fine crackles are discontinuous, high-pitched, crackling, and popping sounds—similar to popping of bubble wrap, or the sound created by rolling hair between fingers near one's ear—heard near the end of inspiration (see Sound Diagram A). Fine crackles are produced by the rapid equalization of gas pressure when collapsed alveoli or terminal bronchioles suddenly snap open (Figure 2-17). Fine crackles usually do not clear after a strong cough. Fine crackles are associated with alveolar collapse (atelectasis), interstitial fibrosis, early pulmonary edema, and pneumonia.

Medium crackles are the same as fine crackles but are medium in pitch and have a moist quality as the disease process worsens.

Coarse crackles (previously called **rhonchi**[†]) are discontinuous, low-pitched, rumbling, bubbling, or gurgling sounds that start early during inspiration and extend into exhalation. These sounds are caused by air moving through excessive airway secretions in the larger airways (see Sound Diagram B). Coarse crackles are commonly associated with severe chronic obstructive pulmonary disease, cystic fibrosis, bronchiectasis, and congestive heart failure (pulmonary edema). Coarse crackles may or may not change in nature after a strong, vigorous cough.

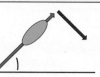

A. Fine Crackles. The green oval shape represents crackles.

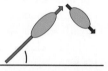

B. Coarse Crackle. The green oval shape represents crackles.

Wheezing

Wheezing is the characteristic sound produced by airway obstruction. Found in all bronchospasm disorders, it is one of the cardinal findings in asthma (Figure 2-17). Wheezes are continuous, high-pitched, musical whistles that are generally heard on expiration (see Sound Diagram). In severe cases, they may be heard during inspiration. In addition to bronchospasm, other common causes of partial or total airway obstruction include bronchospasm, mucosal edema, inflammation, tumors, and foreign bodies.

A partial airway obstruction is often made greater by this mechanism: When the bronchial airway is narrowed, the velocity of air flow through the constricted airway increases, which, in turn, causes the lateral airway wall pressure to decrease. This condition causes the airways to narrow even further—and/or—collapse. As the airways narrow, they vibrate similar to a reed on a woodwind instrument—thereby, producing a wheeze sound (Figure 2-18).

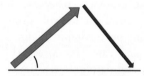

Wheezing
The orange oval shape represents wheezing.

Bronchial breath sounds

Bronchial breath sounds have a harsh, hollow, or tubular quality. They are loud, high in pitch, and about equal in duration during inspiration and expiration. The inspiratory phase is louder (see Figure 2-17 and Sound Diagram). Bronchial breath sounds are associated with alveolar consolidation and atelectasis (Figure 2-19).

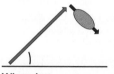

Bronchial breath sound
Note the thickness of the inspiratory and expiratory arrows, which denote loudness.

Stridor

Stridor is a continuous, loud, high-pitched sound caused by an upper obstruction in the trachea or larynx (see Figure 2-17 and Sound Diagram). It is generally heard during inspiration. Stridor is usually loud enough to hear without a stethoscope, as in infantile croup. Stridor indicates a neoplastic or inflammatory condition, including glottic edema, diphtheria, laryngospasm, and papilloma (a benign epithelial neoplasm of the larynx).

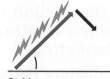

Stridor
The orange shapes represent stridor sounds.

TABLE 2-9 Abnormal Lung Sounds—cont'd

Abnormal Lung Sound	Sound Diagram*

Pleural friction rub

If pleurisy accompanies a respiratory disorder, the inflamed pleural membranes resist movement during breathing and create a peculiar and characteristic sound known as a **pleural friction rub** (see Figure 2-17 and Sound Diagram). It is a continuous, low-pitched, coarse creaking or grating-type sound reminiscent of that made by a creaking shoe. It is usually heard throughout inspiration and expiration over the area where the patient complains of pain. The intensity of a pleural rub often increases with deep breathing. A pleural friction rub does not clear with cough. A pleural friction rub is associated with pleurisy, pneumonia, pulmonary fibrosis, pulmonary infarction, or after thoracic surgery.

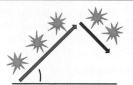

Pleural friction rub
The orange shapes represent pleural friction rub sounds.

Diminished breath sounds

Breath sounds are diminished or distant in any respiratory disorder that reduces the sound intensity of air flow. For example, chronic obstructive pulmonary disease leads to air trapping, an increased function residual capacity, and hypoventilation, which, in turn, result in diminished breath sounds (Figure 2-20). Heart sounds may also be diminished in patients with air trapping.

The intensity of breath sounds is also reduced in any condition that causes shallow or slow breathing patterns—for example, drug overdose, major sedation, or neuromuscular diseases such as Guillain-Barré syndrome or myasthenia gravis. Diminished breath sounds are also found in respiratory disorders that cause hypoventilation by compressing the lung—such as, flail chest, pleural effusion, and pneumothorax.

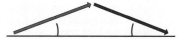

Diminished breath sound
Note the decreased angle on the inspiratory and expiratory arrows, which represent decreased intensity or loudness.

Whispering pectoriloquy

Whispering pectoriloquy is the term used to describe the unusually clear transmission of the whispered voice of a patient as heard through the stethoscope. When the patient whispers "one, two, three," the sounds produced by the vocal cords are transmitted not only toward the mouth and nose but also throughout the lungs. As the whispered sounds travel down the tracheobronchial tree, they remain relatively unchanged, but as the sound disperses throughout the large surface area of the alveoli, it diminishes sharply. Consequently, when the examiner listens with a stethoscope over a normal lung while a patient whispers "one, two, three," the sounds are diminished, distant, muffled, and unintelligible (Figure 2-21).

When a patient who has atelectasis or consolidated lung areas whispers "one, two, three," the sounds produced are prevented from spreading out over a large alveolar surface area. Even though the consolidated area may act as a sound barrier and diminish the sounds somewhat, the reduction in sound is not as great as it would be if the sounds were allowed to dissipate throughout a normal lung. Consequently, the whispered sounds are much louder and more intelligible over the affected lung areas (Figure 2-22).

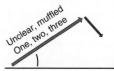

Unclear, muffled One, two, three

Normal vesicular breath sounds—unclear, muffled words ("one, two, three") auscultated.

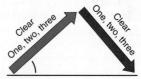

Clear One, two, three   Clear One, two, three

Consolidation and/or atelectasis—clear words ("one, two, three") auscultated.

*For the sound diagram above, the blue upward arrow represents *inhalation*. The red downward arrow symbolizes *exhalation*. The length of the arrow signifies *duration*. The thickness of the arrow denotes *intensity* or *loudness*. The angle between the blue inhalation arrow and the horizontal line symbolizes *pitch* (i.e., fast or slow vibration frequency).

†Historically, coarse crackles have also been called rhonchi, a term not currently recommended. Coarse crackles often produce palpable vibrations called **tactile fremitus**—also known as **rhonchial fremitus**. Coarse crackles are sometimes referred to as a "Death Rattle." It is this abnormal lung sound that every practicing respiratory therapist knows all too well—that is, the patient, whose loud, rumbling, gurgling secretions can be heard across the patient's room, which clearly signals the immediate need for tracheal suctioning or chest physical therapy.

For example, when the normal individual generates a negative intrapleural pressure change of −2 cm H_2O during inspiration, the lungs accept a new volume of about 0.2 L gas. Therefore, the C_L of the lungs and thorax is 0.1 L/cm H_2O:

$$C_L = \frac{\Delta V(L)}{\Delta P(cm\ H_2O)}$$
$$= \frac{0.2\ L\ gas}{2\ cm\ H_2O}$$
$$= 0.1\ L/cm\ H_2O.$$

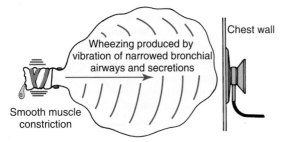

FIGURE 2-18 Wheezing and rhonchi often develop during an asthmatic episode because of smooth muscle constriction, wall edema, and mucous accumulation.

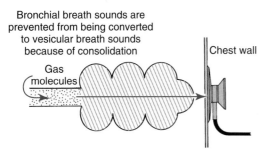

FIGURE 2-19 Auscultation of bronchial breath sounds over a consolidated lung unit.

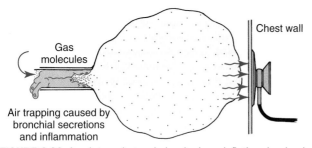

FIGURE 2-20 As air trapping and alveolar hyperinflation develop in obstructive lung diseases, breath sounds progressively diminish.

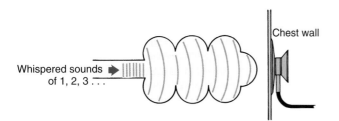

FIGURE 2-21 Whispered voice sounds auscultated over a normal lung are usually faint and unintelligible.

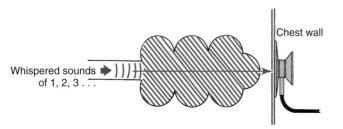

FIGURE 2-22 Whispering pectoriloquy. Whispered voice sounds heard over a consolidated lung are often louder and more intelligible compared with those of a normal lung.

The normal compliance of the lungs is graphically illustrated by the volume-pressure curve (Figure 2-23). When C_L increases, the lungs accept a greater volume of gas per unit pressure change. When C_L decreases, the lungs accept a smaller volume of gas per unit pressure change (Figure 2-24).

Although the precise mechanism is not clear, the fact that certain ventilatory patterns occur when lung compliance is altered is well documented. For example, when C_L decreases, the patient's breathing rate generally increases while the tidal volume simultaneously decreases (Figure 2-25). This type of breathing pattern is commonly seen in restrictive lung disorders such as pneumonia, pulmonary edema, and adult respiratory distress syndrome. This breathing pattern is also commonly seen during the early stages of an acute asthmatic attack when the alveoli are overinflated; C_L progressively decreases as the alveolar volume increases (Figure 2-23) at high lung volumes.

Airway Resistance and Its Effect on the Ventilatory Pattern

Airway resistance (R_{aw}) is defined as the pressure difference between the mouth and the alveoli (**transairway pressure**) divided by the flow rate. Therefore, the rate at which a certain volume of gas flows through the airways is a function of the pressure gradient and the resistance created by the airways to the flow of gas. Mathematically, R_{aw} is calculated as follows:

$$R_{aw} = \frac{\Delta P (cm\,H_2O)}{\dot{V}(L/sec)}.$$

For example, if a patient produces a flow rate of 6 L/sec during inspiration by generating a transairway pressure difference of 12 cm H_2O, R_{aw} would be 2 cm H_2O/L/sec:

$$
\begin{aligned}
R_{aw} &= \frac{\Delta P}{\dot{V}} \\
&= \frac{12\,cm\,H_2O}{6\,L/sec} \\
&= 2\,cm\,H_2O/L/sec.
\end{aligned}
$$

Under normal conditions, the R_{aw} in the tracheobronchial tree is about 1.0 to 2.0 cm H_2O/L/sec. However, in large airway obstructive pulmonary diseases (e.g., bronchitis, asthma), the R_{aw} may be extremely high.[2] An increased R_{aw} has a profound effect on the patient's ventilatory pattern.

When airway resistance increases significantly, the patient's ventilatory rate usually decreases while the tidal volume simultaneously increases (Figure 2-25). This type of breathing pattern is commonly seen in large airway obstructive lung diseases (e.g., chronic bronchitis, bronchiectasis, asthma, cystic fibrosis) during the advanced stages.

The ventilatory pattern adopted by the patient in either a restrictive or an obstructive lung disorder is thought to be based on minimum work requirements rather than gas exchange efficiency. In physics, work is defined as the force multiplied by the distance moved (work = force × distance).

---

[2]For a more in-depth discussion on this topic, see Chapter 3, Pulmonary Function Study Assessments.

TABLE 2-10 Common Assessment Abnormalities

Finding	Description	Possible Etiology and Significance
Inspection		
Pursed-lip breathing	Exhalation through mouth with lips pursed together to slow exhalation.	COPD, asthma. Suggests ↑ breathlessness. Strategy taught to slow expiration, ↓ dyspnea.
Tripod position; inability to lie flat	Leaning forward with arms and elbows supported on overbed table.	COPD, asthma in exacerbation, pulmonary edema. Indicates moderate to severe respiratory distress.
Accessory muscle use; intercostal retractions	Neck and shoulder muscles used to assist breathing. Muscles between ribs pull in during inspiration.	COPD, asthma in exacerbation, secretion retention. Indicates severe respiratory distress, hypoxemia.
Splinting	Voluntary ↓ in tidal volume to ↓ pain on chest expansion.	Thoracic or abdominal incision pain. Chest trauma, pleurisy.
↑ AP diameter	AP chest diameter equal to lateral. Slope of ribs more horizontal (90 degrees) to spine.	COPD, asthma, cystic fibrosis. Lung hyperinflation. Advanced age.
Tachypnea	Rate >20 breaths/min; >25 breaths/min in elderly.	Fever, anxiety, hypoxemia, restrictive lung disease. Magnitude of ↑ above normal rate reflects magnitude of increased work of breathing.
Kussmaul's respiration	Regular, rapid, and deep respirations.	Metabolic acidosis; ↑ in rate aids body in ↑ CO_2 excretion.
Cyanosis	Bluish color of skin best seen in earlobes, under the eyelids, or in nail beds.	↓ Oxygen transfer in lungs, ↓ cardiac output. Nonspecific, unreliable indicator.
Clubbing of fingers	↑ Depth, bulk, sponginess of distal digits of fingers.	Chronic hypoxemia. Cystic fibrosis, lung cancer, bronchiectasis.
Peripheral edema	Pitting edema.	Congestive heart failure, cor pulmonale.
Distended neck veins	Jugular venous distention.	Cor pulmonale, flail chest, pneumothorax.
Cough	Productive or nonproductive.	Bronchial airway and alveolar disease.
Sputum	See Table 2-12.	COPD, asthma, cystic fibrosis, pneumonia.
Abdominal paradox	Inward (rather than normal outward) movement of abdomen during inspiration.	Inefficient and ineffective breathing pattern. Nonspecific indicator of severe respiratory distress.
Palpation		
Tracheal deviation	Leftward or rightward movement of trachea from normal midline position.	Nonspecific indicator of change in position of mediastinal structures. Medical emergency if caused by tension pneumothorax.
Altered tactile fremitus	Increase or decrease in vibrations.	↑ In pneumonia, atelectasis; pulmonary edema; ↓ in pleural effusion, lung hyperinflation; absent in pneumothorax.
Altered chest movement	Unequal or equal but diminished movement of two sides of chest with inspiration.	Unequal movement caused by atelectasis, pneumothorax, pleural effusion, splinting; equal but diminished movement caused by barrel chest, restrictive disease, neuromuscular disease.
Percussion		
Hyperresonance	Loud, lower-pitched sound over areas that normally produce a resonant sound.	Lung hyperinflation (COPD), lung collapse (pneumothorax), air trapping (asthma).
Dullness/flatness	Medium-pitched sound over areas that normally produce a resonant sound.	↑ Density (pneumonia, large atelectasis), ↑ fluid pleural space (pleural effusion).
Auscultation		
Fine crackles	Series of discontinuous short, crackling, and popping sounds, high-pitched sounds heard just before the end of inspiration; result of rapid equalization of gas pressure when collapsed alveoli or terminal bronchioles suddenly snap open; similar sound to that made by rolling hair between fingers just behind ear.	Loss of lung volume (atelectasis), interstitial fibrosis (asbestosis), interstitial edema (early pulmonary edema), alveolar filling (pneumonia), early phase of congestive heart failure.

Continued

TABLE 2-10 Common Assessment Abnormalities—cont'd

Finding	Description	Possible Etiology and Significance
Coarse crackles	Series of discontinuous short, low-pitched bubbling, or gurgling sounds caused by air passing through airway intermittently occluded by mucus, unstable bronchial wall, or fold of mucosa; evident on inspiration and, in more severe cases, expiration; similar sound to blowing through straw under water; increase in bubbling quality with more fluid.	COPD, cystic fibrosis, congestive heart failure, bronchiectasis, pulmonary edema, pneumonia with severe congestion, COPD.
Wheezes	Continuous high-pitched whistling sound caused by rapid vibration of bronchial walls; first evident on expiration but possibly evident on inspiration as obstruction of airway increases; possibly audible without stethoscope.	Bronchospasm (caused by asthma), airway obstruction (caused by mucosal edema, inflammation, foreign body, tumor), COPD.
Bronchial breath sound	A harsh, hollow, or tubular breath sound. They are loud, high in pitch, and about equal in duration during inspiration and expiration. Inspiration is louder.	Alveolar consolidation and alveolar collapse (atelectasis).
Stridor	Continuous, loud, high-pitched sound caused by a partial obstruction of the larynx or trachea. Generally heard during inspiration.	Croup, epiglottitis, vocal cord edema after extubation, foreign body.
Pleural friction rub	A continuous, low-pitched creaking, or grating sound from roughened, inflamed surfaces of the pleura rubbing together. Generally heard during both inspiration and expiration. There is no change with coughing. The patient is usually uncomfortable, especially on deep inspiration.	Pleurisy, pneumonia, pulmonary fibrosis, pulmonary embolism, and thoracic surgery
Diminished breath sounds	Diminished or distant breath sounds.	COPD, drug overdose or major sedation, neuromuscular disease (Guillain-Barré or myasthenia gravis), flail chest, pleural effusion, and pneumothorax
Whispering pectoriloquy	Spoken or whispered syllable more distinct than normal on auscultation.	Alveolar consolidation and alveolar collapse (atelectasis).

AP, Anteroposterior; *COPD*, chronic obstructive pulmonary disease.

In respiratory physiology, the change in pulmonary pressure (force) multiplied by the change in lung volume (distance) may be used to quantify the **work of breathing** (work = pressure × volume).

The patient's usual adopted ventilatory pattern may not be seen in the clinical setting because of secondary heart or lung problems. For example, a patient with chronic bronchitis who has adopted a decreased ventilatory rate and an increased tidal volume because of the increased airway resistance associated with the disorder may demonstrate an increased ventilatory rate and decreased tidal volume in response to a secondary pneumonia (a restrictive lung disorder superimposed on a chronic obstructive lung disorder).

Because the patient may adopt a ventilatory pattern based on the expenditure of energy rather than on the efficiency of ventilation, the examiner cannot assume that the ventilatory pattern acquired by the patient in response to a certain respiratory disorder is the most efficient one in terms of physiologic gas exchange.

Peripheral Chemoreceptors and Their Effect on the Ventilatory Pattern

The **peripheral chemoreceptors** (also called *carotid* and *aortic bodies*) are oxygen-sensitive cells that react to a reduction of oxygen in the arterial blood (PaO_2). The peripheral chemoreceptors are located at the bifurcation of the internal and external carotid arteries (Figure 2-26) and on the aortic arch (Figure 2-27). Although the peripheral chemoreceptors are stimulated whenever the PaO_2 is less than normal, they are generally most active when the PaO_2 falls below 60 mm Hg (SaO_2 of about 90%). Suppression of these chemoreceptors, however, is seen when the PaO_2 falls below 30 mm Hg.

When the peripheral chemoreceptors are activated, an afferent (sensory) signal is sent to the respiratory centers of the medulla by way of the glossopharyngeal nerve (cranial nerve IX) from the carotid bodies and by way of the vagus nerve (cranial nerve X) from the aortic bodies. Efferent (motor) signals are then sent to the respiratory muscles, which results in an increased rate of breathing.

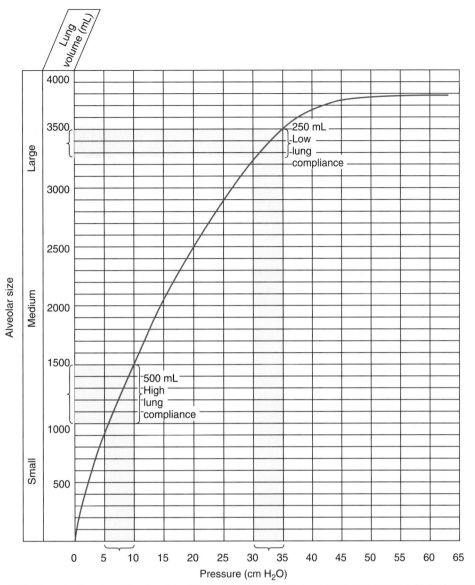

FIGURE 2-23 Normal volume-pressure curve. The curve shows that lung compliance progressively decreases as the lungs expand in response to more volume. For example, note the greater volume change between 5 and 10 cm H_2O (small and medium alveoli) than between 30 and 35 cm H_2O (large alveoli). The yellow volume area between 1000 mL and 1500 mL (the lower left quadrant of the volume-pressure curve) represents the normal tidal volume area.

It should be noted that in patients who have a chronically low PaO_2 (e.g., during the advanced stages of emphysema), the peripheral chemoreceptors are the primary receptor sites for the control of ventilation.

Causes of Hypoxemia. In respiratory disease, a decreased arterial oxygen level (hypoxemia) is the result of a decreased **ventilation-perfusion ratio, pulmonary shunting,** and **venous admixture** (see Chapter 10 for a broader discussion of hypoxemia).

Other Factors That Stimulate the Peripheral Chemoreceptors. Although the peripheral chemoreceptors are primarily activated by a decreased arterial oxygen level, they are also stimulated by a decreased pH (increased H^+ concentration). For example, the accumulation of lactic acid (from anaerobic metabolism) or ketoacids (diabetic acidosis) in the blood increases ventilatory rate almost entirely through the peripheral chemoreceptors. The peripheral chemoreceptors are also activated by hypoperfusion, increased temperature, nicotine, and the direct effect of $PaCO_2$. The response of the peripheral chemoreceptors to $PaCO_2$ stimulation, however, is relatively small compared with the response generated by the **central chemoreceptors.**

Central Chemoreceptors and Their Effect on the Ventilatory Pattern

Although the mechanism is not fully understood, it is now believed that two special respiratory centers in the medulla, the dorsal respiratory group (DRG) and the ventral respiratory group (VRG), are responsible for coordinating **respiration** (Figure 2-28). Both the DRG and VRG are stimulated by an increased concentration of H^+ in the cerebrospinal fluid (CSF). The H^+ concentration of the CSF is

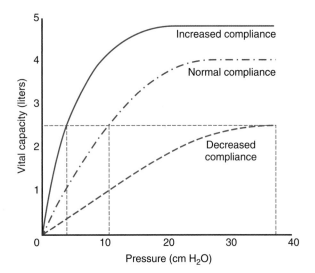

FIGURE 2-24 The effects of increased and decreased compliance on the volume-pressure curve. As the lung compliance decreases, greater pressure change is required to obtain the same volume of 2.5 L (*dotted lines*).

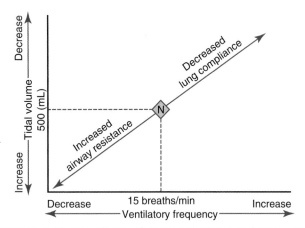

FIGURE 2-25 The effects of increased airway resistance and decreased lung compliance on ventilatory frequency and tidal volume. *N*, Normal resting tidal volume and ventilatory frequency.

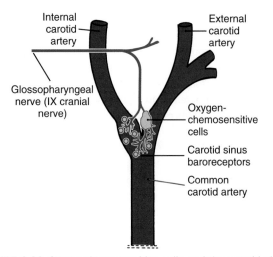

FIGURE 2-26 Oxygen-chemosensitive cells and the carotid sinus baroreceptors are located on the carotid artery.

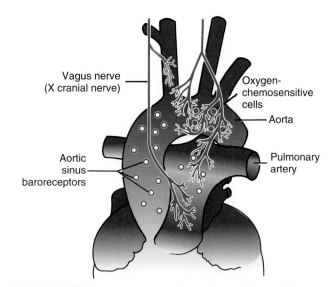

FIGURE 2-27 Oxygen-chemosensitive cells and the aortic sinus baroreceptors are located on the aortic notch and pulmonary artery.

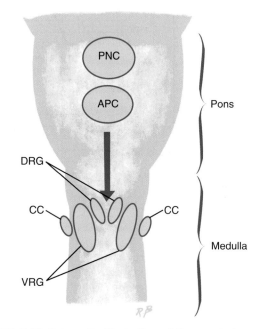

FIGURE 2-28 Schematic illustration of the respiratory components of the lower brain stem (pons and medulla). *APC*, Apneustic center; *CC*, central chemoreceptors; *DRG*, dorsal respiratory group; *PNC*, pneumotaxic center; *VRG*, ventral respiratory group.

monitored by the central chemoreceptors, which are located bilaterally and ventrally in the substance of the medulla. A portion of the central chemoreceptor region is actually in direct contact with the CSF. The central chemoreceptors transmit signals to the respiratory neurons by the following mechanism:

1. When the CO_2 level increases in the blood (e.g., during periods of hypoventilation), CO_2 molecules readily diffuse across the blood-brain barrier and enter the CSF. The blood-brain barrier is a semipermeable membrane that separates circulating blood from the CSF. The blood-brain barrier is relatively impermeable to ions such as H^+ and HCO_3^- but is very permeable to CO_2.

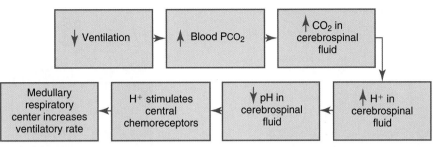

FIGURE 2-29 Sequence of events in alveolar hypoventilation. The central chemoreceptors are stimulated by hydrogen ions (H⁺), which increase in concentration as CO_2 moves into the cerebrospinal fluid.

2. After CO_2 crosses the blood-brain barrier and enters the CSF, it forms carbonic acid:

$$CO_2 + H_2O \Leftrightarrow H_2CO_3^- \Leftrightarrow H^+ + HCO_3^-.$$

3. Because the CSF has an inefficient buffering system, the H⁺ produced from the previous reaction rapidly increases and causes the pH of the CSF to decrease.
4. The central chemoreceptors react to the liberated H⁺ by sending signals to the respiratory components of the medulla, which in turn increases the ventilatory rate.
5. The increased ventilatory rate causes the $PaCO_2$ and subsequently the Pco_2 in the CSF to decrease. Therefore, the CO_2 level in the blood regulates ventilation by its indirect effect on the pH of the CSF (Figure 2-29).

Pulmonary Reflexes and Their Effect on the Ventilatory Pattern

Several reflexes may be activated in certain respiratory diseases and influence the patient's ventilatory rate.

Deflation Reflex. When the lungs are compressed or deflated (e.g., atelectasis), an increased rate of breathing is seen. The precise mechanism responsible for this reflex is not known. Some investigators suggest that the increased rate of breathing may simply result from reduced stimulation of the receptors (the **Hering-Breuer reflex**) rather than the stimulation of specific deflation receptors. Receptors for the Hering-Breuer reflex are located in the walls of the bronchi and bronchioles. When these receptors are stretched (e.g., during a deep inspiration), a reflex response is triggered to decrease the ventilatory rate. Other investigators, however, feel that the deflation reflex does not result from the absence of receptor stimulation of the Hering-Breuer reflex because the deflation reflex is still seen when the bronchi and bronchioles are below a temperature of 8° C. The Hering-Breuer reflex does not occur when the bronchi and bronchioles are below this temperature.

Irritant Reflex. When the lungs are compressed, deflated, or exposed to noxious gases, the irritant receptors are stimulated. The irritant receptors are subepithelial mechanoreceptors located in the trachea, bronchi, and bronchioles. When the receptors are activated, a reflex causes the ventilatory rate to increase. Stimulation of the irritant reflex may also produce a cough and bronchoconstriction.

Juxtapulmonary-Capillary Receptors. The juxtapulmonary-capillary receptors, or J receptors, are located in the interstitial tissues between the pulmonary capillaries and the alveoli. Their precise mechanism of action is not known. When the J receptors are stimulated, a reflex triggers rapid, shallow breathing. The J receptors may be activated by the following:
- Pulmonary capillary congestion
- Capillary hypertension
- Edema of the alveolar walls
- Humoral agents (e.g., serotonin)
- Lung deflation
- Emboli in the microcirculation

Reflexes from the Aortic and Carotid Sinus Baroreceptors. The normal function of the **aortic and carotid sinus baroreceptors**, located near the aortic and carotid peripheral chemoreceptors, is to activate reflexes that cause (1) decreased heart rate and ventilatory rate in response to increased systemic blood pressure and (2) increased heart rate and ventilatory rate in response to decreased systemic blood pressure.

Pain, Anxiety, and Fever

An increased respiratory rate may result from chest pain or fear and anxiety associated with the patient's inability to breathe. Chest pain, fear, and anxiety occur in a number of cardiopulmonary pathologies, such as pleurisy, rib fractures, pulmonary hypertension, and angina. An increased respiratory rate may also be caused by fever. Fever is commonly associated with infectious lung disorders such as pneumonia, lung abscess, tuberculosis, and fungal disease.

Use of the Accessory Muscles of Inspiration

During the advanced stages of chronic obstructive pulmonary disease, the accessory muscles of inspiration are activated when the diaphragm becomes significantly depressed by the increased residual volume and functional residual capacity. The accessory muscles assist or largely replace the diaphragm in creating subatmospheric pressure in the pleural space during inspiration. The major accessory muscles of inspiration are as follows:
- **Scalene**
- **Sternocleidomastoid**
- **Pectoralis major**
- **Trapezius**

Scalenes

The anterior, medial, and posterior **scalene muscles** are separate muscles that function as a unit. They originate on the

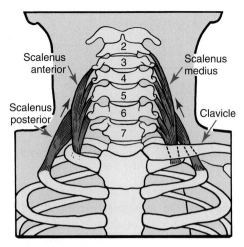

FIGURE 2-30 The scalene muscles (anterior neck). Red arrows indicate upward movement of the ribs.

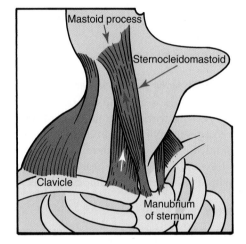

FIGURE 2-31 The sternocleidomastoid muscle. White arrow indicates upward movement of the sternum.

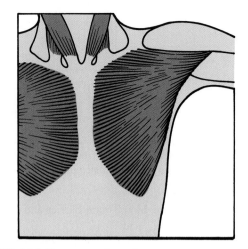

FIGURE 2-32 The pectoralis major muscles (anterior thorax).

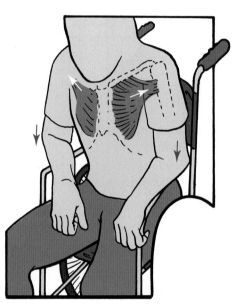

FIGURE 2-33 The way a patient may appear when using the pectoralis major muscles for inspiration. White arrows indicate the elevation of the chest. Downward blue arrows near the patient's elbows indicate how the patient may fix the arms to a stationary object.

transverse processes of the second to sixth cervical vertebrae and insert into the first and second ribs (Figure 2-30). These muscles normally elevate the first and second ribs and flex the neck. When they are used as accessory muscles of inspiration, their primary role is to elevate the first and second ribs.

Sternocleidomastoids

The **sternocleidomastoid muscles** are located on each side of the neck (Figure 2-31), where they rotate and support the head. They originate from the sternum and clavicle and insert into the mastoid process and occipital bone of the skull.

Normally, the sternocleidomastoid pulls from its sternoclavicular origin, rotates the head to the opposite side, and turns it upward. When the sternocleidomastoid muscle functions as an accessory muscle of inspiration, the head and neck are fixed by other muscles, and the sternocleidomastoid pulls from its insertion on the skull and elevates the sternum. This action increases the anteroposterior diameter of the chest. It is often prominent in patients with end-stage chronic obstructive pulmonary disease and other causes of respiratory distress.

Pectoralis Major Muscles

The pectoralis major muscles are powerful, fan-shaped muscles that originate from the clavicle and sternum and insert into the upper part of the humerus. The primary function of the pectoralis muscles is to pull the upper part of the arm to the body in a hugging motion (Figure 2-32).

When operating as an accessory muscle of inspiration, the pectoralis pulls from the humeral insertion and elevates the chest, resulting in an increased anteroposterior diameter. Patients with chronic obstructive pulmonary disease usually secure their arms to something stationary and use the pectoralis major muscles to increase the anteroposterior diameter of the chest (Figure 2-33). This braced position is called the **tripod position**.

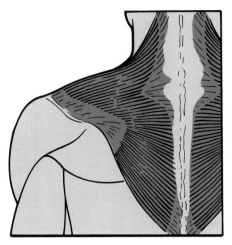

FIGURE 2-34 The trapezius muscles (posterior thorax).

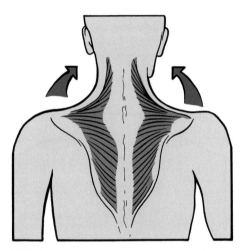

FIGURE 2-35 The action of the trapezius muscle is typified in shrugging the shoulders.

Trapezius

The trapezius is a large, flat, triangular muscle that is situated superficially in the upper part of the back and the back of the neck. The muscle originates from the occipital bone, the ligamentum nuchae, the spinous processes of the seventh cervical vertebra, and all the thoracic vertebrae. It inserts into the spine of the scapula, the acromion process, and the lateral third of the clavicle (Figure 2-34). The **trapezius muscle** rotates the scapula, raises the shoulders, and abducts and flexes the arm. Its action is typified in shrugging the shoulders (Figure 2-35). When used as an accessory muscle of inspiration, the trapezius helps elevate the thoracic cage.

Use of the Accessory Muscles of Expiration

Because of the airway narrowing and collapse associated with chronic obstructive pulmonary disorders, the accessory muscles of exhalation are often recruited when airway resistance becomes significantly elevated. When these muscles actively contract, intrapleural pressure increases and offsets the increased airway resistance. The major accessory muscles of exhalation are as follows:

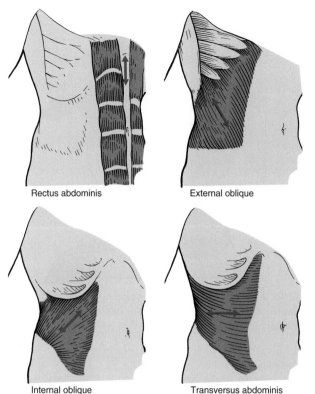

Rectus abdominis   External oblique

Internal oblique   Transversus abdominis

FIGURE 2-36 Accessory muscles of expiration. Arrows indicate the action of these muscles in reducing the volume of the lungs.

- **Rectus abdominis**
- **External oblique**
- **Internal oblique**
- **Transversus abdominis**

Rectus Abdominis

A pair of **rectus abdominis muscles** extends the entire length of the abdomen. Each muscle forms a vertical mass about 4 inches wide, separated by the linea alba. It arises from the iliac crest and pubic symphysis and inserts into the xiphoid process and the fifth, sixth, and seventh ribs. When activated, the muscle assists in compressing the abdominal contents, which in turn push the diaphragm into the thoracic cage (Figure 2-36).

External Obliques

The broad, thin, external oblique muscle is on the anterolateral side of the abdomen. The muscle is the longest and most superficial of all the anterolateral muscles of the abdomen. It arises by eight digitations from the lower eight ribs and the abdominal aponeurosis. It inserts in the iliac crest and into the linea alba. The muscle assists in compressing the abdominal contents. This action also pushes the diaphragm into the thoracic cage during exhalation (Figure 2-36).

Internal Obliques

The internal oblique muscle is in the lateral and ventral part of the abdominal wall directly under the external oblique muscle. It is smaller and thinner than the external oblique. It arises from the inguinal ligament, the iliac crest, and the

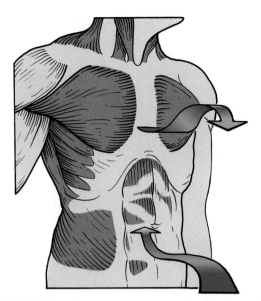

FIGURE 2-37 When the accessory muscles of expiration contract, intrapleural pressure increases, the chest moves outward, and expiratory air flow increases.

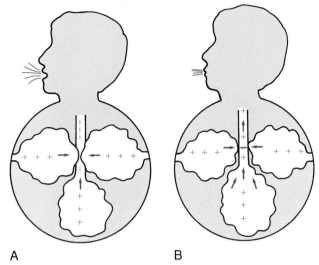

A   B

FIGURE 2-38 A, Schematic illustration of alveolar compression of weakened bronchiolar airways during normal expiration in patients with chronic obstructive pulmonary disease (e.g., emphysema). B, Effects of pursed-lip breathing. The weakened bronchiolar airways are kept open by the effects of positive pressure created by pursed lips during expiration.

lower portion of the lumbar aponeurosis. It inserts into the last four ribs and the linea alba. The muscle assists in compressing the abdominal contents and pushing the diaphragm into the thoracic cage (Figure 2-36).

Transversus Abdominis

The **transversus abdominis muscle** is found immediately under each internal oblique muscle. It arises from the inguinal ligament, the iliac crest, the thoracolumbar fascia, and the lower six ribs. It inserts into the linea alba. When activated, it constricts the abdominal contents (Figure 2-36).

When all four pairs of accessory muscles of exhalation contract, the abdominal pressure increases and drives the diaphragm into the thoracic cage. As the diaphragm moves into the thoracic cage during exhalation, the intrapleural pressure increases and enhances expiratory gas flow (Figure 2-37).

Pursed-Lip Breathing

Pursed-lip breathing occurs in patients during the advanced stages of obstructive pulmonary disease. It is a relatively simple technique that many patients learn without formal instruction. During pursed-lip breathing the patient exhales through lips that are held in a position similar to that used for whistling, kissing, or blowing through a flute. The positive pressure created by retarding the air flow through pursed lips provides the airways with some stability and an increased ability to resist surrounding intrapleural pressures. This action offsets early airway collapse and air trapping during exhalation. In addition, pursed-lip breathing has been shown to slow the patient's ventilatory rate and generate a ventilatory pattern that is more effective in gas mixing (Figure 2-38).

Substernal and Intercostal Retractions

Substernal and intercostal retractions may be seen in patients with severe restrictive lung disorders such as pneumonia or

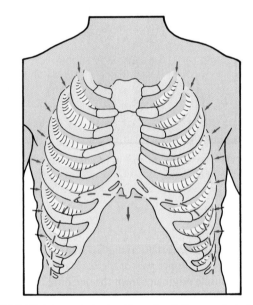

FIGURE 2-39 Intercostal retraction of soft tissues during forceful inspiration.

adult respiratory distress syndrome. In an effort to overcome the low lung compliance, the patient must generate a greater-than-normal negative intrapleural pressure during inspiration. This greater negative intrapleural pressure causes the tissues between the ribs and the substernal area to retract during inspiration (Figure 2-39). Because the thorax of the newborn is very flexible (as a result of the large amount of cartilage found in the skeletal structure), substernal and intercostal retractions are often seen in newborn respiratory disorders—such as, respiratory distress syndrome, meconium aspiration syndrome, transient tachypnea of the newborn, bronchopulmonary dysplasia, and congenital diaphragmatic hernia.

Nasal Flaring

Nasal flaring is often seen during inspiration in infants experiencing respiratory distress. It is likely to be a facial reflex that enhances the movement of gas into the tracheobronchial tree. The dilator naris, which originates from the maxilla and inserts into the ala of the nose, is the muscle responsible for this clinical manifestation. When activated, the dilator naris pulls the alae laterally and widens the nasal aperture, providing a larger orifice for gas to enter the lungs during inspiration (see Chapter 32).

Splinting and Decreased Chest Expansion Caused by Pleuritic and Nonpleuritic Chest Pain

Chest pain is one of the most common complaints among patients with cardiopulmonary problems. It can be divided into two categories: pleuritic and nonpleuritic. Resistance to taking a deep breath is a symptom of pleuritic chest pain, and is called **splinting**.

Pleuritic Chest Pain

Pleuritic chest pain is usually described as a sudden, sharp, or stabbing pain. The pain generally intensifies during deep inspiration and coughing and diminishes during breath holding or splinting. The origin of the pain may be the chest wall, muscles, ribs, parietal pleura, diaphragm, mediastinal structures, or intercostal nerves. Because the visceral pleura, which covers the lungs, does not have any sensory nerve supply, pain originating in the parietal region signifies extension of inflammation from the lungs to the contiguous parietal pleura lining the inner surface of the chest wall. This condition is known as *pleurisy* (Figure 2-40). When a patient with pleurisy inhales, the lung expands, irritating the inflamed parietal pleura and causing pain.

Because of the nature of the pleuritic pain, the patient usually prefers to lie on the affected side to allow greater expansion of the uninvolved lung and help splint the chest.

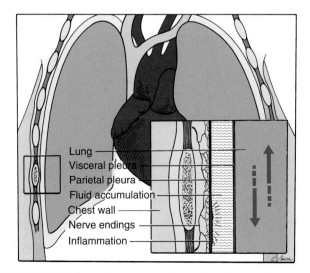

FIGURE 2-40 When the parietal pleura is irritated, the nerve endings in the parietal pleura send pain signals to the brain.

Pleuritic chest pain is a characteristic feature of the following respiratory diseases:
- Pneumonia
- Pleural effusion
- Pneumothorax
- Pulmonary infarction
- Lung cancer
- Pneumoconiosis
- Fungal diseases
- Tuberculosis

Nonpleuritic Chest Pain

Nonpleuritic chest pain is described as a constant pain that is usually located centrally. It is not generally worsened by deep inspiration. The pain may also radiate. Nonpleuritic chest pain is associated with the following disorders:
- Myocardial ischemia
- Pericardial inflammation
- Pulmonary hypertension
- Esophagitis
- Local trauma or inflammation of the chest cage, muscles, bones, or cartilage

Abnormal Chest Shape and Configuration

During inspection, the respiratory care practitioner systematically observes the patient's chest for both normal and abnormal findings. Is the spine straight? Are any lesions or surgical scars evident? Are the scapulae symmetric? Is there a barrel chest deformity? Common chest deformities are listed in Table 2-11.

Abnormal Extremity Findings

The inspection of the patient's extremities should include the following:
- Altered skin color (e.g., cyanotic, pale, red, purple, etc.)
- Presence or absence of digital clubbing
- Presence or absence of peripheral edema
- Presence or absence of distended neck veins

Altered Skin Color

A general observation of the patient's skin color should be routinely performed. For example, does the patient's skin color appear normal—pink, tan, brown, or black? Is the skin cold or clammy? Does the skin and/or mucous membranes appear ashen or pallid? This appearance could be caused by anemia or acute blood loss. Do the patient's eyes, face, trunk, and arms have a yellow, jaundiced appearance (caused by increased bilirubin in the blood and tissue)? Is there redness of the skin or erythema (often caused by capillary congestion, inflammation, or infection)? Does the patient appear cyanotic?

Cyanosis

Cyanosis is common in severe respiratory disorders. *Cyanosis* is the term used to describe the blue-gray or purplish discoloration of the mucous membranes, fingertips, and toes whenever the blood in these areas contains at least 5 g/dL of reduced hemoglobin. When the normal 14 to 15 g/dL of hemoglobin is fully saturated, the PaO_2 is about 97 to

TABLE 2-11 Common Abnormal Chest Shapes and Configurations

Condition	Description
Kyphosis	A "hunchbacked" appearance caused by posterior curvature of the spine
Scoliosis	A lateral curvature of the spine that results in the chest protruding posteriorly and the anterior ribs flattening out
Kyphoscoliosis	The combination of kyphosis and scoliosis (see Figure 25-1)
Pectus carinatum	The forward projection of the xiphoid process and lower sternum (also known as "pigeon breast" deformity)
Pectus excavatum	A funnel-shaped depression over the lower sternum (also called "funnel chest")
Barrel chest	In the normal adult, the anteroposterior diameter of the chest is about half its lateral diameter, or 1:2. When the patient has a barrel chest, the ratio is nearer to 1:1 (Figure 2-41)

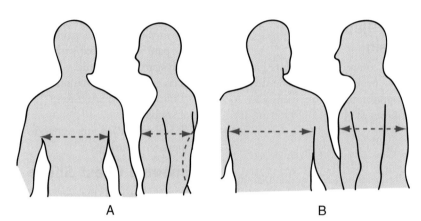

A   B

FIGURE 2-41 A, Normally, the anteroposterior diameter is about half the lateral diameter (a ratio of 1:2). Because of the air trapping and lung hyperinflation in obstructive pulmonary diseases, the natural tendency of the lungs to recoil is decreased and the normal tendency of the chest to move outward prevails. This condition results in an increased anteroposterior diameter and is referred to as the *barrel chest deformity*. The ratio is nearer to 1:1. B, The anteroposterior diameter commonly increases with aging. Therefore, older individuals may have a slight barrel chest appearance in the absence of any pulmonary disease. Normal infants also usually have an anteroposterior diameter near 1:1.

100 mm Hg, and there is about 20 mL/dL of oxygen in the blood. In a cyanotic patient with one third (5 g/dL) of the hemoglobin reduced, the PaO_2 is about 30 mm Hg and there is 13 mL/dL of oxygen in the blood (Figures 2-42 and 2-43).

The detection and interpretation of cyanosis are problematic in clinical practice, and wide individual variations occur among observers. The recognition of cyanosis depends on the acuity of the observer, the light conditions in the examining room, and the pigmentation of the patient. Cyanosis of the nail beds is also influenced by temperature because vasoconstriction induced by cold may slow circulation to the point at which the blood becomes hypoxic (bluish) in the surface capillaries even though the arterial blood in the major vessels is not lacking in oxygen.

Central cyanosis, as observed on the mucous membranes of the lips and mouth, is almost always a sign of hypoxemia and therefore has a definite diagnostic value.

In the patient with polycythemia, cyanosis may be present at a PaO_2 well above 30 mm Hg because the amount of reduced hemoglobin is often greater than 5 g/dL in these patients, even when their total oxygen content is within normal limits. In respiratory disease, cyanosis is the result of (1) a decreased $\dot{V}/\dot{Q}$ ratio, (2) pulmonary shunting, (3) venous admixture, and (4) hypoxemia.

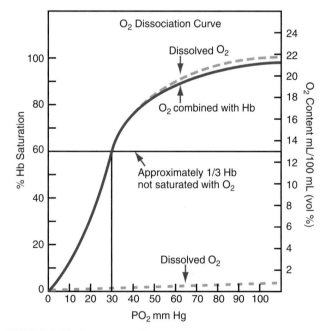

FIGURE 2-42 Cyanosis is likely whenever the blood contains at least 5 g/100 mL of reduced hemoglobin. In the normal individual who has about 15 g of hemoglobin per 100 mL of blood, a PO_2 of about 30 mm Hg produces 5 g/100 mL of reduced hemoglobin. The hemoglobin, however, is still approximately 60% saturated with oxygen.

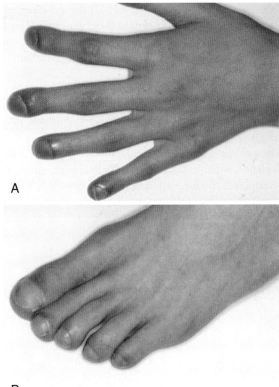

A

B

FIGURE 2-43 Digital clubbing and cyanosis.

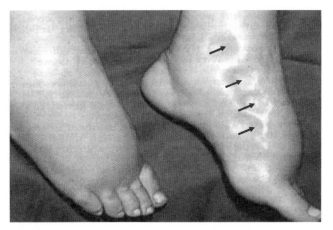

FIGURE 2-44 4+ pitting edema. (From Bloom A, Ireland J: *Color atlas of diabetes*, ed 2, London, 1992, Mosby-Wolfe.)

Digital Clubbing

Digital clubbing is sometimes observed in patients with chronic respiratory disorders. Clubbing is characterized by a bulbous swelling of the terminal phalanges of the fingers and toes. The contour of the nail becomes rounded both longitudinally and transversely, which results in an increase in the angle between the surface of the nail and the dorsal surface of the terminal phalanx (see Figure 2-43).

The specific cause of clubbing is unknown. It is a normal hereditary finding in some families without any known history of cardiopulmonary disease. It is believed that the following factors may be causative: (1) circulating vasodilators, such as bradykinin and the prostaglandins, that are released from normal tissues but are not degraded by the lungs because of intrapulmonary shunting; (2) chronic infection; (3) unspecified toxins; (4) capillary stasis from increased venous back pressure; (5) arterial hypoxemia; and (6) local hypoxia. Successful treatment of the underlying disease may result in at least some resolution of the clubbing and return of the digits to normal.

Peripheral Edema

Bilateral, dependent, **pitting edema** is commonly seen in patients with congestive heart failure, cor pulmonale, and hepatic cirrhosis. To assess the presence and severity of pitting edema, the health-care practitioner places a finger or fingers over the tibia or medial malleolus (2 to 4 inches above the foot), firmly depresses the skin for 5 seconds, and then releases. Normally, this procedure leaves no indentation, although a pit may be seen if the person has been standing all day or is pregnant. If pitting is present, it is graded on the

following subjective scale: 1+ (mild, slight depression) to 4+ (severe, deep depression) (Figure 2-44).

Distended Neck Veins

In patients with left-heart failure (congested heart failure), right-heart failure (cor pulmonale), severe flail chest, pneumothorax, or pleural effusion, the major veins of the chest that return blood to the right side of the heart may be compressed. When this happens, venous return decreases and central venous pressure increases. This condition is manifested by distended neck veins (also called *jugular venous distention;* Figure 2-45). The reduced venous return may also cause the patient's cardiac output and systemic blood pressure to decrease. In severe cases, the veins over the entire upper anterior thorax may be dilated.

Normal and Abnormal Sputum Production

Normal Histology and Mucous Production of the Tracheobronchial Tree

The wall of the tracheobronchial tree is composed of three major layers: an epithelial lining, the lamina propria, and a cartilaginous layer (Figure 2-46).

The epithelial lining, which is separated from the lamina propria by a basement membrane, is predominantly composed of pseudostratified, ciliated, columnar epithelium interspersed with numerous mucus-secreting glands and serous cells. The ciliated cells extend from the beginning of the trachea to—and sometimes including—the respiratory bronchioles. As the tracheobronchial tree becomes progressively smaller, the columnar structure of the ciliated cells gradually decreases in height. In the terminal bronchioles, the epithelium appears more cuboidal than columnar. These cells flatten even more in the respiratory bronchioles (Figure 2-46).

A mucous layer, commonly referred to as the *mucous blanket,* covers the epithelial lining of the tracheobronchial tree (Figure 2-47). The viscosity of the mucous layer progressively increases from the epithelial lining to the inner luminal surface and has two distinct layers: (1) the sol layer, which is

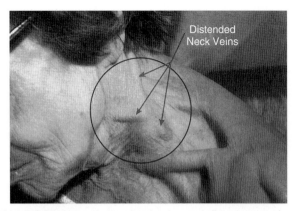

FIGURE 2-45 Distended neck veins (*arrows*). Prominence of sternocleidomastoid muscle is also seen in the lower portion of this photograph.

adjacent to the epithelial lining, and (2) the gel layer, which is the more viscous layer adjacent to the inner luminal surface. The mucous blanket is 95% water. The remaining 5% consists of glycoproteins, carbohydrates, lipids, DNA, some cellular debris, and foreign particles.

The mucous blanket is produced by the goblet cells and the submucosal, or bronchial, glands. The goblet cells are located intermittently between the pseudostratified, ciliated columnar cells distal to the terminal bronchioles.

Most of the mucous blanket is produced by the submucosal glands, which extend deeply into the lamina propria and are composed of different cell types: serous cells, mucous cells, collecting duct cells, mast cells, myoepithelial cells, and clear cells, which are probably lymphocytes. The submucosal

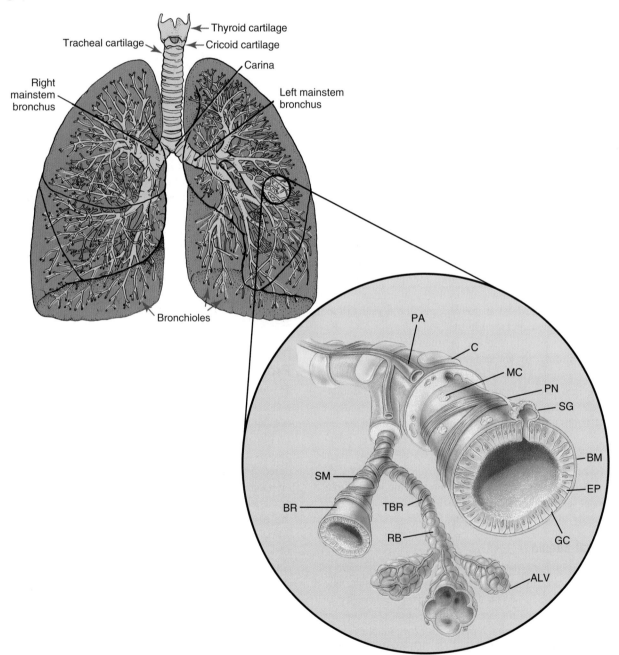

FIGURE 2-46 The normal lung. *ALV*, Alveoli; *BM*, basement membrane; *BR*, bronchioles; *C*, cartilage; *EP*, epithelium; *GC*, goblet cell; *LP*, lamina propria; *MC*, mast cell; *PA*, pulmonary artery; *PN*, parasympathetic nerve; *RB*, respiratory bronchioles; *SG*, submucosal gland; *SM*, smooth muscle; *TBR*, terminal bronchioles.

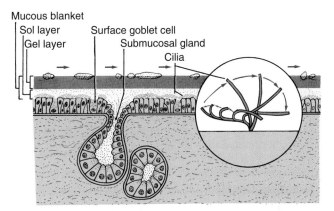

FIGURE 2-47 The epithelial lining of the tracheobronchial tree.

TABLE 2-12 Analysis of Sputum Color and Characteristics

Color/Characteristics	Indications and Conditions
Brown/dark	Old blood
Bright red (hemoptysis)	Fresh blood (bleeding tumor, tuberculosis)
Clear and translucent	Normal
Copious	Large amount
Frank hemoptysis	Massive amount of blood
Green	Stagnant sputum or gram-negative bacteria
Green and foul smelling	Pseudomonas or anaerobic infection
Mucoid (white/gray)	Asthma, chronic bronchitis
Pink, frothy	Pulmonary edema
Tenacious	Secretions that are sticky or adhesive or otherwise tend to hold together
Viscous	Thick, viscid, sticky, or glutinous
Yellow or opaque	Presence of white blood cells, bacterial infection

glands are particularly numerous in the medium-sized bronchi and disappear in the bronchioles. These glands are innervated by parasympathetic (cholinergic) nerve fibers and normally produce about 100 mL of clear, thin bronchial secretions per day.

The mucous blanket is an important cleansing mechanism of the tracheobronchial tree. Inhaled particles stick to the mucus. The distal ends of the cilia continually strike the innermost portion of the gel layer and propel the mucous layer, along with any foreign particles, toward the larynx. At this point, the cough mechanism moves secretions beyond the larynx and into the oropharynx. This mucociliary mechanism is commonly referred to as the *mucociliary transport* or the *mucociliary escalator*. The cilia move the mucous blanket at an estimated average rate of 2 cm/min.

The submucosal layer of the tracheobronchial tree is the lamina propria. Within the lamina propria is a loose, fibrous tissue that contains tiny blood vessels, lymphatic vessels, and branches of the vagus nerve. A circular layer of smooth muscle is also found within the lamina propria. It extends from the trachea down to and including the terminal bronchioles.

The cartilaginous structures that surround the tracheobronchial tree progressively diminish in size as the airways extend into the lungs. The cartilaginous layer is completely absent in bronchioles less than 1 mm in diameter (Figure 2-46).

Abnormal Sputum Production

Excessive sputum production is commonly seen in respiratory diseases that cause an acute or chronic inflammation of the tracheobronchial tree (see Figure 12-1). Depending on the severity and nature of the respiratory disease, sputum production may take several forms. For example, during the early stages of tracheobronchial tree inflammation, the sputum is usually clear, thin, and odorless. As the disease intensifies, the sputum becomes yellow-green and opaque. The yellow-green appearance results from an enzyme (myeloperoxidase) that is released during the cellular breakdown of leukocytes. It may also be caused by retained or stagnant secretions or secretions caused by an acute infection.

Thick and tenacious sputum is commonly seen in patients with chronic bronchitis, bronchiectasis, cystic fibrosis, and asthma. Patients with pulmonary edema expectorate a thin, frothy, pinkish sputum. Technically, this fluid is not true sputum. It results from the movement of plasma and red blood cells across the alveolar-capillary membrane into the alveoli. **Hemoptysis** is the coughing up of blood or blood-tinged sputum from the tracheobronchial tree. In true hemoptysis the sputum is usually bright red and interspersed with air bubbles.

Clinically, hemoptysis may be confused with hematemesis, which is blood that originates from the upper gastrointestinal tract and usually has a dark, coffee-ground appearance. Repeated expectoration of blood-streaked sputum is seen in chronic bronchitis, bronchiectasis, cystic fibrosis, pulmonary embolism, lung cancer, necrotizing infections, tuberculosis, and fungal diseases. A small amount of hemoptysis is common after bronchoscopy, particularly when biopsies are performed. *Massive hemoptysis* is defined as coughing up 400 to 600 mL of blood within a 24-hour period. Death from exsanguination resulting from hemoptysis is rare. Table 2-12 provides a general overview and analysis of the types of sputum commonly seen in the clinical setting.

Cough

A cough is a sudden, audible expulsion of air from the lungs. It is commonly seen in respiratory disease, especially in disorders that cause inflammation of the tracheobronchial tree. In general, a cough is preceded by (1) a deep inspiration, (2) partial closure of the glottis, and (3) forceful contraction of the accessory muscles of expiration to expel air from the lungs. In essence, a cough is a protective mechanism that clears the lungs, bronchi, or trachea of irritants. A cough also prevents the aspiration of foreign material into the lungs. For example, a cough is a common symptom associated with chronic sinusitis and postnasal drip. The effectiveness of a cough depends largely on (1) the depth of the preceding

BOX 2-5 Common Factors That Stimulate the Irritant Receptors

- Inflammation
- Infectious agents
- Excessive secretions
- Noxious gases (e.g., cigarette smoke, chemical inhalation)
- Very hot or very cold air
- A mass of any sort obstructing the airway or compressing the lungs
- Mechanical stimulation (e.g., endotracheal suctioning, compression of the airways)

inspiration and (2) the extent of dynamic compression of the airways.

Although a cough may be voluntary, it is usually a reflex response that arises when an irritant stimulates the irritant receptors (also called *subepithelial mechanoreceptors*). The irritant receptors are located in the pharynx, larynx, trachea, and large bronchi. When stimulated, the irritant receptors send a signal by way of the glossopharyngeal nerve (cranial nerve IX) and vagus nerve (cranial nerve X) to the cough reflex center located in the medulla. The medulla then causes the glottis to close and the accessory muscles of expiration to contract. Box 2-5 lists common factors that stimulate the irritant receptors.

Clinically, a cough is termed *productive* if sputum is produced and *nonproductive* if no sputum is produced.

Nonproductive Cough

Common causes of a nonproductive cough include (1) irritation of the airway, (2) inflammation of the airways, (3) mucous accumulation, (4) tumors, and (5) irritation of the pleura.

Productive Cough

When the cough is productive, the respiratory practitioner should assess the following:

- Is the cough strong or weak? In other words, does the patient have a good or poor ability to mobilize bronchial secretions? A good, strong cough may indicate only deep breathing and cough therapy, whereas an inadequate cough may suggest the need for chest physical therapy or postural drainage.
- A productive cough should be evaluated in terms of its frequency, pitch, and loudness. A brassy cough may indicate a tumor, whereas a barking or hoarse cough indicates croup.
- Finally, the sputum of a productive cough should be monitored and evaluated frequently in terms of amount (teaspoons, tablespoons, cups), consistency (thin, thick, tenacious), odor, and color (Table 2-12).

SELF-ASSESSMENT QUESTIONS

Answers to questions can be found on Evolve. To access additional student assessment questions visit
http://evolve.elsevier.com/DesJardins/respiratory.

1. **Which of the following pathologic conditions increases vocal fremitus?**
   1. Atelectasis
   2. Pleural effusion
   3. Pneumothorax
   4. Pneumonia
      a. 3 only
      b. 4 only
      c. 2 and 3 only
      d. 1 and 4 only

2. **A dull or soft percussion note would likely be heard in which of the following pathologic conditions?**
   1. Chronic obstructive pulmonary disease
   2. Pneumothorax
   3. Pleural thickening
   4. Atelectasis
      a. 1 only
      b. 2 only
      c. 2 and 3 only
      d. 3 and 4 only

3. **Bronchial breath sounds are likely to be heard in which of the following pathologic conditions?**
   1. Alveolar consolidation
   2. Chronic obstructive pulmonary disease
   3. Atelectasis
   4. Fluid accumulation in the tracheobronchial tree
      a. 3 only
      b. 4 only
      c. 1 and 3 only
      d. 2 and 4 only

4. **Wheezing is:**
   1. Produced by bronchospasm
   2. Generally auscultated during inspiration
   3. A cardinal finding of bronchial asthma
   4. Usually heard as high-pitched sounds
      a. 1 only
      b. 1 and 3 only
      c. 2 and 4 only
      d. 1, 3, and 4 only

5. In which of the following pathologic conditions is transmission of the whispered voice of a patient through a stethoscope unusually clear?
   1. Chronic obstructive pulmonary disease
   2. Alveolar consolidation
   3. Atelectasis
   4. Pneumothorax
      a. 1 only
      b. 2 and 3 only
      c. 1 and 4 only
      d. 1, 2, and 3 only

6. An individual's ventilatory pattern is composed of which of the following?
   1. Inspiratory and expiratory force
   2. Ventilatory rate
   3. Tidal volume
   4. Inspiratory and expiratory ratio
      a. 1 and 3 only
      b. 2 and 3 only
      c. 2, 3, and 4 only
      d. 1, 2, and 3 only

7. Which of the following abnormal breathing patterns is commonly associated with diabetic acidosis?
   1. Orthopnea
   2. Kussmaul's respiration
   3. Biot's respiration
   4. Hypoventilation

8. What is the average total compliance of the lungs and chest wall combined?
   1. 0.05 L/cm H_2O
   2. 0.1 L/cm H_2O
   3. 0.2 L/cm H_2O
   4. 0.3 L/cm H_2O

9. When lung compliance decreases, which of the following is seen?
   1. Ventilatory rate usually decreases.
   2. Tidal volume usually decreases.
   3. Ventilatory rate usually increases.
   4. Tidal volume usually increases.
      a. 1 only
      b. 2 only
      c. 3 and 4 only
      d. 2 and 3 only

10. What is the normal airway resistance in the tracheobronchial tree?
    1. 0.5 to 1.0 cm H_2O/L/sec
    2. 1.0 to 2.0 cm H_2O/L/sec
    3. 2.0 to 3.0 cm H_2O/L/sec
    4. 3.0 to 4.0 cm H_2O/L/sec

11. When the systemic blood pressure increases, the aortic and carotid sinus baroreceptors initiate reflexes that cause which of the following?
    1. Increased heart rate
    2. Decreased ventilatory rate
    3. Increased ventilatory rate
    4. Decreased heart rate
       a. 1 only
       b. 2 only
       c. 3 only
       d. 2 and 4 only

12. What is the anteroposterior-transverse chest diameter ratio in the normal adult?
    1. 1:0.5
    2. 1:1
    3. 1:2
    4. 1:3
    5. 1:4

13. Which of the following muscles originate from the clavicle?
    1. Scalene muscles
    2. Sternocleidomastoid muscles
    3. Pectoralis major muscles
    4. Trapezius muscles
       a. 1 only
       b. 2 only
       c. 4 only
       d. 2 and 3 only

14. Which of the following is associated with digital clubbing?
    1. Chronic infection
    2. Local hypoxia
    3. Circulating vasodilators
    4. Arterial hypoxia
       a. 2 only
       b. 2 and 4 only
       c. 2, 3, and 4 only
       d. 1, 2, 3, and 4

15. Which of the following is associated with pleuritic chest pain?
    1. Lung cancer
    2. Pneumonia
    3. Myocardial ischemia
    4. Tuberculosis
       a. 1 only
       b. 2 only
       c. 1 and 3 only
       d. 1, 2, and 4 only

Pulmonary Function Study Assessments

Chapter Objectives

After reading this chapter, you will be able to:

- Describe the following lung volumes and capacities:
  - List the normal lung volumes and capacities of normal recumbent subjects who are 20 to 30 years of age.
  - Describe the residual volume/total lung capacity ratio (RV/TLC ratio).
  - Identify lung volumes and lung capacity findings characteristic of restrictive lung disorders.
  - List the anatomic alterations of the lungs associated with restrictive lung disorders.
  - Identify lung volumes and capacity findings characteristic of obstructive lung disorders.
  - List the anatomic alterations of the lungs associated with obstructive lung disorders.
- Describe the following indirect measurements of the residual volume and lung capacities containing the residual volume:
  - Describe expiratory flow rate and volume measurements and their respective normal values.
  - Describe how the FVC, FEV_1, and FEV_1/FVC ratio ($FEV_{1\%}$) are used to differentiate restrictive and obstructive lung disorders.
  - Identify forced expiratory flow rate findings characteristic of restrictive lung disorders.
  - Identify forced expiratory flow rate findings characteristic of obstructive lung disorders.
  - Describe the pulmonary diffusion capacity (DLCO).
  - Identify DLCO findings characteristic of restrictive lung disorders.
  - Identify DLCO findings characteristic of obstructive lung disorders.
- Describe the following tests used to assess the patient's muscle strength at the bedside:
  - Describe the role of cardiopulmonary exercise testing (CPET) in the pulmonary function laboratory.
  - Identify other diagnostic tests used to measure airway responsiveness in asthma patients.

Key Terms

Air Trapping
Body Plethysmography
Cardiopulmonary Exercise Testing (CPET)
Closed Circuit Helium Dilution Test
Exercise or Cold Air Challenge
Expiratory Reserve Volume (ERV)
Flow-Volume Loop
Forced Expiratory Flow 200–1200 mL of FVC ($FEF_{200-1200}$)
Forced Expiratory Flow 25%–75% ($FEF_{25\%-75\%}$)
Forced Expiratory Flow at 50% ($FEF_{50\%}$)
Forced Expiratory Volume in 1 second (FEV_1)

Forced Expiratory Volume in 1 second/Forced Vital Capacity Ratio (FEV_1/FVC ratio)
Forced Expiratory Volume in 1 second Percentage ($FEV_{1\%}$)
Forced Expiratory Volume Timed (FEV_T)
Forced Vital Capacity (FVC)
Functional Residual Capacity (FRC)
Inhaled Mannitol
Inhaled Methacholine or Histamine
Inspiratory Capacity (IC)
Inspiratory Reserve Volume (IRV)
Lung Capacities
Lung Volumes
Maximum Expiratory Pressure (MEP)
Maximum Inspiratory Pressure (MIP)
Maximum Voluntary Ventilation (MVV)
Obstructive Lung Disorders
Open-Circuit Nitrogen Washout Test
Peak Expiratory Flow Rate (PEFR)
Pulmonary Diffusion Capacity of Carbon Monoxide (DLCO)
Residual Volume (RV)
Residual Volume/Total Lung Capacity Ratio (RV/TLC)
Restrictive Lung Disorders
Tidal Volume (V_T)
Total Expiratory Time (TET)
Total Lung Capacity (TLC)
Vital Capacity (VC)

Chapter Outline

Normal Lung Volumes and Capacities
  Restrictive Lung Disorders: Lung Volume and Capacity Findings
  Obstructive Lung Disorders: Lung Volume and Capacity Findings
  Indirect Measurements of the Residual Volume and Lung Capacities Containing the Residual Volume
Forced Expiratory Flow Rate and Volume Measurements
  Forced Vital Capacity
  Forced Expiratory Volume Timed
  Forced Expiratory Volume in 1 second/Forced Vital Capacity (FEV_1/FVC) Ratio
  Forced Expiratory Flow at 25% to 75%
  Forced Expiratory Flow between 200 and 1200 mL of Forced Vital Capacity
  Peak Expiratory Flow Rate
  Maximum Voluntary Ventilation
  Flow-Volume Loop
Pulmonary Diffusion Capacity
Assessment of Respiratory Muscle Strength
Cardiopulmonary Exercise Testing (CPET)
Other Diagnostic Tests for Asthma
Self-Assessment Questions

TABLE 3-1 General Hierarchy of Expense and Complexity of Pulmonary Function Tests

Cost	Pulmonary Function Test
$	Peak expiratory flow rate (PEFR) determinations
$$	Expiratory only (simple) spirometry*
$$$	Conventional spirometry*
$$$$	Flow-volume loop analysis
$$$$	Complete lung volume studies (open-circuit and closed-circuit)
$$$$	Pulmonary diffusion capacity studies
$$$$	Peak inspiratory and expiratory pressure determinations
$$$$$	Pulmonary mechanic (body plethysmography)
$$$$$	Studies of pulmonary compliance (esophageal balloon)
$$$$$$	Cardiopulmonary exercise tests†

*With and without bronchodilator.
†With and without arterial blood gas analysis.

Pulmonary function studies play a major role in the assessment of pulmonary disease. The results of pulmonary function studies are used to (1) evaluate pulmonary causes of dyspnea, (2) differentiate between obstructive and restrictive pulmonary disorders, (3) assess severity of the pathophysiologic impairment, (4) follow the course of a particular disease, (5) evaluate the effectiveness of therapy, and (6) assess the patient's preoperative status. Pulmonary function studies are commonly subdivided into the following categories: (1) **lung volumes** and **lung capacities**, (2) **forced expiratory flow rate** and **volume measurements**, (3) **pulmonary diffusion capacity measurements**, (4) **test of respiratory muscle strength**, and (5) **cardiopulmonary exercise testing**.

Pulmonary function tests and studies range from the simple and inexpensive in cost to the complex and expensive. The more complex tests are reserved for use in patients with hard-to-diagnose dyspnea, when physical examination, chest imaging studies, and simple pulmonary function studies have not been definitive. A general hierarchy of the increasing expense and complexity of pulmonary function tests is given in Table 3-1.

Normal Lung Volumes and Capacities

As shown in Table 3-2, gas in the lungs is divided into four lung volumes and four lung capacities. The lung capacities represent different combinations of lung volumes. The amount of air the lungs can accommodate varies with age, weight, height, gender, and, to a much lesser extent, race. Prediction formulas for normal values exist that take these variables into account. Lung volumes and capacities change as a result of pulmonary disorders. These changes are classified as either **restrictive lung disorders** or **obstructive lung disorders.**

Restrictive Lung Disorders: Lung Volume and Capacity Findings

Table 3-3 provides some of the more common restrictive anatomic alterations of the lungs and examples of respiratory disorders that cause them. Restrictive lung disorders result in an increased lung rigidity, which in turn decreases lung compliance. When lung compliance decreases, the ventilatory rate increases and the **tidal volume (V_T)** decreases (see Figure 2-23). Table 3-4 presents an overview of the lung volume and capacity findings characteristic of restrictive lung disorders. Restrictive lung volumes and capacities are associated with pathologic conditions that alter the anatomic structures of the lungs distal to the terminal bronchioles (i.e., the alveoli or the lung parenchyma).

Obstructive Lung Disorders: Lung Volume and Capacity Findings

Table 3-5 provides an overview of the lung volumes and capacity findings characteristic of obstructive lung disorders. These lung volume and capacity findings are associated with pathologic conditions that alter the tracheobronchial tree. Table 3-6 provides some of the more common obstructive anatomic alterations of the lungs and examples of respiratory disorders that cause them.

In obstructive lung disorders, the gas that enters the alveoli during inspiration (when the bronchial airways are naturally wider) is prevented from leaving the alveoli during expiration (when the bronchial airways narrow). As a result, the alveoli become overdistended with gas, a condition known as **air trapping**. Figure 3-1 provides a visual comparison of obstructive and restrictive lung disorders.

Indirect Measurements of the Residual Volume and Lung Capacities Containing the Residual Volume

Because the **residual volume (RV)** cannot be exhaled, the RV and the lung capacities that contain the RV—the **functional residual capacity [FRC]** and **total lung capacity [TLC]**—can be measured indirectly by one of the following methods: closed-circuit helium dilution test, open-circuit nitrogen washout test, or body plethysmography. A brief explanation of each of these tests follows:

For the **closed-circuit helium dilution test**, the patient rebreathes both a known volume of gas (V_1) and a known concentration (C_1) of helium (He) for about 7 minutes (Figure 3-2). The concentration of He is normally 10%. During the test, the patient is "switched in" to a closed-circuit system at the end of a normal tidal volume breath—or, at the top of their FRC (see Figure 3-1). A helium analyzer continuously monitors the He concentration, and the exhaled carbon dioxide is chemically removed from the system. The gas in the patient's FRC—which at the beginning of the test contained no He—mixes with the gas in the closed-circuit system. This causes the He to dilute throughout the entire closed-circuit system—the patient's lungs, spirometer, and circuit. When the He concentration changes by 0.2%, or less, over a 1-second period, the test is completed. The He

TABLE 3-2 Lung Volumes and Capacities of Normal Recumbent Subjects 20 to 30 Years of Age

	Male (mL)	Female (mL)
Lung Volume Measurements		
Tidal volume (V_T): The volume of gas that normally moves into and out of the lungs in one quiet breath.	500	400–500
Inspiratory reserve volume (IRV): The volume of air that can be forcefully inspired after a normal tidal volume.	3100	1900
Expiratory reserve volume (ERV): The volume of air that can be forcefully exhaled after a normal tidal volume exhalation.	1200	800
Residual volume (RV): The amount of air remaining in the lungs after a forced exhalation.	1200	1000
Lung Capacity Measurements		
Vital capacity (VC): VC = IRV + V_T + ERV. The volume of air that can be exhaled after a maximal inspiration.	4800	3200
Inspiratory capacity (IC): IC = V_T + IRV. The volume of air that can be inhaled after a normal exhalation.	3600	2400
Functional residual capacity (FRC): FRC = ERV + RV. The lung volume at rest after a normal tidal volume exhalation.	2400	1800
Total lung capacity (TLC): TLC = IC + ERV + RV. The maximal amount of air that the lungs can accommodate.	6000	4200
Residual volume/total lung capacity ratio (RV/TLC × 100): The percentage of TLC occupied by the RV.	$\frac{1200}{6000} = 20\%$ (approx)	$\frac{1000}{4200} = 25\%$ (approx)

TABLE 3-3 Anatomic Alterations of the Lungs Associated with Restrictive Lung Disorders: Pathology of the Alveoli or Lung Parenchyma

Pathology (Anatomic Alteration of the Alveoli)	Examples of Respiratory Disorders Associated with Specific Pathology
Atelectasis	Pneumothorax, pleural effusion, flail chest, or mucous plugging
Consolidation	Pneumonia, acute respiratory distress syndrome, lung abscess, tuberculosis
Increased alveolar-capillary membrane thickness	Pulmonary edema, pneumoconiosis, tuberculosis, fungal disease

TABLE 3-4 Restrictive Lung Disorders: Lung Volume and Capacity Findings

V_T	IRV	ERV	RV	
N or ↓	↓	↓	↓	
VC	IC	FRC	TLC	RV/TLC
↓	↓	↓	↓	N

ERV, Expiratory reserve volume; FRC, functional residual capacity; IC, inspiratory capacity; IRV, inspiratory reserve volume; N, normal; RV, residual volume; TLC, total lung capacity; VC, vital capacity; V_T, tidal volume.

TABLE 3-5 Obstructive Lung Disorders: Lung Volume and Capacity Findings

V_T	IRV	ERV	RV	
N or ↑	N or ↓	N or ↓	↑	
VC	IC	FRC	TLC	RV/TLC ratio
↓	N or ↓	↑	N or ↑	N or ↑

ERV, Expiratory reserve volume; FRC, functional residual capacity; IC, inspiratory capacity; IRV, inspiratory reserve volume; N, normal; RV, residual volume; TLC, total lung capacity; VC, vital capacity; V_T, tidal volume.

TABLE 3-6 Anatomic Alterations of the Lungs Associated with Obstructive Lung Disorders: Pathology of the Tracheobronchial Tree

Pathology (Anatomic Alteration of the Bronchial Airways)	Examples of Respiratory Disorders Associated with Specific Pathology
Excessive mucous production and accumulation	Chronic bronchitis, asthma, respiratory syncytial virus
Bronchospasm	Asthma
Distal airway weakening	Emphysema

concentration at this point is C_2. The final volume of the entire system—the He circuit and lungs (V_2)—can now be calculated by using the following equation:

$$V_1 C_1 = V_2 C_2$$

which can be rearranged to solve for V_2 as follows:

$$V_2 = \frac{V_1 C_1}{C_2}.$$

The FRC can be calculated by subtracting the initial spirometer volume (V_1) from the equilibrium volume (V_2) as follows: FRC = V2 − V1. The RV can be calculated by subtracting the ERV from the FRC: FRC − ERV. The TLC can be determined by adding the VC to the RV: RV + VC.

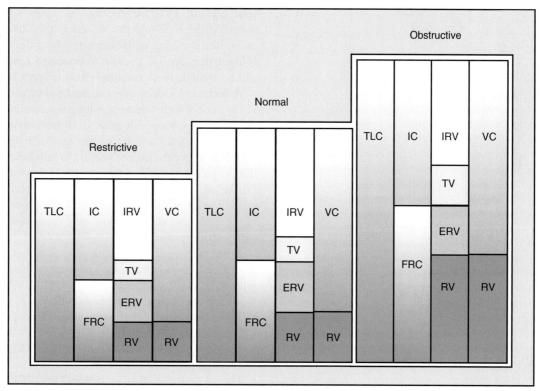

FIGURE 3-1 Visual comparison of lung volumes and capacities in obstructive and restrictive lung disorders. (From Kacmarek RM, Stoller JK, Albert HJ: *Egan's fundamentals of respiratory care*, ed 10, St Louis, 2013, Mosby-Elsevier.)

For the **open-circuit nitrogen washout test**, the patient inhales and exhales 100 percent oxygen through a one-way valve for about 7 minutes (Figure 3-3). At the start of the test, the concentration of nitrogen (N_2) in the alveoli is 79% (C_1). After a few moments into the test, the patient is "switched-in" to the system at the end of a normal tidal volume—or, at the top of their FRC (see Figure 3-1). At this point, the patient inhales 100% oxygen and exhales N_2-rich gas from the FRC. Over the next several minutes, the N_2 in the patient's FRC progressively washes out. During the washout period, the exhaled gas volume is measured, and the average N_2 concentration is measured with a nitrogen analyzer. The test is terminated when the N_2 concentration drops to 1.5% or less. Based on the initial N_2 concentration, and the final N_2 concentration, the volume of air in the patient's lungs at the start of the test—i.e., the FRC—can be calculated as follows:

$$FRC = \frac{F_E N_2 \text{ final} \times \text{Expired Volume} - N_2 \text{ tissue}}{F_A N_2 \text{ alveolar } 1 - F_A N_2 \text{ alveolar } 2}$$

where:

$F_E N_2$ final = fraction of N_2 in volume expired

$F_A N_2$ alveolar 1 = fraction of N_2 in alveolar gas initially (0.79)

$F_A N_2$ alveolar 2 = fraction of N_2 in alveolar gas at end of the test (from an alveolar sample)

N_2 tissue = volume of N_2 washed out of blood and tissues. A correction must be made for the N_2 washed out of the blood and tissue. It is estimated that for each minute of oxygen breathing, about 30–40 mL of N2 is removed from the blood and tissue. This value is subtracted from the total volume of N_2 washed out.

Body plethysmography measures the volume of gas in the lungs (thoracic gas volume [VTG]) indirectly by applying a modification of Boyle's law. The patient sits in an airtight chamber called a body box (Figure 3-4). During the first part of the test, the patient breathes quietly in and out through an open valve (shutter). Once the patient is relaxed, the patient is "switched in" to the system at the end of a normal tidal volume—that is, at the level at which only the FRC remains in the lungs. At this point, the shutter valve is closed and the patient is instructed to pant against the closed shutter. Pressure and volume changes are monitored during this time. The alveolar pressure changes—created by the compression and decompression of the lungs—are estimated at the patient's mouth. Because there is no air flow during this period, and because the temperature is kept constant, the pressure and volume changes can be used to calculate the trapped volume—the FRC—by applying Boyle's law. Body plethysmography is generally considered to be the most precise of the three methods for measuring the RV and FRC.

Body plethysmography can also measure *airway resistance* (R_{aw}) and airway conductance ($1/R_{aw}$).

Forced Expiratory Flow Rate and Volume Measurements

In addition to the volumes and capacities that can be measured by pulmonary function testing, the flow rate and volume at which gas flows out of the lungs can also be measured. Such measurements provide data on the patency of the airways and the severity of the airway impairment.

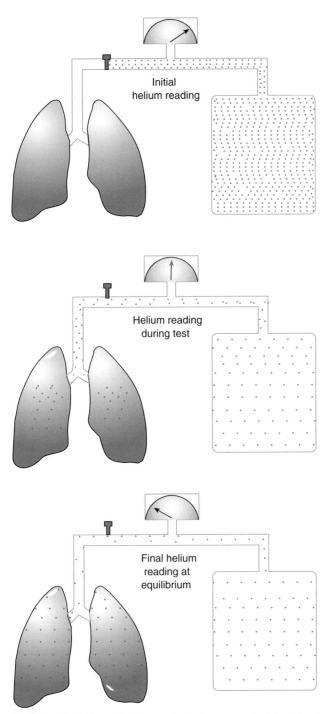

FIGURE 3-2 Helium dilution method for measuring functional residual capacity, residual volume, and total lung capacity. (From Kacmarek RM, Stoller JK, Heuer AJ: *Egan's fundamentals of respiratory care*, ed 10, St Louis, 2013, Mosby-Elsevier.)

Forced Vital Capacity

The **forced vital capacity (FVC)** is the total volume of gas that can be exhaled as forcefully and rapidly as possible after a maximal inspiration. In the healthy individual, the **total expiratory time (TET)** necessary to perform an FVC is 4 to 6 seconds. In obstructive lung disease (e.g., chronic bronchitis or emphysema), the TET increases because of the increased airway resistance and air trapping associated with the disorder. TETs of more than 10 seconds have been reported in these patients. In the normal individual, the FVC equals the

vital capacity (VC). Clinically, the lungs are considered normal if the FVC and the VC are within 200 mL of each other. In the patient with obstructive lung disease, the FVC is lower than the VC because of increased airway resistance and air trapping with maximal effort (Figure 3-5).

A decreased FVC is also a common clinical manifestation in the patient with a restrictive lung disorder (e.g., pneumonia, acute respiratory distress syndrome, atelectasis). This decrease is mainly a result of the fact that restrictive lung disorders reduce the patient's ability to fully expand the lungs, thus reducing the VC necessary to generate a good FVC exhalation. However, the TET required to perform an FVC exhalation is usually normal or even less than normal because of the high lung elasticity (low lung compliance) associated with restrictive disorders.

A number of pulmonary function values can be calculated from a single FVC maneuver. The most common tests are as follows:

- Forced expiratory volume timed (FEV_T)
- Forced expiratory volume in 1 second/forced vital capacity ratio (FEV_1/FVC ratio)
- Forced expiratory flow between 200 and 1200 mL of FVC ($FEF_{200-1200}$)
- Forced expiratory flow at 25% to 75% ($FEF_{25\%-75\%}$)
- Peak expiratory flow rate (PEFR)

Forced Expiratory Volume Timed

The maximum volume of gas that can be exhaled over a specific period is the **forced expiratory volume timed (FEV_T)**. This measurement is obtained from an FVC measurement. Commonly used time periods are 0.5, 1.0, 2.0, 3.0, and 6.0 seconds. The most commonly used time period is 1 second (**forced expiratory volume in 1 second [FEV_1]**). In the normal adult, the percentages of the total volume exhaled during these time periods are as follows: $FEV_{0.5}$, 60%; FEV_1, 83%; FEV_2, 94%; and FEV_3, 97%. In obstructive disease, the FEV_T is decreased because the time necessary to exhale a certain volume forcefully is increased (Figure 3-6). Although the FEV_T may be normal in restrictive lung disorders (e.g., pneumonia, acute respiratory distress syndrome, atelectasis), it is commonly decreased because of the decreased VC associated with restrictive disorders (similar to the FVC in restrictive disorders). The FEV_T progressively decreases with age (about 23 mL per year after age 18).

Forced Expiratory Volume in 1 Second/ Forced Vital Capacity (FEV_1/FVC) Ratio

The **FEV_1/FVC ratio** compares the amount of air exhaled in 1 second with the total amount exhaled during an FVC maneuver. Because the FEV_1/FVC ratio is expressed as a percentage, it is commonly referred to as the **forced expiratory volume in 1 second percentage ($FEV_{1\%}$)**. Simply stated, the FEV_1/FVC ratio provides the percentage of the patient's total volume of air forcefully exhaled (FVC) in 1 second. As discussed earlier in the FEV_T section, the normal adult exhales 83% or more of the FVC in 1 second (FEV_1). Therefore, the FEV_1/FVC ratio should also be 83% or greater under normal circumstances. The $FEV_{1\%}$ progressively decreases with age.

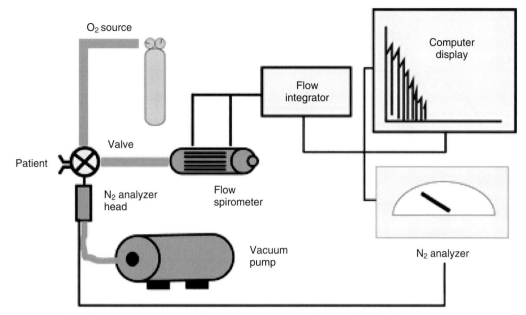

FIGURE 3-3 Open-circuit equipment used for N_2 washout determination of FRC. The patient inspires O_2 from a regulated source and exhales past a rapidly responding N_2 analyzer into a pneumotachometer. FRC is calculated from the total volume of N_2 exhaled and the change in alveolar N_2 from the beginning to the end of the test. (From Mottram CD: *Ruppel's manual of pulmonary function testing*, ed 10, St Louis, Elsevier, 2013.)

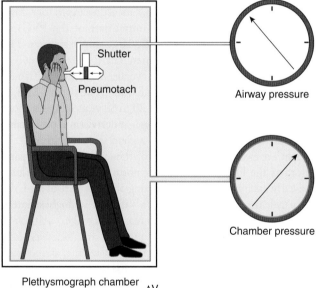

Plethysmograph chamber
$$V(FRC) = P_B \text{ atmospheric} \times \frac{\Delta V}{\Delta P}$$

FIGURE 3-4 Body plethysmography method for measuring lung volumes. V is the change in gas volume in the lungs, as sensed by the chamber pressure manometer. P is the change in pressure produced by the respiratory effort of breathing against the shutter, as sensed by the airway pressure manometer. (From Kacmarek RM, Stoller JK, Heuer AJ: *Egan's fundamentals of respiratory care*, ed 10, St Louis, 2013, Mosby-Elsevier.)

Clinically, the **FVC, FEV₁, and FEV₁%** are commonly used to (1) assess the severity of a patient's pulmonary disorder and (2) to determine whether the patient has either an obstructive or a restrictive lung disorder. The primary pulmonary function study differences between an obstructive and a restrictive lung disorder are as follows:

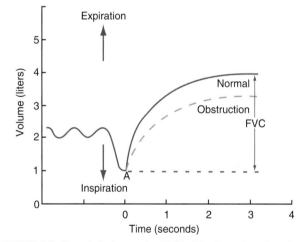

FIGURE 3-5 Forced vital capacity (FVC). A is the point of maximal inspiration and the starting point of an FVC maneuver. Note the reduction in FVC in obstructive pulmonary disease.

- In an obstructive disorder, the FEV_1 and $FEV_{1\%}$ are both decreased. The FVC is often normal.
- In a classic restrictive disorder, the FVC and FEV_1 are decreased and the $FEV_{1\%}$ is normal or increased.

Forced Expiratory Flow 25% to 75%

The **forced expiratory flow 25%-75% ($FEF_{25\%-75\%}$)** is the average flow rate generated by the patient during the middle 50% of an FVC measurement (Figure 3-7). This expiratory maneuver is used to evaluate the status of medium-to-small airways in obstructive lung disorders. The normal $FEF_{25\%-75\%}$ in a healthy man 20 to 30 years of age is about 4.5 L/sec (270 L/min). The normal $FEF_{25\%-75\%}$ in a healthy woman 20 to 30 years of age is about 3.5 L/sec (210 L/min). The $FEF_{25\%-75\%}$ is somewhat effort-dependent because it depends on the FVC exhaled.

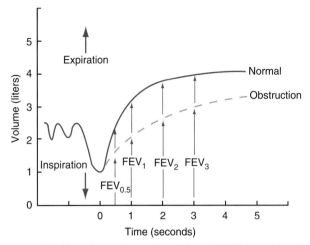

FIGURE 3-6 Forced expiratory volume timed (FEV_T). In obstructive pulmonary disease, more time is needed to exhale a specified volume.

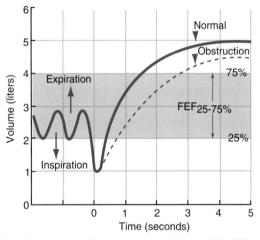

FIGURE 3-7 Forced expiratory flow at 25% to 75% ($FEF_{25\%-75\%}$). This test measures the average rate of flow between 25% and 75% of a forced vital capacity (FVC) maneuver. The flow rate is measured when 25% of the FVC has been exhaled and again when 75% of the FVC has been exhaled. The average rate of flow is derived by dividing the combined flow rates by 2. Note that expiration (in this figure) starts at 1.0 L on the upward axis.

The $FEF_{25\%-75\%}$ progressively decreases in obstructive diseases and with age. The $FEF_{25\%-75\%}$ may also be decreased in moderate or severe restrictive lung disorders. This decrease is believed to be caused primarily by the reduced cross-sectional area of the small airways associated with restrictive lung problems. Clinically, the $FEF_{25\%-75\%}$ is often used to further confirm—or rule out—the presence of an obstructive pulmonary disease in the patient with a borderline $FEV_{1\%}$ value.

Forced Expiratory Flow between 200 and 1200 mL of Forced Vital Capacity

The **forced expiratory flow 200-1200 ($FEF_{200-1200}$)** measures the average flow rate between 200 and 1200 mL of an FVC (Figure 3-8). The first 200 mL of the FVC is usually exhaled more slowly than at the average flow rate because of (1) the normal inertia involved in the respiratory maneuver and (2) the initial slow response time of the pulmonary function

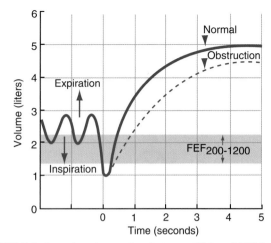

FIGURE 3-8 Forced expiratory flow between 200 and 1200 mL of forced vital capacity (FVC) ($FEF_{200-1200}$). This test measures the average rate of flow between 200 mL and 1200 mL of the FVC. The flow rate is measured when 200 mL has been exhaled and again when 1200 mL has been exhaled. The average rate of flow is derived by dividing the combined flow rates by 2. Note that expiration (in this figure) starts at 1.0 L on the upward axis.

equipment. Because the $FEF_{200-1200}$ measures expiratory flows at high lung volumes (i.e., the initial part of the FVC), it provides a good assessment of the large upper airways. The $FEF_{200-1200}$ is relatively effort-dependent.

The normal $FEF_{200-1200}$ for the average healthy man 20 to 30 years of age is about 8 L/sec (480 L/min). The normal $FEF_{200-1200}$ in the average healthy woman 20 to 30 years of age is about 5.5 L/sec (330 L/min). The $FEF_{200-1200}$ decreases in obstructive lung disorders. The $FEF_{200-1200}$ is a good test to determine the patient's response to bronchodilator therapy. In restrictive lung disorders the $FEF_{200-1200}$ is usually normal because it measures the early expiratory flow rates during the first part of an FVC maneuver (i.e., when the patient's VC is at its highest level). The $FEF_{200-1200}$ progressively decreases with age.

Peak Expiratory Flow Rate

The **peak expiratory flow rate (PEFR)** (also known as the *peak flow rate*) is the maximum flow rate generated during an FVC maneuver (Figure 3-9). The PEFR provides a good assessment of the large upper airways. It is very effort-dependent. The normal PEFR in the average healthy man 20 to 30 years of age is about 10 L/sec (600 L/min). The normal PEFR in the average healthy woman 20 to 30 years of age is about 7.5 L/sec (450 L/min). The PEFR decreases in obstructive lung diseases. In restrictive lung disorders, the PEFR is usually normal because it measures the early expiratory flow rates during the first part of an FVC maneuver (i.e., when the patient's VC is at its highest level). The PEFR progressively decreases with age.

The PEFR can also easily be measured at the patient's bedside with a hand-held peak flowmeter (e.g., Wright peak flowmeter). The hand-held peak flowmeter is used to monitor the degree of airway obstruction on a moment-to-moment basis and is relatively small, inexpensive, accurate, reproducible, and easy for the patient to use. In addition, the

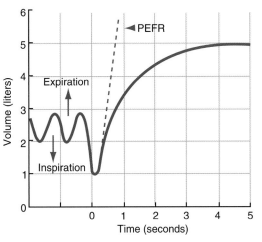

FIGURE 3-9 Peak expiratory flow rate (PEFR). The steepest slope of the $\Delta\dot{V}/\Delta T$ line is the PEFR ($\dot{V}$).

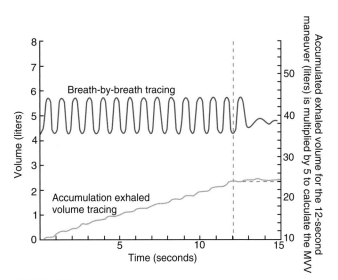

FIGURE 3-10 Volume-time tracing for a maximum voluntary ventilation (MVV) maneuver. *Note:* The patient actually performs the MVV maneuver for only 12 seconds, not 60 seconds.

mouthpieces are disposable, thus allowing the safe use of the same peak flowmeter from one patient to another. PEFR measurements should routinely be performed at the patient's bedside to assess the degree of bronchospasm, effect of bronchodilators, and day-to-day progress. The PEFR results generated by the patient before and after bronchodilator therapy can serve as excellent objective data by which to assess the effectiveness of therapy.

Maximum Voluntary Ventilation

The **maximum voluntary ventilation (MVV)** is the largest volume of gas that can be breathed voluntarily in and out of the lungs in 1 minute (Figure 3-10). The normal MVV in the average healthy man 20 to 30 years of age is about 170 L/min. The normal MVV in the average healthy woman 20 to 30 years of age is about 110 L/min. The MVV progressively decreases in obstructive pulmonary disorders. In restrictive pulmonary disorders, the MVV may be normal or decreased. It is very effort-dependent.

Flow-Volume Loop

The flow-volume loop is a graphic illustration of both a forced vital capacity (FVC) maneuver and a forced inspiratory volume (FIV) maneuver. The FVC and FIV are plotted together as two curves that form what is called a **flow-volume loop**. As shown in Figure 3-11, the upper half of the flow-volume loop (above the zero flow axis) represents the maximum expiratory flow generated at various lung volumes during an FVC maneuver plotted against volume. This portion of the curve shows the flow generated between the TLC and RV. Poor patient effort can be identified on the "flow portion" of the flow-volume loop—for example, the upper half of the flow-volume loop (above the zero flow axis) will decrease, show hesitation, or stop altogether.

The lower half of the flow-volume loop (below the zero flow axis) illustrates the maximum inspiratory flow generated at various lung volumes during a forced inspiration (called a *forced inspiratory volume [FIV]*) plotted against the volume inhaled. This portion of the curve shows the flow generated between the RV and TLC. Depending on the sophistication

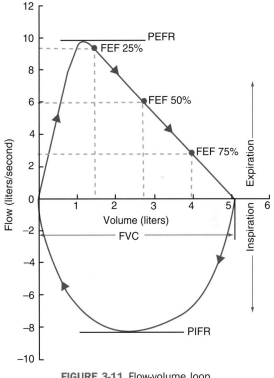

FIGURE 3-11 Flow-volume loop.

of the equipment, several important pulmonary function study values can be obtained, including the following:

- FVC
- FEV_T
- $FEF_{25\%-75\%}$
- $FEF_{200-1200}$
- PEFR
- Peak inspiratory flow rate (PIFR)
- Forced expiratory flow at 50% ($FEF_{50\%}$)
- Instantaneous flow at any given lung volume during forced inhalation and exhalation

In the normal subject the expiratory flow rate decreases linearly during an FVC maneuver, immediately after the PEFR

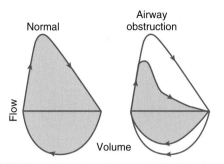

FIGURE 3-12 Flow-volume loop demonstrating the shape change that results from an obstructive lung disorder. The curve on the right represents intrathoracic airway obstruction.

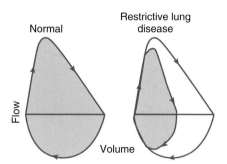

FIGURE 3-13 Flow-volume loop demonstrating the shape change that results from a restrictive lung disorder. Note the symmetric loss of flow and volume.

has been achieved. In the patient with an obstructive lung disease, however, the flow rate decreases in a nonlinear fashion after the PEFR has been reached. This nonlinear flow rate causes a cuplike or scooped-out appearance in the expiratory flow curve when 50% of the FVC has been exhaled. This portion of the flow curve is the FEF$_{50\%}$, or $\dot{V}_{max\,50}$ (Figure 3-12). Table 3-7 summarizes (1) the forced expiratory flow rate and volume measurements and (2) the normal values found in healthy men and women ages 20 to 30 years.

Table 3-8 provides an overview of the expiratory flow rate measurements characteristic of restrictive lung disorders. In restrictive lung disorders, flow and volume are, in general, reduced equally. Clinically, this phenomenon is referred to as *symmetric reduction* in flows and volumes. The flow-volume loop is therefore a small version of normal in restrictive pulmonary disease (Figure 3-13).

Table 3-9 provides an overview of the expiratory flow rate measurements characteristic of obstructive lung disorders. Obstructive lung disorders cause increased airway resistance (R$_{aw}$) and airway closure during expiration. When R$_{aw}$ becomes high, the patient's ventilatory rate decreases and the V$_T$ increases. This ventilatory pattern is thought to be an adaptation to reduce the work of breathing (see Figure 2-23).

Pulmonary Diffusion Capacity

The **pulmonary diffusion capacity of carbon monoxide (DLCO)** measures the amount of carbon monoxide (CO) that moves across the alveolar-capillary membrane. When the patient has a normal hemoglobin concentration, pulmonary capillary blood volume, and ventilatory status, the only limiting factor to the diffusion of CO is the alveolar-capillary membrane. Under normal conditions, the average DLCO value for the resting man is 25 mL/min/mm Hg (STPD). This value is slightly lower in women, presumably because of their smaller normal lung volumes. Table 3-10 provides a general guide to conditions that alter the patient's DLCO.

Assessment of Respiratory Muscle Strength

The most commonly used tests to evaluate the patient's respiratory muscle strength at the bedside are **maximum inspiratory pressure (MIP)** and **maximum expiratory pressure**

(MEP), **forced vital capacity (FVC)**, and **maximum voluntary ventilation (MVV)**.[1]

Maximum inspiratory pressure (MIP), also called *the negative inspiratory force (NIF)*, is the maximum inspiratory pressure the patient is able to generate against a closed airway and is recorded as a negative number in either cm H$_2$O or mm Hg. The MIP can be measured through an endotracheal tube, or by using a mask or mouthpiece, and an external pressure gauge. The MIP primarily measures inspiratory muscle strength—that is, the power of the diaphragm and external intercostal muscles.

In the normal healthy adult, the MIP is about −80 to −100 cm H$_2$O. Ideally, the MIP should be measured at the patient's residual volume. An MIP of −25 cm H$_2$O or less (more negative) usually indicates adequate muscle strength to maintain spontaneous breathing. An MIP of −20 cm H$_2$O or greater (less negative) is a strong indicator for the need for ventilatory support (Protocol 10-1). Unsatisfactory MIP values are commonly seen in patients with neuromuscular disease (e.g., Guillain-Barré syndrome or myasthenia gravis), chronic obstructive pulmonary disease (COPD), and chest wall deformities (e.g., kyphoscoliosis).

Maximum expiratory pressure (MEP) is the highest pressure that can be generated during a forceful expiratory effort against an occluded airway and is recorded as a positive number in either cm H$_2$O or mm Hg. The MEP primarily measures the strength of the abdominal muscles—that is, the rectus abdominis muscles, external abdominis obliquus muscles, internal abdominis obliquus muscles, transversus abdominis muscles, and internal intercostal muscles. Ideally, the MEP is measured at maximal inspiration (near the total lung capacity). The adult normal MEP is greater than 100 cm H$_2$O in the male, and greater than 80 cm H$_2$O in the female. Unsatisfactory MEP values are commonly seen in patients with neuromuscular disease (e.g., Guillain-Barré syndrome or myasthenia gravis), COPD, and high cervical spine fractures. Finally, it should be noted that a low MEP is associated with a poor or inadequate cough effort. Thus, in patients with excessive airway secretions (e.g., chronic bronchitis or cystic fibrosis) a low MEP, accompanied with the inability to effectively mobilize airway secretions, can further complicate the patient's respiratory condition.

---

[1]See page 48 for discussion of FVC, and page 51 for a discussion of MVV.

TABLE 3-7 Normal Forced Expiratory Flow Rate Measurements in Healthy Men and Women 20 to 30 Years of Age

Forced Expiratory Flow Rate Measurement	Men	Women
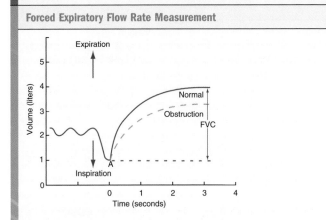 **Forced vital capacity (FVC).** *A* is the point of maximal inspiration and the starting point of an FVC maneuver. Note the reduction in FVC in obstructive pulmonary disease caused by dynamic compression of the airways.	Usually equals vital capacity (VC) (FVC and VC should be within 200 mL of each other)	Usually equals VC (FVC and VC should be within 200 mL of each other)
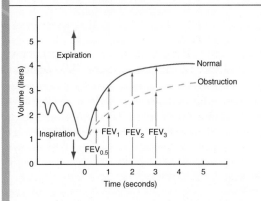 **Forced expiratory volume timed (FEV$_T$):** FEV$_{0.5}$, FEV$_{1.0}$, FEV$_{2.0}$, FEV$_{3.0}$. In obstructive disorders, more time is needed to exhale a specified volume.	FEV$_{0.5}$: 60% FEV$_{1.0}$: 83% FEV$_{2.0}$: 94% FEV$_{3.0}$: 97%	FEV$_{0.5}$: 60% FEV$_{1.0}$: 83% FEV$_{2.0}$: 94% FEV$_{3.0}$: 97%
Forced expiratory volume in 1 second/forced vital capacity ratio (FEV$_1$/FVC); commonly called *forced expiratory volume in 1 second percentage* (FEV$_{1\%}$).	Derived by dividing the predicted FEV$_1$ by the predicted FVC Should be >70%	Derived by dividing the predicted FEV$_1$ by the predicted FVC Should be >70%
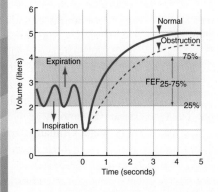 **Forced expiratory flow 25%–75% (FEF$_{25\%-75\%}$).** This test measures the average rate of flow between 25% and 75% of an FVC maneuver. The flow rate is measured when 25% of the FVC has been exhaled and again when 75% of the FVC has been exhaled. The average rate of flow is derived by dividing the combined flow rates by 2.	4.5 L/sec (270 L/min)	3.5 L/sec (210 L/min)

Continued

Forced Expiratory Flow Rate Measurement	Men	Women
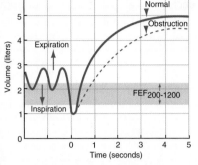	8 L/sec (480 L/min)	5.5 L/sec (330 L/min)
Forced expiratory flow 200–1200 (FEF$_{200-1200}$). This test measures the average rate of flow between 200 mL and 1200 mL of an FVC maneuver. The flow rate is measured when 200 mL has been exhaled and again when 1200 mL has been exhaled. The average rate of flow is derived by dividing the combined flow rates by 2.		
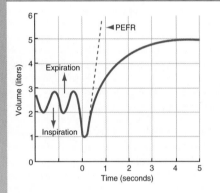	8–10 L/sec (500–600 L/min)	7.5 L/sec (450 L/min)
Peak expiratory flow rate (PEFR). The maximum flow rate (steepest slope of the volume-time trace) generated during an FVC maneuver.		
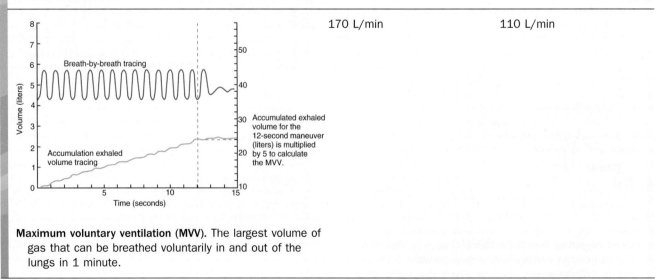	170 L/min	110 L/min
Maximum voluntary ventilation (MVV). The largest volume of gas that can be breathed voluntarily in and out of the lungs in 1 minute.		

TABLE 3-8 Restrictive Lung Disease: Forced Expiratory Flow Rate and Volume Findings

FVC	FEV_T	FEV_1/FVC	$FEF_{25\%-75\%}$
↓	N or ↓	N or ↑	N or ↓

$FEF_{50\%}$	$FEF_{200-1200}$	PEFR	MVV
N or ↓	N or ↓	N or ↓	N or ↓

$FEF_{25\%-75\%}$, Forced expiratory flow 25%–75%; *$FEF_{50\%}$*, forced expiratory flow at 50%; *$FEF_{200-1200}$*, forced expiratory flow 200–1200 mL of FVC; *FEV_1/FVC*, forced expiratory volume in 1 second/forced vital capacity ratio; *FEV_T*, forced expiratory volume timed; *FVC*, forced vital capacity; *MVV*, maximum voluntary ventilation; *N*, normal; *PEFR*, peak expiratory flow rate.

TABLE 3-9 Obstructive Lung Diseases: Forced Expiratory Flow Rate and Volume Findings

FVC	FEV_T	FEV_1/FVC	$FEF_{25\%-75\%}$
↓	↓	↓	↓

$FEF_{50\%}$	$FEF_{200-1200}$	PEFR	MVV
↓	↓	↓	↓

$FEF_{25\%-75\%}$, Forced expiratory flow 25%–75%; *$FEF_{50\%}$*, forced expiratory flow at 50%; *$FEF_{200-1200}$*, forced expiratory flow 200–1200 mL of FVC; *FEV_1/FVC*, forced expiratory volume in 1 second/forced vital capacity ratio; *FEV_T*, forced expiratory volume timed; *FVC*, forced vital capacity; *MVV*, maximum voluntary ventilation; *N*, normal; *PEFR*, peak expiratory flow rate.

TABLE 3-10 Pulmonary Diffusion Capacity of Carbon Monoxide (DLCO)

Obstructive Lung Disorders*	Restrictive Lung Disorders†
N or ↓	N or ↓

N, Normal.

*A decreased DLCO is a hallmark clinical manifestation in emphysema (because of the destruction of the alveolar pulmonary capillaries and decreased surface area for gas diffusion associated with the disease). The DLCO, especially when corrected for alveolar volume (VA), is usually normal in all other obstructive lung disorders.
†This is usually decreased when moderate to severe alveolar atelectasis, alveolar consolidation, or increased alveolar-capillary membrane thickness is present in the restrictive lung disorder.

BOX 3-1 Cardiopulmonary Exercise Testing (CPET) Parameters

Measured and/or Observed Values
- Heart rate (HR)
- Cardiac rhythm
- Electrocardiogram (ECG)
- Blood pressure
- O_2 saturation (SpO_2)
- Breath sounds (e.g., wheezing, crackles)
- Arterial blood gas (ABG)
- Minute ventilation

Derived (Calculated) Values
- Oxygen consumption ($\dot{V}O_2$)
- Maximum oxygen consumption ($\dot{V}O_{2Max}$)
- Heart rate reserve
- CO_2 production ($\dot{V}CO_2$)
- Respiratory quotient (RQ)
- Anaerobic threshold ($\dot{V}O_2$ AT)
- Impairment classification for prolonged physical work
- Oxygen pulse ($\dot{V}O_2 \div HR$)
- Breathing reserve
- Ventilatory equivalent for CO_2

BOX 3-2 Contraindications to Cardiopulmonary Stress Testing

NO significant history of the following:
- Acute myocardial infarction (3–5 days)
- Unstable angina pectoris
- Uncontrolled cardiac arrhythmias, hypertension, or seizure history
- Lightheadedness or syncope
- Uncontrolled congestive heart failure/pulmonary edema
- Uncontrolled asthma
- Pulmonary embolism
- Room air $SpO_2 \leq 85\%$
- Respiratory failure
- Mental impairment limiting cooperation
- Orthopedic/neurologic impairment

Cardiopulmonary Exercise Testing (CPET)

When one considers the fact that *dyspnea on exertion* is a common sign of pulmonary disease, it should be noted that the pulmonary function tests, as described in the foregoing, are all *done at rest*. Tests range from simple and inexpensive (e.g., the 6-minute walk used in pulmonary rehabilitation) to the more complex cardiopulmonary exercise test (CPET), with or without, blood gas analyses. CPET involves treadmill or bicycle ergometer testing while a variety of physiologic parameters are measured and/or calculated (Box 3-1). Contraindications to CPET are listed in Box 3-2.

Although interpretation of CPET variables are beyond the scope of this volume, evaluation of the physiologic data seen with increasing exercise, at or near the anaerobic threshold—where minute ventilation as a function of oxygen consumption increases sharply—can assist in the clinical diagnosis of malignancy and deconditioning, obesity, hyperventilation/anxiety, coronary artery disease, neuromuscular disease, congestive heart failure/valvular heart disease, interstitial lung disease, obstructive pulmonary disease, pulmonary vascular disease, and for the purpose of disability determinations.

Other Diagnostic Tests for Asthma

Because some patients have clinical manifestations associated with asthma, but otherwise normal lung function between asthma episodes, measurements of airway responsiveness to **inhaled methacholine or histamine**, or an indirect challenge test *to* **inhaled mannitol**, or an **exercise or cold air challenge** may be useful in confirming a diagnosis of asthma. These inhalation challenge tests can only be performed when the patient has an FEV_1 of 80% or greater, to avoid electively inducing significant asthma symptoms in an already compromised patient. For more information on asthma, see Chapter 13.

SELF-ASSESSMENT QUESTIONS

Answers to questions can be found on Evolve. To access additional student assessment questions visit **http://evolve.elsevier.com/DesJardins/respiratory**.

1. What is the PEFR in the normal healthy woman 20 to 30 years of age?
   a. 250 L/min
   b. 350 L/min
   c. 450 L/min
   d. 550 L/min

2. A restrictive lung disorder is confirmed when the:
   1. FEV_1 is decreased
   2. FVC is increased
   3. FEV_1/FVC ratio is normal or increased
   4. FEV_1 is increased
      a. 1 only
      b. 4 only
      c. 1 and 3 only
      d. 2 and 4 only

3. Which of the following expiratory maneuver findings are characteristic of restrictive lung disease?
   1. Normal FVC
   2. Decreased $FEF_{25\%-75\%}$
   3. Increased PEFR
   4. Decreased FEV_T
      a. 1 and 3 only
      b. 2 and 4 only
      c. 3 and 4 only
      d. 2 and 3 only

4. In an obstructive lung disorder, which of the following occurs?
   1. FRC is decreased
   2. RV is increased
   3. VC is decreased
   4. IRV is increased
      a. 1 and 3 only
      b. 2 and 3 only
      c. 2 and 4 only
      d. 2, 3, and 4 only

5. Under normal conditions, the average DLCO value for the resting man is which of the following?
   a. 10 mL/min/mm Hg
   b. 15 mL/min/mm Hg
   c. 20 mL/min/mm Hg
   d. 25 mL/min/mm Hg

6. What is the vital capacity of the normal recumbent man 20 to 30 years of age?
   a. 2700 mL
   b. 3200 mL
   c. 4000 mL
   d. 4800 mL

7. What is the normal percentage of the total volume exhaled during an FEV_1?
   a. 60%
   b. 83%
   c. 94%
   d. 97%

8. Which of the following can be obtained from a flow-volume loop study?
   1. FVC
   2. PEFR
   3. FEV_T
   4. $FEF_{25\%-75\%}$
      a. 4 only
      b. 1 and 2 only
      c. 1, 3, and 4 only
      d. 1, 2, 3, and 4

9. An obstructive lung disorder is confirmed when the:
   1. FEV_1 is decreased
   2. FVC is increased
   3. FEV_1 is increased
   4. FEV_1/FVC ratio is decreased
      a. 3 only
      b. 4 only
      c. 1 and 3 only
      d. 1 and 4 only

10. Which of the following anatomic alterations of the lungs is or are associated with a restrictive lung disorder?
    1. Bronchospasm
    2. Atelectasis
    3. Distal airway weakening
    4. Consolidation
       a. 1 only
       b. 3 only
       c. 2 and 4 only
       d. 1 and 3 only

CHAPTER

4 Arterial Blood Gas Assessments

Chapter Objectives

After reading this chapter, you will be able to:
- Identify the respiratory acid-base disturbances.
- Identify the metabolic acid-base disturbances.
- Identify the combined acid-base disturbances
- Describe the PCO_2/pH/HCO_3^- relationship.
- Describe the most common acid-base abnormalities seen in the clinical setting.
- Describe the metabolic acid-base abnormalities including metabolic acidosis, anion gap, and metabolic alkalosis.
- List the causes of metabolic acidosis and metabolic alkalosis.
- Describe the potential common errors in the sampling, analysis, and interpretation of arterial blood gas assessments.

Key Terms

Acute Alveolar Hyperventilation
Acute Alveolar Hyperventilation with Partial Renal Compensation
Acute Alveolar Hyperventilation Superimposed on Chronic Ventilatory Failure
Acute Respiratory Acidosis
Acute Respiratory Alkalosis
Acute Ventilatory Failure
Acute Ventilatory Failure with Partial Renal Compensation
Acute Ventilatory Failure Superimposed on Chronic Ventilatory Failure
Anaerobic Metabolism
Anaerobic Threshold

Anion Gap
Chronic Alveolar Hyperventilation with Complete Renal Compensation
Chronic Ventilatory Failure
Chronic Ventilatory Failure with Complete Renal Compensation
Combined Metabolic and Respiratory Acidosis
Combined Metabolic and Respiratory Alkalosis
Compensated Respiratory Acidosis
Compensated Respiratory Alkalosis
Hyperchloremic Metabolic Acidosis
Hypoxemia
Lactic Acidosis
Law of Electroneutrality
Metabolic Acidosis
Metabolic Acidosis with Complete Respiratory Compensation
Metabolic Acidosis with Partial Respiratory Compensation
Metabolic Alkalosis
Metabolic Alkalosis with Complete Respiratory Compensation
Metabolic Alkalosis with Partial Respiratory Compensation

Chapter Outline

Acid-Base Abnormalities
    The P_{CO_2}/HCO_3^-/pH Relationship
    Common Acid-Base Abnormalities Seen in the Clinical Setting
    Metabolic Acid-Base Abnormalities
Errors Associated with Arterial Blood Gas Measurements
Self-Assessment Questions

Acid-Base Abnormalities

As the pathologic processes of a respiratory disorder intensify, the patient's arterial blood gas (ABG) values are usually altered to some degree. Table 4-1 lists the normal ABG values. Box 4-1 provides an overview of the common respiratory and metabolic acid-base disturbances. In the profession of respiratory care, a basic knowledge and understanding of the acid-base disturbances is an absolute—and unconditional—prerequisite to the assessment and treatment of the patient with a respiratory disorder. Because of the fundamental importance of this subject, this chapter provides the following review:

- The PCO_2/HCO_3^-/pH relationship—an essential cornerstone of ABG interpretations.
- The most common acid-base abnormalities seen in the clinical setting.
- The metabolic acid-base abnormalities.

The PCO_2/HCO_3^-/pH Relationship

To fully understand the clinical significance of the acid-base disturbances listed in Box 4-1, a fundamental knowledge base of the PCO_2/HCO_3^-/pH relationship is essential. The PCO_2/HCO_3^-/pH relationship is graphically illustrated in the PCO_2/HCO_3^-/pH nomogram shown in Figure 4-1.[1]

How to Read the PCO_2/HCO_3^-/pH Nomogram

The thick red bar moving from left to right across the PCO_2/HCO_3^-/pH nomogram represents the normal PCO_2 blood buffer line. This red bar is used to identify the pH and HCO_3^- changes that occur immediately in response to an

---

[1]The PCO_2/HCO_3^-/pH nomogram is an excellent clinical tool to identify acid-base disturbances. See Appendix XIV for a pocket-size PCO_2/HCO_3^-/pH nomogram card that can be cut out, laminated, and used as a handy arterial blood gas reference tool in the clinical setting.

TABLE 4-1 Normal Blood Gas Values

Blood Gas Value*	Arterial	Venous
pH	7.35 to 7.45	7.30 to 7.40
PCO_2	35 to 45 mm Hg	42 to 48 mm Hg
HCO_3^-	22 to 28 mEq/L	24 to 30 mEq/L
PO_2	80 to 100 mm Hg	35 to 45 mm Hg

*Technically, only the oxygen (PO_2) and carbon dioxide (PCO_2) pressure readings are true blood gas values. The pH indicates the balance between the bases and acids in the blood. The bicarbonate (HCO_3^-) reading is an indirect measurement that is calculated from the pH and PCO_2 levels.

BOX 4-1 Acid-Base Disturbance Classifications

Respiratory Acid-Base Disturbances
- Acute alveolar hyperventilation (acute respiratory alkalosis)
- **Acute alveolar hyperventilation with partial renal compensation** (partially **compensated respiratory alkalosis**)
- **Chronic alveolar hyperventilation with complete renal compensation** (compensated respiratory alkalosis)
- Acute ventilatory failure (**acute respiratory acidosis**)
- **Acute ventilatory failure with partial renal compensation** (partially **compensated respiratory acidosis**)
- **Chronic ventilatory failure with complete renal compensation** (compensated respiratory acidosis)
- Acute alveolar hyperventilation superimposed on chronic ventilatory failure
- Acute ventilatory failure superimposed on chronic ventilatory failure

Metabolic Acid-Base Disturbances
- Metabolic acidosis
- Metabolic acidosis with partial respiratory compensation
- Metabolic acidosis with complete respiratory compensation
- Metabolic alkalosis
- Metabolic alkalosis with partial respiratory compensation
- Metabolic alkalosis with complete respiratory compensation

Combined Acid-Base Disturbances
- **Combined metabolic and respiratory acidosis**
- **Combined metabolic and respiratory alkalosis**

---

acute increase or decrease in PCO_2. The purple bar is used to identify the pH and HCO_3^- changes that occur in response to acute **metabolic acidosis** and **metabolic alkalosis** conditions. The colored areas that surround the red and purple bars are used to identify (1) partial and complete renal compensation, (2) partial and complete respiratory compensation, and (3) combined metabolic and respiratory acid-base disturbances (Figure 4-1).

For example, when the pH, PCO_2, and HCO_3^- values all intersect in the light purple area—shown in the upper left-hand corner of the PCO_2/HCO_3^-/pH nomogram—partial renal compensation has occurred in response to a chronically high PCO_2 level. When the HCO_3^- increases enough to move the pH into the light-blue normal bar, complete renal compensation is confirmed. When the pH, PCO_2, and HCO_3^- values all intersect in the green area—shown in the lower right-hand corner of the PCO_2/HCO_3^-/pH nomogram—partial renal compensation has occurred in response to a chronically low PCO_2 level. When the HCO_3^- decreases enough to move the pH into the light-blue normal bar, complete renal compensation is confirmed.

When the pH, PCO_2, and HCO_3^- values all intersect in the orange area—shown immediately below the red bar on the left side of the PCO_2/HCO_3^-/pH nomogram—a combined respiratory and metabolic acidosis is confirmed. When the pH, PCO_2, and HCO_3^- values all intersect in the blue area—shown immediately above the red bar on the right side of the PCO_2/HCO_3^-/pH nomogram—a combined respiratory and metabolic alkalosis is confirmed.

Finally, when the pH, PCO_2, and HCO_3^- values all intersect in the yellow area—shown in the lower left corner of the PCO_2/HCO_3^-/pH nomogram—respiratory compensation has occurred in response to metabolic acidosis. When the pH, PCO_2, and HCO_3^- values all intersect in the pink area—shown in the upper right corner of the PCO_2/HCO_3^-/pH nomogram—respiratory compensation has occurred in response to metabolic alkalosis.

Although it is beyond the scope of this textbook to fully explain how each of the acid-base disturbances listed in Box 4-1 can be identified on the PCO_2/HCO_3^-/pH nomogram, a basic understanding of the following two most commonly encountered PCO_2/HCO_3^-/pH relationships is important: (1) an acute PCO_2 increase and its effects on the pH and HCO_3^- values, and (2) an acute PCO_2 decrease and its effects on the pH and HCO_3^- values.[2]

How Acute PCO_2 Increases Affect the pH and HCO_3^- Values

As mentioned previously, the red normal PCO_2 blood buffer bar shown on the PCO_2/HCO_3^-/pH nomogram is used to identify the pH and HCO_3^- values that will result immediately in response to a sudden increase in PCO_2—for example, as a result of net alveolar hypoventilation. For example, if the patient's $PaCO_2$ were to suddenly increase to 60 mm Hg, the pH would immediately fall to about 7.28 and the HCO_3^- level would increase to about 26 mEq/L. Furthermore, the PCO_2/HCO_3^-/pH nomogram shows that these ABG values represent **acute ventilatory failure (acute respiratory acidosis)**. This is shown by (1) all of the ABG values (i.e., PCO_2, HCO_3^-, and pH) intersect within the red normal PCO_2 blood buffer bar, and (2) the pH and HCO_3^- readings are precisely what is expected for an acute increase in the PCO_2 of 60 mm Hg (Figure 4-2).

---

[2]For a complete review of the role of the PCO_2/HCO_3^-/pH relationship in acid-base balance, see Des Jardins T: *Cardiopulmonary anatomy and physiology: essentials of respiratory care*, ed 6, 2013, Delmar/Cengage Learning.

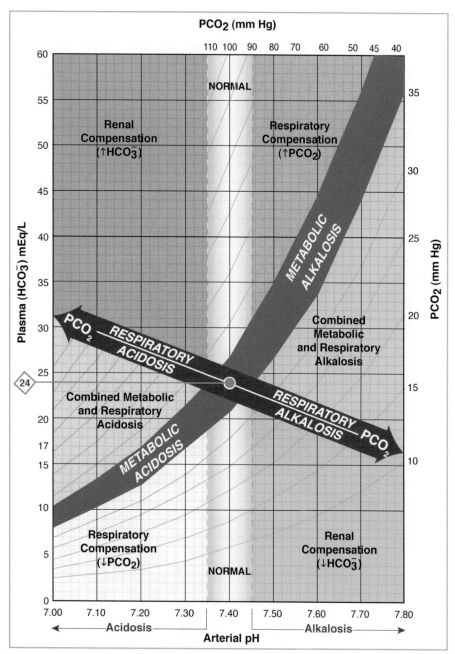

FIGURE 4-1 Nomogram of $PCO_2/HCO_3^-/pH$ relationship. For explanation see text. The green box (with 24) and the green dot in the middle of the red arrow represent the normal pH, PCO_2, and HCO_3^- relationship in the arterial blood. (Used, with permission, from author Terry Des Jardins.)

How Acute PCO_2 Decreases Affect pH and HCO_3^- Values

By contrast, the red normal PCO_2 blood buffer bar shown on the $PCO_2/HCO_3^-/pH$ nomogram is also used to identify the pH and HCO_3^- values that will result immediately in response to a sudden decrease in PCO_2—for example, as a result of alveolar hyperventilation. For example, if the patient's $PaCO_2$ were suddenly to decrease to, say, 25 mm Hg, the pH would immediately increase to about 7.55 and the HCO_3^- level would decrease to about 21 mEq/L. In addition, the $PCO_2/HCO_3^-/pH$ nomogram shows that these ABG values represent **acute alveolar hyperventilation (acute respiratory**

alkalosis). This is shown by (1) all of the ABG values (i.e., PCO_2, HCO_3^-, and pH) intersect within the red normal PCO_2 blood buffer bar, and (2) the pH and HCO_3^- readings are precisely what is expected for an acute increase in the PCO_2 of 25 mm Hg (Figure 4-3).

A Quick Clinical Calculation for the Effect of Acute $PaCO_2$ Changes on pH and HCO_3^-: Rule of Thumb

In addition to using the graphic $PCO_2/HCO_3^-/pH$ nomogram (Figure 4-1), the following simple calculations can also be used to estimate the expected pH and HCO_3^- value

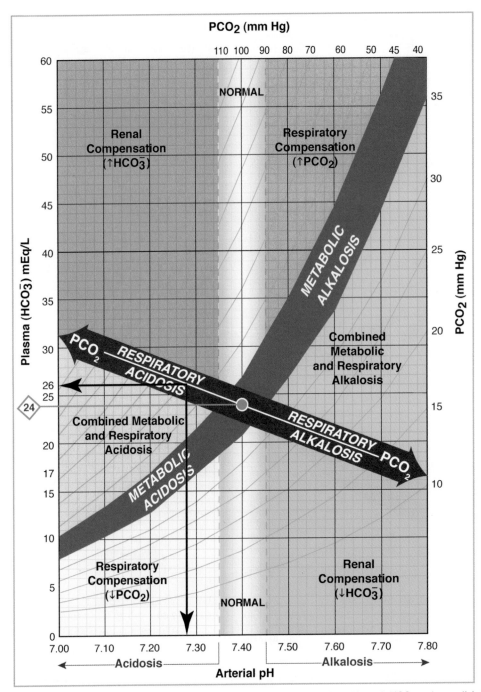

FIGURE 4-2 Acute ventilatory failure is confirmed when the reported PCO₂, pH, and HCO₃⁻ values all intersect within the red-colored respiratory acidosis bar to the left of the light-blue, vertical bar labeled "normal." For example, when the PCO₂ is 60 mm Hg at a time when the pH is 7.28 and the HCO₃⁻ is 26 mEq/L, acute ventilatory failure is confirmed (see black arrows). (Used, with permission, from author Terry Des Jardins.)

changes that will occur in response to a sudden increase or decrease in PaCO₂.

Acute Increases in PaCO₂ (e.g., Acute Hypoventilation). Using the normal ABG values as a baseline (i.e., pH 7.40, PaCO₂ 40 mm Hg, and HCO₃⁻ 24 mEq/L), for every 10 mm Hg the PaCO₂ increases, the pH will decrease about 0.06 units (from 7.4) and the HCO₃⁻ will increase about 1 mEq/L (from 24). Or, by way of another example, for every 20 mm Hg the PaCO₂ increases, the pH will decrease about 0.12 units (from 7.40), and the HCO₃⁻ will increase about 2 mEq/L (from 24). Thus, if the patient's PaCO₂ suddenly increases to, say, 60 mm Hg, the expected pH change would be about 7.28 and the HCO₃⁻ would be about 26 mEq/L.

It should be noted, however, that if the patient's PaO₂ is severely low, lactic acid may also be present, resulting in **a combined metabolic and respiratory acidosis**. In such cases, the patient's pH and HCO₃⁻ values would both be lower than expected for a particular PaCO₂ level.

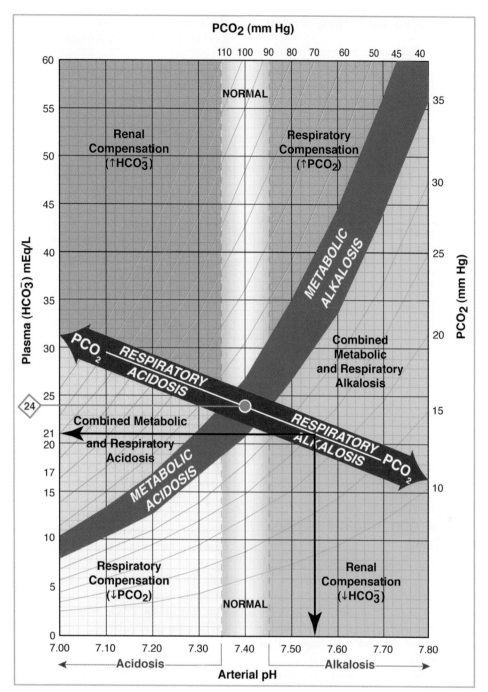

FIGURE 4-3 Acute alveolar hyperventilation is confirmed when the reported PCO_2, pH, and HCO_3^- values all intersect within the red-colored "Respiratory alkalosis" bar. For example, when the reported PCO_2 is 25 mm Hg at a time when the pH is 7.55 and the HCO_3^- is 21 mEq/L, acute alveolar hyperventilation is confirmed (see black arrows). (Used, with permission, from author Terry Des Jardins.)

Acute Decreases in $PaCO_2$ (e.g., Acute Hyperventilation). Using the normal ABG values as a baseline (i.e., pH 7.40, $PaCO_2$ 40 mm Hg, and HCO_3^- 24 mEq/L), for every 5 mm Hg the $PaCO_2$ decreases, the pH will increase about 0.06 units (from 7.40), and the HCO_3^- will decrease about 1 mEq/L. Or, by way of another example, for every 10 mm Hg the $PaCO_2$ decreases, the pH will increase about 0.12 units (from 7.40), and the HCO_3^- will decrease about 2 mEq/L. Thus, if the patient's $PaCO_2$ suddenly decreases to, say, 30 mm Hg, the expected pH change would be around 7.52 and the HCO_3^- would be about 22 mEq/L.

Again, it should be noted that if the patient's PaO_2 is also very low, lactic acid may also be present. In such cases, the patient's pH and HCO_3^- values would both be lower than expected for a particular $PaCO_2$ level.

Table 4-2 provides a summary of the effects of acute $PaCO_2$ changes on pH and HCO_3 levels (see discussion above). Note that the pH and HCO_3 changes with hypoventilation (increased $PaCO_2$) and hyperventilation (decreased $PaCO_2$) *are not equal*. Based on the $PCO_2/HCO_3^-/pH$ relationship presented in Table 4-2, Table 4-3 provides a general rule of thumb—an excellent and handy clinical tool—to

TABLE 4-2 Summary of Acute $PaCO_2$ Changes on pH and HCO_3 Levels

If This Happens	Then this Happens	
$PaCO_2$ increases by 10 mm Hg	pH will decrease by 0.06 units	HCO_3 will Increase by 1 mEq/L
$PaCO_2$ decreases by 10 mm Hg	pH will increase by 0.12 units	HCO_3 will decrease by 2 mEq/L

TABLE 4-3 General Rule of Thumb for the $PaCO_2$/HCO_3^-/pH Relationship

pH (approximate)	$PaCO_2$ (approximate)	HCO_3^- mEq/L (approximate)
7.55	25	21
7.50	30	22
7.45	35	23
7.40	**40**	**24**
7.35	50	25
7.30	60	26
7.25	70	27

determine the expected pH and HCO_3^- changes that occur in response to an acute increase or decrease in the PCO_2 level.

Common Acid-Base Abnormalities Seen in the Clinical Setting

The most common acid-base abnormalities associated with the respiratory disorders presented in this textbook are (1) **acute alveolar hyperventilation** (acute respiratory alkalosis), (2) **acute ventilatory failure** (acute respiratory acidosis), (3) **chronic ventilatory failure** (compensated respiratory acidosis), (4) **acute alveolar hyperventilation superimposed on chronic ventilatory failure** (acute respiratory alkalosis on compensated respiratory acidosis), (5) **acute ventilatory failure superimposed on chronic ventilatory failure** (acute respiratory acidosis on compensated respiratory acidosis), (6) **metabolic alkalosis**, and (7) **metabolic acidosis** (especially lactic acidosis). A brief overview of these common acid-base abnormalities follows.

Acute Alveolar Hyperventilation (Acute Respiratory Alkalosis)

Acute alveolar hyperventilation is defined as a pH above 7.45 and a $PaCO_2$ level below 35 mm Hg and an HCO_3 level down slightly. Table 4-4 provides an example of acute alveolar hyperventilation. The most common cause of acute alveolar hyperventilation is **hypoxemia**. The decreased PaO_2 seen during acute alveolar hyperventilation usually develops from a decreased ventilation-perfusion ratio ($\dot{V}/\dot{Q}$ ratio), capillary shunting (or a relative shunt or shuntlike effect), and venous admixture associated with the pulmonary disorder.

TABLE 4-4 Acute Alveolar Hyperventilation (Acute Respiratory Alkalosis)

ABG Changes	Example
pH: increased	7.55
$PaCO_2$: decreased	29 mm Hg
HCO_3^-: decreasing but normal	23 mEq/L
PaO_2: decreased	61 mm Hg (when pulmonary pathology is present)

The PaO_2 continues to drop as the pathologic effects of the disease intensify. Eventually the PaO_2 may decline to a point low enough (a PaO_2 of about 60 mm Hg) to significantly stimulate the peripheral chemoreceptors, which in turn causes the ventilatory rate to increase (Figure 4-4). The increased ventilatory response in turn causes the $PaCO_2$ to decrease and the pH to increase (Figure 4-5). Box 4-2 lists additional pathophysiologic mechanisms in respiratory disorders that can contribute to an increased ventilatory rate and a reduction in $PaCO_2$.

Acute Ventilatory Failure (Acute Respiratory Acidosis)

Acute ventilatory failure is defined as a pH below 7.35 and a $PaCO_2$ level above 45 mm Hg and an HCO_3 level up slightly. Table 4-5 provides an example of acute ventilatory failure. Acute ventilatory failure is a condition in which the lungs are unable to meet the metabolic demands of the body in terms of CO_2 homeostasis—and, typically, tissue oxygenation. In other words, the patient is unable to provide the muscular, mechanical work necessary to move gas into and out of the lungs to meet the normal CO_2 production of the body. This condition leads to an increased $PACO_2$ and, subsequently, an increased $PaCO_2$. The increased $PACO_2$ causes a decrease in the PAO_2, which, in turn, leads to a decreased PaO_2 in the arterial blood.

Acute ventilatory failure is not associated with a typical ventilatory pattern. For example, the patient may demonstrate apnea, severe hyperpnea, or tachypnea. The bottom line is that acute ventilatory failure can develop in response to any ventilatory pattern that does not provide adequate *alveolar* ventilation. When an increased $PaCO_2$ is accompanied by acidemia (decreased pH), then acute ventilatory failure, or respiratory acidosis, is said to exist. Clinically, this is a medical emergency that may require mechanical ventilation.

Chronic Ventilatory Failure (Compensated Respiratory Acidosis)

Chronic ventilatory failure is defined as a greater-than-normal $PaCO_2$ level with a normal pH status—and, typically, a decreased PaO_2 on room air. Table 4-6 provides an example of chronic ventilatory failure. Although chronic ventilatory failure is most commonly seen in patients with severe chronic obstructive pulmonary disease, it is also seen in several chronic restrictive lung disorders (e.g., severe tuberculosis, kyphoscoliosis). Box 4-3 lists common respiratory diseases

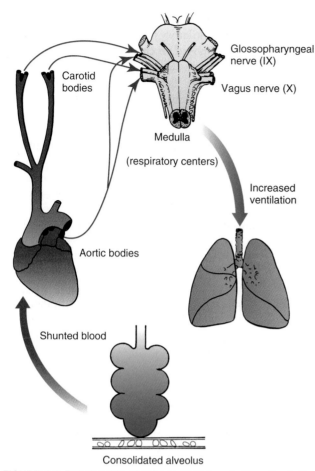

FIGURE 4-4 Relationship of venous admixture to the stimulation of peripheral chemoreceptors in response to alveolar consolidation.

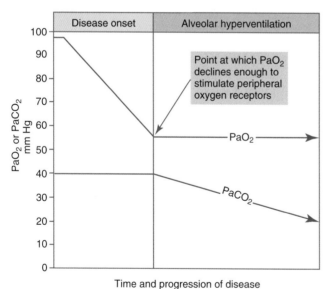

FIGURE 4-5 PaO_2 and $PaCO_2$ trends during acute alveolar hyperventilation.

associated with chronic ventilatory failure during the advanced stages of the disorder.

The basic pathophysiologic mechanisms that produce ABGs associated with chronic ventilatory failure are these: as a respiratory disorder gradually worsens, the work of

TABLE 4-5 Acute Ventilatory Failure (Acute Respiratory Acidosis)

ABG Changes	Example
pH: decreased	7.18
$PaCO_2$: increased	79 mm Hg
HCO_3^-: decreasing but normal	28 mEq/L
PaO_2: decreased	57 mm Hg

TABLE 4-6 Chronic Ventilatory Failure (Compensated Respiratory Acidosis)

ABG Changes	Example
pH: normal	7.36
$PaCO_2$: increased	79 mm Hg
HCO_3^-: increased (significantly)	43 mEq/L
PaO_2: decreased	61 mm Hg

breathing progressively increases to a point at which more oxygen is consumed than is gained. Although the exact mechanism is unclear, the patient slowly develops a breathing pattern that uses the least amount of oxygen for the energy expended. In essence, the patient selects a breathing pattern based on *work efficiency* rather than *ventilatory efficiency*.[3] As a result, the patient's alveolar ventilation slowly decreases, which in turn causes the PaO_2 to decrease and the $PaCO_2$ to increase further (Figure 4-6). As the $PaCO_2$ increases, the pH falls.

When an individual hypoventilates for a long period of time, the kidneys work to correct the decreased pH by retaining HCO_3^-. Renal compensation in the presence of chronic hypoventilation can be shown when the calculated HCO_3^- and pH readings are higher than expected for a particular PCO_2 level. For example, in terms of the absolute $PCO_2/HCO_3^-/pH$ relationship, when the PCO_2 level is about 70 mm Hg, the HCO_3^- level should be about 27 mEq/L and the pH should be about 7.22, according to the normal blood buffer line (Figure 4-2).

If the HCO_3^- and pH levels are greater than these values (i.e., the pH and HCO_3^- readings cross a PCO_2 isobar* above

---

[3]See the discussion of airway resistance and its effect on the ventilatory pattern in Chapter 2.

*The isobars on the $PCO_2/HCO_3^-/pH$ nomogram illustrate the pH changes that develop in the blood as a result of (1) metabolic changes (i.e., HCO_3^- changes) or (2) a combination of metabolic and respiratory (CO_2) changes.

the normal blood buffer line in the upper left-hand corner of the nomogram), renal retention of HCO_3^- (partial renal compensation) has occurred (see Figure 4-2, purple area, upper left quadrant). When the HCO_3^- level increases enough to return the acidic pH to normal, complete renal compensation is said to have occurred (chronic ventilatory failure) (see Figure 4-2, normal area).

Thus, the following should be understood. The lungs play an important role in maintaining the $PaCO_2$, HCO_3^-, and pH levels on a moment-to-moment basis. The kidneys play an important role in maintaining the HCO_3^- and pH levels during long periods of hyperventilation or hypoventilation.

Acute Ventilatory Changes Superimposed on Chronic Ventilatory Failure

Because acute ventilatory changes (i.e., hyperventilation or hypoventilation) are frequently seen in patients who have chronic ventilatory failure (compensated respiratory acidosis), the respiratory therapist must be familiar with and be on the alert for (1) **acute alveolar hyperventilation superimposed on chronic ventilatory failure**, and (2) **acute ventilatory failure superimposed on chronic ventilatory failure**.

Like any other person (healthy or unhealthy), the patient with chronic ventilatory failure can also experience acute periods of hyperventilation. For example, the patient with chronic ventilatory failure can acquire an acute shunt-producing disease (e.g., pneumonia)—and hypoxemia. Some of these patients have the mechanical reserve to increase their alveolar ventilation significantly in an attempt to maintain their baseline PaO_2. However, in regard to the patient's baseline $PaCO_2$ level, the increased alveolar ventilation is often excessive.

When excessive alveolar ventilation occurs, the patient's $PaCO_2$ rapidly decreases. This action causes the patient's $PaCO_2$ to decrease from its normally "high baseline" level. As the $PaCO_2$ decreases, the arterial pH increases. As this condition intensifies, the patient's baseline ABG values can quickly change from chronic ventilatory failure to **acute alveolar hyperventilation superimposed on chronic ventilatory failure**. Table 4-7 provides an example of acute alveolar hyperventilation superimposed on chronic ventilatory failure.

If the clinician does not know the *past history of the patient* with acute alveolar hyperventilation superimposed on chronic ventilatory failure, he or she might initially interpret the ABG values as signifying partially compensated metabolic alkalosis with severe hypoxemia (Box 4-1). However, the clinical situation that offsets this interpretation is the presence of marked hypoxemia. A low oxygen level is not normally seen in patients with pure metabolic alkalosis. Thus, whenever the ABG values appear to reflect partially compensated metabolic alkalosis but the condition is accompanied by significant hypoxemia, the respiratory therapist should be alert to the possibility of *acute alveolar hyperventilation superimposed on chronic ventilatory failure*.

Often patients with chronic ventilatory failure do not have the mechanical reserve to meet the hypoxemic challenge of a respiratory disorder. When these patients attempt to maintain their baseline PaO_2, by increasing their alveolar

---

BOX 4-3 Respiratory Diseases Associated with Chronic Ventilatory Failure during the Advanced Stages

Chronic Obstructive Pulmonary Disorders (Most Common)
- Chronic bronchitis
- Emphysema
- Bronchiectasis
- Cystic fibrosis

Restrictive Respiratory Disorders
- Tuberculosis
- Fungal diseases
- Kyphoscoliosis
- Chronic interstitial lung diseases
- Bronchopulmonary dysplasia

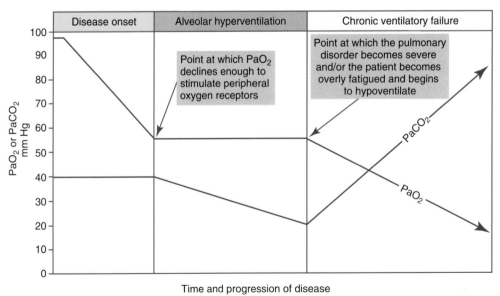

FIGURE 4-6 PaO_2 and $PaCO_2$ trends during acute or chronic ventilatory failure.

TABLE 4-7 Acute Alveolar Hyperventilation Superimposed on Chronic Ventilatory Failure (Acute Hyperventilation on Compensated Respiratory Acidosis)

ABG Changes	Example
pH: increased	7.52
$PaCO_2$: increased	51 mm Hg
HCO_3^-: increased	40 mEq/L
PaO_2: decreased	46 mm Hg

TABLE 4-8 Acute Ventilatory Failure Superimposed on Chronic Ventilatory Failure Acute Hypoventilation on Compensated Respiratory Acidosis)

ABG Changes	Example
pH: decreased	7.28
$PaCO_2$: increased	99 mm Hg
HCO_3^-: increased	45 mEq/L
PaO_2: decreased	34 mm Hg

TABLE 4-9 Overview Examples of Acute Changes in Chronic Ventilatory Failure

Acute Ventilatory Failure on Chronic Ventilatory Failure	Chronic Ventilatory Failure (Baseline Values)	Acute Alveolar Hyperventilation on Chronic Ventilatory Failure
7.28 ←	pH 7.36	→ 7.52
99 ←	$PaCO_2$ 79	→ 51
45 ←	HCO_3^- 43	→ 40
34 ←	PaO_2 61	→ 46

TABLE 4-10 Metabolic Alkalosis

ABG Changes	Example
pH: increased	7.56
$PaCO_2$: normal	44 mm Hg
HCO_3^-: increased	36 mEq/L
PaO_2: normal	94 mm Hg

ventilation, they often consume more oxygen than is gained and/or become fatigued, or experience a combination of both. When this happens, the patient begins to breathe less. This action causes the $PaCO_2$ to increase and eventually to rise above the patient's normally high $PaCO_2$ baseline level. This action causes the patient's arterial pH level to fall or become acidic. In short, the patient's baseline ABG values shift from chronic ventilatory failure to **acute ventilatory failure superimposed on chronic ventilatory failure**. Table 4-8 provides an example of acute ventilatory failure superimposed on chronic ventilatory failure. Table 4-9 provides an overview summary of acute ventilatory failure superimposed on chronic ventilatory failure, and acute alveolar hyperventilation superimposed on chronic ventilatory failure, in relationship to typical baseline ABG values of a patient with chronic ventilatory failure.

Metabolic Acid-Base Abnormalities

Metabolic acid-base disturbances are subdivided into the following two categories: metabolic acidosis and metabolic alkalosis (Box 4-1). An overview of the metabolic acid-base disturbances are presented in the following section.

Metabolic Alkalosis

The presence of other bases not related to either a decreased $PaCO_2$ level or renal compensation can also be identified by using the PCO_2/HCO_3^-/pH nomogram illustrated in Figure 4-1. The presence of metabolic alkalosis is verified when the calculated HCO_3^- and pH readings are both higher than expected for a particular $PaCO_2$ level in terms of the absolute PCO_2/HCO_3^-/pH relationship. For example, according to the normal blood buffer line, an HCO_3^- reading of 35 mEq/L and a pH level of 7.54 would both be higher than expected in a patient who has a $PaCO_2$ level of 40 mm Hg (Figure

4-1). This condition is known as **metabolic alkalosis**. Table 4-10 provides an example of metabolic alkalosis.

Clinically, metabolic alkalosis is seen more often than metabolic acidosis. Indeed, it is the most common metabolic acid-base abnormality seen in most blood gas laboratories. Box 4-4 provides common causes of metabolic alkalosis.

Metabolic Acidosis

The presence of other acids not related to an increased $PaCO_2$ level can also be identified by using the isobars of the PCO_2/HCO_3^-/pH nomogram shown in Figure 4-1. The presence of other acids is verified when the calculated HCO_3^- reading and pH level are both lower than expected for a particular $PaCO_2$ level in terms of the absolute PCO_2/HCO_3^-/pH relationship. For example, according to the normal blood buffer line, an HCO_3^- reading of 15 mEq/L and a pH of 7.20 would both be less than expected in the patient who has a PCO_2 of 40 mm Hg. This condition is referred to as **metabolic acidosis**. Table 4-11 provides an example of metabolic acidosis. Note that if the PaO_2 is normal—which generally rules out lactic acidosis—the precise cause of the metabolic acidosis is not readily known. Box 4-4 provides common causes of metabolic acidosis.

LACTIC ACIDOSIS (Metabolic Acidosis). Because acute hypoxemia is commonly associated with any of the respiratory disorders presented in this textbook, **acute metabolic acidosis** (caused by **lactic acid**) often further compromises the patient's ABG status. This is because oxygenation is inadequate to meet tissue metabolism, so alternate biochemical reactions that do not use oxygen are activated. This is called **anaerobic metabolism** (non–oxygen-using). It is commonly seen in cardiopulmonary exercise testing as occurring at the **anaerobic threshold** (see Chapter 3), where the $\dot{V}CO_2$ increases rapidly as a function of work done (as measured

TABLE 4-11 Metabolic Acidosis

ABG Changes	Example
pH: decreased	7.26
$PaCO_2$: normal	37 mm Hg
HCO_3^-: decreased	16 mEq/L
PaO_2: normal (or decreased if lactic acidosis is present)	94 mm Hg (or 37 mm Hg if lactic acidosis is present)

TABLE 4-12 Lactic Acidosis (Metabolic Acidosis)

ABG Changes	Example
pH: decreased	7.21
$PaCO_2$: normal or decreased	35 mm Hg
HCO_3^-: decreased	14 mEq/L
PaO_2: decreased	34 mm Hg

continuously by the $\dot{V}O_2$). Lactic acid is the end-product of this process. When acidic ions move into the blood, the pH decreases. Thus, whenever moderate to severe acute hypoxemia is present, the possible presence of lactic acid should be suspected. For example, when acute alveolar hyperventilation is caused by a sudden drop in PaO_2, the patient's pH may be lower than expected for a particular decrease in $PaCO_2$ level. Table 4-12 provides an example of lactic acidosis.

Anion Gap. The **anion gap** is used to assess if the patient's metabolic acidosis is caused by either (1) the accumulation of fixed acids (lactic acids, keto acids, or salicylate intoxication) or (2) an excessive loss of HCO_3^-.

The **law of electroneutrality** states that the total number of plasma positively charged ions (cations) must equal the total number of plasma negatively charged ions (anions) in

the body fluids. To calculate the anion gap, the most commonly measured cations are sodium (Na^+) ions. The most commonly measured anions are the chloride (Cl^-) ions and bicarbonate (HCO_3^-) ions. The normal plasma concentrations of these cations and anions are the following:

$$Na^+: 140 \text{ mEq/L}$$
$$Cl^-: 105 \text{ mEq/L}$$
$$HCO_3^-: 24 \text{ mEq/L}$$

The anion gap is the calculated difference between the Na^+ ions and the sum of the HCO_3^- and Cl^- ions:

$$\begin{aligned} \text{Anion gap} &= Na^+ - (Cl^- + HCO_3^-) \\ &= 140 - (105 + 24) \\ &= 140 - 129 \\ &= 11 \text{ mEq/L} \end{aligned}$$

The normal range for the anion gap is 9 to 14 mEq/L. When the anion gap is greater than 14 mEq/L, metabolic acidosis is present—that is, an elevated anion gap caused by the accumulation of fixed acids in the blood. Fixed acids produce H^+ ions that chemically react with—and are buffered by—the plasma HCO_3^-. This action causes (1) the HCO_3^- level to fall, and (2) the anion gap to rise.

Clinically, when the patient demonstrates both metabolic acidosis and an increased anion gap, the source of the fixed acids must be identified for the patient to be appropriately treated. For example, metabolic acidosis caused by lactic acids requires oxygen therapy to reverse the accumulation of the lactic acids. Metabolic acidosis caused by ketone acids requires insulin therapy to help facilitate the movement of glucose into the cells and normalize metabolism.

It is interesting to note that metabolic acidosis caused by an excessive loss of HCO_3^- (e.g., from renal disease or severe diarrhea) does not cause an increase in the anion gap. This is because as the HCO_3^- level decreases, the Cl^- level usually increases to maintain electroneutrality. In short, for every HCO_3^- ion that is lost, a Cl^- anion takes its place (i.e., the law of electroneutrality). This action maintains a normal anion gap. Metabolic acidosis caused by decreased HCO_3^- is commonly called **hyperchloremic metabolic acidosis**.

Thus, when metabolic acidosis is accompanied by an increased anion gap, the most likely cause of the acidosis is the accumulation of fixed acids. When metabolic acidosis is seen with a normal anion gap, the most likely cause of the acidosis is an excessive loss of HCO_3^- (e.g., caused by renal failure or severe diarrhea).

Errors Associated with Arterial Blood Gas Measurements

Because an ABG error can occur before, during, or after the analysis of the sample, the respiratory therapist must always be on alert for ABG results that do not fit the patient's current clinical condition. Accurate and efficient ABG samplings, along with the correct analysis and interpretation of ABG values, are no simple matters, as anyone who has performed these procedures can testify. Fast and precise ABG results are often life-critical!

TABLE 4-13 Common Errors of Arterial Blood Gas Measurements

Preanalytic Errors Include

	pH	PaCO$_2$	PaO$_2$
· Air in syringe or icing plastic syringes	↑	↓	↑
· Venous sample or contamination	↓	↑	↓
· Anticoagulant type or concentration	↑↓	↓	↑
· Metabolic effects (e.g., delay in running the blood sample)	↓	↑	↓
· Misidentification of patient			
· Inappropriately transported sample			

Analytic Errors Include

· Poor quality assurance (QA) and quality control (QC) programs*
  · Malfunctioning PO$_2$ and PCO$_2$ electrodes
  · Out-of-date reagents (cleaning, rinse, and calibration solutions)

Postanalytic Errors Include

· Incorrect patient name/location/demographics on report
· Typographical and transcription errors—e.g., 74 instead of 47 mm Hg
· Incorrect FIO$_2$ or ventilator setting on patient chart
· Incorrect sampling time recorded
· Failure to notify appropriate personnel of critical results—e.g., impending ventilatory failure and/or acute ventilatory failure
· Slow turnaround time for results to get back to the patient's bedside—to be interpreted by the medical staff

Interpretation Errors Include

· The incorrect interpretation of *any* of the acid-base disturbances discussed in this chapter (Box 4-1)
· Interpretation errors can result in serious harm and/or death to the patient—e.g., failure to correctly identify impending ventilatory failure and/or acute ventilatory failure

*Note: Two quick internal checks of blood gas accuracy entail (1) calculating the Henderson-Hasselbalch equation to determine if the measured arterial blood gas (ABG) values correlate, and (2) calculating the alveolar-arterial oxygen gradient for the same purpose. The Henderson-Hasselbalch equation assures that the pH, PCO$_2$, and HCO$_3$ determinations are at least minimally consistent. The alveolar-arterial oxygen gradient assures that the FIO$_2$, PO$_2$, and PCO$_2$ calculations are at least reasonable. For a complete review of these two equations, see Des Jardins T: *Cardiopulmonary anatomy and physiology: essentials of respiratory care*, ed 6, 2013, Delmar/Cengage Learning.

In general, the types of ABG errors can be classified as (1) **preanalytic errors**, (2) **analytic errors**, (3) **postanalytic errors**, and (4) **interpretation errors**. *Preanalytic errors* include errors that occur either before or after the sample analysis—for example, improper sample or data handling. *Analytic errors* include errors that occur during the actual analysis of the ABG sample—for example, blood gas machine malfunctions and poor individual technique. *Postanalytic errors* include the recording of the ABG results after analysis—for example, incorrect patient name or FIO$_2$ setting. *Interpretation errors* are the incorrect classification of any ABG results (Box 4-1). Table 4-13 provides an overview of common errors of ABG measurements.

The "take home message" from this brief section is to be aware of the common sources of ABG errors, and to be ready to repeat the test if the ABG data do not correlate with the clinical situation. Unexpected or questionable ABG results should always be thoroughly investigated. Failure to do so is unacceptable! Noninvasive "reality checks" on ABG results include observation of the patient's sensorium and vital signs, presence or absence of cyanosis, and the timely readings from pulse oximeters and transcutaneous PO$_2$ and PCO$_2$ electrodes.

SELF-ASSESSMENT QUESTIONS

1. During acute alveolar hyperventilation, which of the following occurs?
   1. HCO_3^- decreases.
   2. $PaCO_2$ increases.
   3. HCO_3^- increases.
   4. $PaCO_2$ decreases.
      a. 2 only
      b. 3 only
      c. 1 and 4 only
      d. 2, 3, and 4 only

2. When lactic acidosis is present, which of the following will occur?
   1. pH will likely be lower than expected for a particular $PaCO_2$.
   2. HCO_3^- will likely be higher than expected for a particular $PaCO_2$.
   3. pH will likely be higher than expected for a particular $PaCO_2$.
   4. HCO_3^- will likely be lower than expected for a particular $PaCO_2$.
      a. 2 only
      b. 3 only
      c. 2 and 3 only
      d. 1 and 4 only

3. What is the clinical interpretation of the following ABG values (in addition to hypoxemia)?
   pH: 7.17
   $PaCO_2$: 77 mm Hg
   HCO_3^-: 27 mEq/L
   PaO_2: 54 mm Hg
      a. Acute alveolar hyperventilation superimposed on chronic ventilatory failure
      b. Acute ventilatory failure
      c. Acute alveolar hyperventilation
      d. Acute ventilatory failure superimposed on chronic ventilatory failure

4. A 74-year-old man with a long history of emphysema and chronic bronchitis enters the emergency room in respiratory distress. His respiratory rate is 34 breaths per minute and labored. His heart rate is 115 beats per minute, and his blood pressure is 170/120. What is the clinical interpretation of the following ABG values (in addition to hypoxemia)?
   pH: 7.51
   $PaCO_2$: 68 mm Hg
   HCO_3^-: 52 mEq/L
   PaO_2: 49 mm Hg
      a. Acute alveolar hyperventilation superimposed on chronic ventilatory failure
      b. Acute ventilatory failure
      c. Acute alveolar hyperventilation
      d. Acute ventilatory failure superimposed on chronic ventilatory failure

5. Which of the following is classified as metabolic acidosis?
   a. pH 7.23; $PaCO_2$ 63; HCO_3^- 26; PaO_2 52
   b. pH 7.16; $PaCO_2$ 38; HCO_3^- 13; PaO_2 86
   c. pH 7.56; $PaCO_2$ 27; HCO_3^- 23; PaO_2 101
   d. pH 7.64; $PaCO_2$ 49; HCO_3^- 51; PaO_2 91

6. Which of the following cause metabolic acidosis?
   1. Hypokalemia
   2. Renal failure
   3. Excessive administration of sodium bicarbonate
   4. Hypochloremia
      a. 1 only
      b. 2 only
      c. 1 and 4 only
      d. 2 and 3 only

7. Using the general rule of thumb for the $PaCO_2/HCO_3^-/pH$ relationship, if the $PaCO_2$ suddenly increased to 90 mm Hg in a patient who normally has a pH of 7.40, a $PaCO_2$ of 40 mm Hg, and an HCO_3^- of 24 mEq/L, the pH will decrease to approximately what level?
   a. 7.15
   b. 7.10
   c. 7.05
   d. 7.00

8. Which of the following is classified as metabolic alkalosis?
   a. pH 7.23; $PaCO_2$ 63; HCO_3^- 26; PaO_2 52
   b. pH 7.16; $PaCO_2$ 38; HCO_3^- 13; PaO_2 86
   c. pH 7.56; $PaCO_2$ 27; HCO_3^- 23; PaO_2 101
   d. pH 7.64; $PaCO_2$ 44; HCO_3^- 46; PaO_2 91

9. Lactic acidosis develops from which of the following?
   1. Inadequate tissue oxygenation
   2. Renal failure
   3. An inadequate insulin level
   4. Anaerobic metabolism
   5. An inadequate glucose level
      a. 1 only
      b. 2 only
      c. 1 and 4 only
      d. 3 and 5 only

10. Metabolic alkalosis can develop from which of the following?
   1. Hyperchloremia
   2. Hypokalemia
   3. Hypochloremia
   4. Hyperkalemia
      a. 4 only
      b. 1 and 3 only
      c. 1 and 4 only
      d. 2 and 3 only

11. During acute alveolar hypoventilation, the blood:
   1. HCO_3^- increases
   2. pH decreases
   3. PCO_2 increases
   4. HCO_3^- decreases
      a. 2 only
      b. 4 only
      c. 2 and 3 only
      d. 1, 2, and 3 only

12. During acute alveolar hyperventilation, the blood:
   1. PCO_2 increases
   2. HCO_3^- increases
   3. HCO_3^- decreases
   4. pH increases
      a. 2 only
      b. 4 only
      c. 1 and 3 only
      d. 3 and 4 only

13. In chronic hypoventilation, kidney compensation has likely occurred when the:
   1. HCO_3^- is higher than expected for a particular $PaCO_2$
   2. pH is lower than expected for a particular $PaCO_2$
   3. HCO_3^- is lower than expected for a particular $PaCO_2$
   4. pH is higher than expected for a particular $PaCO_2$
      a. 1 only
      b. 2 only
      c. 1 and 4 only
      d. 3 and 4 only

14. Which of the following represents acute alveolar hyperventilation?
   a. pH 7.56; $PaCO_2$ 51; HCO_3^- 44
   b. pH 7.45; $PaCO_2$ 37; HCO_3^- 25
   c. pH 7.53; $PaCO_2$ 46; HCO_3^- 29
   d. pH 7.54; $PaCO_2$ 26; HCO_3^- 22

15. Which of the following represents compensated metabolic alkalosis?
   a. pH 7.55; $PaCO_2$ 21; HCO_3^- 19
   b. pH 7.52; $PaCO_2$ 45; HCO_3^- 29
   c. pH 7.45; $PaCO_2$ 26; HCO_3^- 18
   d. pH 7.45; $PaCO_2$ 61; HCO_3^- 41

Chapter Objectives

After reading this chapter, you will be able to:

- Describe the two ways in which oxygen is carried in the blood.
- Calculate the oxygen tension–based indices equations.
- Calculate the oxygen saturation– and content–based indices equations.
- Describe the clinical significance of pulmonary shunting.
- List factors that increase and decrease the previously listed oxygen content and transport calculations.
- Discuss how specific respiratory diseases alter the oxygen transport studies.
- Differentiate between hypoxemia and hypoxia.
- Distinguish the classification differences between mild, moderate, and severe hypoxemia.
- Describe the four types of hypoxia.
- List common causes for each of the listed types of hypoxia.
- Describe the pathophysiologic conditions associated with chronic hypoxia.

Key Terms

Alveolar-Arterial Oxygen Tension Difference (P[A-a]O$_2$)
Anemic Hypoxia
Arterial-Venous Oxygen Content Difference (C[a-$\bar{v}$]O$_2$)
Circulatory Hypoxia
Cor Pulmonale
Histotoxic Hypoxia
Hypoxemia
Hypoxia
Hypoxic Hypoxia

Hypoxic Vasoconstriction of the Lungs
Ideal Alveolar Gas Equation (PAO$_2$)
Lactic Acid
Mild Hypoxemia
Moderate Hypoxemia
Oxygen Consumption ($\dot{V}O_2$)
Oxygen Content of Arterial Blood (CaO$_2$)
Oxygen Content of Mixed Venous Blood (C$\bar{v}$O$_2$)
Oxygen Content of Pulmonary Capillary Blood (CcO$_2$)
Oxygen Extraction Ratio (O$_2$ER)
Polycythemia
Pulmonary Shunt Fraction ($\dot{Q}_S/\dot{Q}_T$)
Severe Hypoxemia
Total Oxygen Delivery (DO$_2$)

Chapter Outline

Oxygen Transport Review

Oxygen transport between the lungs and the metabolizing cells is a function of the blood itself and the cardiovascular system (blood vessels and heart). Oxygen is carried in the blood in two ways: (1) as dissolved oxygen in the blood plasma, and (2) bound to the hemoglobin (Hb). Most oxygen is carried to the tissue cells bound to hemoglobin.

Oxygen Dissolved in the Blood Plasma

A small amount of oxygen that diffuses from the alveoli to the pulmonary capillary blood remains in the dissolved form. The term *dissolved* means that the gas molecule (in this case

oxygen) maintains its exact molecular structure and freely moves throughout the plasma of the blood in its normal gaseous state. Clinically, it is the dissolved oxygen that is measured to assess the patient's partial pressure of oxygen (PO$_2$).

At normal body temperature, about 0.003 mL of oxygen will dissolve in each 100 mL of blood for every 1 mm Hg of PO$_2$. Therefore, in the normal individual with an arterial oxygen partial pressure (PaO$_2$) of 100 mm Hg, about 0.3 mL of oxygen exists in the dissolved form in every 100 mL of plasma (0.003 × 100 mm Hg = 0.3 mL). Clinically, this is written as 0.3 volumes percent (vol%), or as 0.3 vol% oxygen. Relative to the total oxygen transport, only a small amount of oxygen is carried to the tissue cells in the form of dissolved oxygen.

Oxygen Bound to Hemoglobin

In the healthy individual, over 98% of the oxygen that diffuses into the pulmonary capillary blood chemically combines with hemoglobin. The normal hemoglobin value for men is 14 to 16 g/100 mL of blood. Clinically, the weight measurement of hemoglobin, in reference to 100 mL of blood, is known as the *grams percent of hemoglobin* (g% Hb). The normal hemoglobin value for women is 12 to 15 g%. The normal hemoglobin value for infants is 14 to 20 g%.

Each gram of hemoglobin (1 g% Hb) is capable of carrying about 1.34 mL of oxygen. Therefore, if the hemoglobin level is 12 g% and the hemoglobin is fully saturated with oxygen (i.e., carrying all the oxygen that is physically possible), about 16.08 vol% will be bound to the hemoglobin:

$$O_2 \text{ bound to Hb} = 1.34 \text{ mL } O_2 \times 12 \text{ g\% Hb}$$
$$= 16.08 \text{ vol\% } O_2 \text{ (16.08 mL oxygen/}$$
$$100 \text{ mL of blood).}$$

Because of normal physiologic shunts (e.g., Thebesian venous drainage and bronchial venous drainage), however, the actual normal hemoglobin saturation is only about 97%. Therefore, the amount of arterial oxygen shown in the calculation must be adjusted by 97% as follows:

$$16.08 \text{ (vol\% } O_2) \times 0.97 = 15.60 \text{ vol\% } O_2.$$

Total Oxygen Content

To calculate the total amount of oxygen in each 100 mL of blood, the dissolved oxygen and the oxygen bound to the hemoglobin must be added together. The following case example summarizes the mathematics required to determine the total oxygen content of the patient's blood.

Case Example

A 44-year-old woman with a long history of asthma arrives in the emergency room in severe respiratory distress. Her vital signs are as follows: respiratory rate 36 breaths/min, heart rate 130 bpm, and blood pressure 160/95 mm Hg. Her hemoglobin concentration is 10 g%, and her PaO_2 is 55 mm Hg (SaO_2 85%). On the basis of these data, the patient's total oxygen content is determined as follows:

1. Dissolved O_2

$$55 \text{ } PaO_2 \times 0.003 \text{ (dissolved } O_2) = 0.165 \text{ vol\% } O_2$$

2. Oxygen bound to hemoglobin

$$10 \text{ g\%} \times 1.34 \times 0.85 \text{ (}SaO_2) = 11.39 \text{ vol\% } O_2$$

3. Total oxygen content

$$11.39 \text{ vol\%} + 0.165 \text{ vol\%} = 11.55 \text{ vol\% } O_2.$$

The total oxygen content can be calculated in the patient's arterial blood (CaO_2), venous blood ($C\bar{v}O_2$), and pulmonary capillary blood, also known as the *oxygen content of capillary blood* (CcO_2). The mathematics for these calculations is as follows:

Ca_{O_2}: oxygen content of arterial blood
$(Hb \times 1.34 \times SaO_2) + (PaO_2 \times 0.003)$

$C\bar{v}O_2$: oxygen content of venous blood
$(Hb \times 1.34 \times S\bar{v}O_2) + (P\bar{v}O_2 \times 0.003)$

Cc_{O_2}: oxygen content of pulmonary capillary blood
$(Hb \times 1.34[1]) + PAO_2[2] \times 0.003$.

As it will be shown later in this chapter, various mathematical manipulations of the CaO_2, $C\bar{v}O_2$, and CcO_2 values are used in several different oxygen transport studies that provide important clinical information regarding the patient's ventilatory and cardiac status.

Oxyhemoglobin Dissociation Curve

As shown in Figure 5-1, the **oxyhemoglobin dissociation curve** (HbO_2 curve), also called the **oxyhemoglobin equilibrium curve**, is the S-shaped curve on a nomogram that illustrates the *percentage of hemoglobin* (left-hand side of the graph) that is chemically connected to oxygen at a specific oxygen pressure (PO_2) (bottom portion of the graph). On the right-hand side of the graph, the precise oxygen content that is carried by the hemoglobin, for a particular oxygen pressure, is provided.

The steep portion of the oxyhemoglobin dissociation curve falls between a 10- and 60-mm Hg, and the flat portion falls between 70 and 100 mm Hg. The steep part of the curve demonstrates that oxygen quickly combines with hemoglobin as the PO_2 increases—or, the converse, quickly breaks away (or dissociates) from the hemoglobin as the PO_2 decreases. It is also interesting to note that very little oxygen combines with hemoglobin between a PO_2 of 60 and 100 mm Hg. In fact, a PO_2 increase from 60 to 100 mm Hg increases the total saturation of hemoglobin by only 7% (from 90% to 97% saturated) (Figure 5-1).

---

[1]It is assumed that the hemoglobin saturation with oxygen in the pulmonary capillary blood is 100%.
[2]See Ideal Alveolar Gas Equation, Appendix VIII.

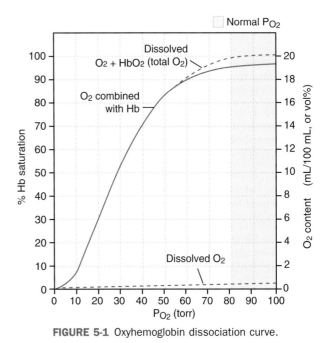

FIGURE 5-1 Oxyhemoglobin dissociation curve.

Oxygenation Indices

A number of oxygen transport measurements are available to assess the oxygenation status of the critically ill patient. Results from these studies can provide important information to adjust therapeutic interventions. The oxygen transport studies can be divided into (1) the oxygen tension–based indices, and (2) the oxygen saturation– and content–based indices.[3]

Oxygen Tension–Based Indices
Arterial Oxygen Tension (PaO_2)

The PaO_2 has withstood the test of time as a good indicator of the patient's oxygenation status. In general, an appropriate PaO_2 on an inspired low oxygen concentration almost always indicates good tissue oxygenation. The PaO_2, however, can be misleading in a number of clinical situations. For example, the PaO_2 may give a "falsely normal" impression when the patient has (1) a low hemoglobin concentration, (2) a decreased cardiac output, (3) peripheral shunting, or (4) been exposed to carbon monoxide. In all these cases, the PaO_2 may be at an appropriate level (normal PaO_2), but the actual oxygen content available for tissue metabolism—the oxygen bound to the hemoglobin—is inadequate.

Alveolar-Arterial Oxygen Tension Difference ($P[A\text{-}a]O_2$)

The **alveolar-arterial oxygen tension difference ($P[A\text{-}a]O_2$)** is the oxygen tension difference between the alveoli and arterial blood. The $P(A\text{-}a)O_2$ is also known as the *alveolar-arterial oxygen tension gradient*. Clinically, the information required for the $P(A\text{-}a)O_2$ is obtained from (1) the patient's calculated alveolar oxygen tension (**PAO_2**), which is derived from the **ideal alveolar gas equation (PAO_2)**, and (2) the patient's PaO_2, which are obtained from an arterial blood gas analysis.

The ideal alveolar gas equation is written as follows:

$$PAO_2 = FIO_2 (P_B - PH_2O) - PaCO_2/RQ$$

where P_B is the barometric pressure, PAO_2 is the partial pressure of oxygen within the alveoli, PH_2O is the partial pressure of water vapor in the alveoli (which is 47 mm Hg), FIO_2 is the fractional concentration of inspired oxygen, $PaCO_2$ is the partial pressure of arterial carbon dioxide, and RQ is the respiratory quotient. The RQ is the ratio of carbon dioxide production ($\dot{V}CO_2$) divided by **oxygen consumption ($\dot{V}O_2$)**. Under normal circumstances, about 250 mL of oxygen/min is consumed by the tissue cells and about 200 mL of carbon dioxide is excreted into the lung. Thus, the RQ is normally about 0.8, but can range from 0.7 to 1.0. Clinically, 0.8 is generally used for the RQ.

If the patient is receiving an FIO_2 of 0.30 on a day when the barometric pressure is 750 mm Hg, and if the patient's $PaCO_2$ is 70 mm Hg and PaO_2 is 60 mm Hg, the $P(A\text{-}a)O_2$ can be calculated as follows:

$$
\begin{aligned}
PAO_2 &= FIO_2 (P_B - PH_2O) - PaCO_2/RQ \\
&= 0.30 (750 - 47) - 70/0.8 \\
&= (703)\,0.30 - 87.5 \\
&= 123.4 \text{ mm Hg.}
\end{aligned}
$$

Using the PaO_2 obtained from the arterial blood gas, the $P(A\text{-}a)O_2$ can now easily be calculated as follows:

$$
\begin{array}{r}
123.4 \text{ mm Hg } (PAO_2) \\
- 60.0 \text{ mm Hg } (PaO_2) \\
\hline
= 63.4 \text{ mm Hg } [P(A\text{-}a)O_2]
\end{array}.
$$

The normal $P(A\text{-}a)O_2$ on room air at sea level ranges from 7 to 15 mm Hg, and it should not exceed 30 mm Hg. Although the $P(A\text{-}a)O_2$ may be useful in patients breathing a low FIO_2, it loses some of its sensitivity in patients breathing a high FIO_2. The $P(A\text{-}a)O_2$ increases at high oxygen concentrations. Because of this, the $P(A\text{-}a)O_2$ has less value in the critically ill patient who is breathing a high oxygen concentration. The normal value on 100% oxygen is between 25 and 65 mm Hg. *The critical value is greater than 350 mm Hg.*

The $P(A\text{-}a)O_2$ increases in response to (1) oxygen diffusion disorders (e.g., chronic interstitial lung diseases), (2) ventilation-perfusion ratio mismatching, (3) right-to-left intracardiac shunting (e.g., a patent ventricular septum), and (4) age.

Arterial-Alveolar Pressure Ratio (PaO_2/PAO_2 Ratio)

The **PaO_2/PAO_2 Ratio** (also called *a-A Ratio or PaO_2/PAO_2 Index*) is the percentage of alveolar oxygen that moves into the arterial blood—not the calculated difference between alveolar and arterial pressure. The normal range for the young adult is 0.75 to 0.95. *Critical value is less than 0.75.* With pulmonary shunting, diffusion defects, and ventilation-perfusion mismatching, the PaO_2/PAO_2 Ratio decreases in proportion to the amount of lung abnormality. Clinically, the PaO_2/PAO_2 Ratio is most reliable when (1) the ratio is less than 0.55, (2) the FIO_2 is greater than 0.30, and (3) the PaO_2 is less than 100 mm Hg. Because of its reliability, the PaO_2/PAO_2 Ratio is useful in following the patient's oxygenation status as the FIO_2 changes. Assuming that the cardiovascular system is stable, the PaO_2/PAO_2 Ratio is an excellent clinical indicator of pulmonary shunting. It also changes minimally with FIO_2 changes and is not affected by $PaCO_2$ changes. It may also be used to predict the FIO_2 needed to obtain a desired PaO_2 level.

Thus, using the data obtained for the case example presented above ($PaO_2 = 60$ mm Hg and $PAO_2 = 123.4$ mm Hg), the patient's PaO_2/PAO_2 Ratio is determined as follows:

$$
\begin{aligned}
PaO_2/PAO_2 \text{ Ratio} &= 60/123.4 \\
&= 0.49.
\end{aligned}
$$

Arterial Oxygen Tension to Fractional Concentration of Oxygen Ratio (PaO_2/FIO_2 Ratio)

The **PaO_2/FIO_2 Ratio** (also called *oxygenation ratio*) is useful in determining the extent of lung diffusion defects—for example, acute respiratory distress syndrome. On room air, the normal PaO_2/FIO_2 Ratio range is between 350 and 450.[4]

---

[3]See Appendix X for a representative example of a cardiopulmonary profile sheet used to monitor the oxygen transport status of the critically ill patient.

[4]The precise normal PaO_2/FIO_2 Ratio range is 380 to 476 (80 mm Hg/0.21 = 380; 100 mm Hg/0.21 = 476).

A PaO_2/FIO_2 Ratio less than 200 indicates poor lung function—for example, *acute respiratory distress syndrome*. The PaO_2/FIO_2 Ratio decreases with ventilation-perfusion mismatching, pulmonary shunting, and diffusion defects.

The PaO_2/FIO_2 Ratio is a relatively easy calculation to use when the PaO_2 is less than 100 mm Hg. For example, a PaO_2 of 75 mm Hg divided by an FIO_2 of 1.0 is 75 (75/1.0 = 75). However, a major limiting factor associated with the PaO_2/FIO_2 Ratio is that changes in $PaCO_2$ can cause false readings. For example, if the $PaCO_2$ increases from 40 to 70 mm Hg during a period of hypoventilation, the PaO_2 decreases by about the same amount (e.g., from 85 to 55 mm Hg). Thus, if the patient was on an FIO_2 of 0.4, the PaO_2/FIO_2 Ratio is 55/0.40 = 138. This low value of 138 indicates that the diffusion of oxygen is more impaired than the actual lung oxygenation status—which, in this case, is: 85/0.40 = 212. Thus, caution should be used when using the PaO_2/FIO_2 Ratio in patients who are hypoventilating and retaining CO_2.

Oxygen Saturation– and Content–Based Indices

The oxygen saturation– and content–based indices can serve as excellent indicators of the individual's cardiac and ventilatory status. These oxygenation studies are derived from the patient's total **oxygen content in the arterial blood (Cao_2)** **mixed venous blood ($C\overline{v}O_2$)**, and **pulmonary capillary blood (Cco_2)**. As explained earlier in this chapter, the CaO_2, $C\overline{v}O_2$, and CcO_2 are calculated using the following formulas:

$$CaO_2 = (Hb \times 1.34 \times SaO_2) + (PaO_2 \times 0.003)$$

$$C\overline{v}O_2 = (Hb \times 1.34 \times S\overline{v}O_2) + (P\overline{v}O_2 \times 0.003)$$

$$CcO_2 = (Hb \times 1.34) + (PAO_2 \times 0.003).$$

Clinically, the most common oxygen saturation– and content–based indices are (1) **total oxygen delivery (DO_2)**, (2) **arterial-venous oxygen content difference ($C[a\text{-}\overline{v}]O_2$)**, (3) **oxygen consumption ($\dot{V}O_2$)**, (4) **oxygen extraction ratio (O_2ER)**, (5) **mixed venous oxygen saturation ($S\overline{v}O_2$)**, and (6) **pulmonary shunt fraction ($\dot{Q}_S/\dot{Q}_T$)**.[5]

Total Oxygen Delivery (DO_2)[6]

Total oxygen delivery (DO_2) is the amount of oxygen delivered to the peripheral tissue cells. The DO_2 is calculated as follows:

$$DO_2 = \dot{Q}_T \times (CaO_2 \times 10)$$

---

[5]The availability of the oxygen saturation– and–content–based indices that require the venous oxygen content—the $C(a\text{-}\overline{v})O_2$, $\dot{V}O_2$, O_2ER, $S\overline{v}O_2$, and $\dot{Q}_S/\dot{Q}_T$—may not be readily available because of the high risk/benefit ratio associated with the insertion of the pulmonary artery catheter needed to obtain venous blood. See pulmonary artery catheter, page 85.

[6]Clinical note: It is important to understand that the formula used to calculate total oxygen delivery is one in which factors are *multiplied* rather than added—in short, small decreases or increases in these factors have a marked influence on the final product. For example, consider the following: An elderly two-pack-per-day smoking gentlemen presents with dyspnea. His PaO_2 is 65 mm Hg on room air. He is mildly anemic (Hb = 9.0 g%) and has an SpO_2 of 90%. His carboxyhemoglobin (3.0%), which in turn makes the SaO_2 87% (90% − 3% = 87%). He is on a beta-blocker for his hypertension, which reduces his cardiac output to 3.0 L/min. In addition, he has mild

---

where $\dot{Q}_T$ is total cardiac output (L/min), CaO_2 is oxygen content of arterial blood (milliliters of oxygen per 100 mL of blood), and the factor 10 is used to convert the CaO_2 to milliliters of oxygen per liter of blood.

Therefore, if the patient has a cardiac output of 4 L/min and a CaO_2 of 15 vol%, the DO_2 is 600 mL of oxygen per minute:

$$\begin{aligned} DO_2 &= \dot{Q}_T \times (CaO_2 \times 10) \\ &= 4\,L/min \times (15\,vol\% \times 10) \\ &= 600\,mL\,O_2/min. \end{aligned}$$

Normally, the DO_2 is about 1000 mL of oxygen/minute. Box 5-1 provides factors that increase and decrease the DO_2.

Arterial-Venous Oxygen Content Difference ($C[a\text{-}\overline{v}]O_2$)[7]

The **arterial-venous oxygen content difference** ($C[a\text{-}\overline{v}]O_2$) is the difference between the CaO_2 and the $C\overline{v}O_2$ ($CaO_2 - C\overline{v}O_2$). Therefore, if the patient's CaO_2 is 15 vol% and the $C\overline{v}O_2$ is 8 vol%, the $C(a\text{-}\overline{v})O_2$ is 7 vol%:

$$\begin{aligned} C(a\text{-}\overline{v})O_2 &= CaO_2 - C\overline{v}O_2 \\ &= 15\,vol\% - 8\,vol\% \\ &= 7\,vol\%. \end{aligned}$$

Normally, the $C(a\text{-}\overline{v})O_2$ is about 5 vol%. The $C(a\text{-}\overline{v})O_2$ is useful in assessing the patient's cardiopulmonary status because oxygen changes in the mixed venous blood ($C\overline{v}O_2$) often occur earlier than oxygen changes in arterial blood gas. Box 5-2 provides factors that increase and decrease the $C(a\text{-}\overline{v})O_2$.

Oxygen Consumption ($\dot{V}O_2$)[8]

Oxygen consumption ($\dot{V}O_2$), also known as *oxygen uptake*, is the amount of oxygen consumed by the peripheral tissue

---

metabolic alkalosis (pH 7.48) from chronic diuretic therapy, which causes a left shift in his oxyhemoglobin dissociation curve. Inserting these figures into the total oxygen delivery formula results in a markedly reduced oxygen delivery (oxygen transport) of about 321 mL of O_2 per minute. Couple this condition with fever and pain, which increase oxygen consumption, and we see real trouble ahead!

[7]The availability of $C(a\text{-}\overline{v})O_2$ may not be readily available because of the high risk/benefit ratio associated with the insertion of the pulmonary artery catheter needed to obtain venous blood. See pulmonary artery catheter, page 85.

[8]The determination of $\dot{V}O_2$ may not be readily available because of the high risk/benefit ratio associated with the insertion of the pulmonary artery catheter needed to obtain venous blood. See pulmonary artery catheter, page 85.

cells during a 1-minute period. The $\dot{V}O_2$ is calculated as follows:

$$\dot{V}O_2 = \dot{Q}_T[C(a\text{-}\bar{v})O_2 \times 10]$$

where $\dot{Q}_T$ is the total cardiac output (L/min), $C(a\text{-}\bar{v})O_2$ is the arterial-venous oxygen content difference, and the factor 10 is used to convert the $C(a\text{-}\bar{v})O_2$ to mL O_2/L.

Therefore, if a patient has a cardiac output of 4 L/min and a $C(a\text{-}\bar{v})O_2$ of 6 vol%, the total amount of oxygen consumed by the tissue cells in 1 minute would be 240 mL:

$$\begin{aligned}\dot{V}O_2 &= \dot{Q}_T[C(a\text{-}\bar{v})O_2 \times 10]\\ &= 4\,L/\min \times 6\,vol\% \times 10\\ &= 240\,mL\,O_2/\min.\end{aligned}$$

Normally, the $\dot{V}O_2$ is about 250 mL of oxygen per minute. It is often reported as a function of body weight (i.e., mL/kg or mL/lb). Box 5-3 provides factors that increase and decrease the $C(a\text{-}\bar{v})O_2$.

Oxygen Extraction Ratio (O_2ER)[9]

The **oxygen extraction ratio (O_2ER)**, also known as the *oxygen coefficient ratio* or *oxygen utilization ratio,* is the amount of oxygen consumed by the tissue cells divided by the total amount of oxygen delivered. The O_2ER is calculated by dividing the $C(a\text{-}\bar{v})O_2$ by the CaO_2. Therefore, if a patient has a CaO_2 of 15 vol% and a $C\bar{v}O_2$ of 10 vol%, the O_2ER would be 33%:

$$\begin{aligned}O_2ER &= \frac{CaO_2 - C\bar{v}O_2}{CaO_2}\\[4pt] &= \frac{15\,vol\% - 10\,vol\%}{15\,vol\%}\\[4pt] &= \frac{5\,vol\%}{15\,vol\%}\\[4pt] &= 0.33\end{aligned}$$

Normally, the O_2ER is about 25%. Box 5-4 provides factors that increase and decrease the O_2ER.

Mixed Venous Oxygen Saturation $(S\bar{v}O_2)$[10]

When a patient has a normal arterial oxygen saturation (SaO_2) and hemoglobin concentration, the **mixed venous oxygen saturation** ($S\bar{v}O_2$) is often used as an early indicator of changes in the patient's $C(a\text{-}\bar{v})O_2$, $\dot{V}O_2$, and O_2ER—which are measures of net tissue oxygenation. The $S\bar{v}O_2$ can signal changes in the patient's $C(a\text{-}\bar{v})O_2$, $\dot{V}O_2$, and O_2ER earlier than arterial blood gases because the PaO_2 and SaO_2 levels are often normal during early tissue oxygenation changes. Normally, the $S\bar{v}O_2$ is about 75%. The $S\bar{v}O_2$ can be measured directly by obtaining a venous blood sample from a pulmonary arterial catheter, or derived as follows:

$$S\bar{v}O_2 = \frac{DO_2 - \dot{V}O_2}{DO_2}$$

---

[9]The determination of O_2ER may not be readily available because of the high risk/benefit ratio associated with the insertion of the pulmonary artery catheter needed to obtain venous blood. See pulmonary artery catheter, page 85.

[10]The $S\bar{v}O_2$ may not be readily available because of the risk/benefit ratio associated with the insertion of the pulmonary artery catheter needed to obtain mixed venous blood.

where the DO_2 is the total oxygen delivery and the $\dot{V}O_2$ is the oxygen consumption. Thus, if the patient has a normal DO_2 of 1000 mL O_2/min, and a normal $\dot{V}O_2$ of 250 mL O_2/min, the $S\overline{v}O_2$ is 0.75:

$$S\overline{v}O_2 = \frac{DO_2 - \dot{V}O_2}{DO_2}$$
$$= \frac{1000 - 250}{1000}$$
$$= \frac{750}{1000}$$
$$= 0.75.$$

Box 5-5 provides factors that increase and decrease the $S\overline{v}O_2$. Table 5-1 summarizes the way various clinical factors alter the patient's DO_2, $\dot{V}O_2$, $C(a\text{-}\overline{v})O_2$, O_2ER, and $S\overline{v}O_2$.

Pulmonary Shunt Fraction ($\dot{Q}_S/\dot{Q}_T$)[11]

Because pulmonary shunting and venous admixture are frequent complications in respiratory disorders, knowledge of the degree of shunting is desirable in developing patient care plans. The amount of intrapulmonary shunting can be calculated by using the classic shunt equation:

$$\frac{\dot{Q}_S}{\dot{Q}_T} = \frac{CcO_2 - CaO_2}{CcO_2 - C\overline{v}O_2}$$

where $\dot{Q}_S$ is the cardiac output that is shunted, $\dot{Q}_T$ is the total cardiac output, CcO_2 is the oxygen content of pulmonary capillary blood, CaO_2 is the oxygen content of arterial blood, and $C\overline{v}O_2$ is the oxygen content of mixed venous blood.

To obtain the data necessary to calculate the patient's intrapulmonary shunt, the following information must be gathered:
- Barometric pressure
- PaO_2

- SaO_2 (arterial oxygen saturation)
- $PaCO_2$
- $P\overline{v}O_2$
- $S\overline{v}O_2$ (mixed venous oxygen saturation)
- Hb concentration
- PAO_2 (partial pressure of alveolar oxygen)[12]
- FIO_2 (fractional concentration of inspired oxygen)

A clinical example of the shunt calculation follows:

Shunt Study Calculation in an Automobile Accident Victim

A 22-year-old man is on a volume-cycled mechanical ventilator on a day when the barometric pressure is 755 mm Hg. The patient is receiving an FIO_2 of 0.60. The following clinical data are obtained:
- Hb: 15 g/dL
- PaO_2: 65 mm Hg (SaO_2: 90%)
- $PaCO_2$: 56 mm Hg
- $P\overline{v}O_2$: 35 mm Hg ($S\overline{v}O_2$: 65%)

With this information the patient's PAO_2, CcO_2, CaO_2, and $C\overline{v}O_2$ can now be calculated. (The clinician should remember that PH_2O represents alveolar water vapor pressure and is always 47 mm Hg.)

1. $PAO_2 = (PB - P_{H_2O}) FIO_2 - PaCO_2 (1.25)$
   $= (755 - 47) 0.60 - 56 (1.25)$
   $= (708) 0.60 - 70$
   $= 424.8 - 70$
   $= 354.8$

2. $CcO_2 = (Hb \times 1.34) + (PAO_2 \times 0.003)$
   $= (15 \times 1.34) + (354.8 \times 0.003)$
   $= 20.1 + 1.064$
   $= 21.164$ (vol% O_2)

3. $CaO_2 = (Hb \times 1.34 \times SaO_2) + (PaO_2 \times 0.003)$
   $= (15 \times 1.34 \times 0.90) + (65 \times 0.003)$
   $= (18.09 + 0.195$
   $= 18.285$ (vol% O_2)

4. $C\overline{v}O_2 = (Hb \times 1.34 \times S\overline{v}O_2) + (P\overline{v}O_2 \times 0.003)$
   $= (15 \times 1.34 \times 0.65) + (35 \times 0.003)$
   $= 13.065 + 0.105$
   $= 13.17$ (vol% O_2)

With this information the patient's intrapulmonary shunt fraction can now be calculated:

$$\frac{\dot{Q}_S}{\dot{Q}_T} = \frac{CcO_2 - CaO_2}{CcO_2 - C\overline{v}O_2}$$
$$= \frac{21.164 - 18.285}{21.164 - 13.17}$$
$$= \frac{2.879}{7.994}$$
$$= 0.36$$

Therefore, 36% of the patient's pulmonary blood flow is perfusing lung alveoli that are not being ventilated.

---

[11]The measurement of $\dot{Q}_S/\dot{Q}_T$ may not be readily available because of the high risk/benefit ratio associated with the insertion of the pulmonary artery catheter needed to obtain venous blood.

[12]See Ideal Alveolar Gas Equation, Appendix VIII.

TABLE 5-1 Clinical Factors That Affect Oxygen Transport Calculations*

Oxygen Transport Study	Equation	Factors That Increase Value	Factors That Decrease Value
Total oxygen delivery (DO_2)	$DO_2 = Q_T \times (CaO_2 \times 10)$	Increased blood oxygenation Increased hemoglobin Increased cardiac output	Decreased blood oxygenation Decreased hemoglobin Decreased cardiac output

Arterial-venous oxygen content difference ($C(a\text{-}\bar{v})O_2$)	$C(a\text{-}\bar{v})O_2$	Decreased cardiac output
		Increased O_2 consumption
		    Exercise
		    Seizures
		    Shivering
		    Hyperthermia
			Increased cardiac output
			Skeletal muscle relaxation
			Induced by drugs
			Peripheral shunting
			Sepsis
			Trauma
			Certain poisons
			Cyanide
			Hypothermia

Oxygen consumption ($\dot{V}O_2$)	$\dot{V}O_2 = \dot{Q}_T[C(a\text{-}\bar{v})O_2 \times 10]$	Exercise Seizures Shivering Hyperthermia	Skeletal muscle relaxation induced by drugs Peripheral shunting Sepsis Trauma Certain poisons Cyanide Hypothermia

Oxygen extraction ratio (O_2ER)	$O_2ER = \dfrac{CaO_2 - C\bar{v}O_2}{CaO_2}$	Increased cardiac output
		Skeletal muscle relaxation induced
		    by drugs
		Peripheral shunting
		Sepsis
		Trauma
		Certain poisons
		Cyanide
		Hypothermia
		Increased hemoglobin
		Increased arterial oxygenation
			Decreased cardiac output
			Increased O_2 consumption
			    Exercise
			    Seizures
			    Shivering
			    Hyperthermia
			Anemia
			Decreased arterial oxygenation

Mixed venous oxygen saturation ($S\bar{v}O_2$)	$S\bar{v}O_2 = \dfrac{DO_2 - \dot{V}O_2}{DO_2}$	Decreased cardiac output
		Increased O_2 consumption
		    Exercise
		    Seizures
		    Shivering
		    Hyperthermia
			Increased cardiac output
			Skeletal muscle relaxation
			    induced by drugs
			Peripheral shunting
			Sepsis
			Trauma
			Certain poisons (cyanide)
			Hypothermia

Pulmonary shunt fraction ($\dot{Q}_S/\dot{Q}_T$)	$\dfrac{\dot{Q}_S}{\dot{Q}_T} = \dfrac{CcO_2 - CaO_2}{CcO_2 - C\bar{v}O_2}$	See Table 5-3	N/A

*The availability of the oxygen saturation– and content–based indices that require the venous oxygen content—the $C(a\text{-}\bar{v})O_2$, $\dot{V}O_2$, O_2ER, $S\bar{v}O_2$, and $\dot{Q}s/\dot{Q}t$—may not be readily available because of the risk/benefit ratio associated with the insertion of the pulmonary arterial catheter needed to obtain mixed venous blood.

TABLE 5-2 Clinical Significance of Pulmonary Shunting

Degree of Pulmonary Shunting (%)	Clinical Significance
Below 10%	Normal lung status
10% to 20%	Indicates a pulmonary abnormality but is not significant in terms of cardiopulmonary support
20% to 30%	May be life threatening, possibly requiring cardiopulmonary support
Greater than 30%	Serious life-threatening condition, almost always requiring cardiopulmonary support

Table 5-2 shows the clinical significance of pulmonary shunting. Table 5-3 summarizes how specific respiratory diseases alter the oxygen saturation– and content–based indices.[13]

Hypoxemia versus Hypoxia

Hypoxemia refers to an abnormally low arterial oxygen tension (PaO_2) and is frequently associated with **hypoxia**, which is an inadequate level of tissue oxygenation (see the following discussion). Although the presence of hypoxemia

[13]*Note in Table 5-3 that virtually every respiratory disorder presented in this textbook causes the $\dot{Q}_S/\dot{Q}_T$ to increase and the DO_2 to decrease.

TABLE 5-3 Oxygenation Index Changes Commonly Seen in Respiratory Diseases

Pulmonary Disorder	Oxygenation Indices					
	$S\bar{v}O_2$	DO_2*	$\dot{V}O_2$	$C(a-\bar{v})O_2$	O_2ER	$\dot{Q}_s/\dot{Q}_T$
Obstructive airway disease	↑	↓	~†	~	↑	↓
Chronic bronchitis						
Emphysema						
Bronchietasis						
Asthma						
Cystic fibrosis						
Croup syndrome						
Infectious pulmonary disease	↑	↓	~	~	↑	↓
Pneumonia						
Lung abscess						
Fungal disorders						
Tuberculosis			~			
Pulmonary edema	↑	↓	~	↑†	↑	↓
Pulmonary embolism	↑	↓	~	↑†	↑	↓
Lung collapse	↑	↓		↑†	↑	↓
Flail chest						
Pneumothorax						
Pleural disease (e.g., hemothorax)						
Kyphoscoliosis	↑	↓	~	~	↑	↓
Pneumoconiosis	↑	↓	~	~	↑	↓
Cancer of the lung	↑	↓	~	~	↑	↓
Adult respiratory distress syndrome	↑	↓	~	~	↑	↓
Idiopathic (infant) respiratory distress syndrome	↑	↓	~	~	↑	↓
Chronic interstitial lung disease	↑	↓	~	~	↑	↓
Sleep apnea	↑	↓	~	↑†	↑	↓
Smoke inhalation						
Without surface burns	↑	↓	~	~	↑	↓
With surface burns	↑	↓	↑	↑	↑	↓
Near drowning (wet)	↑	↓	↑	↑	↑	↓

*The DO_2 may be normal in patients with an increased cardiac output, an increased hemoglobin level (polycythemia), or a combination of both. For example, a normal DO_2 is often seen in patients with chronic obstructive pulmonary disease and polycythemia. When the DO_2 is normal, the patient's O_2ER is usually normal.

†, ~ Unchanged.

†The increased $C(a-\bar{v})O_2$ is associated with a decreased cardiac output.

TABLE 5-4 Hypoxemia Classifications*

Classification	PaO_2 (mm Hg) (Rule of Thumb)
Normal	80–100
Mild hypoxemia	60–80
Moderate hypoxemia	40–60
Severe hypoxemia	<40

*The hypoxemia classifications provided in this table are generally accepted clinical values. Minor variations of these values are found in the literature. As a general rule of thumb, however, the hypoxemia classifications and PaO_2 range(s) presented in this table are useful guidelines.

strongly suggests tissue hypoxia, it does not necessarily mean the absolute existence of tissue hypoxia. For example, the reduced level of oxygen in the arterial blood may be offset by an increased cardiac output or an increased hemoglobin level. However, in sick patients, these compensatory mechanisms are often not available. A good example would be an anemic patient on beta-adrenergic blockers such a propranolol, or an elderly patient with reduced cardiac function.

Hypoxemia is commonly classified as **mild hypoxemia,** **moderate hypoxemia,** or **severe hypoxemia** (Table 5-4). Clinically, the presence of mild hypoxemia generally stimulates the oxygen peripheral chemoreceptors to increase the patient's breathing rate and heart rate (see Figure 2-26).

Hypoxia refers to low or inadequate oxygen for aerobic cellular metabolism. Hypoxia is characterized by tachycardia, hypertension, peripheral vasoconstriction, dizziness, and mental confusion. Table 5-5 provides an overview of the four main types of hypoxia. When hypoxia exists, alternate anaerobic mechanisms are activated in the tissues that produce dangerous metabolites—such as **lactic acid**—as waste products. Lactic acid is a nonvolatile acid and causes the pH to decrease.

Pathophysiologic Conditions Associated with Chronic Hypoxia

Cor Pulmonale

Cor pulmonale is the term used to denote pulmonary arterial hypertension, right ventricular hypertrophy, increased right

TABLE 5-5 Types of Hypoxia

Hypoxia	Descriptions	Common Causes
Hypoxic hypoxia (also called *hypoxemic hypoxia*)	Inadequate oxygen at the tissue cells caused by low arterial oxygen tension (PaO_2)	Low PAO_2 caused by: • Hypoventilation • High altitude Diffusion impairment • Interstitial fibrosis • Interstitial lung disease • Interstitial pulmonary edema • Pneumoconiosis Ventilation-perfusion mismatch Pulmonary shunting
Anemic hypoxia	PaO_2 is normal, but the oxygen-carrying capacity of the hemoglobin is inadequate	Decreased hemoglobin concentration • Anemia • Hemorrhage Abnormal hemoglobin • Carboxyhemoglobin • Methemoglobin
Circulatory hypoxia (also called *stagnant* or *hypoperfusion hypoxia*)	Blood flow to the tissue cells is inadequate; therefore adequate oxygen is not available to meet tissue needs	Slow or stagnant (pooling) peripheral blood flow Arterial-venous shunts
Histotoxic hypoxia	Impaired ability of the tissue cells to metabolize oxygen	Cyanide poisoning

ventricular work, and ultimately right ventricular failure. The three major mechanisms involved in producing cor pulmonale in chronic pulmonary disease are (1) the increased viscosity of the blood associated with **polycythemia**, (2) the increased pulmonary vascular resistance caused by hypoxic vasoconstriction, and (3) the obliteration of the pulmonary capillary bed, particularly in emphysema. Items 1 and 2 are discussed in greater depth in the following paragraphs.

Polycythemia

When pulmonary disorders produce chronic hypoxia, the renal cells release higher than normal amounts of the hormone erythropoietin, which in turn stimulates the bone marrow to increase red blood cell (RBC) production. RBC production is known as *erythropoiesis*. An increased level of RBCs is called *polycythemia*. The polycythemia that results from hypoxia is an adaptive mechanism that increases the oxygen-carrying capacity of the blood.

Unfortunately, the advantage of the increased oxygen-carrying capacity in polycythemia is at least partially offset by the increased viscosity of the blood when the hematocrit reaches 50% to 60%. Because of the increased viscosity of the blood, a greater driving pressure is needed to maintain a given flow.

Hypoxic Vasoconstriction of the Lungs

Hypoxic vasoconstriction of the pulmonary vascular system **(hypoxic vasoconstriction of the lungs)** commonly develops

in response to the decreased PAO_2 that occurs in chronic respiratory disorders. The decreased PAO_2 causes the smooth muscles of the pulmonary arterioles to constrict. The exact mechanism of this phenomenon is unclear. However, the PAO_2 (and not the PaO_2) is known to chiefly control this response.

The early effect of hypoxic vasoconstriction is to direct blood away from the hypoxic regions of the lungs and thereby offset the shunt effect. However, when the number of hypoxic regions becomes significant—as during the advanced stages of emphysema or chronic bronchitis—a generalized pulmonary vasoconstriction develops, causing the pulmonary vascular resistance to increase substantially. Increased pulmonary vascular resistance leads to pulmonary hypertension, increased work of the right side of the heart, right ventricular hypertrophy, and cor pulmonale.

The cor pulmonale associated with chronic respiratory disorders may develop from the combined effects of polycythemia and pulmonary arterial vasoconstriction. Both of these conditions occur as a result of chronic hypoxia. Clinically, cor pulmonale leads to the accumulation of venous blood in the large veins. This condition causes (1) the neck veins to become distended (see Figure 2-45), (2) the extremities to show signs of peripheral edema and pitting edema (see Figure 2-44), and (3) the liver to become enlarged and tender.

SELF-ASSESSMENT QUESTIONS

1. A 46-year-old woman with severe asthma arrives in the emergency room with the following clinical data:
   Hb: 11 g%
   PaO_2: 46 mm Hg
   SaO_2: 70%
   Based on these clinical data, what is the patient's CaO_2?
   a. 6.75 vol% O_2
   b. 10.50 vol% O_2
   c. 12.30 vol% O_2
   d. 15.25 vol% O_2

2. If the patient has a cardiac output of 6 L/min and a CaO_2 of 12 vol%, what is the DO_2?
   a. 210 mL O_2/min
   b. 345 mL O_2/min
   c. 540 mL O_2/min
   d. 720 mL O_2/min

3. If the patient's CaO_2 is 11 vol% and the $C\bar{v}O_2$ is 7 vol%, what is the $C(a-\bar{v})O_2$?
   a. 4 vol% O_2
   b. 7 vol% O_2
   c. 11 vol% O_2
   d. 15 vol% O_2

4. Clinically, the patient's $C(a-\bar{v})O_2$ increases in response to which of the following?
   1. Hypothermia
   2. Decreased cardiac output
   3. Seizures
   4. Cyanide poisoning
      a. 2 only
      b. 4 only
      c. 2 and 3 only
      d. 1 and 4 only

5. If a patient has a cardiac output of 6 L/min and a $C(a-\bar{v})O_2$ of 4 vol%, what is the $\dot{V}O_2$?
   a. 160 mL O_2/min
   b. 180 mL O_2/min
   c. 200 mL O_2/min
   d. 240 mL O_2/min

6. Clinically, the $\dot{V}O_2$ decreases in response to which of the following?
   1. Exercise
   2. Hyperthermia
   3. Body size
   4. Peripheral shunting
      a. 2 only
      b. 4 only
      c. 1 and 3 only
      d. 2, 3, and 4 only

7. If the patient's CaO_2 is 12 vol% and the $C\bar{v}O_2$ is 7 vol%, what is the O_2ER?
   a. 0.27
   b. 0.33
   c. 0.42
   d. 0.53

8. Clinically, the $S\bar{v}O_2$ decreases in response to which of the following?
   a. Increased cardiac output
   b. Seizures
   c. Peripheral shunting
   d. Hypothermia

9. In the patient with severe emphysema, which of the following oxygenation indices are commonly seen?
   1. Decreased $S\bar{v}O_2$
   2. Increased $\dot{V}O_2$
   3. Decreased $C(a-\bar{v})O_2$
   4. Increased O_2ER
      a. 1 only
      b. 3 only
      c. 1 and 4 only
      d. 2 and 3 only

10. In the patient with pulmonary edema, which of the following oxygenation indices are commonly seen?
    1. Increased O_2ER
    2. Decreased $S\bar{v}O_2$
    3. Increased $\dot{V}O_2$
    4. Decreased $\dot{V}O_2$
       a. 2 only
       b. 4 only
       c. 1 and 2 only
       d. 1, 2, and 3 only

Case Study: Gunshot Victim (Questions 11-15)
A 37-year-old woman is on a volume-cycled mechanical ventilator on a day when the barometric pressure is 745 mm Hg. The patient is receiving an FIO_2 of 0.50. The following clinical data are obtained:
Hb: 11 g%
PaO_2: 60 mm Hg (SaO_2 90%)
$P\bar{v}O_2$: 35 mm Hg ($S\bar{v}O_2$ 65%)
$PaCO_2$: 38 mm Hg
Cardiac output: 6 L/min

11. Based on this information, calculate the patient's total oxygen delivery:
    a. 510 mL O_2/min
    b. 740 mL O_2/min
    c. 806 mL O_2/min
    d. 930 mL O_2/min

12. Based on this information, calculate the patient's arterial-venous oxygen content difference:
    a. 2.45 vol% O_2
    b. 3.76 vol% O_2
    c. 4.20 vol% O_2
    d. 5.40 vol% O_2

13. **Based on this information, calculate the patient's intrapulmonary shunt fraction:**
   a. 22%
   b. 26%
   c. 33 %
   d. 37%

14. **Based on this information, calculate the patient's oxygen consumption:**
   a. 170 mL O_2/min
   b. 200 mL O_2/min
   c. 230 mL O_2/min
   d. 280 mL O_2/min

15. **Based on this information, calculate the patient's oxygen extraction ratio:**
   a. 16%
   b. 24%
   c. 26%
   d. 28%

Cardiovascular System Assessments

Chapter Objectives

After reading this chapter, you will be able to:

- Describe the electrocardiogram (ECG) pattern of a normal cardiac cycle.
- Evaluate and identify arrhythmias.
- Describe the noninvasive hemodynamic monitoring assessments.
- Evaluate the basic pathophysiologic mechanisms associated with an increased heart rate (pulse), cardiac output, and blood pressure, and a decreased perfusion state.
- Describe invasive hemodynamic monitoring assessment methods.
- Describe how the hypoxemia, acidemia, or pulmonary vascular obstruction associated with respiratory disease alters the hemodynamic status.

Key Terms

Arterial Catheter
Asystole (Cardiac Standstill)
Atrial Fibrillation
Atrial Flutter
Central Venous Pressure (CVP) Catheter
ECG Patterns
Hemodynamic
Invasive Hemodynamic Monitoring Assessments
Noninvasive Hemodynamic Monitoring Assessments
P Wave
Premature Ventricular Contraction (PVC)
Pulmonary Artery Catheter
Pulmonary Capillary Wedge Pressure (PWCP)

Pulseless Electrical Activity (PEA)
QRS Complex
Sinus Arrhythmia
Sinus Bradycardia
Sinus Tachycardia
T wave
Ventricular Fibrillation
Ventricular Tachycardia

Chapter Outline

The Electrocardiogram
Common Heart Arrhythmias
  Sinus Bradycardia
  Sinus Tachycardia
  Sinus Arrhythmia
  Atrial Flutter
  Atrial Fibrillation
  Premature Ventricular Contractions
  Ventricular Tachycardia
  Ventricular Fibrillation
  Asystole (Cardiac Standstill)
Noninvasive Hemodynamic Monitoring Assessments
  Heart Rate (Pulse), Cardiac Output, and Blood Pressure
  Perfusion State
Invasive Hemodynamic Monitoring Assessments
  Pulmonary Artery Catheter
  Arterial Catheter
  Central Venous Pressure Catheter
Hemodynamic Monitoring in Respiratory Diseases
Self-Assessment Questions

Because the transport of oxygen to the tissue cells and the delivery of carbon dioxide to the lungs are functions of the cardiovascular system, a basic knowledge and understanding of (1) **normal electrocardiogram (ECG) patterns**, (2) **common heart arrhythmias**, (3) **noninvasive hemodynamic monitoring assessments**, (4) **invasive hemodynamic monitoring assessments**, and (5) **determinants of cardiac output** are essential components of patient assessment.[1]

The Electrocardiogram

Because the respiratory care practitioner frequently works with critically ill patients who are on cardiac monitors, a basic

understanding of normal and common abnormal **ECG patterns** is important. An ECG monitors, both visually and on recording paper, the electrical activity of the heart.

Figure 6-1 illustrates the ECG pattern of a **normal cardiac cycle**. The **P wave** reflects depolarization of the atria. The **QRS complex** represents the depolarization of the ventricles, and the **T wave** represents ventricular repolarization.

In normal adults the **heart rate** is between 60 and 100 beats per minute (bpm). In normal infants the heart rate is 130 to 150 bpm. A number of methods can be used to calculate the heart rate. For example, when the rhythm is regular, the heart rate can be determined at a glance by counting the number of large boxes (on the ECG strip) between two QRS complexes and then dividing this number into 300. Therefore, if an ECG strip consistently shows four large boxes between each pair of QRS complexes, the heart rate is

---

[1]See Appendix XV for an example of a cardiopulmonary profile sheet used to monitor the hemodynamic status of the critically ill patient.

75 bpm (300 ÷ 4 = 75). When the rhythm is irregular, the heart rate can be determined by counting the QRS complexes on a 6-second strip and multiplying by 10. The following heart arrhythmias are commonly seen and should be recognized by the respiratory care practitioner.

Common Heart Arrhythmias[2]

Sinus Bradycardia

In **sinus bradycardia** the heart rate is less than 60 bpm. *Bradycardia* means "slow heart." Sinus bradycardia has a normal P-QRS-T pattern, and the rhythm is regular (Figure 6-2). Healthy athletes often demonstrate this finding because of increased cardiac stroke volume and other poorly understood mechanisms. Common pathologic causes of sinus

---

[2]For a complete review of common heart arrhythmias, see Des Jardins T: *Cardiopulmonary anatomy and physiology: essentials of respiratory care,* ed 6, 2013, Delmar/Cengage Learning.

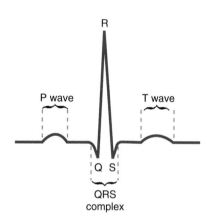

FIGURE 6-1 Electrocardiographic pattern of a normal cardiac cycle.

bradycardia include a weakened or damaged sinoatrial (SA) node, severe or chronic hypoxemia, increased intracranial pressure, obstructive sleep apnea, and certain drugs (most notably the beta-blockers). Sinus bradycardia may lead to decreased cardiac output and blood pressure. In severe cases, sinus bradycardia may lead to a decreased vascular perfusion state and tissue hypoxia. The patient may demonstrate a weak pulse, poor capillary refill, cold and clammy skin, and a depressed sensorium—a clinical condition known as **pulseless electrical activity** (PEA).

Sinus Tachycardia

In **sinus tachycardia** the heart rate is greater than 100 bpm. Tachycardia means "fast heart." Sinus tachycardia has a normal P-QRS-T pattern, and the rhythm is regular (Figure 6-3). Sinus tachycardia is the normal physiologic response to stress and exercise. Common abnormal causes of sinus tachycardia include hypoxemia, severe anemia, hyperthermia, massive hemorrhage, pain, fear, anxiety, hyperthyroidism, and sympathomimetic or parasympatholytic drug administration.

Sinus Arrhythmia

In **sinus arrhythmia** the heart rate varies by more than 10% from beat to beat. The P-QRS-T pattern is normal (Figure 6-4), but the interval between groups of complexes (i.e., the R-R interval) varies. Sinus arrhythmia is a normal rhythm in children and young adults. The patient's pulse will often increase during inspiration and decrease during expiration. No treatment is required unless significant alteration occurs in the patient's arterial blood pressure.

Atrial Flutter

In **atrial flutter** the normal P wave is absent and replaced by two or more regular sawtooth waves. The QRS complex is normal and the ventricular rate may be regular or irregular,

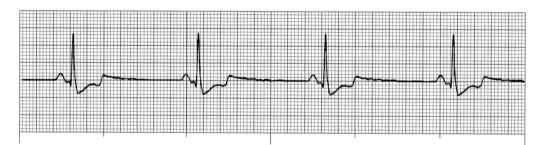

FIGURE 6-2 Sinus bradycardia at about 40 bpm. (From Aehlert B: *ECGs made easy,* ed 5, St Louis, 2013, Mosby.)

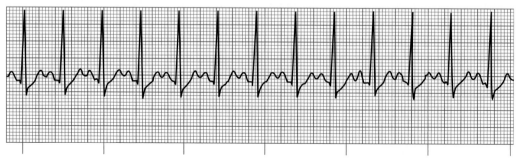

FIGURE 6-3 Sinus tachycardia at about 125 bpm. (From Aehlert B: *ECGs made easy,* ed 5, St Louis, 2013, Mosby.)

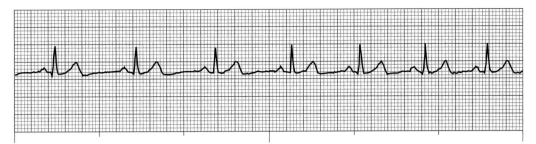

FIGURE 6-4 Sinus arrhythmia at 63 to 81 bpm. (From Aehlert B: *ECGs made easy*, ed 5, St Louis, 2013, Mosby.)

II

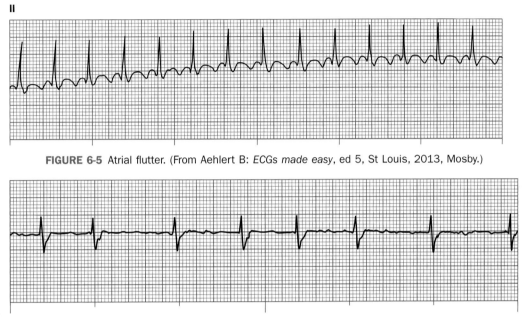

FIGURE 6-5 Atrial flutter. (From Aehlert B: *ECGs made easy*, ed 5, St Louis, 2013, Mosby.)

FIGURE 6-6 Atrial fibrillation with a ventricular response of 63 to 100 bpm. (From Aehlert B: *ECGs made easy*, ed 5, St Louis, 2013, Mosby.)

depending on the relationship of the atrial to the ventricular beats. Figure 6-5 shows an atrial flutter with a regular rhythm with a 2:1 conduction ratio (i.e., two atrial beats for every ventricular beat). The atrial rate is usually constant, between 250 and 350 bpm, whereas the ventricular rate is in the normal range or elevated. Causes of atrial flutter include hypoxemia, a damaged SA node, and congestive heart failure.

Atrial Fibrillation

In **atrial fibrillation** the atrial contractions are disorganized and ineffective, and the normal P wave is absent (Figure 6-6). The atrial rate ranges from 350 to 700 bpm. The QRS complex is normal, and the ventricular rate ranges from 100 to 200 bpm. Causes of atrial fibrillation include hypoxemia and a damaged SA node. Atrial fibrillation may reduce the cardiac output by 20% because of a loss of atrial filling (the so-called "atrial kick"). Atrial fibrillation is frequently seen in sleep apnea (see Chapter 31).

Premature Ventricular Contractions

A **premature ventricular contraction (PVC)** is not preceded by a P wave. The QRS complex is wide, bizarre, and unlike the normal QRS complex (Figure 6-7). The regular heart rate is altered by the PVC. The heart rhythm may be very irregular when there are many PVCs. PVCs can occur at any rate. PVCs often occur in pairs. A PVC may also be seen after every normal heartbeat—an arrhythmia called bigeminal PVCs. A PVC may also be seen after every two normal heartbeats—an arrhythmia called trigeminal PVCs. Common causes of PVCs include intrinsic myocardial disease, hypoxemia, acidemia, hypokalemia, and congestive heart failure. PVCs may also be a sign of theophylline or alpha-stimulant or beta-agonist toxicity.

Ventricular Tachycardia

In **ventricular tachycardia** the P wave is generally indiscernible, and the QRS complex is wide and bizarre in appearance (Figure 6-8). The T wave may not be separated from the QRS complex. The ventricular rate ranges from 150 to 250 bpm, and the rate is regular or slightly irregular. The patient's blood pressure is usually decreased during ventricular tachycardia. In fact, ventricular tachycardia may be without a palpable pulse and a blood pressure of zero. Clinically, the respiratory therapist should note that the treatment and management for ventricular tachycardia—with and without a pulse—is different, but both are medical emergencies.

Ventricular Fibrillation

Ventricular fibrillation is characterized by chaotic electrical activity and cardiac activity. The ventricles literally quiver out of control with no perfusion beat-producing rhythm (Figure 6-9). During ventricular fibrillation, there is no cardiac

II

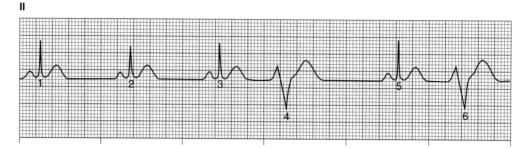

FIGURE 6-7 Sinus rhythm with premature ventricular complexes (PVCs). The fourth and sixth beats are very different in appearance from the normal conducted sinus beats. Beats 4 and 6 are PVCs. They are not preceded by P waves. (From Aehlert B: *ECGs made easy*, ed 5, St Louis, 2013, Mosby.)

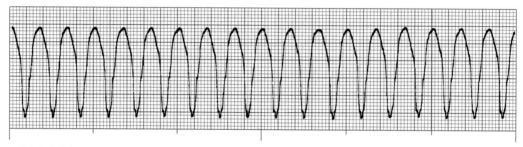

FIGURE 6-8 Ventricular tachycardia. (From Aehlert B: *ECGs made easy*, ed 5, St Louis, 2013, Mosby.)

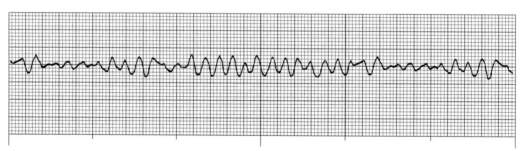

FIGURE 6-9 Ventricular fibrillation. (From Aehlert B: *ECGs made easy*, ed 5, St Louis, 2013, Mosby.)

output or blood pressure, and the patient will die in minutes without treatment.

Asystole (Cardiac Standstill)

Asystole (cardiac standstill) is the complete absence of electrical and mechanical activity. As a result, the cardiac output stops and the blood pressure falls to zero. The ECG tracing appears as a flat line and indicates severe damage to the heart's electrical conduction system (Figure 6-10). Occasionally, periods of disorganized electrical and mechanical activity may be generated during long periods of asystole; this is referred to as an *agonal rhythm* or a *dying heart*. Electric shock (defibrillation) is not effective for this rhythm—cardiopulmonary resuscitation (CPR) and advanced cardiovascular life support (ACLS) medications are required.

Noninvasive Hemodynamic Monitoring Assessments

Hemodynamics describe forces that influence the circulation of blood. The general hemodynamic status of the patient can be monitored noninvasively at the bedside by assessing the heart rate (via an ECG monitor, auscultation, or pulse), blood pressure, and perfusion state. During the acute stages

of respiratory disease, the patient frequently demonstrates the hemodynamic changes described in the following paragraphs.

Heart Rate (Pulse), Cardiac Output, and Blood Pressure

Increased heart rate, pulse, and blood pressure develop frequently during the acute stages of pulmonary disease. This can result from the indirect response of the heart to hypoxic stimulation of the peripheral chemoreceptors, primarily the carotid bodies. When the carotid bodies are stimulated, reflex signals are sent to the respiratory muscles, which in turn activate the so-called *pulmonary reflex,* which triggers tachycardia and an increased cardiac output and blood pressure. The increased cardiac output is a compensatory mechanism that at least partially counteracts the hypoxemia produced by the pulmonary shunting in respiratory disorders.

Other causes of increased cardiac output and blood pressure include severe anemia, high fever, anxiety, massive hemorrhage, certain cardiac arrhythmias, and hyperthyroidism. When the heart rate increases beyond 150 to 175 bpm, cardiac output and blood pressure begin to decline (Starling's relationship).

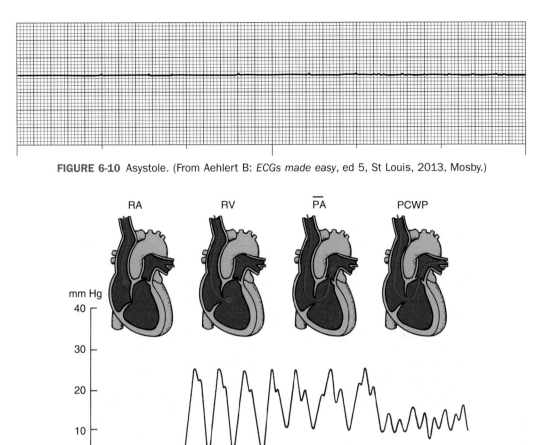

FIGURE 6-10 Asystole. (From Aehlert B: *ECGs made easy*, ed 5, St Louis, 2013, Mosby.)

FIGURE 6-11 Insertion of the pulmonary catheter (shown in blue in the illustration). The insertion site of the pulmonary catheter may be the basilic, brachial, femoral, subclavian, or internal insertion sites. As the catheter advances, pressure readings and waveforms are monitored to determine the catheter's position as it moves through the right atrium (RA), right ventricle (RV), mean pulmonary artery ($\overline{PA}$), and finally into a pulmonary capillary wedge pressure (PCWP) position. Immediately after a PCWP reading, the balloon is deflated to allow blood to flow past the tip of the catheter. When the balloon is deflated, the catheter continuously monitors the pulmonary artery pressure.

Perfusion State

The perfusion state can be evaluated by examining the patient's skin color, capillary refill, and sensorium. Under normal conditions the patient's nail beds and oral mucosa are pink. If these areas appear cyanotic or mottled, poor perfusion and tissue hypoxia is likely to be present. When the nail beds are compressed to expel blood, they should refill and turn pink within 2 seconds when the pressure is released. If the nail beds remain white, perfusion is inadequate. Under normal conditions the patient's skin should be dry and warm. When the skin is diaphoretic (wet), cool, or clammy, local perfusion is inadequate. Finally, when the patient is disoriented as to person, place, and time, a decreased perfusion state and cerebral hypoxia may be present.

Invasive Hemodynamic Monitoring Assessments

Invasive hemodynamic monitoring is used in the assessment and treatment of critically ill patients. Invasive hemodynamic monitoring includes the measurement of (1) intracardiac pressures and flows via a **pulmonary artery catheter**, (2)

arterial pressure via an **arterial catheter**, and (3) central venous pressure via a **central venous catheter**. Monitoring of these parameters provides rapid and precise measurements (assessment data) of the patient's cardiovascular function—which in turn are used to down-regulate or up-regulate the patient's treatment plan in a timely manner.

Pulmonary Artery Catheter

The pulmonary artery catheter (Swan-Ganz catheter) is a balloon-tipped, flow-directed catheter that is inserted at the patient's bedside; the respiratory therapist monitors the pressure waveform as the catheter, with the balloon inflated, is guided by blood flow through the right atrium and right ventricle into the pulmonary artery (Figure 6-11). The pulmonary artery catheter is used directly to measure the (1) right atrial pressure (via the proximal port), (2) pulmonary artery pressure (via the distal port), (3) left atrial pressure (indirectly via the **pulmonary capillary wedge pressure**), (4) cardiac output (via the thermodilution technique), and (5) oxygenation levels in the central venous blood to be used for oxygen transport studies ($C[a\text{-}\overline{v}]O_2$, $\dot{V}O_2$, O_2ER, $S\overline{v}O_2$ and $\dot{Q}_s/\dot{Q}_T$), (see Chapter 5). The insertion of a pulmonary

TABLE 6-1 Hemodynamic Values Measured Directly

Hemodynamic Value	Abbreviation	Normal Range
Central venous pressure	CVP	0–8 mm Hg
Right atrial pressure	RAP	0–8 mm Hg
Mean pulmonary artery pressure	$\overline{PA}$	10–20 mm Hg
Pulmonary capillary wedge pressure (also called *pulmonary artery wedge, pulmonary artery occlusion*)	PCWP PAW PAO	4–12 mm Hg
Cardiac output	CO	4–6 L/min

TABLE 6-2 Hemodynamic Values Calculated from Direct Hemodynamic Measurements

Hemodynamic Value	Abbreviation	Normal Range
Stroke volume	SV	40–80 mL
Stroke volume index	SVI	$40 \pm$ mL/beat/m^2
Cardiac index	CI	3.0 ± 0.5 L/min/m^2
Right ventricular stroke work index	RVSWI	7–12 g/m^2
Left ventricular stroke work index	LVSWI	40–60 g/m^2
Pulmonary vascular resistance	PVR	50–150 dynes $\times$ sec $\times$ cm^{-5}
Systemic vascular resistance	SVR	800–1500 dynes $\times$ sec $\times$ cm^{-5}

catheter is not without risks and can be life threatening. For example, it can lead to arrhythmias, rupture of the pulmonary artery, thrombosis, infection, pneumothorax, and bleeding. Because of the high risk/benefit ratio associated with the insertion of the pulmonary artery catheter, its use is reserved for only the most critically ill patients.

Arterial Catheter

The arterial catheter (referred to as an a-line) is the most commonly used mode of invasive hemodynamic monitoring. It is generally inserted in the radial artery for patient comfort and convenient access. The indwelling arterial catheter allows (1) continuous and precise measurements of systolic, diastolic, and mean blood pressure; (2) accurate information regarding fluctuations in blood pressure; and (3) guidance in the decision to up-regulate or down-regulate therapy—for example, hypotension or hypertension. The arterial catheter is also useful in patients who require frequent or repeated arterial blood gas samples (e.g., the patient being mechanically ventilated). The blood samples are readily available, and the patient is not subjected to the pain of repeated arterial punctures.

Central Venous Pressure Catheter

The **central venous pressure (CVP) catheter** readily measures the CVP and the right ventricular filling pressure. It serves as an excellent monitor of right ventricular function. An increased CVP reading is commonly seen in patients who (1) have left ventricular heart failure (e.g., pulmonary edema), (2) are receiving excessively high positive-pressure

mechanical breaths, (3) have cor pulmonale, or (4) have a severe flail chest, pneumothorax, or pleural effusion.

Table 6-1 summarizes the hemodynamic parameters that can be measured directly. Table 6-2 lists the hemodynamic parameters that can be calculated from results obtained from the direct measurements.

Hemodynamic Monitoring in Respiratory Diseases

Because respiratory disorders can have a profound effect on the cardiopulmonary system, the data generated by the previously described invasive hemodynamic monitors can be used in the assessment and treatment of these patients. For example, respiratory diseases associated with severe or chronic hypoxemia, acidemia, or pulmonary vascular obstruction can increase the pulmonary vascular resistance (PVR) significantly. An increased PVR, in turn, can lead to a variety of secondary hemodynamic changes such as increased CVP, right atrial pressure (RAP), mean pulmonary artery pressure ($\overline{PA}$), right ventricular stroke work index (RVSWI), and decreased cardiac output (CO), stroke volume (SV), stroke volume index (SVI), cardiac index (CI), and left ventricular stroke work index (LVSWI). Table 6-3 lists common hemodynamic changes seen in pulmonary diseases known to alter the patient's hemodynamic status.

TABLE 6-3 Hemodynamic Changes Commonly Seen in Respiratory Diseases

Disorder	CVP	RAP	$\overline{PA}$	PCWP	CO	SV	SVI	CI	RVSWI	LVSWI	PVR	SVR
			Oxygenation Indices									
Chronic obstructive pulmonary disease (COPD) Chronic bronchitis Emphysema Cystic fibrosis Bronchiectasis	↑	↑	↑↑	~*	~	~	~	~	↑	~	↑	~
Pulmonary edema (cardiogenic)	~	↑	↑	↑↑	↓	↓	↓	↓	↑	↓	↑	↓
Pulmonary embolism	↑	↑	↑↑	↓	↓	↓	↓	↓	↑	↓	↑	~
Adult respiratory distress syndrome (ARDS)—severe	~↑	~↑	~↑	~	~	~	~	~	~↑	~	~↑	~
Lung collapse Flail chest Pneumothorax Pleural disease (e.g., hemothorax)	↑	↑	↑	↓	↓	↓	↓	↓	↑	↓	↑	↓
Kyphoscoliosis	↑	↑	↑	~	~	~	~	~	↑	~	↑	~
Pneumoconiosis	↑	↑	↑↑	~	~	~	~	~	↑	~	↑	~
Chronic interstitial lung diseases	↑	↑	↑↑	~	~	~	~	~	↑	~	↑	~
Cancer of the lung (tumor mass)	↑	↑	↑	↓	↓	↓	↓	↓	↑	~	↑	~
Hypovolemia	↓↓	↓	↓	↓	↓	↓	↓	↓	↓	↓	~	↑
Hypervolemia (burns)	↑↑	↑	↑	↑	↑	↑	↑	↑	↑	↑	~	~
Right heart failure (cor pulmonale)	↑↑	↑↑	↓	↓	~	~	~	~	~	~	~	~

CI, Cardiac index; *CO*, cardiac output; *CVP*, central venous pressure; *LVSWI*, left ventricular stroke work index; $\overline{PA}$, mean pulmonary artery pressure; *PCWP*, pulmonary capillary wedge pressure; *PVR*, pulmonary vascular resistance; *RAP*, right atrial pressure; *RVSWI*, right ventricular stroke work index; *SV*, stroke volume; *SVI*, stroke volume index; *SVR*, systemic vascular resistance.

*, ~, Unchanged.

SELF-ASSESSMENT QUESTIONS

Answers to questions can be found on Evolve. To access additional student assessment questions visit
http://evolve.elsevier.com/DesJardins/respiratory.

1. In which of the following arrhythmias is there no cardiac output or blood pressure?
   a. Ventricular flutter
   b. Arial fibrillation
   c. Premature ventricular contractions
   d. Ventricular fibrillation

2. The general hemodynamic status of the patient can be monitored noninvasively at the patient's bedside by assessing which of the following?
   1. Perfusion state
   2. Heart rate
   3. Pulse rate
   4. Blood pressure
      a. 4 only
      b. 2 and 3 only
      c. 2, 3, and 4 only
      d. 1, 2, 3, and 4

3. Cardiac output and blood pressure begin to decline when the heart rate increases beyond which of the following?
   a. 125 to 150 bpm
   b. 150 to 175 bpm
   c. 175 to 200 bpm
   d. 200 to 250 bpm

4. An increased central venous pressure reading is commonly seen in the patient who:
   1. Has a severe pneumothorax
   2. Is receiving high positive-pressure breaths
   3. Has cor pulmonale
   4. Is in left-sided heart failure
      a. 3 only
      b. 4 only
      c. 2, 3, and 4 only
      d. 1, 2, 3, and 4

5. What is the normal range of the mean pulmonary artery pressure?
   a. 0 to 5 mm Hg
   b. 5 to 10 mm Hg
   c. 10 to 20 mm Hg
   d. 20 to 30 mm Hg

6. What is the normal range for the pulmonary capillary wedge pressure?
   a. 0 to 4 mm Hg
   b. 4 to 12 mm Hg
   c. 12 to 20 mm Hg
   d. 20 to 25 mm Hg

7. The hemodynamic indices in patients with chronic obstructive pulmonary disease commonly show which of the following?
   1. Increased central venous pressure
   2. Decreased right atrial pressure
   3. Increased mean pulmonary artery pressure
   4. Decreased pulmonary capillary wedge pressure
   5. Increased cardiac output
      a. 3 only
      b. 1 and 3 only
      c. 2 and 4 only
      d. 3, 4, and 5 only

8. The hemodynamic indices in patients with pulmonary edema commonly show which of the following?
   1. Decreased central venous pressure
   2. Increased right atrial pressure
   3. Decreased mean pulmonary artery pressure
   4. Increased pulmonary capillary wedge pressure
   5. Decreased cardiac output
      a. 1 and 3 only
      b. 2, 3, and 5 only
      c. 2, 4, and 5 only
      d. 1, 2, 4, and 5

9. Atrial flutter is defined as a constant atrial rate of:
   a. 100 to 150 bpm
   b. 150 to 250 bpm
   c. 250 to 350 bpm
   d. 350 to 450 bpm

10. In sinus arrhythmia, the heart rate varies by more than:
   a. 5%
   b. 10%
   c. 15%
   d. 20%

Radiologic Examination of the Chest

Chapter Objectives

After reading this chapter, you will be able to:

- Describe the fundamentals of radiography.
- Differentiate among the standard positions and techniques of chest radiography.
- Define the radiologic terms commonly used during inspection of the chest radiograph.
- Describe the three steps to evaluate technical quality of the radiograph.
- Describe a logical, systematic sequence of radiograph examination.
- Describe the diagnostic values of the following radiologic procedures:
    - Computed tomography (CT)
    - Positron emission tomography (PET)
    - Positron emission tomography and computed tomography scan (PET/CT scan)
    - Magnetic resonance imaging (MRI)
    - Pulmonary angiography
    - Ventilation-perfusion scan
    - Fluoroscopy
    - Bronchography

Key Terms

Air Cyst
Anteroposterior (AP) Radiograph
Bleb
Bronchogram
Bronchography
Bullae
Cardiothoracic Ratio
Cavity
Computed Tomography (CT)
Computed Tomography Pulmonary Angiogram (CTPA)
Consolidation
Fluoroscopy
High Resolution CT (HRCT) Scans
Homogeneous Density
Honeycombing
Infiltrates
Interstitial Density
Lateral Decubitus Radiograph
Lateral Radiograph
Lesion
Lung Window CT Scan
Magnetic Resonance Imaging (MRI)
Mediastinal Window CT Scan
Opacity
Pleural Density
Pleural Mass
Pleural Nodule
Positron Emission Tomography (PET)
Positron Emission Tomography and Computed Tomography Scan (PET/CT Scan)
Posteroanterior (PA) Projection
Pulmonary Angiography
Pulmonary Mass
Pulmonary Nodule
Radiodensity
Radiolucency
Rib Series (Radiograph)
Translucency
Ventilation-Perfusion Scan

Chapter Outline

Fundamentals of Radiography
Standard Positions and Techniques of Chest Radiography
    Posteroanterior Radiograph
    Anteroposterior Radiograph
    Lateral Radiograph
    Lateral Decubitus Radiograph
Inspecting the Chest Radiograph
    Technical Quality of the Radiograph
    Sequence of Examination
    Computed Tomography (CT)
    Positron Emission Tomography (PET)
    Positron Emission Tomography and Computed Tomography scan (PET/CT scan)
    Magnetic Resonance Imaging (MRI)
    Pulmonary Angiography
    Ventilation-Perfusion Scan
    Fluoroscopy
    Bronchography
Self-Assessment Questions

Radiography is the making of a photographic image of the internal structures of the body by passing x-rays through the body to an x-ray film, or radiograph. In patients with respiratory disease, radiography plays an important role in the diagnosis of lung disorders, the assessment of the extent and location of the disease, and the evaluation of the subsequent progress of the disease.

Fundamentals of Radiography

X-rays are created when fast-moving electrons with sufficient energy collide with matter in any form. Clinically, x-rays are produced by an electronic device called an *x-ray tube*.

The x-ray tube is a vacuum-sealed glass tube that contains a cathode and a rotating anode. A tungsten plate approximately a half-inch square is fixed to the end of the rotating anode at the center of the tube. This tungsten plate is called the *target*. Tungsten is an effective target metal because of its high melting point, which can withstand the extreme heat to which it is subjected, and because of its high atomic number, which makes it more effective in the production of x-rays.

When the cathode is heated, electrons "boil off." When a high voltage (70 to 150 kV) is applied to the x-ray tube, the electrons are driven to the rotating anode where they strike the tungsten target with tremendous energy. The sudden deceleration of the electrons at the tungsten plate converts energy to x-rays. Although most of the electron energy is converted to heat, a small amount (less than 1%) is transformed to x-rays and allowed to escape from the tube through a set of lead shutters called a *collimator*. From the collimator the x-rays travel through the patient to the x-ray film.

The ability of the x-rays to penetrate matter depends on the density of the matter. For chest radiographs the x-rays may pass through bone, air, soft tissue, and fat. Dense objects such as bone absorb more x-rays (preventing penetration) than objects that are not as dense, such as blood and the air-filled lungs.

After passing through the patient, the x-rays strike the x-ray film. X-rays that pass through low-density objects strike the film at full force and produce a black image on the film. X-rays that are absorbed by high-density objects (such as bone) either do not reach the film at all or strike the film with less force. Relative to the density of the object, these objects appear as light gray to white on the film.

Standard Positions and Techniques of Chest Radiography

Clinically, the standard radiograph of the chest includes two views: a **posteroanterior (PA) projection** and a lateral projection (either a left or right **lateral radiograph**) with the patient in the standing position. When the patient is seriously ill or immobilized, an upright radiograph may not be possible. In such cases, a supine **anteroposterior (AP) radiograph** is obtained at the patient's bedside. A lateral radiograph is rarely obtainable under such circumstances.

Posteroanterior Radiograph

The standard PA chest radiograph is obtained by having the patient stand (or sit) in the upright position. The anterior aspect of the patient's chest is pressed against a film cassette holder, with the shoulders rotated forward to move the scapulae away from the lung fields. The distance between the x-ray tube and the film is 6 feet. The x-ray beam travels from the x-ray tube, through the patient from back to front, and to the x-ray film.

The x-ray examination is usually performed with the patient's lungs in full inspiration to show the lung fields and related structures to their greatest possible extent. At full inspiration the diaphragm is lowered to approximately the level of the ninth to eleventh ribs posteriorly (Figure 7-1).

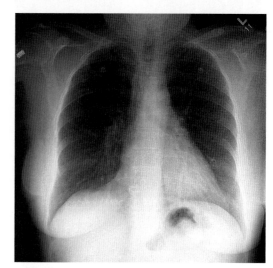

FIGURE 7-1 Standard posteroanterior chest radiograph with the patient's lungs in full inspiration.

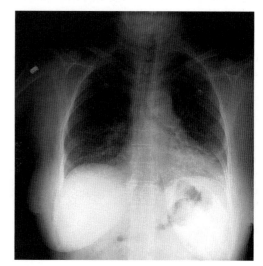

FIGURE 7-2 A posteroanterior chest radiograph of the same patient shown in Figure 7-1 during expiration.

For certain clinical conditions, radiographs are sometimes taken at the end of both inspiration and expiration. For example, in patients with obstructive lung disease an expiratory radiograph may be made to evaluate diaphragmatic excursion and the symmetry or asymmetry of such excursion (Figure 7-2).

Anteroposterior Radiograph

A supine AP radiograph may be taken in patients who are debilitated, immobilized, or too young to tolerate the PA procedure. The AP radiograph is usually taken with a portable x-ray unit at the patient's bedside. The film is placed behind the patient's back, with the x-ray unit positioned in front of the patient, approximately 48 inches from the film.

Compared with the PA radiograph, the AP radiograph has a number of disadvantages. For example, the heart and superior portion of the mediastinum are significantly magnified in the AP radiograph. This is because the heart is positioned in front of the thorax as the x-ray beams pass through the chest in the anterior-to-posterior direction, causing the image of the heart to be enlarged (Figure 7-3).

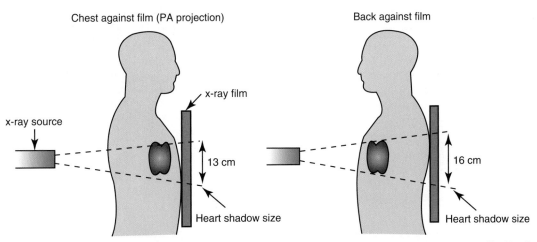

Chest against film (PA projection)

x-ray source

x-ray film

13 cm

Heart shadow size

Back against film

16 cm

Heart shadow size

FIGURE 7-3 Compared with the posteroanterior (PA) chest radiograph, the heart is significantly magnified in the anteroposterior (AP) chest radiograph. In the PA radiograph, the ratio of the width of the heart to the thorax is normally less than 1:2. The reason the heart appears larger in the AP radiograph is that it is positioned in front of the thorax as the x-ray beams pass through the chest in the anterior-to-posterior direction. This allows more space for the heart shadow to "fan out" before it reaches the x-ray film.

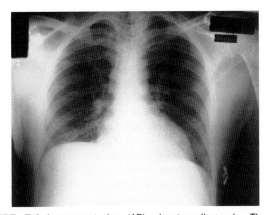

FIGURE 7-4 Anteroposterior (AP) chest radiograph. The diaphragms are elevated, the lower lung lobes appear hazy, the ratio of the width of the heart to the thorax is greater than 2:1 (i.e., the width of the heart is greater than 50% of the width of the thorax), and extraneous object is apparent outside the patient's left lateral chest (probably an EKG lead). X-ray examinations using portable machines are frequently performed on patients too ill to be transported to the radiology department. These films, in the best of circumstances, are of poorer quality than erect films taken with standard x-ray apparatus. The films are usually AP projections taken with the x-ray unit in front of and the film plate behind the patient. Overexposure, underexposure, malpositioning, marginal cutoffs, and motion artifacts are often present. In this setting, major events such as partial pneumothoraces, pleural effusions, and infiltrates in dependent parts of the lung may go unrecognized. Therefore, careful clinical correlation with the patient's pathophysiology and symptomatology is imperative.

The AP radiograph frequently has less resolution and more distortion. Because the patient is often unable to sustain a maximal inspiration, the lower lung lobes frequently appear hazy, erroneously suggesting pulmonary congestion or pleural effusion. Finally, because the AP radiograph is commonly taken in the intensive care unit, extraneous shadows, such as those produced by ventilator tubing and indwelling lines, are often present (Figure 7-4).

Lateral Radiograph

The lateral radiograph is obtained to complement the PA radiograph. It is taken with the side of the patient's chest compressed against the cassette. The patient's arms are raised, with the forearms resting on the head.

To view the right lung and heart, the patient's right side is placed against the cassette. To view the left lung and heart, the patient's left side is placed against the cassette. Therefore, a right lateral radiograph would be selected to view a density or **lesion** that is known to be in the right lung. If neither lung is of particular interest, a left lateral radiograph is usually selected to reduce the magnification of the heart. The lateral radiograph provides a view of the structures behind the heart and diaphragmatic dome. It can also be combined with the PA radiograph to give the respiratory therapist a three-dimensional view of the structures or of any abnormal densities (Figure 7-5).

Lateral Decubitus Radiograph

The **lateral decubitus radiograph** is obtained by having the patient lie on the left or right side rather than standing or sitting in the upright position. The naming of the decubitus radiograph is determined by the side on which the patient lies; thus, a right lateral decubitus radiograph means that the patient's right side is down.

The lateral decubitus radiograph is useful in the diagnosis of a suspected or known fluid accumulation in the pleural space (e.g., a pleural effusion) that is not easily seen in the PA radiograph. A pleural effusion, which is usually more thinly spread out over the diaphragm in the upright position, collects in the gravity-dependent areas while the patient is in the lateral decubitus position, allowing the fluid to be more readily seen (Figure 7-6).

Inspecting the Chest Radiograph

Before the respiratory therapist can effectively identify abnormalities on a chest radiograph, he or she must be able

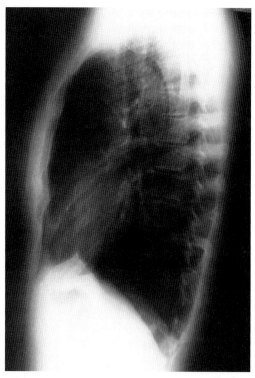

FIGURE 7-5 Lateral radiograph. The patient has an overexpanded lung and chest wall (barrel chest deformity) consistent with his known emphysema.

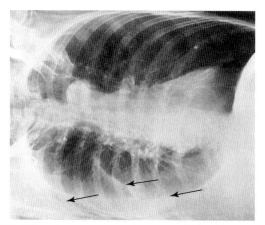

FIGURE 7-6 Right lateral decubitus view. Subpulmonic pleural effusion. Subdiaphragmatic fluid has run up the lateral chest wall, producing a band of soft tissue density. The medial curvilinear shadow (*arrows*) indicates fluid in the lips of the major fissure.

to recognize the normal anatomic structures. Figure 7-7 represents a normal PA chest radiograph with identification of important anatomic landmarks. Figure 7-8 labels the anatomic structures seen on a lateral chest radiograph.

Table 7-1 lists some of the more important radiologic terms used to describe abnormal chest x-ray findings.

Technical Quality of the Radiograph

The *first step* in examining a chest radiograph is to evaluate its technical quality. Was the patient in the correct position when the radiograph was taken? To verify the proper position, check the relationship of the medial ends of the clavicles to the vertebral column. For the PA radiograph the vertebral

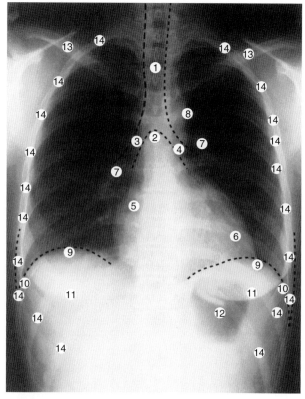

FIGURE 7-7 Normal posteroanterior (PA) chest radiograph. *1*, Trachea (note vertebral column in middle of trachea in this correctly centered and exposed film); *2*, carina; *3*, right main stem bronchus; *4*, left main stem bronchus; *5*, right atrium; *6*, left ventricle; *7*, hilar vasculature; *8*, aortic knob; *9*, diaphragm; *10*, costophrenic angles; *11*, breast shadows; *12*, gastric air bubble; *13*, clavicle; *14*, rib.

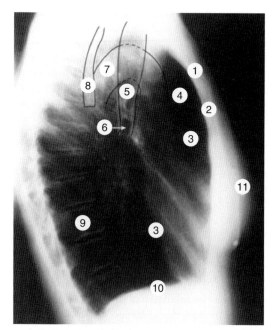

FIGURE 7-8 Normal lateral chest radiograph. *1*, Manubrium; *2*, sternum; *3*, cardiac shadow; *4*, retrosternal air space in the lung; *5*, trachea; *6*, bronchus, on end; *7*, aortic arch (ascending and descending); *8*, scapulae; *9*, vertebral column; *10*, diaphragm; *11*, breast shadow.

TABLE 7-1 Common Radiologic Terms

Term	Definition
Air cyst	A thin-walled radiolucent area surrounded by normal lung tissue
Bleb	A superficial air cyst protruding into the pleura; also called *bullae*
Bronchogram	An outline of air-containing bronchi beyond the normal point of visibility. An air bronchogram develops as a result of an infiltration or consolidation that surrounds the bronchi, producing a contrasting air column on the radiograph—that is, the bronchi appear as dark tubes surrounded by a white area produced by the infiltration or consolidation
Bullae	A large, thin-walled radiolucent area surrounded by normal lung tissue
Cavity	A radiolucent (dark) area surrounded by dense tissue (white). A cavity is the hallmark of a lung abscess. A fluid level may be seen inside a cavity
Consolidation	The act of becoming solid; commonly used to describe the solidification of the lung caused by a pathologic engorgement of the alveoli, as occurs in acute pneumonia
Homogeneous density	Refers to a uniformly dense lesion (white area); commonly used to describe solid tumors, fluid-containing cavities, or fluid in the pleural space
Honeycombing	A coarse reticular (netlike) density commonly seen in pneumoconiosis
Infiltrate	Any poorly defined radiodensity (white area); commonly used to describe an inflammatory lesion
Interstitial density	A density caused by interstitial thickening
Lesion	Any pathologic or traumatic alteration of tissue or loss of function of a part
Opacity	State of being opaque (white); an opaque area or spot; impervious to light rays, or by extension, x-rays; opposite of translucent or radiolucent
Pleural density	A radiodensity caused by fluid, tumor, inflammation, or scarring
Pulmonary mass	A lesion in the lung that is 6 cm or more in diameter; commonly used to describe a pulmonary tumor
Pulmonary nodule	A lesion in the lung that is less than 6 cm in diameter and composed of dense tissue; also called a *solitary pulmonary nodule* or *"coin" lesion* because of its rounded, coinlike appearance
Radiodensity	Dense areas that appear white on the radiograph; the opposite of radiolucency
Radiolucency	The state of being radiolucent; the property of being partly or wholly permeable to x-rays; commonly used to describe darker areas on a radiograph such as an emphysematous lung or a pneumothorax
Translucent (translucency)	Permitting the passage of light (or in this case, x-rays); commonly used to describe darker areas of the radiograph

column should be precisely in the center between the medial ends of the clavicles, and the distance between the right and left costophrenic angles and the spine should be equal. Even a small degree of patient rotation relative to the film can create a false image, erroneously suggesting tracheal deviation, cardiac displacement, or cardiac enlargement.

Second, the exposure quality of the radiograph should be evaluated. Normal exposure is verified by determining whether the spinal processes of the vertebrae are visible to the fifth or sixth thoracic level (T-5 to T-6). X-ray equipment is now available that allows the vertebrae to be seen down to the level of the cardiac shadow. The degree of exposure can be evaluated further by comparing the relative densities of the heart and lungs. For example, because the heart has a greater density than the air-filled lungs, the heart appears whiter than the lung fields. The heart and lungs become more radiolucent (darker) with greater exposure of the radiograph. A radiograph that has been overexposed is said to be "heavily penetrated" or "burned out." Conversely, the heart and lungs on an underexposed radiograph may appear denser and whiter. The lungs may erroneously appear to have **infiltrates,** and there may be little or no visibility of the thoracic vertebrae.

Third, the level of inspiration at the moment the radiograph was taken should be evaluated. At full inspiration the diaphragmatic domes should be at the level of the ninth to eleventh ribs posteriorly. On radiographs taken during expiration, the lungs appear denser, the diaphragm is elevated, and the heart appears wider and enlarged (Figure 7-2).

Sequence of Examination

Although the precise sequence in examining a chest radiograph is not important, the inspection should be done in a systematic manner. Some practitioners prefer an "inside-out" approach to inspecting the chest radiograph, which entails beginning with the mediastinum and proceeding outward to the peripheral extrathoracic soft tissue. Some practitioners prefer the reverse. The following is an "inside-out" method.

Mediastinum

The mediastinum should be inspected for width, contour, and shifts from the midline. The respiratory therapist should inspect the anatomy of the mediastinum, including the trachea, carina, cardiac borders, aortic arch, and superior vena cava (Figure 7-7).

TABLE 7-2 Examples of Factors That Pull or Push Anatomic Structures Out of Their Normal Position in the Chest Radiograph

Structure	Examples of Abnormal Position	Lesion
Mediastinum and hilar region Trachea Carina Heart Major vessels	Leftward shift	Pulled left by left upper lobe tuberculosis, atelectasis, or fibrosis Pushed left by right upper lobe emphysematous bullae, fluid, gas, or tumor
Left diaphragm	Upward shift	Pulled up by left lower lobe atelectasis or fibrosis Pushed up by distended gastric air bubble
Horizontal fissure	Downward shift	Pulled down by right middle lobe or right lower lobe atelectasis Pushed down by right upper lobe neoplasm
Left lung	Rightward shift	Pulled right by right lung collapse, atelectasis, or fibrosis Pushed right by left-sided tension pneumothorax or hemothorax

Trachea

On the PA projection the trachea should appear as a **translucent column** overlying the vertebral column. The diameter of the bronchi progressively tapers a short distance beyond the carina and then disappears (Figure 7-7). A number of clinical conditions can cause the trachea to shift from its normal position. For example, fluid or gas accumulation in the pleural space causes the trachea to shift away from the affected area. Atelectasis or fibrosis usually causes the trachea to shift toward the affected area. The trachea may also be displaced by tumors of the upper lung regions.

Anatomic structures in the chest (e.g., the trachea) move out of their normal position because they are either pushed or pulled in a given direction. In other words, they may be moved up or down or from side to side by lesions pulling or pushing in that direction. Table 7-2 lists examples of factors that push or pull the trachea and other anatomic structures out of their normal position in the chest radiograph.

Heart

On the PA projection the ratio of the width of the heart to the thorax (the **cardiothoracic ratio**) is normally less than 1:2. In other words, the width of the heart should be less than 50% of the width of the thorax. A small portion of the heart should be visible on the right side of the vertebral column. Two bulges should be seen on the right border of the heart. The upper bulge is the superior vena cava; the lower bulge is the right atrium. Three bulges are normally seen on the left side of the heart. The superior bulge is the aorta, the middle bulge is the main pulmonary artery, and the inferior bulge is the left ventricle (Figure 7-7). See Table 7-2 for examples of factors that push or pull the heart out of its normal position in the chest radiograph.

Hilar Region

The right and left hilar regions should be evaluated for change in size or position. Normally, the left hilum is about 2 cm higher than the right (Figure 7-7). An increased density of the hilar region may indicate engorgement of hilar vessels caused by pulmonary hypertension. Vertical displacement of the hilum suggests volume loss from one or more upper lobes of the lung on the affected side. In infectious lung disorders such as histoplasmosis or tuberculosis, the lymph nodes around the hilar region are often enlarged, calcified, or both. Malignant pulmonary lesions, including hilar malignant lymphadenopathy, may also be seen. See Table 7-2 for additional factors that push or pull structures in the hilar region out of their normal position in the chest radiograph.

Lung Parenchyma (Tissue)

The lung parenchyma should be systematically examined from top to bottom, one lung compared with the other. Normally, tissue markings can be seen throughout the lungs (Figure 7-7). The absence of tissue markings may suggest a pneumothorax, recent pneumonectomy, or chronic obstructive lung disease (e.g., emphysema), or may be the result of an overexposed radiograph. An excessive amount of tissue markings may indicate fibrosis, interstitial or alveolar edema, lung compression, or an underexposed radiograph. The periphery of the lung fields should be inspected for abnormalities that obscure the interface of the lung with the pleural space, mediastinum, or diaphragm. See Table 7-2 for additional examples of factors that push or pull the lung tissue out of its normal position in the chest radiograph.

Pleura

The peripheral borders of the lungs should be examined for pleural thickening, presence of fluid (pleural effusion) or air (pneumothorax) in the pleural space, or mass lesions (Figure 7-7). The costophrenic angles should be inspected. Blunting of the costophrenic angle suggests the presence of fluid. A lateral decubitus radiograph may be required to confirm the presence of fluid (Figure 7-6).

Diaphragms

Both the right and left hemidiaphragms should have an upwardly convex, dome-shaped contour. The right and left costophrenic angles should be clear. Normally, the right diaphragm is about 2 cm higher than the left because of the liver below it (Figure 7-7). Chronic obstructive pulmonary diseases (e.g., emphysema), and diseases that cause gas or fluid to accumulate in the pleural space (e.g., pneumothorax or pleural effusion), flatten and depress the normal curvature of the diaphragm. Abnormal elevation of one diaphragm may result from excessive gas in the stomach, collapse of the middle or lower lobe on the affected side, pulmonary infection at the lung bases, phrenic nerve damage, or spinal curvature. See Table 7-2 for additional examples of factors that push or pull the diaphragm out of its normal position in the chest radiograph.

Gastric Air Bubble

The area below the diaphragm should be inspected. A stomach air bubble is commonly seen under the left hemidiaphragm (Figure 7-7). Free air may appear under either diaphragm after abdominal surgery or in patients with peritoneal abscess.

Bony Thorax

The ribs, vertebrae, clavicles, sternum, and scapulae should be inspected. The intercostal spaces should be symmetrical and equal over each lung field (Figure 7-7). Intercostal spaces that are too close together suggest a loss of muscle tone, commonly seen in patients with paralysis involving one side of the chest. In chronic obstructive pulmonary disease, the intercostal spaces are generally far apart because of alveolar hyperinflation. Finally, the ribs should be inspected for deformities or fractures. If a rib fracture is suspected but not seen on the standard chest radiograph, a special **rib series** (radiographs that focus on the ribs) may be necessary.

Extrathoracic Soft Tissues

The soft tissue external to the bony thorax should be closely inspected. If the patient is a female (or an obese man), the outer boundaries of the breast shadows may be seen (Figure 7-7). If the patient has undergone a mastectomy, there will be a relative hyperlucency on the side of the mastectomy. Large breasts can create a significant amount of haziness over the lower lung fields, giving the false appearance of pneumonia or pulmonary congestion. Although nipple shadows are easily identified when they are bilaterally symmetrical, one may become less visible when the patient is slightly rotated. The other nipple then appears abnormally opaque and may be mistaken for a **pulmonary nodule**. Fatty tissue in the chest wall in obese patients may also be seen. After a tracheostomy or pneumothorax, subcutaneous air bubbles (called *subcutaneous emphysema*) often form in the soft tissue, especially if the patient is on a positive-pressure ventilator.

Computed Tomography

The same basic principles used in film radiography apply to **computed tomography (CT)** scanning—namely the absorption of x-rays by tissues that contain anatomic structures and organs of different atomic number. A CT scan provides a series of cross-sectional (transverse) pictures (called *tomograms*) of the structures within the body at numerous levels. The procedure is painless and noninvasive and requires no special preparation. The patient simply lies on the examination table, and this moves the patient through the opening of the CT scanner. The major components of a CT scanner are (1) an x-ray tube, which rotates in a continuous 360-degree motion around the patient to image the body in

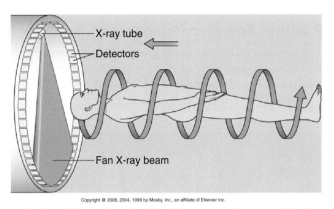

FIGURE 7-9 The principle of spiral computed tomography. The patient moves into the scanner with the x-ray tube continuously rotating and the detectors acquiring information. The rapidity of data acquisition allows a complete examination of the thorax to be performed in a single breath hold. (From Albert RK, Spiro SG, Jett JR: *Clinical Respiratory Medicine*, ed 3, St Louis, 2008, Mosby.)

cross-sectional slices; (2) an array of x-ray detectors opposite the x-ray tube, which record the x-rays that pass through the body; and (3) a computer, which converts the different x-ray absorption levels to cross-sectional images based on the density of the structures being scanned (Figure 7-9). This cross-sectional slice is called an *axial view* or *computerized axial tomogram*.

Up to 250 images, about 1 mm apart, can be generated on a chest CT scan. These "cuts" are often called **high resolution CT (HRCT) scans** (also called *spiral, volume,* or *helical scans*). In essence, each CT scan provides an image of what a "slice" through the body looks like at specific points—similar to cutting a piece of fruit in half and viewing the cross-section of the structures inside the fruit. Dense structures, such as bone, appear white on the tomogram, whereas structures with a relatively low density, such as the lungs, appear dark or black. Therefore, a dense tumor in the lungs would appear as a white object surrounded by dark lungs.

The resolution of a CT scan can be adjusted to primarily view (1) lung tissue—commonly called a **lung window CT scan**—or (2) bone and mediastinal structures—commonly called a **mediastinal window CT scan.** In a mediastinal window CT scan, the lung tissue is overexposed and appears mostly black; the bones and mediastinal organs appear mostly white. Figure 7-10 provides an overview of a normal lung window CT scan. Figure 7-11 shows a close-up of one "slice" of a normal lung window CT scan. Figure 7-12 provides a close-up view of one slice of a normal mediastinal window CT scan.

Finally, for poorly defined lesions evident on the standard radiograph, the CT scan is a useful supplement in determining the precise location, size, and shape of the lesion. The CT scan is especially helpful in confirming the presence of a mediastinal mass, small pulmonary nodules, small lesions of the bronchi, pulmonary cavities, a small pneumothorax, pleural effusion, and small tumors (as small as 0.3 to 0.5 cm). The CT scan can be done with contrast material in the vessels to delineate vascular structures.

Positron Emission Tomography

The **positron emission tomography (PET)** scan shows both the anatomic structures and the metabolic activity of the tissues and organs scanned. Used in conjunction with a chest x-ray and CT scan for comparison, the PET scan is an excellent diagnostic tool for early detection of cancerous lesions. The unique aspect of the PET scan is its ability to evaluate highly metabolic cells that may be cancerous. In other words, the PET scan is able to detect cancerous cells in the tissues of the body before changes develop in the anatomic shape of the organ.

Before undergoing the scan, the patient is injected intravenously with a solution of glucose that has been tagged with a radioactive chemical isotope (generally fluorine-18 fluorodeoxyglucose, or F18-FDG compound). Cancer cells metabolize glucose at extremely high rates. The PET scan measures the way cells burn glucose. When present, the cancer cells rapidly consume the tagged glucose. As the glucose molecules break down, end-products that emit positrons are produced. The positrons collide with electrons that give off gamma rays. The gamma rays are converted to dark spots on the PET scan image. These dark spots are commonly referred to as "hot spots." The presence of a hot spot on a PET scan is likely to confirm a rapidly growing tumor.

Clinically, a PET scan is an excellent tool to rule out suspicious findings (i.e., a possible cancerous area) that are identified on either the chest radiograph or CT scan. For example, Figure 7-13 shows a chest radiograph that identifies two suspicious findings—one small nodule in the right upper lung lobe and a larger density in the left lower lung lobe, just behind the heart. Figure 7-14 shows two CT scans that also identify the two suspicious findings and their precise location. Figures 7-15, 7-16, and 7-17 show PET scans that all confirm a hot spot (likely to be cancer) in the lower left lobe. However, the PET scan shown in Figure 7-18 confirms that the nodule in the right upper lobe is benign (i.e., no hot spot noted).

Although the PET scan is relatively painless (i.e., tantamount to intravenous insertion), it is lengthy. It may take up to 90 minutes to complete the scan. After the injection, the patient quietly rests in a reclining chair for 30 to 60 minutes

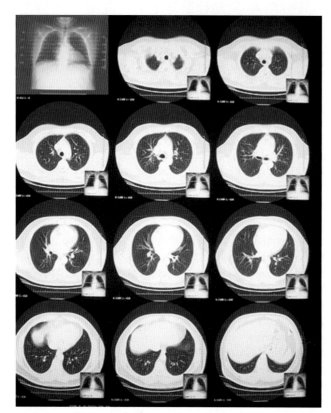

FIGURE 7-10 Overview of normal lung window computed tomography (CT) scan. The apex appears in the two views in the upper right-hand corner of this figure; the diaphragm at the base of the lungs appears in the lower right-hand view.

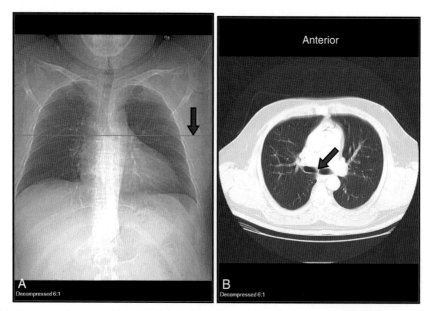

FIGURE 7-11 Close-up of a normal lung window computed tomography (CT) scan. **A,** The red arrow indicates the portion of the chest undergoing CT scanning. **B,** The actual cross-sectional slice or axial view of the chest. Note the carina and both main stem bronchi (arrow).

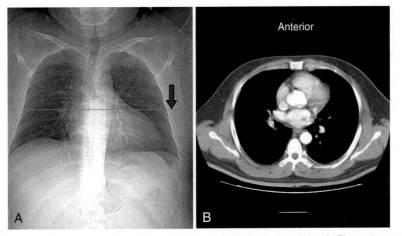

FIGURE 7-12 Close-up of normal computed tomography (CT) mediastinal window. **A,** The red arrow indicates the portion of the chest the CT scan is taken. **B,** The actual cross-sectional slice or axial view of the chest. Note that the lungs are overexposed and appear mostly black. The bone and mediastinal organs appear mostly white.

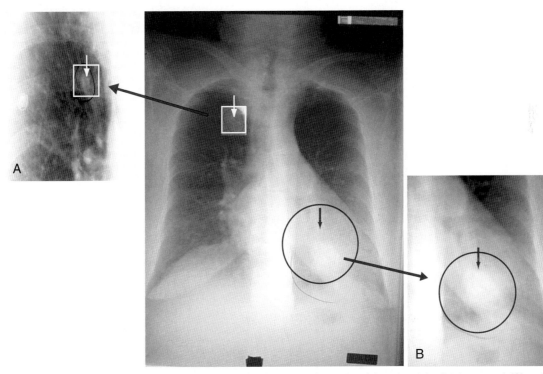

FIGURE 7-13 Chest radiograph identifying two suspicious findings: in the right upper lobe (*white arrows*) (**A**) and in the left lower lobe (**B**), just behind the heart (*red arrows*).

before the scan is performed. This allows time for the body to absorb the compound. This step may be difficult or impossible for patients who are unable to remain motionless for long periods of time. PET scans are very expensive to perform, compared with CT or **magnetic resonance imaging (MRI)** studies.

Positron Emission Tomography and Computed Tomography Scan

As described in the preceding sections, PET and CT are both standard imaging tools used by the radiologist to pinpoint the location of cancer or infection within the body before developing a treatment strategy. Individually, however, each scan has its own benefits and limitations. For example, the

PET scan detects the metabolic activity of growing cancer cells in the body, and the CT scan provides a detailed picture of the pulmonary anatomy that shows the precise location, size, and shape of a tumor or mass. By contrast, because the PET scan and CT scan are done at different times and locations, variations in the patient's body position often make the interpretation of the two images difficult.

Technology has now been developed that allows both the PET scan and the CT scan to be merged together and performed at the same time. The image produced is called a **positron emission tomography and computed tomography scan (PET/CT scan)** (also known as a *PET/CT fusion*). The PET/CT scan provides an image far superior to that afforded by either technology independently. When

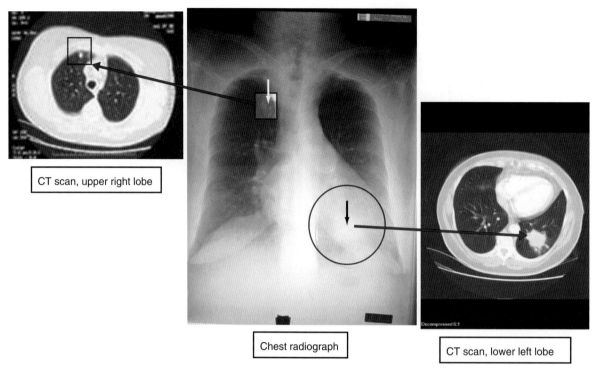

CT scan, upper right lobe

Chest radiograph

CT scan, lower left lobe

FIGURE 7-14 Same chest radiograph as shown in Figure 7-13. Note that the CT scan also identifies the suspicious nodules and their precise location.

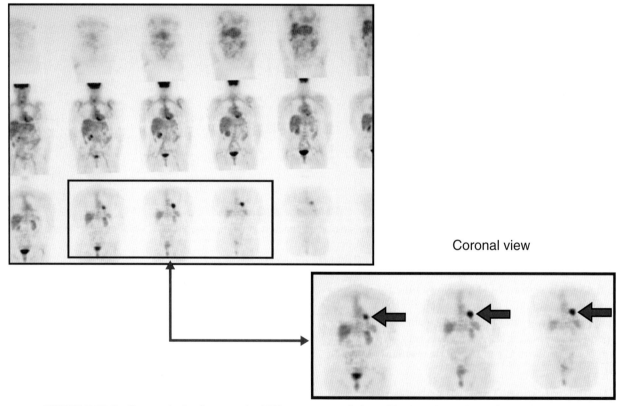

Coronal view

FIGURE 7-15 Positron emission tomography (PET) scan: coronal views. The last three views show a hot spot in left lower lobe.

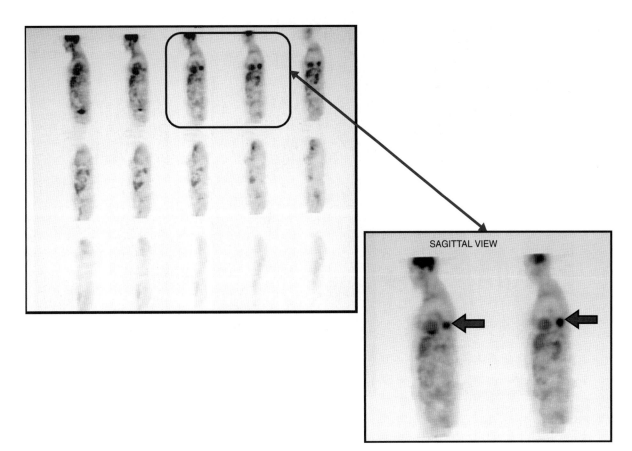

FIGURE 7-16 Positron emission tomography (PET) scan: sagittal view. The encircled images show a hot spot in the lower left lobe.

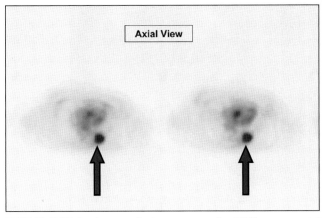

FIGURE 7-17 Positron emission tomography (PET) scan: axial view. A hot spot is further confirmed in left lower lobe.

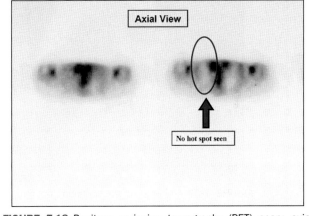

FIGURE 7-18 Positron emission tomography (PET) scan: axial view. This image confirms that the small nodule identified in the upper right lobe in the chest radiograph and computed tomography scan is benign (i.e., no hot spot is evident).

combined, the CT scan provides the anatomic detail regarding the precise size, shape, and location of the tumor, and the PET scan provides the metabolic activity of the tumor or mass. The PET/CT image provides excellent image quality and high sensitivity and specificity in detecting malignant lesions in the chest. Figure 7-19 shows a PET/CT scan alongside a CT scan and a PET scan; all the images show the same malignant nodule in the right upper lung lobe.

The benefits of a combined PET/CT scan include earlier diagnosis, accurate staging and localization, and precise treatment and monitoring. With the high quality and accuracy of the PET/CT image, the patient has a better chance for a favorable outcome, without the need for unnecessary procedures. In addition, the PET/CT scan provides early detection of the recurrence or metastasis of cancer, revealing tumors that might otherwise be obscured by scars from previous surgery and/or radiation therapy. Thus, the combined PET/CT scan provides the radiologist with a more complete overview of what is occurring in the patient's body, both anatomically and metabolically at the same time.

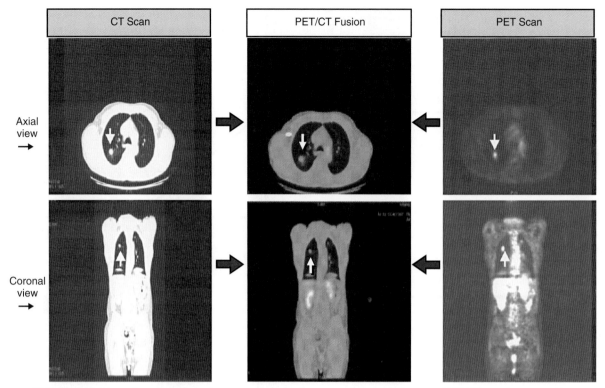

FIGURE 7-19 Merged positron emission tomography and computed tomography scan (PET/CT scan) (*center*). The CT scan, PET/CT fusion, and PET scan are all showing the same malignant nodule in the right upper lobe (*white arrow*). Note: The PET/CT fusion is normally presented in color (e.g., red, blue, yellow).

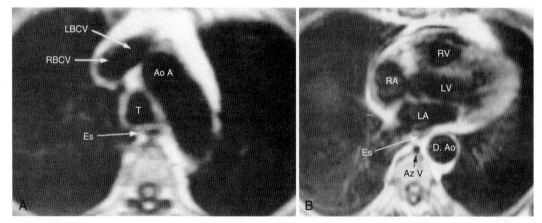

FIGURE 7-20 Anatomy of mediastinum on magnetic resonance imaging (MRI) scan. **A**, *Ao A*, Aortic arch; *Es*, esophagus; *LBCV*, left brachiocephalic vein; *RBCV*, right brachiocephalic vein; *T*, trachea. **B**, *Az V*, Azygos vein; *D. Ao*, descending aorta; *Es*, esophagus; *LA*, left atrium; *LV*, left ventricle; *RA*, right atrium; *RV*, right ventricle. (From Armstrong P, Wilson AG, Dee P: *Imaging of diseases of the chest*, St Louis, 1990, Mosby.)

Magnetic Resonance Imaging

MRI uses magnetic resonance as its source of energy to take cross-sectional (transverse, sagittal, or coronal) images of the body. It uses no ionizing radiation. The patient is placed in the cylindric imager, and the body part in question is exposed to a magnetic field and radiowave transmission. The MRI produces a high-contrast image that can detect subtle lesions (Figure 7-20).

MRI is superior to CT scanning in identifying complex congenital heart disorders, bone marrow diseases, adenopathy, and lesions of the chest wall. MRI is an excellent supplement to CT scanning for study of the mediastinum and hilar region. For most abnormalities of the chest, however, CT scanning is generally better than MRI for motion (patient motion causes loss of resolution in the MRI), spatial resolution, and cost reasons.

Because the magnetic resonance imager generates an intense magnetic field, objects made of ferromagnetic material are strongly attracted to it. Therefore, patients with ferromagnetic cerebral aneurysm clips, metallic artificial joints, or ferromagnetic prosthetic cardiac valves should not undergo MRI because the magnetic force of the imager can cause

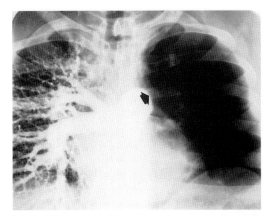

FIGURE 7-21 Abnormal pulmonary angiogram. Radiopaque material injected into the blood is prevented from flowing into the left lung past the pulmonary embolism (*arrow*). No vascular structures are seen distal to obstruction.

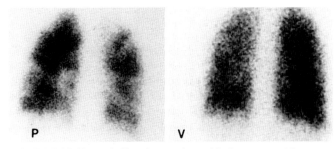

FIGURE 7-22 Fat embolism in a patient with dyspnea and hypoxemia after a recent orthopedic procedure. Perfusion (P) and ventilation (V) radionuclide scans show multiple peripheral subsegmental perfusion defects suggestive of fat embolism. (From Hansell DM, Armstrong P, Lynch DA, McAdams HP: *Imaging of diseases of the chest*, ed 4, Philadelphia, 2005, Elsevier.)

these devices to heat, shift, and harm the patient. The magnetic force of the imager can also interfere with the normal function of cardiac pacemakers and most ventilators.

Pulmonary Angiography

Pulmonary angiography is useful in identifying pulmonary emboli or arteriovenous malformations. It involves the injection of a radiopaque contrast medium through a catheter that has been passed through the right side of the heart and into the pulmonary artery. The injection of the contrast material into the pulmonary circulation is followed by rapid serial pulmonary angiograms. The pulmonary vessels are filled with radiopaque contrast material and therefore appear white. Figure 7-21 shows an abnormal angiogram in which the major blood vessels appear absent distal to pulmonary emboli in the left lung. Today, the spiral (helical) volumetric **computed tomography pulmonary angiogram** (CTPA) (also called a CT pulmonary angiogram) with intravenous contrast has largely replaced pulmonary angiography and is fast becoming the first-line test for diagnosing suspected pulmonary embolism. The CTPA is now a preferred choice of imaging in the diagnosis of a pulmonary embolism, because the only invasive requirement for the scan is an intravenous line.

Ventilation-Perfusion Scan

A **ventilation-perfusion scan** can be used in determining the presence of a pulmonary embolism. The perfusion scan is obtained by injecting small particles of albumin, called *macroaggregates,* tagged with a radioactive material such as iodine-131 or technetium-99m. After injection the radioactive particles are carried in the blood to the right side of the heart, from which they are distributed throughout the lungs by the blood flow in the pulmonary arteries. The radioactive particles that travel through unobstructed arteries become trapped in the pulmonary capillaries because they are 20 to 50 μm in diameter and the diameter of the average pulmonary capillary is approximately 8 to 10 μm.

The lungs are then scanned with a gamma camera that produces a picture of the radioactive distribution throughout the pulmonary circulation. The dark areas show good blood flow, and the white or light areas represent decreased or complete absence of blood flow. The macroaggregates eventually break down, pass through the pulmonary circulation, and are excreted by the liver. The injection of these radioactive particles has no significant effect on the patient's hemodynamics because the patent pulmonary capillaries far outnumber those "embolized" by the radioactive particles. In addition to pulmonary emboli, a perfusion scan defect (white or light areas) may be caused by a lung abscess, lung compression, loss of the pulmonary vascular system (e.g., emphysema), atelectasis, or alveolar **consolidation.**

The perfusion scan is supplemented with a ventilation scan. During the ventilation scan the patient breathes a radioactive gas such as xenon-133 from a closed-circuit spirometer. A gamma camera is used to create a picture of the gas distribution throughout the lungs. A normal ventilation scan shows a uniform distribution of the gas, with the dark areas reflecting the presence of the radioactive gas and therefore good ventilation. White or light areas represent decreased or complete absence of ventilation. See Figure 7-22 for an abnormal perfusion scan and a normal ventilation scan of a patient with a severe pulmonary embolism. An abnormal ventilation scan may also be caused by airway obstruction (e.g., mucous plug or bronchospasm), loss of alveolar elasticity (e.g., emphysema), alveolar consolidation, or pulmonary edema.

This test is slowly being replaced by more sensitive and rapid tests, such as the spiral **computed tomography pulmonary angiogram** (CTPA) scan.

Fluoroscopy

Fluoroscopy is a technique by which x-ray motion pictures of the chest are taken. Fluoroscopy subjects the patient to a larger dose of x-rays than does standard radiography. Therefore, it is used only in selected cases, as in the assessment of abnormal diaphragmatic movement (e.g., unilateral phrenic nerve paralysis) or for localization of lesions to be biopsied during fiber-optic bronchoscopy.

Bronchography

Bronchography entails the instillation of a radiopaque material into the lumen of the tracheobronchial tree. A chest radiograph is then taken, providing a film called a **bronchogram**. The contrast material provides a clear outline of the trachea, carina, right and left main stem bronchi, and segmental bronchi. Bronchography is occasionally used to diagnose bronchogenic carcinoma and determine the presence or extent of bronchiectasis (Figure 7-23). CT of the chest has largely replaced this technique.

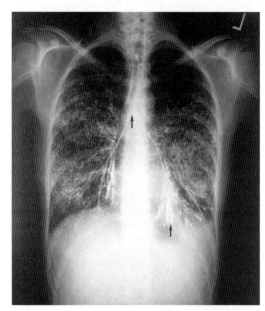

FIGURE 7-23 Bronchogram obtained using contrast medium in a patient with a history of bronchiectasis. Arrows indicate the carina and the dilated and thickened bronchi leading to the posterior basilar segment of the left lower lobe. (From Rau JL Jr, Pearce DJ: *Understanding chest radiographs*, Denver, 1984, Multi-Media Publishing.)

SELF ASSESSMENT QUESTIONS

Answers to questions can be found on Evolve. To access additional student assessment questions visit **http://evolve.elsevier.com/DesJardins/respiratory**.

1. Clinically, the standard radiograph of the chest includes which of the following?
   1. Anteroposterior radiograph
   2. Lateral decubitus radiograph
   3. Lateral radiograph
   4. Posteroanterior radiograph
      a. 1 only
      b. 4 only
      c. 3 and 4 only
      d. 1 and 2 only

2. Compared with the posteroanterior radiograph, the anteroposterior radiograph:
   1. Magnifies the heart
   2. Is usually more distorted
   3. Frequently appears more hazy
   4. Often has extraneous shadows
      a. 2 only
      b. 3 and 4 only
      c. 1, 3, and 4 only
      d. 1, 2, 3, and 4

3. To view the right lung and the heart in the lateral radiograph, the:
   a. Left side of the patient's chest is placed against the cassette
   b. Anterior portion of the patient's chest is placed against the cassette
   c. Right side of the patient's chest is placed against the cassette
   d. Posterior portion of the patient's chest is placed against the cassette

4. A right lateral decubitus radiograph means that the:
   a. Right side of the chest is down
   b. Posterior side of the chest is up
   c. Left side of the chest is down
   d. Anterior side of the chest is up

5. A leftward shift of the mediastinum is commonly seen on the chest radiograph in response to which of the following?
   1. Left upper lobe atelectasis
   2. Right upper lobe gas
   3. Left upper lobe fibrosis
   4. Right upper lobe tumor
      a. 1 and 3 only
      b. 3 and 4 only
      c. 2, 3, and 4 only
      d. 1, 2, 3, and 4

6. The normal exposure of the radiograph is verified by determining whether the spinal processes of the vertebrae are visible to which level?
   a. C-1 to C-3
   b. C-3 to C-5
   c. T-2 to T-4
   d. T-5 to T-6

7. The lung in a radiograph that is described as being "heavily penetrated" is which of the following?
   1. Darker in appearance
   2. More translucent
   3. Whiter in appearance
   4. More opaque in appearance
      a. 3 only
      b. 4 only
      c. 3 and 4 only
      d. 1 and 2 only

8. When the radiograph is taken at full inspiration, the diaphragmatic domes should be at the level of the:
   a. First to fourth ribs posteriorly
   b. Fourth to sixth ribs posteriorly
   c. Sixth to ninth ribs posteriorly
   d. Ninth to eleventh ribs posteriorly

9. Which of the following involves x-ray motion pictures of the chest?
   a. Bronchography
   b. Fluoroscopy
   c. Magnetic resonance imaging
   d. Computed tomography

10. Magnetic resonance imaging is superior to computed tomography scanning for identifying which of the following?
    1. Lesions of the chest
    2. Bone marrow diseases
    3. Congenital heart disorders
    4. Adenopathy
       a. 3 and 4 only
       b. 2 and 3 only
       c. 2, 3, and 4 only
       d. 1, 2, 3, and 4

Other Important Tests and Procedures

Chapter Objectives

After reading this chapter, you will be able to:

- Describe the diagnostic value of the sputum examination.
- Describe the diagnostic tests and procedures presented in this chapter.
- Describe the components of hematology testing.
- Describe the role of platelets.
- Identify the blood chemistry tests commonly monitored in respiratory care.
- Identify the electrolytes commonly monitored in respiratory care.

Key Terms

Acid-Fast Smear and Culture
Alanine Aminotransferase (ALT)
Anergy
Aspartate Aminotransferase (AST)
Basophils
Bilirubin
Blood Chemistry
Blood Urea Nitrogen (BUN)
Bronchoscopy
Bronchoalveolar Lavage
Calcium (Ca^{++})
Chloride (Cl$^-$)
Complete Blood Count (CBC)
Culture and Sensitivity Study
Cytology
Electrolytes
Endobronchial ultrasound (EBUS)
Endoscopic Examinations
Eosinophils
Exudates
Glucose
Gram-Negative Organisms
Gram-Positive Organisms
Gram Staining
Granular Leukocytes
Haemophilus influenzae
Hematocrit (Hct)
Hematology
Hemoglobin (Hb)
Hypochromic Microcytic Anemia
Klebsiella
Lactic Dehydrogenase (LDH)
Legionella pneumophila
Leukocytosis
Lung Biopsy

Lymphocytes
Macrocytic Anemia
Macrophages
Mean Cell Hemoglobin (MCH)
Mean Cell Volume (MCV)
Mean Corpuscular Hemoglobin Concentration (MCHC)
Mediastinoscopy
Monocytes
Mycoplasma pneumoniae
Neutrophils
Nongranular Leukocytes
Normochromic and Normocytic Anemia
Open Lung Biopsy
Platelets
Pleurodesis
Potassium (K$^+$)
Pseudomonas aeruginosa
Red Blood Cell (RBC) Count
Red Blood Cell Indices
Respiratory Syncytial Virus
Serum Creatinine
Serum Glutamic Oxaloacetic Transaminase (SGOT)
Skin Tests
Sodium (Na$^+$)
Sputum Examination
Staphylococcus
Streptococcus
Therapeutic Bronchoscopy
Thoracentesis
Thrombocytopenia
Transbronchial Lung Biopsy
Transudates
Video-Assisted Thoracoscopy Surgery (VATS)
Viral Organisms
White Blood Cell (WBC) Count

Chapter Outline

Sputum Examination
Skin Tests
Endoscopic Examinations
 Bronchoscopy
Thoracentesis
Pleurodesis
Hematology, Blood Chemistry, and Electrolyte Findings
 Hematology
 Blood Chemistry
 Electrolytes
Self-Assessment Questions

As already discussed throughout the first seven chapters of this textbook, the correct assessment associated with patients with pulmonary disease depends on a variety of important diagnostic studies and bedside skills. In addition to the clinical data obtained at the patient bedside (i.e., the patient interview and the physical examinations) and from standard laboratory tests and special procedures (i.e., pulmonary function studies, arterial blood gases, hemodynamic monitoring, and the radiologic examination of the chest), a number of other important tests are often required to diagnose and treat the patient appropriately. Additional important diagnostic studies include the **sputum examination, skin tests, endoscopic examinations, lung biopsy, thoracentesis**, and **hematology, blood chemistry**, and **electrolyte tests**.

Sputum Examination

A sputum sample can be obtained by expectoration, tracheal suction, or **bronchoscopy** (discussed later). In addition to the analysis of the amount, quality, and color of the sputum (previously discussed in Chapter 2), the sputum sample may be examined for (1) culture and sensitivity, (2) Gram stain, (3) acid-fast smear and culture, and (4) cytology.

For a **culture and sensitivity study**, a single sputum sample is collected in a sterile container. This test is performed to diagnose bacterial infection, select an antibiotic, and evaluate the effectiveness of antibiotic therapy. The turnaround time for this test is 48 to 72 hours. **Gram staining** of sputum is performed to classify bacteria into **gram-negative organisms** and **gram-positive organisms**. The results of the Gram stain tests guide therapy until the culture and sensitivity results are obtained. Box 8-1 presents common organisms associated with respiratory disorders. All but the viral organisms can be seen on a Gram stain.

The **acid-fast smear and culture** is performed to determine the presence of acid-fast bacilli (e.g., *Mycobacterium tuberculosis*). A series of three early morning sputum samples is tested. The respiratory therapist should take care in obtaining a clean sample that is not contaminated. **Cytology** examination entails the collection of a single sputum sample in a special container with fixative solution. The sample is evaluated under a microscope for the presence of abnormal cells that may indicate a malignant condition.

The amount, color, and components of the sputum are often important in the assessment and diagnosis of many respiratory disorders, including tuberculosis, pneumonia, cancer of the lungs, and pneumoconiosis. Table 8-1 provides an overview of sputum characteristics that correlate with clinical disease states.

Skin Tests

Skin tests are commonly performed to evaluate allergic reactions or exposure to tuberculous bacilli or fungi. Skin tests entail the intradermal injection of an antigen. A positive test result indicates that the patient has been exposed to the antigen. However, it does not mean that active disease is actually present. A negative test result indicates that the patient has had no exposure to the antigen. A negative test result may also be seen in patients with a depression of cell-mediated immunity (**anergy**), such as that which develops in human immunodeficiency virus (HIV) infections.

Endoscopic Examinations

Bronchoscopy

Bronchoscopy is a well-established diagnostic and therapeutic tool used by a number of medical specialists, including those in intensive care units, special procedure rooms, and outpatient settings. With minimal risk to the patient—and without interrupting the patient's ventilation—the flexible fiberoptic bronchoscope allows direct visualization of the upper airways (nose, oral cavity, and pharynx), larynx, vocal cords, subglottic area, trachea, bronchi, lobar bronchi, and segmental bronchi down to the third or fourth generation. Under fluoroscopic control, more peripheral areas can be examined or treated (Figure 8-1). Bronchoscopy may be diagnostic or therapeutic.

A diagnostic bronchoscopy is usually performed when an infectious disease is suspected and not otherwise diagnosed

---

BOX 8-1 Common Organisms Associated With Respiratory Disorders

Gram-Negative Organisms
Klebsiella
Pseudomonas aeruginosa
Haemophilus influenzae
Legionella pneumophila

Gram-Positive Organisms
Streptococcus (80% of all bacterial pneumonias)
Staphylococcus

Viral Organisms
Mycoplasma pneumoniae
Respiratory syncytial virus

TABLE 8-1 Sputum Correlations

Sputum Characteristics	Correlations
Yellow Sputum	Acute infection
Green Sputum	Associated with old, retained secretions. Green and foul-smelling secretions are frequently found in patients with anaerobic or *Pseudomonas* infection, such as bronchiectasis, cystic fibrosis, and lung abscess
Thick, stringy, and white or mucoid sputum	Bronchial asthma
Brown sputum	Presence of old blood
Red sputum	Fresh blood

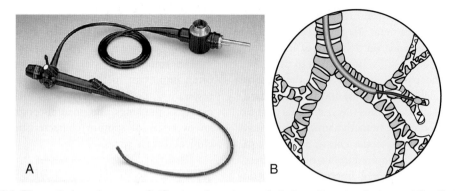

FIGURE 8-1 Fiberoptic bronchoscope. **A,** The transbronchoscopic balloon-tipped catheter and the flexible fiberoptic bronchoscope. Transbronchoscopic tissue biopsies may be obtained with this device. **B,** The catheter is introduced into a small airway and the balloon inflated with 1.5 to 2 mL of air to occlude the airway. Bronchoalveolar lavage is performed by injecting and withdrawing 30-mL aliquots of sterile saline solution, gently aspirating after each instillation. Specimens are sent to the laboratory for analysis. (**A** from Lewis SM, Heitkemper MM, Dirksen SR: *Medical-surgical Nursing: Assessment and Management of Clinical Problems*, ed 6, St Louis, 2004, Mosby. **B** from Meduri GU, Beals DH, Maijub AG, Baselski V: Protected bronchoalveolar lavage. A new bronchoscopic technique to retrieve uncontaminated distal airway secretions, *Am Rev Respir Dis* 143:855, 1991.)

or to obtain a lung biopsy sample when the abnormal lung tissue is located on or near the bronchi. Diagnostic bronchoscopy is indicated for a number of clinical conditions, including further inspection and assessment of (1) abnormal radiographic findings (e.g., question of bronchogenic carcinoma or the extent of a bronchial tumor or mass lesion), (2) persistent atelectasis, (3) excessive bronchial secretions, (4) acute smoke inhalation injuries, (5) intubation damage, (6) bronchiectasis, (7) foreign bodies, (8) hemoptysis, (9) lung abscess, (10) major thoracic trauma, (11) stridor or localized wheezing, and (12) unexplained cough.

A videotape or colored picture of the bronchoscopic procedure may also be obtained to record any abnormalities. When abnormalities are found, additional diagnostic procedures include brushings, biopsies, needle aspirations, and washings. For example, a common diagnostic bronchoscopic technique, termed **bronchoalveolar lavage** (BAL), involves injecting a small amount (30 mL) of sterile saline through the bronchoscope and then withdrawing the fluid for examination of cells. BAL is commonly used to diagnose *Pneumocystis carinii* pneumonia.

Therapeutic bronchoscopy includes (1) suctioning of excessive secretions or mucous plugs, especially when lung atelectasis is present or forming, (2) the removal of foreign bodies or cancer obstructing the airway, (3) selective lavage (with normal saline or mucolytic agents), and (4) management of life-threatening hemoptysis. Although the virtues of therapeutic bronchoscopy are well established, routine respiratory therapy modalities at the patient's bedside (e.g., chest physical therapy, intermittent percussive ventilation, postural drainage, deep breathing and coughing techniques, and positive expiratory pressure therapy) are considered the first line of defense in the treatment of atelectasis from retained secretions. Clinically, therapeutic bronchoscopy is commonly used in the management of bronchiectasis, alveolar proteinosis (with lavage) lung abscess, smoke inhalation and thermal injuries, and lung cancer (see Bronchopulmonary Hygiene Therapy Protocol 9-2, page 123).

Endobronchial Ultrasound

An **endobronchial ultrasound (EBUS)** examination may be performed during a bronchoscopy to help establish the stage of lung cancer and, importantly, establish if—and how—the cancer may have spread. An EBUS can provide an accurate staging of a lung cancer and can help reduce the amount of tissue that needs to be removed during surgery. Traditionally, accurate staging has often required invasive tests such as mediastinoscopy, thoracoscopy, or thoracotomy. An EBUS may provide sufficient information to stage a cancer without these invasive procedures. It can also spare the patient from going through unnecessary surgery when it is determined that the cancer can be better treated in another way, such as chemotherapy or radiation.

During an EBUS procedure, an ultrasound probe is used to send sound waves through the walls of the airways into the surrounding areas, lungs, and mediastinum. When abnormal areas are detected, a small sample of tissue is taken with a small needle guided by the ultrasound (transbronchial needle aspiration). The sample is then sent to a laboratory to determine the presence of cancer or other abnormalities.

There are four primary reasons an EBUS is recommended:
- To detect the presence of tumors or enlarged lymph nodes
- To diagnose tumors within the lung
- To diagnose lymph node abnormalities in the mediastinum or hilum
- To diagnose tumors in the mediastinum

In addition to diagnosing and staging lung cancer, an EBUS examination may also be used to identify infections or help to diagnose other lung conditions such as sarcoidosis.

Mediastinoscopy

Mediastinoscopy is the insertion of a scope through a small incision in the suprasternal notch; the scope is then advanced into the mediastinum. The test is used to inspect and biopsy lymph nodes in the mediastinal area. This procedure is performed to diagnose carcinoma, granulomatous infections, and sarcoidosis. Mediastinoscopy is done in the operating room while the patient is under general anesthesia.

Lung Biopsy

A lung biopsy sample can be obtained by means of a transbronchial needle biopsy or an open-lung biopsy. A **transbronchial lung biopsy** entails passing a forceps or needle through a bronchoscope to obtain a specimen (Figure 8-2). An **open-lung biopsy** involves surgery to remove a sample of lung tissue. An incision is made over the area of the lung from which the tissue sample is to be collected. In some cases, a large incision may be necessary to reach the suspected problem area. After the procedure, a chest tube is inserted for drainage and suction for 7 to 14 days. An **open-lung biopsy** is usually performed when either a bronchoscopic biopsy or a needle biopsy has been unsuccessful or cannot be performed or when a larger piece of tissue is necessary to establish a diagnosis.

An open biopsy requires general anesthesia and is more invasive and thus more likely to cause complications. Overall, the risks include pneumothorax, bleeding, bronchospasm, heart arrhythmias, and infection. A needle lung biopsy is contraindicated in patients with lung bullae, cysts, blood coagulation disorders of any type, severe hypoxia, pulmonary hypertension, or cor pulmonale.

A lung biopsy is usually performed to diagnose abnormalities identified on a chest radiograph or computed tomography (CT) scan that are not readily accessible by other diagnostic procedures, such as bronchoscopy. A lung biopsy is especially useful in investigating peripheral lung abnormalities, such as recurrent infiltrates and pleural or subpleural lesions. Additional conditions under which a lung biopsy may be performed include metastatic cancer to the lung and pneumonia with lung abscess.

The tissues from a lung biopsy are sent to a pathology laboratory for examination of malignant cells. Other samples may be sent to a microbiology laboratory to determine the presence of infection. Lung biopsy results are usually available in 2 to 4 days. In some cases, however, it may take several weeks to confirm (by culture) certain infections, such as tuberculosis.

Video-Assisted Thoracoscopy Surgery

In **video-assisted thoracoscopy surgery (VATS)**, a small incision is made in the chest wall, and a device called a *thoracoscope* is inserted. This device is equipped with a fiberscope that can examine the pleural cavity. The results are displayed on a video monitor (as in bronchoscopy). When pleural lesions are identified, they can be biopsied under video guidance. This procedure is helpful in the diagnosis of tuberculosis, mesothelioma, and metastatic cancer.

Thoracentesis

Thoracentesis (also called *thoracocentesis*) is a procedure in which excess fluid accumulation (pleural effusion) between the chest cavity and lungs (pleural space) is aspirated through a needle inserted through the chest wall (Figure 8-3). A chest radiograph, CT scan, or ultrasound scan may be used to confirm the precise location of the fluid. Once the fluid has been located, thoracentesis may be performed for diagnostic or therapeutic purposes.

Diagnostic thoracentesis may be performed to identify the cause of a pleural effusion. The analysis of the pleural fluid may be useful in the diagnosis and staging of a suspected or known malignancy. A pleural biopsy may also be performed during a thoracentesis to collect a tissue sample from the inner lining of the chest wall. **Therapeutic thoracentesis** may be performed to relieve shortness of breath or pain caused by a large pleural effusion, to remove air trapped between the lung and chest wall, or to administer medication directly into the lung cavity to treat the cause of the fluid accumulation or to treat cancer. The fluid in the lung cavity is classified as either a transudate or an exudate.

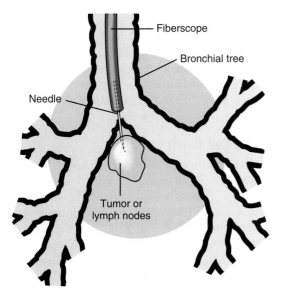

FIGURE 8-2 Transbronchial needle biopsy. The diagram shows a transbronchial biopsy needle penetrating the bronchial wall and entering a mass of subcarinal lymph nodes or tumor. (Redrawn from DuBois RM, Clarke SW: *Fiberoptic bronchoscopy in diagnosis and management*, Orlando, 1987, Grune and Stratton.)

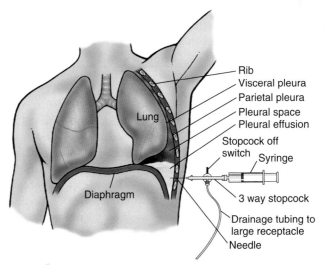

FIGURE 8-3 Thoracentesis. A catheter is positioned in the pleural space to remove accumulated fluid. Pleural fluid is seen as the yellow shadow at the base of the left lung. (From Monahan FD, Neighbors M, Sands JK, Marek JF, Green CJ: *Phipps' medical-surgical nursing health and illness perspectives*, ed 8, St Louis, 2007, Mosby/Elsevier.)

Transudates develop when fluid from the pulmonary capillaries moves into the pleural space. The fluid produced is thin and watery and usually has a low **white blood cell (WBC) count,** a low lactate dehydrogenase (LDH) enzyme level, and a low protein level. The pleural surfaces are not involved in producing the transudate. A transudate may be caused by left ventricular heart failure, cirrhosis, nephrotic syndrome, and peritoneal dialysis.

Exudates may be caused by a variety of conditions, including pulmonary infections (e.g., pneumonia, tuberculosis, and fungal diseases), cancer, chest trauma, pancreatitis, autoimmune disease, or a pulmonary embolism. When an infection is present, the fluid usually has a high WBC count, a high LDH enzyme level, a high protein level, a large amount of cellular debris, and the presence of bacteria or other infectious organisms. When cancer is present, the fluid usually has a high WBC count (often **lymphocytes**), a high LDH enzyme level, and a high protein level. Abnormal cells may also be found. When a pulmonary embolism is present, a large number of red blood cells (RBCs) are usually present and the WBC and protein levels are both low.

The thoracentesis procedure is generally performed while the patient is in an upright position, leaning forward slightly, typically over a bedside table. Using a local anesthetic, the physician inserts a large-bore thoracentesis needle (16 to 19 gauge), or needle-catheter, between the ribs over the fluid accumulation. The needle or catheter is connected to a small tube with a three-way stopcock, which in turn is attached to either a large syringe or a vacuum and collection bottle. Depending on the purpose of the thoracentesis, up to 1500 mL may be withdrawn. Once the fluid has been collected, the needle or catheter is removed and a bandage is placed over the puncture site. The patient is usually instructed to lie on the puncture site side for about an hour to allow the puncture site to seal.

A thoracentesis is usually a safe procedure. However, a chest radiograph is generally obtained shortly after the procedure to ensure that no complications have developed. Complications may include pneumothorax, pulmonary edema (which sometimes occurs when large amounts of fluid are aspirated too rapidly), infection, bleeding, and organ damage.

Pleurodesis

Pleurodesis is performed to prevent the recurrence of a pneumothorax or pleural effusion. Pleurodesis is achieved by injecting any number of agents (called *sclerosing agents* or *sclerosants*) into the pleural space through a chest tube. There is no one sclerosant that is more effective or safer than the others. Common sclerosant chemicals include a slurry of talc, bleomycin, nitrogen mustard, doxycycline, povidone iodine, or quinacrine. The instilled sclerosing agents cause irritation and inflammation (pleuritis) between the parietal and the visceral layers of the pleura. This action causes the pleurae to stick together and thereby prevents subsequent gas or fluid accumulation.

A chemical pleurodesis is considered to be the standard of care for patients with malignant pleural effusions. Because chemical pleurodesis is a painful procedure, the patient is premedicated with a sedative and analgesics. A local anesthetic

may also be instilled into the pleural space or added to the sclerosant. Although complications of pleurodesis are uncommon, risks include the following:
- Infection
- Bleeding
- Acute respiratory distress syndrome
- Collapsed lung (pneumothorax) and respiratory failure

Complications may be specific for each sclerosant.
- Talc and doxycycline can cause fever and pain.
- Quinacrine can cause low blood pressure, fever, and hallucination.
- Bleomycin can cause fever, pain, and nausea.

Pleurodesis may fail because of the following complications:
- Trapped lung, in which the lung is enclosed in scar or tumor tissue
- Formation of isolated pockets (loculation) within the pleural space
- Loss of lung flexibility (elasticity)
- Production of large amounts of pleural fluid
- Extensive spread (metastasis) of pleural cancer
- Improper positioning, blockage, or kinking of the chest tube

Hematology, Blood Chemistry, and Electrolyte Findings

Abnormal hematology, blood chemistry, or electrolyte values assist the respiratory care practitioner and physician in the assessment of cardiopulmonary disorders. Knowledge of these laboratory tests provides a greater understanding of the clinical manifestations of a particular cardiopulmonary disorder.

Hematology

The most frequent laboratory hematology test is the **complete blood count (CBC).** The CBC provides important information about the patient's blood counts, clotting ability, and blood content. The CBC includes the **RBC count, hemoglobin (Hb), hematocrit (Hct),** the total WBC count, and at least an estimate of the platelet count. Various types of anemia (e.g., iron deficiency, pernicious anemia, and sickle cell anemia) are all diagnosed by visual examination of the peripheral blood smear (Table 8-2).

Red Blood Cell Count

The RBCs (erythrocytes) constitute the major portion of the blood cells. The healthy man has about 5 million RBCs in each cubic millimeter (mm^3) of blood. The healthy woman has about 4 million RBCs in each cubic millimeter of blood. Clinically, the total number of RBCs and the RBC indices are useful in assessing the patient's overall oxygen-carrying capacity. The RBC indices are helpful in the identification of specific RBC deficiencies.

White Blood Cell Count

The major functions of the **WBCs** (leukocytes) are to (1) fight against infection, (2) defend the body by phagocytosis against foreign substances, and (3) produce (or at least

TABLE 8-2 Red Blood Cell Indices

Index	Description
Hematocrit (Hct)	The Hct is the volume of red **blood cells (RBCs)** in 100 mL of blood and is expressed as a percentage of the total volume. In the healthy man, the Hct is about 45%; in the healthy woman, the Hct is about 42%. In the healthy newborn, the Hct ranges from 45% to 60%. The Hct is also called the *packed cell volume* (PCV).
Hemoglobin (Hb)	Most of the oxygen that diffuses into the pulmonary capillary blood rapidly moves into the RBCs and chemically attaches to the Hb. Each RBC contains about 280 million Hb molecules. The Hb value is reported in grams per 100 mL of blood (also referred to as grams percent of hemoglobin [g% Hb]). The normal Hb value for men is 14 to 16 g%. The normal Hb value for women is 12 to 15 g%. Hb constitutes about 33% of the RBC weight.
Mean cell volume (MCV)	The MCV is the actual size of the RBCs and is used to classify anemias. It is an index that expresses the volume of a single red cell and is measured in cubic microns. The normal MCV is 87 to 103 μm^3 for both men and women.
Mean corpuscular hemoglobin concentration (MCHC)	The MCHC is a measure of the concentration or proportion of Hb in an average (mean) RBC. The MCHC is derived by dividing the g% Hb by the Hct. For example, if a patient has 15 g% Hb and an Hct of 45%, the MCHC is 33%. The normal MCHC for men and women ranges from 32% to 36%. The MCHC is most useful in assessing the degree of anemia because the two most accurate hematologic measurements (Hb and Hct—not RBC) are used for the test.
Mean cell hemoglobin (MCH)	The MCH is a measure of weight of Hb in a single RBC. This value is derived by dividing the total Hb (g% Hb) by the RBC count. The MCH is useful in diagnosing severely anemic patients but not as good as the MCHC because the RBC is not always accurate. The normal range for the MCH is 27 to 32 pg/RBC.
Types of Anemias Normochromic (normal Hb) and normocytic (normal cell size) anemia	Normochromic anemia is most commonly caused by excessive blood loss. The amount of Hb and the number of RBCs are decreased, but the individual size and content remain normal. Clinically, the laboratory report reveals the following: Hct: below normal Hb: below normal MCV: normal MCHC: normal MCH: normal
Hypochromic (decreased Hb) microcytic (small cell size) anemia	In hypochromic anemia, the size of the RBCs and the Hb content are decreased. This form of anemia is commonly seen in patients with chronic blood loss, iron deficiency, chronic infections, and malignancies. Clinically, the laboratory report reveals the following: Hct: below normal Hb: below normal MCV: below normal MCHC: below normal MCH: below normal
Macrocytic (large cell size) anemia	**Macrocytic anemia** is commonly caused by folic acid and vitamin B_{12} deficiencies. Patients with macrocytic anemia produce fewer RBCs, but the RBCs that are present are larger than normal. Clinically, the laboratory report reveals the following: Hct: below normal Hb: below normal MCV: above normal (because of the larger RBC size) MCHC: above normal (because of the larger RBC size)

TABLE 8-3 Common Causes of White Blood Cell Increase

Cell Type	Causes of Increase
Neutrophil	Bacterial infection, inflammation
Eosinophil	Allergic reaction, parasitic infection
Basophil	Myeloproliferative disorders
Monocyte	Chronic infections, malignancies
Lymphocyte	Viral infections

transport and distribute) antibodies in the immune response. The WBCs are far less numerous than the RBCs, averaging 5000 to 10,000 cells per cubic millimeter of blood. There are two types of WBCs: **granular leukocytes** and **nongranular leukocytes.** Because the general function of the leukocytes is to combat inflammation and infection, the clinical diagnosis of an injury or infection often entails a differential count, which is the determination of the number of each type of cell in 100 WBCs. Box 8-2 shows a normal differential count. Table 8-3 provides an overview of cell types and common causes for their increase (**leukocytosis**).

Granular Leukocytes. The granular leukocytes (also called *granulocytes*) are so classified because of the granules present in their cytoplasm. The granulocytes are further divided into the following three types according to the staining properties of the granules: **neutrophils, eosinophils,** and **basophils.** Because these cells have distinctive multilobar nuclei, they are often referred to as *polymorphonuclear leukocytes.*

Neutrophils. The neutrophils comprise about 60% to 70% of the total number of WBCs. They have granules that are neutral and therefore do not stain with an acid or a basic dye. The neutrophils are the first WBCs to arrive at the site of inflammation, usually appearing within 90 minutes of the injury. They represent the primary defense against bacterial organisms through the process of phagocytosis. The neutrophils are one of several types of cells called *phagocytes* that ingest and destroy bacterial organisms and particulate matter. The neutrophils also release an enzyme called *lysozyme,* which destroys certain bacteria. An increased neutrophil count is associated with (1) bacterial infection, (2) physical and emotional stress, (3) tumors, (4) inflammatory or traumatic disorders, (5) some leukemias, (6) myocardial infarction, and (7) burns.

Early forms of neutrophils are nonsegmented and are called "band" forms. They almost always signify infection if elevated above 10% of the differential. More mature forms of neutrophils have segmented nuclei. They may increase even in the absence of infection (e.g., with stress [exercise] or the use of corticosteroid medication).

Eosinophils. The cytoplasmic granules of the eosinophils stain red with the acid dye eosin. These leukocytes comprise 2% to 4% of the total number of WBCs. Although the precise function of the eosinophils is unknown, they are thought to play a role in the breakdown of protein material. It is known, however, that the eosinophils are activated by allergies (such as an allergic asthmatic episode) and parasitic infections. Eosinophils are thought to detoxify the agents or chemical mediators associated with allergic reactions. An increased eosinophil count may also be associated with lung cancer, chronic skin infections (e.g., psoriasis, scabies), polycythemia, and tumors.

Basophils. The basophils comprise only about 0.5% to 1% of the total white blood count. The granules of the basophils stain blue with a basic dye. The precise function of the basophils is not clearly understood. Increased basophils are primarily associated with certain myeloproliferative disorders. It is thought that the basophils are involved in allergic and stress responses. They are also considered to be phagocytic and to contain heparin, histamines, and serotonin.

Nongranular Leukocytes. There are two groups of nongranular leukocytes, the **monocytes** and **lymphocytes.** The term *mononuclear leukocytes* is also used to describe these cells because they do not contain granules but have spheric nuclei.

Monocytes. The monocytes are the second order of cells to arrive at the inflammation site, usually appearing about 5 hours or more after the injury. After 48 hours, however, the monocytes are usually the predominant cell type in the inflamed area. The monocytes are the largest of the WBCs and comprise about 3% to 8% of the total leukocyte count. The monocytes are short-lived, phagocytic WBCs, with a half-life of about 1 day. They circulate in the bloodstream, from which they move into tissues—at which point they may mature into long-living macrophages (also called *histiocytes*).

Macrophages are large wandering cells that engulf larger and greater quantities of foreign material than the neutrophils. When the foreign material cannot be digested by the macrophages, the macrophages may proliferate to form a capsule that surrounds and encloses the foreign material (e.g., fungal spores). Although the monocytes and macrophages do not respond as quickly to an inflammatory process as the neutrophils, they are considered one of the first lines of inflammatory defense. Therefore, an elevated number of monocytes suggests infection and inflammation. The monocytes play an important role in chronic inflammation and are also involved in the immune response and malignancies.

Lymphocytes. Increased lymphocytes are typically seen in viral infections (e.g., infectious mononucleosis). The lymphocytes are also involved in the production of antibodies, which are special proteins that inactivate antigens. For a better understanding of the importance of the lymphocytes and the clinical significance of their destruction or depletion (e.g., in acquired immunodeficiency syndrome [AIDS]), a brief review of the role and function of the lymphocytes in the immune system is in order.

The lymphocytes can be divided into two categories: B cells and T cells. These cells can be identified with an electron microscope according to certain distinguishing surface marks, called *rosettes:* T cells have a smooth surface; B cells have projections. B cells comprise 10% to 30% of the total lymphocytes; T cells comprise 70% to 90% of the total lymphocytes.

The B cells, which are formed in the bone marrow, further divide into either plasma cells or memory cells. The plasma cells secrete antibodies in response to foreign antigens. The memory cells retain the ability to recognize specific antigens long after the initial exposure and therefore contribute to long-term immunity against future exposures to invading pathogens.

The T cells, which are formed in the thymus, are further divided into four functional categories: (1) cytotoxic T cells (also called *killer lymphocytes* or *natural killer cells*), which attack and kill foreign or infected cells; (2) helper T cells, which recognize foreign antigens and help activate cytotoxic T cells and plasma cells (B cells); (3) inducer T cells, which stimulate the production of the different T-cell subsets; and (4) suppressor T cells, which work to suppress the responses of the other cells and help provide feedback information to the system.

The T cells may also be classified according to their surface antigens (i.e., the T cells may display either T4 antigen or T8 antigen). The T4 surface antigen subset, which comprises 60% to 70% of the circulating T cells, consists mainly of the helper and inducer cells. The T8 surface antigen subset consists mainly of the cytotoxic and suppressor cells.

Sequence of Lymphocyte Responses to Infection. Initially, the macrophages attack and engulf the foreign antigens. This activity in turn stimulates the production of T cells and, ultimately, the antibody-producing B cells (plasma cells). The T4 cells play a pivotal role in the overall modulation of this immune response by (1) secreting a substance called *lymphokine*, which is a potent stimulus to T-cell growth and differentiation; (2) recognizing foreign antigens; (3) causing clonal proliferation of T cells; (4) mediating cytotoxic and suppressor functions; and (5) enabling B cells to secrete specific antibodies.

Because T cells (especially the T4 lymphocytes) have such a central role in this complex immune response, it should not be difficult to imagine the devastating effect that would ultimately follow from the systematic depletion of T lymphocytes. For example, virtually all the infectious complications of AIDS may be explained with reference to the effect that HIV has on the T cells. A decreased number of T cells increases the patient's susceptibility to a wide range of opportunistic infections and neoplasms. In the healthy subject, the T4/T8 ratio is about 2.0. In the patient with HIV/AIDS, the T4/T8 ratio is usually 0.5 or less.

Platelet Count. **Platelets** (also called thrombocytes) are the smallest of the formed elements in the blood. They are round or oval, flattened, and disk-shaped in appearance. Platelets are produced in the bone marrow and possibly in the lungs. Platelet activity is essential for blood clotting. The normal platelet count is 150,000 to 350,000/mm^3.

A deficiency of platelets leads to prolonged bleeding time and impaired clot retention. A low platelet count (**thrombocytopenia**) is associated with (1) massive blood transfusion, (2) pneumonia, (3) cancer chemotherapy, (4) infection, (5) allergic conditions, and (6) toxic effects of certain drugs (e.g., heparin, isoniazid, penicillins, prednisone, streptomycin). A high platelet count (thrombocythemia) is associated with (1) cancer, (2) trauma, (3) asphyxiation, (4) rheumatoid arthritis, (5) iron deficiency, (6) acute infections, (7) heart disease, (8) tuberculosis, and (9) polycythemia vera.

A platelet count of less than 20,000/mm^3 is associated with spontaneous bleeding, prolonged bleeding time, and poor clot retraction. The precise platelet count necessary for hemostasis is not firmly established. Generally, platelet counts greater than 50,000/mm^3 are not associated with spontaneous bleeding. Therefore, various diagnostic or therapeutic procedures, such as bronchoscopy or the insertion of an arterial catheter, are usually safe when the platelet count is greater than 50,000/mm^3.

Blood Chemistry

A basic knowledge of blood chemistry, normal values, and common health problems that alter these values is an important cornerstone of patient assessment. Table 8-4 lists the blood chemistry tests usually monitored in respiratory care.

Electrolytes

For the cells of the body to function properly, a normal concentration of **electrolytes** must be maintained—especially for normal cardiac function. Therefore, the monitoring of electrolytes is extremely important in the patient whose body fluids are being endogenously or exogenously manipulated (e.g., intravenous therapy, renal disease, diarrhea). Table 8-5 lists electrolytes monitored in respiratory care.

TABLE 8-4 Blood Chemistry Tests Commonly Monitored in Respiratory Care

Chemical	Normal Value	Common Abnormal Findings
Glucose	70 to 110 mg/dL	Hyperglycemia (excess glucose level) Diabetes mellitus Acute infection Myocardial infarction Thiazide and loop diuretics Hypoglycemia (low glucose level) Pancreatic tumors or liver disease Pituitary or adrenocortical hyperfunction
Lactic dehydrogenase (LDH)	80 to 120 Wacker units	Increases are associated with the following: Myocardial infarction Chronic hepatitis Pneumonia Pulmonary infarction
Serum glutamic oxaloacetic transaminase (SGOT)	8 to 33 U/mL	Increases are associated with the following: Myocardial infarction Congestive heart failure Pulmonary infarction
Aspartate aminotransferase (AST)	7 to 40 U/L (0.12–0.67 μKat/L)	Increases are associated with the following: Acute aminotransferase hepatitis Liver disease Myocardial infarction Pulmonary infection
Alanine aminotransferase (ALT) (previously called serum glutamic pyruvic transaminase [SGPT])	5 to 36 U/L (0.08–0.6 μKat/L)	Increases are associated with the following: Liver damage Inflammation Shock
Bilirubin	Adult: 0.1 to 1.2 mg/dL Newborn: 1 to 12 mg/dL	Increases are associated with the following; Massive hemolysis Hepatitis
Blood urea nitrogen (BUN)	8 to 18 mg/dL	Increases are associated with acute or chronic renal failure
Serum creatinine	0.6 to 1.2 mg/dL	Increases are associated with renal failure

TABLE 8-5 Electrolytes Commonly Monitored in Respiratory Care

Electrolyte	Normal Value	Common Abnormal Findings	Clinical Manifestations
Sodium (Na$^+$)	136 to 142 mEq/L	Hypernatremia (excess Na$^+$) Dehydration	Desiccated mucous membranes Flushed skin Great thirst Dry tongue

		Hyponatremia (low Na$^+$)
		  Sweating
		  Burns
		  Loss of gastrointestinal secretions
		  Use of some diuretics
		  Excessive water intake
			Abdominal cramps
			Muscle twitching
			Poor perfusion
			Vasomotor collapse
			Confusion
			Seizures

Potassium (K$^+$)	3.8 to 5.0 mEq/L	Hyperkalemia (excess K$^+$)
		  Renal failure
		  Muscle tissue damage
			Irritability
			Nausea
			Diarrhea
			Weakness
			Ventricular fibrillation

TABLE 8-5 Electrolytes Commonly Monitored in Respiratory Care—cont'd

Electrolyte	Normal Value	Common Abnormal Findings	Clinical Manifestations
		Hypokalemia (low K^+) Diuretic therapy Endocrine disorder Diarrhea Reduced intake or loss of K^+ Chronic stress	Metabolic alkalosis Muscular weakness Malaise Cardiac arrhythmias Hypotension
Chloride (Cl⁻)	95 to 103 mEq/L	Hyperchloremia (excess Cl⁻) Renal tubular acidosis Hypochloremia (low Cl⁻) Alkalosis	Deep, rapid breathing Weakness Disorientation Metabolic alkalosis Muscle hypertonicity Tetany Depressed ventilation (respiratory compensation)
Calcium (Ca⁺⁺)	4.5 to 5.4 mEq/L	Hypercalcemia (excess Ca⁺⁺) Malignant tumors Bone fractures Diuretic therapy Excessive use of antacids or milk consumption Vitamin D intoxication Hyperparathyroidism	Lethargy, weakness Hyporeflexia Constipation, anorexia, renal stones Mental deterioration
		Hypocalcemia (low Ca⁺⁺) Respiratory alkalosis Pregnancy Vitamin D deficiency Diuretic therapy Hypoparathyroidism	Paresthesia, cramping of muscles, stridor, convulsions, mental disturbance, Chvostek's sign, Trousseau's sign

SELF-ASSESSMENT QUESTIONS

Answers to questions can be found on Evolve. To access additional student assessment questions visit **http://evolve.elsevier.com/DesJardins/respiratory**.

1. In the healthy woman, what is the hematocrit (Hct)?
   a. 31%
   b. 38%
   c. 42%
   d. 45%

2. Which of the following represent the primary defense against bacterial organisms through phagocytosis?
   a. Eosinophils
   b. Neutrophils
   c. Monocytes
   d. Basophils

3. What is the normal hemoglobin value for men?
   a. 10 to 12 g%
   b. 12 to 14 g%
   c. 14 to 16 g%
   d. 16 to 18 g%

4. What percent of the normal white blood cell count are neutrophils?
   a. 20% to 25%
   b. 40% to 50%
   c. 60% to 70%
   d. 75% to 85%

5. In the healthy man, what is the red blood cell count?
   a. 5,000,000/mm³
   b. 6,000,000/mm³
   c. 7,000,000/mm³
   d. 8,000,000/mm³

6. What is the normal white blood cell count?
   a. 1000 to 5000/mm³
   b. 5000 to 10,000/mm³
   c. 10,000 to 15,000/mm³
   d. 15,000 to 20,000/mm³

7. Which of the following are activated by allergies (such as an allergic asthmatic episode)?
   a. Eosinophils
   b. Neutrophils
   c. Monocytes
   d. Basophils

8. Various clinical procedures such as bronchoscopy or the insertion of an arterial catheter are generally safe when the platelet count is *no lower* than which of the following?
   a. 100,000/mm^3
   b. 75,000/mm^3
   c. 50,000/mm^3
   d. 20,000/mm^3

9. Which of the following are associated with hyperglycemia?
   1. Diabetes mellitus
   2. Myocardial infarction
   3. Thiazide and loop diuretics
   4. Acute infection
      a. 2 and 4 only
      b. 2, 3, and 4 only
      c. 1, 2, and 3 only
      d. 1, 2, 3, and 4

10. Which of the following are clinical manifestations associated with hyponatremia?
    1. Seizures
    2. Confusion
    3. Muscle twitching
    4. Abdominal cramps
       a. 2 and 4 only
       b. 2, 3, and 4 only
       c. 1, 2, and 3 only
       d. 1, 2, 3, and 4

The Therapist-Driven Protocol Program and the Role of the Respiratory Therapist

Chapter Objectives

After reading this chapter, you will be able to:

- Describe the Therapist-Driven Protocol (TDP) program and the role of the respiratory care practitioner.
- Discuss the knowledge base required for a successful TDP program.
- Explain the assessment process skills required for a successful TDP program.
- Describe the essential cornerstone respiratory protocols for a successful TDP program.
- List the common anatomic alterations of the lungs.
- Describe the clinical scenarios—chain of events—activated by the common anatomic alterations of the lungs.
- Identify the most common anatomic alterations associated with the respiratory disorders presented in this textbook.

Key Terms

Aerosolized Medication Therapy Protocol
Anatomic Alterations of the Lung
Atelectasis
Bronchopulmonary Hygiene Therapy Protocol
Bronchospasm
Clinical Practice Guidelines (CPGs)
Clinical Scenarios
Consolidation
Disease-Specific Protocols
Distal Airway and Alveolar Weakening
Excessive Bronchial Secretions
Increased Alveolar-Capillary Membrane Thickness
Lung Expansion Therapy Protocol
Oxygen Therapy Protocol
Pathophysiologic Mechanisms
Patient Protection and Affordable Care Act
Protocol Competency Testing
Therapist-Driven Protocols (TDPs)

Chapter Outline

The "Knowledge Base" Required for a Successful Therapist-Driven Protocol Program
The "Assessment Process Skills" Required for a Successful Therapist-Driven Protocol Program
  Severity Assessment
  The Essential Cornerstones for a Successful Therapist-Driven Protocol Program
Overview Summary of a Good Therapist-Driven Protocol Program
Common Anatomic Alterations of the Lungs
  Clinical Scenarios Activated by Common Anatomic Alterations of the Lungs
Self-Assessment Questions

An emerging consensus voices the concern that the United States health-care system is broken, and new and innovative solutions to the problem must be sought. The **Patient Protection and Affordable Care Act** (PPACA or ACA) came into law in 2010, which proposed to limit payments to hospitals based on quality outcomes, limited hospital readmissions, and established a Center for Medicare and Medicaid innovations within the center for Medicare and Medicaid services. All of this fits nicely into the strategies set in place by "the Therapist-Driven Protocol movement."

Therapist-driven protocols (TDPs) are an integral part of respiratory care health services. According to the American Association for Respiratory Care (AARC), the purposes of respiratory TDPs are to:

- Deliver individualized diagnostic and therapeutic respiratory care to patients
- Assist the physician with evaluating patients' respiratory care needs and optimize the allocation of respiratory care services
- Determine the indications for respiratory therapy and the appropriate modalities for providing high-quality, cost-effective care that improves patient outcomes and decreases length of stay
- Empower respiratory therapists to allocate care using sign-and-symptom based algorithms for respiratory treatment

To further support the AARC's purpose statement on TDPs, the American College of Chest Physicians (ACCP) defines respiratory therapy protocols as follows:

... Patient care plans which are initiated and implemented by credentialed respiratory care workers. These plans are designed and developed with input from physicians, and are approved for use by the medical staff and the governing body of the hospitals in which they are used. They share in common extreme reliance on assessment and evaluation skills. Protocols are by their nature dynamic and flexible, allowing up- or down-regulation of intensity of respiratory services. Protocols allow the respiratory therapist authority to evaluate the patient, initiate care, and to adjust, discontinue, or restart respiratory care procedures on a shift-by-shift or hour-to-hour basis once the protocol is ordered by the physician. They must contain clear strategies for various therapeutic interventions, while avoiding any misconception that they infringe on the practice of medicine.

It must be emphasized that respiratory TDPs provide the respiratory therapist with a wide-ranging flexibility to both assess and treat the patient—but only within preapproved and clearly defined boundaries outlined by the physician, the medical staff, and the hospital. In addition, respiratory TDPs give the therapist specific authority to (1) gather clinical information related to the patient's respiratory status, (2) make an assessment of the clinical data collected, and (3) start, increase, decrease, or discontinue certain respiratory therapies on a moment-to-moment, hour-to-hour, shift-by-shift, or day-to-day basis. The innate beauty of respiratory TDPs is that (1) the physician is always in the "information loop" regarding patient care and (2) therapy can be quickly modified in response to the specific and immediate needs of the patient. Numerous clinical research studies have verified these facts: respiratory TDPs (1) significantly improve respiratory therapy outcomes and (2) appreciably lower therapy costs.

Unfortunately, the implementation of TDPs throughout the United States has been slow. In 2008, the AARC Protocol Implementation Committee conducted a survey to evaluate the barriers to implementation. Over 450 respiratory managers responded to the survey. Despite the overwhelming evidence that protocols clearly improve outcomes and reduce cost, the survey showed that less than 50% of respiratory care was provided by protocols. About 75% of the respondents had at least one protocol in operation. The majority of the hospitals did not have a comprehensive program in place. According to the managers, the medical directors, managers of the department, nurses, and administrators were not perceived as barriers.

The biggest barrier to the implementation of protocols was perceived to be the medical staff. The primary reason for the medical staff's resistance was perceived to be that "staff therapists did not have the skills (e.g., assessment skills) to function under protocols." The AARC Protocol Implementation Committee stated that "[this] perception *must* change...."[1] To address this concern, many respiratory care departments have established mandatory **protocol competency testing** on a periodic basis, to assure that their employees are "TDP safe and ready," up-to-date on *the medical staff*

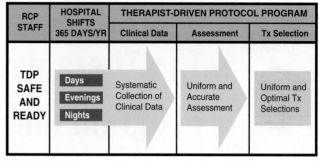

FIGURE 9-1 The promise of a good therapist-driven protocol program.

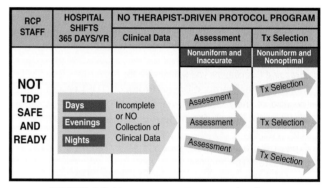

FIGURE 9-2 No assessment program in place.

and specific hospital-approved TDPs used in their place of work. It goes beyond what the respiratory therapy student learns at school, and beyond what is being tested on the National Board for Respiratory Care (NBRC) examinations. It gets right at the issue of *this* therapist's assessment and treatment (i.e., protocol) skills in *this* hospital at *this* point in time.

TDPs must be recognized as different from **Disease-Specific Protocols**, which refer to diagnosis and treatment of individual disease—for example, an "asthma management protocol" such as might be used in an Emergency Department. Respiratory therapists may be asked to be familiar with certain Disease-Specific Protocols, but should be *required* to be competent in the use of *all* the general TDPs (i.e., Oxygen Therapy Protocol, Bronchopulmonary Hygiene Therapy Protocol, Lung Expansion Therapy Protocol, Aerosolized Medication Therapy Protocol, and Mechanical Ventilation Protocol).

The essential components of a good TDP program do not come easy. This is because a strong TDP program promises that the respiratory therapist, who is identified as "TDP safe and ready," be qualified to (1) systematically collect the appropriate clinical data, (2) formulate a uniform and accurate assessment, and (3) select a uniform and optimal treatment within the limits set by the protocol (Figure 9-1). The converse, however, is also true: When the respiratory therapist is *not* "TDP safe and ready," the systematic collection of clinical data is not done at all or is incomplete. As a result, nonuniform or inaccurate assessments are made, resulting in nonuniform or inaccurate treatment selections (Figure 9-2). This inappropriate and ineffective type of respiratory therapy leads to the misallocation of care, the administration of unneeded care, and—most important—the nonprovision of needed patient care. The bottom line is poor-quality patient care and

---

[1]The AARC Protocol Implementation Committee has developed a PowerPoint presentation of the complete survey, which is intended to assist in understanding the barriers and developing successful strategies to implement protocol utilization (www.aarc.org; search for AARC Protocol Implementation Committee).

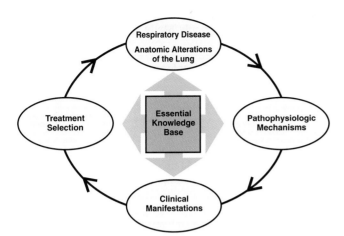

FIGURE 9-3 Foundations for a strong therapist-driven protocol program. Overview of the essential knowledge base for assessment of respiratory disease.

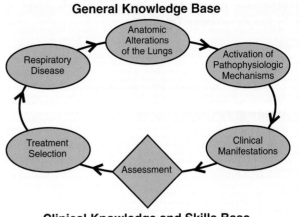

FIGURE 9-4 Overview of TDP program: The way knowledge, assessment, and a therapist-driven protocol program interface between each other.

unnecessary costs. To be sure, the development and implementation of a strong TDP program require a good deal of fundamental knowledge, training, and practice, but the benefits are worth the price. The essential components of a good TDP program are discussed in the following paragraphs.

The "Knowledge Base" Required for a Successful Therapist-Driven Protocol Program

As shown in Figure 9-3, the essential knowledge base for a successful TDP program includes (1) the anatomic alterations of the lungs caused by common respiratory disorders, (2) the major pathophysiologic mechanisms activated throughout the respiratory and cardiac systems as a result of the anatomic alterations, (3) the common clinical manifestations that develop as a result of the activated pathophysiologic mechanisms, and (4) the treatment modalities used to correct them. *In other words, the clinical manifestations demonstrated by the patient do not arbitrarily appear but are the result of anatomic lung alterations and pathophysiologic events.*

Hence, it is essential that the respiratory therapist knows and understands that certain anatomic alterations of the lung will lead to specific—and often predictable—clinical manifestations. Each respiratory disease presented in this textbook describes these four essential knowledge components necessary for TDPs to work. In the clinical setting, this knowledge base enhances the assessment process essential to a good TDP program.

The "Assessment Process Skills" Required for a Successful Therapist-Driven Protocol Program

Using the knowledge base described above, the respiratory therapist must also be competent in performing the actual assessment process. This means that the practitioner can (1) quickly and systematically gather the clinical information demonstrated by the patient, (2) formulate an accurate assessment of the clinical data (i.e., identify the cause and severity of the problem), (3) select an optimal treatment modality, and

(4) document this process quickly, clearly, and precisely. In the clinical setting, the practice—and mastery—of the assessment process is absolutely central and essential to the success of a good TDP program (Figure 9-4). In other words, immediately after the respiratory therapist identifies the appropriate clinical manifestations (clinical indicators), an assessment of the data must be performed, and a treatment plan must be formulated. For the most part, the assessment is primarily directed at the anatomic alterations of the lungs that are causing the clinical indicators (e.g., **bronchospasm**) and the severity of the clinical indicators.

For example, an appropriate assessment for the clinical cause and indicator of wheezing might be bronchospasm—the anatomic alteration of the lungs. If the therapist assesses the cause of the wheezing correctly as bronchospasm, then the correct treatment selection would be a bronchodilator treatment from the **Aerosolized Medication Therapy Protocol**, Protocol 9-4. If, however, the cause of the wheezing is correctly assessed to be excessive airway secretions, then the appropriate treatment plan would entail a specific treatment modality found in the **Bronchopulmonary Hygiene Therapy Protocol**, such as deep breathing and coughing or chest physical therapy, Protocol 9-2.

Table 9-1 illustrates common clinical manifestations (i.e., clinical indicators), assessments, and treatment selections routinely made by the respiratory therapist.

Severity Assessment

The frequency at which a respiratory therapy modality is to be administered is just as important to quality cost-efficient care as the correct selection of a respiratory therapy treatment. Often the frequency of treatment must be up-regulated or down-regulated on a shift-by-shift, hour-to-hour, minute-to-minute, or even (in life-threatening situations) second-to-second basis. Such frequency changes must be made in response to a severity assessment. In a good TDP program, the well-seasoned respiratory therapist routinely and systematically documents many severity assessments throughout each working day. For the new practitioner, however, a

TABLE 9-1 Clinical Manifestations, Assessments, and Treatment Selections Commonly Made by the Respiratory Therapist

Clinical Data (indicators)	Assessments	Treatment Selections
Vital Signs		
↑ Breathing rate, blood pressure, pulse	Respiratory distress	Treat underlying cause
Abnormal Airway Indicators		
Wheezing	Bronchospasm	Bronchodilator treatment
Inspiratory stridor	Laryngeal edema	Racemic epinephrine
Coarse crackles	Secretions in large airways	Bronchial hygiene treatment
Fine and medium crackles	Secretions in distal airways	Treat underlying cause—e.g., congestive heart failure
		Hyperinflation treatment
Cough Effectiveness Indicators		
Strong cough	Good ability to mobilize secretions	None
Weak cough	Poor ability to mobilize secretions	Bronchial hygiene treatment
Abnormal Secretion Indicators		
Amount: >25 mL/24 h	Excessive bronchial secretions	Bronchial hygiene treatment
White and translucent sputum	Normal sputum	None
Yellow or opaque sputum	Acute airway infection	Treat underlying cause
Green sputum	Old, retained secretions and infections	Bronchial hygiene treatment
Brown sputum	Old blood	Bronchial hygiene treatment
Red sputum	Fresh blood	Notify physician
Frothy secretions	Pulmonary edema	Treat underlying cause—e.g., congestive heart failure
		Hyperinflation treatment
Abnormal Lung Parenchyma Indicators		
Bronchial breath sounds	Atelectasis	Hyperinflation treatment, oxygen treatment
Dull percussion note	Infiltrates or effusion	Treat underlying cause
Opacity on chest radiograph	Fibrosis	No specific treatment
Restrictive pulmonary function test values	Consolidation	No specific, effective respiratory care treatment
Depressed diaphragm on x-ray	Air trapping and hyperinflation	Treat underlying cause
Abnormal Pleural Space Indicators		
Hyperresonant percussion note	Pneumothorax	Evacuate air[†] and hyperinflation treatment
Dull percussion note	Pleural effusion	Evacuate fluid[†] and hyperinflation treatment
Abnormalities of Chest Shape and Motion		
Paradoxical movement of the chest wall	Flail chest	Mechanical ventilation[†]
Barrel chest	Air trapping (hyperinflation)	Treat underlying cause—e.g., asthma
Posterior and lateral curvature of spine	Kyphoscoliosis	Bronchial hygiene treatment
Arterial Blood Gases—Ventilatory		
pH ↑, $PaCO_2$ ↓, HCO_3^- ↓	Acute alveolar hyperventilation	Treat underlying cause
pH N, $PaCO_2$ ↓, HCO_3^- ↓↓*	Chronic alveolar hyperventilation	Generally none
pH ↓, $PaCO_2$ ↑, HCO_3^- ↑	Acute ventilatory failure	Mechanical ventilation[†]
pH N, $PaCO_2$ ↑, HCO_3^- ↑↑	Chronic ventilatory failure	Low-flow oxygen, bronchial hygiene
Sudden Ventilatory Changes on Chronic Ventilatory Failure (CVF)		
pH ↑, $PaCO_2$ ↑, HCO_3^- ↑↑, PaO_2 ↓	Acute alveolar hyperventilation on CVF	Treat underlying cause
pH ↓, $PaCO_2$ ↑↑, HCO_3^- ↑ PaO_2 ↓	Acute ventilatory failure on CVF	Mechanical ventilation[†]

TABLE 9-1 Clinical Manifestations, Assessments, and Treatment Selections Commonly Made by the Respiratory Therapist—cont'd

Clinical Data (indicators)	Assessments	Treatment Selections
Metabolic		
pH ↑, PaCO$_2$ N or ↑, HCO$_3^-$ ↑, PaO$_2$ N	Metabolic alkalosis	Give potassium[†]—Hypokalemia
		Give chloride[†]—Hypochloremia
pH ↓, PaCO$_2$ N or ↓, HCO$_3^-$ ↓, PaO$_2$ ↓	Metabolic acidosis	Give oxygen—Lactic acidosis
pH ↓, PaCO$_2$ N or ↓, HCO$_3^-$ ↓, PaO$_2$ N	Metabolic acidosis	Give insulin[†]—Ketoacidosis
pH ↓, PaCO$_2$ N or ↓, HCO$_3^-$ ↓, PaO$_2$ N	Metabolic acidosis	Renal therapy[†]
Indication for Mechanical Ventilation		
pH ↑, PaCO$_2$ ↓, HCO$_3^-$ ↓, PaO$_2$ ↓	Impending ventilatory failure	Mechanical ventilation
pH ↓, PaCO$_2$ ↑, HCO$_3^-$ ↑, PaO$_2$ ↓	Ventilatory failure	Mechanical ventilation
pH ↓, PaCO$_2$ ↑, HCO$_3^-$ ↑, PaO$_2$ ↓	Apnea	Mechanical ventilation
Oxygenation Status		
PaO$_2$ < 80 mm Hg	Mild hypoxemia	Oxygen therapy and treat underlying cause
PaO$_2$ < 60 mm Hg	Moderate hypoxemia	
PaO$_2$ < 40 mm Hg	Severe hypoxemia	
Oxygen Transport Status		
↓ PaO$_2$, anemia, ↓ cardiac output	Inadequate oxygen transport	Oxygen therapy and treat underlying cause

*Significant.
[†]These procedures should be performed only as ordered by the physician. It should be noted that some of the treatment options are not included in respiratory protocols and may not necessarily be administered by respiratory therapists.

predesigned *Severity Assessment Rating Form* may be used to enhance this important part of the assessment process. One excellent, semiquantitative method of accomplishing this is illustrated in Table 9-2. The clinical application of this severity assessment is provided in the following case example:

Severity Assessment Case Example

A 67-year-old man arrived in the emergency room in respiratory distress. The patient was well known to the therapist-driven protocol (TDP) team; he had been diagnosed with chronic bronchitis several years before this admission (3 points). The patient had no recent surgery history, and he was ambulatory, alert, and cooperative (0 points). He complained of dyspnea and was using his accessory muscles of inspiration (3 points). Auscultation revealed bilateral coarse crackles over both lung fields (3 points). His cough was weak and productive of thick gray secretions (3 points). A chest x-ray revealed pneumonia (**consolidation**) in the left lower lung lobe (3 points). On room air his arterial blood gas values were pH 7.52, PaCO$_2$ 54, HCO$_3^-$ 41, and PaO$_2$ 52, suggesting a diagnosis of acute alveolar hyperventilation superimposed on chronic ventilatory failure (3 points).

Using the Severity Assessment Form shown in Table 9-2, the following treatment selection and administration frequency would be appropriate:

Total score: 17
Treatment selection: Chest physical therapy
Frequency of administration: Four times a day; and as needed

The Essential Cornerstones for a Successful Therapist-Driven Protocol Program

Although there are many "assess and treat" respiratory care protocols (now more appropriately called "Assess, Treat, and Teach" protocols) used throughout the health-care industry today, the following respiratory protocols provide the "essential foundation" of a successful TDP program:

- **Oxygen Therapy Protocol (Protocol 9-1)**
- **Bronchopulmonary Hygiene Therapy Protocol (Protocol 9-2)**
- **Lung Expansion Therapy Protocol (Protocol 9-3)**
- **Aerosolized Medication Therapy Protocol (Protocol 9-4)**

Protocols for Mechanical Ventilation and Mechanical Ventilation Weaning are found in Chapter 10, pages 150 to 159. A discussion of the content required for a pulmonary rehabilitation protocol can be found in Chapter 12, pages 187 and 188. The vast majority of the daily work performed by the respiratory therapist involves assessments and treatments associated with these protocols. These respiratory protocols are the essential cornerstones of a good TDP program. For example, a patient experiencing a severe asthmatic episode would probably demonstrate a variety of objective clinical indicators to justify the assessments that call for the administration of oxygen therapy (e.g., to treat hypoxemia), an aerosolized bronchodilator (e.g., to treat bronchospasm), bronchial hygiene therapy (e.g., to mobilize the thick white secretions associated with asthma), and mechanical ventilation (e.g., to treat acute ventilatory failure).

TABLE 9-2 Respiratory Care Protocol Severity Assessment

Item	0 Points	1 Point	2 Points	3 Points	4 Points
Respiratory history	Negative for smoking or history not available	Smoking history <1 pack a day	Smoking history >1 pack a day	Pulmonary disease	Severe or exacerbation
Surgery history	No surgery	General surgery	Lower abdominal	Thoracic or upper abdominal	Thoracic with lung disease
Level of consciousness	Alert, oriented, cooperative	Disoriented, follows commands	Obtunded, uncooperative	Obtunded	Comatose
Level of activity	Ambulatory	Ambulatory with assistance	Nonambulatory	Paraplegic	Quadriplegic
Respiratory pattern	Normal rate 8–20/min	Respiratory rate 20–25/min	Patient complains of dyspnea	Dyspnea, use of accessory muscles, prolonged expiration	Severe dyspnea, use of accessory muscles, respiratory rate > 25, and/or swallow
Breath sounds	Clear	Bilateral crackles	Bilateral fine, medium, or coarse crackles	Bilateral wheezing; fine, medium, or coarse crackles	Absent and/or diminished bilaterally and/or severe wheezing; fine, medium, or coarse crackles
Cough	Strong, spontaneous, nonproductive	Excessive bronchial secretions and strong cough	Excessive bronchial secretions but weak cough	Thick bronchial secretions and weak cough	Thick bronchial secretions but no cough
Chest radiograph	Clear	One lobe: infiltrates, atelectasis, consolidation, or pleural effusion	Same lung, two lobes: infiltrates, atelectasis, consolidation, or pleural effusion	One lobe in both lungs: infiltrates, atelectasis, consolidation, or pleural effusion	Both lungs, more than one lobe: infiltrates, atelectasis, consolidation, or pleural effusion
Arterial blood gases and/or oxygen saturation measured by pulse oximeter (SpO_2)	Normal	Normal pH and $PaCO_2$ but PaO_2 60–80 and/or SpO_2 91% to 96%	Normal pH and $PaCO_2$ but PaO_2 40–60 and/or SpO_2 85% to 90%	Acute respiratory alkalosis, PaO_2 < 40 and/or SpO_2 80% to 84%	Acute respiratory failure, PaO_2 < 80 and/or SpO_2 < 80%

Severity Index

Total Score	Severity Assessment	Treatment Frequency
1–5	Unremarkable	As needed
6–15	Mild	Two or three times a day
16–25	Moderate	Four times a day or as needed
Greater than 26	Severe	Two to four times a day and as needed; alert attending physician

As shown in the algorithms in Protocols 9-1 through 9-4,[2] a step-by-step, branching logic process directs the practitioner to (1) gather clinical data (clinical indicators), (2) make assessment decisions based on the clinical data, and (3) either start, up-regulate, down-regulate, or discontinue treatment modality. In fact, the primary reason a good TDP program works is because a specific treatment modality cannot be started, stopped, or modified unless there are specific—and measurable—clinical indicators identified to justify the assessment and treatment decision.[3]

The treatment selections outlined in each of the above protocols are based on current **American Association for Respiratory Care's (AARC) Clinical Practice Guidelines (CPGs)**, which provide the most recent scientific evidence

[2]Protocols for mechanical ventilation are provided in Chapter 10.

[3]The authors would like to thank the Respiratory Care Department at the Kettering Health Network, in Dayton, Ohio, for providing their Oxygen Therapy Protocol, Bronchopulmonary Hygiene Therapy Protocol, Lung Expansion Protocol, and Aerosolized Medication Therapy Protocol.

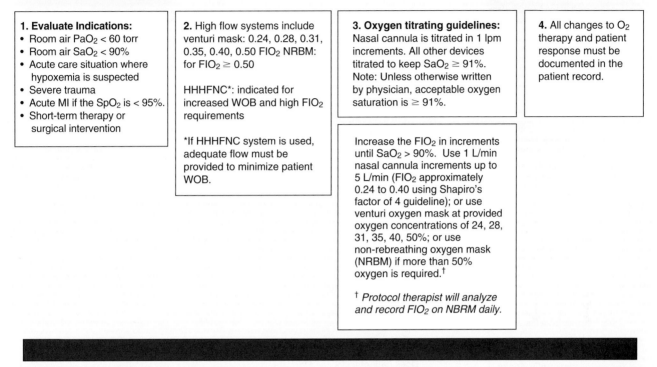

OXYGEN THERAPY PROTOCOL

1. Evaluate Indications:
- Room air PaO_2 < 60 torr
- Room air SaO_2 < 90%
- Acute care situation where hypoxemia is suspected
- Severe trauma
- Acute MI if the SpO_2 is < 95%.
- Short-term therapy or surgical intervention

2. High flow systems include venturi mask: 0.24, 0.28, 0.31, 0.35, 0.40, 0.50 FIO_2 NRBM: for $FIO_2 \geq 0.50$

HHHFNC*: indicated for increased WOB and high FIO_2 requirements

*If HHHFNC system is used, adequate flow must be provided to minimize patient WOB.

3. Oxygen titrating guidelines:
Nasal cannula is titrated in 1 lpm increments. All other devices titrated to keep $SaO_2 \geq 91\%$. Note: Unless otherwise written by physician, acceptable oxygen saturation is $\geq 91\%$.

4. All changes to O_2 therapy and patient response must be documented in the patient record.

Increase the FIO_2 in increments until SaO_2 > 90%. Use 1 L/min nasal cannula increments up to 5 L/min (FIO_2 approximately 0.24 to 0.40 using Shapiro's factor of 4 guideline); or use venturi oxygen mask at provided oxygen concentrations of 24, 28, 31, 35, 40, 50%; or use non-rebreathing oxygen mask (NRBM) if more than 50% oxygen is required.[†]

[†] Protocol therapist will analyze and record FIO_2 on NBRM daily.

Modified from the Respiratory Care Department at the Kettering Health Network, in Dayton, Ohio
* Heated and Humidified High Flow Nasal Cannula

PROTOCOL 9-1

that justifies the administration of a specific treatment modality. Using the evidence-based methods mandated by the scientific community, CPGs provide the indications, contraindications, hazards and complications, assessment of need, assessment of outcome, and appropriate monitoring techniques used for specific therapy modalities. In other words, the CPGs are the gold standards used by the respiratory therapist to start, adjust, or discontinue a specific treatment modality. In Box 9-1 (see page 129), excerpts from the AARC's CPG on oxygen therapy for adults in the acute care facility provide a representative example of a CPG—and, more important, the scientific basis for the Oxygen Therapy Protocol, Protocol 9-1.

Several different treatment selections are listed under each of the protocols. In essence, the various treatment selections serve as a "therapy selection menu." When the patient demonstrates the clinical indicators associated with any of these protocols, the respiratory therapist is expected to select and administer the most efficient and most cost-effective treatment to the patient. As already discussed, the treatment selection decision and the frequency with which the therapy is to be administered are based on (1) the identification of the appropriate clinical indicators, (2) the severity suggested by the clinical information, (3) the patient's ability to perform or tolerate the therapy, and (4) the patient's response to the therapy.

In another example, the implementation of the **Lung Expansion Therapy Protocol**, Protocol 9-3 (see pages 125–126), would probably be indicated after thoracic surgery to prevent, or correct, **atelectasis**. If the patient were unconscious or unable to follow directions, a continuous positive airway pressure (CPAP) mask would be a more appropriate treatment selection (under the Lung Expansion Therapy Protocol) than, say, incentive spirometry—even though both are designed to treat or prevent atelectasis. In this example, the CPAP mask therapy would be more expensive but more appropriate than the less expensive incentive spirometry.

Remember, the treatment portion of a protocol is based on the therapy that will *best* work to correct or offset the anatomic alterations and pathophysiologic mechanisms caused by the respiratory disorder in a timely and cost-efficient manner. Finally, even when the patient is transferred to the intensive care unit, intubated, and placed on a mechanical ventilator, the respiratory therapist must usually still administer one or more of the first four respiratory therapy treatment protocols listed in this section. For example, the patient would probably need CPAP or positive end-expiratory pressure (PEEP) to offset any alveolar atelectasis caused by airway mucous plugs via the Lung Expansion Therapy Protocol. Or, the patient would probably require a bronchodilator agent to offset bronchospasm via the Aerosolized Medication Therapy Protocol.

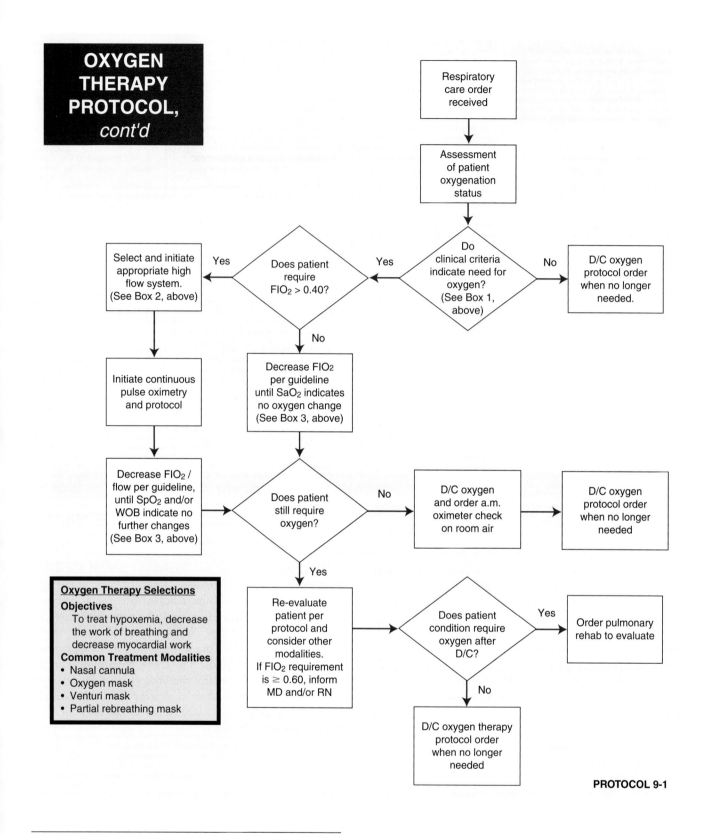

OXYGEN THERAPY PROTOCOL, *cont'd*

Respiratory care order received

↓

Assessment of patient oxygenation status

↓

Do clinical criteria indicate need for oxygen? (See Box 1, above) — No → D/C oxygen protocol order when no longer needed.

Yes ↓

Does patient require FIO₂ > 0.40? — Yes → Select and initiate appropriate high flow system. (See Box 2, above)

No ↓

Decrease FIO₂ per guideline until SaO₂ indicates no oxygen change (See Box 3, above)

Select and initiate appropriate high flow system. (See Box 2, above) ↓

Initiate continuous pulse oximetry and protocol ↓

Decrease FIO₂ / flow per guideline, until SpO₂ and/or WOB indicate no further changes (See Box 3, above) →

Does patient still require oxygen? — No → D/C oxygen and order a.m. oximeter check on room air → D/C oxygen protocol order when no longer needed

Yes ↓

Re-evaluate patient per protocol and consider other modalities. If FIO₂ requirement is ≥ 0.60, inform MD and/or RN →

Does patient condition require oxygen after D/C? — Yes → Order pulmonary rehab to evaluate

No ↓

D/C oxygen therapy protocol order when no longer needed

Oxygen Therapy Selections
Objectives
To treat hypoxemia, decrease the work of breathing and decrease myocardial work
Common Treatment Modalities
• Nasal cannula
• Oxygen mask
• Venturi mask
• Partial rebreathing mask

PROTOCOL 9-1

Overview Summary of a Good Therapist-Driven Protocol Program

Figure 9-5 provides an overview of the essential components of a good TDP program. As illustrated, the implementation of every respiratory care plan must be directly linked to (1) a physician's order, (2) the identification and documentation of specific clinical indicators (obtained from both the patient's chart and physical examination), (3) a bedside respiratory assessment and severity assessment, (4) a treatment selection that is both therapeutic and cost-efficient, and (5) the evaluation of the patient's response to the treatment.

This step-by-step process mandates that the respiratory therapist (1) has a strong knowledge base of the major respiratory disorders, and (2) be competent in the actual assessment process (Figure 9-4). Figure 9-6 provides an assessment form with common examples for each category (i.e., clinical indicators, respiratory assessments, and

BRONCHOPULMONARY HYGIENE THERAPY PROTOCOL

Evaluate indications: (1)
- Difficulty with secretion clearance with sputum production > 25 mL/day
- Evidence of retained secretions
- Mucous plug-induced atelectasis
- Foreign body in airway
- Diagnosis of cystic fibrosis, bronchiectasis, or cavitating lung disease

Assess Outcomes — Goals Achieved? (3)
- Optimal hydration with sputum production > 25 mL/day
- Breath sounds from diminished to adventitious with crackles cleared by cough
- Patient subjective impression of less retention and improved clearance
- Resolution/improvement in chest radiograph
- Improvement in vital signs and measures of gas exchange
- If on ventilator, reduced airway resistance and improved compliance

Care Plan Considerations:
- Discontinue therapy if improvement is observed and sustained over a 24-hour period.
- Patients with chronic pulmonary disease who maintain secretion clearance in their home environment should remain on treatment no less than their home frequency.
- Lung Expansion Therapy Protocol (9-3) should be considered for patients who are at high risk for pulmonary complications as listed in the indications for Lung Expansion Therapy Protocol.

Bronchopulmonary Hygiene Therapy Selections

Objective (2)
To enhance mobilization of bronchial secretions

Common Treatment Modalities
- Increased broncial hydration
  Increased fluid intake
    (6-10 glasses of water a day)
  Bland aerosol therapy
  Ultrasonic nebulization (USN)
- Cough and deep breathing (C & DB)
  Techniques used the enhance C & DB
    Incentive spirometry (IS)
    Intermittent positive-pressure breathing (IPPB)
    Intermittent percussion ventilation (IPV)
    Positive expiratory pressure (PEP) therapy
    Flutter valve
- Chest physical therapy (CPT)
- Postural drainage (PD)
- Percussion and vibration with postural drainage
- Suctioning (Note: in some hospitals suctioning cannot be performed without TPDs or direct physician order)
- Mucolytic therapy (see Protocol 9-4)
  Acetylcysteine—often in combination with a bronchodilator
  Recombinant human deoxyribonuclease (DNase, Pulmozyme)
  Sodium bicarbonate (2% solution)
- Assist physician in bronchoscopy

Modified from the Respiratory Care Department at the Kettering Health Network, in Dayton, Ohio

PROTOCOL 9-2 *cont'd on page 124*

treatment plans). The examples shown in Figure 9-5 can easily be transferred to the subjective-objective evaluation and treatment (SOAP) format. The SOAP format used in the assessment of respiratory diseases is discussed in more detail in Chapter 11.

Common Anatomic Alterations of the Lungs

Although the respiratory therapist may at some time treat one or two cases of every respiratory disorder presented in this textbook, most of the therapist's professional career will be spent caring for patients with only a few of them. For example, the *diagnosis-related group* (DRG) and the most current edition of the *International Statistical Classification of Diseases and Related Health Problems* (ICD-9) identification systems show that more than 80% of the respiratory therapist's work is concerned with intelligent assessment and treatment selection for a relatively short list of respiratory illnesses. This short list of respiratory disorders includes *chronic bronchitis, emphysema, asthma, pneumonia, atelectasis,*

adult respiratory distress syndrome (ARDS), interstitial fibrosis, pulmonary edema/congestive heart failure, and acute and chronic respiratory failure with and without ventilatory support.

From this relatively short list of respiratory disorders identified through the DRG system, the most common anatomic alterations of the lungs treated by the respiratory therapist can be derived—which includes (1) **atelectasis** (e.g., which can occur from mucous plugging, upper abdominal surgery, or pneumothorax), (2) **alveolar consolidation** (e.g., pneumonia), (3) **increased alveolar-capillary membrane thickness** (e.g., ARDS, pneumoconiosis, or pulmonary edema), (4) **bronchospasm** (e.g., asthma), (5) **excessive bronchial secretions** (e.g., chronic bronchitis, asthma, pulmonary edema), and (6) **distal airway and alveolar weakening** (e.g., emphysema). Each of these anatomic alterations of the lung in turn leads to a chain of events that can be summarized in the following clinical scenarios.

Clinical Scenarios Activated by Common Anatomic Alterations of the Lungs

For the purposes of this text, we have chosen to refer to the interrelationship among the major **anatomic alterations of**

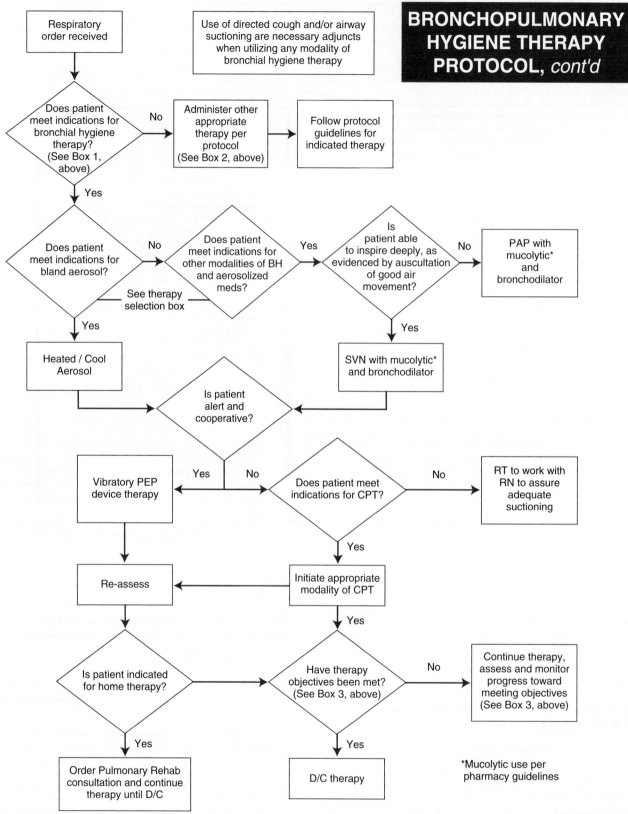

Respiratory order received

Use of directed cough and/or airway suctioning are necessary adjuncts when utilizing any modality of bronchial hygiene therapy

BRONCHOPULMONARY HYGIENE THERAPY PROTOCOL, cont'd

Does patient meet indications for bronchial hygiene therapy? (See Box 1, above) — No → Administer other appropriate therapy per protocol (See Box 2, above) → Follow protocol guidelines for indicated therapy

Yes

Does patient meet indications for bland aerosol? — No → Does patient meet indications for other modalities of BH and aerosolized meds? — Yes → Is patient able to inspire deeply, as evidenced by auscultation of good air movement? — No → PAP with mucolytic* and bronchodilator

See therapy selection box

Yes

Heated / Cool Aerosol

Yes

SVN with mucolytic* and bronchodilator

Is patient alert and cooperative?

Yes / No

Vibratory PEP device therapy

Does patient meet indications for CPT? — No → RT to work with RN to assure adequate suctioning

Yes

Re-assess

Initiate appropriate modality of CPT

Yes

Is patient indicated for home therapy?

Have therapy objectives been met? (See Box 3, above) — No → Continue therapy, assess and monitor progress toward meeting objectives (See Box 3, above)

Yes

Order Pulmonary Rehab consultation and continue therapy until D/C

Yes

D/C therapy

*Mucolytic use per pharmacy guidelines

PROTOCOL 9-2

LUNG EXPANSION PROTOCOL
(Hyperinflation Therapy)

Evaluate Indications: (1)

- Predisposing conditions for pulmonary atelectasis
  - Upper abdominal surgery
  - Thoracic surgery
  - Surgery in patients with COPD
- Pulmonary atelectasis
- Restrictive lung defect
- Neuromuscular conditions

Hyperinflation Therapy Selections (2)

Objective

To prevent or treat alveolar consolidation and atelectasis

Common Treatment Modalities

- Cough and deep breathing (C & DB)
- Incentive spirometry (IS)
- Intermittent positive-pressure breathing (IPPB)
- Continuous positive airway pressure (CPAP)
- Positive end pressure (PEP) and positive end-expiratory pressure (PEEP)

Assess outcomes — Goals achieved? (3)

Absence of or improvement in signs of atelectasis:
- Decreased respiratory rate
- Resolution of fever
- Normal pulse rate
- Absent crackles
- Improvement in previously absent or diminished breath sounds
- Improved chest radiograph
- Improved arterial oxygen tension (PaO_2) and decreased alveolar-arterial oxygen tension gradient, $[P(A–a)O_2]$
- Increased VC and peak expiratory flows
- Return of functional residual capacity (FRC) or VC to preoperative values in absence of lung resection

Improved inspiratory muscle function:
- Attainment of preoperative flow and volume levels
- Increased forced vital capacity (FVC)

Modified from the Respiratory Care Department at the Kettering Health Network, in Dayton, Ohio

PROTOCOL 9-3 *cont'd on page 126*

the lung, the **pathophysiologic mechanisms**, and the clinical manifestations that result as "**clinical scenarios**." Specific anatomic alterations of the lung (such as the ones listed previously) lead to the activation of specific and predictable pathophysiologic mechanisms and to their effects. The more common pathophysiologic mechanisms are listed in Box 9-2. The pathophysiologic mechanisms in turn activate specific and predictable clinical manifestations (Figure 9-3). To enhance the reader's knowledge and understanding of commonly encountered respiratory disorders, clinical scenarios for the anatomic alterations presented in the following paragraphs are provided.[4]

Atelectasis

Figure 9-7 (see page 131) shows the pathophysiologic mechanisms caused by atelectasis (e.g., from a pneumothorax), the clinical manifestations that result, and the treatment protocols used to offset them. The hypoxemia that results from atelectasis is caused by capillary shunting. This type of hypoxemia is often refractory to oxygen therapy. Therefore, the implementation of the *Lung Expansion Therapy Protocol*

may be more beneficial in the treatment of hypoxemia than the *Oxygen Therapy Protocol* in such a patient.

Alveolar Consolidation

Figure 9-8 (see page 132) shows the pathophysiologic mechanisms caused by alveolar consolidation (e.g., pneumonia), the clinical manifestations that result, and the treatment protocols used to offset them. The hypoxemia that develops as a result of consolidation is caused by capillary shunting. This type of hypoxemia is often refractory to oxygen therapy.

Depending on the severity of the alveolar consolidation, the *Lung Expansion Therapy Protocol* or the *Oxygen Therapy Protocol* may be beneficial. In general, however, there is no effective, specific respiratory care treatment modality for alveolar consolidation. With pneumonia, the great temptation for the respiratory therapist is to do too much, such as instituting lung expansion therapy, bronchodilator therapy, and bronchial hygiene therapy. Such treatment protocols generally are not indicated, especially during the early stages of the disease process. Appropriate antibiotics (prescribed by the physician), bed rest, fluids, and supplementary oxygen are all that are usually needed. When pneumonia is in its resolution stage, however, the patient may experience excessive secretions and atelectasis, accompanied by bronchoconstriction. At this time, other treatment modalities may be indicated.

---

[4]The Case Study Discussion Section at the end of each respiratory disease chapter often refers the reader back to these clinical scenarios, correlating various clinical manifestations to specific pathophysiologic mechanisms and alterations of the lungs.

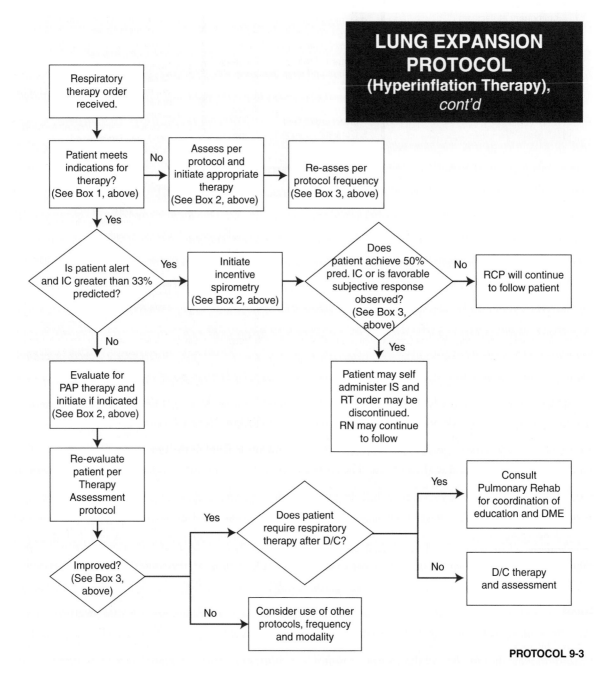

Respiratory therapy order received.

Patient meets indications for therapy? (See Box 1, above)

No → Assess per protocol and initiate appropriate therapy (See Box 2, above) → Re-asses per protocol frequency (See Box 3, above)

Yes ↓

Is patient alert and IC greater than 33% predicted?

Yes → Initiate incentive spirometry (See Box 2, above) → Does patient achieve 50% pred. IC or is favorable subjective response observed? (See Box 3, above)

No → RCP will continue to follow patient

Yes ↓

Patient may self administer IS and RT order may be discontinued. RN may continue to follow

No ↓

Evaluate for PAP therapy and initiate if indicated (See Box 2, above)

↓

Re-evaluate patient per Therapy Assessment protocol

↓

Improved? (See Box 3, above)

Yes → Does patient require respiratory therapy after D/C?

Yes → Consult Pulmonary Rehab for coordination of education and DME

No → D/C therapy and assessment

No → Consider use of other protocols, frequency and modality

PROTOCOL 9-3

(1)
Evaluate indications:

The primary general indication for aerosolized bronchodilator therapy is reversible reactive airway disease. This condition is detected through the following symptoms:

- C/O dyspnea
- Wheezing
- Hyperinflation
- Reduction in airflow (peak flow, FEV_1, FVC, prolonged expiration)

(3)
Assess outcomes — Goals achieved?
- Diminished wheezing and the volume of air moved is increased
- Improvement in airflow (peak expiratory flow rate, PEFR)
- Improved vital signs and measures of gas exchange
- Improved patient appearance with decreased use of accessory muscles

* Note that this protocol is for simple bronchodilator administration for non-ventilated patients. There are a variety of other options such as continuous bronchodilator administration, acute maximum titration of dose, and multiple delivery devices that can be incorporated within this protocol or as a separate protocol depending on site-specific preference.

Modified from the Respiratory Care Department at the Kettering Health Network, in Dayton, Ohio

(2)
AEROSOLIZED MEDICATION THERAPY SELECTIONS*
BRONCHODILATOR AGENTS
Objective
Bronchodilator agents are used to offset bronchial smooth muscle constriction. Common agents used are:
Ultra-Short-Acting Bronchodilator Agents
- Epinephrine (Adrenalin)
- Racemic epinephrine (generic)

Short-Acting Beta$_2$ Agents (SABAs)
- Albuterol (Ventolin HFA, Proventil HFA, ProAir HFA)
- Metaproternol (Generic only)
- Levalbuterol (Xopenex, Xopenex HFA)

Long-Acting Beta$_2$ Agents (LABAs)
- Salmeterol (Serevent Diskus)
- Formoterol (Perforomist, Foradil Aerolizer)
- Arformoterol (Brovana)
- Indacaterol (Arcapta Neohaler)
- Olodaterol (Striverdi Respimat)

Anticholinergic Agents Short Acting
- Ipratropium (Atrovent HFA)

Anticholinergic Agents, Long Acting
- Tiotropium (Spiriva HandiHaler, Spiriva Respimat)
- Aclidinium (Tudorza Pressair)
- Umeclidinium (Incruse Ellipta)

Short-Acting Beta$_2$ Agents (SABAs) and Anticholinergic Agents (Combined)
- Ipratropium and Albuterol (DuoNeb, Combivent)

Long-Acting Beta$_2$ Agents (LABAs) and Anticholinergic Agents (Combined)
- Umeclidinium and Vilanterol (Anoro Ellipta)

ANTI-INFLAMMATORY AGENTS
Objective
Anti-inflammatory agents suppress bronchial inflammation and edema. They also are used for their ability to enhance the responsiveness of B_2 receptor sites to sympathomimetic agents. Common agents used are:
Inhaled Corticosteroids (ICSs)
- Beclomethasone (QVAR)
- Flunisolide (Aerospan HFA)
- Fluticasone (Flovent HFA, Flovent Diskus, Arnuity Ellipta)
- Budesonide (Pulmicort Flexhaler, Pulmicort Respules)
- Mometasone (Asmanex Twisthaler, Asmanex HFA)
- Ciclesonide (Alvesco)

Inhaled Corticosteroids and Long-Acting Beta$_2$ Agents (Combined)
- Fluticasone and Salmeterol (Advair Diskus, Advair HFA)
- Budesonide and Formoterol (Symbicort)
- Mometasone and Formoterol (Dulera)
- Fluticasone and Vilanterol (Breo Ellipta)

MUCOLYTIC AGENTS
Objective
Mucolytic agents are used to enhance the mobilization and thinning of bronchial secretions. Common agents used are:
- Acetylcysteine (Generic only)
- Dornase alfa (Pulmozyme)
- Sodium bicarbonate (2% solution)

* For the complete listing, doses, and administra tion of agents approved by the FDA, visit the Drugs@FDA website (www.accessdata.fda.gov/scripts/cder/drugsatfda/).

PROTOCOL 9-4 *cont'd on page 128*

Increased Alveolar-Capillary Membrane Thickness

Figure 9-9 (see page 132) illustrates the major pathophysiologic mechanisms caused by increased alveolar-capillary membrane thickness (e.g., postoperative ARDS, pulmonary edema, asbestosis, chronic interstitial lung disease), the clinical manifestations that develop, and the treatment protocols used to offset them. The hypoxemia that develops as a result of an increased alveolar-capillary membrane thickness is caused by an alveolar-capillary diffusion block. This type of hypoxemia often responds favorably to the *Oxygen Therapy Protocol* and the *Lung Expansion Protocol*.

Bronchospasm

Figure 9-10 (see page 133) shows the major pathophysiologic mechanisms activated by bronchospasm (e.g., asthma), the clinical manifestations that result, and the appropriate treatment protocols used to offset them. The *Aerosolized Medication Therapy Protocol* (Bronchodilator Therapy) is the primary treatment modality used to offset the anatomic alterations of bronchospasm (the original cause of the pathophysiologic chain of events). The *Oxygen Therapy Protocol* and *Mechanical Ventilation Protocol*[5] are secondary treatment modalities used

---

[5]The mechanical ventilation protocols are presented in Chapter 10.

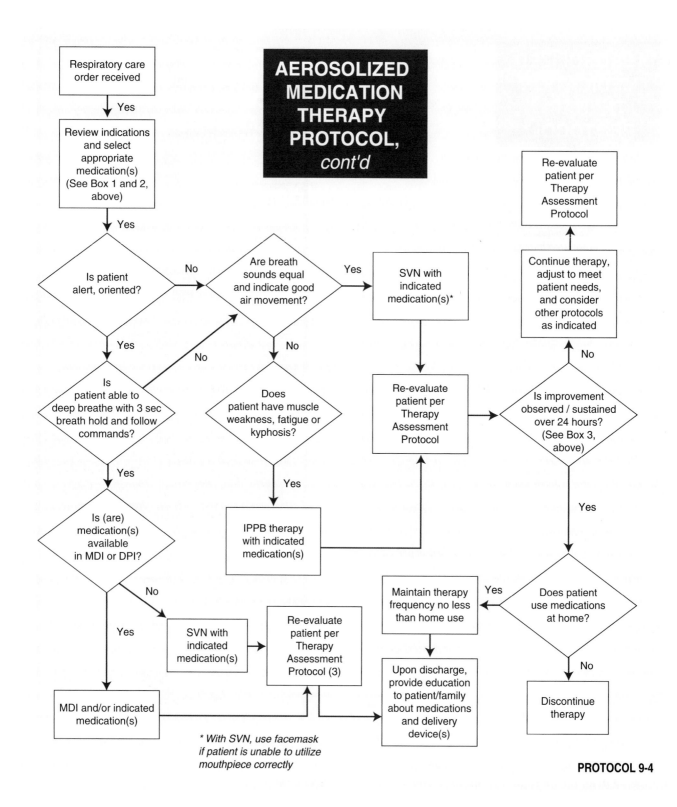

AEROSOLIZED MEDICATION THERAPY PROTOCOL, *cont'd*

Respiratory care order received

↓ Yes

Review indications and select appropriate medication(s) (See Box 1 and 2, above)

↓ Yes

Is patient alert, oriented? — No → Are breath sounds equal and indicate good air movement? — Yes → SVN with indicated medication(s)*

Is patient alert, oriented? ↓ Yes

Is patient able to deep breathe with 3 sec breath hold and follow commands? — No → Are breath sounds equal and indicate good air movement?

Are breath sounds equal and indicate good air movement? ↓ No

Does patient have muscle weakness, fatigue or kyphosis?

↓ Yes

IPPB therapy with indicated medication(s)

Is patient able to deep breathe with 3 sec breath hold and follow commands? ↓ Yes

Is (are) medication(s) available in MDI or DPI? — No → SVN with indicated medication(s) → Re-evaluate patient per Therapy Assessment Protocol (3)

Is (are) medication(s) available in MDI or DPI? ↓ Yes

MDI and/or indicated medication(s)

SVN with indicated medication(s)* ↓

Re-evaluate patient per Therapy Assessment Protocol → Is improvement observed / sustained over 24 hours? (See Box 3, above)

Is improvement observed / sustained over 24 hours? — No → Continue therapy, adjust to meet patient needs, and consider other protocols as indicated → Re-evaluate patient per Therapy Assessment Protocol

Is improvement observed / sustained over 24 hours? ↓ Yes

Does patient use medications at home? — Yes → Maintain therapy frequency no less than home use → Upon discharge, provide education to patient/family about medications and delivery device(s)

Does patient use medications at home? ↓ No

Discontinue therapy

* With SVN, use facemask if patient is unable to utilize mouthpiece correctly

PROTOCOL 9-4

to offset the mild, moderate, or severe clinical manifestations associated with bronchospasm. In other words, when the patient responds favorably to the *Aerosolized Medication Therapy Protocol*, the need for the *Oxygen Therapy Protocol* may be minimal and the *Mechanical Ventilation Protocol* may not be necessary at all.

Excessive Bronchial Secretions

Figure 9-11 (see page 133) illustrates the major pathophysiologic mechanisms caused by excessive bronchial secretions (e.g., chronic bronchitis, cystic fibrosis, asthma), the clinical manifestations that result, and the appropriate treatment protocols used to correct them. The *Bronchopulmonary Hygiene Therapy Protocol* is the primary treatment modality used to offset the anatomic alterations associated with excessive bronchial secretions. When the patient demonstrates chronic ventilatory failure during the advanced stages of respiratory disorders associated with chronic excessive airway secretions (e.g., chronic bronchitis), caution must be taken not to over-oxygenate the patient.

Indications

- Documented hypoxemia. Defined as a decreased PaO_2 in the blood below normal range.
- $PaO_2 < 60$ mm Hg or $SaO_2 < 90\%$ in subjects breathing room air.
- Acute care situations in which hypoxemia is suspected.
- Severe trauma.
- Acute myocardial infarction.
- Short-term therapy or surgical intervention (e.g., postanesthesia recovery, hip surgery).

Contraindications

- No specific contraindications to oxygen therapy exist when indications are present.

Precautions and/or Possible Complications

- $PaO_2 > 60$ mm Hg may depress ventilation in some patients with elevated $PaCO_2$.
- $FIO_2 > 0.50$, may cause absorption atelectasis, oxygen toxicity, and/or ciliary or leukocyte depression.
- Supplemental oxygen should be administered with caution to patients with paraquat poisoning or to those receiving bleomycin.
- During laser bronchoscopy, minimal FIO_2 should be used to avoid intratracheal ignition.
- Fire hazard is increased in the presence of increased oxygen concentration.
- Bacterial contamination associated with nebulizers or humidifiers is a possible hazard.

Assessment of Need

- Need is determined by measurement of inadequate oxygen tension and/or saturation, by invasive or noninvasive methods, and/or the presence of clinical indicators.

Assessment of Outcome

- Outcome is determined by clinical and physiologic assessment to establish adequacy of patient response to therapy.

Monitoring

Patient

- Clinical assessment including cardiac, pulmonary, and neurologic status.
- Assessment of physiologic parameters (PaO_2, SaO_2, SpO_2) in conjunction with the initiation of therapy or:
  Within 12 hours of initiation with $FIO_2 < 0.40$
  Within 8 hours with $FIO_2 \geq 0.40$ (including postanesthesia recovery)
  Within 72 hours in acute myocardial infarction
  Within 2 hours for any patient with principal diagnosis of chronic obstructive pulmonary disease.

Equipment

- All oxygen delivery systems should be checked at least once per day.
- More frequent checks are needed in systems:
  Susceptible to variation in oxygen concentration (e.g., hood, high-flow blending systems)
  Applied to patients with artificial airways
  Delivering a heated gas mixture
  Applied to patients who are clinically unstable or who require $FIO_2 > 0.50$
- Care should be taken to avoid interruption of oxygen therapy in situations including ambulation or transport for procedure.

BOX 9-2 Pathophysiologic Mechanisms Commonly Activated in Respiratory Disorders

- Decreased ventilation/perfusion ($\dot{V}/\dot{Q}$) ratio
- Alveolar diffusion block
- Decreased lung compliance
- Stimulation of oxygen receptors
- Deflation reflex
- Irritant reflex
- Pulmonary reflex
- Increased airway resistance
- Air trapping and alveolar hyperinflation

Distal Airway and Alveolar Weakening

Figure 9-12 (see page 134) illustrates the major pathophysiologic mechanisms caused by distal airway and alveolar weakening (e.g., emphysema), the clinical manifestations that result, and the appropriate treatment protocols used to offset them. Pulmonary rehabilitation and oxygen therapy may be all the practitioner can provide to treat the symptoms associated with distal airway and alveolar weakening. When the patient demonstrates chronic ventilatory failure during the advanced stages of the disorder, caution must be taken with the *Oxygen Therapy Protocol* not to over-oxygenate the patient.

Text continued on p. 134

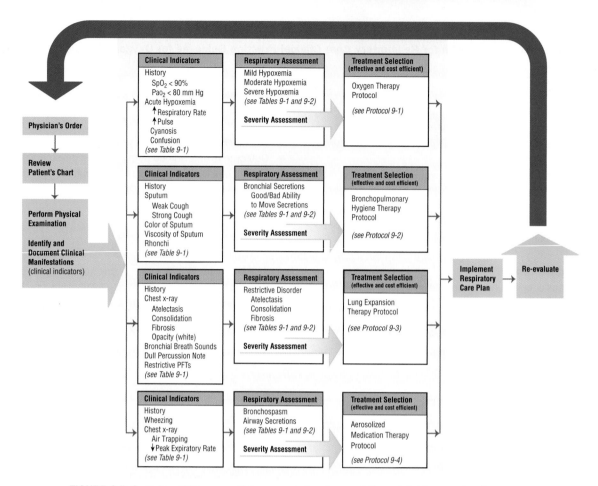

FIGURE 9-5 Overview of the essential components of a good therapist-driven protocol program.

| Patient Identification Box | Date:_____ | Admitting Diagnosis:_____ |
| | Time:_____ | Attending Physician:_____ |

Clinical Indicators (see Table 9-1)			
Oxygen Therapy	**Bronchopulmonary Hygiene Therapy**	**Lung Expansion Therapy**	**Aerosolized Medication**
Examples:	Examples:	Examples:	Examples:

☐ History
☐ SpO₂ < 90%
☐ PaO₂ < 80 mm Hg
☐ Acute hypoxemia
  ☐ ≠ Respiratory rate
  ☐ ≠ Pulse
  ☐ Cyanosis
  ☐ Confusion
  ☐ Other
	☐ History
	☐ Sputum
	  ☐ Weak cough
	  ☐ Color of sputum
	  ☐ Viscosity of sputum
	  ☐ Rhonchi
		☐ History
		☐ Chest x-ray
		  ☐ Atelectasis
		  ☐ Consolidation
		  ☐ Fibrosis
		  ☐ Opacity (white)
		☐ Bronchial breath sounds
		☐ Restrictive PFT values
			☐ History
			☐ Wheezing
			☐ Chest x-ray
			  ☐ Air trapping
			☐ Obstructive PFT values

Respiratory Assessments (see Tables 9-1 and 9-2)			
Oxygen Therapy	**Bronchopulmonary Hygiene Therapy**	**Lung Expansion Therapy**	**Aerosolized Medication**
Examples:	Examples:	Examples:	Examples:
☐ Mild hypoxemia ☐ Moderate hypoxemia ☐ Severe hypoxemia	☐ Excessive sputum production ☐ Thick secretions ☐ Weak cough	☐ Atelectasis ☐ Consolidation ☐ Weak diaphragm	☐ Bronchospasm ☐ Thick secretions ☐ Bronchial edema
Severity Score:_____	Severity Score:_____	Severity Score:_____	Severity Score:_____

Treatment Plans			
Oxygen Therapy (see Protocol 9-1)	**Bronchopulmonary Hygiene Therapy (see Protocol 9-2)**	**Lung Expansion Therapy (see Protocol 9-3)**	**Aerosolized Medication (see Protocol 9-4)**
Examples:	Examples:	Examples:	Examples:
☐ Nasal cannula ☐ Oxygen mask ☐ 28% Venturi mask	☐ Deep breath and cough ☐ Chest physical therapy ☐ Postural drainage	☐ Incentive spirometry ☐ CPAP ☐ PEEP	☐ SABA ☐ LABA ☐ Corticosteroids
Frequency:_____	Frequency:_____	Frequency:_____	Frequency:_____

| Reevaluation Date:_____ | Therapist Signature:_____ |

FIGURE 9-6 Therapist-driven protocol program assessment form.

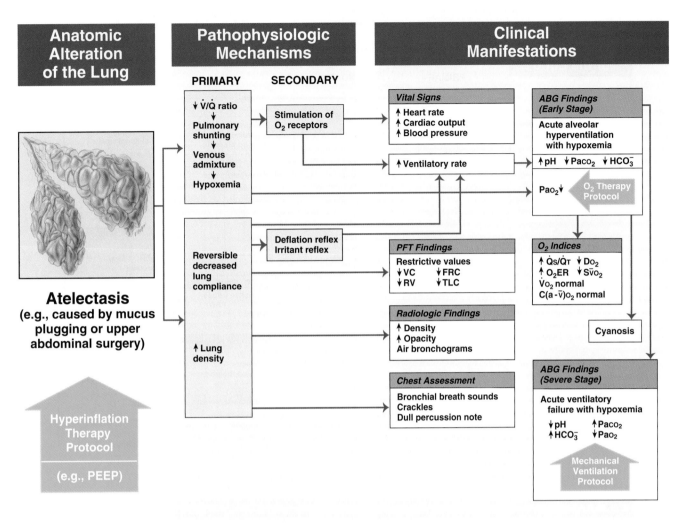

FIGURE 9-7 Atelectasis clinical scenario.

Key to Abbreviations in Figures 9-7 through 9-13

ABG	= Arterial blood gas		MVV	= Maximum voluntary ventilation
ARDS	= Acute respiratory distress syndrome		O_2ER	= Oxygen extraction ratio
CPAP	= Continuous positive airway pressure		PD	= Postural drainage
CPT	= Chest physical therapy		PEEP	= Positive end-expiratory pressure
DO_2	= Total oxygen delivery		PEFR	= Peak expiratory flow rate
ERV	= Expiratory reserve volume		PFT	= Pulmonary function test
FEF	= Forced expiratory flow, midexpiratory phase		$\dot{Q}s/\dot{Q}t$	= Shunt fraction
FEV_1	= Forced expiratory volume in 1 second		RV	= Residual volume
FEV_T	= Forced expiratory volume timed		$S\bar{v}O_2$	= Mixed venous oxygen saturation
FRC	= Functional residual capacity		TLC	= Total lung capacity
FVC	= Forced vital capacity		VC	= Vital capacity
IC	= Inspiratory capacity		$\dot{V}/\dot{Q}$	= Ventilation-perfusion ratio

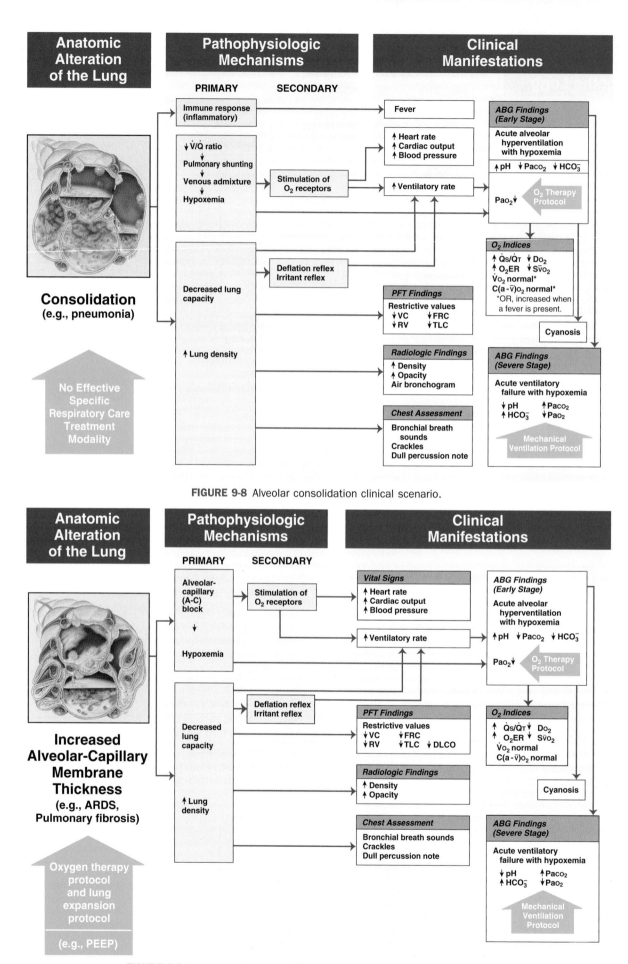

FIGURE 9-8 Alveolar consolidation clinical scenario.

FIGURE 9-9 Increased alveolar-capillary membrane thickness clinical scenario.

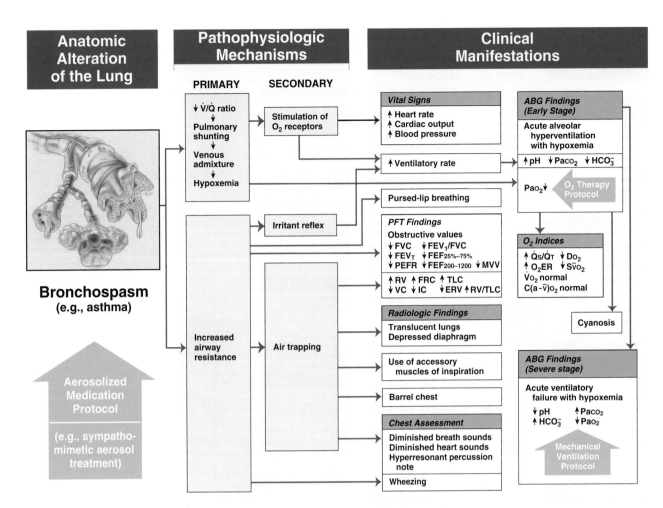

FIGURE 9-10 Bronchospasm clinical scenario.

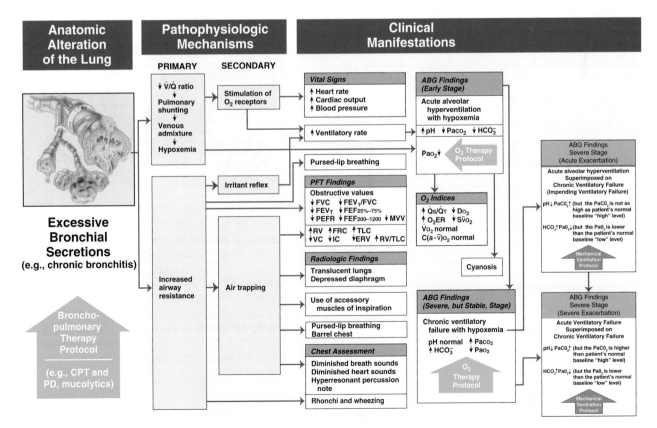

FIGURE 9-11 Excessive bronchial secretions clinical scenario.

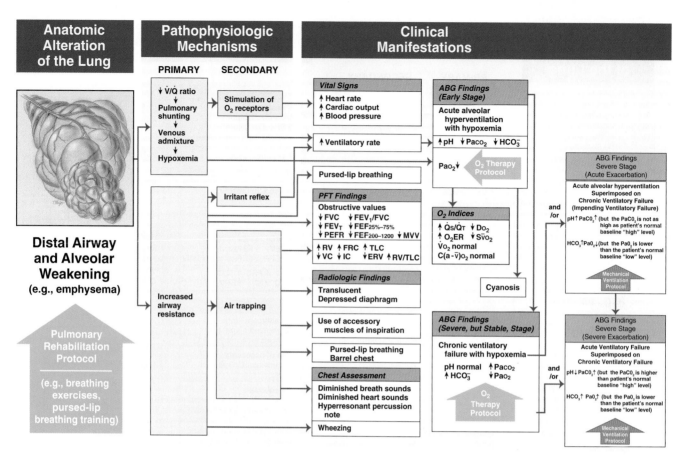

FIGURE 9-12 Distal airway and alveolar weakening clinical scenario.

Overview of Common Anatomic Alterations Associated with Respiratory Disorders

When the respiratory therapist knows and understands the chain of events (clinical scenarios) that develop in response to common anatomic alterations of the lungs, an assessment and an appropriate treatment protocol can be easily determined. Table 9-3 provides an overview of the most common anatomic alterations associated with the respiratory disorders presented in this textbook.

Figure 9-13 provides a three-component overview model of a prototype airway to further enhance the reader's visualization of anatomic alterations of the lungs commonly associated with obstructive respiratory disorders (e.g., asthma, bronchitis, or emphysema) and the treatment plans commonly used to offset them.

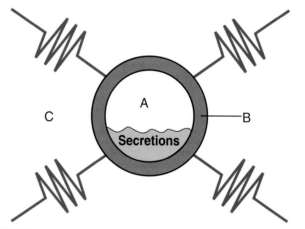

FIGURE 9-13 A three-component model of a prototype airway. Therapy may be directed at any or all components. **A**, Airway lumen; **B**, airway wall; **C**, supporting structures. Therapy for **A** includes deep breathing and coughing, smoking cessation, suctioning, mucolytics, bland aerosols, systemic and parental hydration, and therapeutic bronchoscopy. Therapy for **B** includes bronchodilators, aerosolized antiinflammatory agents, aerosolized antibiotics, and aerosolized decongestants. Therapy for **C** includes pursed-lip breathing exercises (e.g., when the elastic recoil of the lungs is absent in emphysema) and removal of external factors compressing the airway (e.g., bullae, pleural effusion, pneumothorax, tumor masses).

TABLE 9-3 Common Anatomic Alterations of the Lungs Associated With Respiratory Disorders

Respiratory Disorder	Atelectasis	Alveolar Consolidation	Increased Alveolar-Capillary Membrane Thickness	Bronchospasm	Excessive Bronchial Secretions	Distal Airway Weakening
Chronic bronchitis				X*	X	
Emphysema				X	X*	X
Bronchiectasis	X	X		X	X	
Asthma				X	X	
Pneumonia		X	X		X*	
Lung abscess		X			X	
Tuberculosis		X	X			
Fungal diseases		X	X			
Pulmonary edema	X		X		X	
Pulmonary embolism	X			X		
Flail chest	X	X				
Pneumothorax	X					
Pleural diseases	X					
Kyphoscoliosis	X				X*	
Pneumoconiosis			X	X		
Cancer of the lung	X	X			X	
Adult respiratory distress syndrome	X*	X	X			
Chronic interstitial lung diseases			X	X*		
Guillain-Barré syndrome	X*	X*			X*	
Myasthenia gravis	X*	X*			X*	
Meconium aspiration syndrome	X	X			X	
Transient tachypnea of newborn			X		X	
Infant respiratory distress syndrome	X	X			X	
Pulmonary air leak syndromes	X					
Respiratory syncytial virus	X	X			X	
Bronchopulmonary dysplasia	X		X		X	
Diaphragmatic hernia	X					
Cystic fibrosis	X*			X*	X	
Near drowning	X	X	X	X		
Smoke inhalation and thermal injuries	X	X	X	X		
Postoperative atelectasis	X					

*Common secondary anatomic alterations of the lungs associated with this disorder.

SELF-ASSESSMENT QUESTIONS

Ⓔ Answers to questions can be found on Evolve. To access additional student assessment questions visit
http://evolve.elsevier.com/DesJardins/respiratory.

1. Which of the following pathophysiologic mechanisms is or are associated with the "atelectasis" clinical scenario?
   1. Air trapping
   2. Decreased ventilation/perfusion ratio
   3. Deflation reflex
   4. Irritant reflex
      a. 1 and 4 only
      b. 2 and 3 only
      c. 1 and 4 only
      d. 2, 3, and 4 only

2. Which of the following clinical manifestations is or are associated with the "excessive bronchial secretions" clinical scenario?
   1. Translucent radiographs
   2. Increased forced vital capacity
   3. Pursed-lip breathing
   4. Air bronchograms
      a. 1 and 4 only
      b. 1 and 3 only
      c. 2, 3, and 4 only
      d. 1, 2, 3, and 4

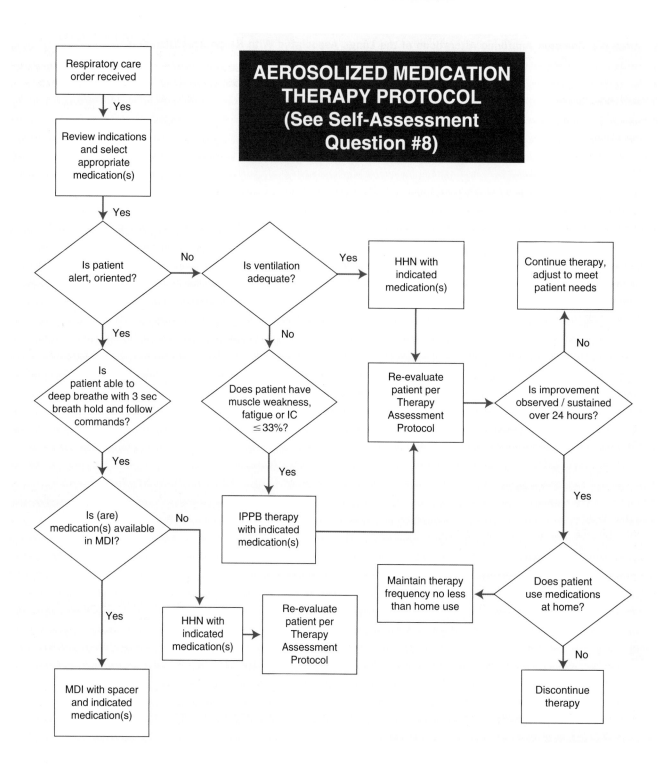

AEROSOLIZED MEDICATION THERAPY PROTOCOL
(See Self-Assessment Question #8)

Respiratory care order received

Yes

Review indications and select appropriate medication(s)

Yes

Is patient alert, oriented? — No → Is ventilation adequate? — Yes → HHN with indicated medication(s)

Yes (from "Is patient alert, oriented?")

Is patient able to deep breathe with 3 sec breath hold and follow commands?

Yes

Is (are) medication(s) available in MDI? — No → HHN with indicated medication(s) → Re-evaluate patient per Therapy Assessment Protocol

Yes

MDI with spacer and indicated medication(s)

(from "Is ventilation adequate?") No

Does patient have muscle weakness, fatigue or IC ≤ 33%?

Yes

IPPB therapy with indicated medication(s)

Re-evaluate patient per Therapy Assessment Protocol

Is improvement observed / sustained over 24 hours? — No → Continue therapy, adjust to meet patient needs

Yes

Does patient use medications at home? — No → Discontinue therapy

(Yes) → Maintain therapy frequency no less than home use

3. Which of the following clinical manifestations is or are associated with the "atelectasis" clinical scenario?
   1. Increased opacity in chest x-ray
   2. Decreased forced vital capacity
   3. Bronchial breath sounds
   4. Diminished heart sounds
      a. 1 and 4 only
      b. 2 and 3 only
      c. 1, 2, and 3 only
      d. 2, 3, and 4 only

4. Which of the following pathophysiologic mechanisms is or are associated with the "bronchospasm" clinical scenario?
   1. Air trapping
   2. Decreased ventilation/perfusion ratio
   3. Increased airway resistance
   4. Irritant reflex
      a. 1 and 4 only
      b. 2 and 3 onl
      c. 2, 3, and 4 only
      d. 1, 2, 3, and 4

5. Which of the following clinical manifestations is or are associated with the "distal airway and alveolar weakening" clinical scenario?
   1. Diminished breath sounds
   2. Decreased residual volume
   3. Pursed-lip breathing
   4. Dull percussion note
      a. 1 and 4 only
      b. 1 and 3 only
      c. 2, 3, and 4 only
      d. 1, 2, 3, and 4

6. According to the American Association for Respiratory Care (AARC), the purpose(s) of respiratory TDPs is/are to:
   1. Deliver individualized diagnostic and therapeutic respiratory care to patients
   2. Assist the physician with evaluating patients' respiratory care needs and optimize the allocation of respiratory care services
   3. Determine the indications for respiratory therapy and the appropriate modalities for providing high-quality, cost-effective care that improves patient outcomes and decreases length of stay
   4. Empower respiratory therapists to allocate care using sign-and-symptom based algorithms for respiratory treatment
      a. 1 only
      b. 3 only
      c. 1, 2, and 3 only
      d. 1, 2, 3, and 4

7. A patient experiencing a severe asthmatic episode would probably demonstrate a variety of objective clinical indicators to justify the assessments that call for the administration of which of the following protocols:
   1. Oxygen Therapy Protocol
   2. Bronchopulmonary Hygiene Therapy Protocol
   3. Aerosolized Medication Therapy Protocol
   4. Lung Expansion Therapy Protocol
      a. 1 and 3 only
      b. 3 and 4 only
      c. 1, 2, and 4 only
      d. 1, 2, and 3 only

8. On the previous page, the Aerosolized Medication Protocol appears with one or more steps left out. Which steps have been omitted?
   1. Discharge training/documentation has been left out
   2. Effect of treatment with MDI/spacer has not been evaluated
   3. Failure to be able to breath hold has not been related to muscle weakness, following the finding of a reduced inspiratory capacity
   4. Use of additional protocols has not been considered in view of the patient's failure to improve on aerosol therapy via small volume nebulizer treatment or intermittent positive-pressure breathing
      a. 1 and 3 only
      b. 2 and 4 only
      c. 2, 3, and 4 only
      d. 1, 2, 3, and 4

9. A patient with recent thoracic surgery, who has developed both left and right lower lung lobe atelectasis, would *most* likely benefit from which of the following protocols?
   a. Oxygen Therapy Protocol
   b. Bronchopulmonary Hygiene Therapy Protocol
   c. Aerosolized Medication Therapy Protocol
   d. Lung Expansion Therapy Protocol

10. An obese 37-year-old male enters the emergency room in respiratory distress. He stated that he had been bedridden for the past 8 days with the flu. He thought he was getting better, but had been short of breath for the past 2 days. His vital signs are: blood pressure 175/125, respiratory rate 25 bpm, heart rate 110 bpm. He has bilateral bronchial breath sounds over the lower lobes and dull percussion notes over the bases. His arterial blood gases show that he has acute alveolar hyperventilation with moderate hypoxemia. His chest x-ray revealed bilateral atelectasis throughout his right and left lower lobes. Which of the following protocols would initially be the *most* beneficial?
    a. Oxygen Therapy Protocol
    b. Bronchopulmonary Hygiene Therapy Protocol
    c. Aerosolized Medication Therapy Protocol
    d. Lung Expansion Therapy Protocol

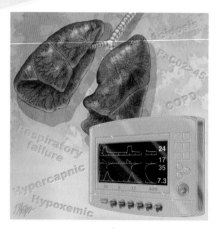

Chapter Objectives

After reading this chapter, you will be able to:

- Define respiratory failure.
- Identify the six major anatomic alterations of the lungs and subsequent clinical scenarios that can lead to respiratory failure.
- Evaluate the two major classifications of respiratory failure.
- Describe hypoxemic respiratory failure (type I) (oxygenation failure).
- Explain respiratory disorders associated with hypoxemic respiratory failure.
- Discuss the pathophysiologic mechanisms of hypoxemic respiratory failure.
- Describe hypercapnic respiratory failure (type II) (ventilatory failure).
- Describe the pathophysiologic mechanisms of hypercapnic respiratory failure.
- Explain respiratory disorders associated with hypercapnic respiratory failure.
- Differentiate the types of ventilatory failure.
- Describe the major components of the mechanical ventilation protocol.

Key Terms

Absolute Shunt
Acute Alveolar Hyperventilation Superimposed on Chronic Ventilatory Failure
Acute Ventilatory Failure
Acute Ventilatory Failure Superimposed on Chronic Ventilatory Failure
Airway Obstruction
Alveolar-Arterial Oxygen Tension Difference [P(A-a)O$_2$]

Alveolar Hypoventilation
Anatomic Shunt
Apnea
Arterial Oxygen Tension (PaO$_2$)
Arterial Oxygen Tension to Fractional Inspired Oxygen Ratio (PaO$_2$/FIO$_2$)
Arterial to Alveolar Oxygen Tension Ratio (PaO$_2$/PAO$_2$ ratio)
Capillary Shunt
Chronic Ventilatory Failure
Clinical Scenarios
Dead Space/Tidal Volume Ratio (V$_D$/V$_T$ ratio)
Diffusion Defects
Hypercapnic Respiratory Failure (Type II)
Hypoxemic (Type I) Respiratory Failure
Impending Ventilatory Failure
Invasive Ventilation
Mechanical Ventilation
Noninvasive Ventilation
Oxygenation Failure
Permissive Hypercapnia
Prophylactic Ventilatory Support
Pulmonary Shunting
Relative Shunt
Respiratory Failure
Severe Refractory Hypoxemia
Shunt-like Effect
Static Lung Compliance
Type III Respiratory Failure
Venous Admixture
Ventilation-Perfusion Mismatch
Ventilatory Failure

Chapter Outline

Introduction
Hypoxemic Respiratory Failure (Type I) (Oxygenation Failure)
    Pathophysiologic Mechanisms of Hypoxemic Respiratory Failure
Hypercapnic Respiratory Failure (Type II) (Ventilatory failure)
    Types of Ventilatory Failure
Mechanical Ventilation
    Standard Criteria for Mechanical Ventilation
    Prophylactic Ventilatory Support
    Key Clinical Indicators for Hypercapnic and Hypoxemic Respiratory Failure
    Ventilatory Support Strategy
    Mechanical Ventilation Protocols
        Ventilator Initiation and Management Protocol
        Ventilator Weaning Protocol
Self-Assessment Questions

Introduction

Respiratory failure is a general term used to describe the inability of the respiratory system to maintain an adequate amount of (1) oxygen (O_2) exchange between the alveoli and the pulmonary capillaries, or (2) carbon dioxide (CO_2) removal out of the lungs, or (3) a combination of both. The arterial blood gas (ABG) criteria for respiratory failure in the normal individual are an arterial partial pressure of oxygen (PaO_2) less than 60 mm Hg, or an arterial partial pressure of carbon dioxide ($PaCO_2$) greater than 50 mm Hg, or a mixture of both. Respiratory failure is a life-threatening clinical condition that the respiratory therapist must be 100% proficient in recognizing, assessing, and managing.

Virtually every respiratory disorder presented in this textbook can result in respiratory failure. This is because, as described earlier in Chapter 9, respiratory disorders can cause one or more abnormal **anatomic alterations of the lung**—which, in turn, activate specific, and very predictable, **pathophysiologic mechanisms and clinical manifestations**—which can progressively worsen if not identified and treated. The interrelationship between the anatomic alterations of the lungs, the pathophysiologic mechanisms, and the clinical manifestations are collectively referred to as "**clinical scenarios.**"

There are six major anatomic alterations of the lungs—which, in turn, cause six different clinical scenarios—that can result in respiratory failure. They are (1) **atelectasis** (e.g., which can occur from mucus plugging, upper abdominal surgery, pneumothorax, or flail chest), (2) **alveolar consolidation** (e.g., caused by pneumonia), (3) **increased alveolar-capillary membrane thickness** (e.g., acute respiratory distress syndrome, pneumoconiosis, or pulmonary edema), (4) **bronchospasm** (e.g., asthma), (5) **excessive bronchial secretions** (e.g., chronic bronchitis), and (6) **distal airway and alveolar weakening** (e.g., emphysema). In severe cases, any one of these six abnormal alterations of the lungs can lead to a clinical scenario that ends in respiratory failure (see clinical scenarios, Figures 9-7 through Figure 9-12, pages 131 to 134).

Respiratory failure is commonly classified as either: (1) **hypoxemic (type I) respiratory failure**, or (2) **hypercapnic (type II) respiratory failure**, or (3) a combination of both. These categories reflect the pathophysiologic basis responsible for the respiratory failure. For example, the term *hypoxemic (type I) respiratory failure* is used when the primary problem is an inadequate oxygenation exchange between the alveoli and the pulmonary capillary system—which results in a decreased PaO_2. The term *hypercapnic (type II) respiratory failure* is used when the primary problem is alveolar hypoventilation—which results in an increased $PaCO_2$ and, without supplemental oxygen, a decreased PaO_2.

In the clinical setting, hypercapnic respiratory failure is commonly called **ventilatory failure**. Based on the $PaCO_2$ and pH values, ventilatory failure is further classified as being either **acute ventilatory failure** (high $PaCO_2$ and low pH) or **chronic ventilatory failure** (high $PaCO_2$ and normal pH). Because acute ventilatory changes (i.e., hyperventilation or hypoventilation) are often seen in patients with chronic ventilatory failure, the patient may also present with either (1) **acute alveolar hyperventilation superimposed on chronic ventilatory failure**, or (2) **acute ventilatory failure superimposed on chronic ventilatory failure**.

The various types of respiratory failure are described in more detail in the following section.

Hypoxemic Respiratory Failure (Type I) (Oxygenation Failure)

Hypoxemic respiratory failure (type I) is used to describe a patient whose primary problem is inadequate oxygenation. Patients with hypoxemic respiratory failure typically demonstrate hypoxemia—a low PaO_2—and a normal, or low $PaCO_2$ value.[1] The low $PaCO_2$ is usually attributable to the alveolar hyperventilation associated with hypoxemia (see Figure 2-26 and Figure 2-27). Box 10-1 provides a listing of common respiratory disorders that can cause hypoxemic respiratory failure. The major pathophysiologic causes of

---

[1]Key clinical indicators of hypoxemic respiratory failure are also reflected by a decreased **arterial oxygen tension (PaO_2)**, an increased alveolar-arterial oxygen tension gradient [$P(A-a)O_2$], a decreased **arterial-to-alveolar oxygen tension ratio (PaO_2/PAO_2 ratio)**, a decreased **arterial oxygen tension to fractional inspired oxygen ratio (PaO_2/FIO_2 ratio)**, and/or an increased pulmonary shunt ($\dot{Q}_S/\dot{Q}_T$). See key clinical indicators of hypoxemic respiratory failure. See Table 10-10, under standard criteria for mechanical ventilation, page 146.

> **BOX 10-1 Respiratory Disorders Associated With Hypoxemic Respiratory Failure (Oxygenation Failure)**
>
> - **Restrictive Pulmonary Disorders***
>   - Pneumonia
>   - Lung abscess
>   - Pulmonary edema
>   - Interstitial lung diseases
>   - Acute respiratory distress syndrome
>   - Alveolar atelectasis
> - **Chronic Obstructive Pulmonary Disorders†**
>   - Emphysema
>   - Chronic bronchitis
>   - Asthma
>   - Cystic fibrosis
> - **Neoplastic Disease***
>   - Cancer of the lung
> - **Newborn and Early Childhood Respiratory Disorders***
>   - Meconium aspiration syndrome
>   - Transient tachypnea of the newborn
>   - Respiratory distress syndrome
>   - Pulmonary air leak syndromes
>   - Respiratory syncytial virus infection
>   - Congenital diaphragmatic hernia
>   - Bronchopulmonary dysplasia§
>   - Croup syndrome†
> - **Other***
>   - Near drowning
>   - Smoke inhalation and thermal injuries

*Primary pulmonary shunting disorders.
†Primarily a decreased $\dot{V}/\dot{Q}$ ratio and alveolar hypoventilation disorders.
§Pulmonary shunting, decreased $\dot{V}/\dot{Q}$ ratio, and alveolar hypoventilation disorders.

hypoxemic respiratory failure are (1) *alveolar hypoventilation*, (2) *pulmonary shunting*, and (3) *ventilation-perfusion* ($\dot{V}/\dot{Q}$) *mismatch*. Although less common, a decrease in inspired oxygen pressure (PIO_2) (e.g., high altitudes or decreased FIO_2) can also cause hypoxemic respiratory failure.

The primary pathophysiologic mechanisms of hypoxemic respiratory failure are discussed in more detail in the following sections.

Pathophysiologic Mechanisms of Hypoxemic Respiratory Failure

Alveolar Hypoventilation

Alveolar hypoventilation is an abnormal condition of the respiratory system that develops when the volume and distribution of alveolar ventilation is not adequate for the body's metabolic needs. It is characterized by an increased $PaCO_2$ level and, without supplemental oxygen, a decreased PaO_2. Common causes of hypoventilation include central nervous system depressants, head trauma, chronic obstructive pulmonary disease, obesity, sleep apnea, and neuromuscular disorders (e.g., myasthenia gravis or Guillain-Barré syndrome). *The results of hypoventilation are hypoxia, hypercapnia, respiratory acidosis, and—in severe cases—pulmonary hypertension with cor pulmonale.* It should be emphasized, however, that even though alveolar hypoventilation causes hypoxemia, the alveoli are still able to efficiently transfer oxygen into the pulmonary capillary blood—assuming the inspired oxygen can be delivered to the alveoli. Thus, treatment primarily consists of ventilatory support.

Pulmonary Shunting

Pulmonary shunting is defined as that portion of the cardiac output that moves from the right side to the left side of the heart without being exposed to alveolar oxygen (PAO_2). Pulmonary shunting is divided into the following two categories: (1) **absolute shunt** (also called **true shunt**) and (2) **relative shunt** (also called **shunt-like effect**). As discussed in more detail in the following section, all forms of pulmonary shunting lead to **venous admixture** and a decreased PaO_2 level.

Absolute Shunt. **Absolute shunts** (also called *true shunt*) are commonly classified under two major categories: **anatomic shunt** and **capillary shunt**.

Anatomic shunts occur when blood flows from the right side of the heart to the left side without coming in contact with an alveolus for gas exchange (Figure 10-1, *B*). In the healthy lung, there is a normal anatomic shunt of about 3% of the cardiac output. This normal shunting is caused by non-oxygenated blood completely bypassing the alveoli and entering (1) the pulmonary vascular system by means of the bronchial venous drainage, and (2) the left atrium by way of the **thebesian veins**. Common causes of anatomic shunt include the following:
- Congenital heart disease
- Intrapulmonary fistula
- Vascular lung tumors.

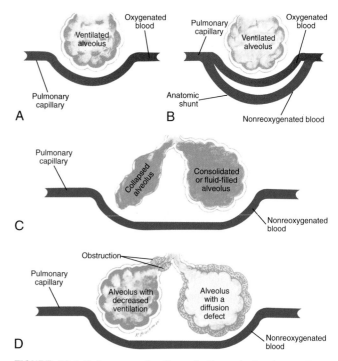

FIGURE 10-1 Pulmonary shunting. **A**, Normal alveolar-capillary unit. **B**, Anatomic shunt. **C**, Types of capillary shunt. **D**, Types of relative or shunt-like effect.

Capillary shunts are caused by (1) alveolar collapse or atelectasis, (2) alveolar fluid accumulation, or (3) alveolar consolidation or pneumonia (Figure 10-1, *C*).

The sum of both the anatomic shunt and capillary shunt make up the **absolute**, or **true**, **shunt**. The patient with absolute shunting responds poorly to oxygen therapy because of the two pathologic mechanisms:
1. In an *anatomic shunt*, the alveolar oxygen does not come in direct contact with the shunted blood—that is, the non-oxygenated blood completely bypasses the ventilated alveoli and mixes downstream with the oxygenated blood.
2. When a *capillary shunt* is present, the non-oxygenated blood passes alveoli that are not ventilated—and, as a result—moves downstream as venous blood and mixes with the oxygenated blood.

The patient with absolute shunting is **refractory** to oxygen therapy. In short, the reduced arterial oxygen level caused by this type of pulmonary shunting cannot be easily treated by increasing the concentration of oxygen for these two major reasons: (1) because of the pathology associated with an absolute shunt, the alveoli are unable to accommodate any form of ventilation, and (2) the blood that bypasses the normal, functional alveoli is unable to carry more oxygen once it has become fully saturated—except for a very small amount of oxygen that dissolves in the plasma ($PO_2 \times 0.003 =$ dissolved O_2).

Relative Shunt. When pulmonary capillary perfusion is in excess of alveolar ventilation, **a relative shunt**, or a **shunt-like effect** is said to be present (Figure 10-1, *D*). *Relative shunt* are caused by an **airway obstruction**, an **alveolar-capillary diffusion defect**, or a combination of both.

Airway obstruction leads to poor ventilation of the distal airways. As a result, the pulmonary capillary blood flow is greater than the alveolar ventilation—in short, a decreased $\dot{V}/\dot{Q}$ ratio exists. This condition results in a relative shunt, or shunt-like effect—which, in turn, causes the PaO_2 to fall (Figure 10-1, *D*). Common respiratory disorders that cause airway obstruction include emphysema, chronic bronchitis, asthma, and cystic fibrosis.

Alveolar-capillary diffusion defects occur when an abnormality in the structure of the alveolar-capillary membranes slows the movement of oxygen between the alveoli and the pulmonary capillary blood. Under these conditions, the pulmonary capillary blood passing by the alveolus does not have enough time to equilibrate with the alveolar oxygen tension. This condition results in a relative shunt, or shunt-like effect—which, in turn, causes the PaO_2 to fall (Figure 10-1, *D*). Common causes of diffusion defects include interstitial pulmonary edema and interstitial lung disorders (e.g., asbestosis, scleroderma, or idiopathic pulmonary fibrosis). A relative shunting may also occur following the administration of drugs that cause an increase in cardiac output or dilation of the pulmonary vessels. Unlike an absolute shunt, which is refractory to oxygen therapy, conditions that cause a shunt-like effect are more easily corrected (at least partially) by oxygen therapy.

Table 10-1 illustrates the type of pulmonary shunting associated with common respiratory disorders.

Venous Admixture. **Venous admixture** is defined as the mixing of shunted, non-oxygenated blood with reoxygenated blood distal to the alveoli—that is, downstream in the pulmonary venous system in route to the left side of the heart (Figure 10-2). When venous admixture occurs, the shunted—non-oxygenated—blood gains oxygen molecules while, at the same time, the reoxygenated blood loses oxygen molecules. This process continues until (1) the PO_2 throughout all the plasma of the newly mixed blood is in equilibrium, and (2) all the hemoglobin molecules carry the same number of oxygen molecules.

The final result of venous admixture is (1) a "downstream" blood mixture that has a higher PO_2 and CaO_2 than the original shunted, non-oxygenated blood, and (2) a lower PO_2 and CaO_2 than the original reoxygenated blood—in other words, a blood mixture with PaO_2 and CaO_2 values somewhere between the original values of the reoxygenated and non-oxygenated blood. The overall final outcome of venous admixture is a reduced PaO_2 and CaO_2 level returning to the left side of the heart. Clinically, it is this oxygen mixture that is evaluated downstream (e.g., from the radial artery) to assess the patient's arterial blood gases.

To calculate a patient's pulmonary shunting, see pulmonary shunt fraction discussion, Chapter 5 (Oxygenation Assessment), page 75.

Ventilation-Perfusion ($\dot{V}/\dot{Q}$) Ratio Mismatch

Under normal conditions, the overall alveolar ventilation is about 4 L/min and pulmonary capillary blood flow is about 5 L/min, making the average overall ratio of ventilation to blood flow about 4:5 or 0.8. This relationship is expressed as the **ventilation-perfusion ratio ($\dot{V}/\dot{Q}$) ratio** (Figure 10-3).

TABLE 10-1 Type of Pulmonary Shunting Associated With Common Respiratory Diseases

Respiratory Diseases	Capillary Shunt	Relative or Shunt-like Effect
Chronic bronchitis		X
Emphysema		X
Asthma		X
Croup/epiglottitis		X
Sleep apnea		X
Bronchiectasis*	X	X
Cystic fibrosis*	X	X
Pneumoconiosis*	X	X
Cancer of the lungs	X	X
Guillain-Barré syndrome	X	X
Myasthenia gravis	X	X
Pneumonia	X	
Lung abscess	X	
Tuberculosis	X	
Fungal diseases	X	
Pulmonary edema	X	
Flail chest	X	
Pneumothorax	X	
Kyphoscoliosis	X	
Interstitial lung disease	X	
Adult respiratory distress syndrome	X	
Pleural diseases	X	
Respiratory distress syndrome	X	
Near drowning	X	
Smoke inhalation	X	
Atelectasis	X	

*Relative or shunt-like effect is most common.

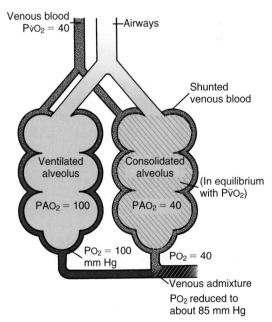

FIGURE 10-2 Venous admixture occurs when reoxygenated blood mixes with nonreoxygenated blood distal to the alveoli. Technically, the PO_2 in the pulmonary capillary system will not equilibrate completely because of the normal $P(A-a)O_2$. The PO_2 in the pulmonary capillary system is normally a few millimeters of mercury less than the PO_2 in the alveoli.

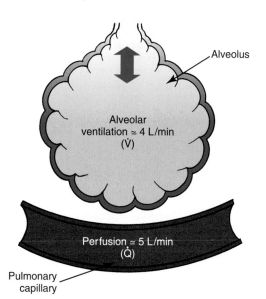

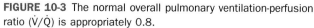

FIGURE 10-3 The normal overall pulmonary ventilation-perfusion ratio ($\dot{V}/\dot{Q}$) is appropriately 0.8.

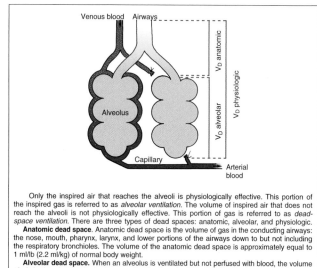

Only the inspired air that reaches the alveoli is physiologically effective. This portion of the inspired gas is referred to as *alveolar ventilation*. The volume of inspired air that does not reach the alveoli is not physiologically effective. This portion of gas is referred to as *dead-space ventilation*. There are three types of dead spaces: anatomic, alveolar, and physiologic.
Anatomic dead space. Anatomic dead space is the volume of gas in the conducting airways: the nose, mouth, pharynx, larynx, and lower portions of the airways down to but not including the respiratory bronchioles. The volume of the anatomic dead space is approximately equal to 1 ml/lb (2.2 ml/kg) of normal body weight.
Alveolar dead space. When an alveolus is ventilated but not perfused with blood, the volume of air in the alveolus is dead space, that is, the air within the alveolus is not physiologically effective in terms of gas exchange. The amount of alveolar dead space is unpredictable.
Physiologic dead space. The physiologic dead space is the sum of the anatomic dead space and the alveolar dead space. Because neither of these two forms of dead space is physiologically effective in terms of gas exchange, the two forms are combined and are referred to as *physiologic dead space*. (See Physiologic Dead-Space Calculation, Appendix IX.)

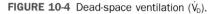

FIGURE 10-4 Dead-space ventilation ($\dot{V}_D$).

In some disorders, such as pulmonary embolism, the lungs receive less blood flow in relation to ventilation. When this condition develops the $\dot{V}/\dot{Q}$ ratio increases. A larger portion of the alveolar ventilation, therefore, will not be physiologically effective and the patient will be said to demonstrate "wasted" or dead-space ventilation (Figure 10-4).

In many lung disorders (e.g., asthma, emphysema, pulmonary edema, or pneumonia), the lungs receive less ventilation in relation to blood flow. When this condition develops, the $\dot{V}/\dot{Q}$ ratio decreases. A decreased $\dot{V}/\dot{Q}$ ratio leads to a **relative shunt**, or **shunt-like effect**, which in turn leads to venous admixture and a decreased PaO_2 (Figure 10-1, *D*).

Dead-Space/Tidal Volume Ratio. In the clinical setting, the patient's alveolar dead space is often expressed as a ratio to tidal volume (V_D/V_T ratio). The V_D/V_T ratio provides a good reference of the patient's wasted ventilation (i.e., both the

anatomic and alveolar dead space) per each breath. The calculation of the V_D/V_T ratio requires both a sample of the patient's arterial CO_2 ($PaCO_2$) and the mixed expired CO_2 ($P_{\bar{E}}CO_2$). The $PaCO_2$ is usually obtained from a routine arterial blood gas sample, and the $P_{\bar{E}}CO_2$ can be collected in a sampling bag or balloon or estimated via capnography. The V_D/V_T ratio uses a modified form of the Bohr equation, which assumes that there is no CO_2 in the inspired gas. The V_D/V_T ratio is written as follows:

$$\frac{V_D}{V_T} = \frac{PaCO_2 - P_{\bar{E}}CO_2}{PaCO_2}$$

where $PaCO_2$ is the arterial CO_2 tension, and the $P_{\bar{E}}CO_2$ is the expired CO_2 tension. Thus, if a patient has a $PaCO_2$ of 40 mm Hg and a $P_{\bar{E}}CO_2$ of 30 mm Hg, the V_D/V_T ratio would be calculated as follows:

$$\frac{V_D}{V_T} = \frac{PaCO_2 - P_{\bar{E}}CO_2}{PaCO_2}$$
$$= \frac{40 - 30}{40}$$
$$= \frac{10}{40}$$
$$= 0.25 \text{ or } 25\%.$$

The V_D/V_T ratio in the normal adult breathing spontaneously ranges between 20% and 40%. For patients receiving **mechanical ventilation**, the normal V_D/V_T ratio ranges between 40% and 60%, because of the "mechanical dead space" added by the endotracheal tube, etc. The V_D/V_T ratio increases with diseases that cause significant dead space, such as pulmonary embolism.

Decreased Partial Pressure of Inspired Oxygen (Decreased PiO₂)

Hypoxemia can also develop from decreases in inspired oxygen. For example, hypoxemia can develop at high altitudes. This is because the partial pressure of inspired air oxygen progressively decreases in response to the falling barometric pressure that occurs at high altitudes. The higher the altitude above sea level, the lower the barometric pressure. The lower the barometric pressure, the lower the inspired partial pressure of oxygen. For example, at an altitude of 18,000 to 19,000 feet, the barometric pressure is about half the sea-level value of 760 mm Hg (380 mm Hg). The barometric pressure on the summit of Mount Everest (altitude: 29,028 feet) is about 250 mm Hg (the atmospheric PO_2 is about 43 mm Hg). It is not uncommon for a mountain climber to use an oxygen mask. At an altitude of about 65,000 feet, the barometric pressure falls below the pressure of water vapor, and tissue fluids begin to "boil" or "vaporize." Airlines correct for the decreased barometric pressure by pressurizing their cabins.[2] However, the individual with chronic hypoxemia may still require supplemental oxygen during the flight.

---

[2]Most commercial jet aircraft fly at cruising altitudes between 30,000 and 40,000 feet. The barometric pressure (P_B) at sea level is about 760 mm Hg (14.7 psi). At 30,000 feet above sea level, the P_B is about 226 mm Hg (4.4 psi); at 40,000 feet, the P_B is about 104 mm Hg (2.7 psi). To prevent people from passing out from the lack of oxygen at these high cruising altitudes, the plane's cabin is pressurized at a comfortable altitude between 6000 and 8000 feet—which provides a P_B between 609 mm Hg (11.8 psi) and 563 mm Hg (10.9 psi), respectively.

Identifying the Pathophysiologic Mechanisms of Acute Hypoxemic Respiratory Failure. To more effectively treat the patient, the **alveolar-arterial oxygen tension difference [P(A-a)O$_2$]** can be used to identify the primary cause of the hypoxemic respiratory failure—*alveolar hypoventilation, pulmonary shunting,* or *$\dot{V}/\dot{Q}$ mismatch*. The clinical determination of the P(A-a)O$_2$ is made by subtracting the PaO$_2$ (obtained from an arterial blood gas) from the PAO$_2$, which is obtained from the **ideal alveolar gas equation**:

$$PAO_2 = FIO_2\,(P_B - PH_2O) - PaCO_2/RQ$$

where P$_B$ is the barometric pressure, PAO$_2$ is the partial pressure of oxygen within the alveoli, PH$_2$O is the partial pressure of water vapor in the alveoli (which is 47 mm Hg), FIO$_2$ is the fractional concentration of inspired oxygen, PaCO$_2$ is the partial pressure of arterial carbon dioxide, and RQ is the respiratory quotient. The RQ is the ratio of carbon dioxide production ($\dot{V}CO_2$) divided by **oxygen consumption** ($\dot{V}O_2$). Under normal circumstances, about 250 mL of oxygen per minute is consumed by the tissue cells and about 200 mL of carbon dioxide is excreted into the lung. Thus, the RQ is normally about 0.8, but can range from 0.7 to 1.0. Clinically, 0.8 is generally used for the RQ. For example, consider the following case example:

Case Example. If a patient is receiving an FIO$_2$ of 0.30 on a day when the barometric pressure is 750 mm Hg, and if the patient's PaCO$_2$ is 70 mm Hg and PaO$_2$ is 60 mm Hg, the P(A-a)O$_2$ can be calculated as follows:

$$
\begin{aligned}
PAO_2 &= FIO_2\,(P_B - PH_2O) - PaCO_2/RQ \\
&= 0.30\,(750 - 47) - 70/0.8 \\
&= (703)\,0.30 - 87.5 \\
&= 123.4 \text{ mm Hg.}
\end{aligned}
$$

Using the PaO$_2$ obtained from the arterial blood gas, the P(A-a)O$_2$ can now easily be calculated as follows:

$$
\begin{array}{r}
123.4 \text{ mm Hg (PAO}_2) \\
- 60.0 \text{ mm Hg (PaO}_2) \\
\hline
63.4 \text{ mm Hg [P(A-a)O}_2]
\end{array}
$$

The normal P(A-a)O$_2$ on room air at sea level ranges from 7 to 15 mm Hg, and it should not exceed 30 mm Hg. Although the P(A-a)O$_2$ may be useful in patients breathing a low FIO$_2$, it loses some of its sensitivity in patients breathing a high FIO$_2$. The P(A-a)O$_2$ increases at high oxygen concentrations. Because of this, the P(A-a)O$_2$ has less value in the critically ill patient who is breathing a high oxygen concentration. The normal P(A-a)O$_2$ for an FIO$_2$ of 1.0 is between 25 and 65 mm Hg. The critical value is greater than 350 mm Hg.

When conditions such as obesity or drug overdose lead to **alveolar hypoventilation** and, subsequent, hypoxemic respiratory failure, the (P[A-a]O$_2$) is normal—thus, indicating that the lungs are normal. In these cases, the treatment management is directed at a ventilatory support strategy. These patients readily respond to ventilator therapy.

When a **$\dot{V}/\dot{Q}$ mismatch** or **pulmonary shunting** is the primary cause of the hypoxemic respiratory failure, the (P[A-a]O$_2$) is elevated. In these cases, the administration of

oxygen is used to identify the specific pathologic basis of the hypoxemic respiratory failure—that is, a $\dot{V}/\dot{Q}$ mismatch or pulmonary shunting. The patient with a $\dot{V}/\dot{Q}$ mismatch shows significant improvement with oxygen therapy—indicating that the patient's $\dot{V}/\dot{Q}$ status has not been permanently altered. By contrast, the patient with an absolute shunt shows little to no improvement with oxygen therapy—even at an FIO$_2$ of 1.0. In these cases, the treatment needs to focus on the cause of the intrapulmonary shunting. For example, therapeutic efforts are directed at opening collapsed alveoli (atelectasis), reducing pulmonary edema, or mobilizing excessive secretions that lead to atelectasis.

Table 10-2 summarizes the major causes of hypoxemic respiratory failure, the pathophysiologic mechanism, the typical P(A-a)O$_2$ findings, and the expected patient response to oxygen therapy.

Hypercapnic Respiratory Failure (Type II) (Ventilatory Failure)

Hypercapnic respiratory failure (type II) term is used when the primary problem is alveolar hypoventilation. Patients with hypercapnic respiratory failure demonstrate an increased PaCO$_2$ and, without supplemental oxygen, a decreased PaO$_2$.[3] The major pathophysiologic mechanisms that result in hypercapnic respiratory failure are (1) alveolar hypoventilation, (2) increased dead-space disease, and (3) $\dot{V}/\dot{Q}$ ratio mismatch. Box 10-2 provides common respiratory disorders associated with hypercapnic respiratory failure.

Types of Ventilatory Failure

In the clinical setting, *hypercapnic respiratory failure* is commonly referred to as **ventilatory failure**. Based on the arterial blood PaCO$_2$ and pH values, ventilatory failure can be further classified as either (1) **acute ventilatory failure** (high PaCO$_2$ and low pH), or (2) **chronic ventilatory failure** (high PaCO$_2$ and normal pH).

In addition, chronic ventilatory failure is often complicated by conditions that cause the patient to either *hyperventilate* or *hypoventilate*—that is, on top of (in addition to) their chronic ventilatory failure. In these cases, the patient is said to have either (1) **acute alveolar hyperventilation superimposed on chronic ventilatory failure**, or (2) **acute ventilatory failure (hypoventilation) superimposed on chronic ventilatory failure**. The different classifications of ventilatory failure are discussed in more detail in the following paragraphs.

Acute ventilatory failure (acute respiratory acidosis) is a condition in which the lungs are unable to meet the metabolic demands of the body in terms of CO$_2$ removal. As a result, the PaCO$_2$ rises and, without supplemental oxygen, the PaO$_2$ falls. When an increased PaCO$_2$ level is accompanied

---

[3]In addition to the patient's arterial blood gas status discussed here, key clinical indicators of hypercapnic respiratory failure are also reflected in the patient's tidal volume (V$_T$), respiratory rate (breaths per minute), maximum inspiratory pressure (MIP), vital capacity (VC), and work of breathing (e.g., minute ventilation and dead-space/tidal volume ratio [V$_D$/V$_T$ ratio]). See Table 10-9, under standard criteria for mechanical ventilation, page 146.

TABLE 10-2 Causes of Hypoxemic Respiratory Failure

Cause of Hypoxemic Respiratory Failure	Pathophysiologic Mechanism	P(A-a)O$_2$ Findings	General Response to Oxygen Therapy	Examples
Alveolar Hypoventilation	Decreased minute ventilation—increased PaCO$_2$, decreased PaO$_2$	Normal	Good—with ventilatory support or increased alveolar ventilation	• Drug overdose • Oversedation • Obesity • Head trauma • Myasthenia gravis • Guillain-Barré syndrome
Pulmonary Shunting	Venous admixture (venous blood mixing with arterial blood)	Increased	Poor	• Atelectasis • Pneumonia • Alveolar fibrosis • ARDS • Pulmonary edema
Ventilation-Perfusion Mismatch	Venous admixture (non-oxygenated blood mixing with arterial blood)	Increased	Good	• Emphysema • Chronic bronchitis • Asthma • Pulmonary embolus
Decrease in Inspired Oxygen (decreased FIO$_2$ or PiO$_2$)	Decreased oxygen concentration or decreased inspired oxygen pressure (e.g., decreased barometric pressure)	Normal	Good	• High altitude • Low oxygen content of gas mixture • Enclosed breathing spaces (suffocation)

ARDS, Acute respiratory distress syndrome.

BOX 10-2 Respiratory Disorders Associated With Hypercapnic Respiratory Failure* (Ventilatory Failure)

- **Pulmonary Disorders**
  - Emphysema
  - Chronic bronchitis
  - Asthma
  - Cystic fibrosis
- **Respiratory Center Depression**
  - Drug overdose
  - Cerebral trauma or infarction
  - Bulbar poliomyelitis
  - Encephalitis
- **Neuromuscular Disorders**
  - Myasthenia gravis
  - Guillain-Barré syndrome
  - Spinal cord trauma
  - Muscular dystrophy
- **Pleural and Chest Wall Disorders**
  - Flail chest
  - Pneumothorax
  - Pleural effusion
  - Kyphoscoliosis
  - Obesity
- **Sleep Apnea**

*It should be noted that any of the pulmonary disorders associated with hypoxemic respiratory failure can—when severe enough—lead to hypercapnic respiratory failure.

TABLE 10-3 Acute Ventilatory Failure (Acute Respiratory Acidosis)

ABG Changes	Example
pH: decreased	7.17
PaCO$_2$: increased	79 mm Hg
HCO$_3^-$: increased (but normal)	28 mEq/L
PaO$_2$: decreased	49 mm Hg*

ABG, Arterial blood gas.
*Moderate to severe hypoxemia.

by acidemia (decreased pH), *acute ventilatory failure*, or *acute respiratory acidosis*, is said to exist. Table 10-3 shows an ABG example of acute ventilatory failure. Clinically, this is a life-threatening medical emergency that requires ventilatory support.

Chronic ventilatory failure (compensated respiratory acidosis) is defined as a greater-than-normal PaCO$_2$ level with a normal pH status. The renal system has compensated for the low pH by adding more bicarbonate (HCO$_3^-$) to the patient's blood. Although chronic ventilatory failure is most commonly seen in patients with severe chronic obstructive pulmonary disease (e.g., chronic bronchitis, emphysema, or cystic fibrosis), it is also seen in several chronic restrictive lung disorders (e.g., obesity, severe tuberculosis, fungal disease, kyphoscoliosis, or interstitial lung disease). Table 10-4 shows an ABG example of chronic ventilatory failure with hypoxemia.

Acute Alveolar Hyperventilation Superimposed on Chronic Ventilatory Failure. Like any other patient (healthy or unhealthy), the patient with chronic ventilatory failure can also acquire an acute shunt-producing disease (e.g., pneumonia or pulmonary edema). For example, when such a patient has the

TABLE 10-4 Chronic Ventilatory Failure (Compensated Respiratory Acidosis)

Baseline ABG Values*	
ABG Changes	Example
pH: normal	7.37
$PaCO_2$: increased	77 mm Hg
HCO_3^-: increased (significantly)	43 mEq/L
PaO_2: decreased	61 mm Hg

ABG, Arterial blood gas.
*Note: Chronic ventilatory failure ABG baseline values are much different than the ABG baseline values of the normal individual (e.g., pH: 7.35–7.45; $PaCO_2$: 35–45; HCO_3^-: 22–26; PaO_2: 80–100).

TABLE 10-5 Acute Alveolar Hyperventilation Superimposed on Chronic Ventilatory Failure*

ABG Changes	Example
pH: increased	7.51
$PaCO_2$: increased (but lower than patient's typical elevated baseline level)	52 mm Hg
HCO_3^-: increased (significantly) (but lower than patient's typical elevated baseline level)	40 mEq/L
PaO_2: decreased (but lower than patient's typical low baseline level)	49 mm Hg

ABG, Arterial blood gas; *COPD*, chronic obstructive pulmonary disease.
*This condition is often seen in patients with acute bronchitis, pneumonia, or pulmonary edema that exacerbate their COPD.

TABLE 10-6 Acute Ventilatory Failure Superimposed on Chronic Ventilatory Failure

ABG Changes	Example
pH: decreased	7.28
$PaCO_2$: increased (but higher than patient's typical elevated baseline level)	97 mm Hg
HCO_3^-: increased (significantly) (but higher than patient's typical elevated baseline level)	44 mEq/L
PaO_2: decreased (but lower than patient's typical low baseline level)	39 mm Hg

ABG, Arterial blood gas.

TABLE 10-7 Examples of Acute Changes Superimposed on Chronic Ventilatory Failure

Acute Ventilatory Failure on Chronic Ventilatory Failure	Chronic Ventilatory Failure (Baseline Values)	Acute Alveolar Hyperventilation on Chronic Ventilatory Failure
7.28 ←	pH 7.37	→ 7.51
97 ←	$PaCO_2$ 77	→ 52
44 ←	HCO_3^- 43	→ 40
39 ←	PaO_2 61	→ 49

mechanical reserve to increase their alveolar ventilation significantly in an attempt to maintain their baseline PaO_2, their $PaCO_2$ often decreases from their normally high baseline level. This action causes their pH to increase. As this condition intensifies, the patient's baseline ABG values can quickly change from chronic ventilatory failure to **acute alveolar hyperventilation superimposed on chronic ventilatory failure** (Table 10-5).

Acute Ventilatory Failure (Hypoventilation) Superimposed on Chronic Ventilatory Failure. When the patient with chronic ventilatory failure does *not* have the mechanical reserve to meet the hypoxemic challenge of a respiratory disorder, the patient begins to breathe less.[4] This action causes the $PaCO_2$ to increase above the patient's already high $PaCO_2$ baseline level. As the $PaCO_2$ suddenly increases, the patient's arterial pH level falls, or becomes acidic. As this condition intensifies, the patient's baseline ABG values change from chronic ventilatory failure to **acute ventilatory failure superimposed on chronic ventilatory failure**—acute on chronic ventilatory failure (Table 10-6).

Table 10-7 provides a summary overview of (1) chronic ventilatory failure, (2) acute hyperventilation superimposed on chronic ventilatory failure, and (3) acute ventilatory failure superimposed on chronic ventilatory failure.

---

[4]Oftentimes, the patient demonstrates acute alveolar hyperventilation superimposed on chronic ventilatory failure before becoming fatigued and acute ventilatory failure superimposed on chronic ventilatory failure develop. Clinically, this condition is called "impending ventilatory failure."

Mechanical Ventilation

Before a decision can be made to commit the patient to any form of mechanical ventilation, the respiratory therapist must first answer these questions: Does the patient demonstrate the standard criteria for mechanical ventilation? Are key clinical indicators of respiratory failure present? Does the patient primarily have hypoxemic respiratory failure, or hypercapnic respiratory failure, or a combination of both? Which ventilatory support strategy would best serve the patient's short-term or long-term ventilatory needs—that is, **noninvasive ventilation** or **invasive ventilation**?

To satisfactorily answer these questions, moreover, it is also essential that the respiratory therapist use good clinical judgment skills—which are based on the ability to (1) collect all the clinical data relevant to the patient's respiratory status, (2) formulate an objective—and measurable—respiratory assessment, (3) select a safe and effective ventilatory support plan, and (4) clearly and correctly document the subjective and objective data, assessment, and ventilatory support plan.

Standard Criteria for Mechanical Ventilation

The four standard criteria for mechanical ventilation are (1) **apnea**, (2) **acute ventilatory failure**, (3) **impending ventilatory failure**, and (4) **severe refractory hypoxemia**. To help determine if the mechanical ventilation should be invasive or noninvasive, the respiratory therapist should establish if the patient is able to protect their own airway for each of these criteria. *Apnea* is defined as the complete absence of spontaneous ventilation—which is an absolute indication for invasive mechanical ventilation. Apnea causes the PaO_2 to rapidly decrease and the $PaCO_2$ to increase. Death will ensue in minutes. *Acute ventilatory failure* is defined as a sudden increase in $PaCO_2$ to greater than 50 mm Hg with an accompanying low pH value (<7.30). *Impending ventilatory failure* occurs when the patient demonstrates a significant increase in the work of breathing, but with only a borderline acceptable arterial blood gas. *Severe refractory hypoxemia* is a critically low oxygenation status that does not respond well to oxygen therapy. Severe refractory hypoxemia is often seen in cases of severe pneumonia, interstitial lung diseases, and acute respiratory distress syndrome. Table 10-8 presents the basic criteria for mechanical ventilation and the primary type of respiratory failure associated with these conditions.

Prophylactic Ventilatory Support

In addition to the four primary criteria for mechanical ventilation, the decision to place the patient on ventilatory support may be based on prophylactic reasons. For example, **prophylactic ventilatory support** is often provided to patients in whom the risk of pulmonary complications, or hypercapnic respiratory failure, or hypoxemic respiratory failure is high. For example, prophylactic ventilatory support is sometimes provided to patients in postanesthesia recovery.

Key Clinical Indicators for Hypercapnic and Hypoxemic Respiratory Failure

There are a variety of key clinical indicators (laboratory and bedside) that can be used to help establish the need for ventilatory support. In addition, these clinical indicators can also be used to determine (1) the primary type of respiratory failure, and (2) the ventilatory strategy that may be used to safely and effectively ventilate the patient. Table 10-9 lists key clinical indicators associated with hypercapnic respiratory failure. Table 10-10 provides key clinical indicators associated with hypoxemic respiratory failure.

Ventilatory Support Strategy

The selection of a ventilatory support strategy is based on the type of respiratory failure the patient demonstrates. For example, *hypoxemic respiratory failure* is treated with various oxygen therapy modalities to manage the patient's oxygenation status. Table 10-11 provides common oxygenation treatments for specific causes of hypoxemia.

By contrast, *hypercapnic respiratory failure* is treated with ventilatory support techniques to manage the patient's PCO_2 levels and acid-base status. Both oxygen and ventilatory support modalities are used when the patient demonstrates both hypoxemic and hypercapnic respiratory failure (sometimes referred to as **Type III respiratory failure**). Either **noninvasive ventilation** or **invasive ventilation** can be used as a ventilatory support strategy.

Noninvasive ventilation (NIV) is defined as any mode of ventilatory support that does not require an invasive artificial airway (i.e., endotracheal tube or tracheostomy tube). As shown in Box 10-3, NIV has many benefits and is often the first choice for ventilatory support. NIV systems include **continuous positive airway pressure (CPAP)** alone (which is a forced vital capacity [FRC]—restoring treatment modality to improve oxygenation, not a method of ventilatory [CO_2] support), or in combination with any mode of **pressure-limited** or **volume-limited ventilation**. Both hypoxemic and hypercapnic type respiratory failure can be managed effectively by NIV.

TABLE 10-9 Key Clinical Indicators of Hypercapnic Respiratory Failure (Ventilatory Failure)

Clinical Indicator*	Normal Value	Critical Value
Alveolar Ventilation		
• $PaCO_2$ (acute change)	35-45 mm Hg	>50 mm Hg and rising
• pH	7.35-7.45	<7.2
Lung Expansion		
• Tidal volume (V_T)	5-8 mL/kg	<3 to 5 mL/kg
• Respiratory rate (breaths/min)	12-20/min	>30/min, or <10/min
Muscle Strength		
• Maximum inspiratory pressure (MIP, cm H_2O)	–80 to 100 cm H_2O	<–20 cm H_2O
• Vital capacity (VC)	65-75 mL/kg	<10 to 15 mL/kg
Work of Breathing		
• Minute ventilation ($\dot{V}E$)	5-6 L/min	>10 L/min
• V_D/V_T (%)	25-40%	>60%

*See a detailed discussion of these clinical indications for hypercapnic respiratory failure in Chapter 3: Pulmonary Function Assessment, and Chapter 4: Arterial Blood Gas Assessment.

TABLE 10-8 Criteria for Instituting Mechanical Ventilation and the Primary Type of Respiratory Failure Associated With These Conditions

Criteria for Instituting Mechanical Ventilation	Primary Type of Respiratory Failure
1. Apnea	
2. Acute Ventilatory Failure	Hypercapnic Respiratory Failure
3. Impending Ventilatory Failure	
4. Severe Refractory Hypoxemia	Hypoxemic Respiratory Failure

TABLE 10-10 Key Clinical Indicators of Hypoxemic Respiratory Failure (Oxygenation Failure)

Clinical Indicator*	Normal Value	Critical Value
Oxygenation Status		
• PaO_2 (mm Hg)	80 to 100	<60 on FIO_2 >0.50
• $P(A-a)O_2$ on 100%	25-65	>350
• PaO_2/PAO_2 ratio	0.75-0.95	<0.15
• PaO_2/FIO_2 ratio	350-450	<200
• $\dot{Q}_S/\dot{Q}_T$ (%)	<5	>20

*See a detailed discussion of these oxygen clinical indications in Chapter 5: Oxygenation Assessment.

TABLE 10-11 Common Oxygen Treatment Modalities for Specific Causes of Hypoxemia

Cause of Hypoxemia	Treatment

• Alveolar Hypoventilation—examples:
  • COPD
  • Drug overdose
	• Ventilatory support—increased alveolar ventilation

• Decreased ventilation/perfusion ratio—examples:
  • COPD
  • Asthma
  • Pulmonary edema
	• Ventilatory support
	• Oxygen
	• CPAP
	• PEEP

• Pulmonary shunting—examples:
  • Pneumonia
  • Atelectasis
  • ARDS
	• Oxygen via:
	  • CPAP
	  • PEEP

• Decreased barometric pressure • High attitude	• Oxygen • Move to lower altitude

ARDS, Acute respiratory distress syndrome; *COPD*, chronic obstructive pulmonary disease; *CPAP*, continuous positive airway pressure; *PEEP*, positive end expiratory pressure.

BOX 10-3 Benefits of Noninvasive Ventilation

- Avoids endotracheal intubation
- Reduces problems associated with intubation—for example, airway trauma, increased risk of aspiration, and nosocomial pneumonia
- Maximizes patient comfort
- Decreases mortality
- Increases alveolar ventilation
- Improves alveolar oxygen (PAO_2) and carbon dioxide ($PACO_2$) status
- Opens and/or prevents alveolar collapse
- Reduces the work of breathing
- Decreases oxygen consumption
- Decreases muscle fatigue

The primary indication for NIV is *hypercapnic respiratory failure* secondary to chronic obstructive pulmonary disease (COPD) exacerbation. NIV is also beneficial for a variety of other respiratory disorders when the patient is able to protect their own airway—including (1) asthma, (2) hypoxemic respiratory failure, (3) community-acquired pneumonia, (4) cardiogenic pulmonary edema, (5) acute respiratory distress syndrome, (6) obesity-hypoventilation syndrome, and (7) neuromuscular diseases such as myasthenia gravis or Guillain-Barré syndrome.

Although NIV is usually a very safe and effective means of ventilatory support, it may be poorly tolerated, contraindicated, or even harmful in patients with (1) respiratory arrest, (2) cardiac arrest, (3) nonrespiratory organ failure—for example, severe encephalopathy, severe gastrointestinal bleeding or hemodynamic instability, (4) upper airway obstruction, (5) excessive or viscous airway secretions, (6) a poor ability to clear secretions, (7) an improperly fitting mask, (8) facial or head trauma or surgery, (9) profound refractory hypoxemia, (10) cardiovascular instability—for example, hypotension, dysrhythmias, or acute myocardial infarction, (11) an inability to cooperate—for example, impaired mental status, somnolence, (12) extreme obesity, or (13) the anticipation of a slowly resolving respiratory condition.

In these cases, invasive ventilation is required.

Invasive mechanical ventilation is defined as mechanical ventilation via an endotracheal tube or tracheostomy tube. Both hypoxemic and hypercapnic type respiratory failure can be managed effectively by invasive mechanical ventilation. Acute respiratory distress syndrome, pulmonary edema, severe asthma, and flail chest are examples of some clinical conditions that often require invasive ventilatory support for the primary purpose of oxygenation.

Mechanical Ventilation Protocols

It is interesting to note that many medical centers have started their therapist-driven protocol (TDP) programs with a Mechanical Ventilation Protocol rather than with one of the relatively simple protocols described in Chapter 9 (e.g., Oxygen Therapy Protocol, Bronchial Hygiene Protocol, Lung Expansion Protocol, or Aerosolized Medical Protocol). The decision to proceed in this manner often appears to be based on humanistic, pathophysiologic, and economic grounds. Indeed, who could defend practices that are unnecessary (if not harmful), uncomfortable, and costly to patients requiring ventilator support?

Although there are a number of good ventilatory management strategies used to treat specific respiratory failure problems, the need for a standardized approach to ventilatory management has required the development of Mechanical Ventilation Protocols. Protocol 10-1 provides an example of a **Ventilator Initiation and Management Protocol**. Protocol 10-2 provides an example of a **Ventilator Weaning Protocol**.[5]

Unquestionably, the high technology, high-risk, high visibility portion of respiratory therapy work is embedded in ventilator management. Much of the success of the TDP movement has occurred because of the dramatic ways in which standardized, data-driven algorithms have improved patient outcomes. Most dramatic outcomes include shortened ventilator weaning times, reduction of nosocomial infections, and reduced complication rates of mechanical ventilation (e.g., barotrauma).

Although most Mechanical Ventilation Protocols require the respiratory therapist to select a ventilator mode on the basis of specific patient needs, it is not the intent of this textbook to fully review or discuss the various ventilator modes and weaning strategies. Table 10-12, however, does provide an overview of common ventilatory management strategies and good starting points used to treat specific pulmonary disorders.

---

[5]The authors would like to thank the Respiratory Care Department at the Kettering Health Network, in Dayton, Ohio, for providing their Ventilator Initiation and Management Protocol and Ventilator Weaning Protocol.

TABLE 10-12 Common Ventilatory Management Strategies Used to Treat Specific Disorders (Good Starting Points)

Disorder	Disease Characteristics	Ventilator Mode	Tidal Volume and Respiratory Rate	Flow Rate	I : E Ratio	FIO₂	General Goals and/or Concerns
Normal Lung Mechanics But patient has apnea (e.g., drug overdose or abdominal surgery)	Normal compliance and airway resistance	Volume ventilation in the AC or SIMV mode Or pressure ventilation—either PRVC or PC	4 to 8 mL/kg of ideal body weight 10-12 breaths/min or slower rates (6-10 breaths/min) when SIMV mode is used	60-80 L/min	1 : 2	Low to moderate	Care to ensure plateau pressure of 30 cm H₂O or less Small tidal volumes (<7 mL/kg) should be avoided, because atelectasis can develop
Chronic Obstructive Pulmonary Disease (e.g., chronic bronchitis or emphysema)	High lung compliance and high airway resistance	Volume ventilation in the AC or SIMV mode Or pressure ventilation—either PRVC or PC Noninvasive positive pressure ventilation (NPPV) by nasal or full face mask is a good alternative during acute exacerbation	Good starting point: 4 to 8 mL/kg and a rate of 10 to 12 breaths/min A smaller tidal volume (8-10 mL/kg) and slightly slower rate (8-10 breaths/min) with increased flow rates to allow adequate expiratory time	60 L/min 60–100 L/min	1 : 2 or 1 : 3	Low to moderate	Air trapping and auto-PEEP can occur when expiratory time is too short. The preferred method of managing auto-PEEP is to increase expiratory time In severe cases, the development of auto-PEEP may be inevitable. With controlled ventilation, a small amount of PEEP to offset auto-PEEP may be cautiously applied Inspiratory flow up to 100 L/min may be helpful in decreasing inspiratory time and increasing expiratory time Tidal volume or rate may be decreased to reduce inspiratory and increasing expiratory time Care to avoid overventilating COPD patients with chronically high PaCO₂ levels

Condition	Characteristics	Mode	Tidal Volume / Rate	Flow	I:E Ratio	FIO2	Comments
Acute Asthmatic Episode	High airway resistance (bronchospasm and excessive thick airway secretions)	The SIMV mode is recommended to avoid patient triggering at an increased rate—leading to a decrease in expiratory time and further air trapping	Good starting point: 8 to 4 to 8 mL/kg and rate of 10-12 breaths/min. When air trapping is extensive, a lower tidal volume (5-6 mL/kg) and slower rate may be required	60 L/min	1:2 or 1:3	Start at 100% and titrate downward as pulse oximetry findings and arterial blood gas values permit	In severe cases, the development of auto-PEEP may be inevitable. With controlled ventilation, a small amount of PEEP to offset auto-PEEP may be cautiously applied
Acute Respiratory Distress Syndrome	Diffuse, uneven alveolar injury	Volume ventilation in the AC or SIMV mode or pressure ventilation—either PRVC or PC	Typically started at low tidal volumes and higher respiratory rate. Initial tidal volume set at 8 mL/kg and adjusted downward to 6 mL/kg. May be as low as 4 mL/kg. Respiratory rates as high as 35 breaths/min may be required	60-80 L/min	1:1 or 1:2. Do what is necessary to meet a rapid respiratory rate	FIO_2 less than 0.6 if possible	The goal is to limit transpulmonary pressure and the resultant barotraumas caused by overdistending portions of the lungs. Maintaining a plateau pressure of 30 cm H_2O or less is preferred. PEEP is usually required with a low tidal volume to prevent atelectasis. The $PaCO_2$ may be allowed to increase (**permissive hypercapnia**). The hypercapnia is not a therapeutic goal, it is a final tradeoff and may be accepted as a lung protective strategy when lower airway pressures are necessary
Postoperative Ventilatory Support (e.g., coronary artery bypass surgery, heart valve and replacement)	Often normal compliance and airway resistance	SIMV with pressure support or AC volume ventilation are acceptable modes or pressure ventilation—either PRVC or PC	Good starting point: 10 to 4 to 8 mL/kg and a rate of 10 to 12 breaths/min	60 L/min	1:2	Low to moderate	PEEP or CPAP of 3 to 5 cm H_2O may be applied to offset the development of atelectasis
Neuromuscular Disorders (e.g., myasthenia gravis or Guillain-Barré syndrome)	Normal compliance and airway resistance	Volume ventilation in the AC or SIMV mode or pressure ventilation—either PRVC or PC	Good starting point: 4 to 8 mL/kg and a rate of 10 to 12 breaths/min	60 L/min	1:2	Low to moderate	PEEP of 3 to 5 cm H_2O may be applied to offset the development of atelectasis

AC, Assist-control; breaths/min, breaths per minute; CPAP, continuous positive airway pressure; PC, pressure control; PEEP, positive end expiratory pressure; PRVC, pressure regulated volume control; SIMV, synchronized intermittent mandatory ventilation.

VENTILATOR INITIATION AND MANAGEMENT PROTOCOL

PURPOSE:
The Respiratory Therapist will utilize the following protocol to determine the most appropriate settings to maintain and manage oxygenation and ventilation for mechanically ventilated patients.

PATIENT TYPE:
All adult patients requiring mechanical ventilation

EQUIPMENT NEEDED:
- Pulse oximeter
- Ventilator
- Stethoscope
- Oxygen analyzer
- Wright respirometer
- NIP manometer
- EKG monitor
- Heated aerosol with appropriate attachments
- $ETCO_2$ analyzer (if available)

LABORATORY DATA NEEDED:
Recent arterial blood gas results, chest x-ray

OVERVIEW

| Patient meets criteria for mechanical ventilation | → | Stabilization of patient's ventilatory status | → | Initiation (A) and adjustment (B) of ventilatory support to meet patient's physical condition | → | Reversal/ stabilization of underlying condition | → | Ventilator Weaning Protocol and extubation |

| STEP 1 | STEP 2 A&B | STEP 3 | STEP 4 (Protocol 10-2) |

STEP 1: CRITERIA FOR MECHANICAL VENTILATION AND CERTIFICATION OF STABILITY SHORT OF MECHANICAL INTUBATION

Assure that the patient meets criteria for mechanical ventilation as below. Assure that the basic underlying pathophysiology has been treated optimally, short of mechanical ventilation. If you have questions, check with attending physician.

Step 1 Indications for mechanical ventilation include:

A. Basic Indications

1. Acute respiratory failure (ARF)

    a. Acute hypoxic respiratory failure with tachypnea, respiratory distress, and persistent hypoxemia despite administration of high FIO_2 via high flow system or in the presence of any of the following:
    1) acute cardiovascular instability
    2) altered mental status
    3) inability to protect lower airway

    b. Acute hypercarbic ventilatory failure with tachypnea, respiratory distress, and persistent hypoxemia despite administration of high FIO_2 via high flow system or in the presence of any of the following:
    1) pH <7.30
    2) acute cardiovascular instability
    3) altered mental status
    4) inability to protect lower airway

2. Apnea

3. Impending Acute Respiratory Failure: Studies have failed to define "impending ventilatory failure." This remains the judgment call of the attending physician.

Modified from the Respiratory Care Department at the Kettering Health Network, in Dayton, Ohio

PROTOCOL 10-1P1

B. Clinical Conditions That May Require Mechanical Ventilation

1. Acute exacerbation of COPD if patient has dyspnea, tachycardia, and acute respiratory acidosis plus at least one of the following:

   a. Acute cardiovascular instability
   b. Altered mental status
   c. Inability to protect lower airway
   d. Copious/viscous secretions
   e. Progressive respiratory acidosis despite non-invasive positive pressure ventilation (mask CPAP)

2. Neuromuscular disease with any of the following:

   a. Acute respiratory acidosis
   b. Progressive decrease in VC to <10-15 mL/kg
   c. Progressive decrease in NIP to < −20 cm H_2O

3. Cardiac or respiratory arrest

4. Postoperative patients requiring ongoing sedation

5. Other complex medical conditions leading to impending acute respiratory failure as determined by the attending physician

6. In the following conditions, **Non-Invasive Positive Pressure Ventilation (NIPPV)** should be attempted before intubation:

   a. Dyspnea / respiratory distress
   b. Acute exacerbation of COPD without other indicators listed above
   c. Acute hypoxemia in immunocompromised patients
   d. Cardiogenic pulmonary edema

STEP 2: INITIATION (A) AND ADJUSTMENT (B) OF VENTILATION SUPPORT
A. DEVICE AND VENTILATOR MODE SELECTION

The following guidelines will be used in <u>selecting the most appropriate ventilator mode</u>:

I. **Volume Control Ventilation** (although no ventilatory mode has been proven better than another, volume control is generally accepted as a traditional method of ventilation – a good place to start).

1. Benefits

   a. Clinician has direct control over Tidal Volume (V_T) and Minute Ventilation ($\dot{V}_E$)
   b. Appropriate starting place for newly intubated patients

2. Limitations

   a. Decreased lung compliance will result in high airway pressures
   b. May not be able to appropriately ventilate patients with very poor lung compliance

3. Modes

   a. **Assist Control (A/C)**

      1) Most effective mode for unloading of respiratory muscles
      2) Can be used with patients with no spontaneous respiratory effort
      3) Should be used as long as hyperventilation is necessary to normalize pH (e.g., renal failure with decreased HCO_3^- or metabolic ketoacidosis)
      4) Things to consider with A/C

         a) Alkalosis – if patient assists at high respiratory rate
         b) Auto PEEP if patient assists at high respiratory rate
         c) Increased PIP if lung compliance decreases or if patient assists at high respiratory rate. Both static and dynamic lung compliance should be calculated and documented at least Q8 hours, regardless of the mode of ventilation (see Section II, 4 b and c)

   b. **Synchronized Intermittent Mechanical Ventilation (SIMV)**

      1) Normal rate SIMV provides unloading of respiratory muscles with less risk of respiratory alkalosis than A/C.
      2) Prevents respiratory muscle atrophy
      3) Things to consider with SIMV

         a) Fatigue / tachypnea if rate set too low
         b) Hypercapnia if rate set too low
         c) High demand valve-imposed WOB in older ventilators

      4) Pressure Support (PS) should be used in conjunction with SIMV if the patient has spontaneous respiratory effort above the set ventilator rate. This helps to overcome the resistance to air flow caused by ventilator tubing and ETT, and avoids increased WOB.
      5) The use of SIMV / PS in the clinical setting has not proven as efficient a weaning mode as compared to T-piece trials and pressure support ventilation. Compared to T-piece trials and PSV, it is associated with the longest weaning time and the lowest success rates.

PROTOCOL 10-1P2

II Pressure Controlled Ventilation (PCV)

1. Benefits

   a. In spontaneously breathing patients, the variable flow characteristic of PCV is more comfortable and may actually decrease WOB – especially in patients with variable respiratory demand.
   b. Patients who are air hungry when being ventilated with low tidal volumes in volume ventilation modes may experience less dyspnea with PCV because of the variable flow and patient-dependent nature of the mode.
   c. Peak airway pressures are able to be controlled and still ventilate the patient.

2. Limitations

   a. V_T is not pre-set and therefore is not guaranteed.
   b. V_T is dependent on lung compliance and is subject to change quickly.
   c. Alarms are essential in PCV to ensure adequate ventilation.
      1) V_T is set 50-100 mL above and below target V_T
      2) Placing exhaled minute ventilation within 1 liter/min. of target $\dot{V}E$

3. Consider placing patient on PCV if:

   a. V_T and V_E are compromised because inspiration terminates when pressure limit is reached in volume control mode.
   b. Patient is spontaneously breathing and appears to be air hungry. PCV may be able to meet patient demand because of its variable flow characteristics.
   c. Patient's oxygenation status requires inverse ratio ventilation (IRV). A physician's order must be received for I:E ratio less than 1:2 (e.g., 1:1.5, 1:1, 2:1, etc.).

4. Compliance

   a. Abnormally low or high lung compliance impairs the lung's ability to effectively exchange gases. Low compliance makes expansion difficult and high compliance induces incomplete exhalation and compromises CO_2 elimination. Changes in lung compliance may greatly impact volumes achieved in pressure control mode.
   b. Dynamic lung compliance should be calculated and documented at least every 6 hours, using the following formula:
      $$C_{dyne} = V_T \text{ (in mL)} \div (PIP - PEEP)$$
   c. **Static lung compliance** should be calculated and documented at least every 6 hours using the following formula:
      $$C_{stat} = V_T \div (P_{plat} - PEEP)$$. Critically low Cstat is <25 mL/cm H_2O.

III Bi-Level Ventilation

1. Benefits

   a. The same as those for PCV
   b. Has been found to result in better gas exchange than CMV (either volume controlled or pressure controlled) in ARDS patients.
   c. Patients requiring Inverse Ratio Ventilation (IRV):
      1) Bi-level may reduce need for sedation and/or paralytics and allow patients to breathe spontaneously.
      2) IRV must be ordered by an attending physician.

2. Limitations

   a. V_T and V_E are not pre-set. They are not guaranteed.
   b. Alarms must be set 50-100 mL above and below target V_T in order to assure adequate ventilation.
   c. Bi-level ventilation is not available on all ventilators.

3. Patients who require PCV may be placed on bi-level as long as an appropriate ventilator is available and the patient's I:E level is 1:2 or greater. It patient requires less than 1:2 I:E (e.g., 1:1.5; 1:1; 2:1, etc.), an order from the attending physician must be obtained.

IV Airway Pressure Release Ventilation (APRV)

1. Benefits

   a. Airway Pressure Release Ventilation (APRV) has been found to result in better gas exchange than CMV (either volume controlled or pressure controlled) in ARDS patients.
   b. APRV may reduce need for sedation and/or paralytics and allow patients to breathe spontaneously.

2. Limitations

   a. V_T and $\dot{V}_E$ are not pre-set. They are not guaranteed.
   b. Alarms must be set 50-100 mL above and below target V_T in order to assure adequate ventilation.
   c. APRV is not available on all ventilators.
   d. APRV can only be initiated with the order of the attending physician.

PROTOCOL 10-1P3

V Pressure Support Ventilation (CPAP/PS)

1. Benefits

   a. Peak flow and V_T are entirely patient dependent.
   b. Prevents respiratory muscle atrophy.

2. Limitations

   a. V_T and $\dot{V}_E$ are not guaranteed, therefore alarms must be set and monitored closely.
   b. Respiratory muscles may become fatigued.

3. Use on patients who

   a. Have stable lung compliance
   b. Are spontaneously breathing
   c. Are hemodynamically stable

4. Things to observe

   a. Sedation levels
   b. Sudden changes in $\dot{V}_E$
   c. Fatigue
   d. Tachypnea
   e. Hypercapnea
   f. Increased WOB

B. Adjustment of Ventilatory Support
The following guidelines will be used in selecting the most appropriate ventilatory settings.

A. **Tidal Volume** (V_T): 6-8 mL/kg ideal body weight

1. Reasons for using small volumes:

   a. Minimizes ventilator-induced lung injury (volutrauma and/or barotrauma)
   b. Improved clinical outcomes for ARDS patients

2. V_T may be increased if:

   a. Patient's demand is not met AND
   b. Plateau pressures are < 30 cm H_2O

3. IBW is calculated using the following formulas:

   a. Females – 100 pounds for the first 5 feet in height + 5 pounds for each additional inch of height, divided by 2.2 to convert pounds to kilograms (kg)

      e.g., a 5'5" female, weighing 250 pounds has an ideal body weight of [100 + (5×5)] / 2.2 100+25 = 125 pounds divided 2.2 = 57 kg and should be placed on V_T of about 340 mL based on 6 mL/kg IBW.

   b. Males – 106 pounds for the first 5 feet of height + 6 pounds for each additional inch in height, divided by 2.2 to convert pounds to kilograms (kg)

      e.g., a 6'1" male, weighing 310 pounds has an ideal weight of [106 + (6×13)] / 2.2 106+78 = 184 pounds divided 2.2 = 85 kg and should be placed on V_T of about 500 mL based on 6 mL/kg IBW.

B. **Pressure Control (PC) Level** (if patient being ventilated in pressure mode as opposed to volume mode):

1. Inspiratory pressure should be set and adjusted to keep V_T within 50 to 100 mL of the selected target of 6 mL/kg IBW.
2. Setting I:E ratio in pressure control ventilation:

   a. I:E ratio should be set between 1:2 and 1:4 for most patients.
   b. When setting I:E, observe patient and waveforms to determine if patient has time for full exhalation.
   c. When traditional I:E ratio has failed to improve patient's ventilation and oxygenation status, inverse ratio ventilation (IRV) may be used, pending physician's approval.
   d. The use of sedation and paralytics may be necessary when a patient is being ventilated with IRV in PC.
   e. If a patient's oxygen status requires ventilation at less than 1:2 I:E ratio (e.g., 1:1.5; 1:1; 2:1, etc.), ventilator settings must be ordered by the attending physician.

PROTOCOL 10-1P4

C. Respiratory Rate (RR)

1. Once V_T or PC level is chosen, frequency is set to provide a $\dot{V}_E$ that achieves adequate pH.
2. As a starting point, RR 12-20/min is considered physiological in adults.

   a. When using small V_T per protocol (6 mL/kg IBW), higher RRs will be needed to achieve adequate $\dot{V}_E$.
   b. ABG should be obtained 30 minutes after initiation of mechanical ventilation. The following formula is used to determine the appropriate RR:

   $$\text{New Rate} = \frac{\text{current vent rate} \times \text{current } P_aCO_2}{^*\text{Desired } P_aCO_2}$$

   For example: 5'8" male has IBW ~ 75 kg and V_T is set at 450 mL and rate 14.
   ABG shows pH = 7.29, PCO$_2$ = 56. Respiratory therapist wishes to reduce P_aCO_2 to 45.

   $$\text{New Rate} = \frac{14 \times 56}{45} = 17$$

   c. If respiratory therapist determines that both V_T and RR should change as a result of the ABG, use the following formulas, instead:

   $$\text{New } \dot{V}_E = \frac{\text{current } \dot{V}_E \times \text{current } P_aCO_2}{^*\text{Desired } P_aCO_2}$$

   $$\text{New RR} = \frac{\text{desired } \dot{V}_E}{\text{New } V_T}$$

For example: 5'2" female has IBW ~ 55 kg and is placed on V_T of 330 and RR of 16. ABG shows pH = 7.25, P_aCO_2 = 62. Plateau pressures = 14 cm H_2O; therefore, the respiratory therapist decides to increase both V_T and RR. The patient's plateau pressure is 20 at a V_T of 400 mL. The respiratory therapist selects V_T of 400 mL. The demand P_aCO_2 is 45 mm Hg.

$$\text{New } \dot{V}_E = \frac{5.28 \times 62}{45} = 7.27$$

$$\text{New RR} = \frac{7.27}{.400} = 18$$

Desired is not necessarily normal P_aCO_2

D. Positive End Expiratory Pressure (PEEP)

1. Application of PEEP in patient with ARDS receiving mechanical ventilation may improve oxygenation and increase lung volume.
2. PEEP is especially important in maintaining lung volumes and recruiting alveoli when ventilating at low tidal volumes.
3. Setting Optimal PEEP: Normally, the alveolar and end-expiratory pressure equilibrates with atmospheric pressure (i.e. zero pressure) and the average pleural pressure is approximately −5 cm H_2O. Under these conditions, the alveolar distending pressure is 5 cm H_2O (alveolar-pleural). This distending pressure is sufficient to maintain a normal end-expiratory alveolar volume to overcome the elastic recoil of the alveoli.

   a. Patients without expiratory flow limitations (no COPD or asthma).

      1) If ICP and cardiovascular status are **stable**, set PEEP at 5 cm H_2O and make changes based on ABG results, FIO_2 requirements, tolerance of PEEP, and cardiovascular response.
      2) If ICP and/or cardiovascular status is **unstable**, set PEEP at 3 cm H_2O and increase only if attending physician agrees that risk of hypoxemia is greater than risk of increased ICP or cardiovascular collapse.

   b. Patients with expiratory flow limitations (COPD/asthma) are subject to intrinsic PEEP.

      1) Prior to changing PEEP to overcome expiratory flow limitations, adjust RR and peak flow to maximize expiratory time.
      2) If patient is not breathing spontaneously (e.g. sedated), calculate intrinsic PEEP and set PEEP at 85% of that value.
      3) If patient is breathing spontaneously and has PRN sedation ordered, work with RN to coordinate intrinsic PEEP measurement with administration of sedation.
      4) If patient is breathing spontaneously so that intrinsic PEEP measurement is impossible, an optimal PEEP study may be performed.

4. Utilizing PEEP to meet oxygenation goals.

   a. Arterial oxygenation is the driving force behind setting optimal PEEP and FIO_2 levels; however, maximizing oxygenation is not the only goal for patients with refractory hyoxemia.

      1) PaO$_2$ of 55-80 with saturation of 88-95% are acceptable therapeutic goals.*
      2) The following guide should be used in determining appropriate combined PEEP and FIO_2 levels:

* Recently, a prediction equation for the "new" FIO_2 setting has been reported by El-Khatib and Chatburn which can easily be determined using a scientific calculator. AJRCCM (2012) 185:685-686. We are currently validating the utility of this approach.

PROTOCOL 10-1P5

PEEP AND FIO$_2$ GUIDELINES																	
PEEP (cm H$_2$O) Combined with FIO$_2$	5 →	5 →	8 →	8 →	10 →	10 →	10 →	12 →	14 →	14 →	14 →	16 →	18 →	18 →	20 →	22 →	24 →
	0.3	0.4	0.4	0.5	0.5	0.6	0.7	0.7	0.8	0.9	0.9	1.0	1.0	1.0	1.0	1.0	1.0

IF MEASURED VALUE IS BELOW GOAL (PaO$_2$ 55-80 AND/OR SATURATION 88-95%) MOVE UP ONE STEP.
IF PEEP > 10 AND FIO$_2$ > 0.60 CALL ATTENDING PHYSICIAN BEFORE PROCEEDING THROUGH TABLE.

Example:

Patient was intubated yesterday for acute ventilatory failure with hypoxemia. Patient placed on the following settings: V$_T$ 500, A/C rate 12, PEEP+5, FIO$_2$ 0.40. ABG has been within normal limits on those settings. This morning, however, oxygen saturation is dropping and CXR indicates patient is in ARDS. By using the chart on the previous page, the ventilatory changes would be as follows:

Increase PEEP to 8 with FIO$_2$ at 0.40. If saturation improves, leave on those settings. If saturation continues to drop or does not improve, proceed to next step on the chart.

Increase FIO$_2$ to 0.50 with PEEP at 8. If saturation improves, leave on those settings. If saturation continues to drop or does not improve, proceed to next step on the chart.

Increase PEEP to 10 with FIO$_2$ 0.50. If saturation improves, leave on those settings. If saturation continues to drop or does not improve, proceed to next step on the chart.

Increase FIO$_2$ to 0.60 with PEEP at 10. At this point, **call physician.**

E. Pressure Support (PS)

1. Pressure support may be used in conjunction with SIMV. In this case, PS increases the patient's spontaneous tidal volume, decreases spontaneous respiratory rate, and decreases work of breathing.
   a. PS can be set to maintain spontaneous V$_T$ to meet the patient's ventilatory requirements while keeping RR < 25.
   b. PS can be set to overcome resistance of airflow cause by ETT, thereby decreasing WOB. In this case, PS should be calculated using the following formula:

   1) $$\frac{(PIP - PEEP) - (Plateau\ Pressure - PEEP)}{Peak\ Flow \div 60}$$

   e.g., PIP 45 cm H$_2$O P$_{plat}$ 24 cm H$_2$O, peak flow 70 L/min

   $$PS = \frac{(45-6) - (24-6)}{70 \div 60} = \frac{39 - 18}{.17} = 17.95\ cm\ H_2O$$

   Therefore, PS should be set at 18 for those conditions.

   2) If Tubing Compensation (TC) is available, it may be used instead of PS to compensate for resistance to airflow caused by tubing. TC makes adjustments breath to breath to ensure proper support levels.
   c. If patient's RR > 25 or WOB is visibly increased, patient should be returned to A/C until underlying condition resolved.
   d. The use of SIMV/PS in the clinical setting has not proven as an efficient weaning mode as compared to T-piece trials and pressure support ventilation. Compared to T-piece trials and PSV, it is associated with the longest weaning and the lowest success rates.
2. Pressure support may be used as a spontaneous ventilatory mode in conjunction with CPAP in patients who do not require a ventilator rate to ensure adequate ventilation.
   a. The difference between the PS level and the CPAP level is the driving pressure and should be set at a level that meets patient's ventilatory demand with RR > 25.
   b. PS may be decreased as the patient's condition and lung compliance improves (see above formula).
   c. Low V$_T$ and/or $\dot{V}_E$ alarms are essential to ensure adequate ventilation in PSV mode.

F. Peak Inspiratory Flow

1. Peak inspiratory flow (PF) should be set at the lowest possible flow to maintain I:E ratio and patient comfort.
   a. Normal I:E is 1:2 to 1:4 for mechanically ventilated patients.
   b. Larger I:E ratio should be used on patients needing additional time for exhalation due to air trapping and intrinsic PEEP.
2. Flow rate may be used to change I:E. This should be monitored with each ventilator check.
3. Decelerating flow pattern should be utilized whenever it is available to assure optimal gas distribution, lower inspiratory pressures, improved patient comfort, and reduced WOB.

PROTOCOL 10-1P6

G. <u>Bi-Level</u>

1. A form of augmented pressure ventilation that allows for unrestricted spontaneous breathing at any moment of the ventilator cycle, thereby promoting patient/ventilator synchrony.

   a. The initial settings of upper PEEP ($PEEP_H$) and lower PEEP ($PEEP_L$) should be based on the set PEEP and the plateau pressure during volume ventilation.

   b. $PEEP_L$ is adjusted to obtain adequate oxygenation (refer to setting PEEP C-4).

   c. $PEEP_H$ is usually set at 12-16 above $PEEP_{L2}$ depending on patient lung compliance. It should be set to ensure V_T of 6 mL/kg IBW.

   d. PS can be added to assist spontaneous breathing in bi-level.

      1) Since PS is delivered above the $PEEP_L$ level, the RCP must calculate the PS level needed.

         e.g., Patient is set on bi-level of 24/5 ($PEEP_L$ 5) for a driving pressure of 19 cm H_2O (the difference between $PEEP_H$ and $PEEP_L$). You have calculated that you need a PS of 8 to overcome resistance to airflow caused by tubing (see formula on previous page). In order for patient's spontaneous breaths taken at $PEEP_H$ to be supported, PS must be set so that peak pressure on PS breaths is 8 cm H_2O higher than $PEEP_H$.

         $PEEP_H - PEEP_L + PS$ needed to overcome resistance = needed PS

         24 cm H_2O − 5 cm H_2O + 8 cm H_2O = 27 cm H_2O

   e. If a patient's oxygen status requires ventilation at less than 1:2 I:E ratio (e.g., 1:1.5; 1:1; 2:1, etc.), ventilator settings must come from the attending physician.

Ventilator Management – General Instructions

A. <u>New Ventilator Protocol Orders</u>

When a new ventilator protocol order is written on a patient who has been on mechanical ventilation for 24 hours or longer and ordered on $V_T > 8$ mL/kg IBW, proceed as follows:

1. Calculate IBW.
2. Calculate desired V_T.
3. Titrate V_T by reducing 1 mL/kg Q2 hours until 8 mL/kg IBW has been achieved.
4. Increase respiratory rate to ensure that $\dot{V}_E$ remains the same.
5. After achieving 8 mL/kg IBW, obtain an ABG after 30 minutes of last change.

B. <u>Monitoring patient response to therapy</u>

1. Respiratory therapist will obtain an ABG 30 minutes after the patient has been placed on initial ventilator protocol settings.
2. Respiratory therapist will obtain an ABG 30 minutes after any significant change in ventilator settings (increase or decrease in $V_T > 100$ mL or increase/decrease respiratory rate ≥ 4 bpm.
3. SpO_2 monitor will be used to titrate PEEP and FIO_2.

STEP 3: REVERSAL / STABILIZATION OF UNDERLYING CONDITION

This depends on its etiology and the knowledge and skills of the caregivers. Review management of each condition (as outlined elsewhere in this volume). Be aware that new conditions may develop while the patient is on the ventilator (see box) and treat accordingly.

- Pneumothorax
- Pleural effusion
- Obstructed endotracheal tube
- Fluid overload
- Cardiac arrhythmias
- Pulmonary embolism
- Ventilator-associated pneumonia
- Congestive heart failure
- Pulmonary edema
- Atelectasis

STEP 4: VENTILATOR WEANING PROTOCOL AND EXTUBATION
See Protocol 10-2

PROTOCOL 10-1P7

MECHANICAL VENTILATION WEANING PROTOCOL

PURPOSE:
The Respiratory Therapist will utilize the following protocol to facilitate timely liberation from mechanical ventilation.

PATIENT TYPE AND CLINICAL INDICATIONS
All adolescent, adult, and geriatric patients requiring mechanical ventilation

OVERVIEW

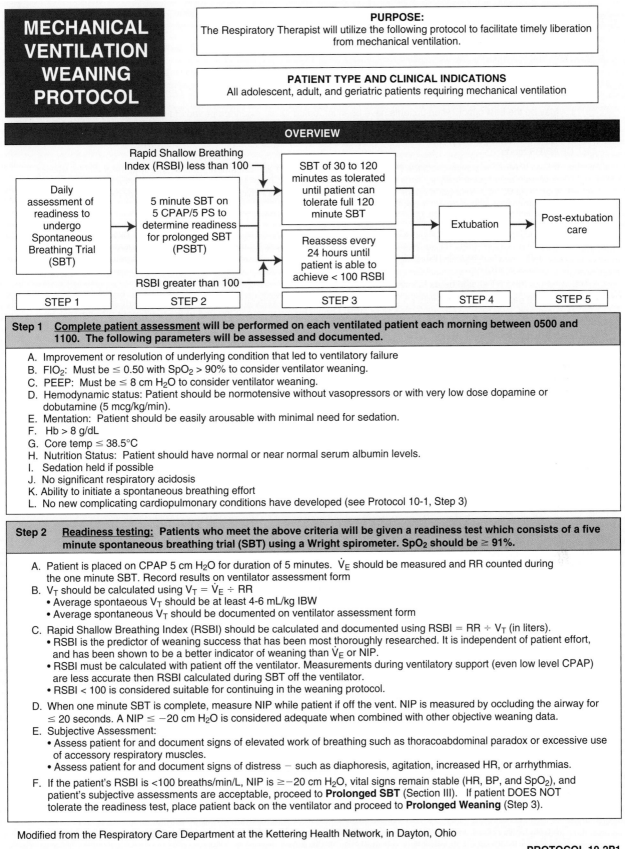

| STEP 1 | STEP 2 | STEP 3 | STEP 4 | STEP 5 |

Daily assessment of readiness to undergo Spontaneous Breathing Trial (SBT) → 5 minute SBT on 5 CPAP/5 PS to determine readiness for prolonged SBT (PSBT) — Rapid Shallow Breathing Index (RSBI) less than 100 / RSBI greater than 100 → SBT of 30 to 120 minutes as tolerated until patient can tolerate full 120 minute SBT / Reassess every 24 hours until patient is able to achieve < 100 RSBI → Extubation → Post-extubation care

---

Step 1 <u>Complete patient assessment</u> **will be performed on each ventilated patient each morning between 0500 and 1100. The following parameters will be assessed and documented.**

A. Improvement or resolution of underlying condition that led to ventilatory failure
B. FIO_2: Must be ≤ 0.50 with $SpO_2 > 90\%$ to consider ventilator weaning.
C. PEEP: Must be ≤ 8 cm H_2O to consider ventilator weaning.
D. Hemodynamic status: Patient should be normotensive without vasopressors or with very low dose dopamine or dobutamine (5 mcg/kg/min).
E. Mentation: Patient should be easily arousable with minimal need for sedation.
F. Hb > 8 g/dL
G. Core temp $\leq 38.5°C$
H. Nutrition Status: Patient should have normal or near normal serum albumin levels.
I. Sedation held if possible
J. No significant respiratory acidosis
K. Ability to initiate a spontaneous breathing effort
L. No new complicating cardiopulmonary conditions have developed (see Protocol 10-1, Step 3)

Step 2 <u>Readiness testing:</u> **Patients who meet the above criteria will be given a readiness test which consists of a five minute spontaneous breathing trial (SBT) using a Wright spirometer. SpO_2 should be $\geq 91\%$.**

A. Patient is placed on CPAP 5 cm H_2O for duration of 5 minutes. $\dot{V}_E$ should be measured and RR counted during the one minute SBT. Record results on ventilator assessment form
B. V_T should be calculated using $V_T = \dot{V}_E \div RR$
   - Average spontaneous V_T should be at least 4-6 mL/kg IBW
   - Average spontaneous V_T should be documented on ventilator assessment form

C. Rapid Shallow Breathing Index (RSBI) should be calculated and documented using $RSBI = RR \div V_T$ (in liters).
   - RSBI is the predictor of weaning success that has been most thoroughly researched. It is independent of patient effort, and has been shown to be a better indicator of weaning than $\dot{V}_E$ or NIP.
   - RSBI must be calculated with patient off the ventilator. Measurements during ventilatory support (even low level CPAP) are less accurate then RSBI calculated during SBT off the ventilator.
   - RSBI < 100 is considered suitable for continuing in the weaning protocol.

D. When one minute SBT is complete, measure NIP while patient if off the vent. NIP is measured by occluding the airway for ≤ 20 seconds. A NIP ≤ -20 cm H_2O is considered adequate when combined with other objective weaning data.
E. Subjective Assessment:
   - Assess patient for and document signs of elevated work of breathing such as thoracoabdominal paradox or excessive use of accessory respiratory muscles.
   - Assess patient for and document signs of distress — such as diaphoresis, agitation, increased HR, or arrhythmias.
F. If the patient's RSBI is <100 breaths/min/L, NIP is ≥ -20 cm H_2O, vital signs remain stable (HR, BP, and SpO_2), and patient's subjective assessments are acceptable, proceed to **Prolonged SBT** (Section III). If patient DOES NOT tolerate the readiness test, place patient back on the ventilator and proceed to **Prolonged Weaning** (Step 3).

Modified from the Respiratory Care Department at the Kettering Health Network, in Dayton, Ohio

PROTOCOL 10-2P1

A. Patients should undergo a Spontaneous Breathing Trial (SBT) of 120 minutes to determine readiness to extubate.

B. Methods of providing SBT

1. Heated, humidified O_2 via T-piece

a. Recent research indicates that post-extubation WOB is the same as or greater than that imposed by the endotracheal tube.

b. May be the best option when patients have been intubated for an extended period of time and airway inflammation and/or edema is likely. Breathing unassisted through the ETT may approximate post-extubation WOB.

2. CPAP of ≤ 5 cm H_2O

3. CPAP/PS mode

a. If the CPAP/PS mode is used, the PS level must be calculated and documented to ensure that the patient does not receive more support than is necessary to overcome the work imposed by the ventilator/ventilator tubing/ETT.

b. Low level PS may be a good option when patient has a small ETT (high resistance to airflow) or excessive secretions increasing airway resistance.

- It is important to note that studies have failed to identify one of these SBT strategies as being statistically better at predicting extubation success than another. What research has proven, however, is the necessity of conducting an SBT. Thirty-seven percent (37%) of patients extubated after satisfying classically applied screening criteria required reintubation. This is up to 3 times greater than that seen among patients extubated after passing SBT.

C. The length of the SBT should be as follows:

1. In surgical patients or patients with no underlying lung disease a 30 minute SBT is usually sufficient. Results must be documented. Weaning parameters, including RSBI should be measured at the end of the trial before placing back on ventilator. Complex patients may benefit from longer PSBT periods. Examples of complex medical patients include, but are not limited to, the following:

a. COPD

b. ARDS

c. Multi-System Organ Failure (MSOF)

d. Patients over 70 years of age (these patients have the highest incidence of reintubation and should complete a full 120 minutes SBT prior to extubation).

D. Use the following to determine response to the PSBT.

1. Criteria to extubate:

a. RR < 30

b. $SpO_2 \geq 92\%$ on $\leq 50\%$ FIO_2. If patient is a COPD patient, will accept SpO_2 of 88%. An SpO_2 less than 92% (88% in COPD patients) for 5 minutes results in termination of the PSBT.

c. No signs of respiratory distress as evidenced by any two of the following:

1) Pulse > 120% of the rate before initiation of SBT

a) e.g., if pulse **before** SBT is 70, pulse should not exceed 84 during PSBT.

b) e.g., if **before** SBT is 112, pulse should not exceed 134 during PSBT.

2) Significant change in cardiac rhythm (PVCs, atrial fib, etc.)

3) Marked use of accessory muscles of respiration

4) Thoraco-abdominal paradox

5) Diaphoresis

6) Marked dyspnea

d. For complex medical patients receiving 120 minutes PSBT, RCP should obtain an ABG at the end of the PSBT, analyze, and document.

1) If ABG results are within normal limits and above criteria are met, patient may be extubated.

2) If ABG results are outside of normal limits, but are normal for the patient, based on documented baseline ABGs and above criteria are met, patient may be extubated.

2. Criteria to call physician before determining if extubation is appropriate.

a. RR 30-35

b. ABG results are outside of satisfactory limits but no baseline is available and patient met above criteria.

3. If the patient does not meet the criteria outlined above, place back on ventilator and allow patient to rest for 24 hours. Begin the assessment / PSBT process again the following day.

Prolonged Weaning: Special Instructions

A. Patients who fail the first SBT should be placed back on the ventilator on full support and reassessed in 24 hours.

B. *Patients who fail the second* SBT should be weaned using the following guidelines:

1. Place on CPAP/PS at a PS level that provides the patient with V_T of 6-8 mL/kg and RR < 30 bpm.

2. Rest for 24 hours on those settings and repeat SBT in the a.m.

3. If SBT failed again, place back on CPAP/PS, but titrate PS level downward by 2 cm H_2O q12 hours as long as respiratory rate remains < 30 bpm.

4. Repeat SBT daily once every 24 hours.

C. SBTs should be documented daily and reported to the attending physician.

PROTOCOL 10-2P2

Step 4 Extubation

A. Criteria to extubate. Attending physician must have pre-approved extubation if criteria met (**ALL** 3 criteria must be met to extubate):

1. Patient tolerates PSBT for 120 minutes.
2. Post PSBT parameters are within normal limits.

   a. RSBI < 100
   b. RR < 30
   c. NIP ≤ -20
   d. VC (if patient able to follow commands) of 10-15 mL/kg IBW

3. ABG drawn at end of PSBT is within normal limits (or normal for the patient based on baseline).

B. Criteria to call physician prior to making the decision to extubate:

1. Patient tolerated PSBT or toleration is marginal (RR 30-35) but one of the following occurs:

   a. Post PSBT parameters do not meet above criteria **OR**
   b. Post PSBT ABG results are outside of normal limits.

C. Criteria to place back on ventilator and wait 24 hours before attempting another PSBT:

1. Patient does not tolerate PSBT

   a. RR > 35
   b. SpO_2 < 92% (88-90% for COPD patient with chronic hypoxemia)
   c. Exhibits marked dyspnea
   d. Arrhythmia which started after initiation of the PSBT.

D. The respiratory therapist may obtain a post-extubation ABG if (s)he feels it is needed to determine the patient's post-extubation status.

STEP 5 Post-Extubation Care

A. Place patient on low flow oxygen to approximate the FIO_2 delivered during the PSBT. Titrate oxygen for SpO_2 > 92% (88-92% for COPD patients with hypoxic drive to breathe).
B. Assess patient's immediate response to extubation by documenting the following:

1. Vital signs (HR and rhythm, RR and respiratory pattern, SpO_2, BP)
2. Breath sounds including presence/absence of stridor

C. If stridor is present, patient should be given stat racemic epinephrine med neb and placed on cool mist aerosol.
D. If stridor persists after one Vaponephrine treatment, notify attending physician immediately. A second Vaponephrine treatment should **NOT** be given immediately (may be given q2 hours).
E. Document extubation and post-extubation assessment on the ventilator assessment form.

Post operative heart patients (CABG and valve surgeries) in the Cardio-Thoracic Care Unit: These patients will be weaned from the ventilator using an expedited form of the SBT/PSBT process.

A. Patient will be received and placed on initial settings as follows:

1. V_T 6-8 mL
2. RR 10-20 as needed to keep $ETCO_2$ 35-45 mm Hg
3. PEEP 3-5 cm H_2O
4. FIO_2 for SpO_2 > 92%
5. May be in AC, PC or SIMV ventilator mode. If patient is on SIMV, set PS to match resistance imposed by ventilator tubing and ETT.

B. No ventilator changes should be made until initial ABG has been drawn and analyzed.
C. As soon as patient begins to wake up and has spontaneous respiratory effort, an SBT may be initiated.
   Any of the following methods may be used:

1. Heated aerosol
2. CPAP
3. CPAP/PS (PS level must be calculated to determine that which overcomes resistance of the ETT and ventilator tubing)
4. CPAP/TC if patient is ventilated by PB 840 ventilator.

D. Weaning parameters will be measured and documented when patient has tolerated PSBT for 30 minutes.
E. Patient may be extubated when 30 minutes SBT is completed and weaning parameters are within normal limits. The respiratory therapist may order an ABG before extubation if (s)he deems it necessary to determine response to PSBT.
F. Post-extubation ABG will be drawn 30-60 minutes after extubation.

TC, tube-compensation.   **PROTOCOL 10-2P3**

SELF-ASSESSMENT QUESTIONS

Answers to questions can be found on Evolve. To access additional student assessment questions visit
http://evolve.elsevier.com/DesJardins/respiratory.

1. Which of the following pulmonary condition(s) respond poorly to oxygen therapy?
   1. Chronic obstructive pulmonary disease
   2. Atelectasis
   3. Asthma
   4. Consolidation
      a. 1 only
      b. 3 only
      c. 2 and 4 only
      d. 1 and 3 only

2. A 68-year-old male presents in the emergency department with paralysis of the lower extremities that has progressively worsened over the past several hours. Arterial blood gases on room air are as follows: pH = 7.12, $PaCO_2$ 86, HCO_3^- 27, PaO_2 39, and SaO_2 70%. Which of the following is indicated?
   a. Oxygen with nonrebreathing mask
   b. Oxygen with continuous positive airway pressure
   c. Bronchodilator therapy
   d. Ventilatory support with oxygen

3. A relative shunt is caused by:
   1. Alveolar-capillary defect
   2. Atelectasis
   3. Airway obstruction
   4. Consolidation
      a. 2 only
      b. 1 and 3 only
      c. 2, 3, and 4 only
      d. 1, 2, 3, and 4

4. A 76-year-old female in the intensive care unit is in respiratory distress. She appears cyanotic and short of breath. Her vital signs are as follows: blood pressure 186/115, heart rate 125, and a respiratory rate of 35 and shallow. Her PaO_2 is 81 on an FIO_2 of 0.40. Her PaO_2/PAO_2 ratio is 0.90 and her $\dot{Q}_s/\dot{Q}_T$ is 4%. Her $PaCO_2$ is 67 and her maximum inspiratory pressure (MIP) is −12 cm H_2O. Based on this information, which of the following is the primary problem?
   a. Hypercapnic respiratory failure
   b. Hypoxemic respiratory failure
   c. Both hypoxemic and respiratory failure
   d. Severe refractory hypoxemia

5. Which of the following indicate(s) the need for ventilatory support?
   1. VC: 65 mL/kg
   2. $\dot{Q}_s/\dot{Q}_T$: <5
   3. MIP: ≥−20 (less negative)
   4. $P(A-a)O_2$: >350
      a. 1 and 3 only
      b. 2 and 4 only
      c. 3 and 4 only
      d. 1, 2, and 3 only

6. One cause of hypoxemic respiratory failure is alveolar hypoventilation. Which of the following best describes the pathophysiologic mechanism of alveolar hypoventilation?
   a. Venous blood mixing with arterial blood
   b. Decreased oxygen concentration
   c. Decreased minute ventilation
   d. Non-oxygenated blood mixing with arterial blood

7. An 81-year-old male with a long history of chronic obstructive pulmonary disease presents in the emergency department in respiratory distress. He is pursed-lip breathing and using his accessory muscles of inspiration. His heart rate is 125 and his blood pressure is 176/105. His arterial blood gases on a 2-L nasal cannula are as follows: pH 7.54, $PaCO_2$ 56, HCO_3^- 46, and PaO_2 41. Based on this information, which of the following best identifies the arterial blood gas status?
   a. Acute ventilatory failure
   b. Acute alveolar hyperventilation
   c. Acute alveolar hyperventilation superimposed on chronic ventilatory failure
   d. Acute ventilatory failure superimposed on chronic ventilatory failure

8. The $P(A-a)O_2$ finding is increased in which of the following conditions?
   1. Alveolar atelectasis
   2. Drug overdose
   3. Consolidation
   4. Obesity
      a. 1 and 3 only
      b. 2 and 4 only
      c. 1 and 2 only
      d. 2 and 3 only

9. A 67-year-old male with chronic obstructive pulmonary disease presented in the emergency department with acute alveolar hyperventilation superimposed on chronic ventilatory failure. He was taken to the intensive care unit and placed on a noninvasive ventilation (NIV) system with supplemental oxygen at an FIO_2 of 0.40. Arterial blood gas values are as follows: pH 7.22, $PaCO_2$ 84, HCO_3^- 33, PaO_2 43, SaO_2 71%. At this time, which of the following would be the most appropriate treatment?
   a. Change the patient to invasive ventilation
   b. Increase the FIO_2
   c. Recommend a sedative
   d. Change the NIV mask

10. A 57-year-old female presents in the coronary care unit in respiratory distress. She is alert and appropriately answering the doctor's questions. Her vital signs are as follows: heart rate 145, blood pressure 170/110, and respiratory rate 32. She appears cyanotic and her breath sounds reveal bilateral crackles. Arterial blood gases on a nonrebreathing oxygen mask are: pH 7.51, $PaCO_2$ 27, HCO_3^- 21, and PaO_2 46. Based on this information, which of the following would you recommend to initially treat the patient?
   a. Invasive ventilation
   b. Continuous positive airway pressure mask
   c. Noninvasive ventilation
   d. Nonrebreathing oxygen mask

CHAPTER 11

Recording Skills: The Basis for Data Collection, Organization, Assessment Skills, and Treatment Plans

Chapter Objectives

After reading this chapter, you will be able to:

- Describe the clinical importance of good charting skills.
- Differentiate among the following types of patient records:
  - Traditional charting
  - Problem-oriented medical records (POMRs), and include SOAPIER progress notes
  - Computer documentation
- Discuss the importance of the Health Insurance Portability and Accountability Act.

Key Terms

Block Chart
Computer-Based Personal Records
Electronic Health Records
Electronic Medical Records

Electronic Patient Medical Charts
Department of Health and Human Services (HHS)
Health Insurance Portability and Accountability Act (HIPAA)
Problem-Oriented Medical Record (POMR)
SOAP
SOAPIER
Source-Oriented Record
Traditional Record

Chapter Outline

Types of Patient Records
  Traditional Chart
  Problem-Oriented Medical Record (POMR)
  Computer Documentation
Health Insurance Portability and Accountability Act
Self-Assessment Questions

Because all health-care workers share information through written or electronic communication, the respiratory therapist must understand the way to document and use the patient's medical records effectively and efficiently. The process of adding documentary information to the patient's chart is called *charting*, *recording*, or *documenting*. Good charting should provide the basic clinical information necessary for critical thinking, or assessment skills—that is, good charting should be an effective way to summarize pertinent clinical data, analyze and assess it (i.e., determine the cause of the clinical data), record the formulation of an appropriate treatment plan, and document the adjustments of the treatment plan (in response to its effectiveness) after it has been implemented.

Good charting enhances communication and continuity of care among all members of the health-care team. There is a definite and direct relationship between effective charting (communication) and the quality of patient care. Good charting also provides a permanent record of past and current assessment data, treatment plans, therapy given, and the patient's response to various therapeutic modalities. This information may be used by various governmental agencies and accreditation teams to evaluate the institution's patient care and prove that care was given appropriately. Accurate and legible records are the only

means by which hospitals can prove that they are providing appropriate care and meeting established standards.

In addition, many health-care reimbursement plans (e.g., Medicare and Medicaid) are based on diagnosis related groups (DRGs). Under these plans, remuneration is based on disease diagnoses. Many private insurance companies use similar illness categories when setting hospital payment rates. Before providing reimbursement, insurance companies carefully review the patient's medical record when assessing whether appropriate and efficient care was given.

Finally, the patient's chart is a legal document that can be called into court. Even though the physician or institution owns the original record, the patient, lawyers, and courts can gain access to it. As an instrument of continuous patient care and as a legal document, the patient's chart therefore should contain all pertinent respiratory care assessments, planning, interventions, and evaluations.

Types of Patient Records

Three basic methods are used to record assessment data: the traditional chart, the **problem-oriented medical record (POMR)**, and computer documentation.

Traditional Chart

The **traditional record** (also called **block chart** or **source-oriented record**) is divided into distinct areas or blocks, with emphasis placed on specific information. The traditional record is commonly seen in the patient's chart as full-colored sheets of block information. Typical blocks of information include the admission sheet, physician's order sheet, progress notes, history and physical examination, medication sheet, nurses' admission information, nursing care plans, nursing notes, graphs and flowsheets, laboratory and x-ray reports, and discharge summary. The order, content, and number of blocks vary among institutions. The traditional chart makes recording easier, but it also makes it more difficult to review a particular event readily and efficiently or to follow the overall progress of the patient, without going back and forth among the blocks.

Problem-Oriented Medical Record (POMR)

The organization of the POMR is based on an objective, scientific, problem-solving method. The POMR is one of the most important medical records used by the health-care practitioner to (1) systematically gather clinical data, (2) formulate an assessment (i.e., the cause of the clinical data), and (3) develop an appropriate treatment plan. A number of good POMR methods are available for recording assessment data. Regardless of the method selected, it is essential that one method be adopted and used consistently.

A good POMR method should take a systematic approach in documenting the following:
- The subjective and objective information collected
- An assessment based on the subjective and objective data
- The treatment plan (with measurable outcomes)
- An evaluation of the patient's response to the treatment plan
- A section to record any adjustments made to the original treatment plan

One of the most common POMR methods is the **SOAPIER** progress note—often abbreviated in the clinical setting to a **SOAP** progress note.[1] *SOAPIER* is an acronym for seven specific aspects of charting that systematically review one health problem.

S *Subjective* information refers to information about the patient's feelings, concerns, or sensations presented by the patient:

"I coughed hard all night long."

"My chest feels very tight."

"I feel very short of breath."

Only the patient can provide subjective information. Some cases may not involve subjective information. For instance, a comatose, intubated patient on a mechanical ventilator is unable to provide subjective data.

O *Objective* information is the data the respiratory therapist can measure, factually describe, or obtain from other professional reports or test results. Objective data include the following:

- Heart rate
- Respiratory rate
- Blood pressure
- Temperature
- Breath sounds
- Cough effort
- Sputum production (volume, consistency, color, and odor)
- Arterial blood gas and pulse oximetry data
- Pulmonary function study results
- X-ray reports
- Hemodynamic data
- Chemistry results

A *Assessment* refers to the practitioner's professional conclusion about the cause of the subjective and objective data presented by the patient. In the patient with a respiratory disorder, the cause is usually related to a specific anatomic alteration of the lung. The assessment, moreover, provides the specific reason as to why the respiratory therapist is working with the patient. For example, the presence of wheezes are objective data (the clinical indicator) to verify the assessment (the cause) of bronchial smooth muscle constriction; an arterial blood gas with a pH of 7.18, a $PaCO_2$ of 80 mm Hg, an HCO_3^- of 29 mm/L, and a PaO_2 of 54 mm Hg are the objective data to verify the assessment of acute ventilatory failure with moderate hypoxemia. The presence of coarse crackles is a clinical indicator to verify the assessment of secretions in the large airways.

P *Plan* is/are the therapeutic interventions selected to remedy the cause identified in the assessment. For example, an assessment of bronchial smooth muscle constriction justifies the administration of a bronchodilator; the assessment of acute ventilatory failure justifies mechanical ventilation.

I *Implementation* is the actual administration of the specific therapy plan. It documents exactly what was done, when, and by whom.

E *Evaluation* is the collection of measurable data regarding the effectiveness of the therapy plan and the patient's response to it. For example, an arterial blood gas assessment may reveal that the patient's PaO_2 did not increase to a safe level in response to oxygen therapy.

R *Revision* refers to any changes that may be made to the original therapy plan in response to the evaluation. For example, if the PaO_2 does not increase appropriately after the implementation of oxygen therapy, the respiratory therapist might continue to increase the patient's FIO_2 until the desired PaO_2 is reached.

For the new practitioner, a predesigned SOAP form is especially useful in (1) the rapid collection and systematic organization of important clinical data, (2) the formulation of an assessment (i.e., the cause of the clinical data), and (3) the development of a treatment plan. For example, consider the case example and SOAP progress note shown in Figure 11-1.

Although the SOAP form may initially appear long and time-consuming, the experienced respiratory therapist and assessor can typically condense and abbreviate SOAP information in a few minutes (primarily at the patient's bedside), in just a few short statements. Typically, a written SOAP

---

[1]The authors fully expect that the student will become proficient in the development of good "SOAP notes" as a result of reading—and studying—this textbook.

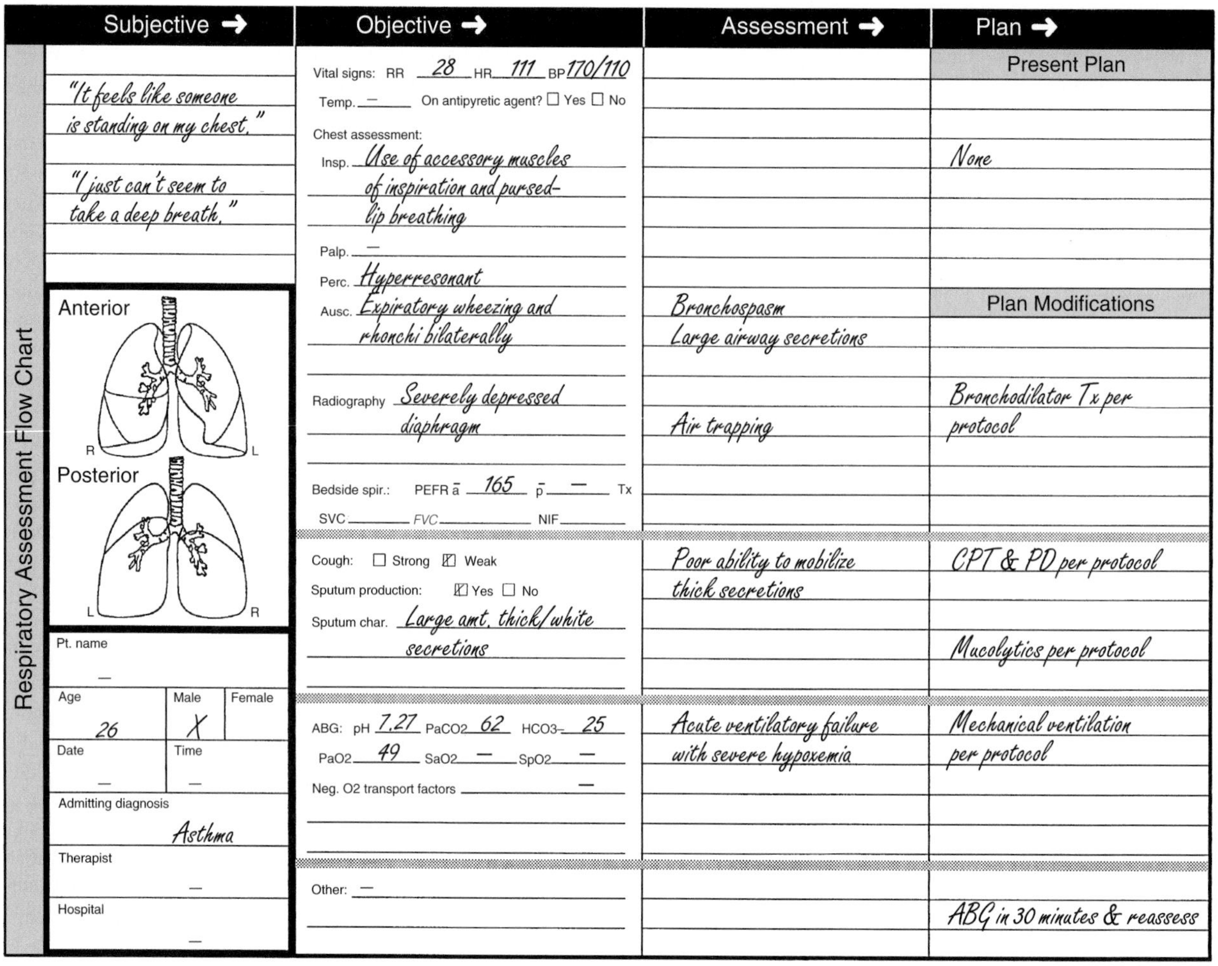

FIGURE 11-1 Completed predesigned SOAP form (see SOAP Case Example below).

The form contains the following handwritten entries organized under four columns: Subjective, Objective, Assessment, and Plan.

Subjective:
- "It feels like someone is standing on my chest."
- "I just can't seem to take a deep breath."

Respiratory Assessment Flow Chart (with Anterior and Posterior lung diagrams)
- Pt. name: —
- Age: 26
- Male: X Female:
- Date: — Time: —
- Admitting diagnosis: Asthma
- Therapist: —
- Hospital: —

Objective:
- Vital signs: RR 28 HR 111 BP 170/110
- Temp. — On antipyretic agent? ☐ Yes ☐ No
- Chest assessment:
  - Insp. Use of accessory muscles of inspiration and pursed-lip breathing
  - Palp. —
  - Perc. Hyperresonant
  - Ausc. Expiratory wheezing and rhonchi bilaterally
- Radiography: Severely depressed diaphragm
- Bedside spir.: PEFR ā 165 p̄ — Tx
  - SVC ___ FVC ___ NIF ___
- Cough: ☐ Strong ☒ Weak
- Sputum production: ☒ Yes ☐ No
- Sputum char. Large amt. thick/white secretions
- ABG: pH 7.27 PaCO2 62 HCO3- 25 PaO2 49 SaO2 — SpO2 —
- Neg. O2 transport factors ___
- Other: —

Assessment:
- Bronchospasm
- Large airway secretions
- Air trapping
- Poor ability to mobilize thick secretions
- Acute ventilatory failure with severe hypoxemia

Plan:
- Present Plan
  - None
- Plan Modifications
  - Bronchodilator Tx per protocol
  - CPT & PD per protocol
  - Mucolytics per protocol
  - Mechanical ventilation per protocol
  - ABG in 30 minutes & reassess

---

form uses only 1 to 3 inches of space in the patient's chart. For example, the information presented in Figure 11-1 may actually be documented in the patient's chart in the following abbreviated form:

S—"It feels like someone is standing on my chest. I can't take a deep breath."

O—Use of acc. mus. of insp.; HR 111, BP 170/110, RR 28 & shallow, pursed-lip; hyperresonance; exp. whz; diaph. & alv. hyperinfl.; PEFR 165; wk. cough; lg. amt. thick/white sec.; pH 7.27, PaCO₂ 62; HCO₃⁻ 27; PaO₂ 49.

A—Bronchospasm; hyperinflation; poor ability to mob. tk. sec.; acute vent. fail. with severe hypox.

P—Bronchodilator Tx/pro.; CPT & PD/pro., mucolytic/pro., mech. vent/pro., ABG 30 min.

After the treatment has been administered, another abbreviated SOAP note should be made to determine whether the treatment plan needs to be up-regulated or down-regulated. For example, if the arterial blood gas data obtained after the implementation of the plan (outlined in the SOAP form) showed that the patient's PaO₂ was still too low, it would be appropriate to revise the original treatment plan by increasing the FIO₂ on the mechanical ventilator. Figure 11-2 illustrates objective data, assessments, and treatment plans commonly associated with respiratory disorders.

SOAP Case Example*

A **26-year-old man** arrived in the emergency room having a **severe asthmatic episode**. On observation, his arms were fixed to the bed rails, he was using his **accessory muscles of inspiration**, and he was using **pursed-lip breathing**. The patient stated that "**it feels like someone is standing on my chest. I just can't seem to take a deep breath.**" His **heart rate** was **111 beats per minute**, and his **blood pressure** was **170/110**. His **respiratory rate** was **28 and shallow**. **Hyperresonant notes** were produced on percussion. **Auscultation** revealed **expiratory wheezing** and **coarse crackles bilaterally**. His **chest x-ray film** revealed a **severely depressed diaphragm** and **alveolar hyperinflation**. His **peak expiratory flow** was **165 L/min**. Even though his **cough effort** was **weak**, he produced a **large amount of thick white secretions**. His **arterial blood gases** showed pH of **7.27**, **PaCO₂** of **62**, **HCO₃⁻ of 25**, and **PaO₂ of 49** (on room air) (Figure 11-1).

*Subjective and objective data presented in bold.

Computer Documentation

Computer-based records (also called **electronic medical records, electronic health records, computer-based personal records,** and **electronic patient medical charts**) are

A

OBJECTIVE DATA — Clinical manifestations (clinical indicators) that commonly develop in response to respiratory disease						ASSESSMENT	PLAN
Chest Assessment				Chest Radiograph	Bedside Spirometry	COMMON CAUSES/ SEVERITY OF CLINICAL INDICATORS	TREATMENT SELECTION (PHYSICIAN ORDERED*)
Inspection	Palpation	Percussion	Auscultation				
• Barrel chest • Use of accessory muscles • Pursed-lip breathing • Cyanosis	May show ↓ chest excursion	May be hyper-resonant	• Wheezes • Prolonged exhalation	May be normal or show over expansion	↓ PEFR ↓ FEV$_1$ SVC > FVC	BRONCHOSPASM e.g., Asthma EXCESSIVE BROCHIAL SECRETIONS e.g., Bronchitis or Cystic Fibrosis BRONCHIAL TUMOR	Bronchodilator therapy Bronchial hygiene therapy General management/ comfort
• Dyspneic • Cyanosis	Usually normal	Usually normal	Inspiratory stridor	Laryngeal narrowing	Not indicated	LARYNGEAL EDEMA e.g., Croup or Post-extubation Edema	Cool, bland aerosol therapy Racemic epinephrine
Sputum production	May be normal	May be normal	Crackles	May be normal	↓ PEFR ↓ FEV$_1$	LARGE AIRWAY SECRETIONS e.g., Bronchitis or Cystic Fibrosis	Bronchial hygiene therapy
• Use of accessory muscles of inspiration • Pursed-lip breathing • Barrel chest • Cyanosis	↓ Tactile and vocal fremitus	Hyper-resonant	• ↓Breath sounds • ↓Heart sounds • Prolonged exhalation	• ↓ Diaphragm • Translucency • Over-expanded	↓ PEFR ↓ FVC ↓ FEV$_1$/FVC	AIR TRAPPING (Hyperinflation) e.g., • COPD • Asthma • Bronchitis • Emphysema	Treat underlying cause, if possible, e.g., • Bronchospasm • Airway secretions
• May appear dyspneic • Cyanosis	↑ Tactile and vocal fremitus	Dull	• Bronchial breath sounds • Crackles • Whispered pectoriloquy	• Opacity	↓ VC	CONSOLIDATION e.g., Pneumonia ATELECTASIS e.g., Post-op or mucus plugs INFILTRATION e.g., Pneumoconiosis	• Antibiotic agents* • Lung expansion Tx • Bronchial hygiene therapy when atelectasis is caused by mucus accumulation/ mucus plugs
• Rapid shallow breath • Cyanosis • Frothy pink secretions	Usually normal	Dull	• Crackles • May be: wheezes	• Enlarged heart • Infiltrates "Butterfly"	↓ VC	PULMONARY EDEMA • Left heart failure	• Lung expansion Tx • Positive inotropic agents* • Diuretics*
• Cyanosis • Rapid shallow breath • Unilateral expansion	• Usually normal • Tracheal shift	Hyper-resonant	Absent or ↓ breath sounds	• Pneumothorax • Translucency • Mediastinum shift • ↓Diaphragm	Not indicated	AIR PRESSURE IN INTRAPLEURAL SPACE GREATER THAN ATMOSPHERE • Tension pneumothorax	Chest tube to evacuate air* Lung expansion Tx
• Cyanosis • Rapid shallow breath • Unilateral expansion	• Usually normal • May be tracheal shift	Dull	↓Breath sounds	• Opacity • Obscured diaphragm	↓ VC	FLUID IN INTRAPLEURAL SPACE • Pleural effusion • Empyema	• Treat underlying cause • Thoracentesis* • Lung expansion Tx
Paradoxical chest movement	Tender	Not indicated	Varies	• Rib fractures • Opacity (e.g., ARDS and/or atelectasis	Not possible	DOUBLE FRACTURES OF THREE OR MORE ADJACENT RIBS • Flail chest	• Stabilization of chest mechanical ventilation* • Lung expansion Tx

FIGURE 11-2 Respiratory care protocol guide. (Used with permission from Terry DesJardins.)

Continued

now commonly used throughout the health-care industry. Common uses of computer documentation include ordering supplies and services for the patient; storing admission data; writing and storing patient care plans (e.g., SOAPs and physician progress notes); writing prescriptions, listing medications, treatments, and procedures; and storing and retrieving diagnostic test results (e.g., x-ray films, pulmonary function studies, and arterial blood gas values). Many health-care facilities have incorporated software for their specific patient care needs. Such computer programs include options for starting individualized patient care plans, using automated card filing systems, documenting acuity levels, and providing a mechanism to electronically record ongoing assessment data. There are literally hundreds of electronic medical chart solutions available today, targeted at every size and type of medical setting.

With all the patient information in a central location, computer documentation provides easy access to patient data. It greatly reduces the chance for errors, and updated patient information can easily be entered in real time. Computer-based records do away with the need to make phone calls to other departments to gather patient information or to order patient supplies or services. In addition, electronic documentation eliminates the need to read through the entire chart to evaluate the patient's progress or to review specific data such as medication listings, treatments, diagnostic test results,

B

	Objective Data	ASSESSMENT	Plan
	(Clinical manifestations or clinical indicators)	COMMON CAUSES/SEVERITY OF CLINICAL INDICATORS	TREATMENT SELECTION (PHYSICIAN ORDERED*)

RESPIRATORY CARE POCKET PROTOCOL CARD	Cough effort: Sputum production: ○ Strong ○ Weak ○ No ○ Yes Sputum characteristics: • Amount > 25 mL/24 hrs. _____ • White and translucent sputum _____ • Yellow/opaque sputum _____ • Green sputum _____ • Brown sputum _____ • Red sputum _____ • Frothy secretion _____	Patient's abiltily to mobilize secretions: ○ Good ○ Poor • Excessive bronchial secretions _____ • Normal sputum _____ • Acute airway infection _____ • Old, retained secretions and infections ___ • Old blood _____ • Fresh blood _____ • Pulmonary edema _____	Bronchial hygiene therapy • Bronchial hygiene therapy • None • Treat underlying cause • Bronchial hygiene therapy • Bronchial hygiene therapy • Notify physician • Treat underlying cause, e.g., CHF

	Arterial blood gas status - Ventilatory
	• pH↑, PaCO$_2$↓, HCO$_3$↓ _____
	
	• pH normal, PaCO$_2$↓, HCO$_3$↓↓* _____
	
	• pH↓, PaCO$_2$↑, HCO$_3$↑ _____
	• pH normal, PaCO$_2$↑, HCO$_3$↑↑ _____
		• Acute alveolar hyperventilation _____
		
		• Chronic alveolar hyperventilation _____
		
		• Acute ventilatory failure _____
		• Chronic ventilatory failure _____
			• Treat underlying cause, if possible.
			  Ex: pneumonia, pain.
			• Generally none (occurs normally
			  at high altitude)
			• Mechanical ventilation*
			• Low flow oxygen, bronchial hygiene,
			  nocturnal ventilation

	Sudden ventilatory changes or chronic ventilatory failure:
	• pH↑, PaCO$_2$↓, HCO$_3$↑↑, PaO$_2$↓ _____
	
	• pH↑, PaCO$_2$↑↑, HCO$_3$↑, PaO$_2$↓ _____
		• Acute alveolar hyperventilation on
		  chronic ventilatory failure _____
		• Acute ventilatory failure on
		  chronic ventilatory failure _____
			• Treat the underlying cause, if possible.
			  Ex: pneumonia
			• Mechanical ventilation*

	Indicators for mechanical ventilation: • pH↑, PaCO$_2$↓, HCO$_3$↓, PaO$_2$↓ but pt is fatigued _____ • pH↓, PaCO$_2$↑, HCO$_3$↑, PaO$_2$↓ hypoventilation _____ • pH↓, PaCO$_2$↑, HCO$_3$↓, PaO$_2$↓ apnea _____	• Impending ventilatory failure • Ventilatory failure • Apnea	• Mechanical ventilation*

	Metabolic
	• pH↑, PaCO$_2$ normal or ↑, HCO$_3$↑, PaO$_2$ normal _____
	
	• pH↓, PaCO$_2$ normal or ↓, HCO$_3$↓, PaO$_2$↓ _____
	
	• pH↓, PaCO$_2$ normal or ↓, HCO$_3$↓, PaO$_2$ normal _____
	• pH↓, PaCO$_2$ normal or ↓, HCO$_3$↓, PaO$_2$ normal _____
		• Metabolic alkalosis:
		  • Hypokalemia _____
		  • Hypochloremia _____
		• Metabolic acidosis:
		  • Lactic acidosis _____
		
		  • Ketoacidosis _____
		  • Renal failure _____
			• Potassium administration*
			• Chlorine administration*
			
			• Oxygen administration, cardiovascular
			  support*
			• Insulin administration*
			• Renal failure management*

	Ventilatory and metabolic:
	• pH↓, PaCO$_2$↑, HCO$_3$↓ _____
	
	• pH↑, PaCO$_2$↓, HCO$_3$↑ _____
		• Combined metabolic and
		  respiratory acidosis
		
		• Combined metabolic and
		  respiratory alkalosis
			• Mechanical ventilation*
			• Treat the underlying cause of metabolic
			  acidosis (see above)
			• Treat the underlying cause for acute
			  alveolar hyperventilation
			• Treat the underlying cause for metabolic
			  alkalosis (see above)

	Oxygenation status: • PaO$_2$ < 80mm Hg _____ • PaO$_2$ < 60mm Hg _____ • PaO$_2$ < 40mm Hg _____	• Mild hypoxemia • Moderate hypoxemia • Severe hypoxemia	• Oxygen therapy • Treat the underlying cause of hypoxemia

	Negative oxygen transport indicators:
	○ ↓PaO$_2$ ○ Anemia
	○ Blood loss ○ ↓Cardiac output
	○ CO poisoning ○ Abnormal Hb
		Oxygen transport status:
		○ Adequate ○ Inadequate
			• Treat the underlying cause,
			  if possible, e.g.,
			  ○ Oxygen therapy ○ Blood replacement*
			  ○ Positive inotropic agents*

* Significant

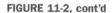

FIGURE 11-2, cont'd

and procedures. The patient's clinical information is permanently recorded, and other health-care departments can review it and communicate with one another.

Basic computer knowledge and skills are usually taught through the institution's in-service education department. Each nursing station usually has multiple data entry stations, laptops, and tablets available for charting. Printers are also readily accessible throughout institutions and clinics. The entire patient record or just a part of it may be retrieved and printed. Today, many health-care practitioners use hand-held bedside computer documentation systems. Bedside computer devices, referred to as *point-of-care (POC) systems*, commonly include specific clinical prompts for data entry, which result in records that are more accurate and complete.

Good charting skills are essential to critical thinking and patient assessment—they provide the basic means to collect clinical data, analyze it, assess it, and formulate a treatment plan. Furthermore, good charting skills document the effectiveness of patient care and adjustments of the treatment plan in response to its effectiveness. Without good charting systems and skills, the practitioner merely administers health-care without a predetermined (and recorded) goal.

Historically, respiratory therapists have focused on treating patients with specific disease entities and implementing physicians' orders. Little planning was done by respiratory therapist to individualize their treatments for a specific patient. Today, a systematic problem-solving approach to respiratory care, based on broad theoretic knowledge, combined with technical expertise and communication skills, is essential, and is the focus of this textbook.

Health Insurance Portability and Accountability Act

In 2003, the **Department of Health and Human Services (HHS)** proposed national rules that outlined the ways in which a patient's medical files should be used or shared with others. These rules were adopted as federal standards after the passage of the **Health Insurance Portability and Accountability Act** (HIPAA). Today, HIPAA requires that all health-care practitioners who have access to patient medical records prove that they have a plan to protect the privacy of the records. In essence, the HIPAA regulations protect the patient's privacy with specific rules outlining when, how, and what type of health-care information can be shared. HIPAA gives the patient the right to know about—and to control—how his or her personal medical records will be used. The following provides a general overview of the HIPAA regulations:

- Both the health-care provider and a representative of the insurance company must explain to the patient how they plan to disclose any medical records.
- Patients may request copies of all their medical information and make appropriate changes to it. Patients may also ask for a history of any unusual disclosures.
- The patient must give formal consent should anyone want to share any health information.
- The patient's health information is to be used only for health purposes. Without the patient's consent, medical records cannot be used by either (1) a bank to determine whether to give the patient a loan or (2) a potential employer to determine whether to hire the patient.
- When the patient's health information is disclosed, only the minimum necessary amount of information should be released.
- Records dealing with a patient's mental health get an extra level of protection.
- The patient has the right to complain to the HHS about violations of HIPAA rules.

One disadvantage of the HIPAA regulations, according to many health-care practitioners, is that the health-care provider must allocate large sums of money to comply with the HIPAA rules—dollars that might be better spent elsewhere. Critics also argue that this cost will probably be passed on to the consumer. In addition, many health-care providers believe that the quality of patient care will be compromised as a result of HIPAA, making it more difficult for various health-care practitioners to obtain vital information regarding patient care. For example, consider the potential HIPAA-related problems for a health-care team in a Miami, Florida, hospital that is trying to obtain the pharmaceutical history—in a timely fashion—of an elderly, unconscious car accident victim whose medical records are in a Detroit, Michigan, hospital. Proponents of the HIPAA regulations argue that this is the tradeoff made to ensure the privacy of an individual's health-care information. Regardless of the pros or cons of the HIPAA regulations, the respiratory therapist—like all other health-care providers—must comply with the current HIPAA regulations.

SELF-ASSESSMENT QUESTIONS

Ⓔ Answers to questions can be found on Evolve. To access additional student assessment questions visit **http://evolve.elsevier.com/DesJardins/respiratory**.

1. **What is the process of adding written information to the patient's chart called?**
   1. Recording
   2. Critical thinking
   3. Documenting
   4. Charting
      a. 2 only
      b. 3 and 4 only
      c. 1 and 3 only
      d. 1, 3, and 4 only

2. **The admission sheet, physician's order sheet, and history sheet are all what type of patient records?**
   1. Source-oriented record
   2. Problem-oriented medical record
   3. Block chart
   4. Traditional chart
      a. 2 only
      b. 4 only
      c. 3 and 4 only
      d. 1, 3, and 4 only

3. **Which of the following is based on a sequential, objective, scientific, problem-solving method?**
   1. Source-oriented record
   2. Problem-oriented medical record
   3. Block chart
   4. Traditional chart
      a. 1 only
      b. 2 only
      c. 4 only
      d. 3 and 4 only

4. According to the respiratory care protocol guide (per Figure 11-2), bronchial breath sounds and dull percussion notes are associated with which of the following clinical assessments?
   1. Air trapping
   2. Bronchospasm
   3. Atelectasis
   4. Consolidation
      a. 2 only
      b. 3 only
      c. 1 and 2 only
      d. 3 and 4 only

5. Good charting should be an effective way to do the following:
   A. _____
   _____
   B. _____
   _____
   C. _____
   _____
   D. _____
   _____
   _____
   _____

6. A good problem-oriented medical record (POMR) should include a systematic approach that documents the following:
   A. _____
   _____
   B. _____
   _____
   C. _____
   _____
   _____
   D. _____
   _____
   _____
   E. _____
   _____
   _____

7. Define the following components of a SOAP progress note, and list one or more examples.
   S _____
   _____
   _____
   Example(s): _____
   _____
   O _____
   _____
   _____
   Example(s): _____
   _____
   _____

A _____
   _____
   _____
   Example(s): _____
   _____
   P _____
   _____
   _____
   Example(s): _____
   _____

8. According to the respiratory care protocol guide (per Figure 11-2), what are the three major indicators (assessments) for mechanical ventilation?
   A. _____
   _____
   _____
   B. _____
   _____
   C. _____
   _____
   _____

9. A patient arterial blood gas values reveal pH of 7.56, $PaCO_2$ of 24, HCO_3^- of 20, and PaO_2 of 52. Based on the blood gas values, identify the indication(s) for initiation of mechanical ventilation.
   Answer: _____
   _____

10. Case: A 36-year-old woman is in the emergency room in respiratory distress. Her heart rate is 136 beats/min, and her blood pressure is 165/120. Her respiratory rate is 32 breaths/min, and her breathing is labored. The patient states that "It feels like a rope is around my neck." Expiratory wheezing and rhonchi are auscultated bilaterally. Her arterial blood gas values reveal a pH of 7.56, a $PaCO_2$ of 28, HCO_3^- of 21, and a PaO_2 of 47 (on room air). Her cough effort is strong, and she is producing a moderate amount of thin white secretions. Her peak expiratory flow rate is 185 L/min, and her chest x-ray film demonstrates a moderately depressed diaphragm and alveolar hyperinflation.
    With this clinical information, provide SOAP documentation for the patient (use Figure 11-2 for assistance).
    S _____
    _____
    _____
    O _____
    _____
    _____
    A _____
    _____
    _____
    P _____
    _____
    _____
    _____

Obstructive Lung Disease

Obstructive lung diseases are characterized by a variety of pathologic conditions—such as bronchial inflammation, excessive airway secretions, mucous plugging, bronchospasm, and distal airway weakening—that cause a reduction of airflow into and out of the lungs. Gas flow reduction is especially decreased during exhalation. The most common obstructive lung disorders are **chronic bronchitis**, **emphysema**, and **asthma**.

As shown in the Venn diagram[1], although chronic bronchitis (subset 3), emphysema (subset 4), and asthma (subset 9) may appear alone, they often appear in combination. For example, when chronic bronchitis and emphysema appear together as one disease complex (subset 5), the patient is said to have **chronic obtructive pulmonary disease (COPD).**

Asthma is represented by subset 9, which by definition is associated with reversible airflow obstruction and, therefore, is not considered as COPD. In some cases, however, it is

virtually impossible to differentiate patients with partially reversible airflow obstruction from the patient with chronic bronchitis or emphysema who have partially reversible airflow obstruction and hyper-reactivity. Thus, asthma patients with unremitting asthma are classified as having COPD (subset 6, 7, and 8).

Chronic bronchitis and **emphysema** with airflow obstruction are commonly seen together (subset 5 and called COPD), and some patients may also have asthma associated with these two disorders (subset 8). Patients with asthma exposed to chronic irritation, as from cigarette smoke, may develop a chronic productive cough, a feature associated with chronic bronchitis (subset 6). Such patients are said to have asthmatic bronchitis, or the asthmatic form of COPD. Patients with **chronic bronchitis** and/or **emphysema**, without airflow obstruction are not classified as having COPD (subsets 1, 2, and 11). The patient demonstrating overlapping signs and symptoms of both asthma and emphysema (subset 7) is discussed on pages 210–211.

Finally, other obstructive lung disorders include **cystic fibrosis**, and **bronchiectasis** (less common) and are not generally included in this definition (subset 10).

---

[1]A Venn diagram or set diagram is a diagram that shows all possible logical relations between a finite collection of sets (aggregation of things). The Venn diagrams were first conceived around 1880 by John Venn. They are used to teach elementary set theory, as well as illustrate simple set relationships in probability, logic, statistics, linguistics and computer science.

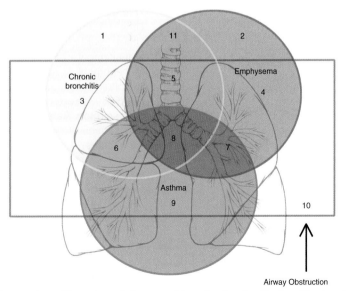

The Venn diagram shown above illustrates all the possible subsets of patients with chronic bronchitis, emphysema, or asthma (see description of subsets above).

Chapter Objectives

After reading this chapter, you will be able to:

- Describe the American Thoracic Society (ATS) guidelines for chronic obstructive pulmonary disease (COPD), chronic bronchitis, and emphysema.
- Describe the Global Initiative for Chronic Obstructive Lung Disease (GOLD) *definition* of COPD.
- Explain the anatomic alterations of the lungs associated with chronic bronchitis and emphysema.
- Describe the etiology and epidemiology of COPD.
- Discuss the risk factors associated with COPD.
- Describe the GOLD guidelines for the *diagnosis* and *assessment* of COPD.
- Identify the key distinctive differences between chronic bronchitis and emphysema—the "pink puffer" and the "blue bloater."
- Describe the cardiopulmonary clinical manifestations associated with chronic bronchitis and emphysema (COPD).
- Describe the GOLD *global strategy* for the diagnosis, management, and prevention of COPD.
- Describe the clinical strategies, rationales, and cost implications of the SOAPs presented in the case studies.

Key Terms

All-Cause Readmission Prevention Program (ACRPP)
Alpha$_1$-Antitrypsin Deficiency
American Thoracic Society (ATS)
Asthma and COPD Overlap Syndrome (ACOS)
"Blue Bloater"
Centriacinar Emphysema
Centrilobular Emphysema
Chronic Bronchitis
Chronic Obstructive Pulmonary Disease (COPD)
COPD Assessment Test (CAT)
Emphysema
Hoover's sign
Global Initiative for Chronic Obstructive Lung Disease (GOLD)
Modified British Medical Research Council (mMRC)
Breathlessness Scale
MM Alpha$_1$-Antitrypsin Phenotype
MZ Alpha$_1$-Antitrypsin Phenotype
Panacinar Emphysema

Panlobular Emphysema
"Pink Puffer"
Pulmonary Rehabilitation
Pulmonary Rehabilitation Protocol
Transitional Care Specialists
ZZ Alpha$_1$-Antitrypsin Phenotype

Chapter Outline

Introduction
Anatomic Alterations of the Lungs Associated with Chronic Bronchitis
Anatomic Alterations of the Lungs Associated with Emphysema
Etiology and Epidemiology
Risk Factors
Diagnosis and Assessment of Chronic Obstructive Pulmonary Disease
  Pulmonary Function Testing
  Severity Assessment of COPD
Key Distinguishing Features between Emphysema and Chronic Bronchitis
Cardiopulmonary Clinical Manifestations Associated with Chronic Bronchitis and Emphysema (COPD)
General Management of Chronic Obstructive Pulmonary Disease
  Global Initiative for Chronic Obstructive Lung Disease
Overview of the Cardiopulmonary Clinical Manifestations Associated with Chronic Bronchitis and Emphysema (COPD)
  Therapeutic Options
  Other Pharmacologic Treatment Options
  Other Treatments Options
  Management of Stable COPD
  Management of Acute COPD Exacerbations
  Hospital Management of COPD Acute Exacerbations
  Hospital Management of COPD Acute Exacerbations Respiratory Care Treatment Protocols
  Implications of the GOLD Guidelines for Respiratory Care
Case Studies
  Chronic Bronchitis
  Emphysema
  Example of Classic Chronic Obstructive Pulmonary Disease (COPD)
Self-Assessment Questions

Introduction

The **American Thoracic Society (ATS)** guidelines for **chronic obstructive pulmonary disease (COPD), chronic bronchitis**, and **emphysema** provide the following definitions:

Chronic obstructive pulmonary disease is a preventable and treatable disease state characterized by airflow limitation that is not fully reversible. The airflow limitation is usually progressive, is associated with an abnormal inflammatory response of the lungs to noxious particles or gases, and is primarily caused by cigarette smoking. Although COPD affects the lungs, it also produces significant systemic consequences.

Chronic bronchitis is defined clinically as chronic productive cough for 3 months in each of 2 successive years in a patient in whom other causes of productive chronic cough have been excluded.

Emphysema is defined pathologically as the presence of permanent enlargement of the air spaces distal to the terminal bronchioles, accompanied by destruction of bronchiole walls and without obvious fibrosis.

In patients with COPD, both chronic bronchitis and emphysema are present. However, the relative contribution of each to the disease process is often difficult to discern. Note that the ATS definition for *chronic bronchitis* is based on the major clinical manifestations associated with the disease (i.e., productive cough). Also note that the ATS definition for *emphysema* is based on the pathology, or the anatomic alterations of the lung associated with the disorder.

The **Global Initiative for Chronic Obstructive Lung Disease** (GOLD) now provides the following working definition:[1]

Chronic obstructive pulmonary disease (COPD) is a preventable and treatable disease with some significant extrapulmonary effects that may contribute to the severity in individual patients. Its pulmonary component is characterized by airflow limitation that is not fully reversible. The airflow limitation is usually progressive and associated with an abnormal inflammatory response of the lung to noxious particles or gases.

Note that the GOLD definition does not use the terms *chronic bronchitis* and *emphysema*. GOLD explains that *chronic bronchitis* is defined as the presence of cough and sputum production for at least 3 months in each of 2 consecutive years (i.e., clinical manifestations), and is not always associated with airflow limitation. GOLD also points out that *emphysema* is defined as destruction of the alveoli and is a pathologic term (i.e., anatomic alteration of the lung) that is sometimes—and incorrectly—used to describe only *one* of several structural abnormalities present in patients with COPD.[2]

---

[1]Modified from GOLD, Global Strategy for the Diagnosis, Management, and Prevention of Chronic Obstructive Pulmonary Disease, Revised 2014. (www.goldcopd.org). GOLD is recognized as a worldwide leading authority for the diagnosis, management, and prevention of COPD.

[2]It should be noted that a chapter on the diagnosis of **Asthma and COPD Overlap syndrome (ACOS)** is in preparation by the Science Committee of the Global Initiative for Asthma (GINA) and the Global Initiative for Chronic Obstructive Lung Disease (GOLD). It is expected to be available with the release of GINA 2014 document Global Strategy for Asthma Management and Prevention in the spring of 2014 (www.ginasthma.org). A full chapter with references will be posted on the GOLD website when it is available. It will also appear in full in the Appendix of the 2015 GOLD update (www.goldcopd.org).

The bottom line is this: even though chronic bronchitis and emphysema can each develop alone, they often occur together as one disease entity. When this happens, the disease entity is called *chronic obstructive pulmonary disease—that is, COPD*. In other words, *COPD* is a term referring to two lung diseases—chronic bronchitis and emphysema—occurring simultaneously. Patients with COPD demonstrate a variety of clinical manifestations associated with both disorders, although the relative contribution of each respiratory disorder is often difficult to ascertain. For this reason the treatment of chronic bronchitis, emphysema, or a combination of both disorders (COPD) is very similar in clinical practice.

Anatomic Alterations of the Lungs Associated with Chronic Bronchitis

The conducting airways (particularly the bronchi) are the primary structures that undergo change in chronic bronchitis. As a result of chronic inflammation the bronchial walls are narrowed by vasodilation, congestion, and mucosal edema. This condition is often accompanied by bronchial smooth muscle constriction. In addition, continued bronchial irritation causes the submucosal bronchial glands to enlarge and the number of goblet cells to increase, resulting in excessive mucus production. The number and function of cilia lining the tracheobronchial tree are diminished, and the peripheral bronchi are often partially or totally occluded by inflammation and mucous plugs, which in turn leads to hyperinflated alveoli (Figure 12-1). Figure 12-2 shows two microscopic views of chronic bronchitis.

To summarize, the following major pathologic or structural changes are associated with chronic bronchitis:
- Chronic inflammation and thickening of the walls of the peripheral airways.
- Excessive mucous production and accumulation.
- Partial or total mucous plugging of the airways.
- Smooth muscle constriction of bronchial airways (bronchospasm)—a variable finding.
- Air trapping and hyperinflation of alveoli may occur in late stages.

Anatomic Alterations of the Lungs Associated with Emphysema

Emphysema is characterized by a weakening and permanent enlargement of the air spaces distal to the terminal bronchioles and by destruction of the alveolar walls. As these structures enlarge and the alveoli coalesce, many of the adjacent pulmonary capillaries also are affected, and this results in a decreased surface area for gas exchange across the alveolar-capillary membrane. Furthermore, the distal airways, weakened in the process, tend to collapse during expiration in response to increased intrapleural pressure. This traps gas in the alveoli. There are two major types of emphysema: Panacinar (panlobular) emphysema and centriacinar (centrilobular) emphysema.

In **panacinar emphysema**, or **panlobular emphysema** there is an abnormal weakening and enlargement of all alveoli distal to the terminal bronchioles, including the respiratory

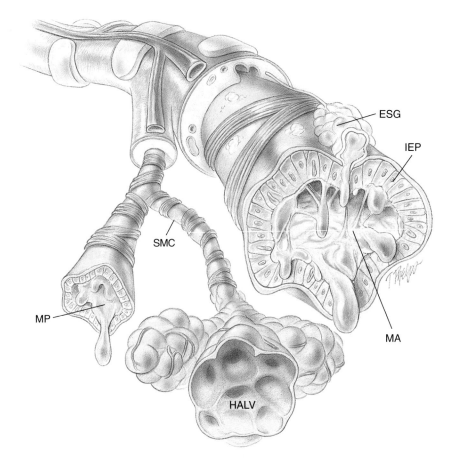

FIGURE 12-1 Chronic bronchitis, one of the most common airway diseases. *SMC*, Smooth muscle constriction; *ESG*, enlarged submucosal gland; *HALV*, hyperinflation of alveoli (distal to airway obstruction); *IEP*, inflammation of epithelium; *MA*, mucous accumulation; *MP*, mucous plug.

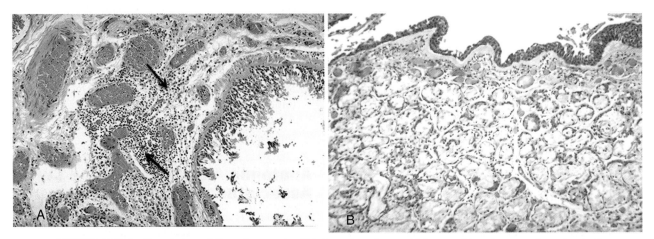

FIGURE 12-2 A, Chronic bronchitis, microscopic. This bronchus *(lower right corner)* has increased numbers of chronic inflammatory cells *(arrows)* in the submucosal bronchial region. (Figure was obtained from: Klatt: Robbins and Cotran Atlas of Pathology, 2nd edition, 2010, Elsevier/Saunders.) **B**, Chronic bronchitis. The lumen of the bronchus is above. Note the marked thickening of the mucous gland layer (approximately twice normal) and squamous metaplasia of lung epithelium. (Figure was obtained from: Robbins Basic pathology, by Kumar, Abbas, and Aster, 2013, Elsevier/Saunders.)

bronchioles, alveolar ducts, alveolar sacs, and alveoli—the entire acinus is affected by dilatation and destruction. The alveolar-capillary surface area is significantly decreased (Figure 12-3). Panlobular emphysema is commonly found in the lower parts of the lungs and is sometimes associated with a deficiency of the protease inhibitor alpha$_1$-antitrypsin.

Panlobular emphysema is one of the more severe types of emphysema and therefore the most likely to produce significant clinical manifestations.

In **centriacinar emphysema**, or **centrilobular emphysema**, the pathology involves the respiratory bronchioles in the proximal portion of the acinus. The respiratory

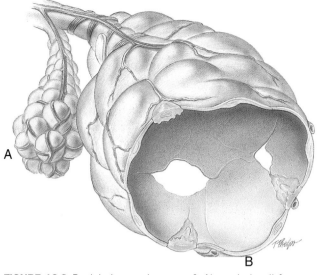

FIGURE 12-3 Panlobular emphysema. **A**, Normal alveoli for comparison purposes. **B**, Panlobular emphysema: Abnormal weakening and enlargement of all air spaces distal to the terminal bronchioles.

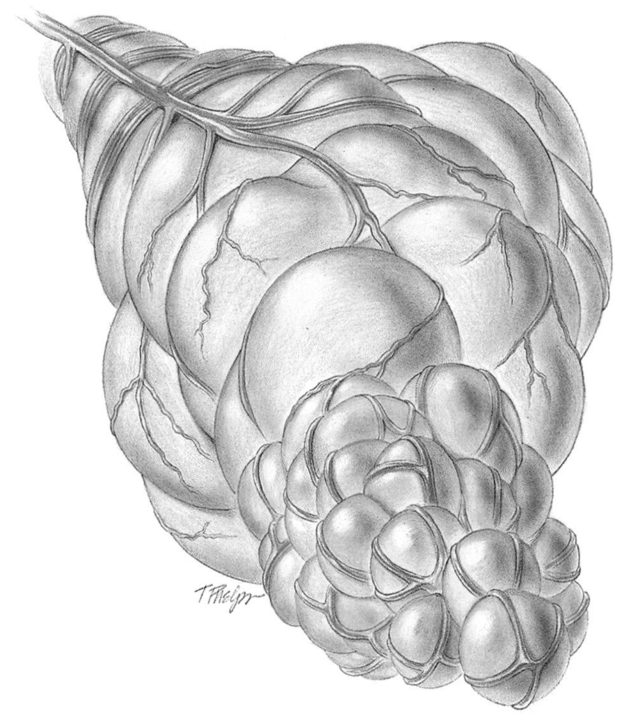

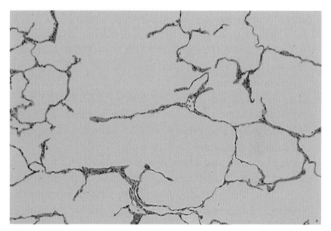

FIGURE 12-4 Centrilobular emphysema. Abnormal weakening and enlargement of the respiratory bronchioles and alveoli in the proximal portion of the acinus.

bronchiolar walls enlarge, become confluent, and are then destroyed. A rim of parenchyma remains relatively unaffected (Figure 12-4). Centriacinar emphysema is the most common form of emphysema and is strongly associated with cigarette smoking and with chronic bronchitis. Figure 12-5 shows a microscopic view of pulmonary emphysema.

To summarize, the following are the major pathologic or structural changes associated with emphysema:

- Permanent enlargement and destruction of the air spaces distal to the terminal bronchioles.
- Destruction of the alveolar-capillary membrane.
- Weakening of the distal airways, primarily the respiratory bronchioles.
- Air trapping and hyperinflation.

Etiology and Epidemiology

Although the precise incidence of COPD is not known, it is estimated that 10 to 15 million people in the United States have chronic bronchitis, emphysema, or a combination of both. Most authorities agree that COPD is underdiagnosed. It is felt that if you take into account the people who have not been "officially" diagnosed with COPD, the incidence would be over 20 million people in the United States. It is generally accepted that more people have chronic bronchitis than emphysema. For example, the National Center for Health Statistics estimates that in the United States about 9.5 million people have chronic bronchitis and 4.1 million people have emphysema. COPD claims more that 138,000 Americans each year. It is the third leading cause of death in the United States. Recent data show that COPD prevalence and mortality is now about equal in men and women, which likely reflects the changing patterns of smoking.

FIGURE 12-5 Pulmonary emphysema, microscopic. There is loss of alveolar ducts and alveoli with emphysema, and the remaining air spaces become dilated. There is less surface area for gas exchange. Emphysema leads to loss of lung parenchyma, loss of elastic recoil, increased lung compliance, and increased pulmonary residual volume with increased total lung capacity, mainly from an increased residual volume. (Figure was obtained from: Klatt: Robbins and Cotran Atlas of Pathology, 2nd edition, 2010, Elsevier/Saunders.)

Risk Factors

According to GOLD, although the current understanding of the risk factors associated with COPD is incomplete, the following factors influence the development and progression of COPD:

- **Genes—Alpha$_1$–antitrypsin deficiency** (also known as alpha$_1$-proteinase inhibitor deficiency, A$_1$AD, AATD, ATT deficiency, AP$_1$ deficiency, and alpha-1 inherited emphysema) is a genetic disorder affecting the lung, liver, and rarely, the skin. Alpha$_1$-antitrypsin is made in the liver and one of its functions is to protect the lungs from neutrophil elastase, an enzyme that can break down connective tissue. When the alpha$_1$-antitrypsin deficiency level is low, the elastase is free to attack and destroy the elastic tissue of the lungs. A severe deficiency of alpha$_1$-antitrypsin poses a strong risk factor for early onset of emphysema—especially **panacinar emphysema** (see Figure 12-3). The premature development of emphysema is the hallmark of alpha$_1$-antitrypsin deficiency. Cigarette smoking significantly increases the risk factor for early onset emphysema in patients with alpha$_1$-antitrypsin deficiency—for example, the onset of dyspnea around 30 years of age.

The normal level of alpha$_1$-antitrypsin ranges between 150 to 350 mg/dL (1.5 to 3.5 g/L) when measured via radial immunodiffusion. Patients with normal levels of alpha$_1$-antitrypsin are referred to genetically as having an **MM phenotype** or simply an M phenotype (homozygote). The phenotype associated with severely low serum concentrations is the **ZZ phenotype**, or simply Z. The heterozygous offspring of parents with the M and Z phenotypes have an **MZ phenotype**. The **MZ phenotype** results in an intermediate deficiency of alpha$_1$-antitrypsin. The precise effect of the intermediate level of alpha$_1$-antitrypsin is unclear. It is strongly recommended, however, that individuals with this phenotype do not smoke or work in areas having significant environmental air pollution. Although alpha$_1$-antitrypsin deficiency is considered to be rare, it is estimated that 80,000 to 100,000 individuals in the United States have severe deficiency of alpha$_1$-antitrypsin.

- **Age**—As a person ages, the risk of COPD increases. Although the precise connection between age and COPD is unclear, it is suggested it may be related to the sum of cumulative exposures throughout life.
- **Lung Growth and Development**—Any condition that affects lung growth during gestation and childhood (e.g., low birth weight, respiratory infections) has the potential for increasing an individual's risk for developing COPD.
- **Exposure to Particles**
  - **Tobacco** smoke—Cigarette smoking is the most commonly encountered risk factor for COPD worldwide. Other types of tobacco (e.g., pipe, cigar, water pipe) are added risk factors for COPD. Passive exposure to cigarette smoke may also cause COPD. Smoking during pregnancy may affect lung growth and development of the fetus.
  - **Occupational exposure**—Organic and inorganic dusts and chemical agents and fumes (e.g., asbestos, coal dust, moldy hay, bird droppings, or paints) may cause COPD.
  - **Indoor Air Pollution**—Wood, animal dander and dung, crop residues, and coal, commonly burned in open fires or poorly functioning stoves, may lead to very high levels of indoor pollution. Research data continues to grow that indoor pollution from biomass cooking and heating in poorly ventilated areas is an important risk factor for COPD. It is estimated that about 3 billion people around the world use biomass and coal as their primary source of energy for cooking, heating, and basic household needs.
  - **Outdoor Air Pollution**—Although high levels of air pollution (e.g., silicates, sulfur dioxide, the nitrogen oxides, and ozone) are known to be harmful to individuals with existing heart and lung disease, the role of outdoor pollution in causing COPD is unclear.
- **Socioeconomic Status**—Poverty is clearly a risk factor for COPD, although the precise components associated with poverty and COPD are unclear. Likely factors include exposure to indoor and outdoor air pollutants, crowding, poor nutrition, and infection. Current CDC data (2012) strongly indicates that the risk of developing COPD is inversely related to an individual's socioeconomic status.
- **Asthma/Bronchial HyperReactivity**—Asthma may be a risk factor for the development of COPD.
- **Chronic Bronchitis**—May be a risk factor for the development of COPD. In other words, chronic bronchitis may lead to emphysema. When both chronic bronchitis and emphysema are present, the patient is said to have COPD.
- **Respiratory Infections**—A history of severe childhood respiratory infections is associated with decreased lung function and increased respiratory complications in adulthood. Susceptibility to respiratory infections may lead to COPD.
- **Tuberculosis**—Has been shown to be a risk factor for COPD.

Diagnosis and Assessment of Chronic Obstructive Pulmonary Disease

According to GOLD, the diagnosis of COPD should be considered for any patient who is over 40 years of age and who has dyspnea, chronic cough or sputum production, and/or a history of exposure to risk factors for the disease—especially cigarette smoking. The primary indicators and their descriptions for considering a COPD diagnosis are listed in Table 12-1. Although these indicators are not diagnostic by themselves, the presence of any combination of these clinical markers significantly increases the possibility of a diagnosis of COPD. A **pulmonary function test** (PFT) is required to confirm the airflow limitation (see below).

Pulmonary Function Testing

The three main pulmonary function tests used to measure the severity of airflow limitation in the COPD patient are the spirometric **forced vital capacity (FVC), forced expiratory volume in 1 second (FEV$_1$),** and **forced expiratory volume in 1 second/forced vital capacity ratio (FEV$_1$/FVC ratio)**. Clinically, the FEV$_1$/FVC ratio is also commonly called the **forced expiratory volume 1 second percentage (FEV$_1$%)**. Figure 12-6 illustrates a normal FEV$_1$ and an FEV$_1$ that is typically seen in the spirogram of patients with mild to moderate COPD.

An FEV$_1$/FVC ratio of less than 0.70 usually indicates the presence of airway obstruction. A diagnosis of COPD is

TABLE 12-1 Primary Indicators of COPD in Patients Over age 40

Indicator	Description
Dyspnea	Progressive shortness of breath over time, worse with exercise.
	Persistent
Chronic Cough	Can be intermittent or unproductive
Chronic Sputum Production	Any display of persistent sputum production may suggest COPD
History of Exposure to Risk Factors	Tobacco smoke
	Smoke from home cooking and/or heating fuels
	Work-related dusts and/or chemicals
Family History of COPD	Alpha$_1$-antitrypsin deficiency

Note: The above indicators are not diagnostic themselves. However, the presence of multiple key indicators increases the likelihood of a diagnosis of COPD. A pulmonary function study is required to establish a diagnosis of COPD. (Modified from GOLD, Global Strategy for the Diagnosis, Management, and Prevention of Chronic Obstructive Pulmonary Disease, Revised 2014; www.goldcopd.org.)

TABLE 12-2 Modified Medical Research Council Questionnaire for Assessing the Severity of Breathlessness

Score	Circle the score box that best applies to you (one box only)
0	I only get breathless with strenuous exercise.
1	I get short of breath when hurrying on level ground or walking up a slight hill.
2	On level ground, I walk slower than people of the same age because of breathlessness, or have to stop for breath when walking at my own pace.
3	I stop for breath after walking about 100 meters or after a few minutes on level ground.
4	I am too breathless to leave the house or I am breathless when dressing.

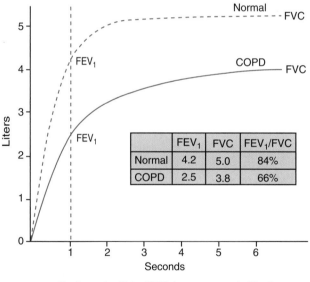

	FEV$_1$	FVC	FEV$_1$/FVC
Normal	4.2	5.0	84%
COPD	2.5	3.8	66%

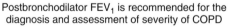

Postbronchodilator FEV$_1$ is recommended for the diagnosis and assessment of severity of COPD

FIGURE 12-6 Normal spirogram and spirogram typical of patients with mild to moderate chronic obstructive pulmonary disease.

made when the patient demonstrates (1) any combination of the COPD indicators (see Table 12-1), (2) an FEV$_1$/FVC ratio of less than 0.70 and an FEV$_1$ less than 80%, and (3) there is no alternative explanation for the symptoms and airflow obstruction (e.g., bronchiectasis, vocal cord paralysis, and tracheal stenosis).

Other important PFT values associated with COPD include the following:

- Decreased inspiratory capacity (IC) and vital capacity (VC).

- Increased total lung capacity (TLC), functional residual capacity (FRC), and residual volume (RV), and residual volume/total lung capacity ratio (RV/TLC).
  - These PFT values confirm alveolar hyperinflation.
- The carbon monoxide diffusing capacity (DLCO) decreases in proportion to the severity of emphysema. The DLCO is normal in pure chronic bronchitis.

Severity Assessment of COPD

According to GOLD, before an effective treatment plan for COPD can be constructed, a thorough COPD assessment must first be performed. The primary goals of COPD assessment are to determine (1) the severity of the disease, (2) the impact the disease has on the patient's health status, and (3) the risk of future events—that is, number of exacerbations and hospital admissions, and death. To achieve this goal, GOLD recommends assessing the following aspects of the disease independently:

- Symptoms
- Severity assessment based on degree of airflow limitation
- Risk of exacerbations
- Comorbidities

Symptom Evaluation—There are several validated questionnaires available to assess symptoms in patients with COPD. GOLD recommends using either the **COPD Assessment Test (CAT)**, or the **Modified British Medical Research Council (mMRC) Breathlessness Scale**. The mMRC questionnaire relates well to other health conditions and predicts future mortality risks. An mMRC score of less than one is classified as a low-risk patient; a score greater than two is considered a high-risk patient. Table 12-2 shows an mMRC questionnaire.

The CAT is an eight-item one-dimensional assessment of health status in COPD. This questionnaire is applicable worldwide and there are validated translations available in a wide range of languages (see example of CAT questionnaire at http://www.catestonline.org). A score less than 10 is classified as a low-risk patient; a score greater than 10 is identified as a high-risk patient.

TABLE 12-3 Severity of Airflow Limitation in COPD Based on Post-Bronchodilator FEV$_1$

(Only in Patients with FEV$_1$/FVC Ratio < 0.70)		
GOLD 1	Mild	FEV$_1$ ≥80% predicted
GOLD 2	Moderate	FEV$_1$ 50%–79% predicted
GOLD 3	Severe	FEV$_1$ 30%–49% predicted
GOLD 4	Very Severe	FEV$_1$ 29% or less than predicted

(Modified from GOLD, Global Strategy for the Diagnosis, Management, and Prevention of Chronic Obstructive Pulmonary Disease, Revised 2014; www.goldcopd.org.)

Severity of Airflow Limitation Evaluation—As shown in Table 12-3, GOLD has established a classification of airflow limitation severity in COPD. This classification defines the severity of the disease according to airflow limitation. The PFT measurements used to evaluate the patient's airflow limitation are the *forced expiratory volume in one second (FEV$_1$)* and the *forced expiratory volume in one second (FEV$_1$) to forced vital capacity ratio (FEV$_1$/FVC ratio)*.

Note: The Centers for Medicare and Medicaid Services (CMS) now require pulmonary rehabilitation patients to qualify for service based on airway limitation severity. Only patients with GOLD 3 or 4 severities qualify for CMS reimbursement at present.

Risk of Exacerbations Assessment—According to GOLD, an exacerbation of COPD is defined as *an acute event, characterized by a worsening of the patient's respiratory symptoms, that is beyond normal day-to-day variations and leads to a change in medication*. The best forecaster of having a risk of exacerbation is the patient's past history—a history of two or more exacerbations per year is considered a high risk for more exacerbations. A worsening FEV$_1$ increases the occurrence of exacerbations in COPD patients and risk of death.

Comorbidities Assessment—Because COPD often develops in middle-aged chronic tobacco smokers, the patient often has a variety of other health problems related to either smoking or aging. Diseases commonly associated with COPD include cardiovascular disease, osteoporosis, depression and anxiety, skeletal muscle dysfunction, the metabolic syndrome, and lung cancer.

Combined COPD Assessment

GOLD recommends combining all the above assessments— that is, the symptoms assessment, airflow limitations assessment, and risk of exacerbations assessment. Combining these three areas helps to determine the impact of COPD on the patient, and improves the ability to develop and manage a treatment plan that is specifically designed to meet the individual patient's needs.

GOLD recommends using a *scoring rubric*[3] *measurement* system to objectively assess the patient's COPD related symptoms, the severity of airflow limitation, and the risk of exacerbations. A representative example of a Combined

COPD Assessment Rubric Scoring Tool, similar to the one developed by GOLD, is shown in Figure 12-7.

How to Use the Combined COPD Scoring Rubric

To assign a patient to either Group A, B, C, or D (see Figure 12-7)—and to subsequently develop and manage a treatment plan that is specifically designed to meet the individual patient's needs—follow these steps:

1. First evaluate the patient's **Symptoms** with the mMRC or CAT score to determine if the patient belongs on the "left" side of the box—Less Symptoms (mMRC 0–1 or CAT < 10); or the "right" side of the box—More Symptoms (mMRC ≥ or CAT ≥ 10).

2. Next, evaluate the **Risk of Exacerbations** to determine if the patient belongs on the "lower" part of the box (Low Risk), or the "upper" part of the box (High Risk). This can be established by either of the following two methods:

   a. **GOLD Classification of Airflow Limitation**— Determine the GOLD grade of airflow limitation. GOLD 1 and 2 indicate Low Risk, whereas GOLD 3 and 4 indicate High Risk.

   b. **Number of Exacerbations during Last 12 Months**— Identify the number of exacerbations the patient experienced during the last 12 months. Zero to one exacerbation indicates Low Risk, whereas two or more exacerbations indicate High Risk.

Finally, it should be noted that in some COPD patients, the above two methods of assessing the risk of exacerbation will not lead to the same severity of risk. In these cases, select the highest risk according to either the GOLD grade or the exacerbation history. For example, consider the case in Box 12-1.

Additional Screening Methods Used to Diagnosis COPD

The following are additional diagnostic procedures that may be helpful in the diagnosis and assessment of COPD:

BODE index—To evaluate the patient's extrapulmonary manifestations associated with COPD more closely, the BODE index may also be used. The **BODE index** and BODE score, which is short for "**B**ody-mass index, airflow **O**bstruction, **D**yspnea and **E**xercise capacity index in chronic obstructive pulmonary disease," is a multidimensional 10-point scale that provides better prognostic information than the FEV$_1$ alone. Changes in the BODE index can also be used to evaluate the patient's response to therapy.

Chest Radiographs

A chest radiograph has a poor sensitivity in establishing a diagnosis of COPD. However, it is useful in eliminating other cardiopulmonary disorders—such as pulmonary fibrosis, bronchiectasis, and cardiomegaly. Radiographic features associated with COPD in the advanced stages include:

- Increased radiolucency of the lungs, rapidly tapering vascular shadows, flat diaphragms, a long and distended heart shadow, widened intercostal spaces, and flattened rib angles on a frontal radiograph. These findings are caused by hyperinflation.
- Bullae, which are radiolucent areas on the lung greater than 1 cm in diameter and surrounded by hairline

---

[3]A scoring *rubric* is defined as an explicit set of criteria used for assessing a particular type of work or performance.

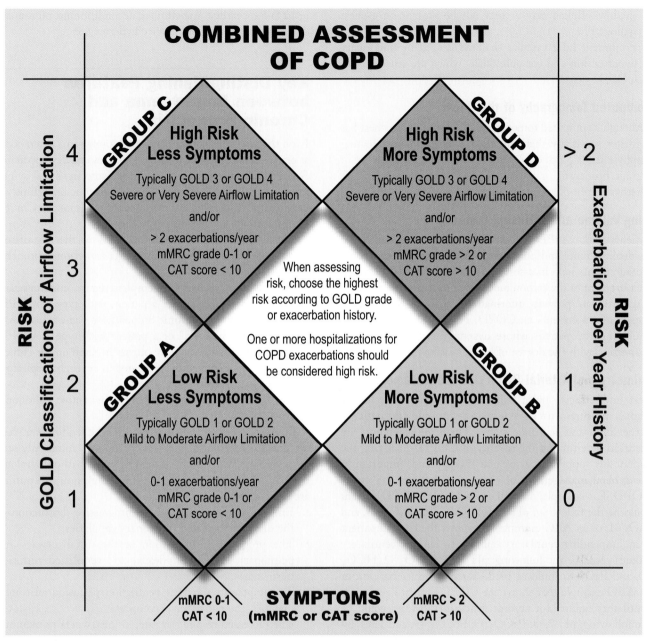

FIGURE 12-7 Combined Assessment of COPD. (Modified from GOLD, Global Strategy for the Diagnosis, Management, and Prevention of Chronic Obstructive Pulmonary Disease, Revised 2014; www.goldcopd.org.)

BOX 12-1 Combined COPD Assessment Case Example

A 73-year-old male patient has a symptom CAT score of 16, and FEV$_1$ of 55% (GOLD grade of 2) of predicted, and a history of three exacerbations within the last 12 months.

Using the Combined COPD Assessment Rubric (Figure 12-7):

- The symptom CAT score indicates that the patient is more symptomatic (CAT ≥ 10) and, therefore, should be placed on the right side of the box—which contains Group B and Group D.
- The GOLD grade of 2 (moderate airflow limitation) indicates Low Risk—which suggests the patient should be placed in Group B.

- However, the patient had three exacerbations in the last 12 months. This indicated High Risk, and outweighs the Low Risk assessment (GOLD grade of 2).
- Therefore, the patient belongs in Group D (see Figure 12-7).

The treatment plan for this patient should be directed at High Risk COPD patient with More Symptoms.

shadows. Bullae may or may not be present on a chest radiograph.

- Prominent hilar vascular shadows caused by pulmonary hypertension and cor pulmonale, which are secondary to COPD.

Computed Tomography of the Chest

Although a computed tomography (CT) scan of the chest has a greater sensitivity than the chest radiograph in detecting emphysema, it is not effective for confirming the presence of chronic bronchitis or asthma. The CT scan can determine whether the emphysema is centriacinar or panacinar.

Lung Volume and Diffusing Capacity

Patients with COPD exhibit air trapping (e.g., increased residual volume and functional residual capacity). These measurements help in assessing the severity of COPD. The measurement of the carbon monoxide diffusing lung capacity (DLCO) can provide information regarding the overall impact of emphysema on COPD. The DLCO is helpful in evaluating the patient whose dyspnea may appear out of proportion with the degree of his/her airflow limitation.

Oximetry and Arterial Blood Gas Measurement

Rest and exercise pulse oximetry and arterial blood gas (ABG) measurements are helpful in determining the patient's oxygenation and acid-base status. These measurements are useful in determining the severity of COPD, qualifying the patient for supplemental oxygen therapy and, importantly, the general management of acute exacerbations and stable COPD. For example, an ABG of a "stable" COPD patient could be the following: pH 7.36, $PaCO_2$ 79, HCO_3^- 43, and PaO_2 61; or an ABG example that shows the COPD patient is in "impending ventilatory failure" (or chronic ventilatory failure) could be the following: pH 7.52, $PaCO_2$ 52, HCO_3^- 40, and PaO_2 46 (mild or moderate acute exacerbation); or an ABG example that shows the COPD patient is in "acute ventilatory failure" (or chronic ventilatory failure) could be the following: pH 7.28, $PaCO_2$ 99, HCO_3^- 45, and PaO_2 34 (severe acute exacerbation). (See Chapter 4 for further discussion).

Alpha₁-Antitrypsin Deficiency Screening

When a younger patient (<45 years old) presents with a history and clinical indicators associated with COPD, an alpha₁-antitrypsin deficiency screen should be considered. A serum concentration below 15% to 20% of normal value is highly suggestive of emphysema caused by alpha₁-antitrypsin deficiency.

Exercise Testing

The objective assessment of exercise impairment, measured by means of a reduction in self-paced walking distance, or by an incremental exercise test in the laboratory, is a powerful evaluation of the patient's health and employment status and is a valid predictor of prognosis. More complex cardiopulmonary exercise tests (e.g., aerobic stress tests) are helpful in the differential diagnosis of dyspnea, and may reveal congestive heart failure, cardiac arrhythmias, deconditioning, pulmonary embolic disease, and pulmonary hypertension.

Key Distinguishing Features between Emphysema and Chronic Bronchitis

Even though chronic bronchitis and emphysema often occur as one disease complex called COPD, they can develop alone. A complete presentation of all the specific signs and symptoms associated with emphysema and chronic bronchitis are provided in the Overview of the Cardiopulmonary Clinical Manifestations section on pages 180–185.

An abbreviated and handy overview of the key distinguishing features between emphysema and chronic bronchitis is provided as follows:

Clinically, the patient with emphysema is sometimes classified as a **"pink puffer,"** or a patient with type A COPD; and the patient with chronic bronchitis is sometimes classified as a **"blue bloater,"** or a patient with type B COPD. These general, older terms are primarily based on the clinical manifestations commonly associated with each respiratory disorder.

"Pink Puffer" (Type A Chronic Obstructive Pulmonary Disease)

The term *pink puffer* is derived from the reddish complexion and the "puffing" (pursed-lip breathing) commonly seen in the patient with emphysema. The major pathophysiologic mechanisms responsible for the red complexion and puffing are the following:

- Emphysema is caused by the progressive destruction of the distal airways and pulmonary capillaries.
- The progressive elimination of the distal airways and pulmonary capillaries leads to ventilation-perfusion mismatches.
- To compensate for these ventilation-perfusion ratio mismatches, the patient hyperventilates.
- The increased respiratory rate, in turn, works to maintain a relatively normal arterial oxygenation level and causes a ruddy or flushed skin complexion. During the end stage of emphysema, however, the patient's oxygenation status decreases and the carbon dioxide level increases.
- Thus, the patient with emphysema, who has both a red complexion and a rapid respiratory rate, is called a *pink puffer*.

In addition to the marked dyspnea and ruddy complexion, the pink puffer tends to be thin (because of the muscle wasting and weight loss associated with the increased work of breathing), has a barrel chest (because of hyperinflated lungs), uses accessory muscles of inspiration, and exhales through pursed lips.

"Blue Bloater" (Type B Chronic Obstructive Pulmonary Disease)

The term *blue bloater* is derived from the cyanosis—the bluish color of the lips and skin—commonly seen in the patient with chronic bronchitis. The bluish complexion is caused by the following:

- Unlike emphysema, the pulmonary capillaries in the patient with chronic bronchitis are not damaged. The patient with chronic bronchitis responds to the increased airway obstruction by decreasing ventilation and increasing cardiac output—that is, a decreased ventilation-perfusion ratio.
- The chronic hypoventilation and increased cardiac output (decreased ventilation-perfusion ratio) leads to a decreased arterial oxygen level, an increased arterial carbon dioxide level, and a compensated (normal) pH—or chronic ventilatory failure arterial blood gas values (also called *compensated respiratory acidosis*). The respiratory drive is depressed in patients with chronic ventilatory failure.
- The persistent low ventilation-perfusion ratio and depressed respiratory drive both contribute to a chronically reduced arterial oxygenation level and polycythemia that, in turn, causes cyanosis. In addition, the blue bloater tends to be stocky and overweight, has a chronic productive cough, and frequently has swollen ankles and legs and distended neck veins as a result of pulmonary hypertension and right-sided heart failure (cor pulmonale).

Table 12-4 provides an overview of the more common distinguishing features between emphysema and chronic bronchitis.

The clinical features of emphysema and chronic bronchitis are not always clear-cut because many patients have a combined disease process, COPD. This is especially the case during the late stages of emphysema and chronic bronchitis.[4]

---

[4]It should be noted that the current definition for these respiratory disorders (i.e., chronic bronchitis and emphysema), even if occurring as a singular disease, is often called COPD if there is airflow limitation.

TABLE 12-4 Key Features Distinguishing Emphysema from Chronic Bronchitis*

Clinical Manifestation	Emphysema (Type A COPD: Pink Puffer)	Chronic Bronchitis (Type B COPD: Blue Bloater)
Inspection		
Body build	Thin	Stocky, overweight
Barrel chest	Common, classic sign	Normal
Respiratory pattern	Hyperventilation and marked dyspnea; often occurs at rest Late stage: diminished respiratory drive and hypoventilation	Diminished respiratory drive Hypoventilation common, with resultant hypoxia and hypercapnia
Pursed-lip breathing	Common	Uncommon
Cough	Uncommon	Common; classic sign
Sputum	Uncommon	Common; classic sign Copious amounts, purulent
Cyanosis	Uncommon (reddish skin)	Common
Peripheral edema	Uncommon	Common Right-sided heart failure
Neck vein distention	Uncommon	Common Right-sided heart failure
Use of accessory muscles	Common	Uncommon
Auscultation	Decreased breath sounds, decreased heart sounds, prolonged expiration	Wheezes, crackles, depending on severity of disease
Percussion	Hyper resonance	Normal
Laboratory Tests		
Chest radiograph	Hyperinflation, narrow mediastinum, normal or small vertical heart, low flat diaphragm, presence of blebs or bullae	Congested lung fields, densities, increased bronchial vascular markings, enlarged horizontal heart
Polycythemia	Uncommon	Common
Infections	Occasionally	Common
Pulmonary Function Study		
DLCO and DL/VA	Decreased	Often normal
Other		
Pulmonary hypertension	Uncommon	Common
Cor pulmonale	Uncommon	Common Right-sided heart failure

*The clinical features of emphysema and chronic bronchitis are not always clear-cut because many patients have a combined disease process (COPD—this is especially the case during the late stages of emphysema and chronic bronchitis).

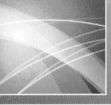

OVERVIEW of the Cardiopulmonary Clinical Manifestations Associated with Chronic Bronchitis and Emphysema (COPD)[a]

The following clinical manifestations result from the pathophysiologic mechanisms caused (or activated) by Excessive Bronchial Secretions (see Figure 9-11) and Bronchospasm (see Figure 9-10)—the major anatomic alterations of the lungs associated with chronic bronchitis (see Figures 12-1 and Figure 12-2); and the clinical manifestations activated by distal airway and alveolar weakening (see Figure 9-12)—the major anatomic alterations of the lungs associated with emphysema (see Figures 12-3, 12-4 and 12-5).

CLINICAL DATA OBTAINED AT THE PATIENT'S BEDSIDE

Vital Signs	Chronic Bronchitis and Emphysema
Heart rate and respiratory rate	Stable patients: normal vital signs
	Exacerbations: usually acute increase in heart rate and respiratory rate (tachypnea)
	Classic signs of hypoxemia

Chest Assessment Findings	Emphysema	Chronic Bronchitis
Inspection		
General body build	Thin, underweight	Stocky, overweight
Altered sensorium—anxiety, irritability	Common during severe stage	Common during moderate and severe stage
	Classic sign of hypoxemia	Classic sign of hypoxemia
Barrel chest	Classic sign	Occasionally
Digital clubbing	Late stage	Common
Cyanosis	Uncommon—often reddish skin	Common
Peripheral edema and venous distention	End-stage emphysema	Common
		Because polycythemia and cor pulmonale are common in chronic bronchitis, the following are often seen:
		• Distended neck veins
		• Pitting edema
		• Enlarged and tender liver
Use of accessory muscles	Common, especially during exacerbations	Uncommon
		End stage in some chronic bronchitis
Hoover's sign	Common—severe stage	Uncommon
The inward movement of the lower lateral chest wall during each inspiration—indicates severe hyperinflation		
Pursed-lip breathing	Common	Uncommon
Cough	Uncommon during mild and moderate stage	Classic sign
		More severe in the mornings
	Some coughing during severe stage with infection	
Sputum	Uncommon	Common
	Little, mucoid	Classic sign; copious amounts, purulent (see sputum examination)
Palpation of the chest	Decreased tactile fremitus	Normal
	Decreased chest expansion	
	Point of maximal impulse (PMI) often shifts to the epigastric area	

Continued

---

[a]Chronic bronchitis and emphysema frequently occur together as a disease complex referred to as chronic obstructive pulmonary disease (COPD). Patients with COPD typically demonstrate clinical manifestations of both chronic bronchitis and emphysema.

Chest Assessment Findings	Emphysema	Chronic Bronchitis
Percussion of the chest	Hyperresonance Decreased diaphragmatic excursion	Normal
Auscultation of the chest	Diminished breath sounds Prolonged expirations Diminished heart sounds	Crackles Wheezes

CLINICAL DATA OBTAINED FROM LABORATORY AND SPECIAL PROCEDURES

Pulmonary Function Test Findings
Moderate to Severe Chronic Bronchitis and Emphysema (Obstructive Lung Pathophysiology)

Pulmonary function tests are the cornerstone to the diagnostic evaluation of patients with suspected COPD. The most important values measured are the forced expiratory volume in one second (FEV_1), the forced vital capacity (FVC), and the FEV_1/FVC ratio.

FORCED EXPIRATORY VOLUME AND FLOW RATE FINDINGS

FVC	FEV_T	FEV_1/FVC ratio	$FEF_{25\%-75\%}$
↓	↓	↓	↓

$FEF_{50\%}$	$FEF_{200-1200}$	PEFR	MVV
↓	↓	↓	↓

LUNG VOLUME AND CAPACITY FINDINGS

V_T	IRV	ERV	RV^b
N or ↑	N or ↓	N or ↓	Normal or ↑

VC	IC	FRC^b	TLC^b	RV/TLC ratio^b
↓	N or ↓	↑	N or ↑	N or ↑

Diffusion Capacity (DLCO)^c

Emphysema	Chronic Bronchitis
Decreased	Normal
A decreased DLCO is a classic diagnostic sign of emphysema	

Arterial Blood Gases
Chronic Bronchitis and Emphysema

MILD TO MODERATE STAGES (GOLD 1 AND 2)

Acute Alveolar Hyperventilation with Hypoxemia^d (Acute Respiratory Alkalosis)

pH	$PaCO_2$	HCO_3^-	PaO_2	SaO_2 or SpO_2
↑	↓	↓ (but normal)	↓	↓

SEVERE STAGES (GOLD 3 AND 4)

Chronic Ventilatory Failure with Hypoxemia^e (Compensated Respiratory Acidosis)

pH	$PaCO_2$	HCO_3^-	PaO_2	SaO_2 or SpO_2
N	↑	↑ (significantly)	↓	↓

ACUTE VENTILATORY CHANGES SUPERIMPOSED ON CHRONIC VENTILATORY FAILURE^f

Because acute ventilatory changes are frequently seen in patients with chronic ventilatory failure, the respiratory therapist must be familiar with—and alert for—the following two dangerous arterial blood gas findings:

- Acute alveolar hyperventilation superimposed on chronic ventilatory failure that should further alert the respiratory therapist to document the following important ABG assessment: possible *impending acute ventilatory failure.*
- Acute ventilatory failure (acute hypoventilation) superimposed on chronic ventilatory failure.

---

^{b}Air trapping, and a subsequent increase in the RV and FRC, is uncommon in patients with only chronic bronchitis.

^{c}The most accurate way to express DLCO as the DLCO corrected for alveolar volume (D_L/V_A). This measure is always reduced in severe emphysema and reflects the loss of alveolar-capillary membrane.

^{d}See Figure 4-3 and related discussion for the acute pH, $PaCO_2$, and HCO_3^- changes associated with acute alveolar hyperventilation.

^{e}See Figure 4-2 and related discussion for the pH, PaCO2, and HCO_3^- changes associated with chronic ventilatory failure.

^{f}See Table 4-9 and related discussion for the pH, $PaCO_2$, and HCO_3^- changes associated with acute ventilatory changes superimpoosed on chronic ventilatory failure.

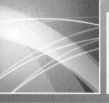

Oxygenation Indices[g] for Chronic Bronchitis and Emphysema
Moderate to Severe Stages

$\dot{Q}s/\dot{Q}\tau$	DO_2[h]	$\dot{V}O_2$	$C(a\text{-}\bar{v})O_2$	O_2ER	$S\bar{v}O_2$
↑	↓	N	N	↑	↓

Hemodynamic Indices[i] for Chronic Bronchitis and Emphysema
Moderate to Severe Stages

CVP	RAP	$\overline{PA}$	PCWP	CO	SV
↑	↑	↑	N	N	N

SVI	cardiac index	RVSWI	LVSWI	PVR	SVR
N	N	↑	N	↑	N

Laboratory Tests and Procedures

Test	Emphysema	Chronic Bronchitis
Hematocrit and hemoglobin	Normal—mild to moderate stage Elevated—late stage	Polycythemia common during early and late stages
Electrolytes (abnormal)	Late stage: • Hypochloremia (Cl^-) when chronic ventilatory failure is present • Hypernatremia (Na^+)	Early and late stages: • Hypochloremia (Cl^-) (when chronic ventilatory failure is present) • Hypernatremia (Na^+)
Sputum examination (culture)	Normal	Streptococcus pneumoniae Haemophilus influenzae Moraxella catarrhalis

Radiology Findings

Test	Chronic Bronchitis
Chest radiograph	Lungs may be clear if only large bronchi are affected.

Chronic Bronchitis

Lungs may be clear if only large bronchi are affected.

Occasionally

• Translucent (dark) lung fields
• Depressed or flattened diaphragms

Common

• Right ventricle (cor pulmonale) and/or left ventricle enlargement

No radiographic abnormalities may be present in chronic bronchitis if only the large bronchi are affected. This often explains why the diagnosis is delayed. Although the situation is uncommon, if the more peripheral bronchi are involved, air trapping may occur. This is revealed on x-ray film as areas of translucency or areas that are darker in appearance. In addition, because of the increased functional residual capacity, the diaphragms may be depressed or flattened and are seen as such on the radiograph (Figure 12-8).

Because bronchial wall thickening is common in chronic bronchitis, increased, diffuse, fibrotic-appearing lung markings are often seen. This is commonly referred to as a "dirty chest x-ray."

[g]DO_2, Total oxygen delivery; $C(a\text{-}\bar{v})O_2$, arterial-venous oxygen difference; O_2ER, oxygen extraction ratio; $\dot{Q}s/\dot{Q}\tau$, pulmonary shunt fraction; $S\bar{v}O_2$, mixed venous oxygen saturation; $\dot{V}O_2$, oxygen consumption.

[h]The DO_2 may be normal in patients who have compensated to the decreased oxygenation status with (1) an increased cardiac output, (2) an increased hemoglobin level, or (3) a combination of both. When the DO_2 is normal, the O_2ER is usually normal.

[i]CO, Cardiac output; CVP, central venous pressure; LVSWI, left ventricular stroke work index; $\overline{PA}$, mean pulmonary artery pressure; PCWP, pulmonary capillary wedge pressure; PVR, pulmonary vascular resistance; RAP, right atrial pressure; RVSWI, right ventricular stroke work index; SV, stroke volume; SVI, stroke volume index; SVR, systemic vascular resistance.

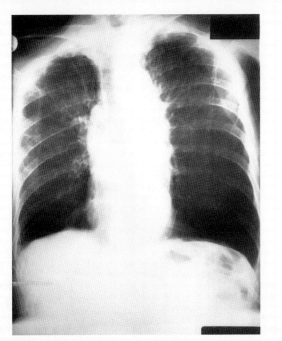

FIGURE 12-8 Chest x-ray film from a patient with chronic bronchitis. Note the translucent (dark) lung fields at the bases, depressed diaphragms, and long and narrow heart.

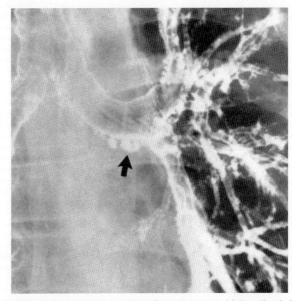

FIGURE 12-9 Chronic bronchitis. Bronchogram with localized view of left hilum. Rounded collections of contrast lie adjacent to bronchial walls and are particularly well demonstrated below the left main stem bronchus (*arrow*) in this film. They are caused by contrast in dilated mucous gland ducts. (From Hansel DM, Armstrong P, Lynch DA, McAdams HP, eds: *Imaging of the diseases of the chest*, ed 4, St Louis, 2005, Mosby.)

Test	
	Chronic Bronchitis
	Finally, because right and left ventricular enlargement and failure are commonly associated with chronic bronchitis, in the late stage an enlarged heart may be seen on the chest radiograph.
Bronchogram Computed tomography (CT) scan	Although rarely done today, small spikelike protrusions ("train tracks" appearance of airways) from the larger bronchi could often be seen on the bronchograms of patients with chronic bronchitis. It is believed that the spikes result from pooling of the radiopaque medium in the enlarged ducts of the mucous glands (Figure 12-9).
	Since the advent of the computed tomography (CT) examination, bronchograms are seldom done today on patients with chronic bronchitis. A "thin-section" CT exam is even more helpful.
	Emphysema
Chest radiograph	Common
	· Translucent (dark) lung fields.
	· Depressed or flattened diaphragms.
	· Long and narrow heart (pulled downward by diaphragms).
	· Increased retrosternal air space (lateral radiograph).
	Occasionally
	· Cor pulmonale (signs of cardiomegaly).
	· Emphysematous bullae.

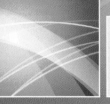

OVERVIEW of the Cardiopulmonary Clinical Manifestations Associated with Chronic Bronchitis and Emphysema (COPD)—cont'd

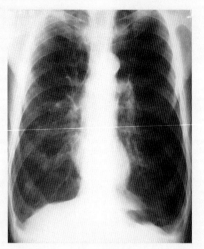

FIGURE 12-10 Chest x-ray film of a patient with emphysema. The heart often appears long and narrow as a result of being drawn downward by the descending diaphragm.

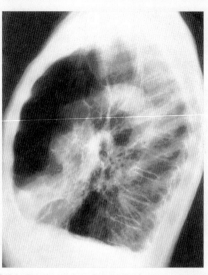

FIGURE 12-11 Emphysema. Lateral chest radiograph demonstrates a characteristically large retrosternal radiolucency with increased separation of the aorta and sternum measuring 4.6 cm, 3 cm below the angle of Louis and extending down to within 3 cm of the diaphragm anteriorly. Both costophrenic angles are obtuse, and both hemidiaphragms are flat. (From Hansel DM, Armstrong P, Lynch DA, McAdams HP, eds: *Imaging of the diseases of the chest*, ed 4, St Louis, 2005, Mosby.)

Chest radiograph cont'd

Emphysema

Because of the decreased lung recoil and air trapping in emphysema, the functional residual capacity increases and the radiographic density of the lungs decreases. Consequently, the resistance to x-ray penetration is not as great, causing areas of translucency or areas that are darker in appearance. Because of the increased functional residual capacity, the diaphragm is depressed or flattened (a hallmark of lung hyperinflation) and the heart often appears long and narrow (Figure 12-10).

The lateral chest radiograph characteristically shows an increased retrosternal air space (more than 3.0 cm from the anterior surface of the aorta to the back of the sternum measured 3.0 cm below the manubriosternal junction), and flattened diaphragms (Figure 12-11). Because right ventricular enlargement and cor pulmonale sometimes develop as secondary problems during the advanced stages of emphysema, an enlarged heart may be seen on the chest radiograph (Figure 12-12).

Occasionally, emphysematous bulla may be seen on the chest radiograph or CT scan. Bullae appear as air-containing cystic spaces whose walls are usually of hairline thickness. They can range in size from 1 to 2 cm in diameter up to an entire hemithorax (Figure 12-13). These large, radiolucent, air-filled sacs are generally found at the apices or at the bases of the lung. Bullae may become so large that they cause respiratory insufficiency by compressing the remaining relatively normal lung. Figure 12-14 shows a CT scan of emphysematous blebs.

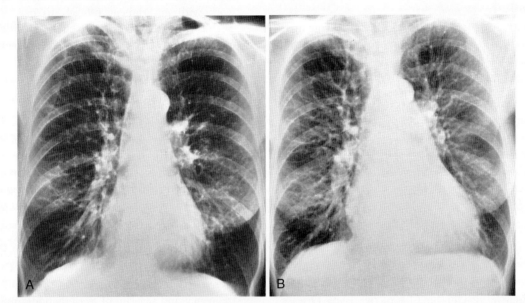

FIGURE 12-12 Cor pulmonale. **A**, A 50-year-old man with chronic airflow obstruction. Lungs are large in volume, the diaphragm is flat, and vascular attenuation is evident at the right apex. These features suggest emphysema, and this diagnosis was supported by a low carbon monoxide diffusion capacity. Lung "markings" are increased peripherally, particularly in the left midzone. **B**, The patient became chronically hypoxic and, with respiratory infections, hypercapnic. One of these episodes was associated with cor pulmonale when the patient became edematous, and the heart and hilar and pulmonary parenchymal vessels became enlarged. The emphysematous right upper zone shows fewer vascular markings and is relatively transradient. The diaphragm is less depressed and more curved than before. (From Hansell DM, Armstrong P, Lynch DA, McAdams HP, eds: *Imaging of the diseases of the chest*, ed 4, St Louis, 2005, Mosby.)

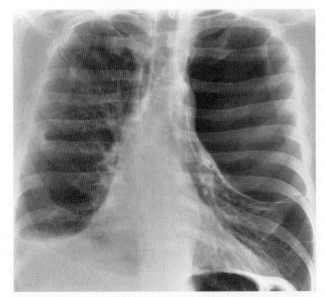

FIGURE 12-13 Giant emphysematous bulla. Air-containing mass fills most of the left hemithorax. (From Eisenberg RL, Johnson NM. *Comprehensive Radiographic Pathology*, ed 5, Philadelphia, 2011, Elsevier.)

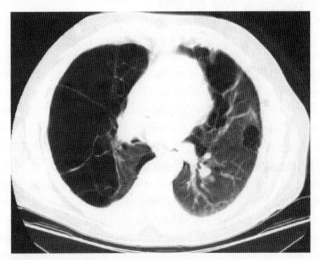

FIGURE 12-14 Emphysematous blebs. CT scan shows the destruction of lung parenchyma. (From Eisenberg RL, Johnson NM. *Comprehensive Radiographic Pathology*, ed 5, Philadelphia, 2011, Elsevier.)

General Management of Chronic Obstructive Pulmonary Disease

Global Initiative for Chronic Obstructive Lung Disease

GOLD provides an outstanding COPD management program that can easily be adapted to local health-care systems and resources. Educational tools, such as laminated cards or computer-based learning programs, can be developed that are tailored to these systems and resources. As of this writing, the GOLD program includes the following publications:

- *Global Initiative for Chronic Obstructive Lung Disease: Global Strategy for the Diagnosis, Management, and Prevention of Chronic Obstructive Pulmonary Disease* (Revised 2014)
- *Global Initiative for Chronic Obstructive Lung Disease: Pocket Guide to COPD Diagnosis, Management, and Prevention. A Guide for Health-Care Professionals* (Revised 2014)
- COPD diagnosis and Management At-A-Glance Desk Reference (2014)
- *Spirometry for Health-Care Providers. Global Initiative for Chronic Obstructive Lung Disease (GOLD)* (Revised 2010)
- Spirometry for Health-Care Providers: Quick Guide, Global Initiative for Chronic Obstructive Lung Disease (GOLD) (2014)
- Diagnosis of Diseases of Chronic Airflow Limitation: Asthma COPD and Asthma—COPD Overlap Syndrome (ACOS) (2014)
- GOLD PowerPoint set (2014)

All of these publications are available at the following Internet site: www.goldcopd.org

Overview of the GOLD Management Program for COPD

The GOLD management program for COPD is subdivided into the following three categories: Therapeutic Options, Management of Stable COPD, and Management of COPD Exacerbations. To obtain the complete report of the GOLD management program for COPD, go to www.goldcopd.org. The key points discussed under each of these headings are presented over the following pages:

Therapeutic Options

Therapeutic options for patients with COPD include the following:

Smoking cessation—Has the greatest influence in improving the natural history of COPD. All patients who smoke should be strongly encouraged to quit. Pharmacotherapies for smoking cessation include the following:

- **Nicotine Replacement Products**—Nicotine replacement therapy in any form (nicotine gum, inhaler, nasal spray, transdermal patch, sublingual tablet, or lozenge) is helpful in reducing the desire to smoke.
- **Other Pharmacologic Agents** (e.g., varenicline, bupropion, and nortriptyline)—Have been shown to increase long-term quit smoking rates when used as one element in a supportive intervention program.

Smoking Prevention—Efforts to encourage comprehensive tobacco-control policies and programs that have clear, consistent, and repeated nonsmoking messages have been developed by the U.S. Public Health Services and other health-care organizations. Coordinated efforts to work with government officials to pass legislation to establish smoke-free schools, public facilities, and work environments and encourage patients to keep smoke-free homes are important and ongoing.

Occupational Exposure—Primary prevention is emphasized by the elimination or reduction of exposure to harmful substances in the workplace.

Indoor and Outdoor Air Pollution—Avoidance of indoor air pollution from burning biomass fuel for cooking and heating in poorly ventilated dwellings is stressed. COPD patients are encouraged to monitor public announcements of air quality and to avoid vigorous exercise outdoors or to remain indoors during pollution episodes.

Physical Activity—COPD patients should be informed of the benefits from regular exercise. Exercise conditioning programs are an integral part of pulmonary rehabilitation.

Pharmacologic Therapy for Stable COPD—This therapy is administered to reduce symptoms, decrease the frequency and severity of exacerbations, and to improve health status and exercise tolerance. The treatment program needs to be individualized to each patient based on the severity of symptoms, airflow limitation, and severity of exacerbations. The classes of medications most commonly used to treat patients with COPD are shown in Table 12-5. The drug selection within each class is based on the availability of medication and the patient's response.

Bronchodilators. These agents are central to symptom management of COPD. GOLD provides the following guidelines for these agents:

- Inhaled bronchodilators are preferred over oral bronchodilators.
- The choice between $beta_2$-agonist, anticholinergics, theophylline, or combination therapy depends on the availability of medications and each patient's individual response in regard to symptoms and side effects.
- Bronchodilators are prescribed on an "as needed" or on a regular basis to prevent or reduce symptoms.
- Long-acting inhaled bronchodilators are convenient and more effective at maintaining symptom relief than short-acting bronchodilators.
- Long-acting inhaled bronchodilators reduce exacerbations and related hospitalizations and improve symptoms and health status. Tiotroprium has been shown to improve the effectiveness of pulmonary rehabilitation.
- Combining different classes of bronchodilator agents may improve the efficacy and reduce the risk of side effects—as opposed to increasing the dose of a single bronchodilator.

Inhaled Corticosteroids—Although controversial, inhaled corticosteroids may be helpful in patients with COPD with an $FEV_1 < 60\%$ predicted. Inhaled corticosteroids may improve symptoms, lung function, and quality of life, and decrease the frequency of exacerbations. Some adverse aspects of inhaled corticosteroids include (1) increased risk of pneumonia, and (2) withdrawal-induced

TABLE 12-5 Medications Commonly Used in the Treatment of Chronic Obstructive Pulmonary Disease (COPD)*

Generic Name	Brand Name
Short-Acting Beta₂ Agents (SABAs)	
Albuterol	Proventil HFA, Ventolin HFA, ProAir HFA
Metaproterenol	Generic only
Levalbuterol	Xopenex, Xopenex HFA, Generic
Long-Acting Beta₂ Agents (LABAs)	
Salmeterol	Serevent Diskus
Formoterol	Perforomist, Foradil Aerolizer
Arformoterol	Brovana
Indacaterol	Arcapta Neohaler
Olodaterol	Striverdi Respimat
Anticholinergic Agents, Short-Acting	
Ipratropium	Atrovent HFA
Anticholinergic Agents, Long-Acting	
Tiotropium	Spiriva HandiHaler, Spiriva Respimat
Aclidinium	Tudorza Pressair
Umeclidinium	Incruse Ellipta
SABAs & Anticholinergic Agents (Combined)	
Ipratropium and Albuterol	DuoNeb, Combivent Respimat
LABAs & Anticholinergic Agents (Combined)	
Umeclidinium and Vilanterol	Anoro Ellipta
Inhaled Corticosteroids & Long-Acting Beta₂ Agents (Combined)	
Fluticasone and Salmeterol	Advair Diskus (250/50 mcg only)
Budesonide and Formoterol	Symbicort (60/4.5 mcg only)
Fluticasone and Vilanterol	Breo Ellipta
Systemic Corticosteroids	
Methylprednisolone	Medrol, Solu-Medrol
Hydrocortisone	Solu-Cortef
Xanthine Derivatives Used as Bronchodilators in COPD	
Theophylline	Theochron, Elxophyllin, Theo-24
Oxtriphylline	Oxtriphylline
Aminophylline	Generic
Dyphylline	Lufyllin
Phosphodiesterase-4 Inhibitor	
Roflumilast	Daliresp

*For the complete listing, doses, and administration of agents approved by the FDA, visit the Drugs@FDA website (www.accessdata.fda.gov/scripts/cder/drugsatfda/).

exacerbation. It is not recommended to use only inhaled corticosteroids for a long period of time.

Combination Inhaled Corticosteroid and Long-Acting Beta₂-Agonist Therapy—The combining of inhaled corticosteroids and long-acting beta₂ agents is more effective than either individual drug in improving lung function, overall health status, and reducing exacerbations in patients with moderate to very severe COPD. However, the combination therapy is associated with an increased risk of pneumonia.

Long-Term Oral Corticosteroids—These agents are not recommended.

Phosphodiesterase-4 Inhibitors (roflumilast)—Roflumilast is helpful in GOLD 3 and GOLD 4 patients with a history of exacerbations and chronic bronchitis, and who are being treated with oral corticosteroids. The helpful effects are also seen when roflumilast is added to long-acting bronchodilators.

Methylxanthines—These agents are not as effective or as well tolerated as inhaled long-acting bronchodilators. Thus, they are not recommended. However, the addition of theophylline to salmeterol (a long-acting bronchodilator) has been shown to produce a greater increase in FEV_1 and relief of breathlessness than salmeterol alone.

Other Pharmacologic Treatment Options

Vaccines—Influenza vaccines can decrease exacerbations and death in COPD patients. Pneumococcal polysaccharide vaccine is recommended for COPD patients 65 years and older, and has been shown to reduce community-acquired pneumonia in patients under age 65 with an $FEV_1 < 40\%$ predicted.

Alpha₁-Antitrypsin Augmentation Therapy—This therapy is not recommended for patients with COPD that is not related to alpha₁-antitrypsin deficiency.

Antibiotics—Only recommended for infectious exacerbations. Long-term use of antibiotics remains controversial (see Appendix III).

Mucolytic Agents (e.g., acetylcysteine)—Acetylcysteine may provide some benefit in patients with viscous sputum. In general, the overall benefits are very small, and are rarely used in the outpatient setting, if at all.

Antitussives—Not recommended.

Vasodilators—The use of nitric oxide is contraindicated in stable COPD. The administration of *endothelium-modulating agents* for the management of pulmonary hypertension associated with COPD is not recommended.

Other Treatment Options

Rehabilitation—All stages of COPD benefit from exercise training programs. These programs improve exercise tolerance and symptoms of dyspnea and fatigue. The minimum length of an effective rehabilitation program is 6 weeks. When the exercise training is maintained at home, the patient's health status remains above pre-rehabilitation levels, and the frequency of hospital admissions is reduced.

Transitional Care Specialists

In 2008, there were more than 800,000 hospitalizations for COPD in the United States. The average length of stay per case was 9.0 days, with an average cost of $7,500 per admission. From this group, 69% were insured by Medicare, and 10% were covered by Medicaid. There were 67% discharged home. However, it needs to be pointed out that the average COPD patient has one or two exacerbations per year with a wide patient-to-patient variation. In the current "Pay for Performance" reimbursement environment, the Centers for Medicare and Medicaid Services (CMS) have instituted a program that penalizes hospitals for adverse events and unnecessary re-admissions for any cause.

Transitions of any kind in medical care are "accidents waiting for time to happen," for example, the dropped signals and messages that occur at shift change. The very nature of many pulmonary conditions is their chronicity, and the goal of good transitional care is to slow, if not to prevent this "revolving door" phenomenon. Although the implications of the recently mandated Medicare **All-Cause Readmission Prevention Program (ACRPP)** may appear daunting, it might well prove to be a true blessing in disguise. In short, a new and important role for the advanced respiratory therapist of the future is emerging—the **Transitional Care Specialist**. With the initial thrust of the Medicare program being so heavily tilted toward patients with respiratory conditions (e.g., COPD, pneumonia, and congestive heart failure), the idea that the respiratory therapist might join certified nurse practitioners and physician's assistants in orchestrating patient locus-of-care transitions is extremely attractive.

Although **pulmonary rehabilitation** has a long track record of preventing pulmonary readmissions, the new paradigm presents fresh challenges for comprehensive respiratory care, with the respiratory therapist and an energized pulmonary rehabilitation program acting as effective change agents. How the respiratory therapist moves into this clear area of need may well determine the future of pulmonary rehabilitation programs, many of which are currently on shaky financial grounds at present.

A typical **pulmonary rehabilitation protocol** will follow guidelines established by expert organizations in a 2007 Joint ACCP/AACVPR Evidence-Based Practice Guideline.[5] Currently, recommended content of such programs are evidence-based on research, and include patient education, exercise training of the muscles of ambulation, endurance training, strengthening of both upper and lower extremities with high-intensity exercise, appropriate use of supplemental oxygen therapy including its use in exercise, and (where appropriate) use of noninvasive ventilation. Scientific evidence does *not* support the routine use of inspiratory muscle training, use of anabolic agents (steroids), psychosocial interventions *alone*, and nutritional supplementation. Consideration of the use of pulmonary rehabilitation in the comprehensive treatment of other chronic respiratory diseases is strongly urged.

---

[5]Ries AI, Bauldoff GS, Casaburi R et al: Pulmonary Rehabilitation—Joint ACCP/AACVPR Evidence Based Clinical Practice Guidelines. Chest 131:4s-42s, 2007.

Oxygen Therapy—The long-term administration of oxygen (>15 hours per day) to COPD patients who have chronic ventilatory failure with severe resting hypoxemia has been shown to increase survival. Long-term oxygen therapy is recommended for patients who have the following:

- PaO_2 at or below 55 mm Hg; or an SaO_2 at or below 88%—with or without hypercapnia that has occurred two times over a 3-week period; or
- PaO_2 between 55 mm Hg and 60 mm Hg, or an SaO_2 of 88% if there is evidence of pulmonary hypertension, peripheral edema suggesting congestive cardiac failure, or polycythemia (hematocrit > 55%).
- See Oxygen Therapy Protocol, Protocol 9-1.

Ventilatory Support—The combination of noninvasive ventilation with long-term oxygen therapy may be of some benefit in some patients; especially in those patients with significant daytime hypercapnia. There are good benefits of continuous positive airway pressure (CPAP) in both survival and risk of hospital admission (see Ventilator Protocols, page 150).

Surgical Treatments—Lung volume reduction surgery (LVRS) is most helpful in patients with upper-lobe predominant emphysema and low exercise capacity before treatment. In selected patients, lung transplantation has been shown to improve quality of life and functional capacity.

Treatment of Comorbid Conditions—The GOLD guidelines suggest that treatment of obstructive sleep apnea in patients with COPD (the so-called "crossover syndrome") has benefits. Other comorbid conditions that should be addressed to ensure optimal care of COPD include: obesity, gastro-esophageal reflux (GERD), congestive heart failure, and conditions where immune mechanisms are suppressed.

Palliative Care, End-of-Life Care, and Hospice Care—Are important components of management of COPD patients during the advanced stages.

Management of Stable COPD

GOLD recommends using the clinical data obtained from a Combined Assessment of COPD Rubric Scoring System (i.e., severity of airflow limitation, patient symptoms, and future risk of exacerbation) as the basis for developing a safe and effective treatment plan (see Figure 12-7). Examples of applying the Combined Assessment of COPD in the clinical setting is provided in the case studies presented at the end of the chapter.

Nonpharmacologic Treatment

The nonpharmacologic treatment plan for COPD is based on the patient's assessment of symptoms and exacerbation risk (Table 12-6). *Smoking cessation* is described as the most important nonpharmacologic treatment for **all** COPD patients who smoke. *Physical activity* is recommended for **all** patients with COPD. *Rehabilitation* generally provides benefits for COPD patients. *Vaccination* decisions are individualized, based on local policies, availability, and affordability.

TABLE 12-6 Nonpharmacologic Management of COPD

Patient Group (See Fig. 12-7)	Essential	Recommended	Depending on Local Guidelines
A	Smoking cessation (can include pharmacologic treatment)	Physical activity	Flu vaccination Pneumococcal vaccination
B, C, D	Smoking cessation (can include pharmacologic treatment) Pulmonary Rehabilitation	Physical activity	Flu vaccination Pneumococcal vaccination

(Modified from GOLD, Global Strategy for the Diagnosis, Management, and Prevention of Chronic Obstructive Pulmonary Disease, Revised 2014; www.goldcopd.org.)

BOX 12-2 The GOLD Guidelines for Bronchodilators in the Treatment of COPD

According to GOLD, the following is recommended for bronchodilators in the treatment of COPD:

- For both beta$_2$-agonists and anticholinergic medications, long-acting agents are preferred over short-acting agents.
- When the patient's COPD symptoms have not improved after the administration of a single agent, the combined use of short- or long-acting agonists and anticholinergics may be considered.
- Inhaled bronchodilators are preferred over oral bronchodilators because they have better efficacy and have fewer side effects.
- Because of relatively low efficacy and greater side effects, the use of theophylline is not recommended, unless other bronchodilators are not available for long-term care.

(Modified from GOLD, Global Strategy for the Diagnosis, Management, and Prevention of Chronic Obstructive Pulmonary Disease, Revised 2014; www.goldcopd.org.)

Pharmacologic Treatment

As shown in Table 12-7, GOLD recommends an initial pharmacological management of COPD program based on the assessment of the patient's symptoms and risk. Box 12-2 provides the GOLD recommended guidelines for bronchodilators in the treatment of COPD. Box 12-3 shows the GOLD recommended guidelines for the use of corticosteroids and phophodiesterase-4 inhibitors.

Management of Acute COPD Exacerbations

According to GOLD, an exacerbation of COPD is defined as *an acute event characterized by a worsening of the patient's respiratory symptoms that is beyond normal day-to-day variations and leads to a change in medication.*

The prognosis in exacerbations of COPD is grim, suggesting that 10% to 20% of such patients will die within 3 months of admission, and as many as 40% in 1 year if significant CO_2 retention ($PaCO_2 \geq 50$ mm Hg) is present. Although an exacerbation of COPD can be caused by a variety of factors, the most common cause (estimated at 70% to 80%) appears to be respiratory tract infections (viral or bacterial). Other conditions that may mimic and/or aggravate exacerbations, and indeed are among the primary causes of death in hospital patients, include pneumonia, pulmonary embolism, congestive heart failure, cardiac arrhythmia, pneumothorax, and pleural effusion. Intentional or inadvertent interruption of maintenance therapy can also lead to COPD exacerbation.

The assessment of an acute exacerbation is based on the patient's medical history, the changes in the current signs and symptoms of severity, and on laboratory tests. Box 12-4 provides common assessment criteria that can be applied to the patient's medical history. Box 12-5 provides common signs of severity that can be helpful to the assessment of the COPD patient's exacerbation. Table 12-8 provides common laboratory tests that are used to further assess the severity of a COPD exacerbation.

Hospital Management of COPD Acute Exacerbations

The primary treatment goals for an acute COPD exacerbation are (1) to reduce the severity of the current exacerbation, and (2) to prevent the reoccurrence of future exacerbations. Box 12-6 provides a general overview of the therapeutic components of hospital management for an acute COPD exacerbation.

Respiratory Care Treatment Protocols

Oxygen Therapy Protocol

Supplemental oxygen should be administered with a target SaO_2 of 88-92%. Venturi masks (high-flow devices) offer more precise control of FIO_2 than nasal cannulas. Long-term oxygen therapy is recommended for patients who have the following:

- PaO_2 at or below 55 mm Hg, or an SaO_2 at or below 88% with or without hypercapnia that has occurred two times over a 3-week period; or
- PaO_2 between 55 mm Hg and 60 mm Hg, or an SaO_2 of 88% if there is evidence of pulmonary hypertension, peripheral edema suggesting congestive cardiac failure, or polycythemia (hematocrit > 55%).

Oxygen therapy is used to treat hypoxemia, decrease the work of breathing, and decrease myocardial work (see Oxygen Therapy Protocol, Protocol 9-1).

Mechanical Ventilation Protocol

Ventilatory support for COPD exacerbations can be provided by either **noninvasive ventilation** (e.g., pressure/volume-limited ventilation via a nasal or facial mask) or **invasive ventilation** (e.g., oral-tracheal tube or tracheostomy).

TABLE 12-7 Initial Pharmacologic Therapy for Stable COPD*

Patient Group (See Fig. 12-7)	First Choice	Second Choice	Alternative Choice†
A	Short-acting anticholinergic PRN Or Short-acting beta₂-agonist PRN	Long-acting anticholinergic Or Long-acting beta₂-agonist Or Short-acting beta₂-agonist & short-acting anticholinergic	Theophylline
B	Long acting anticholinergic Or Long-acting beta₂-agonist	Long-acting anticholinergic & long-acting beta₂-agonist	Short-acting beta₂-agonist and/or short-acting anticholinergic
C	Inhaled corticosteroids & long-acting beta₂-agonist, or long-acting anticholinergic	Long-acting anticholinergic & long-acting beta₂-agonist	Phosphodiesterase-4 inhibitor Short-acting beta₂-agonist and/or short-acting anticholinergic Theophylline
D	Inhaled corticosteroids & long-acting beta₂-agonist, or long-acting anticholinergic	Inhaled corticosteroid & long-acting anticholinergic Or Inhaled corticosteroid & long-acting beta₂-agonist & long-acting anticholinergic Or Inhaled corticosteroid & long-acting beta₂-agonist & phosphodiesterase-4 inhibitor Or Long-acting anticholinergic & long-acting beta₂-agonist Or Long-acting anticholinergic & phosphodiesterase-4 inhibitor	Acetylcysteine Short-acting beta₂-agonist and/or short-acting anticholinergic Theophylline

*Medications listed below are in alphabetical order, and therefore not necessarily in order of preference.
†Medications in this column can be used alone or in combination with other options in the first and second column.
(Modified from GOLD, Global Strategy for the Diagnosis, Management, and Prevention of Chronic Obstructive Pulmonary Disease, Revised 2014; www.goldcopd.org.)

BOX 12-3 The GOLD Guidelines for Corticosteroids and Phosphodiesterase-4 Inhibitors in the Treatment of COPD

- Oral corticosteroids are now recommended for short-term therapeutic trial in patients with COPD. A dose of 40 mg prednisone per day for 5 days is recommended.
- Inhaled corticosteroids for long-term care are recommended for (1) COPD patients with severe and very severe airflow limitations, and (2) for patients with frequent exacerbations that are not satisfactorily controlled by long-acting bronchodilators.
- Long-term monotherapy with inhaled corticosteroids is not recommended in COPD, since inhaled corticosteroids work better when combined with long-acting beta₂-agonists.

- The administration of the phosphodiesterase-4 inhibitor *roflumilast* is recommended to help reduce the number of flare-ups or worsening of COPD symptoms (exacerbations). Roflumilast is not a bronchodilator and should not be used for treating sudden shortness of breath. It is indicated for patients with severe and very severe airflow limitation caused by excessive airway secretions linked to chronic bronchitis. It is not recommended for patients with primary emphysema.

(Modified from GOLD, Global Strategy for the Diagnosis, Management, and Prevention of Chronic Obstructive Pulmonary Disease, Revised 2014; www.goldcopd.org.)

If possible, the use of *noninvasive mechanical ventilation (NIV)* is usually the first ventilatory support technique among patients hospitalized for acute exacerbations of COPD.

Benefits of NIV include the following:

- Avoidance of endotracheal intubation.
- Reduction of problems associated with intubation.
- Comfort of the patient during ventilation.
- Reduction of muscle fatigue.
- The improvement of alveolar and arterial oxygen and carbon dioxide levels.
- The reduction of work of breathing.

TABLE 12-8 Common Laboratory Tests for the Assessment of COPD Exacerbations

Lab Test	Description

Pulse oximetry & arterial blood gas analysis	• A pulse oximeter is helpful in tracking and/or adjusting supplemental oxygen therapy. Portable, inexpensive home units are now available.
	• An arterial blood gas is vital in showing if the following is present:
	  • Impending ventilatory failure (see page 145)
	  • Acute alveolar hyperventilation on chronic ventilatory failure (impending ventilatory failure (see page 145)
	• Assessment of the acid-base status is necessary before initiating mechanical ventilation

Chest radiograph	• The chest radiograph is helpful in eliminating an alternative diagnosis.
ECG	• The ECG is useful in the diagnosis of coexisting cardiac problems.
Complete blood count (CBC)	• A CBC may identify polycythemia (hematocrit > 55%), anemia, and/or leukocytosis.
Sputum culture	• Purulent sputum during an exacerbation can be sufficient indication for starting empirical antibiotic therapy. • *Hemophilus influenza, Streptococcus pneumonia*, and *Moraxella catarrhalis* are the most commonly seen bacterial pathogens associated with exacerbation of COPD. • In GOLD 3 and GOLD 4 patients, *Pseudomonas aeruginosa* becomes important. • When an infectious exacerbation does not respond to the initial antibiotic treatment, a sputum culture and an antibiotic sensitivity test should be performed.
Biochemical tests	• Biochemical test abnormalities including electrolyte disturbances and hyperglycemia. However, these abnormalities can also be due to associated comorbidities. Recent work has suggested that simultaneous elevation of C-reactive protein (CRP), fibrinogen, and white blood cell count were associated with a three- to four-fold increased risk of exacerbation in individuals with stable COPD.
Spirometry	• Spirometry is not recommended during an exacerbation because it can be difficult to perform, measurements are sometimes not accurate, and a decrease in pulmonary function is variable.

(Modified from GOLD, Global Strategy for the Diagnosis, Management, and Prevention of Chronic Obstructive Pulmonary Disease, Revised 2014; www.goldcopd.org.)

BOX 12-4 Common Assessment Criteria Applied to the Patient's Medical History

- Severity of the patient's airflow limitation
  - GOLD 1, 2, 3, or 4
- Duration of worsening of new clinical manifestations
- Number of previous exacerbation episodes and/or hospitalizations during last 12 months
- Complicating comorbidities
  - Cardiovascular disease
  - Osteoporosis
  - Depression and anxiety
  - Skeletal muscle dysfunction
  - Metabolic syndrome
  - Lung cancer
- Resumption of tobacco smoking
- Present treatment program (completeness, patient compliance)
- Need for mechanical ventilation during past hospitalizations

(Modified from GOLD, Global Strategy for the Diagnosis, Management, and Prevention of Chronic Obstructive Pulmonary Disease, Revised 2014; www.goldcopd.org.)

The indications for invasive mechanical ventilation include the following:

- Unable to tolerate NIV.
- Respiratory or cardiac arrest.
- Massive aspiration.
- Severe ventricular arrhythmias.
- Severe hypoxemia in patients unable to tolerate NIV.

BOX 12-5 Common Signs of Severity During the Assessment of COPD Exacerbation

- Use of accessory respiratory muscles
- Cough and sputum production
- Pursed-lip breathing
- Paradoxical chest wall movements
- Impending and/or acute ventilatory failure superimposed on chronic ventilatory failure (ABG)
- Lower than normal baseline SpO_2
- Development of peripheral edema
- Hemodynamic instability
- Deterioration of mental status

(Modified from GOLD, Global Strategy for the Diagnosis, Management, and Prevention of Chronic Obstructive Pulmonary Disease, Revised 2014; www.goldcopd.org.)

Because acute ventilatory failure superimposed on chronic ventilatory failure is often seen in patients with COPD exacerbation, ventilatory support is justified when the acute ventilatory failure is thought to be reversible; for example, when acute pneumonia exists as a complicating factor (see Mechanical Ventilation Protocol 10-1 and Mechanical Ventilation Weaning Protocol 10-2).

Aerosolized Medication Therapy Protocol

As outlined earlier by GOLD, pharmacologic therapy is administered to the COPD patient in an effort to reduce symptoms, decrease the frequency and severity of exacerbations, and to improve health status and exercise tolerance. The medications selected are based on the severity of

BOX 12-6 Therapeutic Management of Acute COPD Exacerbation in the Hospital Setting

Respiratory Support
- Oxygen Therapy
- Ventilatory Support

Pharmacologic Treatment
- Short-acting Bronchodilators (see Table 12-5)
- Corticosteroids
  - Systemic corticosteroids in COPD exacerbations shorten recovery time, improve FEV_1 and PaO_2, and length of hospital stay.
- Antibiotics
  - Antibiotics should be administered to patients with exacerbations of COPD who demonstrate any of the following (see Appendix III):
    - The three cardinal symptoms: increased dyspnea, increased sputum volume, and increased sputum purulence

- Increased sputum purulence and one other of the cardinal symptoms listed above
- Increased sputum purulence
- The need for mechanical ventilation
- Adjunct Therapies

Depending on the patient's clinical condition, the following may be considered:
- Appropriate fluid balance
- Diuretics
- Anticoagulants
- Treatment of comorbidities
- Nutritional considerations
- Stop smoking techniques

(Modified from GOLD, Global Strategy for the Diagnosis, Management, and Prevention of Chronic Obstructive Pulmonary Disease, Revised 2014; www.goldcopd.org).

symptoms, the degree of airflow limitation, the severity of exacerbations, the presence of ventilatory failure, comorbidities (cardiovascular disease, osteoporosis, etc.), and general health (see Aerosolized Medication Therapy Protocol, Protocol 9-4, and Table 12-7).

Bronchopulmonary Hygiene Therapy Protocol

Selected patients who have excessive secretions or an ineffective cough may benefit from a number of techniques used to enhance the mobilization of bronchial secretions such as: postural drainage, positive expiratory pressure therapy, forced expiratory techniques, and flutter valve therapy (see Bronchopulmonary Hygiene Therapy Protocol, Protocol 9-2).

Implications of the GOLD Guidelines for Respiratory Care

IMPORTANT: As the GOLD Guidelines for COPD become implemented in care settings where the respiratory therapist is employed, he or she should be aware that the Guidelines set a *standard of care* to an even greater extent than do Therapist-driven protocol (TDPs). As such, the GOLD Guidelines almost certainly will be used as the basis for malpractice litigation and reimbursement denial—that is if and when they are violated. The role of the respiratory therapist to guard against this (to the extent that he or she can) cannot be over-emphasized.

CASE STUDY Chronic Bronchitis

Admitting History and Physical Examination

This 71-year-old man has worked in a cotton mill in South Carolina for the past 37 years. He smoked 40 cigarettes a day for 30 years (60 pack/year), and he also chews tobacco regularly. He sought medical assistance in the chest clinic because of a worsening chronic cough. He described it as a "smoker's cough" and stated that it was present about 4 to 5 months of the year. For the past 3 years, his cough occasionally produced grayish-yellow sputum during the winter months. The sputum was thick and yellow. He stated that he recently was more short of breath during moderate exercise. He attributed this to "getting older." The patient stated he had not been taking any pulmonary medications.

On physical examination the patient was in mild respiratory distress. He was obese (270 lb). He occasionally generated a strong productive cough during the visit. His sputum appeared grayish-yellow. Auscultation of the chest revealed medium bilateral crackles and scattered wheezes. On a 1 L/min nasal cannula, an arterial blood gas assessment showed pH 7.36, $PaCO_2$ 87 mm Hg, HCO_3^- 48 mEq/L, PaO_2 64 mm Hg, and SaO_2 91%. The chest radiograph revealed hyperinflation.

Pulmonary function tests (PFTs) showed a decrease in the FEV_1/FVC (65%) and a decreased FEV_1 (55% of predicted)—GOLD 2 (see Table 12-3). The patient's mMRC was 1 (Table 12-2). He had no reported exacerbations during the past 12 months. Based on the Combined Assessment of COPD Rubric Scoring System, the patient identified as a GOLD Group A patient classification (low risk, less symptoms) (see Figure 12-7).

The respiratory therapist's assessment at this time was documented in the patient's chart as follows:

Respiratory Assessment and Plan

S "Smoker's cough," sputum production, dyspnea.

O Strong productive cough. Sputum: Yellow-gray. Breath sounds: Medium bilateral crackles throughout and scattered wheezes. On a 1 L/min nasal cannula ABG: pH—7.36, $PaCO_2$—87, HCO_3^-—48, PaO_2—64, and SaO_2 91% x-ray: hyperinflation. PFTs: FEV_1/FVC ratio (65% of predicted), FEV_1 (55% of predicted)—GOLD 2. mMRC: 1. Exacerbations: 0.

A • Combined Assessment: Group A—Low Risk, Low Symptoms (GOLD 2, mMRC 1, exacerbations 0).
   • Mild acute exacerbation (history, physical examination, PFT).
  • Bronchospasm (wheezes).
  • Moderate airway secretions (medium crackles).
  • Good ability to mobilize secretions (strong cough and sputum production).
  • Chronic ventilatory failure with mild hypoxemia (ABG).

P **Bronchopulmonary Hygiene Therapy Protocol** (cough and deep breathing, prn). Patient education on smoking. Refer to Smoking Cessation Clinic. **Aerosolized Medication Protocol** (a pressurized meter dose inhaler [pMDI] short-acting anticholinergic—ipratropium bromide, prn). Continue **Oxygen Therapy Protocol** (1 L/min nasal cannula).

At discharge, the patient was advised to stop smoking and seek medical assistance if his sputum became progressively more thick and yellow or his dyspnea became worse. The physician also prescribed a long-acting beta₂-agonist (see Table 12-7, Group A) and a pneumococcal polysaccharide vaccine. The Smoking Cessation Clinic prescribed slow-release nicotine patches, and the patient attended a weeklong smoking cessation program (see Table 12-6, Group A). The patient did well, and at the 6-month follow-up visit he was no longer smoking. At this time, the patient stated that he had not had his "smoker's cough" or produced any sputum in weeks.

Ten Months Later

Emergency Room History and Physical Examination

The patient presented in the emergency room and was clearly not doing well. He was back to his three-packs-per-day cigarette smoking habit, and he had been physically inactive and gained 30 pounds (to a weight of 300 lb) over the past 10 months. He stated that he frequently coughed and the cough was more troublesome in the early morning. The patient also reported that his cough was now routinely productive—about 3 to 4 tablespoons of thick yellow and green sputum daily. He complained of dyspnea during light exercise (e.g., stair climbing produced shortness of breath). On some days, his

increased work of breathing was more noticeable than on others. He denied hemoptysis, chest pain, orthopnea, fever, chills, or leg edema.

Despite the patient's history, on observation, his ankles *were* swollen, with pitting edema of 3+. His neck veins were distended. He was cyanotic. Vital signs were as follows: blood pressure 165/90, heart rate 116 beats/min, and respiratory rate 26 breaths/min. His oral temperature was 98.4° F. Auscultation of the chest revealed bilateral posterior basilar wheezes and coarse crackles, which partially cleared with coughing. Expectorated sputum was copious, purulent, and yellow and green.

A bedside spirometry showed an FEV_1/FVC ratio of 51% and an FEV_1 of 37%—GOLD 3 (see Table 12-3). The patient's Modified British Medical Research Council Breathlessness Scale mMRC was 2 (see Table 12-2). He had one exacerbation 10 months earlier—for a total of two per year at this point in time (see first SOAP above). Based on the Combined Assessment of COPD Rubric Scoring System, the patient was placed in GOLD Group D (High Risk, More Symptoms) (see Figure 12-7).

On a 1 L/min nasal cannula, his arterial blood gas values were pH 7.51, $PaCO_2$ 51 mm Hg, HCO_3^- 39 mEq/L, PaO_2 41 mm Hg, SaO_2 84%. His resting SpO_2 on room air was 83% and improved to 89% on 2 L/min via nasal cannula. His chest x-ray showed diffuse, fibrotic-appearing lung markings, and a moderately enlarged right side of the heart. His hemoglobin was 17.8 g%.

At this time, the respiratory therapist recorded the following SOAP note in the patient's chart.

Respiratory Assessment and Plan

S Complains of productive cough and exertional dyspnea (history).

O Bibasilar wheezes and coarse crackles, cyanosis, obesity. Neck veins distended. 3+ leg edema. Vital signs: HR 116, BP 165/90, RR 26/min. Cough: productive with copious yellow and green sputum. PFT: FEV_1/FVC (51%), FEV_1 (37% of predicted)—GOLD 3. mMRC 2. Exacerbations one/yr. CXR: diffuse fibrotic lung markings and cardiomegaly (possible cor pulmonale). ABG on a 1 L/min nasal cannula, pH 7.51, $PaCO_2$ 51, HCO_3^- 39, PaO_2 41, SaO_2 84%. SpO_2 on 2 L/min O_2: 89%. Hemoglobin 17.8 g%.

A • Acute exacerbation of chronic bronchitis.
  • Combined Assessment: GOLD Group D—High Risk, More Symptoms. GOLD 3, mMRC 2, exacerbations two/yr. Worsening since last assessment 10 months previously.
    • Acute exacerbation (history, physical examination, PFT).
  • Acute alveolar hyperventilation superimposed on chronic ventilatory failure with moderate to severe hypoxemia (ABG, SpO_2).
    • Impending ventilatory failure.
  • Bronchospasm (wheezes).
  • Excessive mucus accumulation (sputum, coarse crackles).
  • Infection (yellow and green sputum).
  • Tobacco addiction (history).

P **Aerosolized Medication Therapy Protocol**—med neb with short-acting anticholinergic agonist (e.g., 0.5 mL ipratropium bromide in 2.5 mL normal saline q1 hr). **Bronchopulmonary Hygiene Therapy Protocol** (cough and deep breathing under supervision four times daily, cautious trial of CPT with postural drainage to lower lobes, three times a day). Continue **Oxygen Therapy Protocol** (1 L/min nasal cannula; monitor SpO_2). Call physician about impending ventilatory failure and chest x-ray report of cardiomegaly. Also check to see whether the doctor wants to schedule a complete pulmonary function test. Again, advise and facilitate smoking cessation program. Request pulmonary rehabilitation and evaluate.

Discussion

In the first portion of this case study, clearly some of the clinical manifestations caused by **Excessive Airway Secretions** (see Figure 9-11) were present. These findings were documented in the first SOAP note when the therapist charted the presence of a productive cough; coarse crackle sounds, and pulmonary function findings that indicated airway obstruction. Unfortunately, the first SOAP note (and for that matter the initial admitting history) provided no clue as to the time-course of the patient's complaints. Was he stable or worsening? The first part of this case also illustrates a definite role for the modern respiratory therapist. Such a professional may well be working in outpatient settings (e.g., urgent care centers or emergency departments) that necessitate the evaluation and treatment of patients such as this one.

Before writing the first SOAP, the therapist appropriately placed the patient in Group A on the Combined Assessment of COPD Rubric Scoring System, based on the fact that the patient demonstrated an FEV_1/FVC ratio of 65%, an FEV_1 of 55%, an mMRC of 1, and no recent exacerbations. In addition, because the patient was placed in Group A (Low Risk, Low Symptoms), the initial **Aerosolized Medication Protocol** to include the short-acting anticholinergic bronchodilator (ipratropium bromide, prn)—and the long-acting beta$_2$-agonist at discharge—was appropriate according to the GOLD standard guidelines (see Table 12-7).

During the second portion of this case, there were more of the classic clinical manifestations associated with chronic bronchitis. For example, the patient's **Excessive Bronchial Secretions** (see Figure 9-11) not only resulted in hypoxia and cyanosis secondary to a decreased $\dot{V}/\dot{Q}$ ratio and pulmonary shunting, but also produced increased airway resistance that resulted in coarse crackles and a further worsening of the patient's pulmonary function performance.

In the second SOAP, the respiratory therapist correctly placed the patient in Group D (High Risk, More Symptoms) on the Combined Assessment of COPD Rubric Scoring System based on this clinical data: FEV_1/FVC—51%, FEV_1—37% of predicted, GOLD, 3, mMRC 2, and two exacerbations during the past 12 months. Again, because the patient was placed in Group D—and because he was in acute exacerbation—the **Aerosolized Medication Protocol**

included a short-acting anticholinergic bronchodilator, which was appropriate per GOLD Acute COPD Exacerbation Guidelines (see Table 12-8). At discharge, the stable patient should be prescribed an inhaled corticosteroid and a long-acting beta$_2$-agonist, or long-acting anticholinergic agent (see Table 12-7). In addition, a prescription for roflumilast might be considered to help reduce the number of flare-ups or exacerbations associated with excessive airway secretions (see Box 12-3). Referral should then have been made (if possible) to pulmonary rehabilitation (see Table 12-6).

It should also be noted this case study started with the patient's persistent smoking and with increased symptoms and worsening of his obstructive pulmonary disease (dyspnea and productive cough). At the emergency room visit, the findings on the chest radiograph also suggested cor pulmonale, which often occurs in severe bronchitis. His pulmonary function was worsening, and he had acute alveolar hyperventilation superimposed on chronic ventilatory failure with moderate to severe hypoxemia. Impending ventilatory failure was a serious concern.

In addition to treating the acute symptoms with **Aerosolized Medication Protocol** (see Protocol 9-4) and **Bronchopulmonary Hygiene Therapy Protocol** (see Protocol 9-2), the respiratory therapist does not give up on the longer term and extremely important goal of modifying behavior (smoking cessation) in the patient. A complete pulmonary function test in the near future would further define the patient's disease process, both in its nature and severity. Such data are often helpful to the patient's understanding of just how ill he is and may constitute a "teachable moment" for the physician and therapist. Pulmonary function testing is not, however, recommended during an acute exacerbation (see Table 12-8, page 191).

Note to the reader: Not mentioned in this case is the sense of the "time-course" of the patient's symptoms (Acute? Subacute? Progressive? Stable?). We will discuss the importance of this newer part of a "good SOAP" note as we move along. For now, we ask the reader to begin thinking of respiratory disease in an *evolving sense*. Doing so imparts a sense of appropriate urgency to the case, in a way that words like "GOLD," "severe," "worsening," etc., cannot do well.

Although the patient was discharged from the hospital 5 days after his last admission, he unfortunately died from another acute exacerbation of chronic bronchitis, ventilatory failure, and cardiac arrest 3 weeks later. Interestingly, if this patient had been admitted for this terminal episode in 2014, the hospital would not have been reimbursed under the new Affordable Health-Care Act. The Affordable Health-Care Act (2012) has selected several medical conditions (e.g., acute myocardial infarction, congestive heart failure, pneumonia, and COPD) in which readmission to the hospital—*for any reason within 30 days after discharge*—will not be eligible *at all* for Medicare reimbursement to the hospital. Although this is currently cause for great consternation (and for which no durable remedies have yet been identified), it is a fact of life as this textbook goes to press. Note that three of the four conditions listed above—congestive heart failure, pneumonia, and COPD—have strong, if not exclusive cardiopulmonary components! At present, respiratory care departments would do well to consider "their piece of the pie"—that is, to try to identify preventable respiratory causes for readmission of such patients.

This should give the reader pause and an urge to err on the side of completeness: For example, why was it not insisted upon that this patient receive pulmonary rehabilitation, a tobacco addiction consultation, and perhaps a respiratory home care visit?

CASE STUDY Emphysema

Admitting History and Physical Examination

This 27-year-old man was admitted to the hospital with the chief complaint of dyspnea on exertion. He had a 3-year history of recurrent respiratory problems that had necessitated several hospitalizations of several days' duration in the past. A diagnosis of alpha$_1$-antitrypsin deficiency had been made in the outpatient clinic. This was his third hospitalization in the last 12 months. Recently, his respiratory status had deteriorated to the point where he had to stop working. He had been employed for several years as a cook in a fast-food restaurant, where he was continuously exposed to a smoky environment. He had never smoked. On questioning, the patient related that he had been very short of breath for the past 6 weeks. He further stated that he was unable to walk up one flight of stairs without stopping, and his walking tolerance had decreased—he was walking slower and required frequent stops when walking at his normal pace.

On physical examination the patient appeared anxious. He was sweating profusely and was in moderate respiratory distress. He demonstrated a regular heart rate of 120 beats/min, blood pressure of 140/70, respiratory rate of 32 breaths/min, and an oral temperature of 100° F. Inspection of the chest revealed suprasternal notch retraction, with some use of the accessory muscles of inspiration. The lungs were hyperresonant to percussion, and breath sounds were diminished. His I:E ratio was 1:4. He had a barrel chest and his nail beds were moderately cyanotic. The patient was slightly confused and unable to concentrate well.

The chest x-ray showed moderate to severe hyperinflation of the lungs. Some infiltrates were present in the lower lung regions, and possible infiltrates were also noted in the right upper lobe. The radiology report suggested the presence of a pneumonic process superimposed on chronic lung disease.

Bedside spirometry showed an FEV$_1$/FVC ratio of 45% and a FEV$_1$ of 25% of predicted—GOLD 4 (see Table 12-3). The patient's mMRC was 2 (see Table 12-2). He had three exacerbations during the past 12 months. Based on the Combined Assessment of COPD Rubric Scoring System, the patient was placed in Group D (High Risk, More Symptoms) (see Figure 12-7).

His arterial blood gases while on 1 L/min O$_2$ via nasal cannula were pH 7.53, PaCO$_2$ 66 mm Hg, HCO$_3^-$ 53 mEq/L, PaO$_2$ 48 mm Hg, SaO$_2$ 87%. Laboratory studies revealed a hemoglobin of 16.5 g/dL and a white blood count of 15,000/mm^3. Sputum gram stains were positive for a variety of pathogenic and nonpathogenic organisms. His serum alpha$_1$-antitrypsin level as an outpatient had recently been 30 mg/dL (normal = 150 to 350 mg/dL).

The respiratory assessment read as follows:

Respiratory Assessment and Plan

S "I'm short of breath with any exercise at all." Cough for past 6 weeks.

O HR 120, BP 140/70, RR 32, and temp 100° F. Use of accessory muscles of inspiration, increased AP diameter, cyanosis. Hyperresonant percussion note and diminished breath sounds. I:E ratio 1:4. Lower lung infiltrates, hyperinflation of lungs on CXR. PFT: FEV$_1$/FVC ratio (45%), FEV$_1$ (25% of predicted)—GOLD 4. mMRC 3. Exacerbations three/yr. ABGs on 1 L/min nasal cannula: pH 7.53, PaCO$_2$ 66, HCO$_3^-$ 53, PaO$_2$ 48, SaO$_2$ 87%. Elevated WBC, gram positive organisms in the sputum, alpha$_1$-antitrypsin: 30 mg/dL.

A • Panacinar emphysema (history, alpha$_1$-antitrypsin deficiency).
   • Combined Assessment: Group D—High Risk, More Symptoms. (GOLD4, mMRC 3, exacerbations three/yr.).
      • Acute exacerbation (history, physical examination, PFT).
   • Acute alveolar hyperventilation on chronic ventilatory failure with moderate/severe hypoxemia (ABGs).
      • Impending ventilatory failure.
   • Pulmonary hyperinflation (x-ray, diminished breath sounds, barrel chest).
   • Probable pneumonitis (x-ray).

P Notify doctor about acute ventilatory failure stat. Place NIV via pressure-limited ventilator on standby. **Oxygen Therapy Protocol** (Venturi mask at FIO$_2$ 0.28). Monitor and evaluate per ICU standing orders (SpO$_2$, vital signs). **Aerosolized Medication Protocol** (e.g., med/neb treatment with short-acting agonist bronchodilator (e.g., 2.5 mg albuterol q1 hr)—watch for worsening of tachycardia. Check ABG in 30 min.

The hospital course was relatively smooth. The Venturi oxygen mask therapy, at an FIO$_2$ of 0.28, was enough to increase the patient's PaO$_2$ to an acceptable level. Within an hour the patient's arterial blood gases were pH 7.36, $PaCO_2$ 61mm Hg, HCO_3^- 34 mEq/L, PaO_2 76 mm Hg, and SaO_2 93%. The patient's heart rate, respiratory rate, and blood pressure returned to normal over the next hour.

Blood serologies suggested *Mycoplasma pneumoniae* infection. Intravenous antibiotics were prescribed. The patient was managed conservatively and improved steadily. When he appeared to have had the maximum benefit from the hospitalization, he was discharged with an oxygen concentrator, a portable "stroller," and an oxygen-conserving device. He was instructed to use O_2 at 1 L/min at rest and 2.5 L/min with exercise for 18 to 24 hours a day. Arrangements were made to have him enroll in an alpha$_1$-antitrypsin therapy trial and attend pulmonary rehabilitation classes. He was urged to secure employment elsewhere, in a clean air environment.

Discussion

This fascinating (but fortunately rare) form of emphysema is one in which "pure" emphysema is the dominant pathology. In patients with alpha$_1$-antitrypsin deficiency, chronic bronchitis may be present, but it is much less common than is the usual, cigarette smoking–induced COPD. In this condition the patient's deficiency of the protease inhibitor alpha$_1$-antitrypsin resulted in WBC-mediated protease destruction of his pulmonary parenchyma. Note the slow, insidious onset of his symptoms.

The respiratory therapist accurately placed the patient in Group D (High Risk, More Symptoms) on the Combined Assessment of COPD Rubric Scoring System. The clinical data that supported this decision was as follows: an FEV$_1$/FVC ratio of 45% and a FEV$_1$ of 25% of predicted, the GOLD classification of 4 (see Table 12-3), the mMRC of 2 (see Table 12-2), and the fact that the patient had three exacerbations during the past 12 months (see Figure 12-7).

In this case, because there was no wheezing noted on auscultation, it may not have been absolutely necessary to activate the **Aerosolized Medication Protocol** to give this patient an inhaled bronchodilator, per GOLD acute COPD exacerbation guidelines (see Table 12-8). However, given the fact that the ABG findings confirmed acute alveolar hyperventilation on chronic ventilatory failure—which indicates impending ventilatory failure—an initial dose of a short-acting agonist bronchodilator was justified. Furthermore, because this patient was placed in Group D, a prescription for inhaled corticosteroids and a long-acting beta$_2$ agent should be considered at discharge (see Table 12-7).

The patient's emphysema or **Distal Airway and Alveolar Weakening** (see Figure 9-12) was complicated by additional anatomic alterations of the lungs (i.e., **Alveolar Consolidation** [see Figure 9-8]). The alveolar consolidation was reflected in the patient's immune-inflammatory response (fever and increased WBC), alveolar infiltrates (x-ray), low PaO_2 (caused by a decreased $\dot{V}/\dot{Q}$ ratio and intrapulmonary shunting), and abnormal vital signs (see Figure 9-8). The effects of distal airway and alveolar weakening were reflected in the patient's increased AP diameter, use of accessory muscles of inspiration, hyperresonant percussion note, diminished breath sounds, PFT results, and the chest x-ray film, which showed *alveolar hyperinflation* (see Figures 12-8, 12-10, and 12-11).

The selection of a good program of oxygen supplementation was certainly indicated. Note the selection of a Venturi oxygen mask, which allowed for a safe and precise FIO_2 control regardless of the patient's respiratory rate or tidal volume. Pneumococcal and influenza prophylaxis were certainly indicated in this case. Frequent intravenous administration of alpha$_1$-antitrypsin replacement represents modern therapy in the treatment of this unusual disease, as does counseling the patient that he should not knowingly expose himself to irritants such as those present in the smoky environment of his workplace. Replacement alpha$_1$-antitrypsin therapy does not repair the alveolar damage that has already occurred but is thought to stabilize the condition. Roflumilast is not currently recommended for patients with primary emphysema (see Box 12-3).

CASE STUDY Example of Classic Chronic Obstructive Pulmonary Disease (COPD)

Admitting History and Physical Examination

A 78-year-old man was brought to this Chicago, Illinois emergency room by his adult son. The son stated that his father had a long history of cardiopulmonary problems with chronic productive cough and had been diagnosed as having COPD about 15 years ago. Over the past 10 years, the patient had been admitted to this hospital on several occasions for COPD exacerbations.

Bedside spirometry showed an FEV$_1$/FVC ratio of 45% and a FEV$_1$ of 25% of predicted—GOLD 4 (see Table 12-3). The patient's mMRC was 2 (see Table 12-2). He had three exacerbations during the past 12 months. Based on the Combined Assessment of COPD Rubric Scoring System, the patient was placed in Group D (High Risk, More Symptoms) (see Figure 12-7).

At the time of his last hospital discharge (7 months ago), the patient's electronic records showed that his baseline FEV$_1$/FVC ratio was 55% and his FEV$_1$ was 35% of predicted—GOLD 3 (see Table 12-3). His DLCO was 60% of predicted. At the time of this hospitalization his mMRC was 3 (see Table 12-2). It was noted that the patient was experiencing his second exacerbation within the past year.

Based on the Combined Assessment Rubric Scoring System, the patient was classified as a Group D patient (High Risk, More Symptoms) (see Figure 12-7). On a 1 L/min oxygen cannula, his baseline arterial blood gas values at his previous hospital discharge had been as follows: pH 7.37, $PaCO_2$ 93 mm Hg, HCO_3^- 52 mEq/L, PaO_2 63 mm Hg, and SaO_2 90%.

The patient had a long history of cigarette smoking, as well as working many long hours in smoke-filled rhythm-and-blues clubs throughout the Chicago area for over 55 years. The patient had been a rhythm-and-blues guitar player since the late 1950s. He had worked with many of the greats—including Muddy Waters, Buddy Guy, KoKo Taylor, Lonnie Brooks, and Candy Foster and the Shades of Blue. The patient stated that although he no longer worked in smoke-filled bars, he still smoked two to three packs of cigarettes per day. The patient's son stated that when he had checked in on his father earlier that day, he realized that his father was very confused and disoriented. The son immediately transported his father to the emergency room. The patient had "run out" of previously prescribed medications about 2 months earlier. He also stated that he "could not afford" most of them.

On examination the patient appeared to be in moderate to severe respiratory distress. He was anxious, confused, and disoriented. The patient stated that he could not take a deep enough breath. His vital signs were as follows: respiratory rate, 35 breaths/min; heart rate, 145 beats/min, blood pressure, 145/90, and temperature, 37°C. The patient was moderately overweight and had a barrel chest. His skin appeared cyanotic. He had a frequent weak cough. He produced a moderate amount of purulent, gray-yellow sputum with each cough. In an upright position, he used accessory muscles of inspiration. Exhalations were prolonged with pursed-lip breathing. He had 3+ pitting edema of his legs, ankles, and feet. His neck veins were distended. The patient had clubbing of his fingers and toes.

Palpation revealed decreased chest expansion. Hyperresonant percussion notes were present over both lung fields. Auscultation revealed diminished heart and breath sounds, with bilateral wheezes and coarse crackles heard over all lung fields. An x-ray taken in the emergency room with a portable film showed lung hyperinflation, depressed diaphragms, increased bronchial vascular markings, and an apparent enlargement of the heart. Bedside spirometry was attempted, but the patient was too weak and confused to generate a good expiratory maneuver. Arterial blood gas values on a 2 L/min oxygen cannula were pH 7.24, $PaCO_2$ 110 mm Hg, HCO_3^- 46 mEq/L, PaO_2 47 mm hg, SaO_2 77%. Laboratory results reveal a hemoglobin level of 19 g%.

The respiratory therapist working in the emergency room documented the following assessment:

Respiratory Assessment and Plan

S "I can't take a deep breath."
O Moderate to severe respiratory distress. Vital signs: RR 35, HR 145, BP 145/90, T 37° C. Barrel chest, cyanotic, frequent weak cough, moderate amount of purulent, gray-yellow sputum, using accessory muscles of inspiration,

prolonged exhalation, pursed-lip breathing, 3+ pitting edema of legs, ankles, and feet. Distended neck veins, digital clubbing. Decreased chest expansion. AUS: diminished heart and breath sounds. Bilateral wheezes and coarse crackles in all lung fields. PFT baseline (7 months earlier): FEV_1/FVC ratio—55%, FEV—35% of predicted—GOLD 3, DLCO—60% of predicted, mMRC 3. Exacerbations: Two/yr. CXR: hyperinflation, depressed diaphragms, increased bronchial vascular markings, and an enlarged heart. ABG values on 2 L/min O_2: pH 7.24, $PaCO_2$ 110, HCO_3^- 46, PaO_2 47, SaO_2 77%. Hemoglobin 19 g%.

A • Combined Assessment: Group D—High Risk, More Symptoms (GOLD 3, mMRC 3, exacerbations 2/yr.).
    • Acute exacerbation (history, physical examination, PFT).
    • History of poor medication compliance, persistent smoking.
  • Acute ventilatory failure superimposed on chronic ventilatory failure with moderate to severe hypoxemia (ABGs).
  • Bronchospasm (wheezing).
  • Excessive airway secretions (COPD history, coarse crackles, purulent, gray-yellow secretions).
    • Pulmonary infection (yellow sputum).
  • Poor ability to mobilize secretions (weak cough effort).
  • Air trapping (hyperresonant percussion notes, hyperinflation on x-ray film, barrel chest).
  • Probable cor pulmonale (swollen feet, ankles, and legs; enlarged heart on x-ray).
P Notify physician stat regarding acute ventilatory failure superimposed on chronic ventilatory failure. Possible cor pulmonale. Recommend **Mechanical Ventilation Protocol** and **Oxygen Therapy Protocol**. Start **Bronchopulmonary Hygiene Therapy Protocol** (chest physical therapy four times daily, suctioning prn). Start **Aerosolized Medication Protocol** (e.g., short-acting beta$_2$-agonist such as albuterol) until physician can be reached. If physician agrees to intubation and mechanical ventilation, administer in-line short-acting beta$_2$-agonist—for example albuterol, two puffs, three times daily.

Discussion

This case nicely demonstrates the clinical manifestations associated with both chronic bronchitis and emphysema—that is, COPD. The clinical manifestations of chronic bronchitis seen in this case include chronic productive cough, cor pulmonale (swollen lower extremities and distended neck veins), coarse crackles and wheezing on auscultation, digital clubbing, and polycythemia (elevated hemoglobin level).

That the patient's bronchitis was accompanied by emphysema was indicated by his DLCO of 60% of predicted, the use of his accessory muscles of inspiration, his hyperresonant percussion note, and the presence of his pursed-lip breathing. The fact that he was in hypoxemic, hypercapnic respiratory failure—and that he required ventilatory support—does not help to separate the two diagnoses. These arterial blood gas abnormalities can be seen in either condition. The clinical manifestations (clinical scenarios) in this case are caused by the anatomic alteration of the lungs associated with both chronic bronchitis (see clinical scenarios shown in Figure 9-10 [bronchospasm] and Figure 9-11 [excessive bronchial secretions]) and emphysema (see clinical scenario shown in Figure 9-12 [distal airway and alveolar weakening]).

The respiratory therapist appropriately placed the patient in Group D (High Risk, More Symptoms) on the Combined Assessment of COPD Rubric Scoring System. The justification to do this was based on the patient's FEV_1/FVC of 55%, FEV_1 of 35% of predicted, the GOLD classification of 3, the mMRC of 2, and the fact that the patient had two exacerbations during the past 12 months (see Figure 12-7).

Treatment in this case was first driven by the selection of a **Ventilator Management Protocol**—the patient demonstrated hypoxemic, hypercapnic respiratory failure, and clearly required ventilator support (see Chapter 10). With this in place, the **Oxygen Therapy Protocol** and elements of the **Bronchopulmonary Hygiene** and **Aerosolized**

Medication Protocols were begun with standard protocol specifics. Because the patient was in acute COPD exacerbation, the **Aerosolized Medication Protocol** appropriately included an in-line short-acting beta$_2$-agonist (albuterol [e.g., ProAir], two puffs, three times daily) per the GOLD COPD exacerbation guidelines. In addition, the administration of systemic corticosteroids may have been considered in this case to help shorten the patient's recovery time and improve his FEV_1 and PaO_2 level (see Table 12-8). Once stable, an inhaled corticosteroid, and a long-acting beta$_2$-agonist or long-acting anticholinergic should be prescribed (see Table 12-7). In addition, a prescription for roflumilast might be considered to help reduce the number of flare-ups or exacerbations associated with excessive airway secretions (see Box 12-3).

Unfortunately, this patient did not do well, and became ventilator-dependent. He died in a skilled nursing facility 3 months later, still "missing his smokes" and listening to rhythm-and-blues on his iPod.

SELF-ASSESSMENT QUESTIONS

Answers to questions can be found on Evolve. To access additional student assessment questions visit
http://evolve.elsevier.com/DesJardins/respiratory.

1. **In chronic bronchitis:**
   1. The bronchial walls are narrowed because of vasoconstriction
   2. The bronchial glands are enlarged
   3. The number of goblet cells is decreased
   4. The number of cilia lining the tracheobronchial tree is increased
      a. 1 only
      b. 2 only
      c. 3 only
      d. 3 and 4 only

2. **Which of the following bacteria are commonly found in the tracheobronchial tree of patients with chronic bronchitis?**
   1. *Staphylococcus*
   2. *Haemophilus influenzae*
   3. *Klebsiella*
   4. *Streptococcus pneumonia*
      a. 1 only
      b. 2 only
      c. 3 and 4 only
      d. 2 and 4 only

3. **In chronic bronchitis, the patient commonly demonstrates which of the following?**
   1. Increased FVC
   2. Decreased FEV_1/FVC ratio
   3. Increased VC
   4. Decreased FEV_1
      a. 2 only
      b. 1 and 3 only
      c. 2 and 4 only
      d. 3 and 4 only

4. **The patient with severe chronic bronchitis (late stage) commonly has which of the following arterial blood gas values?**
   1. Normal pH
   2. Decreased HCO_3^-
   3. Increased $PaCO_2$
   4. Normal PaO_2
      a. 1 only
      b. 1 and 3 only
      c. 2 and 3 only
      d. 3 and 4 only

5. **Patients with severe chronic bronchitis may demonstrate which of the following?**
   1. Peripheral edema
   2. Distended neck veins
   3. An elevated hemoglobin concentration
   4. An enlarged liver
      a. 3 only
      b. 2 and 4 only
      c. 2, 3, and 4 only
      d. 1, 2, 3, and 4

6. **What type of emphysema creates an abnormal enlargement of all structures distal to the terminal bronchioles?**
   a. Centrilobular emphysema
   b. Alpha$_1$–protease inhibitor deficiency emphysema
   c. ZZ phenotype emphysema
   d. Panlobular emphysema

7. **What is the normal range of alpha$_1$-antitrypsin?**
   a. 0 to 150 mg/dL
   b. 150 to 350 mg/dL
   c. 350 to 500 mg/dL
   d. 500 to 750 mg/dL

8. The DLCO of patients with severe emphysema is:
   a. Increased
   b. Decreased
   c. Normal
   d. The DLCO test is not used to assess emphysema patients.

9. Patients with severe emphysema commonly demonstrate which of the following oxygenation indices?
   1. Decreased $S\bar{v}O_2$
   2. Increased O_2ER
   3. Decreased DO_2
   4. Increased $C(a\text{-}\bar{v})O_2$
      a. 1 only
      b. 3 only
      c. 4 only
      d. 1, 2, and 3 only

10. Which phenotype is associated with the lowest serum concentration of alpha$_1$-antitrypsin?
    a. MM phenotype
    b. MZ phenotype
    c. ZZ phenotype
    d. M phenotype

11. Which of the following pulmonary function study findings are associated with severe emphysema?
    1. Increased FRC
    2. Decreased PEFR
    3. Increased RV
    4. Decreased FVC
       a. 3 and 4 only
       b. 2 and 3 only
       c. 2, 3, and 4 only
       d. 1, 2, 3, and 4

12. The patient with severe COPD commonly demonstrates which of the following hemodynamic indices?
    1. Decreased CVP
    2. Increased $\overline{PA}$
    3. Decreased RVSWI
    4. Increased PVR
       a. 1 only
       b. 3 only
       c. 2 and 4 only
       d. 1 and 2 only

13. Because acute ventilatory changes are often seen in patients with chronic ventilatory failure (compensated respiratory acidosis), the respiratory therapist must be alert for this problem in patients with severe COPD. Which of the following arterial blood gas values represent(s) acute alveolar hyperventilation superimposed on chronic ventilatory failure?
    1. Increased pH
    2. Increased $PaCO_2$
    3. Increased HCO_3^-
    4. Increased PaO_2
       a. 2 only
       b. 2 and 4 only
       c. 1 and 3 only
       d. 1, 2, and 3 only

14. The lung parenchyma in the chest radiograph of a patient with emphysema appears:
    1. Opaque
    2. White
    3. More translucent than normal
    4. Dark
       a. 2 only
       b. 1 and 3 only
       c. 2 and 3 only
       d. 3 and 4 only

15. What is the single most common etiologic factor in emphysema?
    a. Alpha$_1$-antitrypsin deficiency
    b. Cigarette smoking
    c. Infection
    d. Sulfur dioxide

Chapter Objectives

After reading this chapter, you will be able to:
- Describe the role of the national and international guidelines in the management of asthma.
- Describe the anatomic alterations of the lungs associated with asthma.
- Describe the etiology and epidemiology of asthma.
- List risk factors associated with asthma.
- Describe the cardiopulmonary clinical manifestations associated with asthma.
- Describe the general management of asthma.
- Describe the clinical strategies and rationales of the SOAPs presented in the case study.

Key Terms

Allergic or Atopic Asthma
Allergic Bronchopulmonary Aspergillosis (ABPA)
Anaphylaxis
Anticholinergic Agents
Aspirin Induced Asthma (AIA)
Asthma and Chronic Obstructive Pulmonary Disease (COPD)
Overlap Syndrome (ACOS)
Asthma Control
Beta 2 Agonist
Charcot-Leyden Crystals
Controller Medications
Curshmann's Spirals
Difficult-To-Treat Asthma
Dust Mites
Environmental Factors
Eosinophils
Exercise-Induced Bronchoconstriction (EIB)
Fractional Concentration of Exhaled Nitric Oxide ($F_E NO$)
Host Factors
IgE-Mediated Allergic Reaction
Inhaled Corticosteroids (ICSs)
Leukotriene Modifiers
Long-Acting Beta$_2$-Agonists (LABAs)
Monoclonal Antibody
Nonsteroidal Anti-inflammatory Drugs (NSAIDs)
Sick Building Syndrome (SBS)
Occupational Asthma
Occupational Sensitizers
Pulsus Paradoxus
Radioallergosorbent Test (RAST)
Remodeling
Respiratory Infectious Disease Panel (RIDP)
Respiratory Syncytial Virus (RSV)
Reliever (Rescue) Medications
Short-Acting Beta$_2$-Agonists (SABAs)
Status Asthmaticus
Valved Holding Chamber (VHC)

Chapter Outline

Introduction

Hippocrates first recognized asthma more than 2000 years ago. Today, asthma remains one of the most common diseases encountered in clinical medicine. The burdens associated with asthma in the United States—and worldwide—are enormous. Although the precise annual numbers are not known, it is estimated that asthma is linked to a multitude of lost school days, countless missed work days, numerous doctor visits, frequent hospital outpatient visits, and recurrent emergency department visits and hospitalizations.

A relatively new role of the respiratory therapist is that of **asthma educator.*** In this function, the therapist's goal is to be sure that the patient and the family are cognizant of their role and functions in the care of this usually chronic and often serious condition. The asthma educator must serve as

---

*The specialty credentialing exam to earn the AE-C (certified asthma educator) credential is available for respiratory therapists and other health-care professionals through the National Asthma Educator Certification Board (http://www.naecb.com/).

a "change agent," and his or her effect as a convincing, empathetic communicator will be tested. Toward this end, we have greatly expanded this chapter from previous editions.

Fortunately, over the past two decades several new and important advances have been made by expert panels in the development of evidence-based clinical guidelines directed toward the education, prevention, diagnosis, and management of asthma. These guidelines are based on an extensive scientific foundation that has provided our current understanding of the pathophysiologic mechanisms, clinical manifestations, and treatment recommendations used to control asthma.

Updated clinical guidelines are developed and disseminated on a regular basis by (1) "**The National Asthma Education and Prevention Program (NAEPP)**: Expert Panel Report 3 (EPR-3), Guidelines for the Diagnosis and Management of Asthma—Full Report," and (2) the **Global Initiative for Asthma (GINA)**. The information presented in this chapter is consistent with current NAEPP and GINA guidelines.

National Asthma Education and Prevention Program (NAEPP)[1]

The first evidence-based asthma guidelines were published in 1991 by NAEPP, under the coordination of the **National Heart, Lung, and Blood Institute (NHLBI)** of the **National Institutes of Health (NIH)**. These guidelines were updated in 1997, 2002, and 2007. Today, the guidelines are structured around the following four components of care: (1) assessment and monitoring of asthma, (2) patient education, (3) control of factors contributing to asthma severity, and (4) pharmacologic treatments. The NAEPP "stepwise asthma management charts" have been widely used and now specify optimal treatment for specific age groups 0 to 4 years, 5 to 11 years, and 12 years and older.

The NAEPP guidelines include:
- Six steps of asthma management based upon degree of asthma control
- Four levels of asthma :intermittent and 3 levels of persistent: mild, moderate, severe
- Adjustments to management based upon asthma control
- Use of actions plans for children and adults are recommended.

Free download of EPR-3 summary and the complete guidelines are available at www.nhlbi.nih.gov/guidelines/asthma/

Global Initiative for Asthma (GINA)[2]

The **Global Initiative for Asthma (GINA)** was established in 1993 in collaboration between the United States (the National Heart, Lung and Blood Institute [NHLBI], the National Institutes of Health [NIH][3]) and the **World Health Organization (WHO)**. GINA works with a network of asthma experts and researchers, health-care professionals, professional organizations, and public health-care officials from around the world. GINA gathers and disseminates asthma-related information while also ensuring that a system is in place to incorporate the results of scientific investigations into asthma care. GINA's specific goals are the following:
- Increase awareness of asthma and its public health consequences
- Promote identification of reasons for the increased prevalence of asthma
- Promote study of the association between asthma and the environment
- Reduce asthma morbidity and mortality
- Improve management of asthma
- Improve availability and accessibility of effective asthma therapy

Collectively, by using the evidence-based guidelines provided by NAEPP, along with the extensive information gathered worldwide from asthma experts and researchers, GINA now provides an outstanding—and user-friendly—evidence-based guideline program for the management of asthma. As of this writing, the GINA program publications include (available on line at www.ginasthma.org):
- **Global Strategy for Asthma Management and Prevention** (2014). This is an evidence-based strategy for asthma management and prevention, with citations from the scientific literature.
- **Pocket Guide for Asthma Management and Prevention for Adults and Children Older Than 5 Years** (2014). This is a quick-reference guide for physicians, nurses, and respiratory therapists, with key information about patient management and education.
- **Global Strategy for The Diagnosis and Management of Asthma in Children 5 years and Younger** (2014). This consists of an evidence-based strategy for asthma diagnosis and management in the youngest patients, with citations from the scientific literature.
- **Pocket Guide for Asthma Management and Prevention in Children 5 Years and Younger** (2014). This document provides a quick-reference guide for physicians, nurses, and respiratory therapists who are treating asthma in the youngest patients.
- **At-a-Glance Asthma Management Reference** (2014). This four-page pocket-size card puts key principles of evidence-based treatment for asthma at the health-care professional's fingertips for quick reference in clinical decision-making situations.

Anatomic Alterations of the Lungs

Asthma is described as a lung disorder characterized by (1) reversible bronchial smooth muscle constriction,

---

[1]Expert Panel Response 3 (EPR-3): Guidelines for the diagnosis and management of asthma, 2007. Available at: www.nhlbi.nih.gov/guidelines/asthma/asthgdln.htm.
[2]Global Initiative for Asthma (GINA): *Global strategy for asthma management and prevention*, 2014, GINA. The GINA publications are available at www.ginasthma.org.

[3]National Heart, Lung and Blood Institute (NHLBI), the National Institutes of Health (NIH) (http://www.cdc.gov/nchs/index.htm).

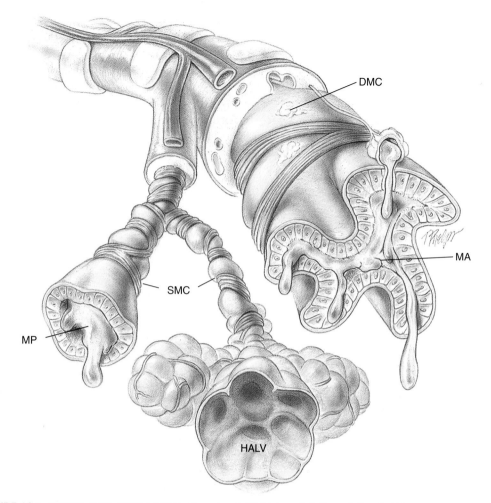

FIGURE 13-1 Asthma. *DMC*, Degranulation of mast cell; *HALV*, hyperinflation of alveoli; *MA*, mucous accumulation; *MP*, mucous plug; *SMC*, smooth muscle constriction (bronchospasm).

(2) airway inflammation, and (3) increased airway responsiveness to an assortment of stimuli. During an asthma attack, the smooth muscles surrounding the small airways constrict. Over time the smooth muscle layers hypertrophy and can increase to three times their normal thickness (Figure 13-1).

The airway mucosa becomes infiltrated with **eosinophils** and other inflammatory cells, which in turn causes airway inflammation and mucosal edema. Microscopic crystals, called **Charcot-Leyden crystals**, are formed from the breakdown of eosinophils in patients with allergic asthma (Figure 13-2). The crystals are slender and pointed at both ends and have a pair of hexagonal pyramids joined at their bases. They vary in size and may be as large as 50 μm in length. The goblet cells proliferate, and the bronchial mucous glands enlarge. The airways become filled with thick, whitish, tenacious mucus. Extensive mucous plugging and atelectasis may develop.

As a result of smooth muscle constriction, bronchial mucosal edema, and excessive bronchial secretions, air trapping and alveolar hyperinflation develop (Figure 13-1). If chronic inflammation develops over time, these anatomic alterations become irreversible, resulting in loss of airway caliber. In addition, the cilia are often damaged, and the basement membrane of the mucosa may become thicker

than normal (fibrosis). This whole process is referred to as "**remodeling**."

A remarkable feature of bronchial asthma, however, is that many of the pathologic anatomic alterations of the lungs that occur during an asthmatic attack are completely *absent* between asthmatic episodes, and that (at least in mild to moderate cases), remodeling does not occur to any great extent.

In summary, the major pathologic or structural changes observed during an asthmatic episode are as follows:

- Smooth muscle constriction of bronchial airways (bronchospasm)
- Excessive production of thick, whitish bronchial secretions
- Mucous plugging
- Hyperinflation of alveoli (air trapping)
- In severe cases, atelectasis caused by mucous plugging
- Bronchial wall inflammation leading to fibrosis (in severe cases, caused by remodeling)

Etiology and Epidemiology

According to the latest information from the **Center for Disease Control and Prevention (CDC)** and the **National Center for Health Statistics (CDC/NCHS)**, the

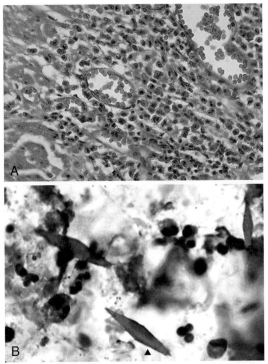

FIGURE 13-2 A, At high magnification, numerous eosinophils are recognized by their bright-red cytoplasmic granules, in this case of bronchial asthma. **B**, In another patient with an acute asthmatic episode, Charcot-Leiden crystals (▲), which are derived from the breakdown of eosinophil granules, are seen microscopically (stained purplish-red). (From: Klatt: Robbins and Cotran Atlas of Pathology, 2nd edition, 2010, Elsevier/Saunders.)

prevalence of asthma in the United States has increased from 7.3% in 2001 to 8.4% in 2010. About 1 in 11 children have asthma; and 1 in 12 adults have asthma. It is estimated that 25.7 million people in the United States suffer from asthma.

In 2009, the CDC reported that there were 479,000 asthma-related hospitalizations, 1.9 million asthma-related emergency department visits, and 8.9 million asthma-related doctor visits. In the United States, alone, asthma costs are over $56 billion per year. The CDC further reported that about 9 people die from asthma each day in the United States—over 3200 each year. Asthma is nearly twice as prevalent in young boys as young girls. In the adult, however, asthma is more common in women than in men.

The **World Health Organization (WHO)**[4] estimates that about 235 million people worldwide suffer from asthma. Low-income and middle-income countries accounts for more than 80% of the mortality. Worldwide, asthma is the most common chronic disease among children. Clearly, the impact of asthma on health, quality of life, and the economy is substantial.

Risk Factors in Asthma

Asthma authorities are not in full agreement as to how the risk factors for asthma should be categorized—for example, under the heading of extrinsic versus intrinsic asthma, or allergic versus nonallergic asthma, or atopic versus nonatopic asthma (Box 13-1). Regardless of this debate, the experts are—for the most part—in agreement that the risk factors for asthma can be divided into (1) **host factors**—which are primarily genetic—that result in the development of (intrinsic) asthma, or (2) **environmental factors** that trigger the clinical manifestations of (extrinsic) asthma, or a combination of both (Box 13-2).

Host Factors

Genetics—There are several persistent and intermittent genetic phenotypes of asthma. Although the genetic factors associated with asthma are varied, and not fully understood, the search for genetic links to asthma has primarily focused on the following four areas: (1) the production of allergen-specific immunoglobulin E (IgE) antibodies, (2) airway hyperresponsiveness, (3) inflammatory mediators, and (4) the T-helper cells (Th1 and Th2), which are an important part of the immune system. The T-helper cells are lymphocytes that recognize foreign pathogens, or in the case of autoimmune disease, normal tissue. Th1 cells are involved in what is called "cell-mediated" immunity, which usually deals with infections by viruses and certain bacteria. They are the body's first line of defense against pathogens that invade the body cells. They tend to be inflammatory. Th2 cells are involved in what is called "humoral-mediated" immunity, which deals with bacteria, toxins, and allergens. They are responsible for stimulating the production of antibodies in response to extracellular pathogens. They tend not to be inflammatory.

Obesity—Asthma is more commonly seen in obese people (body mass index >30 kg/m²). In addition, asthma is more difficult to control in obese patients. Obese patients also have more problems with lung function and more comorbidities compared with normal weight patients with asthma.

Sex and Gender—Before the age of 14 years, the prevalence of asthma is nearly two times greater in boys than in girls. Asthma severity in boys generally peaks around age 5 to 7 years and lessens dramatically during puberty. As children become older, the prevalence of asthma narrows between the sexes—as many girls experience the onset of asthma during puberty. In adulthood, the prevalence of asthma is greater in women than in men.

Environmental Factors

Allergens—Outdoor and indoor air pollution. Outbreaks of asthma exacerbations have been reported in areas of increased levels of air pollution, especially when the environmental air is laden with pollutant particulates less than 5 μm in diameter. The role of outdoor air pollution in causing asthma remains controversial. Similar associations have been reported in relation to indoor pollutants, such as smoke and fumes from gas and biomass fuels used for heating and cooling, molds, and cockroach infestation.

Infections—Although bacterial infections may cause asthma, viral upper and lower airway infections are more likely to contribute to asthma. For example, intrinsic asthma is commonly seen in children after **respiratory syncytial**

4http://www.who.int/en/.

BOX 13-1 Commonly Used Categories for Risk Factors in Asthma

Extrinsic Asthma (Allergic or Atopic Asthma)

When an asthmatic episode can clearly be linked to exposure to a specific allergen (antigen), the patient is said to have *extrinsic asthma* (also called **allergic or atopic asthma**). Common indoor allergens include house dust mites, furred animal dander (e.g., dogs, cats, and mice), cockroach allergen, fungi, molds, and yeast. Outdoor allergens include pollens, fungi, molds, and yeast. In addition, there are a number of occupational substances associated with asthma.

Extrinsic asthma is an immediate (Type I) anaphylactic hypersensitivity reaction. It occurs in individuals who have atopy, a hypersensitivity condition associated with genetic predisposition and an excessive amount of IgE antibody production in response to a variety of antigens. From 10% to 20% of the general population are atopic and therefore have a tendency to develop an IgE-mediated allergic reaction such as asthma, hay fever, allergic rhinitis, and eczema. Such individuals develop a wheal-and-flare reaction to a variety of skin test allergens, called a *positive skin test result.* **Extrinsic asthma is family-related and usually appears in children and in adults younger than 30 years old. It often disappears after puberty.**

Because extrinsic asthma is associated with an antigen antibody–induced bronchospasm, an immunologic mechanism plays an important role. As with other organs, the lungs are protected against injury by certain immunologic mechanisms. Under normal circumstances these mechanisms function without any apparent clinical evidence of their activity. In patients susceptible to extrinsic or allergic asthma, however, the hypersensitive immune response actually creates the disease by causing acute and chronic inflammation.

Immunologic mechanisms (Figure 13-3, A-C)

1. When a susceptible individual is exposed to a certain antigen, lymphoid tissue cells form specific IgE (reaginic) antibodies. The IgE antibodies attach themselves to the surface of mast cells in the bronchial walls (Figure 13-3, *A*).

2. Reexposure or continued exposure to the same antigen creates an antigen-antibody reaction on the surface of the mast cell, which in turn causes the mast cell to degranulate and release chemical mediators such as histamine, eosinophil chemotactic factor of anaphylaxis (ECF-A), neutrophil chemotactic factors (NCFs), leukotrienes (formerly known as *slow-reacting substances of anaphylaxis [SRS-A]*), *prostaglandins*, and *platelet activating factor (PAF)* (Figure 13-3, *B*).

3. *The release of these chemical mediators stimulates parasympathetic nerve endings in the bronchial airways, leading to reflex bronchoconstriction and mucous hypersecretion. Moreover, these chemical mediators increase the permeability of capillaries, which results in the dilation of blood vessels and tissue edema* (Figure 13-3, *C*).

The patient with extrinsic asthma may demonstrate an early asthmatic (allergic) response, a late asthmatic response, or a biphasic asthmatic response. The early asthmatic response begins within minutes of exposure to an inhaled antigen and resolves in about 1 hour. A late asthmatic response begins several hours after exposure to an inhaled antigen but lasts much longer. The late asthmatic response may or may not follow an early asthmatic response. An early asthmatic response followed by a late asthmatic response is called a *biphasic response.*

Intrinsic Asthma (Nonallergic or Nonatopic Asthma)

When an asthmatic episode cannot be directly linked to a specific antigen or extrinsic inciting factor, it is referred to as intrinsic asthma (also called nonallergic or nonatopic asthma) (Figure 13-4). The etiologic factors responsible for intrinsic asthma are elusive. Individuals with intrinsic asthma are not hypersensitive or atopic to environmental antigens and have a normal serum IgE level. The onset of intrinsic asthma usually occurs after the age of 40 years, and typically there is no strong family history of allergy.

In spite of the general distinctions between extrinsic and intrinsic asthma, a significant overlap exists. Distinguishing between the two is often impossible in a clinical setting. Precipitating factors known to cause intrinsic asthma are referred to as nonspecific stimuli. Some of the more common *nonspecific* **stimuli associated with intrinsic asthma are discussed in the main text.**

BOX 13-2 Risk Factors for Asthma

Host Factors

- Genes
  - That is, genes predisposing the patient to IgE-mediated allergic reaction; airway hyperresponsiveness; or a group of inflammatory mediators (e.g., cytokines, chemokines)
- Obesity
- Sex and gender

Environmental Factors

- Allergens
  - Indoor: Domestic mites, furred animals (dogs, cats, mice), cockroach allergen, fungi, molds, yeast
  - Outdoor: Pollens, fungi, molds, yeasts
- Infections (primarily viral)
- Occupational sensitizers and hobbies/leisure activity hazards
- Tobacco smoke
- Outdoor/Indoor air pollution
- Diet: especially in the case of food allergies

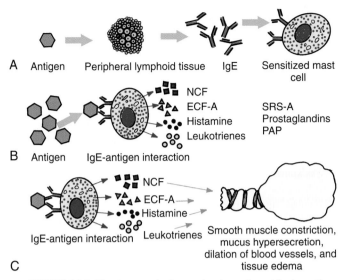

A

Antigen → Peripheral lymphoid tissue → IgE → Sensitized mast cell

B

Antigen → IgE-antigen interaction → NCF, ECF-A, Histamine, Leukotrienes / SRS-A Prostaglandins PAP

C

IgE-antigen interaction → NCF, ECF-A, Histamine, Leukotrienes → Smooth muscle constriction, mucus hypersecretion, dilation of blood vessels, and tissue edema

FIGURE 13-3 The immunologic mechanisms in extrinsic asthma (see Box 13-2).

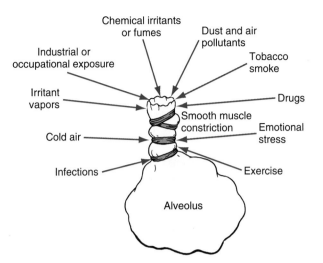

FIGURE 13-4 Some factors known to trigger intrinsic asthma (see Box 13-2).

virus (**RSV**), parainfluenza virus, or rhinovirus infection. These conditions often produce a pattern of symptoms that parallel many features of childhood asthma. For example, it is estimated that about 40% of children with RSV infection will continue to wheeze or have asthma into later childhood.

Occupational sensitizers (occupational asthma). Occupational asthma is defined as asthma caused by exposure to an agent encountered in the work environment. More than 300 different substances have been associated with occupational asthma. Occupational asthma is seen predominantly in adults. It is estimated that **occupational sensitizers** cause about 1 in 10 cases of asthma among adults of working age. High-risk work environments for occupational asthma include farming and agricultural work, painting (including spray painting), cleaning work, and plastic manufacturing. Most occupational asthma is immunologically mediated and has a latency period of months to years after the onset of exposure. Although the cause is not fully understood, it is known that an IgE-mediated allergic reaction and cell-mediated allergic reactions are often involved. Box 13-3 shows additional agents known to cause occupational asthma. It should also be noted that many leisure-time activities can cause asthma by exposing individuals to harmful particles and fumes. For example, severe asthmatic episodes have been triggered by hobbies associated with sawdust and sealants (e.g., commonly found in a woodworker's shop) and the various fumes that can be inhaled by car enthusiasts (e.g., car exhaust, paints, polishes, cleaning products, scented air fresheners, etc.).

Tobacco smoke—Exposure to tobacco smoke—both prenatally and after birth—is associated with a greater risk of developing asthma-like clinical manifestations in early childhood. Infants of smoking parents are four times more likely to develop wheezing illnesses in the first year of life. In fact, the concern of exposing children to tobacco smoke has resulted in several states enacting legislation that prohibits smoking in motor vehicles when children are passengers.

BOX 13-3 Agents Associated with Occupational Asthma

Animal and Plant Proteins
- Flour, amylase
- *Bacillus subtilis* enzymes (detergent manufacturing)
- Colophony, such as pine resin (electrical soldering, cosmetics, adhesives)
- Soybean dust
- Midges, parasites (fish food manufacturing)
- Coffee bean dust, meat tenderizer, tea, shellfish, amylase, egg proteins, pancreatic enzymes, papain
- Storage mites, *Aspergillus*, indoor ragweed, grass (granary workers)
- Psyllium, latex (hospital workers)
- Ispaghula, psyllium (laxative manufacturing)
- Poultry droppings, mites, feathers
- Locusts, dander, urine proteins
- Wood dust, such as western red cedar, oak, mahogany, zebrawood, redwood, Lebanon cedar, African maple, eastern white cedar
- Grain dust, molds, insects, grain
- Silk worm moths and larvae

Inorganic Chemicals
- Persulfate (beauticians)
- Nickel salts
- Platinum salts, vanadium

Organic Chemicals
- Ethanolamine diisocyanate (automobile painting)
- Disinfectants, such as sulfathiazole, chloramines, formaldehyde, and glutaraldehyde
- Latex (hospital workers)
- Antibiotics, piperazine, methyldopa, salbutamol, cimetidine (manufacturing)
- Ethylene diamine, phthalic anhydride
- Toluene diisocyanate, dephenylene, tetramines, trimellitic anhydride, hexamethyl tetramine, acrylates (plastics industry)

Diet—Research has suggested that infants given formulas of intact cow's milk or soy protein have a higher incidence of wheezing symptoms in early childhood compared with infants given breast milk. Studies have also indicated that certain characteristics of Western diets, such as the following, have been associated with asthma:

- Increased use of processed foods
- Decreased antioxidants (in the form of fruits and vegetables)
- Increased n-6 polyunsaturated fatty acid (also called omega-6 fatty acid—which can be found in margarine, vegetable oil, and eggs)
- Decreased n-3 polyunsaturated fatty acid (also called omega-3 fatty acid—which can be found in fish oil) consumption.

Foods that clearly cause an allergy and/or asthma symptoms (usually demonstrated by oral challenges) should of course be avoided.

Other Risk Factors

Drugs—Asthma exacerbations are associated with the ingestion of aspirin and other **nonsteroidal antiinflammatory drugs (NSAIDs)**. It is estimated that as much as 20% of the asthmatic population may be sensitive to aspirin and NSAIDs. Beta-blocking drugs administered orally (e.g., propranolol, metoprolol), or intraocular medications for glaucoma, are also associated with asthma exacerbations.

Food additives and preservatives—Sulfites (common food and drug preservatives found in such foods as processed potatoes, shrimp, dried fruits, beer, wine, and sometimes lettuce in salad bars) have often been associated with causing severe asthma exacerbations. About 5% of the asthmatic population is sensitive to foods and drinks that contain sulfites. The synthetic lemon yellow dye **tartrazine** may provoke an asthmatic episode.

Exercise-induced bronchoconstriction (EIB)—Asthma is sometimes associated with vigorous exercise. (See more on exercise-induced bronchoconstriction under Challenges in the Differential Diagnosis of Asthma, page 207). In children, exercise is a common trigger of asthma symptoms. Research has shown that the drying and cooling of the airways during exercise is the primary trigger mechanism. Running in cold air is the activity that causes the most bronchospasm, whereas swimming in a warm environment causes the fewest asthma symptoms (assuming the water is non-chlorinated and the pool area is well ventilated).

Gastroesophageal reflux—Gastroesophageal reflux disease (GERD), or regurgitation, appears to significantly contribute to bronchoconstriction in some patients. The precise mechanism of this relationship is not known. The patient may complain of burning, substernal pain, belching, and a bitter, acid taste, particularly when lying down. Incidentally, unrecognized GERD is one of the most common causes of a hard-to-diagnose cough; unrecognized sinusitis is the other most common cause.

Sleep (nocturnal asthma)—Patients with asthma often have more breathing difficulty late at night or in the early morning as serum cortisol levels drop at night. Precipitating factors associated with nocturnal asthma include gastroesophageal reflux and retained airway secretions (caused by a suppressed cough reflex during sleep). Additional precipitating factors include exposure to irritants or allergens in the bedroom, and prolonged time between medication doses. Eradication of nocturnal asthma is one measure of good asthma control.

Emotional stress—In some patients, the exacerbation of asthma appears to correlate with emotional stress and other psychological factors. This is most likely mediated by histamine release from circulating mast cells.

Perimenstrual asthma (catamenial asthma)—Clinical manifestations associated with asthma often worsen in women during the premenstrual and menstrual periods. The symptoms often peak 2 to 3 days before menstruation begins. Premenstrual asthma correlates with the late luteal phase of ovarian activity, the phase during which circulating progesterone and estrogen levels are low.

Allergic bronchopulmonary aspergillosis (ABPA)—is characterized by an exaggerated response of the immune system—a hypersensitivity response—to the *Aspergillus* fungus (see Chapter 19) associated in patients with asthma and cystic fibrosis. ABPA can cause airway inflammation and bronchospasm. Patients with ABPA often have symptoms of poorly controlled asthma, such as wheezing, cough, shortness of breath, and reduced exercise tolerance.

Diagnosis of Asthma

The diagnosis of asthma can often be challenging. For example, the diagnosis of asthma in early childhood is based primarily on the assessment of the child's symptoms and physical findings—and good clinical judgment. In the older child and the adult, a complete history and physical examination—along with the demonstration of reversible and variable air-flow obstruction—will in most cases confirm the diagnosis of asthma. In the elderly patient, asthma is often undiagnosed because of the presence of comorbid diseases that complicate the diagnosis.

Furthermore, the diagnosis of asthma is often missed in the patient who acquires asthma in the workplace. This form of asthma is called **occupational asthma** (Box 13-3). Because occupational asthma usually has a slow and insidious onset, the patient's asthma is often misdiagnosed as chronic bronchitis or chronic obstructive pulmonary disease (COPD). As a result, the asthma is either not treated at all or treated inappropriately. Finally, even though asthma can usually be distinguished from COPD, in some patients—those who have chronic respiratory clinical manifestations and fixed air-flow limitations—it is often very difficult to differentiate between the two disorders—that is, asthma or COPD.

GINA provides general guidelines to help in the clinical diagnosis of asthma, which are based on the patient's *symptoms* and *medical history*. There are many signs and symptoms that should increase the suspicion of asthma. These include wheezing and a history of any of the following:

- Recurrent cough
- Recurrent wheeze
- Recurrent difficult breathing
- Recurrent chest tightness

Other indicators are the occurrence or worsening of symptoms at night or in a seasonal pattern. The presence of eczema, hay fever, or a family history of asthma or atopic disease may also be an indicator. Another sign is if an individual has colds that "go to the chest" or that take more than 10 days to clear up. There are also situations in which asthma-related symptoms may worsen, such as exposure to:

- Animals with fur
- Aerosol chemicals
- Changes in temperature
- Domestic dust mites
- Drugs (aspirin, beta-blockers)
- Exercise
- Pollens
- Respiratory (viral) infections
- Smoke
- Strong emotional expression

These symptoms often diminish the response to appropriate asthma control therapy.

Diagnostic and Monitoring Tests for Asthma

Although there are a variety of methods available to assess and monitor a patient's air-flow limitation, the following three tests have gained a widespread acceptance for patients over 5 years of age: **forced expiratory volume in 1 second (FEV$_1$), forced expiratory volume in 1 second to forced vital capacity ratio (FEV$_1$/FVC ratio)**, and **peak expiratory flow rate (PEFR)**. These tests measure the severity, reversibility, and variability of air-flow limitations.

Forced expiratory volume in 1 second (FEV$_1$): An increase in FEV$_1$ of $\geq$12% (or $\geq$200 mL) after administration of a bronchodilator suggests reversible air-flow limitation consistent with asthma.

Forced expiratory volume in 1 second to forced vital capacity ratio (FEV$_1$/FVC ratio): Because many lung disorders can cause a reduction in the FEV$_1$, a better measure of air-flow limitation is the ratio of FEV$_1$ to the FVC. Normally, the FEV$_1$/FVC ratio is greater than 0.75 to 0.80. Any value less than these values indicate air-flow limitation, and asthma should be suspected.

Peak expiratory flow rate (PEFR): An improvement of 60 L/min (or $\geq$20% of the prebronchodilator [PEFR] after inhalation of a bronchodilator), or diurnal variation in PEFR of more than 20% (with twice-daily readings, more than 10%), suggests a diagnosis of asthma. It should be noted that serial PEFR monitoring at home is based on the patient's "personal best" values, not necessarily standard predicted values.

Other Diagnostic Tests for Asthma

Because patients often have normal lung function between asthmatic episodes, measurements of airway responsiveness to *inhaled methacholine* or *histamine*, or an indirect challenge test to *inhaled mannitol*, or an *exercise or cold air challenge* may be useful in confirming a diagnosis of asthma. These inhalation challenge tests can only be performed when the patient

has an FEV$_1$ of 80% or greater, to avoid electively inducing significant asthma symptoms in a compromised patient.

In addition, the presence of allergies (including a positive skin test with allergens or measurement of specific IgE in serum—called the **radioallergosorbent test (RAST)** determination) increases the probability of a diagnosis of asthma, and can help identify risk factors that cause asthma symptoms in individual patients.

Clinicians are now able to judge the control of airway inflammation caused by asthma by measuring **fractional concentration of exhaled nitric oxide (F$_E$NO)**. In adults, the normal F$_E$NO is less than 25 ppb. The normal F$_E$NO in children is less than 20 ppb. The F$_E$NO levels rise with airway inflammation; a high F$_E$NO (greater than 50 parts per billion) suggests a need to increase the patient's controller medication. A common cause of an increased F$_E$NO is a patient's lack of compliance with their prescribed inhaled corticosteroid therapy.

Challenges in the Differential Diagnosis of Asthma

GINA describes the challenges associated with diagnosing asthma among several types of patients, including children 5 years old and younger, older children and adults, and the elderly—and, furthermore, the problems in identifying patients with cough-variant asthma, exercise-induced bronchoconstriction, occupational asthma, and distinguishing asthma from COPD, and the Asthma-COPD Overlap Syndrome (ACOS) (see page 210).

Children 5 Years Old and Younger—This group is challenging because episodes of respiratory symptoms such as wheezing and coughing are common in children who do not have asthma—especially in children younger than 3 years of age. Not all young children who wheeze have asthma. The younger the child, the more likely the cause of the wheeze is not asthma. Common alternative diagnoses of a wheeze include the following:

- Infections (e.g., recurrent viral lower respiratory tract infections or chronic rhino-sinusitis)
- Congenital problems (e.g., cystic fibrosis, bronchopulmonary dysplasia, congenital malformation of the upper airway, or congenital heart disease)
- Mechanical problems (e.g., foreign body aspiration)

A helpful method in confirming the diagnosis of asthma in children 5 years or younger is a trial of treatment with short-acting bronchodilators and inhaled glucocorticosteroids. A marked clinical improvement during the treatment and deterioration when the treatment is stopped supports the diagnosis of asthma. Box 13-4 provides additional signs and symptoms that support the diagnosis of childhood asthma.

Older Children and Adults—A careful history and physical examination, together with the demonstration of reversible and variable air-flow obstruction (preferably by spirometry), will in most cases confirm the diagnosis of asthma. Possible alternative diagnoses include the following:

- Upper airway obstruction or inhaled foreign bodies
- Vocal cord dysfunction
- Congestive heart failure (pulmonary edema)

BOX 13-4 Signs and Symptoms of Childhood Asthma

- Frequent episodes of wheezing—more than once a month
- Activity-induced cough or wheeze
- Cough, particularly at night during periods without viral infections
- Absence of seasonal variation in wheeze
- Symptoms that persist after age 3 years
- Symptoms occur or worsen in the presence of:
  - Aeroallergens (house **dust mites**, companion animals, cockroach, fungi)
  - Exercise
  - Pollen
  - Respiratory (viral) infections
  - Strong emotional expression
  - Tobacco smoke
- The child's colds repeatedly "go to the chest" or take more than 10 days to clear up
- Symptoms improve when asthma medication is given

(Modified from The Global Strategy for Asthma Management and Prevention in Children 5 Years or Younger. Available from www.ginasthma.org.)

The Elderly—Elderly persons who have asthma are frequently undiagnosed. Wheezing, breathlessness, and cough caused by left ventricular heart failure are sometimes called "cardiac asthma," which is a misleading term and should be discouraged. The presence of asthma symptoms during exercise and at night may add to the diagnostic confusion, because these symptoms are consistent with either asthma or left ventricular heart failure. In addition, the use of beta-blockers (e.g., for cardiac conditions and glaucoma), which can cause bronchospasm, are commonly used by the elderly. A thorough history and physical examination, together with an electrocardiogram (ECG), echocardiogram, and chest x-ray, can usually clarify the patient's asthmatic status. Finally, it is often very difficult to distinguish asthma from COPD in the elderly, and may require a trial period with bronchodilators and glucocorticosteroids.

Cough-variant asthma—Some patients have a chronic cough as their primary—if not their only—symptom. It is especially common in children and is most often seen at night. Evaluations during the day are often normal. In these cases, tests directed at the patient's airway hyperresponsiveness, and the search for possible sputum and blood eosinophils, may be helpful in confirming the diagnosis of asthma.

Exercise-induced bronchoconstriction (EIB)—For some patients, physical activity is the only cause of asthma symptoms. Exercise-induced bronchoconstriction typically develops after 5 to 10 minutes of exercise or after completing exercise—in fact, it rarely occurs during exercise. The patient's asthma symptoms, and sometimes a troublesome cough, usually resolve spontaneously within 30 to 45 minutes. Some forms of exercise, such as running, are more potent triggers for bronchoconstriction. Although exercise-induced bronchoconstriction may develop in any climatic condition, it is most common when the patient is breathing dry, cold air; and less common in hot, humid climates. The rapid improvement of postexercise asthma symptoms after inhaled bronchodilator use, or the prevention of asthma symptoms by using a bronchodilator **or mast cell stabilizer** (such as cromolyn sodium) before exercise, supports the diagnosis of exercise-induced asthma. An 8-minute running or 6-minute walk protocol followed by spirometry can also be used to further establish a firm diagnosis of asthma.

Occupational asthma—Asthma acquired in the workplace is a frequently missed diagnosis. Because of the insidious onset of occupational asthma, it is often misdiagnosed as chronic bronchitis or COPD and, therefore, treated inappropriately or not at all. The development of a constant cough, wheezes, and rhinitis should raise suspicion—especially in the nonsmoker. The diagnosis of occupational asthma requires a defined history of occupational exposure to sensitizing agents; the absence of asthma symptoms before beginning employment; a documented relationship between the asthma symptoms and the workplace—an improvement in the asthma symptoms when away from the workplace, and a worsening of the asthma symptoms upon return to the workplace.

Sick building syndrome (SBS)—SBS is a condition characterized by fatigue, loss of concentration, headache, dizziness, nausea, dry and irritated eyes, ear/nose or throat irritation, dry or itchy skin, and respiratory problems reported by people working or living in certain buildings, and there is no specific identifiable cause. Risk factors include the following:

- Poor heating, ventilation, and air conditioning (HVAC) systems which fail to provide adequate fresh air exchanges per hour.
- Low humidity.
- Initial emissions from new components and fittings of a building—the "new smell."
- Volatile organic compounds (e.g., formaldehyde, cleaning products, or manufactured plastic and wood products).
- High temperature or changes in temperature throughout the day.
- Airborne particles, such as dust, carpet fibers, or fungal spores.
- Airborne chemical pollutants, such as those from cleaning materials or furniture, or ozone produced by photocopiers and printers.
- Physical factors, such as electrostatic charges.
- Poor standards of cleanliness in the working environment.
- Poor lighting that causes glare or flicker on visual display units (VDUs).
- Improper use of display screen equipment.
- Tobacco smoke.
- Psychological factors, such as stress or low staff morale.

Distinguishing Asthma from COPD—Because both asthma and COPD are obstructive airway disorders that include underlying airway inflammation, the ability to distinguish asthma from COPD can be difficult. A symptom-based questionnaire for differentiating COPD and asthma may be helpful in these patients (also see Asthma-COPD Overlap Syndrome [ACOS], page 210).

OVERVIEW of the Cardiopulmonary Clinical Manifestations Associated with Asthma

The following clinical manifestations result from the pathophysiologic mechanisms caused (or activated) by Bronchospasm (see Figure 9-10) and Excessive Bronchial Secretions (see Figure 9-11)—the major anatomic alterations of the lungs associated with an asthmatic episode (Figure 13-1).

CLINICAL DATA OBTAINED AT THE PATIENT'S BEDSIDE

The Physical Examination

Vital Signs

Increased Respiratory Rate (Tachypnea)

Several pathophysiologic mechanisms operating simultaneously may lead to an increased ventilatory rate:

- Stimulation of peripheral chemoreceptors (hypoxemia)
- Decreased lung compliance and increased ventilatory rate relationship
  - When lungs are hyperinflated, the patient must work harder to breathe at the flat portion of the volume-pressure curve (see Figure 2-23)
  - Anxiety

Increased Heart Rate (Pulse) and Blood Pressure

Use of Accessory Muscles during Inspiration

Use of Accessory Muscles during Expiration

Pursed-Lip Breathing

Substernal Intercostal Retractions

Substernal, supraclavicular, and intercostal retractions during inspiration may be seen, particularly in children.

Increased Anteroposterior Chest Diameter (Barrel Chest)

Cyanosis

Cough and Sputum Production

During an asthmatic episode the patient may produce an excessive amount of thick, whitish, tenacious mucus. At other times, because of large numbers of eosinophils and other white blood cells, the sputum may be purulent.

Pulsus Paradoxus

When an asthmatic episode produces severe alveolar air trapping and hyperinflation, pulsus paradoxus is a classic clinical manifestation. Pulsus paradoxus is defined as systolic blood pressure that is more than 10 mm Hg lower on inspiration than on expiration. This exaggerated waxing and waning of arterial blood pressure can be detected by using a manual blood pressure cuff or, in severe cases, by palpating the strength of the pulse. Pulsus paradoxus during an asthmatic attack is believed to be caused by the major intrapleural pressure swings that occur during inspiration and expiration—and is associated with a severe life-threatening condition. See discussion below:

Decreased Blood Pressure during Inspiration

During inspiration the patient frequently recruits accessory muscles of inspiration. The accessory muscles help produce an extremely negative intrapleural pressure, which in turn enhances intrapulmonary air flow. The increased negative intrapleural pressure, however, also causes blood vessels in the lungs to dilate and blood to pool. Consequently, the volume of blood returning to the left ventricle decreases. This causes a reduction in cardiac output and arterial blood pressure during inspiration.

Increased Blood Pressure during Expiration

During expiration, the patient often activates the accessory muscles of expiration in an effort to overcome the increased airway resistance. The increased power produced by these muscles generates a greater positive intrapleural pressure. Although increased positive intrapleural pressure may help offset the airway resistance, it also works to narrow or squeeze the blood vessels of the lung. This increased pressure on the pulmonary blood vessels enhances left ventricular filling and results in an increased cardiac output and arterial blood pressure during expiration.

Chest Assessment Findings

- Expiratory prolongation (I:E ratio >1:3)
- Decreased tactile and vocal fremitus
- Hyperresonant percussion note
- Diminished breath sounds
- Diminished heart sounds
- Wheezing
- Crackles

CLINICAL DATA OBTAINED FROM LABORATORY AND SPECIAL PROCEDURES

Pulmonary Function Test Findings
Moderate to Severe Asthmatic Episode
(Obstructive Lung Pathology)

FORCED EXPIRATORY VOLUME AND FLOW RATE FINDINGS

FVC	FEV_T	FEV_1/FVC ratio	$FEF_{25\%-75\%}$
↓	↓	↓	↓

$FEF_{50\%}$	$FEF_{200-1200}$*	PEFR	MVV
↓	↓	↓	↓

*Note: The $FEF_{200-1200}$ is rarely used in pediatrics.

LUNG VOLUME AND CAPACITY FINDINGS

V_T	IRV	ERV	RV
N or ↑	N or ↓	N or ↓	↑

VC	IC	FRC	TLC	RV/TLC ratio
↓	N or ↓	↑	N or ↑	N or ↑

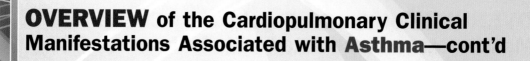

Arterial Blood Gases

MILD TO MODERATE ASTHMATIC EPISODE

Acute Alveolar Hyperventilation with Hypoxemia*
(Acute Respiratory Alkalosis)

pH	$PaCO_2$	HCO_3^-	PaO_2	SaO_2 or SpO_2
↑	↓	↓	↓	↓
		(but normal)		

SEVERE ASTHMATIC EPISODE (STATUS ASTHMATICUS)

Acute Ventilatory Failure with Hypoxemia†
(Acute Respiratory Acidosis)

pH†	$PaCO_2$	$HCO_3^{-\dagger}$	PaO_2	SaO_2 or SpO_2
↓	↑	↑	↓	↓
		(but normal)		

Oxygenation Indices§
Moderate to Severe Stages

$\dot{Q}s/\dot{Q}T$	$DO_2^{\parallel}$	$\dot{V}O_2$	$C(a-\bar{v})O_2$	O_2ER	$S\bar{v}O_2$
↑	↓	N	N	↑	↓

*See Figure 4-3 and related discussion for the acute pH, $PaCO_2$, and HCO_3^- changes associated with acute alveolar hyperventilation.

†See Figure 4-2 and related discussion for the acute pH, $PaCO_2$, and HCO_3^- changes associated with acute ventilatory failure.

†When tissue hypoxia is severe enough to produce lactic acid, the pH and HCO_3^- values will be lower than expected for a particular $PaCO_2$ level.

ABNORMAL LABORATORY TESTS AND PROCEDURES
Sputum Examination

- Eosinophils
- Charcot-Leyden crystals
- Casts of mucus from small airways (**Curschmann spirals**)
- IgE level (elevated in extrinsic asthma)

ASTHMA, COPD, AND ASTHMA-COPD OVERLAP SYNDROME (ACOS)

In May 2014, the Science Committees of both GINA and GOLD published a section on the diagnosis of Asthma, COPD, and **Asthma-COPD Overlap Syndrome (ACOS)**. This document is based on a detailed review of available literature and consensus. It provides an approach to distinguishing between asthma, COPD and the overlap of asthma and COPD—for which the term *Asthma COPD Overlap Syndrome (ACOS)* is proposed. Rather than attempting to provide a formal definition of ACOS, this document presents the clinical manifestations that identify and characterize ACOS, assigning equal weight to features of asthma and COPD. Box 13-5 provides the highlights of the distinguishing features of asthma, COPD, and ACOS:

§ $C(a-\bar{v})O_2$, Arterial-venous oxygen difference; DO_2, total oxygen delivery; O_2ER, oxygen extraction ratio; $\dot{Q}s/\dot{Q}T$, pulmonary shunt fraction; $S\bar{v}O_2$, mixed venous oxygen saturation; $\dot{V}O_2$, oxygen consumption.

∥The DO_2 may be normal in patients who have compensated to the decreased oxygenation status with (1) an increased cardiac output, (2) an increased hemoglobin level, or (3) a combination of both. When the DO_2 is normal, the O_2ER is usually normal.

BOX 13-5

Distinguishing Features of Asthma, COPD, and ACOS*			
Features	**ACOS**	**Favors Asthma**	**Favors COPD**
Age of onset	Usually age >40 years, but may have had symptoms in childhood or early adult.	○ Onset before 20 years	○ Onset after 40 years
Pattern of respiratory symptoms	Respiratory symptoms including exertional dyspnea are persistent, but variability may be prominent	○ Variation in symptoms over minutes, hours or days ○ Symptoms worse during the night or early morning ○ Symptoms triggered by exercise, emotions including laughter, dust or exposure to allergens	○ Persistence of symptoms despite treatment ○ Good and bad days but always daily symptoms and exertional dyspnea ○ Chronic cough and sputum preceded onset of dyspnea, unrelated to triggers
Lung function	Airflow limitation not fully reversible, but often with current or historical variability	○ Record of variable airflow limitation (spirometry, peak expiratory flow)	○ Record of persistent airflow limitation (post-bronchodilator $FEV_1/FVC < 0.7$)

*To read and/or download the complete document ACOS, go to either one of the following web sites: www.ginasthma.org, or http://www.goldcopd.org/.

Continued

BOX 13-5—cont'd

		Distinguishing Features of Asthma, COPD, and ACOS*	
Features	ACOS	Favors Asthma	Favors COPD
Lung function between symptoms	Persistent airflow limitation	○ Lung function normal between symptoms ○ Previous doctor diagnosis of asthma ○ Family history of asthma, and other allergic conditions	○ Lung function abnormal between symptoms ○ Previous doctor diagnosis of COPD, chronic bronchitis or emphysema ○ Heavy exposure to a risk factor: tobacco smoke, biomass fuels
Past history or family history	Frequently a history of doctor-diagnosed asthma (current or previous), allergies and a family history of asthma, and/or a history of noxious exposures		
Time course	Symptoms are partly but significantly reduced by treatment. Progression is usual and treatment needs are high	○ No worsening of symptoms over time. Symptoms vary either seasonally or from year to year ○ May improve spontaneously or have an immediate response to BD or to ICS over weeks	○ Symptoms slowly worsening over time (progressive course over years) ○ Rapid-acting bronchodilator treatment provides only limited relief
Chest X-ray	Similar to COPD	○ Normal	○ Severe hyperinflation

Directions. The area shaded in blue list features that, when present, best distinguish between asthma and COPD. For a patient, count the number of checked features in each column. If three or more features are checked for either asthma or COPD, that diagnosis is suggested. If there are similar numbers of checked features in each column, the diagnosis of ACOS should be considered.

RADIOLOGIC FINDINGS

Chest Radiograph (During an Asthmatic Episode)

· Increased anteroposterior diameter ("barrel chest")
· Translucent (dark) lung fields
· Depressed or flattened diaphragm

As the alveoli become enlarged during an asthmatic attack, the residual volume and functional residual capacity increase. This condition decreases the radiographic density of the lungs.

Consequently, the chest radiograph shows lung shadows that are translucent or darker than normal in appearance. Because of the increased residual volume, functional residual capacity, and total lung capacity, the diaphragms are depressed and flattened (Figure 13-5).

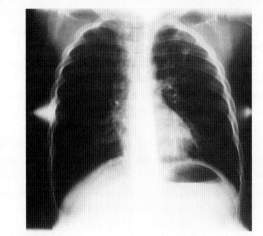

FIGURE 13-5 Chest x-ray film of a 2-year-old patient during an acute asthma attack.

General Management of Asthma

Using the evidence-based information developed by the **National Asthma Education and Prevention Program** (NAEPP), and the extensive research and input provided by leading asthma experts from around the world, the **Global Initiative for Asthma (GINA)** now provides an excellent—and user-friendly—clinical guideline program for the management and prevention of asthma. The complete GINA guidelines are readily available at the following website: www.ginasthma.org. The complete NAEPP guidelines for the diagnosis and management of asthma are available at the following website: www.nhibi.nih.gov/guidelines/asthma/asthgdln.htm. Because they correlate well, the following overview of asthma management is consistent with *both* the NAEPP and GINA guidelines.

The primary goals of asthma management are to:

· Attain and maintain "control" of the clinical manifestations associated with asthma
· Maintain normal activity levels, including exercise
· Maintain pulmonary function as close to normal as possible

- Prevent asthma exacerbations
- Avoid adverse effects from asthma medications
- Prevent asthma mortality

The above goals of asthma care are based on an understanding that asthma is a chronic inflammatory disorder of the airways characterized by recurrent episodes of wheezing, breathlessness, chest tightness, and coughing. Asthma can be effectively controlled by (1) intervening to suppress and reverse the bronchial inflammation, and (2) by treating the bronchoconstriction and related symptoms. In addition, early intervention to stop exposure to risk factors may help to control asthma and reduce medication needs. Based on the current scientific understanding of asthma, GINA provides the following five interrelated components to manage asthma:

- Component 1: Develop Patient/Doctor Partnership
- Component 2: Identify and Reduce Exposure to Risk Factors
- Component 3: Assess, Treat, and Monitor Asthma
- Component 4: Manage Asthma Exacerbations
- Component 5: Special Considerations

The key points of these components of asthma therapy are described below.

GINA Component 1: Develop Patient/Doctor Partnership

The effective management of asthma requires the development of a partnership between the professional(s)—and the patient or parents/caregivers, in the case of young children with asthma. The aim of this partnership is guided self-management—that is, to give the individual with asthma the ability to control their own condition with guidance from health-care professionals. The partnership is formed and strengthened as patients and their health-care professionals discuss and agree on the goals of treatment, the development of a personalized asthma action plan, and the periodic review of the patient's treatment and level of asthma control.

Education should be an integral part of all interactions between health-care professionals and patients, and is relevant to patients with asthma of all ages. Personal written asthma action plans help individuals with asthma make changes to their treatment in response to changes in their level of asthma control, as indicated by symptoms and/or peak expiratory flow, in accordance with written predetermined guidelines. Again, it should be emphasized, in children with asthma the patient/doctor partnership is primarily with the parents, not the patient.

GINA Component 2: Identify and Reduce Exposure to Risk Factors

To improve the control of asthma and reduce medication needs, the patient should take the necessary steps to avoid or reduce exposure to the risk factors (commonly called "triggers") that cause asthma. It is important to develop strategies to avoid the risk factors such as staying away from tobacco smoke as well as foods, drugs, and additives known to trigger symptoms. Also, efforts should be made to reduce or avoid exposure to occupational sensitizers. See "Risk Factors in Asthma" (pages 203).

GINA Component 3: Assess, Treat, and Monitor Asthma

According to GINA, the goal of asthma treatment—which is to achieve and maintain clinical control—can be reached by most patients by means of a continuous cycle that involves (1) **assessing asthma control**, (2) treating to achieve control, and (3) monitoring and maintaining control.

Assessing Asthma Control

Each patient should be evaluated to determine his or her (1) current treatment regimen, (2) adherence to the current treatment schedule, and (3) level of asthma control. As a general rule, when asthma is controlled, most asthmatic episodes can be prevented, the troublesome day and night symptoms are avoided, and the patient can remain physically active. A good protocol for identifying the level of controlled, partly controlled, and uncontrolled asthma in a given week is provided in Table 13-1.

Control versus Severity

It should be noted that in previous NAEPP and GINA guidelines, the management of asthma was implemented according to its "severity classification." Unfortunately, the severity classification system was often erroneous and misleading for a number of reasons, including the fact that (1) the asthma severity approach involved both the severity of the underlying disease and its responsiveness to treatment, (2) asthma severity is not a static feature of an individual patient and the degree of severity may change over months or years, and (3) asthma severity is a poor method in predicting what treatment would be required and what the patient's response to the treatment might be.

For these reasons, both the NAEPP and GINA have concluded (2012) that the assessment of the patient's level of "asthma control" is more relevant and useful—and now is recommended. The assessment of asthma control includes both the control of the asthma symptoms and the control of the expected future risks to the patient—such as, exacerbations, accelerated decline in lung function, and side effects of treatment (Table 13-1). In general, good clinical control of asthma has been shown to result in a reduced number of clinical exacerbations.

Treating to Achieve Control—the Notion of "Step Therapy"

Based on the patient's current level of asthma control—and current treatment regimen—one of five possible treatment steps can be assigned to the patient. For example, Figure 13-6 provides an overview of the management approach based on control for children older than 5 years, adolescents, and adults.[5] As can be seen, **Step 1** through **Step 5** progressively increases treatment medication options and intensity. In short, if the patient's asthma symptoms are not controlled on the current treatment program (e.g., Step 2), then the treatment should be up-regulated to Step 3, Step 4, or Step 5 until control is achieved. When asthma control has been

---

[5]For the management of asthma in children 5 years and younger, see the Global Strategy for the Diagnosis and Management of Asthma in Children 5 Years and Younger, at http://www.ginasthma.org.

TABLE 13-1 Classification of Asthma by Level of Control

	A: Assessment of Current Level of Asthma Control		
Characteristic	Controlled (All of the Following)	Partly Controlled (Any Measure Present)	Uncontrolled
Daytime symptoms	None (2 or less/week)	More than 2/week	Three or more features of partly controlled asthma*,†
Limitation of activities	None	Any	
Nocturnal Symptoms/awakening	None	Any	
Need for reliever/rescue treatment	None (2 or less/week)	>2/week	
Lung function (PEFR or FEV_1)†	Normal	<80% predicted or personal best (if known)	

B: Assessment of Future Risk
· Risk of exacerbations, instability, rapid decline in lung function, side effects
· Features that are associated with increased risk of adverse events in the future include:
· Poor clinical control
· Frequent exacerbations in past year*
· Ever admission to critical care for asthma
· Low FEV_1
· Exposure to cigarette smoke
· High-dose medications

*Any exacerbation should prompt review of maintenance treatment to ensure that it is adequate.
†By definition, an exacerbation in any week makes that an "uncontrolled asthma" week.
†Without administration of bronchodilator (lung function is not a reliable test for children 5 years and younger).
Modified from Global Initiative for Asthma (GINA): *Global strategy for asthma management and prevention*, 2014, GINA (www.ginasthma.org).

maintained for at least 3 months, the treatment regimen can be stepped down with the aim of establishing the lowest step and dose of treatment that maintains control.

Step 2 is usually the assigned treatment regimen for most patients initially diagnosed with asthma symptoms, or those not yet on medications. However, if the patient's asthma clinical manifestations are very symptomatic, **Step 3** may be implemented. If the asthma symptoms are still uncontrolled at this treatment regimen, **Step 4** should be assigned. Patients who do not reach an acceptable level of control at Step 4 are considered to have "**difficult-to-treat asthma**." **Step 5**—which adds oral glucocorticosteroids to the other controller medications and should be considered if the patient's asthma symptoms remain severely uncontrolled on Step 4. The patient should be counseled about the potential side effects of glucocorticosteroids. The addition of anti-IgE treatment to other controller medications in Step 5 has been shown to improve control of allergic asthma.

Common **controller medications** used in the treatment of asthma are presented in Table 13-2. Table 13-3 provides an overview of common reliever medications used to manage acute exacerbations of asthma.

Monitoring to Maintain Control

When asthma control has been achieved, ongoing monitoring is essential to maintain control and establish the lowest step and dose of treatment, which minimizes cost and maximizes the safety of treatment. Asthma control should be monitored by the health-care professional and, ideally, by the patient at regular intervals, using a simplified scheme as shown in Table 13-3. A popular monitoring system is the Asthma Action Plan, using green, yellow, and red zones (Figure 13-7). If the asthma symptoms are not controlled on the current treatment regimen, step up treatment. If the asthma symptoms are partly controlled, consider stepping up treatment. If the asthma symptoms are controlled and maintained for at least 3 months, step down with a gradual, stepwise reduction in treatment. The goal is to reduce the treatment regimen to the least medications necessary to maintain control. Finally, it should be noted that monitoring is still necessary even after control is achieved—because asthma is an episodic disease.

GINA Component 4: Manage Asthma Exacerbations

An asthma exacerbation (also called an asthma attack or asthma episode) is defined as a progressive increase in shortness of breath, cough, wheezing, or chest tightness or a combination of these symptoms. Exacerbations are characterized by decreased expiratory air flow that can be quantified by measurements of the PEFR or FEV_1. These measurements are more reliable indicators of severity of air-flow limitation than the degree of the symptoms. Table 13-4 provides a clinical scale to classify the severity of asthma exacerbations. Severe asthma exacerbations are potentially life threatening, and their monitoring and treatment requires close supervision.

The primary therapies for asthma exacerbations include the repetitive administration of rapid-acting inhaled bronchodilators, the early introduction of systemic glucocorticosteroids, oxygen therapy, and the continuous nebulization of short-acting beta$_2$ agents in status asthmaticus. The primary goals of the treatments are to relieve air-flow obstruction and hypoxemia as quickly as possible, and to plan the prevention of future exacerbations. GINA provides a general management of asthma exacerbations protocol in the acute care setting (Figure 13-8).

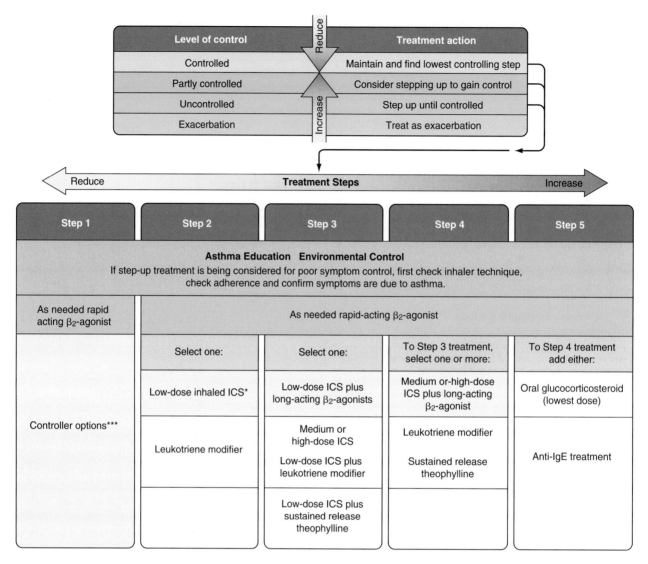

ICS = Inhaled glucocorticosteroids
** Receptor antagonist or synthesis inhibitor
*** Recommended treatment (colored boxes) based on group mean data. Individual patient needs, preferences and circumstances (including costs) should be considered

Alternative reliever treatments included inhaled anticholinergics, short-acting oral β₂-agonists, some long-acting β₂-agonists and short-acting theophylline. Regular dosing with short- and long-acting β₂-agonists is not advised unless accompanied by regular use of an inhaled glucocorticosteroid.

FIGURE 13-6 Management Approach Based on Control for Children Older than 5 Years, Adolescents and Adults. Modified from Global Strategy for Asthma Management and Prevention (2014). GINA (www.ginasthma.org).

GINA Component 5: Special Considerations

Special considerations in managing asthma are required for the following:

Pregnancy—During pregnancy the severity of asthma often changes, and patients often require close monitoring and adjustment of medications. Acute exacerbations should be treated aggressively to avoid fetal hypoxia. The treating physician must balance the consequences of unchecked or poorly controlled asthma in a pregnant woman with the potential adverse effects of asthma medications.[6] Beta-agonists

inhibit uterine contractions and should be minimized in a pregnant woman's asthma management after 35 weeks' gestation.

Obesity—Asthma is more difficult to control in obese patients. Weight loss in the obese patient improves asthma control, lung function, and reduces medication needs.

Surgery—Airway hyperresponsiveness, air-flow limitation, and mucus hypersecretion predispose patients with asthma to intraoperative and postoperative respiratory complications—especially with thoracic and upper abdominal surgeries. A 3- to 5-day pulse of oral steroids is generally recommended before elective surgery for asthmatics.

[6]Current (2007) NAEPP Guidelines suggest careful maternal and fetal monitoring, smoking cessation, and proper control of environmental asthma triggers, patient education, and judicious use of pharmacologic agents. The general consensus is that the side effects of appropriately elected medications are less than the risk of asthma itself. The NAEPP Expert Panel recommends a stepwise approach to the management of nonacute asthma in

pregnant women, with caution being urged for the use of theophylline, LABAs, and oral corticosteroids. Recommended agents in cases of acute maternal asthma include inhaled SABAs, inhaled anticholinergic agents, inhaled corticosteroids (preferably budesonide), and in severe cases, intravenous magnesium sulfate. Supplemental oxygen to keep the $SpO_2 > 95\%$ and the $PaO_2 > 70$ mm Hg is also important, usually via nasal cannula at 3 to 4 L/min.

TABLE 13-2 Controller Medications Used to Treat Asthma*

Generic Name	Brand Name
Long-Acting Beta₂ Agents (LABAs)	
Salmeterol	Serevent Diskus
Inhaled Corticosteroids (ICSs)	
Beclomethasone	QVAR
Flunisolide	Aerospan HFA
Fluticasone	Flovent HFA, Flovent Diskus, Arnuity Ellipta
Budesonide	Pulmicort Flexhaler, Pulmicort Respules
Mometasone	Asmanex Twisthaler, Asmanex HFA
Ciclesonide	Alvesco
Inhaled Corticosteroids & Long-Acting Beta₂ Agents (Combined)	
Fluticasone and Salmeterol	Advair Diskus, Advair HFA
Budesonide and Formoterol	Symbicort
Mometasone and Formoterol	Dulera
Leukotriene Inhibitors (Antileukotrienes)	
Zafirlukast	Accolate
Montelukast	Singulair
Zileuton	Zyflo, Zyflo CR
Monoclonal Antibody	
Omalizumab	Xolair
Xanthine Derivatives	
Theophylline	Theochron, Elxophyllin, Theo-24
Oxtriphylline	Chledyl SA
Aminophylline	Generic
Dyphylline	Lufyllin

*For the complete listing, doses, and administration of agents approved by the FDA, visit the Drugs@FDA website (www.accessdata.fda.gov/scripts/cder/drugsatfda/).

TABLE 13-3 Reliever Medications (Rescue Medications) Used to Treat Asthma*

Generic Name	Brand Name
Ultra-short-Acting Bronchodilator Agents	
Epinephrine	Adrenalin
Racemic epinephrine	Generic
Short-Acting Beta₂ Agents (SABAs)	
Albuterol	Proventil HFA, Ventolin HFA, ProAir HFA, AccuNeb HFA, Generic
Metaproterenol	Generic
Levalbuterol	Xopenex, Xopenex HFA, Generic
Systemic Corticosteroids	
Methylprednisolone	Medrol, Solu-Medrol
Hydrocortisone	Solu-Cortef

*For the complete listing, doses, and administration of agents approved by the FDA, visit the Drugs@FDA website (www.accessdata.fda.gov/scripts/cder/drugsatfda/).

Rhinitis, Sinusitis, and Nasal Polyps—Upper airway disease can adversely influence airway function in some patients with asthma.

Occupational Asthma—Once a diagnosis of occupational asthma has been established, complete avoidance of the relevant exposure is an important component of management.

Respiratory Infections—Concomitant respiratory infections provoke wheezing and increased symptoms in patients with asthma. Respiratory infections are commonly found in children with asthma exacerbation.

Gastroesophageal Reflux—There is significant evidence that gastroesophageal reflux is more common in patients with asthma and obstructive sleep apnea than the general population.

Aspirin-Induced Asthma (AIA)—Up to 28% of adults with asthma suffer from asthma exacerbations in response to aspirin and other NSAIDs. This syndrome is more common in severe asthma. Complete avoidance of drugs that cause asthma symptoms is the standard management. AIA is rarely seen in children with asthma.

Anaphylaxis and Asthma—Anaphylaxis is a serious allergic reaction to a previously encountered antigen. It is a potentially life-threatening condition that can both mimic and complicate severe asthma with significant airway swelling. Symptoms of anaphylaxis include flushing, upper and lower airway involvement manifested by stridor, hoarseness, dyspnea, wheezing, pain with swallowing, cough, or apnea. In addition, dizziness or syncope with or without hypotension; and gastrointestinal problems such as nausea, vomiting, cramping, and diarrhea may be present. Causes of anaphylaxis include the administration of allergenic extracts in immunotherapy, food intolerance (e.g., nuts, fish, shellfish, eggs, and milk), avian-based vaccines, insect stings or bites, latex hypersensitivity, drugs (β-lactam antibiotics, aspirin and NSAIDs, and angiotensin converting enzyme [ACE] inhibitors), and exercise. Effective treatment of anaphylaxis requires early recognition of the event. Treatment for anaphylaxis includes bronchodilators (e.g., albuterol), oxygen, intramuscular epinephrine, injectable antihistamine, intravenous hydrocortisone, insertion of an oropharyngeal or nasopharyngeal airway, and intravenous fluids.

Respiratory Care Treatment Protocols

Aerosolized Medication Protocol

Inhaled beta₂ agents, anticholinergic agents, and corticosteroids agents via a metered dose inhaler (pMDI) spacer, dry powder inhaler (DPI), or small volume nebulizer (SVN) are commonly used in the treatment of asthma to induce bronchial smooth muscle relaxation (see Aerosolized Medication Protocol, Protocol 9-4). Continuous nebulization of albuterol is often used in the management of status asthmaticus to prevent acute ventilatory failure.

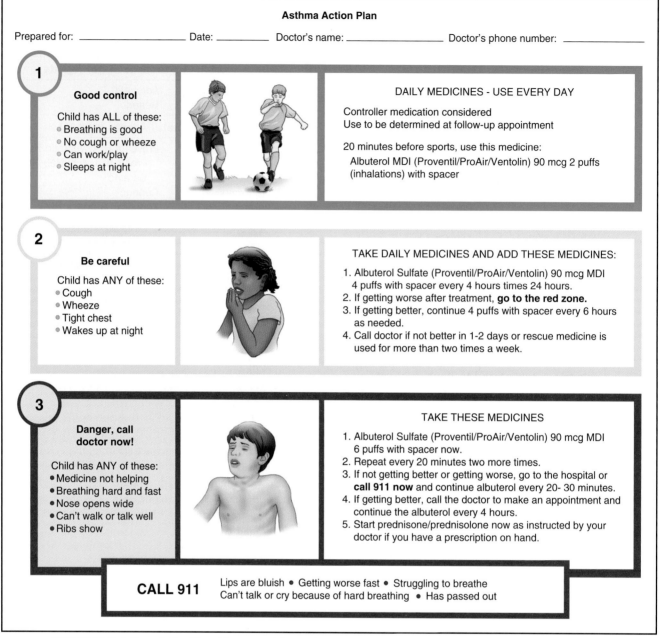

FIGURE 13-7 Asthma Action Plan. (Courtesy of Dayton Children's Hospital Dayton, Ohio for providing their Asthma Action Plan.)

Oxygen Therapy Protocol

Oxygen therapy may be required to treat hypoxemia, decrease the work of breathing, and decrease myocardial work. The hypoxemia that develops in asthma is usually caused by the ventilation-perfusion mismatch and shunt-like effect associated with bronchospasm and increased airway secretions. Hypoxemia caused by this shunt-like effect can at least partly be corrected by oxygen therapy (see Oxygen Therapy Protocol, Protocol 9-1).

Bronchopulmonary Hygiene Therapy Protocol

Because of the excessive mucous production and secretion accumulation associated with asthma, a number of bronchial hygiene treatment modalities may be used to enhance the mobilization

of bronchial secretions (see Bronchopulmonary Hygiene Therapy Protocol, Protocol 9-2). These modalities should be attempted with patients with acute asthma when they can effectively move enough air to deep breathe and cough.

Mechanical Ventilation Protocol

Because acute ventilatory failure is associated with **status asthmaticus**, continuous mechanical ventilation may be required to maintain an adequate ventilatory status.

Status asthmaticus is defined as a severe asthmatic episode that does not respond to conventional pharmacologic therapy. When the patient becomes fatigued, the ventilatory rate decreases. Clinically, the patient demonstrates a progressive decrease in PaO_2 and pH and a steady increase in $PaCO_2$ (acute ventilatory failure). Noninvasive ventilatory assistance

TABLE 13-4 Classification of Severity of Acute Asthma Exacerbations*

	Mild	Moderate	Severe	Respiratory Arrest Imminent
Symptoms				
Breathlessness	While walking	While talking (infant: softer, shorter cry; difficulty feeding)	While at rest (infant: stops feeding)	
	Can lie down	Prefers sitting	Sits upright	
Talks in	Sentences	Phrases	Words	
Alertness	May be agitated	Usually agitated	Usually agitated	Drowsy or confused
Signs				
Respiratory rate	Increased	Increased	Often >30/min	
		Normal rates of breathing in awake children:		
		Age — Normal Rate		
		<2 mo — <60/min		
		2-12 mo — <50/min		
		1-5 yr — <40/min		
		6-8 yr — <30/min		
Use of accessory muscles; suprasternal retractions	Usually not	Commonly	Usually	Paradoxical thoracoabdominal movement
Wheeze	Moderate, often only end-expiratory	Loud; throughout exhalation	Usually loud; throughout inhalation and exhalation	Absence of wheeze
		Normal pulse rates in awake children:		
Pulse/min	<100	100-120	>120	Bradycardia
		Age — Normal Rate		
		2-12 mo — <160/min		
		1-2 yr — <120/min		
		2-8 yr — <110/min		
Pulsus paradoxus	Absent <10 mm Hg	May be present 10-25 mm Hg	Often present >25 mm Hg (adult) 20-40 mm Hg (child)	Absence suggests respiratory muscle fatigue
Functional Assessment				
PEFR (% predicted or % personal best)	80%	~50%-80%	<50% predicted or personal best or response lasts <2 h	
PaO$_2$ (on air)	Normal (ABG usually necessary)	>60 mm Hg (ABG usually necessary)	<60 mm Hg: possible cyanosis	
and/or PaCO$_2$	<42 mm Hg (ABG usually necessary)	<42 mm Hg (ABG usually necessary)	≥42 mm Hg: possible respiratory failure	
SaO$_2$ % (on air) at sea level	>95% (ABG usually necessary)	91%-95%	<91%	
	Hypercapnia (hypoventilation) develops more readily in young children than in adults and adolescents			

PEFR, Peak expiratory flow rate.

*The presence of several parameters, but not necessarily all, indicates the general classification of the exacerbation. Many of these parameters have not been systematically studied, so they serve only as general guides.

From Expert Panel Response 3 (EPR 3): Guidelines for the diagnosis and management of asthma, 2007. Available at: www.nhlbi.nih.gov/guidelines/asthma/asthgdln.htm.

(continuous positive airway pressure [CPAP] or bilevel positive airway pressure [BPAP]*) may be indicated to provide expiratory resistance, while also providing frequent or continuous aerosolized bronchodilator therapy. If ventilation does not improve and hypercarbia is not reversed, intubation and mechanical ventilation becomes necessary (see Mechanical Ventilation Protocol, Protocol 10-1 and Mechanical Ventilation Weaning Protocol, Protocol 10-2).

*BPAP should not be confused with BiPAP, which is the brand name of a single manufacturer, and is just one of many devices that can be used for BPAP.

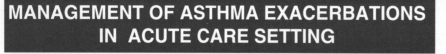

MANAGEMENT OF ASTHMA EXACERBATIONS IN ACUTE CARE SETTING

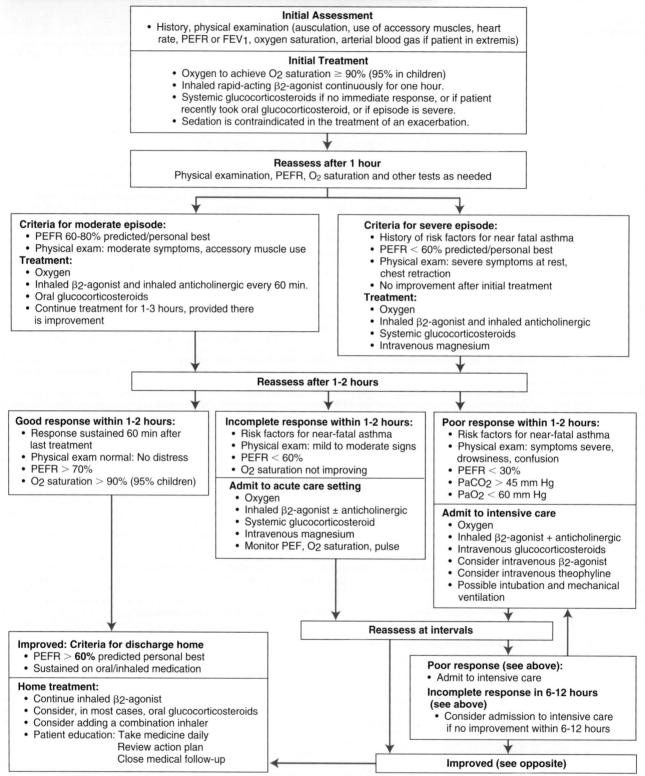

FIGURE 13-8 Management of Asthma Exacerbations in Acute Care Setting. (Modified from Global Initiative for Asthma (GINA): *Global strategy for asthma management and prevention*, 2014, GINA [www.ginasthma.org]).

A 7-year-old girl was admitted to the emergency department (ED) in severe respiratory distress. Her history of wheezing dated back to age 6 months, when she was hospitalized with viral bronchiolitis. Over the past 3 years she was hospitalized in different hospitals on a number of occasions and was usually managed satisfactorily with aerosolized albuterol and oral steroids. She began coughing and wheezing the night before admission and became progressively worse during the night. Her cough was nonproductive. At 8.00 AM, she was brought to the ED after she did not get relief from her albuterol MDI at home.

Physical examination revealed an extremely anxious, well-developed female child in acute respiratory distress. She stated in short, terse phrases: "It's hard…for me…to breathe." Her vital signs were as follows: blood pressure 128/84, pulse 148 beats/min, and respiratory rate 30 breaths/min. Her temperature was 99.1°F. Her SpO_2 was 88% on room air upon arrival. She was actively using her accessory muscles of respiration. On auscultation, her breath sounds were decreased bilaterally with faint expiratory wheezes and coarse crackles.

The ED physician ordered three back-to-back SVN treatments with a combination of albuterol and ipratropium bromide. The patient's level of distress prompted a need to begin bronchodilator treatment with oxygen without attempting serial peak flow measurements. Post-treatment PEFR was less than 70 L/min. (Her personal best was about 200 to 250 L/min.) The patient was then placed on 2 L/min nasal cannula oxygen and a capillary blood gas (CBG) was drawn: pH 7.27, $PaCO_2$ 52 mm Hg, HCO_3^- 22 mEq/L, PaO_2 76 mm Hg, and SaO_2 91%. A chest x-ray examination was ordered but not performed. The physician ordered a respiratory care consultation and stated that she did not want to commit the patient to a ventilator at this time if possible. The physician asked that aggressive noninvasive pulmonary care be tried first. At this time the respiratory therapist documented the following.

Respiratory Assessment and Plan

S Patient air hungry and stated in chopped phrases, "It's hard for me to breathe"

O Vital signs: on arrival BP 128/84, R 148, RR 30, T 99.1°. SpO_2 88% on room air. Using accessory muscles, subcostal, intercostals, and supraclavicular retractions. Decreased breath sounds bilaterally at bases & faint expiratory wheezes and coarse crackles. PEFR: less than 70 L/min after three back-to-back albuterol-ipratropium SVN treatments. Oral prednisolone was given. Several fluid boluses are given. CBGs pH 7.27, $PaCO_2$ 52, HCO_3^- 22, PaO_2 76, and SaO_2 91% on 2 L/min post-treatment. No CXR yet.

A • Severe exacerbation (per NAEPP severity scale) of previously partly controlled asthma

- Respiratory distress (increased heart rate, blood pressure, respiratory rate)
- Bronchospasm (decreased air entry, wheezing, decreased PEFR, history)
- Excessive airway secretions (coarse crackles)
- Acute ventilatory failure (acute respiratory acidosis) with moderate to severe hypoxemia (CBG)
- Metabolic acidosis also likely (both pH and HCO_3^- are both lower than expected for a $PaCO_2$ of 52). Likely caused by lactic acid due to low SpO_2.

P **Oxygen Therapy Protocol** Monitor SpO_2 with oximeter; provide oxygen via continuous medication nebulizer and supplemental cannula as needed. **Aerosolized Medication Therapy Protocol** (continuous med. neb. with albuterol and ipratropium bromide.) Monitor PEFR and breath sounds. **Bronchopulmonary Hygiene Therapy Protocol** (cough and deep breathe as tolerated). Monitor breath sounds. Repeat CBG in 30 minutes. Continuous cardiac monitoring in place. Respiratory Therapy to remain in ED at bedside. Consider noninvasive ventilation if patient does not continue to improve.

In addition to this plan, the patient was treated vigorously with intravenous steroids (Solu-Medrol) and intravenous magnesium sulfate. The chest x-ray results showed depressed diaphragms, hyperinflation bilaterally with patchy atelectasis.

A **Respiratory Infectious Disease Panel (RIDP)**[7] was ordered to rule out viral infection or mycoplasma pneumonia.

After 3 hours of continuous albuterol aerosol with oxygen, the patient began to slowly improve—that is, bilateral aeration was better and the respiratory distress symptoms began to subside. On a 2-L/min oxygen cannula, the patient's capillary blood gas showed pH 7.38, $PaCO_2$ 44 mm Hg, HCO_3^- 24 mEq/L, PaO_2 78 mm Hg, and SpO_2 94%. Asthma scores improved from poor to fair, allowing the patient to be weaned from the continuous albuterol and ipratropium bromide after 6 hours to q2h albuterol medication nebulizer treatments. The RIDP showed the patient was positive for Rhinovirus.

Over the next 30 hours the patient was weaned from q2h to q4h, then to q6h albuterol MDI treatments based on the respiratory care asthma protocol. Oxygen requirements subsided after 20 hours of inpatient care. The patient was instructed in proper MDI and **valved holding chamber (VHC)** technique. With each treatment the patient was encouraged to deep breathe and cough. Oral corticosteroids continued daily and inhaled corticosteroids via MDI and valved holding chamber were also ordered as a daily controller for home therapy. Peak flow measurements were now reaching 150 to 180 L/min post-MDI.

---

[7]The RIDP includes detection of the following: Adenovirus, Coronavirus 229E, Coronavirus HKU1, Coronavirus NL63, Coronavirus OC43, Human Metapneumovirus, Human Rhinovirus (1, 2, 3, and 4), Enterovirus, Influenza A (H1-2009, H1, H3), Influenza B, Parainfluenza (1, 2, 3, and 4), Respiratory Syncytial Virus, *Bordetella pertussis*, *Chlamydophila pneumoniae*, and *Mycoplasma pneumoniae*.

The patient was instructed in asthma trigger prevention, and a personalized asthma action plan was reviewed with the patient and family. The parents verbalized their understanding of controller and reliever medications in the prevention and management their child's asthma. Follow-up was scheduled with the primary care physician within 2 days.

Discussion

Asthma is a potentially fatal disease—largely because its severity is often unrecognized in the home or outpatient setting. Even mild asthmatics can occasionally have a severe, life-threatening attack. Overuse of reliever medications (albuterol), with underutilization of controller medications (inhaled corticosteroids) is also associated with increased severity of attacks. The clinical manifestations presented in this case can all be easily traced back through the **Bronchospasm clinical scenario** (see Figure 9-10) and **Excessive Airway Secretions clinical scenario** (see Figure 9-11). For example, the patient's increased blood pressure, heart rate, and respiratory rate can all be followed back to the hypoxemia caused by the $\dot{V}/\dot{Q}$ mismatch and pulmonary shunting activated by **Bronchospasm** and **Excessive Bronchial Secretions** (see Figures 9-10 and 9-11). The patient's anxiety and possible previous use of beta$_2$-agonists may also have contributed to her abnormal vital signs (tachycardia). *However, anxiety with an asthma attack should always be attributed to hypoxemia until proven otherwise.*

In addition, the decreased PEFR, use of accessory muscles, diminished breath sounds, and wheezing and coarse crackles reflect the increased airway resistance and air trapping caused by the **Bronchospasm** (see Figure 9-10) and **Excessive Airway Secretions** (see Figure 9-11). The fact that the patient's capillary blood gas values showed acute ventilatory failure confirmed that the patient was in the severe stages of an asthmatic episode and that mechanical ventilation could be required if the patient failed to respond to the vigorous respiratory care provided.

In the first SOAP presented above for this case, the respiratory therapist chose a fairly aggressive approach to both the **Oxygen Therapy Protocol** (Protocol 9-1) and the **Aerosolized Medication Therapy Protocol** (Protocol 9-4). Use of a nasal cannula to deliver supplemental oxygen, titrated to an SpO$_2$ of 92% to 94%, often causes less anxiety than the use of a face mask in children. Frequent monitoring of capillary blood gases and SpO$_2$ levels was appropriate.

Also note the use of continuous albuterol inhalation in the **Aerosolized Medication Therapy Protocol**. Because of the severity of the patient's asthmatic episode, the aggressive administration of albuterol, the short-acting bronchodilator agent, was clearly a correct selection according to GINA guidelines.

Adults may not tolerate aggressive albuterol administration because of coexistent cardiac disease; adults must be monitored closely for development of arrhythmias or myocardial ischemia (ST segment elevation). In an acute asthmatic attack, albuterol should be nebulized with oxygen to minimize hypoxic cardiac complications. The manner in which any therapy modality is up-regulated may be (1) a different aerosolized drug or procedure, (2) a larger dose of a drug or therapy, or (3) more frequent use of such drugs or therapy. In this case, the continuous larger dose was successful.

Among the lessons to be learned here is that some asthmatic episodes may initially worsen despite appropriate and vigorous therapy. This patient received optimal emergent treatment of her severe asthma attack but her recovery required several hours of continuous albuterol and intravenous medications, particularly magnesium sulfate and Solu-Medrol. Intravenous aminophylline in the emergency treatment of acute asthma is controversial and rarely used in children. Care must be taken to avoid theophylline toxicity, and symptoms of toxicity often do not reflect serum concentrations of the drug. Almost continuous assessment by the respiratory therapist is necessary if more invasive therapy (including induced sedation, paralysis, and mechanical ventilation) is to be avoided.

The acutely ill asthmatic requires almost continuous monitoring and frequent SOAP notes if the patient care team is to be constantly apprised of the patient's progress. (The one such note recorded here is but a small portion of the more than 14 notes that we found on analysis of the patient's medical record from her ED admission alone.) Current best practice would require that the first SOAP assessment would have included a statement about the patient's preadmission asthma control status, which in this case, would have been (at best) "partly controlled" per GINA (see page 212).

SELF-ASSESSMENT QUESTIONS

Answers to questions can be found on Evolve. To access additional student assessment questions visit http://evolve.elsevier.com/DesJardins/respiratory.

1. During an asthmatic episode, the smooth muscles of the bronchi may hypertrophy as much as:
   a. Two times normal thickness
   b. Three times normal thickness
   c. Four times normal thickness
   d. Five times normal thickness

2. Asthma is associated with which of the following?
   1. Increase in goblet cells
   2. Damage to cilia and deduced mucous clearance
   3. Increase in bronchial gland size
   4. Decrease in eosinophils
      a. 1 and 3 only
      b. 2 and 4 only
      c. 1, 2, and 3 only
      d. 2, 3, and 4 only

3. Which of the following have gained a widespread acceptance for assessing and monitoring a patient's air-flow limitation?
   1. PEFR
   2. $FEF_{200-1200}$
   3. FEV_1
   4. FEV_1/FVC ratio
      a. 1 and 3 only
      b. 2 and 4 only
      c. 1, 3, and 4 only
      d. 2, 3, and 4 only

4. A patient clinical history presents the following: daytime asthma symptoms more than two per week; no limitation in activities; no nocturnal symptoms or awakening; the need for reliever/rescue medications once per week, and a normal PEFR and FEV_1. Which of the following would best classify this patient's level of asthma control?
   a. Controlled
   b. Partly controlled
   c. Uncontrolled
   d. Severe exacerbation

5. Which of the following can be used to help confirm the diagnosis of asthma?
   1. Exercise challenge
   2. Response to inhaled mannitol
   3. Response to inhaled histamine
   4. Response to inhaled methacholine
      a. 1 and 3 only
      b. 2 and 4 only
      c. 2, 3, and 4 only
      d. 1, 2, 3, and 4

6. When pulsus paradoxus appears during an asthma attack:
   1. Left ventricle filling decreases during inspiration
   2. Cardiac output increases during expiration
   3. Left ventricle filling increases during expiration
   4. Cardiac output increases during inspiration
      a. 1 only
      b. 2 only
      c. 3 and 4 only
      d. 1 and 2 only

7. During an asthmatic episode, which of the following abnormal lung volume and capacity findings are found?
   1. Increased FRC
   2. Decreased ERV
   3. Increased VC
   4. Decreased RV
      a. 1 only
      b. 2 only
      c. 1 and 2 only
      d. 3 and 4 only

8. Which of the following chest assessment findings is/are commonly found during an asthmatic episode?
   1. Loud heart sounds
   2. Hyperresonant percussion note
   3. Expiratory prolongation
   4. Increased tactile and vocal fremitus
      a. 2 and 3 only
      b. 1 and 4 only
      c. 1, 2, and 4 only
      d. 1, 2, 3, and 4

9. Patients commonly exhibit which of the following arterial blood gas values early during an acute mild to moderate asthmatic episode?
   1. Increased pH
   2. Increased $PaCO_2$
   3. Decreased HCO_3^-
   4. Decreased PaO_2
      a. 1 and 3 only
      b. 2 and 4 only
      c. 1, 2, and 3 only
      d. 1, 3, and 4 only

10. How long must asthma be controlled before the treatment regimen can be stepped down—with the aim of establishing the lowest step and dose of treatment that maintains control?
    a. At least 2 weeks
    b. At least 1 month
    c. At least 2 months
    d. At least 3 months

14 | Bronchiectasis

Chapter Objectives

After reading this chapter, you will be able to:

- Describe the anatomic alterations of the lungs associated with bronchiectasis.
- Discuss the etiology and epidemiology of bronchiectasis.
- Identify the common classifications used to group the causes of bronchiectasis and include specific examples under each classification.
- Describe the various diagnostic tests used to identify the presence of bronchiectasis.
- Describe the cardiopulmonary clinical manifestations associated with bronchiectasis.
- Describe the general medical and surgical management of bronchiectasis.
- Describe the respiratory care modalities used in the treatment of bronchiectasis.
- Describe and evaluate the clinical strategies and rationales of the SOAPs presented in the case study.

Key Terms

Acquired Bronchial Obstruction
Congenital Anatomic Defects

Cylindrical (Tubular) Bronchiectasis
Cystic (Saccular) Bronchiectasis
High-frequency Chest Compression Devices
Kartagener's Syndrome
Lung Mapping
Primary Ciliary Dyskinesia
Varicose (Fusiform) Bronchiectasis

Chapter Outline

Anatomic Alterations of the Lungs
    Varicose Bronchiectasis (Fusiform Bronchiectasis)
    Cylindrical Bronchiectasis (Tubular Bronchiectasis)
    Cystic Bronchiectasis (Saccular Bronchiectasis)
Etiology and Epidemiology
Overview of the Cardiopulmonary Clinical Manifestations
    Associated With Bronchiectasis
General Management of Bronchiectasis
Respiratory Care Treatment Protocols
Medications Commonly Prescribed by the Physician
Case Study: Bronchiectasis
Self-Assessment Questions

Anatomic Alterations of the Lungs

Bronchiectasis is characterized by chronic dilation and distortion of one or more bronchi—usually as a result of extensive inflammation and destruction of the bronchial wall cartilage, blood vessels, elastic tissue, and smooth muscle components. One or both lungs may be involved. Bronchiectasis is commonly limited to a lobe or segment and is frequently found in the lower lobes. The smaller bronchi, with less supporting cartilage, are predominantly affected.

Because of bronchial wall destruction, normal mucociliary clearance is impaired. This results in the accumulation of copious amounts of bronchial secretions and blood that often become foul-smelling because of secondary colonization with anaerobic organisms. Thoracic infection and irritation may lead to secondary bronchial smooth muscle constriction and fibrosis. The small bronchi and bronchioles distal to the affected areas become partially or totally obstructed with secretions. This condition leads to one or both of the following anatomic alterations: (1) hyperinflation of the distal alveoli as a result of expiratory check-valve obstruction or (2) atelectasis, consolidation, and fibrosis as a result of complete bronchial obstruction.

Based on gross anatomic appearance, the long-accepted Reid classification subdivides bronchiectasis into the following three different patterns:
- Varicose (fusiform)
- Cylindrical (tubular)
- Cystic (saccular)

Varicose Bronchiectasis (Fusiform Bronchiectasis)

In **varicose (fusiform) bronchiectasis**, the bronchi are dilated and constricted in an irregular fashion similar to varicose veins, ultimately resulting in a distorted, bulbous shape (Figure 14-1, *A*).

Cylindrical Bronchiectasis (Tubular Bronchiectasis)

In **cylindrical (tubular) bronchiectasis**, the bronchi are dilated and rigid and have regular outlines similar to a tube. X-ray examination shows that the dilated bronchi fail to

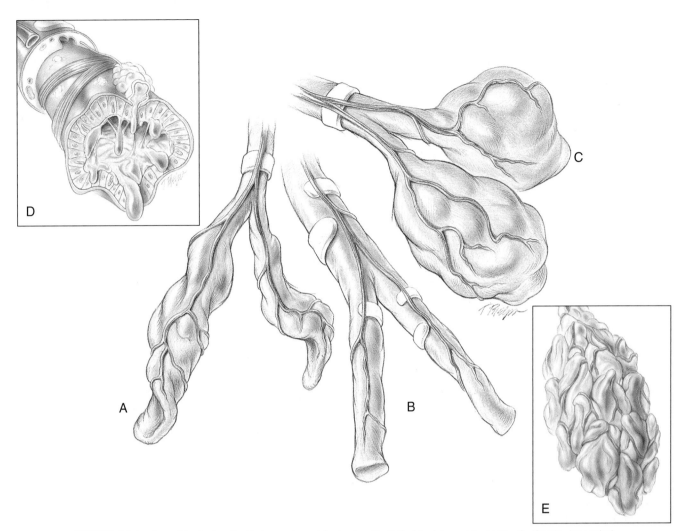

FIGURE 14-1 Bronchiectasis. **A**, Varicose bronchiectasis. **B**, Cylindrical bronchiectasis. **C**, Cystic (saccular) bronchiectasis. Also illustrated are excessive bronchial secretions (**D**) and atelectasis (**E**), which are both common anatomic alterations of the lungs in this disease.

taper for 6 to 10 generations and then appear to end abruptly because of mucous obstruction (Figure 14-1, *B*).

Cystic Bronchiectasis (Saccular Bronchiectasis)

In **cystic (saccular) bronchiectasis,** the bronchi progressively increase in diameter until they end in large, cystlike sacs in the lung parenchyma. This form of bronchiectasis causes the greatest damage to the tracheobronchial tree. The bronchial walls become composed of fibrous tissue alone—cartilage, elastic tissue, and smooth muscle are all absent (Figure 14-1, *C*).

The following are the major pathologic or structural changes associated with bronchiectasis:
- Chronic dilation and distortion of bronchial airways
- Excessive production of often foul-smelling sputum (Figure 14-1, *D*)
- Bronchospasm
- Hyperinflation of alveoli (air trapping)
- Atelectasis (Figure 14-1, *E*)
- Consolidation and parenchymal fibrosis
- Hemoptysis secondary to bronchial arterial erosion

Etiology and Epidemiology

Most causes of bronchiectasis include some combination of bronchial obstruction and infection. In developed countries, cystic fibrosis is the most common cause of bronchiectasis. The prevalence of noncystic fibrosis bronchiectasis (NCFB) in developed nations is relatively low. For example, in the United States, the incidence of NCFB is about 4.2 per 100,000 young adults. The low incidence of NCFB in developed countries is most often attributed to early medical management (e.g., antibiotic therapy). In other populations, however, such as Polynesia, Alaska, Australia, and New Zealand, the occurrence of NCFB is as high as 15 per 1000 children.

The most common cause of NCFB is pulmonary infection. Although this is not a well-defined entity, it is believed that a possible mechanism for postinfectious NCFB is a significant lung infection during early childhood—which causes anatomic alterations of the developing lung that allows persistent bacterial infections. As a result, the continuous bacterial infections lead to bronchiectasis.

Also at risk for chronic pulmonary infection and NCFB are individuals with a mucociliary disorder (**primary ciliary dyskinesia**) or an immunodeficiency disorder involving low levels of immunoglobulin G (IgG), IgM, and IgA. In addition, NCFB is also associated with patients who have rheumatoid arthritis, inflammatory bowel disease (most often in those with chronic ulcerative colitis), and chronic obstructive pulmonary disease (COPD). Finally, other etiologic factors associated with NCFB include foreign-body aspirations, tumors, hilar adenopathy, bronchial airway mucoid impaction, tracheobronchial abnormalities, vascular abnormalities, lymphatic abnormalities, advanced age, malnutrition, socioeconomic disadvantage, and alpha$_1$-antitrypsin deficiency.

The causes of bronchiectasis are commonly classified into the following categories:
- Acquired bronchial obstruction
- Congenital anatomic defects
- Immunodeficiency states
- Abnormal secretion clearance
- Miscellaneous disorders (e.g., alpha$_1$-antitrypsin deficiency)

Table 14-1 provides the common classifications used to group the causes of bronchiectasis, specific examples under each classification, and diagnostic tests used to identify the presence of bronchiectasis.

Diagnosis

A routine chest radiograph may reveal such findings as over-inflated lungs or marked volume loss, increased opacities, dilated fluid-filled airways, crowding of the bronchi, and atelectasis. Although bronchoscopy is rarely performed today, bronchograms can confirm cylindrical, cystic, or varicose bronchiectasis as well as crowding of the bronchi, loss of bronchovascular markings and, in more severe cases, honeycombing, air-fluid levels, and fluid-filled nodules. Bronchoscopy was once the gold standard for the diagnosis of NCFB.

Today, the high resolution computed tomography (HR-CT) scan has virtually replaced bronchography as the best tool for diagnosing NCFB. The diagnosis is made on the basis of an internal diameter of a bronchus that is wider than its adjacent pulmonary artery, a failure of the bronchi to taper, and the visualization of bronchi in the outer 1 to 2 cm of the lung fields. The HR-CT scan is used to better clarify the findings from chest radiograph and standard CT scans, and mapping airway abnormalities that cannot be identified on routine films of the chest.

Spirometry testing can be used to determine if the bronchiectasis is primarily an obstructive or restrictive lung pathophysiology, and arterial blood gas measurements can confirm if the patient has mild, moderate, or severe bronchiectasis.

TABLE 14-1 Causes of Bronchiectasis

Category	Specific Examples	Diagnostic Tests
Acquired Bronchial Obstruction		
Foreign-body aspiration	Peanuts; chicken bone; teeth	Chest imaging; fiberoptic bronchoscopy
Tumors	Laryngeal papillomatosis; airway adenoma; endobronchial teratoma	Chest imaging; fiberoptic bronchoscopy
Hilar adenopathy	Tuberculosis; histoplasmosis; sarcoidosis	PPD; chest imaging; fiberoptic bronchoscopy
COPD	Chronic bronchitis	Pulmonary function tests
Rheumatic disease	Relapsing polychondritis (RP); tracheobronchial amyloidosis	Clinical syndrome of RP/cartilage biopsy; biopsy for amyloid
Mucoid impaction	Allergic bronchopulmonary aspergillosis; bronchocentric granulomatosis (BG); postoperative mucoid impaction	Total and aspergillus specific IgE; specific aspergillus IgG; aspergillus skin test; chest imaging; biopsy for BG
Foreign-body aspiration	Peanut; chicken bone; tooth	Chest imaging; fiberoptic bronchoscopy
Congenital Anatomic Defects That May Cause Bronchial Obstruction		
Tracheobronchial abnormalities	Bronchomalacia; bronchial cyst; cartilage deficiency (Williams-Campbell syndrome); tracheobronchomegaly (Mounier-Kuhn syndrome); ectopic bronchus; tracheoesophageal fistula	Chest CT imaging
Vascular abnormalities	Pulmonary (intralobar) sequestration; pulmonary artery aneurysm	Chest CT imaging
Lymphatic abnormalities	Yellow-nail syndrome	History of dystrophic, slow growing nails

TABLE 14-1 Causes of Bronchiectasis—cont'd

Category	Specific Examples	Diagnostic Tests
Immunodeficiency States		
IgG deficiency	Congenital (Bruton's type) agammaglobulinemia; selective deficiency of subclasses (IgG2, IgG4); acquired immune globulin deficiency; common variable hypogammaglobulinemia; Nezelof's syndrome; "bare lymphocyte" syndrome	Quantitative immunoglobulin levels; immunoglobulin subclass levels; impaired response to immunization with pneumococcal vaccine
IgA deficiency	Selective IgA deficiency ± ataxia-telangiectasia syndrome	Quantitative immunoglobulin levels
Leukocyte dysfunction	Chronic granulomatous disease (NADPH oxidase dysfunction)	Dihydrorhodamine 123 (DHR) oxidation test; nitroblue tetrazolium test; genetic testing
Other rare humoral immunodeficiencies (CXCR4 mutation, CD40 deficiency, CD40 ligand deficiency, and others)	WHIM syndrome; Hypergammaglobulinemia M	Neutrophil count; quantitative immunoglobulin levels
Abnormal Secretion Clearance		
Ciliary defects of airway mucosa	**Kartagener's syndrome**; ciliary dyskinesis (formally called impaired ciliary motility syndrome)	Chest x-ray showing situs inversus; bronchial biopsy; ciliary motility studies; electron microscopy of sperm or respiratory mucosa
Cystic fibrosis (mucoviscidosis)	Typical early childhood syndrome; later presentation with predominantly sinopulmonary symptoms	Sweat chloride; genetic testing
Young's syndrome	Obstructive azoospermia with sinopulmonary infections	Sperm count
Miscellaneous Disorders		
Alpha$_1$-antitrypsin deficiency	Absent or abnormal antitrypsin synthesis and function	Alpha$_1$-antitrypsin level
Recurrent aspiration pneumonia	Alcoholism; neurologic disorders; lipoid pneumonia	History; chest imaging
Rheumatic disease	Associated with rheumatoid arthritis and Sjögren's syndrome	Rheumatoid factor; antiSSA/antiSSB; salivary gland MRI or biopsy
Inflammatory bowel disease	Crohn's disease; ulcerative colitis	History; lower gastrointestinal endoscopy; imaging studies; colonic biopsy
Inhalation of toxic fumes and dusts	Ammonia; nitrogen dioxide, or other irritant gases; smoke; talc; silicates	Exposure history; chest imaging
Chronic organ rejection following transplantation	Bone marrow, lung and heart lung transplantation; associated with obliterative bronchiolitis	History; PFT; chest CT imaging with inspiratory and expiratory views

COPD, Chronic obstructive pulmonary disease; *CT*, computed tomography; *Ig*, immunoglobulin; *MRI*, magnetic resonance imaging; *PFT*, pulmonary function test; *PPD*, percussion and postural drainage.

Modified from Wolters Kluwer Health/UpToDate.com: *Causes of bronchiectasis in children and clinical manifestations and diagnosis of bronchiectasis in adults.* Accessed March 1, 2013.

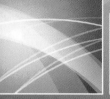

OVERVIEW of the Cardiopulmonary Clinical Manifestations Associated with Bronchiectasis

The following clinical manifestations result from the pathophysiologic mechanisms caused (or activated) by Excessive Bronchial Secretions (see Figure 9-11), Bronchospasm (see Figure 9-10), Atelectasis (see Figure 9-7), Consolidation (see Figure 9-8), and Increased Alveolar-Capillary Membrane Thickness (see Figure 9-12)—the major anatomic alterations of the lungs associated with bronchiectasis (Figure 14-1).

CLINICAL DATA OBTAINED AT THE PATIENT'S BEDSIDE

Depending on the amount of bronchial secretions and the degree of bronchial destruction and fibrosis/atelectasis associated with bronchiectasis, the disease may create an obstructive or a restrictive lung disorder or a combination of both. If the majority of the bronchial airways are only partially obstructed, the bronchiectasis manifests primarily as an obstructive lung disorder. If, by contrast, the majority of the bronchial airways are completely obstructed, the distal alveoli collapse, atelectasis results, and the bronchiectasis manifests primarily as a restrictive disorder. Finally, if the disease is limited to a relatively small portion of the lung—as it often is—the patient may not have any of the following typical clinical manifestations of bronchiectasis.

The Physical Examination
Vital Signs
Increased Respiratory Rate (Tachypnea)
Several pathophysiologic mechanisms operating simultaneously may lead to an increased frequency of breathing (respiratory rate—RR):
- Stimulation of peripheral chemoreceptors (hypoxemia)
- Decreased lung compliance and increased ventilatory rate relationship
- Anxiety

Increased Heart Rate (Pulse) and Blood Pressure
Use of Accessory Muscles during Inspiration
Use of Accessory Muscles during Expiration
Pursed-Lip Breathing (When Pathology is Primarily Obstructive in Nature)
Increased Anteroposterior Chest Diameter (Barrel Chest) (When Pathology is Primarily Obstructive in Nature)
Cyanosis
Digital Clubbing
Peripheral Edema and Venous Distention
Because polycythemia and cor pulmonale are associated with severe bronchiectasis, the following may be seen:
- Distended neck veins
- Pitting edema
- Enlarged and tender liver

Cough, Sputum Production, and Hemoptysis
Chronic cough with production of large quantities of foul-smelling sputum is a hallmark of bronchiectasis. A 24-hour collection of sputum is usually voluminous and tends to settle into several different layers. Streaks of blood are seen frequently in the sputum, presumably originating from necrosis of the bronchial walls and erosion of bronchial blood vessels. Frank hemoptysis may also occur from time to time, but it is rarely life threatening. Because of the excessive bronchial secretions, secondary bacterial infections are frequent. *Haemophilus influenzae, Streptococcus, Pseudomonas aeruginosa,* and various anaerobic organisms are commonly cultured from the sputum of patients with bronchiectasis.

The productive cough seen in patients with bronchiectasis is triggered by the large amount of secretions that fill the tracheobronchial tree. The stagnant secretions stimulate the subepithelial mechanoreceptors, which in turn produce a vagal reflex that triggers the cough. The subepithelial mechanoreceptors are found in the trachea, bronchi, and bronchioles, but they are predominantly located in the upper airways.

Chest Assessment Findings
When the bronchiectasis pathology is primarily obstructive in nature:
- Decreased tactile and vocal fremitus
- Hyperresonant percussion note
- Diminished breath sounds
- Wheezing
- Crackles

When the bronchiectasis pathology is primarily restrictive in nature (over areas of atelectasis and consolidation):
- Increased tactile and vocal fremitus
- Bronchial breath sounds
- Crackles
- Whispered pectoriloquy
- Dull percussion note

CLINICAL DATA OBTAINED FROM LABORATORY TESTS AND SPECIAL PROCEDURES

Pulmonary Function Test Findings
Moderate to Severe Bronchiectasis
(When Primarily Obstructive Lung Pathophysiology)

FORCED EXPIRATORY VOLUME AND FLOW RATE FINDINGS

FVC	FEV_T	FEV_1/FVC ratio	$FEF_{25\%-75\%}$
↓	↓	↓	↓

$FEF_{50\%}$	$FEF_{200-1200}$	PEFR	MVV
↓	↓	↓	↓

LUNG VOLUME AND CAPACITY FINDINGS

V_T	IRV	ERV	RV
N or ↑	N or ↓	N or ↓	↑

VC	IC	FRC	TLC	RV/TLC ratio
↓	N or ↓	↑	N or ↑	N or ↑

Pulmonary Function Test Findings
Moderate to Severe Bronchiectasis
(When Primarily Restrictive Lung Pathophysiology)

FORCED EXPIRATORY FLOW RATE FINDINGS

FVC	FEV_T	FEV_1/FVC ratio	$FEF_{25\%-75\%}$
↓	N or ↓	N or ↑	N or ↓

$FEF_{50\%}$	$FEF_{200-1200}$	PEFR	MVV
N or ↓	N or ↓	N or ↓	N or ↓

LUNG VOLUME AND CAPACITY FINDINGS

V_T	IRV	ERV	RV
N or ↓	↓	↓	↓

VC	IC	FRC	TLC	RV/TLC ratio
↓	↓	↓	↓	N

Arterial Blood Gases
Bronchiectasis

MILD TO MODERATE STAGES

Acute Alveolar Hyperventilation with Hypoxemia*
(Acute Respiratory Alkalosis)

pH	$PaCO_2$	HCO_3^-	PaO_2	SaO_2 or SpO_2
↑	↓	↓	↓	↓
		(but normal)		

SEVERE STAGE

Chronic Ventilatory Failure with Hypoxemia[†]
(Compensated Respiratory Acidosis)

pH	$PaCO_2$	HCO_3^-	PaO_2	SaO_2 or SpO_2
N	↑	↑	↓	↓
		(significantly)		

ACUTE VENTILATORY CHANGES SUPERIMPOSED ON CHRONIC
Ventilatory Failure[‡]

Because acute ventilatory changes are frequently seen in patients with chronic ventilatory failure, the respiratory therapist must be familiar with—and alert for—the following two dangerous arterial blood gas (ABG) findings:

- Acute alveolar hyperventilation superimposed on chronic ventilatory failure—which should further alert the respiratory therapist to document the following important ABG assessment: possible *impending acute ventilator failure*
- Acute ventilatory failure (acute hypoventilation) superimposed on chronic ventilatory failure

---

*See Figure 4-3 and related discussion for the acute pH, $PaCO_2$, and HCO_3^- changes associated with acute alveolar hyperventilation.
[†]See Figure 4-2 and related discussion for the pH, $PaCO_2$, and HCO_3^- changes associated with chronic ventilatory failure.
[†]See TABLE 4-7 and related discussion for the pH, $PaCO_2$, and HCO_3^- changes associated with acute ventilatory changes superimposed on chronic ventilatory failure.

Oxygenation Indices*
BRONCHIECTASIS MODERATE TO SEVERE STAGES

$\dot{Q}s/\dot{Q}T$	DO_2[†]	$\dot{V}O_2$	$C(a-\bar{v})O_2$	O_2ER	$S\bar{v}O_2$
↑	↓	N	N	↑	↓

Hemodynamic Indices[‡]
Bronchiectasis Moderate to Severe Stages

CVP	RAP	$\overline{PA}$	PCWP	CO	SV
↑	↑	↑	N	N	N

SVI	CI	RVSWI	LVSWI	PVR	SVR
N	N	↑	N	↑	N

ABNORMAL LABORATORY TESTS AND PROCEDURES
Hematology

- Increased hematocrit and hemoglobin
- Elevated white blood count (WBC) if patient is acutely infected

SPUTUM CULTURE RESULTS AND SENSITIVITY

- *Streptococcus pneumoniae*
- *Haemophilus influenzae*
- *Pseudomonas aeruginosa*
- Anaerobic organisms

RADIOLOGIC FINDINGS
Chest Radiograph

When the bronchiectasis is primarily obstructive in nature

- Translucent (dark) lung fields
- Depressed or flattened diaphragms
- Long and narrow heart (pulled down by diaphragms)
- Enlarged heart (when heart failure is present)
- Tram-tracks
- Areas of consolidation and/or atelectasis may or may not be seen

When the pathophysiology of bronchiectasis is primarily obstructive in nature, the lungs become hyperinflated, leading to an increased functional residual capacity and depressed diaphragms. Because right and left ventricular enlargement

---

*$C(a-\bar{v})O_2$, Arterial-venous oxygen difference; DO_2, total oxygen delivery; O_2ER, oxygen extraction ratio; $\dot{Q}s/\dot{Q}T$, pulmonary shunt fraction; $S\bar{v}O_2$, mixed venous oxygen saturation; $\dot{V}O_2$, oxygen consumption.
[†]The DO_2 may be normal in patients who have compensated to the decreased oxygenation status with (1) an increased cardiac output, (2) an increased hemoglobin level, or (3) a combination of both. When the DO_2 is normal, the O_2ER is usually normal.
[†]*CI*, Cardiac index; *CO*, cardiac output; *CVP*, central venous pressure; *LVSWI*, left ventricular stroke work index; *$\overline{PA}$*, mean pulmonary artery pressure; *PCWP*, pulmonary capillary wedge pressure; *PVR*, pulmonary vascular resistance; *RAP*, right atrial pressure; *RVSWI*, right ventricular stroke work index; *SV*, stroke volume; *SVI*, stroke volume index; *SVR*, systemic vascular resistance.

and failure may develop as secondary problems during the advanced stages of bronchiectasis, an enlarged heart may be seen on the chest radiograph.

Although the chest radiograph is not as valuable as the CT scan in identifying a specific type of bronchiectasis (i.e., cystic, varicose, or cylindrical), a careful analysis of chest radiographs usually reveals abnormalities in the majority of cases. For example, tram-track opacities (also called tram-lines) may be seen in cylindrical bronchiectasis. Tram-tracks are parallel, or curved opacity lines of varying length caused by bronchial wall thickening. Figure 14-2 shows the x-ray of a patient with gross cystic bronchiectasis and overinflated lungs.

When the bronchiectasis is primarily restrictive in nature
- Atelectasis and consolidation
- Infiltrates (suggesting pneumonia)
- Increased opacity

In generalized bronchiectasis, such as commonly seen in cystic fibrosis, there is usually overinflation of the lungs. However, when the bronchiectasis is localized, the chest radiograph often reveals a restrictive pathology such as atelectasis, consolidation, or infiltrates. When atelectasis and consolidation develop as a result of bronchiectasis, an increased opacity and reduced lung volume are seen in these areas on the radiograph. For example, Figure 14-3 illustrates a marked volume loss in a patient with left lower lobe bronchiectasis.

BRONCHOGRAM

In the past, **bronchography** (the injection of an opaque contrast material into the tracheobronchial tree) was routinely performed on patients with bronchiectasis. Figure 14-4, for example, is a bronchogram of cylindrical bronchiectasis. Figure 14-5, is a bronchogram of cystic (saccular) bronchiectasis. Figure 14-6 shows a bronchogram of varicose bronchiectasis— the bronchi are dilated and constricted in an irregular fashion and terminate in a distorted, bulbous shape. Today, CT scan of the chest has largely replaced this technique.

COMPUTED TOMOGRAPHY (CT SCAN)

With this technique, increased bronchial wall opacity is often seen. The bronchial walls may appear as follows:
- Thick
- Dilated
- Characterized by ring lines or clusters
- Signet ring–shaped
- Flame-shaped

The CT scan changes may include many findings that are similar to those seen on the chest radiograph. The bronchial walls may appear thick, dilated, or as rings of opacities arranged in lines or clusters. A characteristic appearance in

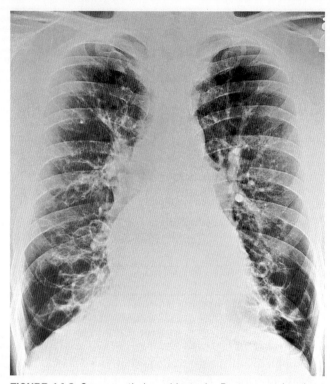

FIGURE 14-2 Gross cystic bronchiectasis. Posteroanterior chest radiograph showing overinflated lungs. There are multiple ring opacities, most obvious at the lung bases, ranging from 3 to 15 mm in diameter. (From Hansell DM, Armstrong P, Lynch DA, McAdams HP, eds: *Imaging of diseases of the chest*, ed 4, Philadelphia, 2005, Elsevier.)

bronchiectasis is the end-on signet ring opacity produced by the ring shadow of a dilated airway with its accompanying artery (Figure 14-7).

The specific type of bronchiectasis can be confirmed with the CT scan. For example, Figure 14-8 confirms the presence of cylindrical bronchiectasis. Figure 14-9 shows varicose bronchiectasis and Figure 14-10 shows cystic bronchiectasis. Airways that are filled with secretions produce rounded or flame-shaped opacities that can be identified by following them through adjacent sections to unfilled airways. The CT scan also confirms atelectasis, consolidation, fibrosis, scarring, and hyperinflation.

Finally, it should be mentioned that the CT scan is an excellent tool to use for what is known as **Lung Mapping**—that is, the ability to map out and determine precisely where chest physical therapy would be delivered, or exactly where surgical resection of lung should be performed.

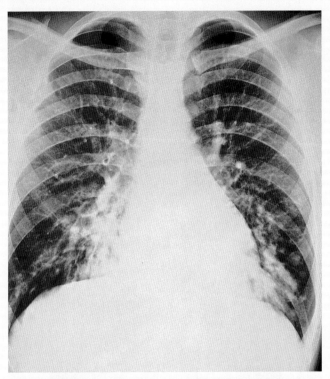

FIGURE 14-3 Left lower lobe bronchiectasis. The marked volume loss of the left lower lobe is indicated by a depressed hilum, vertical left main stem bronchus, mediastinal shift, and left-sided transradiancy. (From Hansell DM, Armstrong P, Lynch DA, McAdams HP, eds: *Imaging of diseases of the chest*, ed 4, Philadelphia, 2005, Elsevier.)

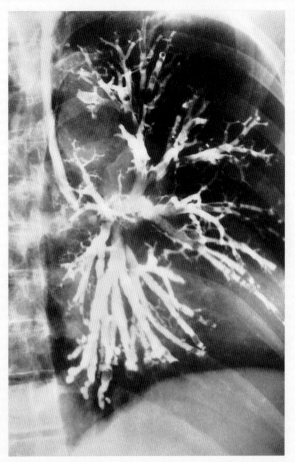

FIGURE 14-4 Cylindrical bronchiectasis. Left posterior oblique projection of a left bronchogram showing cylindrical bronchiectasis affecting the whole of the lower lobe except for the superior segment. Few side branches fill. Basal airways are crowded together, indicating volume loss of the lower lobe, a common finding in bronchiectasis. (From Hansell DM, Armstrong P, Lynch DA, McAdams HP, eds: *Imaging of diseases of the chest*, ed 4, Philadelphia, 2005, Elsevier.)

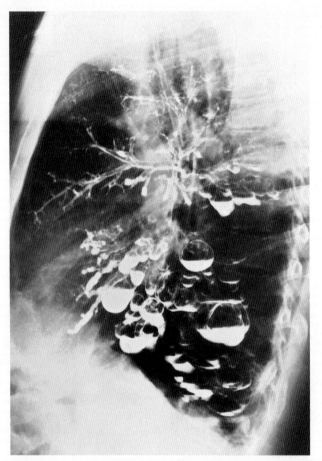

FIGURE 14-5 Cystic (saccular) bronchiectasis. Right lateral bronchogram showing cystic bronchiectasis affecting mainly the lower lobe and posterior segment of the upper lobe. (From Hansell DM, Armstrong P, Lynch DA, McAdams HP, eds: *Imaging of diseases of the chest,* ed 4, Philadelphia, 2005, Elsevier.)

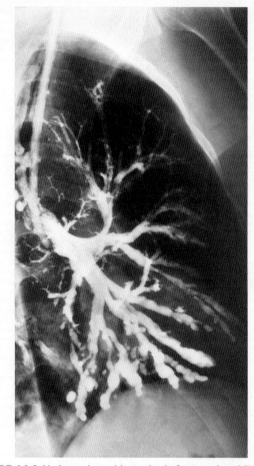

FIGURE 14-6 Varicose bronchiectasis. Left posterior oblique projection of left bronchogram in a patient with the ciliary dyskinesia syndrome. All basal bronchi are affected by varicose bronchiectasis. (From Hansell DM, Armstrong P, Lynch DA, McAdams HP, eds: *Imaging of diseases of the chest,* ed 4, Philadelphia, 2005, Elsevier.)

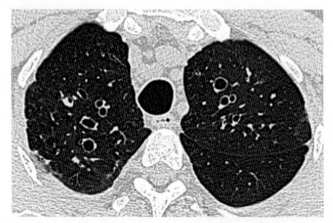

FIGURE 14-7 Signet ring sign in patient with cystic fibrosis. (From Hansell DM, Armstrong P, Lynch DA, McAdams HP, eds: *Imaging of diseases of the chest,* ed 4, Philadelphia, 2005, Elsevier.)

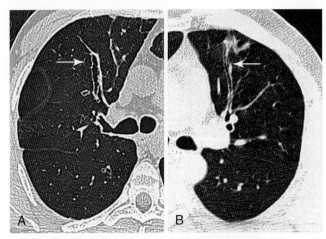

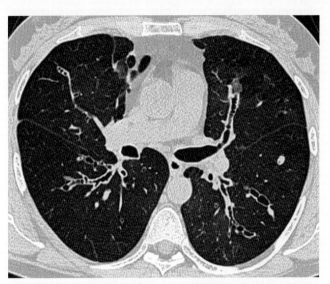

FIGURE 14-8 Cylindrical bronchiectasis. Examples from two patients. Airways parallel to the plane of section in anterior segment of an upper lobe show changes of cylindrical bronchiectasis; bronchi are wider than normal and fail to taper as they proceed toward the lung periphery (arrow). (From Hansell DM, Armstrong P, Lynch DA, McAdams HP, eds: *Imaging of diseases of the chest*, ed 4, Philadelphia, 2005, Elsevier.)

FIGURE 14-9 Varicose bronchiectasis. Patient with allergic bronchopulmonary aspergillosis and cystic fibrosis. The bronchiectatic airways have a corrugated, or beaded, appearance. (From Hansell DM, Armstrong P, Lynch DA, McAdams HP, eds: *Imaging of diseases of the chest*, ed 4, Philadelphia, 2005, Elsevier.)

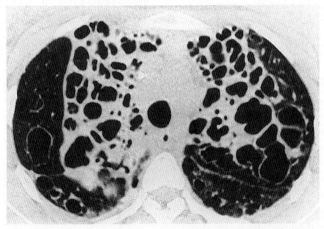

FIGURE 14-10 Cystic bronchiectasis (advanced) in the upper lobes. (From Hansell DM, Armstrong P, Lynch DA, McAdams HP, eds: *Imaging of diseases of the chest*, ed 4, Philadelphia, 2005, Elsevier.)

General Management of Bronchiectasis

The general treatment plan is aimed at controlling pulmonary infections, airway secretions, and airway obstruction and preventing complications. Daily chest percussion, postural drainage, and effective coughing exercises to remove bronchial secretions are routine parts of the treatment. Antibiotics, bronchodilators, and expectorants are often prescribed during periods of exacerbation. Childhood vaccinations and yearly influenza vaccinations help reduce the prevalence of some infections. The avoidance of upper respiratory infections, smoking, and polluted environments also helps reduce susceptibility to pneumonia in these patients. Surgical lung resection may be indicated for those patients who respond poorly to therapy or experience massive bleeding.

Respiratory Care Treatment Protocols

Oxygen Therapy Protocol

Oxygen therapy is used to treat hypoxemia, decrease the work of breathing, and decrease myocardial work. The hypoxemia that develops in bronchiectasis is usually caused by the pulmonary shunting associated with the disorder. The hypoxemia may not respond well to oxygen therapy when true or capillary pulmonary shunting is present (see Oxygen Therapy Protocol, Protocol 9-1).

Bronchopulmonary Hygiene Therapy Protocol

A number of bronchial hygiene treatment modalities may be used to enhance the mobilization of bronchial secretions—which include the following:

- Directed cough
- Exercise breathing programs
- Autogenic breathing
- Forced expiration
- Chest physical therapy (CPT) (postural drainage [PD], hand or mechanical chest clapping)
- Suctioning
- Positive expiratory pressure (PEP)
- Oscillatory PEP (e.g., flutter valve acapella device)
- High frequency chest wall compression

Chest percussion has become more practical with the advent of **high frequency chest compression devices** such as the "pneumovest." However, such compression devices are expensive, and chest wall pain may limit their usefulness (see Bronchopulmonary Hygiene Therapy Protocol, Protocol 9-2).

Lung Expansion Therapy Protocol

Attempts to keep distal lung units inflated may involve the use of deep breathing and coughing and incentive spirometry (see Lung Expansion Therapy Protocol, Protocol 9-3).

Aerosolized Medication Therapy Protocol

Both sympathomimetic and parasympatholytic agents are commonly used in selected patients with bronchiectasis to induce bronchial smooth muscle relaxation, particularly in patients with spirometrically-proven reversible airway obstruction (see Aerosolized Medication Therapy Protocol, Protocol 9-4 and Appendix II).

Finally, it should be noted that the use of corticosteroids is discouraged. The role of aerosolized antibiotics, such as tobramycin, aztreonam, and colistin, is not yet clear in NCFB. These agents may cause bronchospasm and are not approved for use in bronchiectasis by the FDA.

Mechanical Ventilation Protocol

Invasive and noninvasive mechanical ventilation may be necessary to provide and help improve alveolar ventilation and eventually return the patient to spontaneous breathing. Because acute ventilatory failure superimposed on chronic ventilatory failure is often seen in patients with severe bronchiectasis, continuous mechanical ventilation is justified when the acute ventilatory failure is thought to be reversible—for example, when acute pneumonia exists as a complicating factor (see Mechanical Ventilation Protocol, Protocol 10-1 and Mechanical Ventilation Weaning Protocol, Protocol 10-2).

Medications Commonly Prescribed by the Physician

Expectorants

Expectorants sometimes are ordered when oral liquids and aerosol therapy alone are not sufficient to facilitate expectoration (see Appendix II, Expectorants). Their clinical effectiveness is doubtful.

Antibiotics

Antibiotics are commonly administered to treat associated respiratory tract infections (see Appendix III, Antibiotics)

Admitting History and Physical Examination

A 31-year-old obese male patient consulted his physician regarding an increasingly productive cough. He reported a "bad case" of right lower lobe pneumonia 7 years ago and several episodes of pulmonary infection since that time. On those occasions he usually received an antibiotic, and until 6 months ago the infections responded readily to treatment. However, 6 months ago he noticed that his chronic cough had become increasingly severe, and for the first time his cough became productive. Recently, he had produced as much as a cup of thick, tenacious, yellow-white sputum per day. Within the past 2 to 3 days, he noticed a small amount of dark blood mixed with the sputum. He also noticed some dyspnea on exertion, but this had not been particularly troublesome. The past medical history revealed chronic sinusitis since adolescence but was otherwise unremarkable.

Physical examination revealed a well-developed male adult in no apparent distress. Vital signs were within normal limits. His oral temperature was 98.4°F. He coughed frequently during the examination and produced a moderate amount of thick, yellow, blood-streaked sputum. Coarse crackles were heard over the right lower lung fields posteriorly. His SpO_2 on room air while at rest was 85%.

Laboratory results showed a mild leukocytosis but were otherwise normal. An outpatient sputum culture indicated the presence of *H. influenzae*. A CT scan of the chest revealed cystic dilations of the right lower lobe bronchus. The respiratory therapist assigned to assess and treat the patient at this time recorded the following in the patient's chart.

Respiratory Assessment and Plan

S   Productive cough, hemoptysis, worse in past 6 months. Mild dyspnea on exertion.

O   Vital signs: normal. Afebrile. SpO_2 85%. Observed moderate amount of mucopurulent, blood-streaked sputum. Coarse crackles over RLL. Outpatient sputum culture: *H. influenzae*. CT scan suggests saccular dilation of RLL bronchi.

A   • Postpneumonic bronchiectasis RLL (history and CT scan)

   • Excessive airway secretions and sputum production (coarse crackles and sputum expectoration)

   • Acute bronchial infection and hemoptysis (yellow, blood-streaked sputum, culture results)

   • Moderate hypoxemia (SpO_2)

P   **Oxygen Therapy Protocol** (O_2 via 2 L/min nasal cannula). **Aerosolized Medication** and **Bronchopulmonary Hygiene Protocols** (med. neb. with albuterol premix solution, followed by cough and deep breathing, q6h).

The physician prescribed antibiotics and administered pneumococcal vaccine. The patient was discharged from the hospital after 3 days with considerable improvement. However, he was still producing a small amount of thin clear sputum. He was instructed to seek prompt medical attention

for all future pulmonary infections. His wife was instructed in manual chest percussion and postural drainage techniques.

About 6 months later, the patient arrived at the emergency department complaining of a productive cough, pain on the left side of the chest (made worse by deep breathing), shaking chills and fever for 3 days, and noticeable swelling of both ankles. Since his previous visit, he had been doing his manual CPT and PD only one or two times per week. He had gained 30 pounds, and had taken a new job as a painter's apprentice. He admitted to smoking an occasional cigarette. There had been no known recent infectious disease exposure.

Physical examination revealed a young man in obvious respiratory distress. His vital signs were blood pressure 160/100, heart rate 110 beats/min and regular, respiratory rate 20 breaths/min, and oral temperature 101.5°F. His sputum was foul-smelling (a fecal odor), thick, and yellow-green. His cough was strong. Auscultation revealed coarse crackles over both bases. There was mild clubbing of fingers and toes. The physician wrote "bronchiectasis" in the working diagnosis section of the patient's chart.

Although a CT scan was ordered, it had not yet been taken. The patient's WBC was 23,500 mm^3, with 80% segmented neutrophils and 10% bands. Room air ABG showed pH 7.51, $PaCO_2$ 28 mm Hg, HCO_3^- 21 mEq/L, PaO_2 45 mm Hg, and SaO_2 87%. His SpO_2 at rest on room air was 86%; it fell to 78% when he got out of bed to go to the bathroom.

The respiratory therapist recorded the following note in the patient's emergency department chart.

Respiratory Assessment and Plan

S   Cough, pleuritic left-sided chest pain, chills, fever, leg swelling. 30 lb weight gain. Smoking.

O   HR 110; RR 20; BP 160/100; T 101.5°F;. Sputum thick, yellow-green, foul-smelling. Coarse crackles both bases. Strong cough. Clubbing of digits. WBC 23,500 (80% neutrophils, 10% bands). Room air ABG; pH 7.51; $PaCO_2$ 28; HCO_3^- 21; PaO_2 45, and SaO_2 87%; SpO_2 (room air, rest) 86%, falls to 78% with mild exertion.

A   • Bronchiectasis (old chart record)

   • Excessive airway secretions (thick sputum, coarse crackles)

   • Good ability to mobilize secretions (strong cough)

   • Infection likely (fever, yellow-green sputum, leukocytosis)

   • Acute alveolar hyperventilation with moderate hypoxemia (ABG)

   • Postural drainage therapy and smoking cessation noncompliance (history)

P   Review CXR. **Oxygen Therapy Protocol** (2 L/min per nasal cannula). **Aerosolized Medication Protocol** and **Bronchopulmonary Hygiene Protocols** (med. neb. albuterol 0.5 mL, followed by CPT and PD q4 h). Obtain sputum for Gram stain and culture. Check I&O. Repeat ABG in AM. Review deep breathing and cough, flutter valve, and pulmonary rehabilitation strategies with patient and his wife. Train in use of "pneumovest" chest percussion device. Offer smoking cessation and weight reduction programs.

Discussion

The main challenge facing the respiratory therapist caring for the patient with bronchiectasis is the efficient removal of excessive bronchopulmonary secretions. Over the years, postural drainage and percussion, good systemic hydration, and judicious use of antibiotics have been the hallmarks of therapy. More recently, intermittent (rare) use of mucolytics, percussive ventilation, and **Lung Expansion Therapy** (see Protocol 9-3) has become more common. Pneumococcal prophylaxis is, of course, important, as is prompt attention to parenchymal pulmonary infections such as pneumonia. The clinical distinction between chronic bronchiectasis and cystic fibrosis is a subtle one at the bedside, and the latter condition must always be ruled out in patients with bronchiectasis. The goal of long-term therapy in bronchiectasis is prevention of lung parenchyma–destroying pulmonary infections and avoidance of frequent hospitalizations. Hemoptysis is often a sign of more deep-seated infection requiring antibiotic therapy. At the time of the second admission, severe infection was suspected, and intravenous antibiotic therapy was started.

The clinical manifestations throughout this case were all based on the clinical scenario associated with **excessive airway secretions** (see Figure 9-11). For example, the thick yellow sputum resulted in decreased V/Q ratios, venous admixture, and hypoxemia. These pathophysiologic mechanisms caused clinical manifestations of coarse crackles, an increase in blood pressure and heart rate, and acute alveolar hyperventilation with moderate hypoxemia.

Digital clubbing associated with hypoxemia is another clinical manifestation of bronchiectasis. After the first assessment, the **Oxygen Therapy Protocol, Aerosolized Medication Protocol**, and **Bronchopulmonary Hygiene Therapy Protocol** were all administered appropriately (see Protocol 9-1, Protocol 9-2, and Protocol 9-4). The therapist's review of the chest x-ray allowed him to target the postural drainage therapy. Low-flow oxygen per nasal cannula, aerosolized bronchodilators (albuterol), chest percussion, and postural drainage therapy were selected from these protocols and applied with good results.

Finally, during the second admission, patient noncompliance was evident (i.e., weight gain, resumption of smoking, employment in a dusty workplace, failure to continue CPT and PD), which further complicated the patient's respiratory disorder. In response to the patient's condition, the whole respiratory care regimen was up-regulated by an increase in frequency of treatments, with a strong emphasis on the patient's responsibility for his own care. In both of these admissions, no note of the patient's state of systemic or secretion hydration was made. This is an important factor worth noting.

SELF-ASSESSMENT QUESTIONS

Answers to questions can be found on Evolve. To access additional student assessment questions visit **http://evolve.elsevier.com/DesJardins/respiratory**.

1. **In which of the following forms of bronchiectasis are the bronchi dilated and constricted in an irregular fashion?**
   1. Fusiform
   2. Saccular
   3. Varicose
   4. Cylindrical
      a. 2 only
      b. 3 only
      c. 2 and 4 only
      d. 1 and 3 only

2. **Which of the following is or are common causes of acquired bronchiectasis?**
   1. Hypogammaglobulinemia
   2. Pulmonary tuberculosis
   3. Kartagener's syndrome
   4. Cystic fibrosis
      a. 1 only
      b. 2 only
      c. 3 only
      d. 3 and 4 only

3. **In the primarily obstructive form of bronchiectasis, the patient commonly demonstrates which of the following?**
   1. Decreased FRC
   2. Increased FEF 25%-75%
   3. Decreased PEFR
   4. Increased FEV_T
      a. 1 only
      b. 3 only
      c. 1 and 4 only
      d. 2 and 4 only

4. **Which of the following radiologic findings is or are associated with bronchiectasis that is primarily obstructive in nature?**
   1. Atelectasis
   2. Depressed or flattened diaphragms
   3. Long and narrow heart
   4. Translucent lung fields
      a. 1 and 2 only
      b. 3 and 4 only
      c. 1 and 4 only
      d. 2, 3, and 4

5. **Which of the following is considered the hallmark of bronchiectasis?**
   a. Chronic cough and large quantities of foul-smelling sputum
   b. Abnormal bronchogram
   c. Acute ventilatory failure superimposed on chronic ventilatory failure
   d. Presentation as both a restrictive and obstructive pulmonary disorder

6. **Which of the following is or are commonly cultured in the sputum of patients with bronchiectasis?**
   1. *Streptococcus pneumoniae*
   2. *Pseudomonas aeruginosa*
   3. *Haemophilus influenzae*
   4. *Klebsiella*
      a. 3 only
      b. 4 only
      c. 1, 2, and 3 only
      d. 1, 2, 3, and 4

7. **When the pathophysiology of bronchiectasis is primarily obstructive in nature, the patient demonstrates which of the following clinical manifestations?**
   1. Decreased tactile and vocal fremitus
   2. Bronchial breath sounds
   3. Dull percussion note
   4. Rhonchi and wheezing
      a. 2 only
      b. 3 only
      c. 1 and 4 only
      d. 2 and 4 only

8. **Which of the following diagnostic procedures is or are used to positively diagnose bronchiectasis?**
   1. Arterial blood gases
   2. Bronchography
   3. Oxygenation indices
   4. Computed tomography
      a. 2 only
      b. 3 only
      c. 1 and 3 only
      d. 2 and 4 only

9. **Which of the following is or are causes of bronchiectasis are related to abnormal secretion clearance?**
   1. Pertussis
   2. Cystic fibrosis
   3. Kartagener's syndrome
   4. Measles
      a. 1 only
      b. 2 only
      c. 3 and 4 only
      d. 2 and 3 only

10. **Which of the following hemodynamic indices is or are associated with bronchiectasis?**
    1. Decreased central venous pressure
    2. Increased mean pulmonary artery pressure
    3. Decreased right ventricular stroke work index
    4. Increased right atrial pressure
       a. 2 only
       b. 3 only
       c. 2 and 4 only
       d. 1 and 3 only

11. **Which of the following respiratory care protocols may be of importance in the outpatient care of patients with bronchiectasis?**
    1. Oxygen Therapy Protocol
    2. Bronchopulmonary Hygiene Therapy Protocol
    3. Lung Expansion Therapy Protocol
    4. Aerosolized Medication Therapy Protocol
       a. 2 and 3 only
       b. 2 only
       c. 1 and 2 only
       d. 1, 2, 3, and 4 only

Chapter Objectives

After reading this chapter, you will be able to:

- Describe the anatomic alterations of the lungs associated with cystic fibrosis.
- Describe the etiology and epidemiology of cystic fibrosis.
- Describe how the cystic fibrosis gene is inherited.
- Discuss the screening and diagnosis of cystic fibrosis.
- Discuss the cardiopulmonary clinical manifestations associated with cystic fibrosis.
- Describe the general management of cystic fibrosis.
- Describe the clinical strategies and rationales of the SOAPs presented in the case study.
- Define key terms and complete self-assessment questions at the end of the chapter and on Evolve.

Key Terms

Amniocentesis
Cystic Fibrosis Transmembrane Conductance Regulator (CFTR)
Electrical Potential Difference
Genetic Counseling
Immunoreactive Trypsin Test (IRT)
Inhaled Tobramycin (TOBI)
Ivacaftor
Lung or Heart Transplantation

Meconium Ileus
Nasal Potential Difference (NPD)
Pilocarpine
Standard Mendelian Pattern
Sweat Test

Chapter Outline

Anatomic Alterations of the Lungs
Etiology and Epidemiology
  How the Cystic Fibrosis Gene is Inherited
Screening and Diagnosis
  Newborn Screening
  Sweat Test
  Molecular Diagnosis (Genetic Testing)
  Nasal Potential Difference
  Prenatal Testing
  Stool Fecal Fat Test
Overview of the Cardiopulmonary Clinical Manifestations Associated with Cystic Fibrosis
General Management of Cystic Fibrosis
  Respiratory Care Treatment Protocols
  Other Medications and Special Procedures Prescribed by the Physician
Case Study: Cystic Fibrosis
Self-Assessment Questions

Anatomic Alterations of the Lungs[1]

Although the lungs of patients with cystic fibrosis (CF) appear normal at birth, abnormal structural changes can develop quickly. Initially, the patient has bronchial gland hypertrophy and metaplasia of goblet cells. This condition leads to the excessive production and accumulation of thick, tenacious mucus in the tracheobronchial tree secondary to inadequate hydration of the periciliary fluid layer (sol layer). Because the mucus is thick and inflexible, impairment of the normal mucociliary clearing mechanism ensues, and many small bronchi and bronchioles become partially or totally obstructed (mucous plugging). Partial obstruction leads to overdistention of the alveoli, and complete obstruction leads to patchy areas of atelectasis and, in some cases, bronchiectasis (see Chapter 14). The anatomic alterations of the lungs

associated with CF may result in both restrictive and obstructive lung characteristics, but excessive bronchial secretions, bronchial obstruction, and hyperinflation of the lungs are the predominant features of CF in the advanced stages.

The abundance of stagnant mucus in the tracheobronchial tree also serves as an excellent culture medium for bacteria, particularly *Staphylococcus aureus, Haemophilus influenzae,* and *Pseudomonas aeruginosa.* Some gram-negative bacteria are also commonly associated with CF, such as *Stenotrophomonas maltophilia and Burkholderia cepacia complex.* The infection stimulates additional mucous production and further compromises the mucociliary transport system. This condition may lead to secondary bronchial smooth muscle constriction. Finally, as the disease progresses, the patient may develop signs and symptoms of recurrent pneumonia, chronic bronchitis (Chapter 12), bronchiectasis (Chapter 14), and lung abscesses (Chapter 17).

As illustrated in Figure 15-1, the major respiratory pathologic or structural changes associated with CF are as follows:

- Excessive production and accumulation of thick, tenacious mucus in the tracheobronchial tree secondary to inadequate hydration of the periciliary fluid layer.

---

[1]CF does not affect the lungs exclusively. It also affects the function of exocrine glands in other parts of the body. In addition to being characterized by abnormally viscid secretions in the lungs, the disease is clinically manifested by pancreatic insufficiency and high chloride concentrations in the sweat.

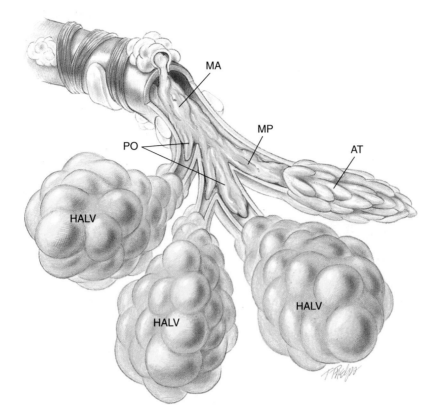

FIGURE 15-1 Cystic fibrosis. *AT*, Atelectasis; *HALV*, hyperinflation of alveoli; *MA*, mucous accumulation; *MP*, mucous plug; *PO*, partial obstruction of the airways.

- Partial bronchial obstruction (mucous plugging)
- Hyperinflation of the alveoli
- Total bronchial obstruction (mucous plugging)
- Atelectasis
- Bronchiectasis

Etiology and Epidemiology

CF is the most common fatal inherited disorder in childhood. CF is an autosomal recessive gene disorder caused by mutations in a pair of genes located on chromosome 7. Under normal conditions, every cell in the body (except the sex cells) has 46 chromosomes—23 pairs (one half inherited from the father and the other half from the mother). Over 2400 different mutations in the gene that encodes for the **cystic fibrosis transmembrane conductance regulator (CFTR)** have been described.

One genetic defect linked to CF involves the absence of three base pairs in codon 508 (ΔF508) that codes for phenylalanine on chromosome 7 (band q31.2). Because of the loss of these three base pairs, the CFTR protein becomes dysfunctional. This is the most common genetic mutation associated with CF and accounts for 70% to 75% of the patients with CF tested.

The abnormal expression of the CFTR results in abnormal transport of sodium and chloride ions across many types of epithelial surfaces, including those lining the bronchial airways, intestines, pancreas, liver ducts, and sweat glands. As a result, thick, viscous mucus accumulates in the lungs, and mucus blocks the passageways of the pancreas, preventing enzymes from the pancreas from reaching the intestines. This condition inhibits the digestion of protein and fat, which in turn leads to deficiencies of fat-soluble vitamins A, D, E, and K. In addition, diarrhea, malnutrition, and failure to thrive are also common problems. Some infants with CF are born with a blockage of the intestine—a condition called **meconium ileus.** Most men with CF are infertile (azospermic) as a result of a missing or an underdeveloped vas deferens. Fertility is decreased in women with CF secondary to thick cervical mucus.

How the Cystic Fibrosis Gene is Inherited

Because CF is a recessive gene disorder, the child must inherit two copies of the defective CF gene—one from each parent (cystic fibrosis carriers)—to have the disease. Even though the carrier of the CF gene may be identified through genetic testing, the carrier (heterozygote) does not demonstrate evidence of the disease. However, if both parents carry the CF gene, the possibility of their children having CF (regardless of gender) follows the **standard Mendelian pattern:** there is a 25% chance that each child will have CF, a 25% chance that each child will be completely normal (and not carry the gene), and a 50% chance that each child will be a carrier. Thus, when both patients carry a CF gene mutation, there is a one in four chance that the child will have CF (Figure 15-2). It is estimated that more than 10 million Americans are unknowing, symptomless carriers of a mutant CF gene.

According to the Cystic Fibrosis Foundation, CF affects about 30,000 children and adults in the United States, and

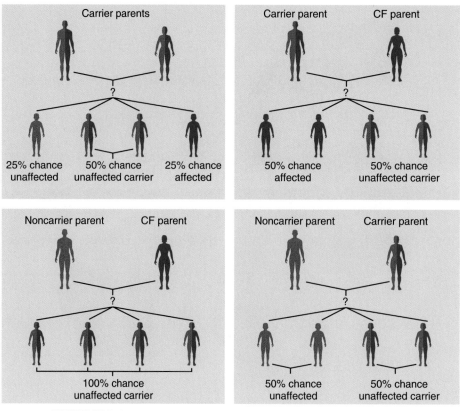

FIGURE 15-2 Standard Mendelian pattern of inheritance of cystic fibrosis.

about 70,000 worldwide. About 1000 new cases of CF are diagnosed each year in the United States. More than 90% of the patients are diagnosed by newborn screening. Over 50% of the patient population with CF is age 18 years or older. The median age of survival for individuals with CF is in the late 30s, but many patients with CF live into their 40s and beyond.[2] CF occurs most often in Caucasians (1:3000). The occurrence in Hispanics is 1:9200, Native Americans 1:10,900, African-Americans 1:15,000, and Asian-Americans 1:30,000. Death is usually caused by pulmonary complications.

Screening and Diagnosis

The diagnosis of CF is based on newborn screening, clinical manifestations associated with CF, family history of CF, and laboratory findings. Box 15-1 provides common clinical indicators that justify evaluation for CF.

The following two criteria must be met to diagnose CF:
1. Clinical symptoms consistent with CF in at least one organ system—for example, pulmonary system, sinus disease, pancreatic disease, meconium ileus, biliary disease, and male infertility.
2. Clinical evidence of cystic fibrosis *transmembrane conductance regulator* (CFTR) dysfunction—any of the following:
   - Elevated **sweat chloride** >60 mEq/L (on two occasions)
   - Molecular diagnosis (**Genetic Testing**). Presence of two disease-causing mutations in CFTR
   - Abnormal nasal potential difference

---

[2]CF Foundation (www.cff.org).

Newborn Screening

Newborn screening for CF has been a part of the newborn genetic testing protocol in all 50 states since 2011. Most infants with CF have an elevated blood level of immunoreactive trypsin (also called trypsin–like immunoreactivity and serum trypsin), which can be measured by radioimmunoassay or by an enzyme-linked immunoassay. The **immunoreactive trypsin level (IRT)** is measured from the blood dots collected on all newborn infants on the Guthrie cards.

The CF screening protocol varies among states and will identify over 90% of infants with CF. The most common protocol is to perform DNA screening for 32 to 85 of the most common CF mutations on 2% to 5% of the samples with the highest IRT levels. Detection of at least one CF mutation is considered a positive screen and is referred to a CF Center in most states for further testing.

The diagnosis of CF is established by a positive sweat test and/or genetic analysis for CF mutations. A negative or normal sweat test identifies the newborn as a CF carrier. All families of infants identified through newborn screening programs should receive genetic counseling. These newborn screening programs now identify 95% of infants with CF. It should be remembered that it is always appropriate to sweat test an individual of any age with symptoms consistent with the possible diagnosis of CF.

Sweat Test

The **sweat test** (sometimes called the sweat chloride test) is the gold standard diagnostic test for CF. The sweat test is a reliable test for the identification of about 98% of patients with CF. This test measures the amount of sodium and

BOX 15-1 Clinical Indicators Justifying the Initial Evaluation for Cystic Fibrosis

Pulmonary
Wheezing
Chronic cough
Sputum production
Frequent respiratory infections (*Staphylococcus aureus, Pseudomonas aeruginosa, Haemophilus influenzae*)
Abnormal chest radiograph and/or computed tomography (CT) scan
Nasal polyps
Parasinusitis
Digital clubbing
Gastrointestinal Disorders
    Failure to thrive
    Foul-smelling, greasy stools
    Voracious appetite
    Milk and formula intolerance
    Rectal prolapse
    Meconium ileus
    Meconium peritonitis
    Distal intestinal obstruction syndrome
    Pancreatic insufficiency
    Pancreatitis
    Hepatobiliary
    Hepatomegaly
    Focal biliary cirrhosis
    Prolonged neonatal jaundice
    Cholelithiasis
    Nutritional deficits
    Fat-soluble vitamin deficiency (vitamins A, D, E, K)
    Hypoproteinemia
    Hypochloremia (metabolic alkalosis)
Infertility (male)
    Obstructive azoospermia

chloride in the patient's sweat. During the procedure a small amount of a colorless, odorless sweat-producing chemical called **pilocarpine** is applied to the patient's arm or leg—usually the forearm. An electrode is attached to the chemically prepared area, and a mild electric current is applied to stimulate sweat production (Figure 15-3). The test is usually done twice.

Although the sweat glands of patients with CF are microscopically normal, the glands secrete up to four times the normal amount of sodium and chloride. The actual volume of sweat, however, is no greater than that produced by a normal individual. In both infants and adults, a sweat chloride concentration greater than 60 mEq/L is considered to be a diagnostic sign of CF. Box 15-2 provides an overview for sweat test interpretations for infants 6 months or younger and infants greater than 6 months, children, and adults.

All patients with the following characteristics should undergo a sweat test to help confirm the diagnosis of CF:
- Infants with positive CF newborn screening results (performed after 2 weeks of age and >2 kg if asymptomatic)
- Infants with symptoms suggestive of CF (Box 15-1)
- Older siblings (including adults) with symptoms suggestive of CF
- Members of the patient's family with confirmed CF

BOX 15-2 Sweat Test Interpretations

Infants Six Months or Younger
≤29 mmol/L: Normal (Cystic fibrosis very unlikely)
30 to 59 mmol/L: Intermediate (Possible cystic fibrosis)
≥60 mmol/L: Abnormal (Diagnosis of cystic fibrosis)

Infants Older than Six Months, Children, and Adults
≤39 mmol/L: Normal (Cystic fibrosis very unlikely)
40 to 59 mmol/L: Intermediate (Possible cystic fibrosis)
>60 mmol/L: Abnormal (Diagnosis of cystic fibrosis)

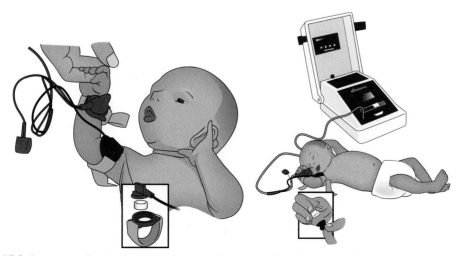

FIGURE 15-3 Sweat test. During the procedure a small amount of a colorless, odorless sweat-producing chemical called pilocarpine is applied to the patient's arm or leg—usually the forearm. An electrode is attached to the chemically prepared area, and a mild electric current is applied to stimulate sweat production. (Used with permission from Wescor, Inc—an ELITech Group Company.)

Molecular Diagnosis (Genetic Testing)

With a sample of the patient's blood or cheek cells, a **genetic test** (also called a *genotype test, gene mutation test,* or *mutation analysis*) can be performed to analyze deoxyribonucleic acid (DNA) for the presence of CFTR gene mutations. Intermediate results of sweat chloride testing should be further investigated with a DNA analysis using a **CFTR multimutation method**. The sweat chloride test should also be repeated.

Most of the diagnostic laboratories in the United States are able to screen for at least 30 to 100 of the most common mutations—including gene mutation **Delta F508** (ΔF508), which is the very most common gene mutation associated with CF. When two CF gene mutations are detected, and the sweat test is intermediate or positive, the diagnosis of CF is confirmed. Although genetic testing for CF is considered a valuable diagnostic tool, it does have its limitations. For example, some individuals have CFTR mutations but demonstrate no typical clinical manifestations of CF. In addition, some patients may have CFTR mutations, but the mutations cannot be identified without special gene analysis methods. It is estimated that genetic testing can confirm CF in about 90% to 96% of the patients tested.

Nasal Potential Difference

The impaired transport of sodium (Na^+) and chloride (Cl^-) across the epithelial cells lining the airways of the patient with CF can be measured. As the Na^+ and Cl^- ions move across the epithelial cell membrane they generate what is called an **electrical potential difference**—the amount of energy required to move an electrical charge from one point to another. In the nasal passages this electrical potential difference is called the **nasal potential difference (NPD)**. The NPD can be measured with a surface electrode over the nasal epithelial cells lining the inferior turbinate. An increased (i.e., more negative) NPD strongly suggests CF. The NPD is recommended for patients with clinical features of CF who have borderline or normal sweat test values and nondiagnostic CF genotyping.

Prenatal Testing

Both the American College of Obstetrics and Gynecology and the American College of Medical Genetics recommend that pregnant females be offered screening for CF mutations using a 32 to 85 mutation panel. Females who test positive for a CF mutation then have the option of having the father of the fetus tested. If both of the parents test positive for a CF mutation then the fetus has a one in four chance of having CF.

If desired, the fetus can be tested for CF by **amniocentesis** after the first trimester. The amniotic fluid is obtained by ultrasound guided needle aspiration of amniotic fluid from around the fetus. Fetal cells are tested for the presence of CF mutations and identified as CF affected, CF carrier, or normal. Because most genetic screening only tests for 32 to 85 of over 2400 mutations associated with CF, a negative or normal result does not entirely rule out the possibility of the person carrying one of the less common CF mutations. Infants have been born with CF when both parents have been normal by genetic screening.

Genetic counseling is very important in all cases of prenatal testing for CF to explain this uncertainty or residual risk to prospective parents. Amniocentesis and genetic analysis of fetal cells can be used to diagnose a large number of genetic disorders and chromosomal abnormalities in the fetus.

Stool Fecal Fat Test

The stool fecal fat test measures the amount of fat in the infant's stool and the percentage of dietary fat that is not absorbed by the body. The test is used to evaluate how the liver, gallbladder, pancreas, and intestines are functioning. Fat absorption requires bile from the gallbladder, enzymes from the pancreas, and normal intestines. Under normal conditions the fat malabsorption is less than 7 g of fat per 24 hours. An elevated stool fecal fat value (i.e., decreased fat absorption) is associated with a variety of disorders, including CF. Fecal elastance is an easier test of pancreatic function as it only requires a small stool sample for analysis. Infants with CF and pancreatic insufficiency will have a fecal elastance of less than 50 µg/g of stool (normal is greater than 300 µg/g of stool).

OVERVIEW of the Cardiopulmonary Clinical Manifestations Associated with Cystic Fibrosis

The following clinical manifestations result from the pathophysiologic mechanisms caused (or activated) by Atelectasis (see Figure 9-7), Bronchospasm (see Figure 9-10), and Excessive Bronchial Secretions (see Figure 9-11)—the major anatomic alterations of the lungs associated with CF (Figure 15-1).

CLINICAL DATA OBTAINED AT THE PATIENT'S BEDSIDE
The Physical Examination
Vital Signs
Increased Respiratory Rate (Tachypnea)
Several pathophysiologic mechanisms operating simultaneously may lead to an increased ventilatory rate:
- Stimulation of peripheral chemoreceptors (hypoxemia)
- Decreased lung compliance–increased ventilatory rate relationship
- Anxiety
- Increased temperature

Increased Heart Rate (Pulse) and Blood Pressure
Use of Accessory Muscles during Inspiration
Use of Accessory Muscles during Expiration
Pursed-Lip Breathing
Increased Anteroposterior Chest Diameter (Barrel Chest)
Cyanosis
Digital Clubbing
Peripheral Edema and Venous Distention
Because polycythemia and cor pulmonale are associated with severe cystic fibrosis, the following may be seen:
- Distended neck veins
- Pitting edema
- Enlarged and tender liver

Cough, Sputum Production, and Hemoptysis
Chest Assessment Findings
- Decreased or increased tactile and vocal fremitus
- Hyperresonant percussion note
- Diminished breath sounds
- Diminished heart sounds
- Bronchial breath sounds (over atelectasis)
- Crackles
- Wheezes

Spontaneous Pneumothorax
Spontaneous pneumothorax is commonly seen in patients with CF. The incidence is greater than 20% in adults with CF. When a patient with CF has a pneumothorax, there is about a 50% chance that it will recur. The respiratory therapist must be alert for the signs and symptoms of this complication (e.g., pleuritic pain, shoulder pain, sudden shortness of breath). Precipitating factors include advanced lung disease, excessive exertion, high altitude, and positive-pressure breathing (see Pneumothorax, Chapter 23)

CLINICAL DATA OBTAINED FROM LABORATORY TESTS AND SPECIAL PROCEDURES

Pulmonary Function Test Findings
Moderate to Severe Cystic Fibrosis
(Obstructive Lung Pathophysiology)*

FORCED EXPIRATORY VOLUME AND FLOW RATE FINDINGS

FVC	FEV_T	FEV_1/FVC ratio	$FEF_{25\%-75\%}$
↓	↓	↓	↓

$FEF_{50\%}$	$FEF_{200-1200}$	PEFR	MVV
↓	↓	↓	↓

LUNG VOLUME AND CAPACITY FINDINGS

V_T	IRV	ERV	RV
N or ↑	N or ↓	N or ↓	↑

VC	IC	FRC	TLC	RV/TLC ratio
↓	N or ↓	↑	N or ↑	N or ↑

Arterial Blood Gases

MILD TO MODERATE STAGES OF CYSTIC FIBROSIS
Acute Alveolar Hyperventilation with Hypoxemia[†]
(Acute Respiratory Alkalosis)

pH	$PaCO_2$	HCO_3^-	PaO_2	SaO_2 or SpO_2
↑	↓	↓ (but normal)	↓	↓

SEVERE STAGE OF CYSTIC FIBROSIS
Chronic Ventilatory Failure with Hypoxemia[†]
(Compensated Respiratory Acidosis)

pH	$PaCO_2$	HCO_3^-	PaO_2	SaO_2 or SpO_2
N	↑	↑ (significantly)	↓	↓

---

*CF is primarily an obstructive lung disorder. However, when extensive total lung obstruction (from mucous plugging) and atelectasis is present throughout the lungs, restrictive pulmonary function testing values will likely appear.
[†]See Figure 4-3 and related discussion for the acute pH, $PaCO_2$, and HCO_3^- changes associated with acute alveolar hyperventilation.
[†]See Figure 4-2 and related discussion for the pH, $PaCO_2$, and HCO_3^- changes associated with chronic ventilatory failure.

ACUTE VENTILATORY CHANGES SUPERIMPOSED ON CHRONIC VENTILATORY FAILURE‡

Because acute ventilatory changes are frequently seen in patients with chronic ventilatory failure, the respiratory therapist must be familiar with—and alert for—the following two dangerous arterial blood gas (ABG) findings:

- Acute alveolar hyperventilation superimposed on chronic ventilatory failure—which should further alert the respiratory therapist to record the following important ABG assessment: possible *impending acute ventilatory failure*
- Acute ventilatory failure (acute hypoventilation) superimposed on chronic ventilatory failure

Oxygenation Indices*
Moderate to Severe Stages

$\dot{Q}s/\dot{Q}T$	DO_2†	$\dot{V}O_2$	$C(a\text{-}\bar{v})O_2$	O_2ER	$S\bar{v}O_2$
↑	↓	N	N	↑	↓

Hemodynamic Indices§
Moderate to Severe Stages

CVP	RAP	$\overline{PA}$	PCWP	CO	SV
↑	↑	↑	N	N	N

SVI	CI	RVSWI	LVSWI	PVR	SVR
N	N	↑	N	↑	N

ABNORMAL LABORATORY TESTS AND PROCEDURES
Hematology

- Increased hematocrit and hemoglobin
- Increased white blood cell count

ELECTROLYTES

- Hypochloremia (chronic ventilatory failure)
- Increased serum bicarbonate (chronic ventilatory failure)

---

*$C(a\text{-}\bar{v})O_2$, Arterial-venous oxygen difference; DO_2, total oxygen delivery; O_2ER, oxygen extraction ratio; $\dot{Q}s/\dot{Q}T$, pulmonary shunt fraction; $S\bar{v}O_2$, mixed venous oxygen saturation; $\dot{V}O_2$, oxygen consumption.

†The DO_2 may be normal in patients who have compensated to the decreased oxygenation status with (1) an increased cardiac output, (2) an increased hemoglobin level, or (3) a combination of both. When the DO_2 is normal, the O_2ER is usually normal.

‡See TABLE 4-7 and related discussion for the pH, $PaCO_2$, and HCO_3^- changes associated with acute ventilatory changes superimposed on chronic ventilatory failure.

§*CI*, Cardiac index; *CO*, cardiac output; *CVP*, central venous pressure; *LVSWI*, left ventricular stroke work index; $\overline{PA}$, mean pulmonary artery pressure; *PCWP*, pulmonary capillary wedge pressure; *PVR*, pulmonary vascular resistance; *RAP*, right atrial pressure; *RVSWI*, right ventricular stroke work index; *SV*, stroke volume; *SVI*, stroke volume index; *SVR*, systemic vascular resistance.

SPUTUM EXAMINATION

- Increased white blood cells
- Gram-positive bacteria
  - *Staphylococcus aureus*
  - *Haemophilus influenzae*
- Gram-negative bacteria
  - *Pseudomonas aeruginosa*
  - *Stenotrophomonas maltophilia*
  - *Burkholderia cepacia complex*

RADIOLOGIC FINDINGS
Chest Radiograph

- Translucent (dark) lung fields
- Depressed or flattened diaphragms
- Right ventricular enlargement (cor pulmonale)
- Areas of atelectasis and fibrosis
- Tram-tracks
- Bronchiectasis (often a secondary complication)
- Pneumothorax (spontaneous)
- Abscess formation (occasionally)

During the late stages of CF, the alveoli become hyperinflated, which causes the residual volume and functional residual capacity to increase. Because this condition decreases the density of the lungs and therefore reduces the resistance to x-ray penetration, the chest radiograph appears darker. Tram-track opacities (also called Tram-lines) may be seen on chest x-rays. Tram-tracks are parallel, or curved opacity lines of varying length caused by bronchial wall thickening. As the patient's residual volume and functional residual capacity increase, the diaphragm moves downward and appears flattened or depressed on the radiograph (Figure 15-4).

Figure 15-5 presents four serial chest radiographs of the progression of CF over 26 years. Because right ventricular enlargement and failure often develop as secondary problems

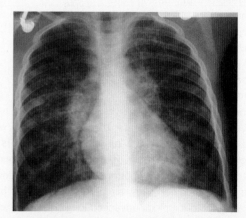

FIGURE 15-4 Chest x-ray of a patient with cystic fibrosis. Note the lung overinflation, the diffuse infiltrates, and the large main pulmonary artery segment, reflecting pulmonary hypertension.

during the advanced stages of CF, an enlarged heart may be identified on the radiograph. In some patients, areas of atelectasis, abscess formation, or a pneumothorax may be seen. Finally, computed tomography (CT) and positron emission tomography (PET) scans may be helpful when borderline radiographic findings are present.

COMMON NONRESPIRATORY CLINICAL MANIFESTATIONS

Meconium Ileus

Meconium ileus is an obstruction of the small intestine of the newborn that is caused by the impaction of thick, dry, tenacious meconium, usually at or near the ileocecal valve. This results from a deficiency in pancreatic enzymes and is the earliest manifestation of CF. The disease is suspected in newborns who demonstrate abdominal distention and fail to pass meconium within 12 hours after birth. Meconium ileus may occur in as many as 25% of infants with CF.

MECONIUM ILEUS EQUIVALENT

Meconium ileus equivalent is an intestinal obstruction (similar to meconium ileus in neonates) that occurs in older children and young adults with CF.

MALNUTRITION AND POOR BODY DEVELOPMENT

In CF, the pancreatic ducts become plugged with mucus, which leads to fibrosis of the pancreas. The pancreatic insufficiency that ensues inhibits the digestion of protein and fat. This condition leads to a deficiency of vitamins A, D, E, and K. Vitamin K deficiency may be the cause of easy bruising and bleeding. About 80% of all patients with CF have vitamin deficiencies and therefore show signs of malnutrition and poor body development throughout life.

NASAL POLYPS AND SINUSITIS

Nasal polyps are seen in between 10% and 30% of patients with CF. The polyps are usually multiple and may cause nasal obstruction; in some cases, they cause distortion of the normal facial features. Between 90% and 100% of patients with CF have sinusitis.

INFERTILITY

About 99% of men with CF are sterile. Women with CF who become pregnant may not be able to carry the infant to term. An infant who is carried to term will either have CF or be a carrier (Figure 15-2).

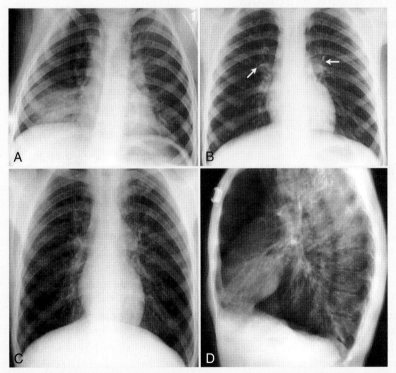

FIGURE 15-5 Cystic fibrosis. Serial chest imaging over a 26-year period showing the progressive changes of cystic fibrosis. **A,** At 3 years of age, the patient had right middle lobe pneumonia. **B,** Mild hyperinflation and bronchial wall thickening (*arrow*) present at age 7 years. **C,** At age 15 years, the patient demonstrates progressive hyperinflation, bronchiectasis, and enlargement of the hila on the chest radiograph. **D,** Lateral chest radiograph at 29 years shows typical findings of end stage cystic fibrosis. Note marked hyperinflation and "barrel chest" deformity, severe bronchiectasis, and tubular opacities consistent with mucous plugs. (From Hansell DM, Armstrong P, Lynch DA, McAdams HP: *Imaging of diseases of the chest,* ed 4, Philadelphia, 2005, Elsevier.)

General Management of Cystic Fibrosis

The management of CF entails an interdisciplinary approach. The primary goals are to prevent pulmonary infections, reduce the amount of thick bronchial secretions, improve air flow, and provide adequate nutrition. The patient and the patient's family should be instructed regarding the disease and the way it affects bodily functions. They should be taught home care therapies, the goals of these therapies, and the way to administer medications. Patients with CF commonly are best managed by a pulmonary rehabilitation team. Such teams include a respiratory therapist, a physical therapist, a respiratory nurse specialist, an occupational therapist, a dietitian, a social worker, and a psychologist. A pediatric pulmonologist, pulmonologist, or an internist trained in CF care and respiratory rehabilitation outlines and orchestrates the patient's therapeutic program.

Patients with CF should have regular medical checkups for comparative purposes to determine their general health, weight, height, pulmonary function abilities, and sputum culture results. In addition, oral time-released pancreatic enzymes, such as pancreatic lipase, are prescribed for patients with CF to aid food digestion. Patients are also encouraged to replace body salts either by heavily salting their food or by taking sodium supplements. Supplemental multivitamins and minerals are also important.

Respiratory Care Treatment Protocols

Oxygen Therapy Protocol

Oxygen therapy is used to treat hypoxemia, decrease the work of breathing, and decrease myocardial work in patients with CF with advanced pulmonary disease or during acute exacerbations. The hypoxemia may not respond well to oxygen therapy when true or capillary pulmonary shunting is present (see Oxygen Therapy Protocol, Protocol 9-1).

Bronchopulmonary Hygiene Therapy Protocol

Because of the excessive mucous production and accumulation associated with CF, a number of respiratory therapy modalities are used to enhance the mobilization of bronchial secretions. Aggressive and vigorous bronchial hygiene should be performed regularly on patients both while in the hospital and at home. Because many patients with CF require bronchial hygiene therapy at least twice a day for 20 to 30 minutes, manual chest physiotherapy and postural drainage can be overwhelming for the caretaker.

Several options for hospital or home care include use of a mechanical percussor with chest physiotherapy and postural drainage, use of a high-frequency chest compression vest, or use of intrapulmonary percussive ventilation to move thick bronchial secretions and improve compliance with prescribed care. Positive Expiratory Pressure (PEP) or Flutter-valve therapy is also effective bronchial hygiene techniques, which can also be employed with deep breathing and coughing (Figure 15-6) (see Bronchopulmonary Hygiene Therapy Protocol, Protocol 9-2).

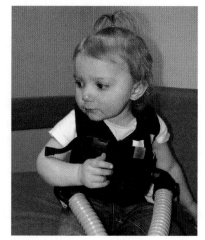

FIGURE 15-6 An 18-month-old female patient with cystic fibrosis wearing a high-frequency chest compression (HFCC) vest (the inCourage System). Today, HFCC is a commonly used bronchopulmonary hygiene treatment for airway clearance in patients with cystic fibrosis.

Lung Expansion Therapy Protocol

Lung expansion therapy may be administered to help offset the alveolar atelectasis associated with CF. Deep breathing and effective cough is key to reversing consolidation caused by mucous plugging (see Lung Expansion Therapy Protocol, Protocol 9-3).

Aerosolized Medication Protocol

A variety of bronchodilators (both beta$_2$-adrenergic agonists and anticholinergic drugs) and mucolytic agents are commonly used to induce bronchial smooth muscle relaxation and mucous thinning.

- **Bronchodilators**—Inhaled bronchodilators are routinely administered to all patients with CF, especially during the following situations:
  - Immediately before the patient receives chest physical therapy or exercise to help mobilize airway secretions.
  - Immediately before the patient receives inhalation of nebulized hypertonic saline, antibiotics, and/or DNase (dornase alpha) to offset bronchial constriction that can occur with use of these agents and to help improve the penetration and distribution of the drugs throughout the airways.

Recommended bronchodilators include beta$_2$-adrenergic agonists—such as the short-acting agent *albuterol*, or long-acting agents such as *salmeterol* or *formoterol*. The anticholinergic agent *ipratropium bromide* and the longer-acting *tiotropium* are also used to treat patients with CF.

- Mucolytic Agents
  - **Inhaled DNase (dornase alpha)** (Pulmozyme®) has been shown to be especially helpful in the management of patients with moderate to severe CF. This aerosolized agent is an enzyme that breaks down the DNA of the thick bronchial mucus associated with chronic bacterial infections with CF. Dornase alpha has shown good results in improving the lung function of patients with CF while reducing the frequency and severity of respiratory infections (Figure 15-7).

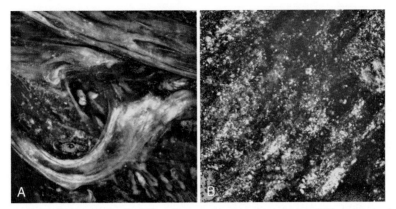

FIGURE 15-7 Illustration of the mode of action of dornase alpha in reducing DNA polymers in cystic fibrosis sputum. Confocal micrograph showing cystic fibrosis sputum stained (with YOYO-1) for DNA before (**A**) and after (**B**) treatment with dornase alpha in vitro. The long DNA polymers are degraded into short units after dornase treatment. (From Gardenhire DS: *Rau's respiratory care pharmacology*, ed 8, Philadelphia, Elsevier, 2012.)

- **Inhaled hypertonic saline** may be administered to help hydrate thick mucus in the airways of patients with CF who are 6 years of age or older, have a chronic cough, and have a reduced FEV_1. A typical treatment regimen is, first, the administration of a bronchodilator (e.g., albuterol), followed by 4 mL of a 3% to 7% saline solution, twice a day.
- **Inhaled N-acetylcysteine** has not been clinically proven to be effective in treating patients with CF. In addition, because of its potential to cause airway inflammation and/or bronchospasm and inhibit ciliary function—along with its disagreeable odor and relatively high cost—its use is not recommended. (see Aerosolized Medication Protocol, Protocol 9-4 and Appendix II).

Mechanical Ventilation Protocol

Because acute ventilatory failure superimposed on chronic ventilatory failure is occasionally seen in patients with severe CF, mechanical ventilation may be required to maintain an adequate ventilatory status. Continuous mechanical ventilation is justified when the acute ventilatory failure is thought to be reversible—for example, when pneumonia complicates the condition. Noninvasive ventilation, such as bilevel positive-pressure ventilation by facial mask, is generally preferred to intubation when feasible (see Mechanical Ventilation Protocol, Protocol 10-1 and Mechanical Ventilation Weaning Protocol, Protocol 10-2).

Other Medications and Special Procedures Prescribed by the Physician

Antibiotics

Antibiotics are commonly administered to prevent or combat chronic respiratory tract infections. Antibiotics are administered orally, via inhalation, or intravenously depending on the infecting organism and the severity of the exacerbation. For example, *azithromycin* is often recommended for patients 6 years and older who are infected with *Pseudomonas aeruginosa* and have evidence of airway inflammation, such as a chronic cough or a reduction in FEV_1. Inhaled antibiotics widely used to treat *P. aeruginosa* in CF include inhaled **tobramycin**

(TOBI)[6] and inhaled **aztreonam** (**Cayston**). Several other inhaled antibiotics are under study for the treatment of *P. aeruginosa* in CF at this time, such as amikacin, colistin, ciprofloxacin, and levofloxacin.

Unfortunately, a major drawback of long-term use of antibiotics is the development of bacteria that become resistant to antibiotic therapy. Moreover, the long-term use of antibiotics may lead to fungal infections of the mouth, oral pharynx, and tracheobronchial tree (see Appendix II, Antibiotic Agents).

Ibuprofen

High-dose *ibuprofen* is recommended in children and young adolescents with mild CF, and who have good lung function (an $FEV_1 > 60\%$ predicted) and no contradictions (e.g., gastrointestinal bleeding or renal impairment). Ibuprofen has been shown to reduce bronchial inflammation without hindering bacterial clearance—reducing the decline in the patient's FEV_1 per year—with no remarkable side effects except painless gastrointestinal bleeding in 1% to 2% of patients. High-dose ibuprofen is thought to work by decreasing neutrophil migration and inflammation in the lungs. The initiation of ibuprofen is not recommended after the age of 13 years.

Inhaled Corticosteroids and Systemic Glucocorticoids

In patients with CF, but without airway reactivity or allergic bronchopulmonary aspergillosis, the administration of *inhaled corticosteroids* has not shown any clear benefits and, therefore, is *not* recommended. However, inhaled corticosteroids may be beneficial in patients with CF who demonstrate airway reactivity. *Systemic glucocorticoids* are *not* recommended in children and adolescents with CF. The benefits of systemic glucocorticoids are outweighed by the adverse effects on growth retardation, glucose metabolism, development of CF-related diabetes, and cataract risks.

---

[6]To help make sure the patient with CF benefits from TOBI, it is important they take TOBI correctly. TOBI is specifically made to be inhaled using: (1) a pump called the DeVilbiss Pulmo-Aide air compressor, and (2) a breathing device called the PARI LC PLUS Reusable nebulizer.

Lung or Heart-Lung Transplantation

Several large organ transplant centers are currently performing **lung or heart-lung transplantations** in selected patients with CF whose general body condition is good. According to the Cystic Fibrosis Foundation, about 1700 lung transplants were performed in 2011 in the United States. Nearly 2800 patients with CF have received lung transplants since 1990. Over the past 5 years, between 150 and 200 patients with CF have received lung transplants each year.

The success of lung transplantation in patients with CF is as good as or better than in patients with other lung diseases (e.g., emphysema). Over 90% of patients with CF are alive 1 year after transplantation, and 80% are alive after 5 years. Transplanted lungs do not have CF, because they come from people with normal lungs. However, the patient still has CF in the trachea, sinuses, pancreas, intestines, sweat glands, and reproductive tract. The new lungs do not "get" CF, but may become infected with the "CF organisms" from the trachea. The immunosuppressive drugs required post-transplant may decrease the recipient's ability to fight infections caused by *Pseudomonas aeruginosa* and *Burkholderia cepacia complex*. Many lung transplant centers will not accept CF patients who have *B. cepacia* because of demonstrated lower survival rates.[7]

Progress and Future Treatments

Much of the current research in CF is focused on correcting the cellular defects in CF. Small molecules (medications that work when taken by mouth) that can help CF mutated cells function more normally are being studied to improve the ability to treat CF. These medications are designed to treat the underlying cellular defects in CF rather than secondary complications of CF, which have been the focus of medical therapy of CF for the past 50 years.

Correctors are drugs which help mutated CFTR reach the epithelial cell surface where the CFTR protein normally functions as a transmembrane regulator of chloride movement out of the cell and sodium transport into the cell. **Potentiators** are drugs which help mutated CFTR function more effectively at the epithelial cell surface transporting chloride out of the cell and inhibiting the movement of sodium into the cell. Correctors are often designed to work on a specific CF mutation or class of mutations (such as mutations that alter proper folding of the CFTR protein, ΔF508 is this type of mutation). Potentiators improve the function of mutated CFTR that has reached the epithelial cell surface (gating mutations, G551D is this type of mutation) and are somewhat less mutation specific.

Ivacaftor (**Kalydeco®**) is a new oral potentiator molecule that has been proven effective to improve cell function and clinical status in patients with CF with the G551D mutation. It was approved by the FDA in 2013 for patients with CF over 6 years of age with the G551D mutation. Ivacaftor is the first drug developed that targets the underlying causes of CF, the faulty CF gene G551D, and its defective CFTR protein. Ivacaftor appears to be remarkably effective for this mutation, significantly reducing sweat test values and improving lung function and weight gain. Unfortunately, the G551D mutation only occurs in 3% to 5% of all patients with CF. All patients with CF should have CFTR genotyping performed to determine if they carry the G551D mutation and could benefit from this breakthrough drug.

Ivacaftor is currently being studied to determine if it is effective in treating other CFTR gating mutations. Because very little CFTR reaches the epithelial cell surface in ΔF508 cells, a two drug approach using both a corrector and a potentiator appears necessary. Clinical trials using this two drug approach were underway in 2013 and the results of these studies are eagerly awaited by the 80% of patients with CF who have at least one ΔF508 mutation. There are also many other compounds being studied which would help correct the CFTR defect for other classes of CF mutations. The Cystic Fibrosis Foundation is committed to its mission to find a cure for all patients with CF as soon as possible. The future for patients with CF has never looked brighter.

---

[7]CF Foundation (www.cff.org).

Admitting History

A 27-year-old man has a long history of respiratory problems caused by CF. Even though his medical records are incomplete, he reported on admission that his parents told him that he had experienced several episodes of pneumonia during his early years. He is an adopted child and therefore does not know his biologic family history. His parents are actively involved in his general care, which entails the home care suggestions and therapeutic procedures presented by the pulmonary rehabilitation team. He takes supplemental multivitamins and timed-release oral pancreatic enzymes regularly, as prescribed by his doctor.

During his teens he had fewer respiratory symptoms than he has today and was able to lead a relatively normal life. During that time, he took up water-skiing and became proficient in the slalom event. He is known to most of his associates as a "wonder." Although he qualifies for disability income because of his continual shortness of breath, he is able to do various small jobs, which always relate to water-skiing. He is well known throughout the water-skiing circuit as an excellent chief judge at national and regional tournaments. In addition, he is a certified driver for jump-trick and slalom events and recently has become involved in selling water-ski tournament ropes and handles, which provides him with a small additional income.

Over the past 3 years, his cough has become more persistent and increasingly productive, with about a cupful of sputum noted daily. Over the same period, he has noted becoming short of breath when climbing stairs. Even though the man has a normal appetite, he has lost a great deal of weight over the past 2 years. On admission, he reported a history of severe shortness of breath. He denied experiencing any recent changes in bowel habits, despite his weight loss, but said that he has noticed a tendency to pass rather pale stools. Much to the chagrin of his doctor, 3 years ago he began smoking about 10 cigarettes a day, his reason being that the cigarettes "help him cough up the sputum."

Physical Examination

On examination the patient appeared pale, cyanotic, and thin. He had a barrel chest and was using his accessory muscles of respiration. Clubbing of the fingers was present. He demonstrated a frequent, productive cough. His sputum was sweet-smelling, thick, and yellow-green. His neck veins were distended, and he showed mild-to-moderate peripheral edema. He stated that he had not been this short of breath in a long time.

He had a blood pressure of 142/90, a heart rate of 108 beats/min, and a respiratory rate of 28 breaths/min. He was afebrile. Palpation of the chest was unremarkable. Expiration was prolonged. Hyperresonant notes were elicited bilaterally during percussion. Auscultation revealed diminished breath sounds and heart sounds. Coarse crackles were heard throughout both lung fields. During his last medical checkup (about 10 months before this admission) a pulmonary function test (PFT) had been conducted. Results revealed moderate-to-severe airway obstruction. No blood gases were analyzed.

His chest x-ray examination on this admission revealed hyperlucent lung fields, depressed hemidiaphragms, and mild cardiac enlargement (Figure 15-8). His hemoglobin level was 18 g%. His ABGs on 1.5 L/min oxygen by nasal cannula were as follows: pH 7.51, $PaCO_2$ 58 mm Hg, HCO_3^- 43 mEq/L, PaO_2 66 mm Hg, and SaO_2 94%. On the basis of these clinical data, the following SOAP was documented:

Respiratory Assessment and Plan

S "I've not been this short of breath in a long time."

Skin: pale, cyanotic; barrel chest, and use of accessory muscles of respiration; digital clubbing; cough frequent and productive; sputum: sweet-smelling, thick, yellow-green; distended neck veins and peripheral edema; vital signs: BP 142/90, HR 108, RR 28, T° normal; bilateral hyperresonant percussion notes; diminished breath sounds; coarse crackles; CXR: hyperlucency, flattened diaphragms, and mild cardiac enlargement; ABGs (1.5 L/min O_2 by nasal cannula): pH 7.51, $PaCO_2$ 58, HCO_3^- 43, PaO_2 66; and SaO_2 94%.

A • Respiratory distress (general appearance, vital signs)
   • Excessive tracheobronchial tree secretions (productive cough, coarse crackles)
   • Infection likely (yellow-green sputum)
   • Hyperinflated alveoli (barrel chest, use of accessory muscles, CXR)
   • Acute alveolar hyperventilation superimposed on chronic ventilatory failure with mild hypoxemia (history, ABGs)
   • Possible impending acute ventilatory failure
   • Cor pulmonale (distended neck veins, peripheral edema, CXR)

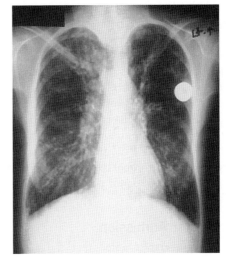

FIGURE 15-8 Chest x-ray from a 27-year-old man with cystic fibrosis.

P **Bronchopulmonary Hygiene Therapy Protocol** (cough and deep breathe Tx q4 h), sputum culture). **Oxygen Therapy Protocol** (2 L/min by nasal cannula). Monitor possible impending ventilatory failure closely (pulse oximetry, vital signs, ABGs).

48 Hours after Admission

The respiratory therapist from the Consult Service noted that the patient was still in respiratory distress. The man stated that he could not get enough air to sleep even 10 minutes. He appeared cyanotic and was using his accessory muscles of respiration. His vital signs were as follows: blood pressure 147/95, heart rate 117 beats/min, respiratory rate 32 breaths/min, and temperature 37°C (98.6°F).

He coughed frequently, and although his cough was weak, he produced large amounts of thick, green sputum. Hyperresonant notes were produced during percussion over both lung fields. On auscultation, breath sounds and heart sounds were diminished. Coarse crackles and wheezing were heard throughout both lung fields. No recent chest x-ray was available. A sputum culture obtained at admission suggested the presence of *Pseudomonas aeruginosa*. On a 2 L/min oxygen cannula, his SpO_2 was 92% and his ABGs were as follows: pH 7.55, $PaCO_2$ 54 mm Hg, HCO_3^- 45 mEq/L, PaO_2 57 mm Hg, and SaO_2 93%.

On the basis of these clinical data, the following SOAP was documented:

Respiratory Assessment and Plan

S "I can't get enough air to sleep 10 minutes!"
Cyanosis and use of accessory muscles of respiration; vital signs: BP 147/95, HR 117, RR 32, T 37°C (98.6°F); cough: frequent, weak, and productive of large amounts of thick, green sputum; *Pseudomonas aeruginosa* cultured; bilateral hyperresonant notes and diminished breath sounds; coarse crackles and wheezes; On a 2 L/min oxygen cannula, SpO_2 92%; ABGs: pH 7.55, $PaCO_2$ 54, HCO_3^- 45, PaO_2 57, SaO_2 93%.

A • Continued respiratory distress (general appearance, vital signs, use of accessory muscles)
 • Excessive bronchial secretions (cough, sputum, coarse crackles)
 • Poor ability to mobilize secretions (weak cough)
 • Acute alveolar hyperventilation superimposed on chronic ventilatory failure with mild-to-moderate hypoxemia (ABGs)
 • Possible impending ventilatory failure

P Start **Aerosolized Medication Protocol** (0.5 mL albuterol in 2 mL NS, followed by 2 mL DNase q4 h). Up-regulate **Bronchopulmonary Hygiene Therapy** per protocol (CPT and PEP therapy q2 h). Up-regulate **Oxygen Therapy Protocol** (venturi oxygen mask at FIO_2 0.35). Continue to monitor possible impending ventilatory failure closely.

64 Hours after Admission

The respiratory therapist noted that the patient was in obvious respiratory distress. The patient said he could not find a position that allowed him to breathe comfortably. He appeared cyanotic, was using pursed-lip breathing, and using his accessory muscles of respiration. His vital signs were as follows: blood pressure 145/90, heart rate 120 beats/min, respiratory rate 22 breaths/min, and oral temperature 38°C (100.5°F). Chest palpation was normal, but bilateral hyperresonant percussion notes were elicited. Auscultation revealed coarse crackles and wheezing bilaterally. No recent chest radiograph was available. ABGs on an FIO_2 of 0.4 venturi mask, were as follows: pH 7.27, $PaCO_2$ 83 mm Hg, HCO_3^- 36 mEq/L, PaO_2 37 mm Hg, and SaO_2 73%.

On the basis of these clinical data, the following SOAP was entered in the patient's chart:

Respiratory Assessment and Plan

S "I can't get into a comfortable position to breathe."
Cyanosis; pursed-lip breathing and use of accessory muscles of respiration; vital signs: BP 145/90, HR 120, RR 22, T 38°C (100.5°F); bilateral hyperresonant percussion notes, coarse crackles, and wheezing; ABGs on FIO_2 of 0.4: pH 7.27, $PaCO_2$ 83, HCO_3^- 36, PaO_2 37, SaO_2 73%.

A • Continued respiratory distress (general appearance, vital signs, use of accessory muscles, pursed-lip breathing)
 • Acute ventilatory failure superimposed on chronic ventilatory failure with severe hypoxemia (ABGs, vital signs)
 • Lactic acidosis likely
 • Excessive bronchial secretions (cough, sputum, breath sounds)

P Contact physician stat. Consider noninvasive **Mechanical Ventilation Protocol**. Continue **Aerosolized Medication and Bronchial Hygiene Therapy Protocol** (after patient has been placed on ventilator). Up-regulate **Oxygen Therapy Protocol** (initially, FIO_2 0.50 and reevaluate when patient is placed on ventilator). Monitor closely.

Discussion

The science of respiratory care has advanced over the years, and the prognosis for patients with this multisystem genetic disorder has improved. In this patient's lifetime, the following therapeutic landmarks can be noted:

1. Vigorous use of chest physical therapy (percussion and postural drainage), including percussion aids
2. The proven benefits of new drugs, such as DNase (Pulmozyme®) and ivacaftor (Kalydeco®)
3. Positive expiratory pressure (PEP) therapy
4. Lung transplantation (when all else fails)

This patient had received at least three of these treatments and was in the hands of caring parents. His own stubborn nature and interest in athletics were clearly helpful in his prolonged survival. Important to note are the circumstances surrounding his admission, especially the fact that he had experienced hemoptysis, dyspnea, and weight loss during the several years preceding his admission. Note also that he had started smoking cigarettes.

In this case study, the patient's chief complaints purposely have been buried in the admitting history. The reader should have discerned that the patient was coughing productively and had dyspnea, and weight loss. The recommended therapeutic strategy arises from recognition of these four presenting complaints. Note also that on admission the patient had neck vein distention and peripheral edema, suggesting cor pulmonale. If the experience with chronic obstructive pulmonary disease can be extrapolated to patients with CF, this is a bad prognostic sign and one that clearly calls for intensification of the therapeutic regimen, probably from the time of the first assessment and treatment plan selection.

Note that on the initial physical examination, the patient demonstrated **excessive bronchial secretions** and a productive cough; no baseline ABGs existed with which to compare his current values (see **Bronchospasm**, Figure 9-10). Thus, the observation of an elevated $PaCO_2$ should initially be taken very, very seriously.

At the time of the second evaluation the patient clearly was not improving. The up-regulation of **Bronchopulmonary Hygiene Therapy** (see Protocol 9-2) and addition of the **Aerosolized Medication Protocol** at this point was appropriate (the increased chest physical therapy, along with PEP therapy, q2 h, and Pulmozyme® therapy). A repeat chest x-ray study would not be out of order at this time. At that time, more might have been made of the enlargement of pulmonary artery seen in Figure 15-8. One could argue that

the Aerosolized Medication Protocol and more aggressive bronchopulmonary hygiene should have been started earlier, including the use of mucolytics.

The third assessment clearly suggests that the patient was deteriorating despite vigorous noninvasive therapy. At this point, the patient was placed on an FIO_2 of 0.5, and the stat call to the physician regarding the acute ventilatory failure was appropriate. The addition of mechanical ventilation at this time would prevent fatigue, allow deep tracheal suctioning, and facilitate repeat therapeutic bronchoscopy if it were to become necessary.

After this initial downhill course, the patient was placed on a ventilator and slowly improved. Over the next 7 days, he was weaned from noninvasive mechanical ventilation. The therapist should note that despite all the "good" things the patient and family did to treat his illness, the patient's initiation of smoking clearly could be a "last-straw" phenomenon. The patient should be placed on a smoking-cessation program. His outpatient program should have been reevaluated, and more closely monitored, and possibly up-regulated as to modality selection and frequency. These steps are as important for the long-term prognosis as is the skill of the practitioner caring for him during this episode of acute ventilatory failure.

SELF-ASSESSMENT QUESTIONS

Answers to questions can be found on Evolve. To access additional student assessment questions visit **http://evolve.elsevier.com/DesJardins/respiratory**.

1. Which of the following organisms is or are commonly found in the tracheobronchial tree secretions of patients with cystic fibrosis?
   1. Staphylococcus
   2. Haemophilus influenzae
   3. Streptococcus
   4. Pseudomonas aeruginosa
      a. 1 only
      b. 2 only
      c. 1 and 4 only
      d. 1, 2, and 4 only

2. When two carriers of cystic fibrosis produce children, there is a:
   1. 75% chance that the baby will be a carrier
   2. 25% chance that the baby will be completely normal
   3. 50% chance that the baby will have cystic fibrosis
   4. 25% chance that the baby will have cystic fibrosis
      a. 1 only
      b. 3 only
      c. 2 and 4 only
      d. 1 and 2 only

3. The cystic fibrosis gene is located on which chromosome?
   a. 5
   b. 6
   c. 7
   d. 8

4. In cystic fibrosis the patient commonly demonstrates which of the following?
   1. Increased FEV_T
   2. Decreased MVV
   3. Increased RV
   4. Decreased FEV_1/FVC ratio
      a. 1 only
      b. 3 only
      c. 3 and 4 only
      d. 2, 3, and 4 only

5. During the advanced stages of cystic fibrosis, the patient generally demonstrates which of the following?
   1. Bronchial breath sounds
   2. Dull percussion notes
   3. Diminished breath sounds
   4. Hyperresonant percussion notes
      a. 1 and 3 only
      b. 2 and 4 only
      c. 1 and 4 only
      d. 1, 3, and 4 only

6. About 80% of all patients with cystic fibrosis demonstrate a deficiency in which of the following vitamins?
   1. A
   2. B
   3. D
   4. E
   5. K
      a. 3 and 4 only
      b. 1, 4, and 5 only
      c. 2, 3, and 4 only
      d. 1, 3, 4, and 5 only

7. Which of the following agents targets the underlying cause of cystic fibrosis, the faulty gene G551D, and its defective CFTR protein?
   a. Aztreonam
   b. Ivacafor
   c. Inhaled DNase
   d. N-acetylcysteine

8. Which of the following is or are mucolytic agents?
   1. DNase
   2. Pulmozyme
   3. Tobramycin
   4. Dornase alpha
      a. 1 only
      b. 2 only
      c. 3 and 4 only
      d. 1, 2, and 4 only

9. With regard to the secretion of sodium and chloride, the sweat glands of patients with cystic fibrosis secrete up to:
   a. 2 times the normal amount
   b. 4 times the normal amount
   c. 7 times the normal amount
   d. 10 times the normal amount

10. Which of the following clinical manifestations are associated with severe cystic fibrosis?
   1. Decreased hemoglobin concentration
   2. Increased central venous pressure
   3. Decreased breath sounds
   4. Increased pulmonary vascular resistance
      a. 1 and 3 only
      b. 2 and 3 only
      c. 3 and 4 only
      d. 2, 3, and 4 only

CHAPTER

16 Pneumonia

Chapter Objectives

After reading this chapter, you will be able to:
- List the anatomic alterations of the lungs associated with pneumonia.
- Describe the causes and classifications of pneumonia.
- List the cardiopulmonary clinical manifestations associated with pneumonia.
- Describe the general management of pneumonia.
- Describe the clinical strategies and rationales of the SOAPs presented in the case study.

Key Terms

Acquired Pneumonia Classifications
Adenovirus
Anaerobic Organisms
Aspiration
Aspiration Pneumonia
Aspiration Pneumonitis
Atypical Organisms
Avian Influenza A
Bacteroides asaccharolyticus
Bacteroides melaninogenicus
Chlamydia pneumoniae
Chlamydia psittaci
Community-Acquired Pneumonia (CAP)
Consolidated
Coronavirus
Croup
Cytomegalovirus
"Double Pneumonia"
Dysarthria
Dysphagia
Dysphonia
Enterobacter species
Escherichia coli
Fungal Infections
Fusobacterium necrophorum
Gastroesophageal Reflux Disease (GERD)
Gram-Negative Organisms
Gram-Positive Organisms
Haemophilus influenzae
Hospital-Acquired Pneumonia
Influenza Virus
Klebsiella
Legionella pneumophila

Lipoid Pneumonitis
Lobar Pneumonia
Mendelson's Syndrome
Moraxella catarrhalis
Multiple Drug–Resistant *Staphylococcus aureus* (MDRSA)
Mycoplasma pneumoniae
Nursing Home–Acquired Pneumonia
Parainfluenza Viruses
Peptostreptococcus Species
Pneumocystis carinii
Porphyromonas endodontalis
Porphyromonas gingivalis
Pseudomonas aeruginosa
Respiratory Syncytial Virus (RSV)
Rickettsial Infections
Rubella
Serratia Species
Severe Acute Respiratory Syndrome (SARS)
Silent Aspiration
Staphylococcus
Streptococcus
Swallowing Mechanics
Tuberculosis
Varicella
Ventilator-Associated Pneumonia
Walking Pneumonia

Chapter Outline

Anatomic Alterations of the Lungs
Etiology and Epidemiology
Community-Acquired Pneumonia
Community-Acquired Atypical Pneumonia
   Hospital-Acquired Pneumonia
   (Nosocomial Pneumonia)
Aspiration Pneumonia
Chronic Pneumonia
Necrotizing Pneumonia and Lung Abscess
Pneumonia in the Immunocompromised Host
Overview of Cardiopulmonary Clinical Manifestations
   Associated with Pneumonia
General Management of Pneumonia
   Respiratory Care Treatment Protocols
Case Study: Pneumonia
Self-Assessment Questions

Anatomic Alterations of the Lungs

Pneumonia[1], or pneumonitis with consolidation, is the result of an inflammatory process that primarily affects the gas exchange area of the lung. In response to the inflammation, fluid (serum) and some red blood cells (RBCs) from adjacent pulmonary capillaries pour into the alveoli. This process of fluid transfer is called *effusion*. Polymorphonuclear leukocytes move into the infected area to engulf and kill invading bacteria on the alveolar walls. This process has been termed *surface phagocytosis*. Increased numbers of macrophages also appear in the infected area to remove cellular and bacterial debris. If the infection is overwhelming, the alveoli become filled with fluid, RBCs, polymorphonuclear leukocytes, and macrophages. When this occurs, the lungs are said to be **consolidated** (Figure 16-1). Figure 16-2 provides a microscopic view of bacterial pneumonia. Atelectasis is often associated with patients who have **aspiration pneumonia.**

The major pathologic or structural changes associated with pneumonia are as follows:
- Inflammation of the alveoli
- Alveolar consolidation
- Atelectasis (e.g., aspiration pneumonia)

---

[1]As of this writing, pneumonia is one of several conditions in which readmission to the hospital for any cause will result in possible significant financial penalties to the hospital for patients on Medicare (for more on this, see Chapter 12). Accordingly, careful evaluation of all such patients, particularly the elderly, should be made for comorbid conditions—especially those with chronic heart and lung disease, swallowing difficulties, and problems with cognition.

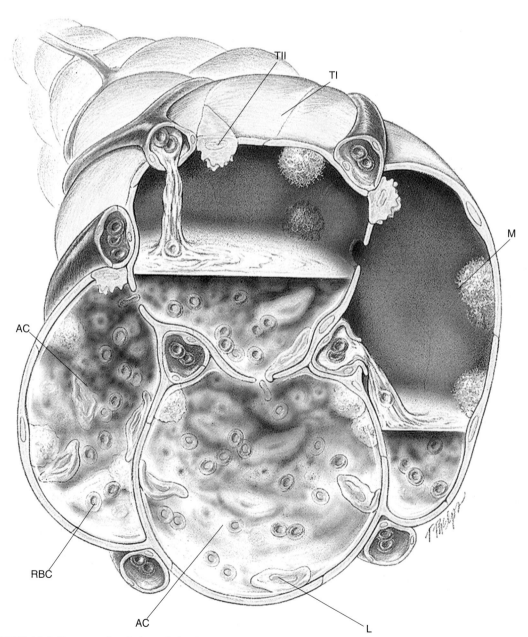

FIGURE 16-1 Cross-sectional view of alveolar consolidation in pneumonia. *AC,* Alveolar consolidation; *L,* leukocyte; *M,* macrophage; *RBC,* red blood cell; *TI,* type I cell.

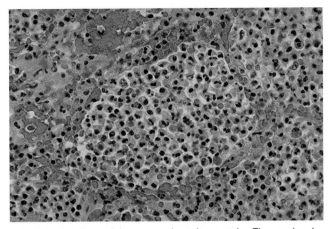

FIGURE 16-2 Bacterial pneumonia, microscopic. These alveolar exudates are mainly composed of neutrophils. The surrounding alveolar walls have capillaries that are congested (dilated and filled with red blood cells). Such an exudative process is typical of bacterial infection. This exudate gives rise to the productive cough of purulent yellow sputum seen with bacterial pneumonias. The alveolar structure is still maintained, which is why even an extensive pneumonia often resolves with minimal residual destruction or damage to the pulmonary parenchyma. In patients with compromised lung function from underlying obstructive or restrictive lung disease or cardiac disease, however, even limited pneumonic consolidation can be life threatening. (From Klatt E: *Robbins and Cotran atlas of pathology*, ed 2, Philadelphia, 2009, Saunders.)

Etiology and Epidemiology

Pneumonia and influenza combined are the eighth leading cause of death among Americans and the sixth leading cause of death over the age of 65 years. It is estimated that about 50,000 Americans die of pneumonia each year. Pneumonia and influenza are especially life threatening in individuals whose lungs are already damaged by chronic obstructive pulmonary disease (COPD), asthma, or smoking. The risk of death from pneumonia or influenza is also higher among people with heart disease, diabetes, or a weakened immune system.

Causes of pneumonia include bacteria, viruses, fungi, protozoa, parasites, tuberculosis, anaerobic organisms, aspiration, and the inhalation of irritating chemicals such as chlorine. Pneumonia is an insidious disease because its symptoms vary greatly, depending on the patient's specific underlying condition and the type of organism causing the pneumonia. Pneumonia often mimics a common cold or the flu (e.g., the signs and symptoms develop quickly). For example, the patient may suddenly experience chills, shivering, high fever, sweating, chest pain (pleurisy), and a dry and nonproductive cough. Often what initially appears to be a cold or the flu, however, can in fact be a much more serious pulmonary infection. The early recognition and treatment of pneumonia provide the best chance for a full recovery.

The terms **bronchopneumonia**, **lobar pneumonia**, or **interstitial pneumonia** often refer to the anatomic location of the inflammation (Figure 16-3). *Bronchopneumonia* is characterized by a patchy pattern of infection that is limited to the segmental bronchi and surrounding lung parenchyma. Bronchopneumonia usually involves both lungs and is seen

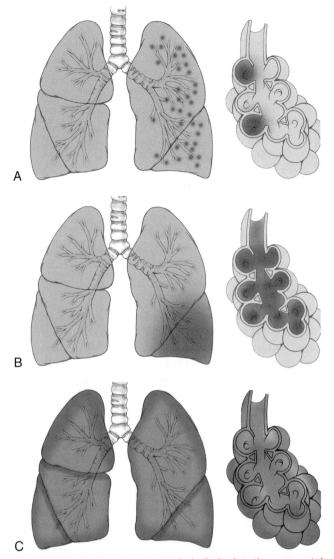

FIGURE 16-3 A, Bronchopneumonia is limited to the segmental bronchi and surrounding lung parenchyma. **B,** Lobar pneumonia is a widespread or diffuse alveolar inflammation and consolidation. Lobar pneumonia is often the end result of severe bronchopneumonia in which the infection spreads from one lung segment to another until the entire lung lobe is involved. **C,** Interstitial pneumonia is usually diffuse and is commonly associated with infections with *Mycoplasma pneumonia* or viruses.

more often in the lower lobes of the lung. *Lobar pneumonia* is a widespread or diffuse alveolar inflammation and consolidation. Lobar pneumonia is typically the end result of a severe or long-term bronchopneumonia in which the infection has spread from one lung segment to another until the entire lung lobe is involved. *Interstitial pneumonia* is usually a diffuse and often bilateral inflammation that primarily involves the alveolar septa and interstitial space. In contrast to alveolar pneumonia caused by bacteria, the polymorphonuclear leukocytes do not migrate into the alveoli—they remain in the alveolar interstitial spaces. *Mycoplasma pneumonia* and other viruses cause interstitial pneumonias. Fortunately, most interstitial pneumonias cause only minor permanent alveolar damage and usually resolve without consequences.

When both lungs are involved, the condition is sometimes called **double pneumonia** by laypersons. Although the lay term "**walking pneumonia**" has no clinical significance, it is often used to describe a mild case of pneumonia. For example, patients infected with *Mycoplasma pneumoniae*, who generally have mild symptoms and remain ambulatory, are sometimes told that they have "walking pneumonia." Box 16-1 provides common risk factors for pneumonia. Because the distinction between lobar pneumonia and bronchopneumonia can often be hazy, it is generally best to classify pneumonias either by the specific etiologic agent or, when no specific pathogen can be identified, by the clinical setting in which the pneumonia occurs; for example, hospital-acquired pneumonia or community-acquired pneumonia (CAP). Box 16-2 provides an overview of seven different clinical settings, and the respective pathogens, associated with pneumonia. The importance of promptly obtaining a sample of sputum for a Gram stain and culture analysis early in the course of the clinical illness cannot be overemphasized. A more in-depth discussion of these pathogens is presented in the following sections.[2]

Community-Acquired Pneumonia

Community-acquired pneumonia (CAP) refers to a pneumonia acquired from normal social contact (i.e., in the community) as opposed to being acquired while in hospitals or

---

[2]It is important to note that the infective causes of pneumonia described in this chapter include all those grouped by the Centers of Medicare and Medicaid Services (CMS), in its Specifications Manual for National Inpatient Quality Measures Discharges (2013-2014). Pneumonia is one of three conditions that CMS is monitoring for excessive readmissions as an indicator of inappropriate, resource-wasteful care. At present, the other two conditions are COPD and congestive heart failure (CHF). The penalties for excessive all-cause readmissions of patients with these conditions will increase to 3% of the hospital's yearly total Medicare/Medicaid income for the year in question, by 2014. Accordingly, all caregivers must practice meticulous, evidence-based respiratory care if hospitals are to survive economically. Particularly crucial will be the care of the Transitional Care Specialist, briefly discussed in Chapter 12.

(Modified from Damjanov I: *Pathology for the health professions*, ed 4, St Louis, 2012, Elsevier/Saunders.)

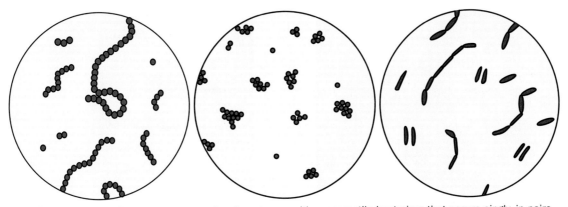

FIGURE 16-4 A, The *Streptococcus* organism is a gram-positive, nonmotile bacterium that occurs singly, in pairs, and in short chains. **B,** The *Staphylococcus* organism is a gram-positive, nonmotile coccus that is found singly, in pairs, and in irregular clusters. **C,** Bacilli are rod-shaped microorganisms and are the major gram-negative organisms responsible for pneumonia.

extended-care facilities (e.g., nursing homes). Common causes of a CAP are discussed as follows:

Streptococcal pneumonia. *Streptococcus pneumoniae* (commonly called pneumococcal pneumonia) accounts for more than 80% of all the bacterial pneumonias (Figure 16-4, *A*). The organism is a gram-positive, nonmotile coccus that is found singly, in pairs (called *diplococci*), and in short chains. The cocci are enclosed in a smooth, thick polysaccharide capsule that is essential for virulence. There are more than 80 different types of *S. pneumoniae*. Serotype 3 organisms are the most virulent. Streptococci are generally transmitted by aerosol from a cough or sneeze of an infected individual. Most strains of *S. pneumoniae* are sensitive to penicillin and its derivatives. *S. pneumoniae* is also commonly cultured from the sputum of patients having an acute exacerbation of chronic bronchitis.

Staphylococcal pneumonia. There are two major groups of **Staphylococcus:** (1) *Staphylococcus aureus,* which is responsible for most "staph" infections in humans, and (2) *Staphylococcus albus* and *Staphylococcus epidermidis,* which are part of the normal skin flora. The staphylococci are gram-positive cocci found singly, in pairs (called *diplococci*), and in irregular clusters (Figure 16-4, *B*). Staphylococcal pneumonia often follows a predisposing virus infection and is seen most often in children and immunosuppressed adults. *S. aureus* is commonly transmitted by aerosol from a cough or sneeze of an infected individual and indirectly via contact with contaminated floors, bedding, clothes, and the like. Staphylococci are a common cause of **hospital-acquired pneumonia or nosocomial pneumonia** (discussed later in this chapter) and are becoming increasingly antibiotic resistant—thus the term **multiple drug–resistant S. aureus (MDRSA)** organisms (some centers shorten this acronym to *MRSA*).

Haemophilus influenzae. *Haemophilus influenzae* is a common inhabitant of human pharyngeal flora. *H. influenzae* is one of the smallest gram-negative bacilli, measuring about 1.5 mm in length and 0.3 mm in width (Figure 16-4, *C*). It appears as coccobacilli on Gram stain. There are six types of *H. influenzae,* designated A to F, but only type B is commonly pathogenic. Pneumonia caused by *H. influenzae* type B is seen most often in children aged 1 month to 6 years old. *H. influenzae* type B is almost always the cause of acute

epiglottitis. The organism is transmitted via aerosol or contact with contaminated objects. It is sensitive to cold and does not survive long after expectoration. *H. influenzae* is commonly cultured from the sputum of patients having an acute exacerbation of chronic bronchitis. Additional risk factors for *H. influenzae* infection include COPD, defects in B-cell function, functional and anatomic asplenia, and human immunodeficiency virus (HIV) infection.

Legionella pneumophila. In July 1976, a severe pneumonia-like disease outbreak occurred at an American Legion convention in Philadelphia. The causative agent eluded identification for many months, despite the concerted efforts of the nation's top epidemiologic experts. When the organism finally was recovered from a patient, it was found to be an unusual and fastidious gram-negative bacillus with atypical concentrations of certain branched-chain lipids. The initial isolate was designated as *Legionella pneumophila.* More than 20 *Legionella* species have now been identified.

Most of the species are free-living in soil and water, where they act as decomposer organisms. The organism also multiplies in standing water such as contaminated mud puddles, large air-conditioning systems, and water tanks. The organism is transmitted when it becomes airborne and enters the patient's lungs as an aerosol. No convincing evidence suggests that the organism is transmitted from person to person. The organism can be detected in pleural fluid, sputum, or lung tissue by direct fluorescent antibody microscopy. Although it is rarely found outside the lungs, the organism may be found in other tissues. The disease is most commonly seen in middle-aged men who smoke.

Enterobacteriaceae (*Klebsiella pneumonia*) (Friedländer's Bacillus). *K. pneumoniae* organisms have long been associated with lobar pneumonia, particularly in men older than 40 years and in chronic alcoholics of both genders. *Klebsiella* is a gram-negative bacillus that is found singly, in pairs, and in chains of varying lengths. It is a normal inhabitant of the human gastrointestinal tract. The organism can be transmitted directly by aerosol or indirectly by contact with freshly contaminated articles. *K. pneumoniae* is a common nosocomial, or hospital-acquired, disease. It is typically transmitted by routes such as clothing, intravenous solutions, foods, and the hands of health-care workers. The mortality of patients

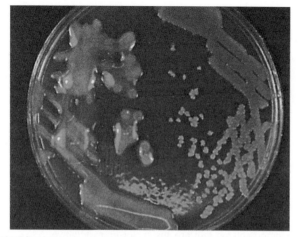

FIGURE 16-5 *Pseudomonas aeruginosa* isolated from the sputum of patients with cystic fibrosis characteristically grows in a very mucoid colonial form (*left*), with the normal colonial form (*right*) for comparison. (From Goering R, Dockrell H, Zuckerman M, Roitt I, Chiodini P: *Mims' medical microbiology*, ed 4, Philadelphia, 2012, Saunders.)

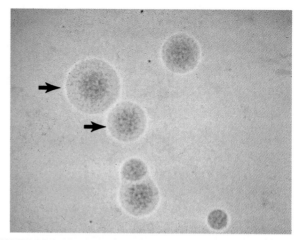

FIGURE 16-6 *Mycoplasma pneumoniae. Mycoplasma pneumoniae* is a small bacterium that lacks a cell wall. (From VanMeter K, Hubert R, VanMeter W: *Microbiology for the healthcare professional*, St Louis, 2010, Mosby.)

with *K. pneumoniae* is very high because septicemia is a frequent complication.

Pseudomonas aeruginosa is a highly mobile, gram-negative bacillus. It is often found in the gastrointestinal tract, burns, and catheterized urinary tract and is a contaminant in many aqueous solutions. *P. aeruginosa* is frequently cultured from the respiratory tract of patients who are chronically ill and tracheostomized, and is a leading cause of **hospital-acquired pneumonia** (see page 257). This makes *P. aeruginosa* a particular problem for the respiratory therapist. Risk factors include neutropenia, HIV infection, preexisting lung disease, endotracheal intubation, and previous antibiotic use. Because the *Pseudomonas* organism thrives in dampness, it is often cultured from contaminated respiratory therapy equipment. The organism is commonly transmitted by aerosol or by direct contact with freshly contaminated articles. *P. aeruginosa* grows in a very mucoid colonial form and the sputum from patients with *Pseudomonas* infection is frequently green and sweet smelling (Figure 16-5).

Community-Acquired Atypical Pneumonia

The clinical presentation of the patient with community-acquired atypical pneumonia is often subacute. The patient typically presents with a variety of both pulmonary and extrapulmonary findings (e.g., respiratory symptoms such as cough *plus* headache, general fatigue, or diarrhea). Common causes of community-acquired atypical pneumonia are discussed as follows:

The **mycoplasma** organism is the most common cause of an acquired atypical pneumonia. The mycoplasma are tiny, cell wall–deficient organisms (Figure 16-6). They are smaller than bacteria but larger than viruses. The pneumonia caused by the mycoplasmal organism is commonly described as a *primary atypical pneumonia.* The term *atypical* refers to the fact that (1) the organism escapes identification by standard

bacteriologic tests, (2) there is generally only a moderate amount of sputum, (3) there is an absence of alveolar consolidation, (4) there is only a moderate elevation of white cell count, and (5) there is a lack of alveolar exudate.

The mycoplasma organism causes symptoms similar to both bacterial and viral pneumonia, although the symptoms develop more gradually and are often milder. Chills and fever are early symptoms. The patient typically presents with a mild fever, and patchy inflammatory changes in the lungs that are mostly confined to the alveolar septa and pulmonary interstitium. A common symptom of mycoplasma pneumonia is a cough that tends to come in violent attacks, producing only a small amount of white mucus. Some patients experience nausea or vomiting. In some cases, the patients may experience a profound weakness that lasts for a long time. *Mycoplasma pneumonia* is commonly seen among children and young adults. This type of pneumonia spreads easily in areas where people congregate, such as child-care centers, schools, and homeless shelters. Patients with *M. pneumoniae* often are said to have "**walking pneumonia**" because the condition is mild (i.e., slight fever, fatigue, and a characteristic dry, hacking cough) and the patient is usually ambulatory.

Chlamydia **spp.** *pneumonia* (*Chlamydia pneumonia, Chlamydia psittaci, Chlamydia trachomatis*) and ***Coxiella burnetii*** (Q fever) closely resemble the clinical manifestations of those caused by *M. pneumoniae.* Chlamydia is a type of bacteria that may be found in the cervix, urethra, rectum, throat, and respiratory tract. Chlamydia is also found in the feces of a variety of birds (e.g., parrots, parakeets, lorikeets, cockatoos, chickens, pigeons, ducks, pheasants, turkeys). The clinical manifestations of *C. psittaci* closely resemble those caused by *M. pneumoniae.*

Viruses account for about 50% of all pneumonias, and several are associated with a community-acquired atypical pneumonia. Although most viruses attack the upper airways, some can produce pneumonia. Most of these pneumonias are not life threatening and last only a short time. Viral pneumonia tends to start with flulike signs and symptoms. The early symptoms are a dry (nonproductive) cough, headache, fever, muscle pain, and fatigue. As the disease progresses, the patient may become short of breath, cough, and produce a small amount of clear or white sputum. *Viral pneumonia always carries the risk of development of a secondary bacterial pneumonia.*

Viruses are minute organisms not visible by ordinary light microscopy. They are parasitic and depend on nutrients inside cells for their metabolic and reproductive needs. About 90% of acute upper respiratory tract infections are caused by viruses. Respiratory viruses are the most common cause of pneumonia in young children, peaking between the ages of 2 and 3 years. By school age, *M. pneumoniae* become more prevalent (see previous section).

Common viruses associated with community-acquired atypical pneumonia include *respiratory syncytial virus, parainfluenza virus* (children); *influenza A and B* (adults); *adenovirus* (military recruits), and *human metapneumovirus*. These viruses are discussed in more detail as follows.

The **respiratory syncytial virus (RSV)** (see Chapter 37) is a member of the paramyxovirus group. Parainfluenza, mumps, and **rubella** viruses also belong to this group. RSV is most often seen in children less than 12 months of age and in older adults with underlying heart or pulmonary disease. Almost all children will be infected with RSV by their second birthday. The infection is rarely fatal in infants. RSV often goes unrecognized but may play an important role as a forerunner to bacterial infections. Early attempts to develop an RSV vaccine have been unsuccessful. The virus is transmitted by aerosol and by direct contact with infected individuals. RSV infections are most commonly seen in patients during the late fall, winter, or early spring months. Many times the virus is misdiagnosed in older children, who are given antibiotics that do not produce improvement.

The **parainfluenza viruses** are also members of the paramyxovirus group and therefore are related to mumps, rubella, and RSV. There are five types of parainfluenza viruses: types 1, 2, 3, 4A, and 4B. Types 1, 2, and 3 are the major causes of infections in humans. Type 1 is considered a **croup** type of virus. Types 2 and 3 are associated with severe infections. Although type 3 is seen in persons of all ages, it usually is seen in infants younger than 2 months of age; types 1 and 2 are seen most often in children between the ages of 6 months and 5 years. Types 1 and 2 typically occur in the fall, whereas type 3 infection most often is seen in the late spring and summer. Parainfluenza viruses are transmitted by aerosol droplets and by direct person-to-person contact. The parainfluenza viruses are known for their ability to spread rapidly among members of the same family.

The **influenza viruses A and B** are the most common causes of viral respiratory tract infections. In the United States, influenza A and B commonly occur in epidemics during the winter months. Children, young adults, and older individuals are most at risk. Influenza is transmitted from person to person by aerosol droplets. Often the first sign of an epidemic is an increase in school absenteeism. The virus survives well in conditions of low temperatures and low humidity. It also has been found in horses, swine, and birds. Influenza viruses have an incubation period of 1 to 3 days and usually cause upper respiratory tract infections. Epidemiologists fear a pandemic of influenza, stating it is an issue of "when" and "where" rather than "if." The recent epidemic of H1N1 ("swine flu") is a case in point.

The **adenovirus** serotypes 4, 7, 14, and 21 cause viral infections and pneumonia in all age groups. Serotype 7 has been related to fatal cases of pneumonia in children. Adenoviruses are transmitted by aerosol. Pneumonia caused by adenoviruses generally occurs during the fall, winter, and spring.

The **human metapneumovirus (hMPV)** is a negative single-stranded RNA virus associated with a family of viruses that also includes respiratory syncytial (RSV) virus and parainfluenza virus. After the respiratory RSV, hMPV is the second most common cause of lower respiratory infections in young children. In comparison to RSV, the hMPV tends to occur in older children and is less severe. Most patients with hMPV infection have mild symptoms including cough, runny nose or nasal congestion, sore throat, and fever. More severe cases demonstrate wheezing, difficulty breathing, hoarseness, cough, and pneumonia.

Hospital-Acquired Pneumonia

Hospital-acquired pneumonia (also called *nosocomial pneumonia*) is an infection whose development is caused by the hospital environment. Common causes of hospital-acquired pneumonias include **Enterobacteriaceae** (*Klebsiella* spp., *Serratia marcescens, Escherichia coli*), **Pseudomonas spp.**, and **Staphylococcus aureus** (usually methicillin-resistant) (see descriptions of these pathogens above).

Ventilator-acquired pneumonia (VAP) (also called *ventilator-associated pneumonia*) can also be included under the nosocomial pneumonia category. A ventilator-acquired pneumonia is defined as a pneumonia that develops more than 48 to 72 hours after endotracheal intubation. Common ventilator-associated infections include *P. aeruginosa, Enterobacter, Klebsiella,* and *S. aureus* (see descriptions of these pathogens above). Concern that the occurrence of VAP is preventable lies as the root of possible reimbursement penalties for hospitals in which it occurs.

Aspiration Pneumonia

Common pathogenic agents associated with *aspiration pneumonia* include anaerobic oral flora (*Bacteroides, Prevotella, Fusobacterium, Peptostreptococcus*), admixed with aerobic bacteria such as *S. pneumonia, S. aureus, H. influenza,* and *P. aeruginosa.*

Aspiration of gastric fluid with a pH of 2.5 or less causes a serious and often fatal form of pneumonia. Aspiration of oropharyngeal secretions and gastric fluids are the major causes of anaerobic lung infections (see discussion of anaerobic bacterial infections earlier). **Aspiration pneumonitis** is commonly missed because acute inflammatory reactions may not begin until several hours after aspiration of the gastric fluid. The inflammatory reaction generally increases in severity for 12 to 26 hours and may progress to acute respiratory distress syndrome (ARDS), which includes interstitial and intraalveolar edema, intraalveolar hyaline membrane formation, and atelectasis. In the absence of a secondary bacterial infection, the inflammation usually becomes clinically insignificant in approximately 72 hours. In 1946, Mendelson first described the clinical manifestations of tachycardia, dyspnea, and cyanosis associated with the aspiration of acid stomach contents. The clinical picture he described is now known as **Mendelson's syndrome** and is usually confined to aspiration pneumonitis in pregnant women.

Aspiration pneumonia is broadly defined as the pulmonary result of the entry of material from the stomach or upper respiratory tract into the lower airways. There are at least three distinctive forms of aspiration pneumonia, classified according to the nature of the aspirate, the clinical presentation, and management guidelines, as follows:

1. Toxic injury to the lung (such as that caused by gastric acid)
2. Obstruction (by foreign body or fluids)
3. Infection

Aspiration is the presumed cause of nearly all cases of anaerobic pulmonary infections. Studies suggest that anaerobic bacteria are the most common causative agents of lung abscesses; they are also commonly isolated in cases of empyema.

There is a difference between the aspiration of gastric contents and the aspiration of food. Aspiration of gastric contents causes initial hypoxemia regardless of the pH level of the aspirate. Consequently, oximetry is a good measurement if aspiration is suspected. If the pH of the aspirate is relatively high (greater than 5.9), the initial injury is rapidly reversible. Such aspiration occurs in patients who receive antacids or proton pump inhibitors (PPIs). If the pH is low (pH of unbuffered gastric contents normally ranges from 1 to 1.5), parenchymal damage may occur, with inflammation, edema, and hemorrhage. When food is aspirated, obliterative bronchiolitis with subsequent granuloma formation occurs.

Gastroesophageal reflux disease (GERD) is the regurgitation of stomach contents into the esophagus. GERD causes disruption in nerve-mediated reflexes in the distal esophagus, resulting in alteration of the primary and secondary peristaltic wave and reflux. Therefore "to-and-fro" peristalsis can result from spasticity at the distal esophageal sphincter and retropulsion of middle and upper esophageal contents. This may result in aspiration, although not necessarily.

GERD is three times more prevalent in patients with asthma than in other patients. In other words, GERD is a frequently unrecognized cause of asthma. Presumably, acid reflux into the esophagus causes vagal stimulation, resulting in a reflexive increase in bronchial tone in patients with asthma. Recent literature suggests that asymptomatic reflux does not contribute to worsening lung function, although it and chronic sinusitis are the two most unrecognized causes of chronic cough. GERD causes chronic cough in 10% to 20% of patients.

Normal **swallowing mechanics** has four phases, as follows:

1. Oral preparatory
2. Oral
3. Pharyngeal
4. Esophageal

The first two phases are considered voluntary stages (cerebral). These phases occur as the food or liquid is prepared for entry to the pharynx and esophagus. The airway is open while food is prepared in the oral cavity. Adequate tongue function is important for the manipulation and propulsion of the prepared food or liquid (called a *bolus*) into the pharynx. Spillage of liquid into the pharynx during the chewing of food is usually not a problem in patients with good airway protection.

The pharyngeal phase (involuntary brain stem function) of swallowing involves numerous physiologic actions that direct the bolus into the esophagus:

- Elevation and retraction of the velopharyngeal port (velum closure)
- Pharyngeal muscle contraction
- Elevation and forward excursion of the larynx (epiglottic closure)
- Closure of the laryngeal vestibule, false vocal folds, and true vocal folds (laryngeal closure)
- Relaxation of the upper esophageal sphincter (UES)

Airway closure progresses inferiorly to superiorly in the larynx as the food bolus is directed laterally around the airway and into the esophagus.

Respiration is halted during the pharyngeal phase for an approximately 1-second apneic period, although duration varies with bolus volume and viscosity. Bolus transit in the esophageal phase (under both brain stem and intrinsic neural control) lasts 8 to 20 seconds. In this phase, the UES relaxes to receive the bolus with a peristaltic wave from the pharyngeal superior constrictor muscles, forcing the bolus through the relaxed UES. The primary peristalsis propels the bolus through the esophagus and lower esophageal sphincter and into the stomach.

Six cranial nerves carry motor signals generated by cerebral and brain stem swallowing centers:

- V (trigeminal)
- VII (facial)
- IX (glossopharyngeal)
- X (vagus)
- XI (spinal accessory [minor involvement])
- XII (hypoglossal)

The relationship between respiration and swallowing is not random. Expiration before and after the pharyngeal phase in normal swallowing is believed to serve as an inherent closure and clearance mechanism against penetration of food or liquids into the airway entrance.

Dysphagia is the result of an abnormal swallow that can involve the oral, pharyngeal, and esophageal phases. Penetration into the laryngeal vestibule occurs when food or liquid (or both) enters the larynx but does not pass through the vocal cords into the trachea. Aspiration is the passage of food or liquid into the trachea via the vocal cords.

Diagnostic tests for dysphagia include the modified barium swallow (MBS), video-fluoroscopy, video-fiberoptic endoscopy, and the modified Evan's blue dye tests. The Evan's blue dye test involves instilling a deep blue dye into the gastrointestinal tract and seeing if it can be suctioned from the trachea. If it can, it suggests a communication between the two structures, such as a fistula. The MBS and video-fluoroscopy tests are most definitive for identification of the particular phase of the swallow that is dysfunctional. The modified Evan's blue dye test can be unreliable (as much as 40% of the time) as a test suggesting aspiration in a patient who is tracheostomized. Both false-positive and false-negative test results occur.

A compromised respiratory system can cause dysphagia and, conversely, dysphagia may cause respiratory complications. COPD can result in a slowed oral and pharyngeal transit time, reduced coordination and strength of the oral and pharyngeal musculature, and reduced airway clearance by coughing.

Treatment of dysphagia is specific to the nature of the disorder. Varied methods of presentation of foods and liquids, bolus volumes and consistency, postural movements, and food temperature can affect the dynamics of the relation between respiration and swallowing. Large volumes of liquid requiring uninterrupted swallowing result in longer apneic periods and can be difficult for patients with shortness of breath and dyspnea. Small-volume bites and swallows make sense in this setting.

Unilateral cerebrovascular accidents (strokes) and hemorrhage tend to cause hypopharyngeal hemiparesis. Difficulty in swallowing (with impairment of the oral phase) and aspiration of thin fluids therefore may follow. The facial and tongue weakness can result in poor bolus control in the oral cavity.

Silent aspiration is defined as aspiration that does not evoke clinically observable adverse symptoms such as overt coughing, choking, and immediate respiratory distress. Some patients have silent aspiration after a stroke. Evidence also suggests that some sequelae of stroke include laryngopharyngeal sensory deficits with no subjective or objective evidence of dysphagia, such as choking, gagging, or cough.

Some patients with severe and bilateral sensory deficits develop aspiration pneumonia. The clinical findings of **dysphonia**, **dysarthria**, abnormal gag reflex, abnormal volitional cough, cough after swallow, and voice change after swallow all significantly relate to aspiration and are predictors of silent aspiration. Conversely, a normal reflex cough after a stroke indicates an intact laryngeal cough reflex, a protected airway, and low risk for developing aspiration pneumonia with oral feeding. The cough reflex is significantly reduced in older patients.

Patients with a tracheostomy are at high risk for silent aspiration. Perhaps 55% to 70% of intubated or tracheostomy patients aspirate. A tracheostomy tube has a direct effect on the pharyngeal phase of a swallow because of the alteration of normal respiratory function (exhalation timing) as well as the anatomic alteration and the physical resistance imposed by the tracheostomy tube itself. Normal laryngeal elevation is reduced, particularly with the cuff inflated, which leads to inadequate airway closure and increased pharyngeal residue.

Poor sensory response to material entering the larynx contributes to the slowing of an uncoordinated laryngeal closure. The protective cough may be lessened because of the impaired laryngeal sensation. Subglottic air pressure (coordinated exhalation with swallow) helps prevent entry of material into the trachea and is reduced in patients with a tracheostomy. An inflated cuffed tracheostomy can cause complications that can anchor the larynx to the anterior wall of the neck and desensitize the pharynx. Delayed triggering of the swallowing response and increased pharyngeal residue are prevalent.

Recommendations for oral feeding include considerations of dietary consistency, specifically defined for solids and liquids; skilled supervision with oral intake; safe swallowing strategies; positioning requirements; cuff deflation; and tracheal occlusion issues. It may be necessary to coordinate mealtime with ventilator weaning attempts to optimize more positive pressure generation to aid in expelling laryngeal residue and creating subglottic pressure.

The dynamic changes a patient may experience clinically necessitate a coordinated team approach, including physical, occupational, and respiratory therapists; a speech-language pathologist; registered dietitian; and nurse. This approach allows for effective management of tracheostomy and nontracheostomy patients and avoidance of aspiration.

Chronic Pneumonia

Chronic pneumonia is typically a localized lesion in patients with a normal immune system, with or without regional lymph node involvement. Patients with chronic pneumonia usually have granulomatous inflammation, which is often due to bacteria (e.g., *M. tuberculosis*) or fungi. In patients whose immune system is compromised (e.g., patients with HIV), the dissemination of the causative organism throughout the body is the usual presentation. Tuberculosis is by far the most important organism within the category of chronic pneumonias. The World Health Organization (WHO) estimates that tuberculosis causes 6% of all deaths worldwide, *making it the most common cause of death resulting from a single infectious agent.*

Chronic pneumonias associated with **granulomas** include tuberculosis and fungal diseases of the lung. Tuberculosis (see Chapter 18) is an infectious disease caused by *Mycobacterium tuberculosis*. *M. tuberculosis* is a slender, rod-shaped aerobic organism. Predisposing factors of tuberculosis include homelessness, drug abuse, and acquired immunodeficiency syndrome (AIDS). The initial response of the lung is an inflammatory reaction that is similar to any acute pneumonia.

Because most fungi are aerobes, the lung is a prime site for fungal infections (see Chapter 19). Primary fungal pathogens include *Histoplasma capsulatum*, *Coccidioides immitis*, and *Blastomyces dermatitidis*.

In addition, the opportunistic yeast pathogens *Candida albicans*, *Cryptococcus neoformans*, and *Aspergillus* may also cause pneumonia in certain patients. For example, *C. albicans*, which occurs as normal flora in the oral cavity, genitalia, and large intestine, is rarely seen in the tracheobronchial tree or lung parenchyma. In patients with AIDS, however, *C. albicans* commonly causes an infection of the mouth, pharynx, esophagus, vagina, skin, and lungs. A *C. albicans* infection of the mouth is called *thrush*; it is characterized by a white, adherent, patchy infection of the membranes of the mouth, gums, cheeks, and throat.

C. neoformans proliferates in pigeon droppings, which have a high nitrogen content, and readily scatters into the air and dust. Today, the highest rate of cryptococcosis occurs among patients with AIDS and persons undergoing steroid therapy. The molds of the genus *Aspergillus* may be the most pervasive of all fungi—especially *Aspergillus fumigatus*. *Aspergillus* is found in soil, vegetation, leaf detritus, food, and compost heaps. Persons who breathe the air of granaries, barns, and silos are at the greatest risk. *Aspergillus* infection usually occurs in the lungs. *Aspergillus* is almost always an opportunistic infection and lately has posed a serious threat to patients with AIDS. When fungal organisms are inhaled, the initial response of the lung is an inflammatory reaction similar to that produced by any acute pneumonia (see Chapter 19).

Nocardia are gram-positive, rod-shaped bacteria that can be found worldwide in soils that are rich with organic matter. It has a total of 85 species. Nocardia is also found in healthy gingiva and periodontal pockets. Most *Nocardia* infections occur as an opportunistic infection in patients with weak immune systems, such as small children, the elderly, and the immunocompromised (most common in patients with HIV).

Actinomyces species are normally present in the gingival area and are common opportunistic pathogens of humans, particularly in the oral cavity (e.g., infections associated with dental procedures and oral abscesses). In rare cases, these bacteria can cause *actinomycosis*, a disease characterized by the formation of abscesses in the mouth, lungs, or the gastrointestinal tract.

Necrotizing Pneumonia and Lung Abscess

Necrotizing pneumonia and lung abscess refers to localized pus formation and necrosis within the pulmonary parenchyma, resulting in one or more large cavities (discussed in detail in Chapter 17, Lung Abscess). Necrotizing pneumonia often coexists with a lung abscess, making the distinction between the two difficult. Common causative pathogens include (1) anaerobic organisms, which entered the lungs via aspiration of infective material (e.g., carious teeth, discharge from infected sinuses or tonsils); (2) aspiration of gastric contents (usually mixed with infectious pathogens from the oropharynx); (3) complications of necrotizing bacterial pneumonia (e.g., *S. aureus*, *Streptococcus pyogenes*, *K. pneumonia*, *Pseudomonas* spp., and rarely, type 3 pneumococci); (4) bronchial obstruction (e.g., bronchogenic carcinoma obstruction, which can lead to the aspiration of blood and tumor fragments); (5) septic embolism (e.g., septic thrombophlebitis or infective endocarditis of the right side of the heart); and (6) anaerobic bacteria (e.g., species of *Prevotella*, *Fusobacterium*, *Bacteroides*, *Peptostreptococcus*, and microaerophilic streptococci). See Chapter 17, Lung Abscess.

Pneumonia in the Immunocompromised Host

Cytomegalovirus (CMV), a member of the herpesvirus family, is the most common viral pulmonary complication of AIDS. CMV infection commonly coexists with *Pneumocystis carinii* infection.

Pneumocystis jirovecii (also known as *Pneumocystis carinii*) is an opportunistic, often fatal, form of pneumonia seen in patients who are profoundly immunosuppressed. Although the *Pneumocystis* organism has been identified as a protozoan, recent information suggests that it is more closely related to fungi. *Pneumocystis* can normally be found in the lungs of humans, but it does not cause disease in healthy hosts, only in individuals whose immune systems are critically impaired. Currently, *Pneumocystis pneumonia* is the major pulmonary infection seen in patients with AIDS and HIV infection.

In vulnerable hosts the disease spreads rapidly throughout the lungs. Before AIDS, *P. carinii* pneumonia was seen primarily in patients with malignancy, in organ transplant recipients, and in patients with diseases requiring treatment with large doses of immunosuppressive agents. Today, most cases of *P. carinii* pneumonia are seen in patients with AIDS. The early clinical manifestations of *Pneumocystis* in patients with AIDS are indistinguishable from those of any other pneumonia. Typical signs and symptoms include progressive exertional dyspnea, a dry cough that may or may not produce mucoid sputum, difficulty in taking a deep breath (not caused by pleurisy), and fever with or without sweats. The therapist may hear normal breath sounds on auscultation or end-inspiratory crackles. The chest x-ray film may be normal at first; later it will show bilateral interstitial infiltrates, which may progress to alveolar filling and "white out" of the chest x-ray film.

Mycobacterium avium **complex (MAC)** is a serious opportunistic infection that is caused by the following two similar bacteria: *Mycobacterium avium* and *Mycobacterium intercellulare*. MAC is found in the soil and dust particles. MAC is commonly found in patients with AIDS. The mode of infection is usually inhalation or ingestion. MAC can spread through the bloodstream to infect lymph nodes, bone marrow, the liver, the spleen, spinal fluid, the lungs, and the intestinal tract. Typical symptoms of MAC include fever, night sweats, weight loss, fatigue, anemia, diarrhea, and enlarged spleen.

Invasive Aspergillosis is a general term used for a wide variety of infections caused by the fungi of the genus *Aspergillus*. The most common forms are allergic bronchopulmonary aspergillosis, pulmonary aspergilloma, and invasive aspergillosis. Most humans inhale *Aspergillus* spores every day. However, in individuals who are immunocompromised, an aspergillosis pneumonia often develops.

Invasive Candidiasis is a general term describing fungal infections caused by a variety of species of the genus *Candida*, most often by *Candida albicans*, a yeastlike fungus. These fungi are normally found in the mouth, vagina, and intestines of healthy individuals. Under normal circumstances, the normal bacteria in these areas keep the amount of *Candida* species in balance. However, in patients with a weakened immune system (such as people with HIV/AIDS), the fungi can invade tissue that normally would be resistant to infection—thus, producing an opportunistic infection. *Candida* infections can involve any part of the body. In some cases, the fungus enters the bloodstream and causes invasive disease affecting internal body organs such as the kidneys, spleen, lungs, liver, eyes, meninges, brain, and heart valves.

Other Causes
Rickettsiae

Rickettsiae are small, pleomorphic coccobacilli. Most rickettsiae are intracellular parasites possessing both ribonucleic acid (RNA) and deoxyribonucleic acid (DNA). There are several pathogenic members of the *Rickettsia* family: *Rickettsia rickettsii* (Rocky Mountain spotted fever), *Rickettsia akari* (rickettsialpox), *Rickettsia prowazekii* (typhus), and *Rickettsia burnetii*, also called *Coxiella burnetii* (Q fever).

All species of the genus *Rickettsia* are unstable outside of cells except for *R. burnetii* (Q fever), which is extremely resistant to heat and light. Q fever can cause pneumonia as well as a prolonged febrile illness, an influenza-like illness, and endocarditis. The organism is commonly transmitted by arthropods (lice, fleas, ticks, mites). It may also be transmitted by cattle, sheep, and goats and possibly in raw milk.

Varicella (Chickenpox)

The **varicella** virus usually causes a benign disease in children aged 2 to 8 years, and complications of varicella are not common. In some cases, however, varicella has been noted to spread to the lungs and cause a serious secondary pneumonitis. The mortality rate of varicella pneumonia is about 20%.

Rubella (Measles)

Measles virus spreads from person to person by the respiratory route. Respiratory complications are often encountered in measles because of the widespread involvement of the mucosa of the respiratory tract (e.g., excessive bronchial secretions and infection).

Severe Acute Respiratory Syndrome

In 2002, China reported the first case of **severe acute respiratory syndrome (SARS)**. Shortly after this report, the disease was documented in numerous countries, including Vietnam, Singapore, and Indonesia. Both the United States and Canada have reported imported cases. Health officials believe that the cause of SARS is a newly recognized virus strain called a **coronavirus.** Other viruses, however, are still under investigation as potential causes. Coronaviruses are a group of viruses that have a halolike or corona-like appearance when observed under an electron microscope. Known forms of coronavirus cause common colds and upper respiratory tract infections. SARS is highly contagious on close personal contact with infected individuals. It spreads through droplet transmission by coughing and sneezing. SARS might be transmitted through the air or from objects that have become contaminated.

The incubation period for SARS is typically 2 to 7 days. Initially, the patient usually develops a fever (>100.4 °F or >38.0 °C), followed by chills, headaches, general feeling of discomfort, and body aches. Toward the end of the incubation period, the patient with SARS usually develops a dry, nonproductive cough, shortness of breath, and malaise. In severe causes hypoxemia develops. According to the Centers for Disease Control and Prevention (CDC), 10% to 20% of patients with SARS require mechanical ventilation. In spite of this fact, death from SARS is rare. No specific treatment recommendations exist at this time. The CDC, however, recommends that patients with SARS receive the same treatment used for any patient with serious community-acquired atypical pneumonia of unknown cause.

Lipoid Pneumonitis

The aspiration of mineral oil, used medically as a lubricant, has also been known to cause pneumonitis–**lipoid pneumonitis.** The severity of the pneumonia depends on the type of oil aspirated. Oils from animal fats cause the most serious reaction, whereas oils of vegetable origin are relatively inert. When mineral oil is inhaled in an aerosolized form, an intense pulmonary tissue reaction occurs.

Avian Influenza A

Avian influenza A (also called *bird flu* and *H5N1*) is a subtype of the A strain virus and is highly contagious in birds. Historically, bird flu has not been known to infect humans. However, in Hong Kong in 1997 the first avian influenza virus to infect humans directly was reported. This outbreak was linked to chickens and classified as avian influenza A (H5N1). Since the Hong Kong outbreak, the bird flu virus has been reported in parts of Europe, Turkey, Romania, the Near East, and Africa. Many of the infected people have died. Experts are concerned that if the avian flu virus continues to spread, a worldwide pandemic outbreak could occur. People with bird flu may develop life-threatening complications, such as viral pneumonia and ARDS (the most common cause of bird flu–related deaths).

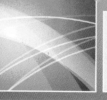

OVERVIEW of the Cardiopulmonary Clinical Manifestations Associated with Pneumonia

The following clinical manifestations result from the pathologic mechanisms caused (or activated) by Alveolar Consolidation (see Figure 9-8), Increased Alveolar-Capillary Membrane Thickness (see Figure 9-9), and Atelectasis (see Figure 9-7)—the major anatomic alterations of the lungs associated with pneumonia (Figure 16-1).

During the resolution stage of pneumonia, Excessive Bronchial Secretions (see Figure 9-11) may also play a part in the clinical presentation.

CLINICAL DATA OBTAINED AT THE PATIENT'S BEDSIDE

The Physical Examination

Vital Signs

Increased Respiratory Rate (Tachypnea)

Several pathophysiologic mechanisms operating simultaneously may lead to an increased ventilatory rate:

- Stimulation of peripheral chemoreceptors (hypoxemia)
- Decreased lung compliance–increased ventilatory rate relationship
- Stimulation of J receptors
- Pain, anxiety, fever

Increased temperature (bacteria >101° F and viral <101° F)

Increased Heart Rate (Pulse) and Blood Pressure

Chest Pain (Pleuritic) and Decreased Chest Expansion

Cyanosis

Cough, Sputum Production, and Hemoptysis

Initially the patient with pneumonia usually has a nonproductive barking or hacking cough. As the disease progresses, however, the cough becomes productive. When the disease progresses to this point, the patient often expectorates small amounts of purulent, blood-streaked, or rusty sputum. This is caused by fluid moving from the pulmonary capillaries into the alveoli in response to the inflammatory process. As fluid crosses into the alveoli, some RBCs may also move into the alveoli and produce the blood-streaked or rusty appearance of the fluid (Figure 16-1). Some of the fluid that moves in the alveoli may also work its way into the bronchioles and bronchi. As the fluid accumulates in the bronchial tree, the subepithelial receptors in the trachea, bronchi, and bronchioles are stimulated and initiate a cough reflex. Because the bronchioles and the smaller bronchi are deep in the lung parenchyma, the patient with pneumonia initially has a dry, hacking cough, and fluid cannot be easily expectorated until secretions reach the larger bronchi.

Chest Assessment Findings

- Increased tactile and vocal fremitus
- Dull percussion note
- Bronchial breath sounds
- Crackles
- Pleural friction rub (if process extends to pleural surface)
- Whispered pectoriloquy

CLINICAL DATA OBTAINED FROM LABORATORY TESTS AND SPECIAL PROCEDURES

Pulmonary Function Test Findings (Restrictive Lung Pathophysiology)*

FORCED EXPIRATORY VOLUME AND FLOW RATE FINDINGS[†]

FVC	FEV_T	FEV_1/FVC ratio	$FEF_{25\%-75\%}$
↓	N or ↓	N or ↑	N or ↓

$FEF_{50\%}$	$FEF_{200-1200}$	PEFR	MVV
N or ↓	N or ↓	N or ↓	N or ↓

LUNG VOLUME AND CAPACITY FINDINGS

V_T	IRV	ERV	RV	
N or ↓	↓	↓	↓	

VC	IC	FRC	TLC	RV/TLC ratio
↓	↓	↓	↓	N

Arterial Blood Gases

MILD TO MODERATE STAGES

Acute Alveolar Hyperventilation with Hypoxemia[†]
(Acute Respiratory Alkalosis)

pH	$PaCO_2$	HCO_3^-	PaO_2	SaO_2 or SpO_2
↑	↓	↓ (but normal)	↓	↓

SEVERE STAGE

Acute Ventilatory Failure with Hypoxemia[§]
(Acute Respiratory Acidosis)

pH[‖]	$PaCO_2$	HCO_3^- [‖]	PaO_2	SaO_2 or SpO_2
↓	↑	↑ (but normal)	↓	↓

---

*The pulmonary function tests (PFTs) here are for a typical case of interstitial or alveolar-filling pneumonia, not complicated with excessive airway secretions, bronchospasm, etc.

[†]The decreased forced expiratory volumes and flow rate findings are primarily caused by the low vital capacity associated with the disorder.

[†]See Figure 4-3 and related discussion for the acute pH, $PaCO_2$, and HCO_3^- changes associated with acute alveolar hyperventilation.

[§]See Figure 4-2 and related discussion for the acute pH, $PaCO_2$, and HCO_3^- changes associated with acute ventilatory failure.

[‖]When tissue hypoxia is severe enough to produce lactic acid, the pH and HCO_3^- values will be lower than expected for a particular $PaCO_2$ level.

Oxygenation Indices[¶]

$\dot{Q}_S/\dot{Q}_T$	DO_2[#]	$\dot{V}O_2$[**]	$C(a\text{-}\bar{v})O_2$[**]	O_2ER	$S\bar{v}O_2$
↑	↓	N	N	↑	↓

[¶]$C(a\text{-}\bar{v})O_2$, Arterial-venous oxygen difference; DO_2, total oxygen delivery; O_2ER, oxygen extraction ratio; $\dot{Q}_S/\dot{Q}_T$, pulmonary shunt fraction; $S\bar{v}O_2$, mixed venous oxygen saturation; $S\bar{v}O_2$, oxygen consumption.

[#]The DO_2 may be normal in patients who have compensated to the decreased oxygenation status with (1) an increased cardiac output, (2) an increased hemoglobin level, or (3) a combination of both. When the DO_2 is normal, the O_2ER is usually normal.

[**]May be increased in the patient with a fever caused bacterial pneumonia.

ABNORMAL LABORATORY TEST AND PROCEDURE RESULTS

Sputum examination findings (see discussion of etiology in this chapter, Box 16-1)

RADIOLOGIC FINDINGS

Chest Radiograph

- Increased density (from consolidation and atelectasis)
- Air bronchograms
- Pleural effusions

The radiographic signs vary considerably depending on the causative agent and the stage of the pneumonia process. In general, pneumonia (alveolar consolidation) appears as an area of increased density that may involve a small lung segment, a lobe, or one or both lungs (Figures 16-3 and 16-7). The process may appear patchy or uniform throughout the area. As the alveolar consolidation intensifies, alveolar density increases and air bronchograms may be seen (Figure 16-8). A pleural effusion may be identified on the chest radiograph (see Chapter 24).

COMPUTED TOMOGRAPHY SCAN

Alveolar consolidation and air bronchograms can also be seen on the computed tomography (CT) scan (Figure 16-9).

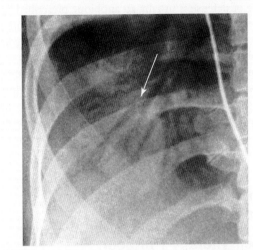

FIGURE 16-8 Air bronchogram (shown in chest radiograph). The branching linear lucencies within the consolidation in the right lower lobe are particularly well demonstrated in this example of staphylococcal pneumonia. (From Hansell DM, Armstrong P, Lynch DA, McAdams HP, eds: *Imaging of diseases of the chest*, ed 4, Philadelphia, 2005, Elsevier.)

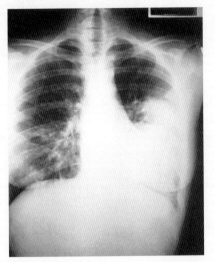

FIGURE 16-7 Chest radiograph of a 20-year-old woman with severe pneumonia of the left lung and patchy pneumonia in the right middle and lower lobes.

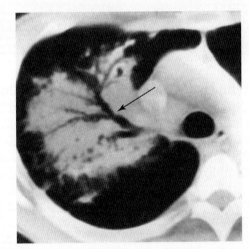

FIGURE 16-9 Air bronchograms shown by computed tomography in a patient with pneumonia. (From Hansell DM, Armstrong P, Lynch DA, McAdams HP, eds: *Imaging of diseases of the chest*, ed 4, Philadelphia, 2005, Elsevier.)

General Management of Pneumonia

The treatment of pneumonia is based on (1) the specific cause of the pneumonia, and (2) the severity of symptoms demonstrated by the patient. For bacterial pneumonia, the first line of defense is usually an antibiotic prescribed by the attending physician (see Appendix III, Antibiotics). Although there are a few viral pneumonias that may be treated with antiviral medications, the recommended treatment is usually the same as for the flu—bed rest and plenty of fluids. In addition, over-the-counter medications are often helpful to reduce fever, treat aches and pains, and depress the dry cough associated with pneumonia. In severe pneumonia, hospitalization may be required. The following is an overview of the treatments used for pneumonia.

Respiratory Care Treatment Protocols

Oxygen Therapy Protocol

Oxygen therapy is used to treat hypoxemia, decrease the work of breathing, and decrease myocardial work. Because of the hypoxemia associated with pneumonia, supplemental oxygen may be required. The hypoxemia that develops in pneumonia is most commonly caused by alveolar consolidation and capillary shunting associated with the disorder. Hypoxemia caused by capillary shunting is at least partially refractory to oxygen therapy (see Oxygen Therapy Protocol, Protocol 9-1).

Lung Expansion Therapy Protocol

Lung expansion therapy may be administered to attempt to offset the atelectasis associated with some pneumonias, but its effects are not consistently good (see Lung Expansion Therapy Protocol, Protocol 9-3).

Thoracentesis

Diagnostic and therapeutically, thoracentesis may be used if a pleural effusion is present (see Chapter 24). From a diagnostic standpoint, fluid samples may be examined for the following:

- Color
- Odor
- RBC count
- Protein
- Glucose
- Lactic dehydrogenase (LDH)
- Amylase
- pH
- Wright's, Gram, and acid-fast bacillus (AFB) stains
- Aerobic, anaerobic, tuberculosis, and fungal cultures
- Cytology

Therapeutic thoracentesis may be used to encourage lung reexpansion when atelectasis is part of the clinical presentation.

CASE STUDY Pneumonia

Admitting History and Physical Examination

A 47-year-old man was deer hunting in northern Michigan with some friends. They spent considerable time outdoors in inclement weather and indulged freely in alcoholic beverages during the afternoons and evenings. Previously the man had been essentially healthy. He smoked one pack of cigarettes a day.

Returning home, he felt listless and thought that he was "coming down with a cold." That night, he noticed a mild, nonproductive cough. He had a headache and some pain in the right side of his chest on deep inspiration and noticed that he was somewhat short of breath when he climbed one flight of stairs. During the night, he woke up and felt very chilled, then very warm. His wife put her hand on his forehead and was certain that he had a "high fever." Because he felt miserable, they went to the emergency room of the nearest hospital.

On physical examination, his vital signs were as follows: blood pressure 150/88, pulse 116 beats/min, respiratory rate 28 beats/min, and temperature (oral) 39.9 °C. He was in moderate distress. Percussion of the chest revealed dullness on the right lower side, and on inspiration there were fine crackles heard in that area. The breath sounds were described as "bronchial." The chest radiograph showed pneumonic consolidation of the right lower lung field. On room air, his arterial blood gas (ABG) values were pH 7.53, $PaCO_2$ 27 mm Hg, HCO_3^- 21 mEq/L, PaO_2 62 mm Hg and SaO_2 93%.

The respiratory therapist assigned to assess and treat the patient charted the following SOAP note.

Respiratory Assessment and Plan

S "I feel miserable." Mild dyspnea.

O Alert, cooperative, acutely ill. Mild nonproductive cough. Vital signs: T 39.9 °C, BP 150/88, P 116, RR 28. Dull to percussion over RLL, along with crackles and bronchial breath sounds. CXR: Pneumonic consolidation RLL. ABG on room air: pH 7.53, $PaCO_2$ 27, HCO_3^- 21, PaO_2 62 and SaO_2 93%.

A • RLL consolidation (pneumonia presumed)
   • Acute alveolar hyperventilation with mild hypoxemia (ABG)

P **Oxygen Therapy Protocol:** Monitor SpO_2. (Titrate O_2 per NC as needed to keep SpO_2 >90%.)

The patient was started on oxygen (2 L/min) via a nasal cannula. The physician prescribed intravenous antibiotic therapy.

Over the next 72 hours, the patient steadily improved, although he felt nauseated and vomited three times. On the fourth hospital day, however, the patient complained of increased shortness of breath. He started to cough up large amounts (3 to 4 tablespoons every 2 hours) of foul-smelling, greenish-yellow sputum. He also complained of choking on his secretions, a bitter taste in his mouth, belching (aspiration likely), mild substernal discomfort, and chills.

On physical examination, the patient appeared anxious. His vital signs were blood pressure 120/82, pulse 140 bpm, respiratory rate 20 beats/min, and oral temperature 40 °C. His sputum was thick, yellow-green, and foul smelling. His cough was strong. He had bronchial breath sounds and coarse, nonclearing, crackles over the right mid-portion of the anterior chest and over both lower lobes posteriorly. There was mild cyanosis of the nail beds. The abdominal examination was unremarkable. There was no peripheral edema. A chest x-ray examination showed new infiltrates in the right middle lung field and left lower lobe. The opaque infiltrate obstructed the view of the heart and was described by the radiologist as consolidation. On 2 L/min O_2 nasal cannula, his ABGs were as follows: pH 7.50, $PaCO_2$ 29 mm Hg, HCO_3^- 21 mEq/L, PaO_2 36 mm Hg, and SaO_2 81%.

At this time the respiratory therapist charted the following SOAP progress note.

Respiratory Assessment and Plan

S Increased dyspnea. Symptoms of belching and substernal chest pain.

O Anxious appearance. BP 120/82, HR 140, RR 20, T 40 °C. Cyanotic. Strong productive cough (foul-smelling, yellow-green sputum). Bronchial breath sounds, coarse crackles, persistent crackles in right middle anterior chest and both bases. CXR: RML and LLL infiltrate and consolidation. ABG (on 2 L/min): pH 7.50, $PaCO_2$ 29, HCO_3^- 21, PaO_2 36, and SaO_2 81%.

A • Aspiration complicating community-acquired pneumonia, involving RML and LLL (history, CXR)
   • Alveolar consolidation (CXR)
   • Excessive airway secretions (thick, yellow-green sputum)
   • Good ability to mobilize secretions (strong cough)
   • Acute alveolar hyperventilation with severe hypoxemia (ABG)

P **Oxygen Therapy Protocol:** Increase FIO_2 to 0.60 via HAFOE mask. **Bronchopulmonary Hygiene**

Protocol: DB&C instruction, prn oropharyngeal suctioning. Trial P&D to lower lobes and RML q shift as tolerated. **Aerosolized Medication Protocol:** 2.0 mL 10% acetylcysteine with 0.5 mL albuterol q4 h. ABG in 1 hour.

Discussion

A history of cold exposure in conjunction with the use of alcoholic beverages before the onset of pneumonia is not uncommon. The first part of this case begins with a classic presentation for community-acquired pneumonia with alveolar consolidation (see **Alveolar Consolidation**, Figure 9-8). For example, the fever and tachycardia represent a normal functioning immune response, and the tachycardia and tachypnea reflect the body's response to shunt-induced hypoxemia. The auscultation of crackles and bronchial breath sounds also reflects the patient's pulmonary consolidation. An attempt at improving his oxygenation, although not successful, was certainly in order. It was hoped that by providing an oxygen-enriched gas to both normal and partially consolidated alveoli, the effects of pulmonary shunting would be at least partially offset.

The second SOAP presents the complication of the patient's community-acquired pneumonia with aspiration pneumonitis. Alcoholics frequently have gastritis or esophagitis, and the patient's eructation (belching) and pyrosis (heartburn) were clues to the development of that complication. At this time there were new clinical manifestations associated with **Excessive Bronchial Secretions** (see Figure 9-11). For example, the patient demonstrated a cough, sputum, and coarse crackles. The **Bronchopulmonary Hygiene Therapy Protocol** (e.g., mucolytic with a bronchodilator, DB&C, suctioning, and P&D) was appropriate. A trial of **Lung Expansion Therapy** (see Protocol 9-3) was not given in this case. However, **Atelectasis** (see Figure 9-7) often complicates aspiration pneumonia, and such a trial would not have been inappropriate.

In cases of pneumonia, the respiratory therapist is often tempted to do too much. Typically, volume expansion therapy, bronchodilator aerosol therapy, and bland aerosol therapy have all been ordered for affected patients, even in the acute, consolidative stage of their pneumonia. Often, however, all that is needed is the appropriate selection of antibiotics, rest, fluids, and supplementary oxygen. When the pneumonia "breaks up" (resolution stage) or is complicated by aspiration (as in this case), **Excessive Bronchial Secretions** (see Figure 9-11) and even **Bronchospasm** (see Figure 9-10) may appear. When this happens, use of other protocol modalities is necessary.

SELF-ASSESSMENT QUESTIONS

Answers to questions can be found on Evolve. To access additional student assessment questions visit **http://evolve.elsevier.com/DesJardins/respiratory**.

1. Which of the following is also known as Friedländer's bacillus?
   a. *Haemophilus influenzae*
   b. *Pseudomonas aeruginosa*
   c. *Legionella pneumophila*
   d. *Klebsiella*

2. Which of the following accounts for more than 80% of all the bacterial pneumonias?
   a. *Klebsiella* pneumonia
   b. Streptococcal pneumonia
   c. *Chlamydia* pneumonia
   d. Staphylococcal pneumonia

3. Which of the following is associated with Q fever?
   a. *Mycoplasma pneumoniae*
   b. *Rickettsia*
   c. Ornithosis
   d. Varicella

4. Mendelson's syndrome is a term associated with which of the following?
   a. Lipoid pneumonitis
   b. Rubella
   c. Varicella
   d. Aspiration pneumonia

5. Which of the following is the most common viral pulmonary complication of AIDS?
   a. *Aspergillus*
   b. *Cryptococcus*
   c. *Pneumocystis carinii*
   d. Cytomegalovirus

6. Which of the following infects almost all children by age two?
   a. *Klebsiella*
   b. *Haemophilus influenzae* type B
   c. Respiratory syncytial virus
   d. *Pseudomonas aeruginosa*

7. Which of the following is almost always the cause of acute epiglottitis?
   a. *Haemophilus influenzae* type B
   b. *Klebsiella*
   c. *Streptococcus*
   d. *Mycoplasma pneumoniae*

8. Which of the following related to mumps, rubella, and RSV?
   a. *Streptococcus*
   b. Parainfluenza virus
   c. *Mycoplasma pneumoniae*
   d. Adenovirus

9. In the absence of a secondary bacterial infection, lung inflammation caused by the aspiration of gastric fluids usually becomes insignificant in approximately how many days?
   a. 2 days
   b. 3 days
   c. 5 days
   d. 7 days

10. Which of the following findings is/are associated with pneumonia?
    1. Decreased tactile and vocal fremitus
    2. Increased $C(a-\bar{v})O_2$
    3. Decreased functional residual capacity
    4. Increased vital capacity
       a. 1 only
       b. 3 only
       c. 2 and 4 only
       d. 1 and 3 only

Chapter Objectives

After reading this chapter, you will be able to:

- List the anatomic alterations of the lungs associated with lung abscess.
- Describe the causes of lung abscess.
- List the cardiopulmonary clinical manifestations associated with lung abscess.
- Describe the general management of lung abscess.
- Describe the clinical strategies and rationales of the SOAPs presented in the case study.

Key Terms

Anaerobic Gram-Negative Bacilli
Anaerobic Gram-Positive Cocci
Bacteroides fragilis
Flash Burn
Fusobacterium

Peptococci
Peptostreptococci
Prevotella melaninogenica
Staphylococci

Chapter Outline

Anatomic Alterations of the Lungs
Etiology and Epidemiology
Overview of the Cardiopulmonary Clinical Manifestations
   Associated with Lung Abscess
General Management of Lung Abscess
   Medications and Procedures Commonly Prescribed by the
      Physician
   Respiratory Care Treatment Protocols
Case Study: Lung Abscess
Self-Assessment Questions

Anatomic Alterations of the Lungs

A *lung abscess* is defined as a necrosis of lung tissue that in severe cases leads to a localized air- and fluid-filled cavity. A lung abscess is also known as "necrotizing pneumonia" or "lung gangrene." The fluid in the cavity is a collection of purulent exudate that is composed of liquefied white blood cell remains, proteins, and tissue debris. The air- and fluid-filled cavity is encapsulated in a so-called *pyogenic membrane* that consists of a layer of fibrin, inflammatory cells, and granulation tissue.

During the early stages of a lung abscess, the pathology is indistinguishable from that of any acute pneumonia. Polymorphonuclear leukocytes and macrophages move into the infected area to engulf any invading organisms. This action causes the pulmonary capillaries to dilate, the interstitium to fill with fluid, and the alveolar epithelium to swell from the edema fluid. In response to this inflammatory reaction, the alveoli in the infected area become consolidated (Figure 17-1).

As the inflammatory process progresses, tissue necrosis involving all the lung structures occurs. In severe cases the tissue necrosis ruptures into a bronchus and allows a partial or total drainage of the liquefied contents from the cavity. An air- and fluid-filled cavity also may rupture into the intrapleural space via a bronchopleural fistula and cause pleural effusion and empyema (see Chapter 24, Pleural Diseases). This may lead to inflammation of the parietal pleura, pleuritic chest pain, atelectasis, and decreased chest expansion. After a period of time, fibrosis and calcification of the tissues around the cavity encapsulate the abscess (see Figure 17-1).

The major pathologic or structural changes associated with a lung abscess are as follows:

- Alveolar consolidation
- Alveolar-capillary and bronchial wall destruction
- Tissue necrosis
- Cavity formation
- Fibrosis and calcification of the lung parenchyma
- Bronchopleural fistulas and empyema
- Atelectasis
- Excessive airway secretions

Etiology and Epidemiology

Lung abscesses most commonly occur as a complication of aspiration pneumonia—i.e., the pathologic events that follow shortly after aspirating either acidic gastric fluids or a variety of anaerobic organisms that are normally found in oropharyngeal secretions. Anaerobic organisms often colonize in the small grooves and spaces between the teeth and gums in patients with poor oral hygiene; they are frequently associated with gingivitis and dead or abscessed teeth. Aspiration often occurs in the patient with a decreased level of consciousness. Predisposing factors include (1) alcohol abuse, (2) seizure disorders, (3) general anesthesia, (4) head trauma, (5) cerebrovascular accidents, and (6) swallowing disorders. Anatomically,

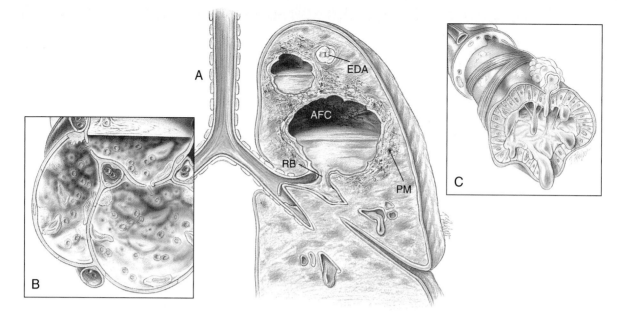

FIGURE 17-1 Lung abscess. **A**, Cross-sectional view of lung abscess. **B**, Consolidation. **C**, Excessive bronchial secretions are common secondary anatomic alterations of the lungs. *AFC*, Air-fluid cavity; *EDA*, early development of abscess; *PM*, pyogenic membrane; *RB*, ruptured bronchus (and drainage of the liquefied contents of the cavity).

lung abscesses most commonly develop in lung regions that are dependent in the recumbent position (e.g., the posterior segments of the upper lobes or the superior segments of the lower lobes). The right lung is more commonly involved than the left.

The aspiration of acidic gastric fluids is associated with immediate injury to the tracheobronchial tree and lung parenchyma—often likened to a **flash burn.** Common anaerobic organisms found in the normal flora of the mouth, gingival crevice, upper respiratory tract, and gastrointestinal tract include the following:

- **Anaerobic gram-positive cocci**
  - **Peptostreptococci**
  - **Peptococci**
- **Anaerobic gram-negative bacilli**
  - *Bacteroides fragilis*
  - *Prevotella melaninogenica*
  - *Fusobacterium species*

Although less frequent, other organisms known to cause a lung abscess are *Klebsiella, Staphylococcus, Mycobacterium tuberculosis* (including the atypical organisms *Mycobacterium kansasii* and *Mycobacterium avium*), *Histoplasma capsulatum, Coccidioides immitis, Blastomyces,* and *Aspergillus fumigatus.* Parasites that may cause lung abscess formation include *Paragonimus westermani, Echinococcus,* and *Entamoeba histolytica.* On rare occasions, a lung abscess may also be caused by *Streptococcus pneumoniae, Pseudomonas aeruginosa,* or *Legionella pneumophila.* Although these pathogens can be the sole cause of a lung abscess, they most often are isolated in mixed infections with anaerobes. Box 17-1 summarizes organisms known to cause lung abscess.

A lung abscess may also develop as a result of (1) bronchial obstruction with secondary cavitating infection (e.g., distal to bronchogenic carcinoma or an aspirated foreign body), (2) vascular obstruction with tissue infarction (e.g., septic embolism, vasculitis), (3) interstitial lung disease with

---

BOX 17-1 Organisms Known to Cause Lung Abscess

Common Organisms Associated with Aspiration
- Anaerobic gram-positive cocci
  - Peptostreptococci
  - Peptococci
- Anaerobic gram-negative bacilli
  - *Bacteroides fragilis*
  - *Prevotella melaninogenica*
  - *Fusobacterium* species

Less Common Organisms
Klebsiella
Staphylococci
Mycobacterium tuberculosis (plus atypical organisms *Mycobacterium kansasii* and *Mycobacterium avium*)
Histoplasma capsulatum
Coccidioides immitis
Blastomyces
Aspergillus fumigatus

Parasites
Paragonimus westermani
Echinococcus
Entamoeba histolytica

Rare Causes
Streptococcus pneumoniae
Pseudomonas aeruginosa
Legionella pneumophila

---

cavity formation (e.g., pneumoconiosis [silicosis], Wegener's granulomatosis, and rheumatoid nodules), (4) bullae or cysts that become infected (e.g., congenital or bronchogenic cysts), or (5) penetrating chest wounds that lead to an infection (e.g., bullet wound).

The following clinical manifestations result from the pathologic mechanisms caused (or activated) by Alveolar Consolidation (see Figure 9-8) and, when the abscess is draining, by Excessive Bronchial Secretions (see Figure 9-11). These are the major anatomic alterations of the lungs associated with lung abscess (see Figure 17-1).

CLINICAL DATA OBTAINED AT THE PATIENT'S BEDSIDE

The Physical Examination

Vital Signs

Increased Respiratory Rate (Tachypnea)

Several pathophysiologic mechanisms operating simultaneously may lead to an increased ventilatory rate:

- Stimulation of peripheral chemoreceptors (hypoxemia)
- Decreased lung compliance–increased ventilatory rate relationship
- Stimulation of J receptors
- Pain, anxiety, fever

Increased Heart Rate (Pulse) and Blood Pressure

Pleuritic Chest Pain, Decreased Chest Expansion

Cyanosis

Cough, Sputum Production, and Hemoptysis

During the early stages, when the lung abscess is in the inflammatory pneumonia-like phase, the patient generally has a nonproductive barking or hacking cough. If the abscess progresses into an air- and fluid-filled cavity and ruptures through a bronchus, the patient may suddenly cough up large amounts of sputum. Foul-smelling brown or gray sputum indicates a putrid infection that is caused by numerous organisms, including anaerobes. An odorless green or yellow sputum indicates a nonputrid infection caused by a single aerobic organism. Blood-streaked sputum is common in patients with a lung abscess. Occasionally, frank hemoptysis is seen.

Chest Assessment Findings

- Increased tactile and vocal fremitus
- Crackles

The following may be heard directly over the abscess:

- Dull percussion note
- Bronchial breath sounds
- Diminished breath sounds
- Whispered pectoriloquy
- Pleural friction rub (if abscess is near pleural surface)

CLINICAL DATA OBTAINED FROM LABORATORY TESTS AND SPECIAL PROCEDURES

Pulmonary Function Test Findings
Severe and Extensive Cases (Restrictive Lung Pathophysiology)

FORCED EXPIRATORY VOLUME AND FLOW RATE FINDINGS*

FVC	FEV_T	FEV_1/FVC ratio	$FEF_{25\%-75\%}$
↓	N or ↓	N or ↑	N or ↓

$FEF_{50\%}$	$FEF_{200-1200}$	PEFR	MVV
N or ↓	N or ↓	N or ↓	N or ↓

LUNG VOLUME AND CAPACITY FINDINGS

V_T	IRV	ERV	RV
N or ↓	↓	↓	↓

VC	IC	FRC	TLC	RV/TLC ratio
↓	↓	↓	↓	N

Arterial Blood Gases

MILD TO MODERATE LUNG ABSCESS

Acute Alveolar Hyperventilation with Hypoxemia[†]
(acute respiratory alkalosis)

pH	$PaCO_2$	HCO_3^-	PaO_2	SaO_2 or SpO_2
↑	↓	↓ (but normal)	↓	↓

SEVERE LUNG ABSCESS

Acute Ventilatory Failure with Hypoxemia[†]
(acute respiratory acidosis)

pH[§]	$PaCO_2$	HCO_3^- [§]	PaO_2	SaO_2 or SpO_2
↓	↑	↑ (but normal)	↓	↓

Oxygenation Indices[||]

$\dot{Q}_S/\dot{Q}_T$	DO_2[¶]	$\dot{V}O_2$	$C(a-\bar{v})O_2$	O_2ER	$S\bar{v}O_2$
↑	↓	N	N	↑	↓

*The decreased forced expiratory volumes and flow rate findings are primarily caused by the low vital capacity associated with the disorder.
[†]See Figure 4-3 and related discussion for the acute pH, $PaCO_2$, and HCO_3^- changes associated with acute alveolar hyperventilation.
[‡]See Figure 4-2 and related discussion for the acute pH, $PaCO_2$, and HCO_3^- changes associated with acute ventilatory failure.
[§]When tissue hypoxia is severe enough to produce lactic acid, the pH and HCO_3^- values will be lower than expected for a particular $PaCO_2$ level.
[||]$C(a-\bar{v})O_2$, Arterial-venous oxygen difference; DO_2, total oxygen delivery; O_2ER, oxygen extraction ratio; $\dot{Q}_S/\dot{Q}_T$, pulmonary shunt fraction; $S\bar{v}O_2$, mixed venous oxygen saturation; $\dot{V}O_2$, oxygen consumption.
[¶]The DO_2 may be normal in patients who have compensated to the decreased oxygenation status with (1) an increased cardiac output, (2) an increased hemoglobin level, or (3) a combination of both. When the DO_2 is normal, the O_2ER is usually normal.

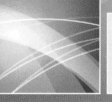

ABNORMAL LABORATORY TEST AND PROCEDURE RESULTS

Sputum Examination—Most Common Organisms (see the discussion in Etiology and Box 17-1). Many of these organisms are "slow growers" and may take some time to be identified completely on culture media.

Anaerobic Organisms

Anaerobic Gram-Positive Cocci

- Peptostreptococci
- Peptococci

Anaerobic Gram-Negative Bacilli

- *Bacteroides fragilis*
- *Prevotella melaninogenica*
- *Fusobacterium species*

RADIOLOGIC FINDINGS

Chest Radiograph

- Increased opacity
- Cavity formation
- Cavities with air-fluid levels
- Fibrosis and calcification
- Pleural effusion

The chest radiograph typically reveals localized consolidation during the early stages of lung abscess formation. Later, the characteristic radiographic appearance of a lung abscess appears after (1) the infection ruptures into a bronchus, and/or (2) tissue destruction and necrosis have occurred, and/or (3) partial evacuation of the purulent contents has occurred. The abscess usually appears on the radiograph as a circular radiolucency that contains an air-fluid level, surrounded by a dense wall of lung parenchyma (Figure 17-2).

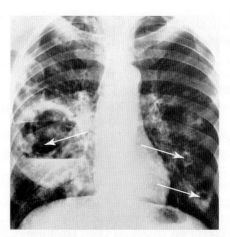

FIGURE 17-2 Reactivation tuberculosis with a large cavitary lesion containing an air-fluid level in the right lower lobe (see arrow). Smaller cavitary lesions are also seen in other lobes (See arrows). (From Hansell DM, Armstrong P, Lynch DA, McAdams HP, eds: *Imaging of diseases of the chest*, ed 4, Philadelphia, 2005, Elsevier.)

General Management of Lung Abscess

Medications and Procedures Commonly Prescribed by the Physician

Treatment varies based on the severity of the pneumonia and the lung abscess. Treatment includes appropriate (usually intravenous) antimicrobial therapy coupled with prompt drainage and surgical debridement. When treated properly, most patients with a lung abscess show improvement. In acute cases, the size of the abscess quickly decreases and eventually closes altogether. In severe or chronic cases, the patient's improvement may be slow or insignificant, even with appropriate therapy.

The standard treatment for a lung abscess caused by an anaerobic pathogen is *clindamycin*. Other drugs that may be used are any combination of *beta-lactam–beta-lactamase inhibitors* (e.g., ampicillin-sulbactam), *penicillin* plus *metronidazole*, or a *carbapenem*. When the lung abscess is caused by methicillin-resistant Staphylococcus aureus (MRSA), *linezolid* is recommended. An alternative to linezolid is *vancomycin*; followed by *ceftaroline*, *trimethoprim-sulfamethoxazole*, and *telavancin*.

Respiratory Care Treatment Protocols

Oxygen Therapy Protocol

Oxygen therapy is used to treat hypoxemia, decrease the work of breathing, and decrease myocardial work. The hypoxemia that develops in lung abscess is usually caused by pulmonary capillary shunting. Hypoxemia caused by capillary shunting is often refractory to oxygen therapy (see Oxygen Therapy Protocol, Protocol 9-1).

Bronchopulmonary Hygiene Therapy Protocol

Because of the excessive production and accumulation of mucus associated with a ruptured lung abscess, a number of bronchial hygiene treatment modalities may be used to enhance the mobilization of bronchial secretions (see Bronchopulmonary Hygiene Therapy Protocol, Protocol 9-2).

Lung Expansion Therapy Protocol

Because of the alveolar consolidation and atelectasis associated with a lung abscess, lung expansion may be tried to offset these anatomic alterations of the lungs (see Lung Expansion Therapy Protocol, Protocol 9-3).

CASE STUDY Lung Abscess

Admitting History and Physical Examination

This 64-year-old unemployed man sought medical attention because of an increasingly severe cough that produced moderate amounts of foul-smelling sputum. He had undergone splenectomy for removal of a ruptured spleen 1 year previously. He reported that on several occasions recently he had a slight fever and that his appetite was poor; he had lost about 6 lb. For the past 3 days he had noticed some right-sided chest pain, and his cough had become very productive. The patient denied cigarette smoking.

Physical examination showed a small and poorly nourished male in moderate distress, coughing throughout the interview. The patient's vital signs were blood pressure 160/90, heart rate 120 beats/min, respiratory rate breaths (22 breaths/min), and oral temperature 100.6° F. There was brawny discoloration of the legs below the knees. His teeth were in deplorable condition, and he had marked halitosis. Examination of the chest revealed dullness to percussion, course crackles, and bronchial breath sounds in the right lower lobe (RLL).

His frequent cough produced large amounts of foul-smelling brown and gray sputum and was weak. The chest radiograph film showed a 4-cm diameter cavity in the RLL with a clear air-fluid level. Patches of alveolar consolidation surrounded the cavity. There was no evidence of air trapping. Sputum for a culture and sensitivity study was obtained, but the results were still pending. On room air, his arterial blood gas values were as follows: pH 7.51, $PaCO_2$ 29 mm Hg, HCO_3^- 22 mEq/L, PaO_2 61 mEq/L, and SaO_2 93%. A broad-spectrum intravenous antibiotic therapy was begun. The respiratory therapist assigned to his case recorded the following:

Respiratory Assessment and Plan

S "I can't stop coughing." Complains of low-grade fever, loss of appetite, weight loss (6 lb).

O Cachectic. BP 160/90, HR 120, RR 22, T 100.6° F orally. Teeth carious. Flat to percussion over RLL. Coarse crackles and bronchial breath sounds over RLL. Chest radiograph: 4-cm diameter cavity with fluid level and consolidation RLL. Room air arterial blood gases: pH 7.51, $PaCO_2$ 29, HCO_3^- 22, PaO_2 61, SaO_2 93%. Excessive amount of foul-smelling, thick brown and gray sputum. Weak cough.

A • Acute infection (fever)
  • Malnourished (inspection)
  • Lung abscess and consolidation, RLL (on chest radiograph)
  • Acute alveolar hyperventilation with mild hypoxemia (arterial blood gases)
  • Excessive and thick airway secretions (sputum, coarse crackles)
  • Poor ability to mobilize secretions (weak cough)

P **Oxygen Therapy Protocol**: 2 L/min per nasal cannula. SpO_2 spot check to verify appropriateness of O_2 therapy. O_2 titration if necessary. **Bronchopulmonary Hygiene Therapy Protocol**: Postural drainage to right lower lobe q6h. **Aerosolized Medication Protocol**: Trial period of med. nebs.: 2.0 mL acetylcysteine with 0.5 mL albuterol 0.5 hours before postural drainage q6h for 3 days, and then reevaluate.

After reviewing the results of sputum culture sensitivity studies, which were positive for peptostreptococci, the physician started the patient on intravenous clindamycin. Over the next 5 days, the patient's general condition improved; his cough and sputum production decreased remarkably but not completely, and his sputum was no longer thick. His room air SpO_2 increased to 94%, and he no longer had acute alveolar hyperventilation. A chest radiograph revealed that his lung abscess was slightly reduced in size compared with the chest radiograph taken on the day of his admission, and his pneumonia had improved significantly. A complete pulmonary function test (PFT) study revealed a mild reduction in lung volumes, capacities, and expiratory flow rates. Social Service worked with him on two occasions during his hospitalization and scheduled a home follow-up appointment 4 weeks after discharge. An oral surgery consultation was obtained and extraction of the patient's carious teeth was scheduled. The patient was instructed on deep-breathing and coughing techniques and general bronchial hygiene. He was discharged on the morning of the sixth day and was prescribed a month-long course of oral clindamycin.

Discussion

This case illustrates some of the classic clinical manifestations of a lung abscess. For example, the **Alveolar Consolidation** surrounding the abscess (see Figure 9-8), which was identified on the chest radiograph likely played a role in producing the patient's fever and increasing his heart rate, blood pressure, and respiratory rate. In addition, the pneumonic consolidation also contributed to the patient's alveolar hyperventilation and hypoxemia, the bronchial breath sounds, and the reduced lung volumes and capacities and flow rates identified on his PFT.

The clinical manifestations associated with **Excessive Bronchial Secretions** (see Figure 9-11) also were seen in this case. Not only did the excessive airway secretions contribute to the patient's hypoxemia, secondary to the decreased $\dot{V}/\dot{Q}$ ratio and pulmonary shunting, but they also contributed to the increased airway resistance (caused by the secretions) that resulted in the coarse crackles, sputum production, and reduced air-flow rates seen on the PFT.

The primary treatments started by the respiratory therapist were directed to the patient's excessive secretions. **Lung Expansion Therapy** (see Protocol 9-3) was not employed. One could argue that it should have been, given the infiltrates seen on the chest radiographic film, which could have represented atelectasis just as well as pneumonia. The appropriate respiratory care of patients with lung abscesses closely resembles that of those with bronchiectasis (see Chapter 14) and pneumonia (see Chapter 16). Identification of this patient's lung abscess in the RLL allowed targeted chest physical therapy to be given. Having a Social Service representative instruct the patient about his personal hygiene was entirely appropriate. Finally, extraction of his carious teeth, as suggested by the Dental Service, will hopefully eradicate this source of infection once and for all.

SELF-ASSESSMENT QUESTIONS

Answers to questions can be found on Evolve. To access additional student assessment questions visit **http://evolve.elsevier.com/DesJardins/respiratory**.

1. **Which of the following is or are anaerobic organisms?**
   1. *Blastomyces*
   2. *Peptococcus*
   3. *Coccidioides immitis*
   4. *Bacteroides*
      a. 1 and 2 only
      b. 2 and 4 only
      c. 3 and 4 only
      d. 2, 3, and 4 only

2. **Which of the following is or are predisposing factors to the aspiration of gastrointestinal fluids (and anaerobes)?**
   1. Seizure disorders
   2. Head trauma
   3. Alcoholic binges
   4. General anesthesia
      a. 1 and 4 only
      b. 2 and 3 only
      c. 2, 3, and 4 only
      d. 1, 2, 3, and 4

3. **Which of the following is or are associated with the formation of a lung abscess?**
   1. Bullae or cysts that become infected
   2. Interstitial lung disease with cavity formation
   3. Bronchial obstruction with secondary cavitating infection
   4. Penetrating chest wounds that lead to an infection
      a. 1 only
      b. 3 only
      c. 2 and 4 only
      d. 1, 2, 3, and 4

4. **Anatomically, a lung abscess most commonly forms in which part(s) of the lung?**
   1. Posterior segment of the upper lobe
   2. Lateral basal segment of the lower lobe
   3. Anterior segment of the upper lobe
   4. Superior segment of the lower lobe
      a. 1 only
      b. 3 only
      c. 1 and 4 only
      d. 2 and 3 only

5. **Which of the following pulmonary function findings may be associated with a severe and extensive lung abscess?**
   1. Decreased FVC
   2. Increased PEFR
   3. Decreased RV
   4. Increased FRC
      a. 3 only
      b. 2 and 4 only
      c. 3 and 4 only
      d. 1 and 3 only

18 Tuberculosis

Chapter Objectives

After reading this chapter, you will be able to:

- List the anatomic alterations of the lungs associated with tuberculosis.
- Describe the causes of tuberculosis.
- List the cardiopulmonary clinical manifestations associated with tuberculosis.
- Describe the general management of tuberculosis.
- Describe the clinical strategies and rationales of the SOAP presented in the case study.

Key Terms

Acid-Fast Bacilli
Acid-Fast Bacteria
Caseous Granuloma
Caseous Lesion
Directly Observed Therapy (DOT)
Disseminated Tuberculosis
Dormant Tuberculosis (Latent Tuberculosis)
Ethambutol
Fluorescent Acid-Fast Stain
Ghon Complex
Ghon Nodules
Granuloma
Induration
Isolation Procedures
Isoniazid (INH)
Mantoux Tuberculin Skin Test
Miliary Tuberculosis
Mycobacterium avium
Mycobacterium kansasii
Mycobacterium tuberculosis

Nontuberculous Acid-Fast Mycobacteria
Post-primary Tuberculosis
Primary Tuberculosis
Prophylactic Use of INH
Purified Protein Derivative (PPD) Skin Test
Pyrazinamide
Respiratory Isolation
Rifampin
Sputum Smear
Streptomycin
Tubercle
Ziehl-Neelsen Stain

Chapter Outline

Anatomic Alterations of the Lungs
    Primary Tuberculosis
    Postprimary Tuberculosis
    Disseminated Tuberculosis
Etiology and Epidemiology
Diagnosis
    Mantoux Tuberculin Skin Test
    Acid-Fast Staining
    Sputum Culture
    QuantiFERON-TB Gold Test
Overview of the Cardiopulmonary Clinical Manifestations Associated with Tuberculosis
General Management of Tuberculosis
    Pharmacologic Agents Used to Treat Tuberculosis
    Respiratory Care Treatment Protocols
Case Study: Tuberculosis
Self-Assessment Questions

Anatomic Alterations of the Lungs

Tuberculosis (TB) is a contagious chronic bacterial infection that primarily affects the lungs, although it may involve almost any part of the body. Clinically, TB is classified as either **primary tuberculosis, postprimary tuberculosis,** or **disseminated tuberculosis.**

Primary Tuberculosis

Primary TB (also called the *primary infection stage*) follows the patient's first exposure to the TB pathogen, Mycobacterium tuberculosis—a rod-shaped bacterium with a waxy capsule. Primary TB begins when the inhaled bacilli implant in the alveoli. As the bacilli multiply over a 3- to

4-week period, the initial response of the lungs is an inflammatory reaction that is similar to acute pneumonia (see Figure 16-1). In other words, a large influx of polymorphonuclear leukocytes and macrophages moves into the infected area to engulf—but not fully kill—the bacilli. This action also causes the pulmonary capillaries to dilate, the interstitium to fill with fluid, and the alveolar epithelium to swell from the edema fluid. Eventually the alveoli become consolidated (i.e., filled with fluid, polymorphonuclear leukocytes, and macrophages). Clinically, this phase of TB coincides with a positive tuberculin reaction—a positive purified protein derivative (PPD) skin test result (see discussion of diagnosis later in this chapter).

Unlike pneumonia however, the lung tissue that surrounds the infected area slowly produces a protective cell wall called

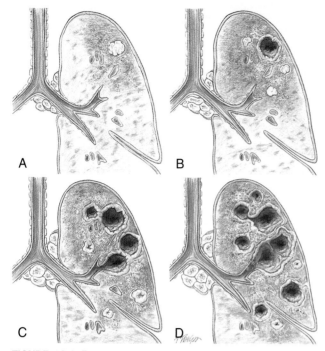

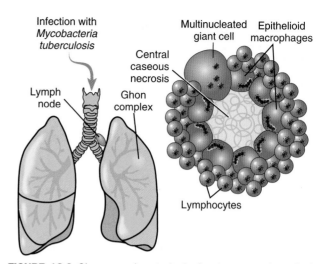

FIGURE 18-2 Ghon complex, typical of pulmonary tuberculosis, consists of a parenchymal focus and hilar lymph node lesions. The detailed section of the diagram shows the typical features of tuberculous granuloma: central caseous necrosis surrounded by epithelioid cells, multinucleated giant cells, and lymphocytes. (From Damjanov I: *Pathology for the health professions*, Philadelphia, 2012, Saunders.)

FIGURE 18-1 Tuberculosis. **A**, Early primary infection. **B**, Cavitation of a caseous tubercle and new primary lesions developing. **C**, Further progression and development of cavitations and new primary infections. Note the subpleural location of some of these lesions. **D**, Severe lung destruction caused by tuberculosis.

a **tubercle**, or **granuloma**. In essence, the tubercles work to encapsulate, or trap the TB bacilli in a nutshell-like structure (Figure 18-1, *A*). Although the initial lung lesions may be difficult to identify on a chest radiograph, the lesions may be seen as small, sharply defined opacities. When detected on a chest radiograph, these initial lung lesions are called **Ghon nodules**. As the disease progresses, the combination of tubercles and the involvement of the lymph nodes in the hilar region is known as the **Ghon complex** (Figure 18-2).

Structurally, a tubercle consists of a central core containing caseous necrosis and TB bacilli (also called caseous lesion or caseous granuloma). The central core is surrounded by enlarged epithelioid macrophages, lymphocytes, and multinucleated giant cells. A tubercle takes about 2 to 10 weeks to form. The function of the tubercle is to contain the TB bacilli, thus preventing the further spread of infectious TB organisms. Unfortunately, the central core of the tubercle has the potential to break down from time to time, especially in a patient with a depressed immune system. The patient is potentially contagious at this stage. In most cases however, the TB bacilli are effectively contained within the tubercles.

Once the bacilli are controlled—either by the patient's immunologic defense system (which contains the TB bacilli in a tubercle) or by antituberculosis drugs—the healing process begins. Tissue fibrosis and calcification of the lung parenchyma slowly replace the tubercle. This tissue fibrosis and calcification cause lung tissue retraction and scarring. In some cases the calcification and fibrosis cause the bronchi to distort and dilate—that is, to develop bronchiectasis.

Finally, when the bacilli are isolated within tubercles and immunity develops, the TB bacilli may remain dormant for

months, years, or life. Individuals with **dormant TB** (also called **latent TB**) do not feel sick or have any TB-related symptoms. They are still infected with TB but do not have clinically active TB. The only indication of a TB infection is a positive reaction to the tuberculin skin test (Mantoux test discuss later), or TB blood test, and the finding of possible residual scarring on the chest radiograph. Individuals with dormant (latent) TB are not infectious and cannot spread the TB bacilli to others.

Postprimary Tuberculosis

Postprimary TB (also called *reactivation TB, reinfection TB,* or *secondary TB*) is a term used to describe the reactivation of TB months or even years after the initial infection has been controlled. Even though most patients with primary TB recover completely from a clinical standpoint, it is important to note that live tubercle bacilli can remain dormant for decades. A positive tuberculin reaction generally persists even after the primary infection stage has been controlled. At any time, TB may become reactivated, especially in patients with depressed immune systems. Most new TB cases are associated with the following risk factors:

- Malnourished individuals
- People in institutional housing (e.g., nursing homes, prisons, homeless shelters)
- People living in overcrowded conditions
- Immunosuppressed patients (e.g., organ transplant patients, cancer patients)
- Human immunodeficiency virus (HIV)–infected patients (TB is a leading cause of death in HIV patients)
- Alcohol abuse

If the TB infection is uncontrolled, further growth of the caseous granuloma tubercle develops. The patient progressively experiences more severe symptoms, including violent coughing episodes, greenish or bloody sputum (possibly mixed with TB bacilli), low-grade fever, anorexia, weight loss, extreme fatigue, night sweats, and chest pain. It is this gradual wasting of the body that provided the basis for an earlier name for TB—*consumption*. The patient is highly contagious at this stage. In severe cases, a tubercle cavity may rupture and allow air and infected material to flow into the pleural space or the tracheobronchial tree. Pleural complications are common in TB (Figure 18-1, *C*).

Disseminated Tuberculosis

Disseminated TB (also called *extrapulmonary TB*, **miliary TB**, and *tuberculosis—disseminated*) refers to infection from TB bacilli that escape from a tubercle and travel to other sites throughout the body by means of the bloodstream or lymphatic system. In general, the TB bacilli that gain entrance to the bloodstream usually gather and multiply in portions of the body that have a high tissue oxygen tension. The most common location is the apex of the lungs. Other oxygen-rich areas in the body include the regional lymph nodes, kidneys, long bones, genital tract, brain, and meninges (Figure 18-3).

Genital TB in males damages the prostate gland, epididymis, seminal vesicles, and testes; and in females, the fallopian tubes, ovaries, and uterus. The spine is a frequent site of TB infection, although the hip, knee, wrist, and elbow can also be involved. Tubercular meningitis is caused by an active brain lesion seeding TB bacilli into the meninges. *Endobronchial TB* may develop via direct extension to the bronchi from an adjacent tubercle cavity or the spread of the TB bacilli via infected sputum.

TB *complications* include hemoptysis, pneumothorax, bronchiectasis, extensive pulmonary destruction, malignancy, and chronic pulmonary aspergillosis. Over time, the tuberculosis infection may cause mental deterioration, permanent retardation, blindness, and deafness.

When a large number of bacilli are freed into the bloodstream, the result can be the presence of numerous small tubercles—about the size of a pinhead—scattered throughout the body. This condition is termed *miliary TB*.

Tuberculosis primarily results in a chronic restrictive pulmonary disorder. The major pathologic or structural changes of the lungs associated with TB (mainly postprimary TB) are as follows:

- Alveolar consolidation
- Alveolar-capillary membrane destruction
- Caseous tubercles or granulomas
- Cavity formation
- Fibrosis and secondary calcification of the lung parenchyma
- Distortion and dilation of the bronchi
- Increased bronchial secretions

Etiology and Epidemiology

Tuberclosis is one of the oldest diseases known to man and remains one of the most widespread diseases in the world. Unmistakable evidence has been provided from mummies dating back to the Stone Age, ancient Egypt, and ancient Peru that TB is a long-lived human disease. In early writings,

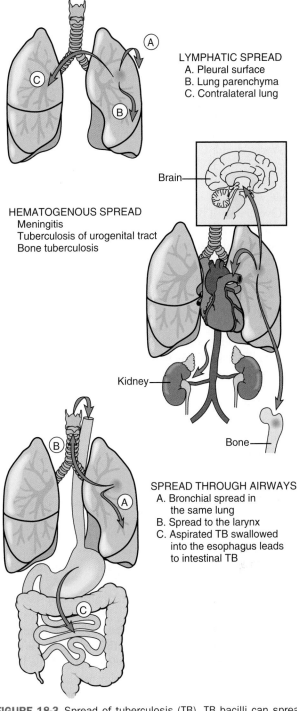

LYMPHATIC SPREAD
A. Pleural surface
B. Lung parenchyma
C. Contralateral lung

HEMATOGENOUS SPREAD
Meningitis
Tuberculosis of urogenital tract
Bone tuberculosis

Brain

Kidney

Bone

SPREAD THROUGH AIRWAYS
A. Bronchial spread in the same lung
B. Spread to the larynx
C. Aspirated TB swallowed into the esophagus leads to intestinal TB

FIGURE 18-3 Spread of tuberculosis (TB). TB bacilli can spread through the lymphatics, blood vessels, or bronchi. TB bacillis spread by the blood usually accounts for tuberculosis in distal sites, such as the urogenital tract, bone, or the brain. Expectorated bacilli may be swallowed and cause intestinal tuberculosis. (From Damjanov I: *Pathology for the health professions,* Philadelphia, 2012, Saunders.)

the disease was variously called "consumption," "Captain of the Men of Death," and "white plague." In the nineteenth century, the disease was named *tuberculosis,* a term that derives mainly from the tubercle formations found during postmortem examinations of victims of the disease.

According to the Centers for Disease Control and Prevention (CDC), there were 9945 new cases of TB reported in the United States in 2012—the lowest since the reporting of TB began in 1953. There were 569 deaths from TB in 2010, the most recent year for which these data are available. Compared to 2000 data, when 776 deaths from TB occurred, this represents a 27% decrease in TB deaths over a decade. Today, the majority of new TB cases in the United States occur in foreign-born individuals emigrating from countries with high rates of endemic TB.

Tuberculosis is still very prevalent globally. According to the World Health Organization (WHO) 2011 report, TB is second only to HIV/AIDS as the greatest killer worldwide that is caused by an infectious agent. In 2011, 8.7 million people were diagnosed with TB, and 1.4 million died from TB. Over 95% of TB deaths occur in low-and middle-income countries. Tuberculosis is among the top three causes of death for women aged 15 to 44 worldwide. Tuberculosis is a leading killer of people living with HIV, causing one quarter of all deaths. Multi-drug resistant TB (MDR-TB) is present in virtually every country surveyed. Approximately one third of the world's population (about 2.3 billon people) has latent TB (i.e., infected by TB bacteria, but not ill and who cannot transmit the TB spore). However, it is important to note that live TB bacilli can remain dormant in the lungs for years—and, if the opportunity arises, progress into reactivation TB (e.g., during immunosuppressed periods).

In spite of the widespread presence of TB around the world, the WHO reports that the estimated number of people falling ill from TB each year is slowly declining, and that the world is on track to achieve their Millennium Development Goal to reduce the spread of TB by 2015. In fact, the TB death rate has dropped 41% between 1990 and 2011.

In humans, TB is primarily caused by the bacteria called *Mycobacterium tuberculosis*. The mycobacteria are long, slender, straight, or curved rods. The *M. tuberculosis* organism is almost exclusively transmitted within aerosol droplets produced by coughing, sneezing, or laughing of an individual with active TB. This accounts for the use of strict **isolation procedures** in acutely ill patients hospitalized and suspected of having active tuberculosis. In fact, it has been shown that in very fine aerosolized spray droplets (0.5 to 1.0 μm), the TB bacilli can remain suspended in the air for several hours after a cough or sneeze. When inhaled, some of the bacilli may be trapped in the mucus of the nasal passages and removed. The smaller bacilli, however, can easily be inhaled into the bronchioles and alveoli. The TB bacilli are highly aerobic organisms and thrive best in areas of the body with high oxygen tension—especially in the apex of the lung.

People living in closed small rooms with limited access to sunlight and fresh air are especially at risk. Other possible ways of contracting TB include the ingestion of unpasteurized milk from cattle infected with the TB pathogen (usually *Mycobacterium bovis*) or in rare cases, direct inoculation through the skin (e.g., a laboratory accident during a postmortem examination).

Diagnosis

The most frequently used diagnostic methods for TB are the **Mantoux tuberculin skin test**, acid-fast bacilli (AFB) sputum

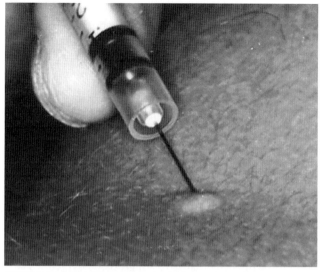

FIGURE 18-4 The Mantoux test, which consists of an intradermal injection of a small amount of a purified protein derivative (PPD) of the tuberculin bacillus. An induration of 10 mm or greater is considered positive. A positive reaction is fairly sound evidence of recent or past infection or disease. (From Price SA, Wilson LM: *Pathophysiology: clinical concepts of disease processes*, ed 6, St. Louis, 2002, Elsevier.)

cultures, and chest radiographs. Recently a new blood test for TB, called the QuantiFERON-TB Gold (QFT-G) test, has been approved.

Mantoux Tuberculin Skin Test

The most widely used tuberculin test is the Mantoux test, which consists of an intradermal injection of a small amount of a **purified protein derivative (PPD)** of the tuberculin bacillus (Figure 18-4). The skin is then observed for **induration** (a wheal) after 48 hours and 72 hours, with results interpreted as follows:

- An induration less than 5 mm is a negative result.
- An induration of 5 to 9 mm is considered suspicious, and retesting is required.
- An induration of 10 mm or greater is considered a positive result. A positive reaction is fairly sound evidence of recent or past infection or of disease.

It should be stressed, however, that a positive reaction does not necessarily confirm that a patient has active TB, but only that the patient has been exposed to the bacillus and has developed cell-mediated immunity to it.

Acid-Fast Staining

Because the *M. tuberculosis* organism has an unusual, waxy coating on the cell surface, which makes the cells impervious to staining, an **acid-fast bacteria** (AFB) test (also called a **sputum smear**) is performed instead. Several variations of the acid-fast stain are currently in use. The frequently used **Ziehl-Neelsen stain** reveals bright red acid-fast bacilli against a blue background (Figure 18-5, *A*). Another popular technique involves a **fluorescent acid-fast stain** that reveals luminescent yellow-green bacilli against a dark brown background. The fluorescent acid-fast stain is becoming the

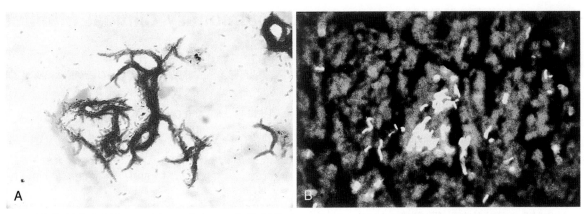

FIGURE 18-5 Acid-fast staining techniques. **A**, Ziehl-Neelsen staining of *Mycobacterium tuberculosis* from sputum. The red rods are *M. tuberculosis*. **B**, A fluorescent acid-fast stain of *M. tuberculosis* from sputum. Organisms appear yellow (fluorescent). (From Murray PR, Rosenthal KS, Pfaller MA: *Medical microbiology*, ed 5, St Louis, 2005, Mosby.)

acid-fast test of choice because it is easier to read and provides a striking contrast (Figure 18-5, *B*).

Sputum Culture

Because a variety of nontuberculous strains of *Mycobacterium* can show up on an AFB smear, a sputum culture is often necessary to differentiate *M. tuberculosis* from other acid-fast organisms. For example, common **nontuberculous acid-fast mycobacteria** associated with chronic obstructive pulmonary disease (COPD) are Mycobacterium avium and Mycobacterium kansasii. Sputum cultures can also identify drug-resistant bacilli and their sensitivity to antibiotic therapy. *M. tuberculosis* grows very slowly. It takes up to 6 weeks for colonies to appear in culture. When the TB bacterium was first studied, it was given the misleading prefix *Myco*, which gave the impression that the TB pathogen was fungal in nature. The bacterium growing in agars appeared as colonies and was similar to fungal colonies (Figure 18-6). However, they are unrelated; TB is caused by a bacterium and not a fungus.

QuantiFERON-TB Gold Test

In 2005 the U.S. Food and Drug Administration (FDA) approved the QFT-G test. The QFT-G test is a whole-blood test used for diagnosing *M. tuberculosis* infection, including latent TB infection. Samples of the patient's blood are mixed with antigens (substances that can generate an immune response) and controls. The QFT-G test contains synthetic antigens that represent two *M. tuberculosis* proteins (ESAT-6 and CFP-10). The mixture is then allowed to incubate for

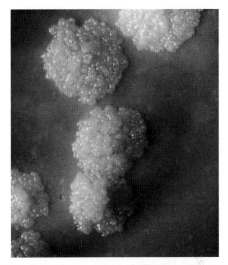

FIGURE 18-6 Cultural appearance of *Mycobacterium tuberculosis*. (Copyright 2009 from Cowan, MK: *Microbiology: a systems approach*, ed 2, Reproduced with permission of The McGraw-Hill Companies, New York.)

16 to 24 hours. After this period the mixture is measured for the presence of interferon-gamma (IFN-gamma). In patients infected with *M. tuberculosis*, the white blood cells will release IFN-gamma when in contact with the TB antigens. An elevated IFN-gamma level is diagnostic of TB. Additional clinical evaluations, such as AFB stain of the sputum smear and chest radiograph, are recommended to further support a positive QFT-G finding.

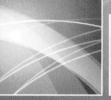

OVERVIEW of the Cardiopulmonary Clinical Manifestations Associated with Tuberculosis

The following clinical manifestations result from the pathophysiologic mechanisms caused (or activated) by Alveolar Consolidation (see Figure 9-8) and Increased Alveolar-Capillary Membrane Thickness (see Figure 9-9)—the major anatomic alterations of the lungs associated with tuberculosis (Figure 18-1).

CLINICAL DATA OBTAINED AT THE PATIENT'S BEDSIDE

The Physical Examination

Vital Signs

Increased Respiratory Rate (Tachypnea)

Several pathophysiologic mechanisms operating simultaneously may lead to an increased ventilatory rate:

- Stimulation of peripheral chemoreceptors
- Decreased lung compliance–increased ventilatory rate relationship
- Pain, anxiety, fever

Increased Heart Rate (Pulse) and Blood Pressure

Chest Pain, Decreased Chest Expansion

Cyanosis

Digital Clubbing

Peripheral Edema and Venous Distention

Because polycythemia and cor pulmonale are associated with severe tuberculosis (TB), the following may be seen:

- Distended neck veins
- Pitting edema
- Enlarged and tender liver

Cough, Sputum Production, and Hemoptysis

Chest Assessment Findings

- Increased tactile and vocal fremitus
- Dull percussion note
- Bronchial breath sounds
- Crackles, wheezing
- Pleural friction rub (if process extends to pleural surface)
- Whispered pectoriloquy

CLINICAL DATA OBTAINED FROM LABORATORY TESTS AND SPECIAL PROCEDURES

Pulmonary Function Test Findings*
(Severe and Extensive Cases) (Restrictive Lung Pathology)

FORCED EXPIRATORY VOLUME AND FLOW RATE FINDINGS

FVC	FEV_T	FEV_1/FVC ratio	$FEF_{25\%-75\%}$
↓	N or ↓	N or ↑	N or ↓

$FEF_{50\%}$	$FEF_{200-1200}$	PEFR	MVV
N or ↓	N or ↓	N or ↓	N or ↓

*Pulmonary function test (PFT) findings are usually normal in most cases of TB.

LUNG VOLUME AND CAPACITY FINDINGS

V_T	IRV	ERV	RV	
N or ↓	↓	↓	↓	

VC	IC	FRC	TLC	RV/TLC ratio
↓	↓	↓	↓	N

Arterial Blood Gases

MODERATE TUBERCULOSIS

Acute Alveolar Hyperventilation with Hypoxemia*
(Acute Respiratory Alkalosis)

pH	$PaCO_2$	HCO_3^-	PaO_2	SaO_2 or SpO_2
↑	↓	↓ (but normal)	↓	↓

EXTENSIVE TUBERCULOSIS WITH PULMONARY FIBROSIS

Chronic Ventilatory Failure with Hypoxemia†
(Compensated Respiratory Acidosis)

pH	$PaCO_2$	HCO_3^-	PaO_2	SaO_2 or SpO_2
N	↑	↑ (significantly)	↓	↓

ACUTE VENTILATORY CHANGES SUPERIMPOSED ON CHRONIC VENTILATORY FAILURE†

Because acute ventilatory changes are frequently seen in patients with chronic ventilatory failure, the respiratory therapist must be familiar with—and alert for—the following two dangerous arterial blood gas findings:

- Acute alveolar hyperventilation superimposed on chronic ventilatory failure—which should further alert the respiratory therapist to record the following important ABG assessment: possible *impending acute ventilatory failure*.
- Acute ventilatory failure (acute hypoventilation) superimposed on chronic ventilatory failure.

Oxygenation Indices§
Moderate to Severe Stages

$\dot{Q}_S/\dot{Q}_T$	DO_2‖	$\dot{V}O_2$	$C(a-\bar{v})O_2$	O_2ER	$S\bar{v}O_2$
↑	↓	N or ↑¶	N or ↑¶	↑	↓

*See Figure 4-3 and related discussion for the acute pH, $PaCO_2$, and HCO_3^- changes associated with acute alveolar hyperventilation.
†See Figure 4-2 and related discussion for the pH, $PaCO_2$, and HCO_3^- changes associated with chronic ventilatory failure.
†See TABLE 4-7 and related discussion for the pH, $PaCO_2$, and HCO_3^- changes associated with Acute Ventilatory Changes Superimposed on Chronic Ventilatory Failure.
§$C(a-\bar{v})O_2$, Arterial-venous oxygen difference; DO_2, total oxygen delivery; O_2ER, oxygen extraction ratio; $\dot{Q}_S/\dot{Q}_T$, pulmonary shunt fraction; $S\bar{v}O_2$, mixed venous oxygen saturation; $\dot{V}O_2$, oxygen consumption.
¶Increased if febrile
‖The DO_2 may be normal in patients who have compensated to the decreased oxygenation status with (1) an increased cardiac output, (2) an increased hemoglobin level, or (3) a combination of both. When the DO_2 is normal, the O_2ER is usually normal.

Hemodynamic Indices*
Severe Tuberculosis

CVP	RAP	$\overline{PA}$	PCWP	CO	SV
↑	↑	↑	N	N	N

SVI	CI	RVSWI	LVSWI	PVR	SVR
N	N	↑	N	↑	N

ABNORMAL LABORATORY TEST AND PROCEDURE RESULTS

- Positive tuberculosis skin test (PPD)
- Positive sputum acid-fast bacillus (AFB) stain test
- Positive ABF sputum culture
- Postive QuantiFERON-TB Gold Test

RADIOLOGIC FINDINGS
Chest Radiograph

- Increased opacity
- Ghon nodule
- Ghon complex
- Cavity formation
- Cavitary lesion containing an air-fluid level (see Figure 17-2)
- Pleural effusion

- Calcification and fibrosis
- Retraction of lung segments or lobe
- Right ventricular enlargement

Chest radiography is most valuable in the diagnosis of pulmonary TB. During the initial primary infection stage, peripheral pneumonic infiltrates (Ghon nodules) can be identified. As the disease progresses, the combination of tubercles and involvement of the lymph nodes in the hilar region (the Ghon complex) can be seen. In severe cases, cavity formation and pleural effusion are seen (Figure 18-7). Healed lesions appear fibrotic or calcified. Retraction of the healed lesions or segments also is revealed on chest radiographs. In patients with post primary TB of the lungs, lesions involving the apical and posterior segments of the upper lobes are often seen. In disseminated miliary tuberculosis, the lungs may show myriad 2- to 3-mm granulomatous foci. The radiographic result is widespread fine nodules that are uniformly distributed and equal in size (Figure 18-8). Finally, because right-sided heart failure (cor pulmonale) may develop as a secondary problem during the advanced stages of TB, an enlarged heart may be seen on the chest radiograph.

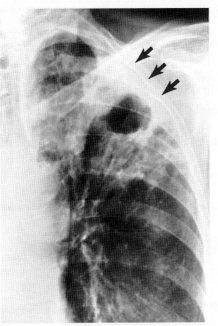

FIGURE 18-7 Cavitary reactivation tuberculosis showing a left upper lobe cavity and localized pleural thickening (*arrows*). (From Hansell DM, Armstrong P, Lynch DA, McAdams HP, eds: *Imaging of diseases of the chest*, ed 4, Philadelphia, 2005, Elsevier.)

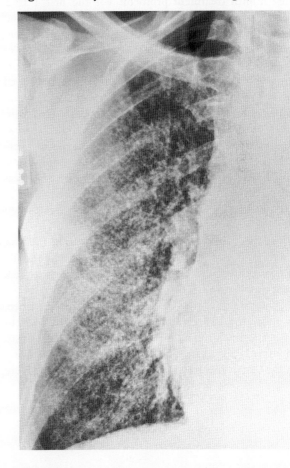

FIGURE 18-8 Miliary tuberculosis showing widespread uniformly distributed fine nodulation of the lung. (From Hansell DM, Armstrong P, Lynch DA, McAdams HP, eds: *Imaging of diseases of the chest*, ed 4, Philadelphia, 2005, Elsevier.)

*CO, Cardiac output; CVP, central venous pressure; LVSWI, left ventricular stroke work index; $\overline{PA}$, mean pulmonary artery pressure; PCWP, pulmonary capillary wedge pressure; PVR, pulmonary vascular resistance; RAP, right atrial pressure; RVSWI, right ventricular stroke work index; SV, stroke volume; SVI, stroke volume index; SVR, systemic vascular resistance.

General Management of Tuberculosis

Because the tubercle bacillus can exist in open cavitary lesions, in closed lesions, and within the cytoplasm of macrophages, a drug that may be effective in one of these environments may be ineffective in another. In addition, some of the TB bacilli are drug-resistant. Because of this problem, several drugs usually are prescribed *concurrently* for individuals with TB. Because toxicity is associated with some of the antituberculosis drugs, frequent examinations are performed to identify toxicity manifested in the kidneys, liver, eyes, and ears.

Pharmacologic Agents Used to Treat Tuberculosis

The standard pharmacologic agents used to treat *M. tuberculosis* consist of two to four drugs for 6 to 9 months. Examples of these protocols are as follows:

- **Six-month treatment protocol:** For the first 2 months (called the *induction phase*) the patient takes a daily dose of **isoniazid (INH), rifampin, pyrazinamide,** and either **ethambutol** or **streptomycin.** For the next 4 months the patient takes isoniazid and rifampin daily or twice weekly.
- **Nine-month treatment protocol:** For the first 1 to 2 months the patient takes a daily dose of isoniazid and rifampin, followed by twice-weekly isoniazid and rifampin until the full 9-month period has been completed.

Isoniazid (INH) and rifampin (Rifadin) are first-line agents prescribed for the entire 9 months. Isoniazid is considered to be the most effective first-line antituberculosis agent. Rifampin is bactericidal and is most commonly used with isoniazid. Although patients with TB usually are not contagious after a few weeks of treatment, a full course of treatment is necessary to kill all the bacteria. The **prophylactic use of isoniazid** is often prescribed as a daily dose for 1 year in individuals who have been exposed to the TB bacilli or who demonstrate a positive tuberculin reaction (even when the acid-fast sputum stain is negative).

When the TB bacterium is resistant to one or more of these agents, at least three or more antibiotics must be added to the treatment regimen and the duration should be extended. A major problem with TB therapy is noncompliance on the part of the patient to take the TB medication as prescribed. Even under the best circumstances, it is very difficult to maintain a regimen of multiple TB antibiotics on a daily basis for months. Unfortunately, most TB patients are not living under the best of circumstances. In addition, failure to adhere to an antibiotic regimen often leads to antibiotic resistance in the slow-growing microorganism. In fact, many *M. tuberculosis* isolates are now found to be multiple drug–resistant TB (MDRTB).

In response to the problem of noncompliance, it is recommended that all such patients with TB be treated by **directly observed therapy (DOT)**—that is, the ingestion of medication is directly observed by a responsible individual. In communities where DOT has been used, the rate of drug-resistant TB and the rate of TB relapse have been shown to decrease.

A new strain of drug-resistant *M. tuberculosis* was identified in Africa in 2006. It is especially lethal for HIV-infected individuals and has been named *extensively drug-resistant TB* (XDRTB).

Respiratory Care Treatment Protocols

Oxygen Therapy Protocol

Oxygen therapy is used to treat hypoxemia, decrease the work of breathing, and decrease myocardial work. Because of the hypoxemia associated with TB, supplemental oxygen may be required. The hypoxemia that develops in patients with lung abscess is usually caused by pulmonary capillary shunting. Hypoxemia caused by capillary shunting is often refractory to oxygen therapy (see Oxygen Therapy Protocol, Protocol 9-1).

Bronchopulmonary Hygiene Therapy Protocol

Because of the excessive mucus production and accumulation sometimes associated with severe TB, a number of bronchial hygiene treatment modalities may be used to enhance the mobilization of bronchial secretions (see Bronchopulmonary Hygiene Therapy Protocol, Protocol 9-2).

Mechanical Ventilation Protocol

Because acute ventilatory failure is occasionally associated with TB, mechanical ventilation may be required to maintain an adequate ventilatory status. Continuous mechanical ventilation is justified when the acute ventilatory failure is thought to be reversible—for example, when pneumonia complicates the condition (see Mechanical Ventilation Protocol 10-1 and Mechanical Ventilation Weaning Protocol 10-2).

Respiratory Isolation Protocol

Patients hospitalized with active tuberculosis are kept in **respiratory isolation** until three sputum AFB smears are negative, taken over three consecutive days.

Admitting History and Physical Examination

This 60-year-old male patient had been in good health until about 4 months before admission when he first noted the onset of night sweats, occasionally accompanied by chills. About 3 months ago he noted that his appetite was decreasing, and he lost about 25 pounds after that time.

Approximately 3 weeks before his admission, he noted that his long-standing "smoker's cough" had become more productive. For the 2 weeks before admission, his daily sputum production had increased to about a cup of thick yellow sputum with an occasional fleck or two of blood. There was a concomitant increase in dyspnea. About 10 days before admission, he had a gradual onset of moderately sharp left-sided chest pain. It was aggravated by deep breathing but did not radiate.

The past history gave little useful information. About 35 years previously, he was told during a routine medical exam that he had a positive TB skin test but that he had no pulmonary problems. Subsequently he had had several chest x-ray examinations in mobile chest x-ray units, once for an insurance application. The last x-ray examination was performed 5 years ago.

For the previous 35 years, he had been employed in a foundry as a "cone maker" and "shaker." He volunteered the information that he worked in a "dusty" environment and that he had worn a protective mask only for the previous few months. His family history was noncontributory. He and his wife lived in the same house with his married daughter and two young granddaughters.

Physical examination revealed a thin man who appeared to be both chronically and acutely ill. His vital signs were blood pressure 132/90, heart rate 116 beats/min, respiratory rate 32 breaths/min, and oral temperature 102.4° F. His room air SpO_2 was 90%. He was coughing up large amounts of yellow, blood-streaked sputum. There was marked dullness to percussion in both apical areas, and diffuse inspiratory and expiratory coarse crackles were present in the right upper and middle lobes. A chest x-ray film demonstrated extensive bilateral apical calcification, cavity formation in the right upper lobe, and diffuse infiltrate and consolidation in the right middle lobe. He was admitted to the hospital and placed in respiratory isolation. The following initial respiratory assessment was entered into the patient's chart.

Respiratory Assessment and Plan

S Productive cough, slight hemoptysis; moderate dyspnea. History of left-sided chest pain for 10 days.

O Febrile to 102.4° F. RR 32, HR 116, BP 132/90. Room air SpO_2 90%. Productive cough: large amounts yellow, blood-streaked sputum. Inspiratory and expiratory coarse crackles in right upper and middle lobes. CXR: Apical calcification; RUL cavity; RML infiltrate/consolidation.

A • Probable tuberculosis (patient possibly infectious)
  • Excessive airway secretions (yellow sputum, cough)
  • Mild hypoxemia (SpO_2 90%)

P Flag chart: Continue respiratory isolation pending AFB smear results. Obtain sputum for routine, anaerobic, and acid-fast cultures and cytology—induce if necessary. Obtain baseline ABG on room air. **Bronchopulmonary Hygiene Therapy Protocol:** C&DB q2h. Based on ABG results, titrate oxygen therapy per **Oxygen Therapy Protocol**. Discuss need for bedside spirogram with physician.

Discussion

Two primary clinical scenarios were activated in this case. First, the **Alveolar Consolidation** (see Figure 9-8) identified on the chest x-ray film reflected the patient's challenged immune response. This was further manifested by the objective data noted at the patient's bedside—fever, dull percussion notes, and increased heart rate, blood pressure, and respiratory rate. In addition, the alveolar consolidation undoubtedly contributed to the patient's pulmonary shunting and mild hypoxemia (see Figure 9-8).

Secondly, clinical manifestations associated with **Excessive Bronchial Secretions** (see Figure 9-11) also were present in this patient: daily cough, yellow sputum production, and coarse crackles. His oxygen desaturation was mild (SpO_2 = 90%), and a room air ABG and subsequent oxygen titration (presumably with low-flow oxygen by nasal cannula) were appropriate.

As expected, the patient produced sputum containing acid-fast organisms. The attending physician prescribed isoniazid, rifampin, and streptomycin for 2 months, followed by an outpatient course of isoniazid and rifampin for 4 months. The patient also was instructed regarding several different **Bronchopulmonary Hygiene Therapy** (see Protocol 9-2) to perform at home. He remained in the hospital for 14 days, until three consecutive sputum AFB smears were negative, and he was no longer febrile. The patient did well through 1 year of follow-up.

SELF-ASSESSMENT QUESTIONS

Answers to questions can be found on Evolve. To access additional student assessment questions visit **http://evolve.elsevier.com/DesJardins/respiratory**.

1. **Which of the following are known as the first stage of tuberculosis?**
   1. Reinfection tuberculosis
   2. Primary tuberculosis
   3. Secondary tuberculosis
   4. Primary infection stage
      a. 2 only
      b. 3 only
      c. 1 and 3 only
      d. 2 and 4 only

2. **What is the name of the protective wall that surrounds and encases lung tissue infected with tuberculosis?**
   1. Miliary tuberculosis
   2. Reinfection tuberculosis
   3. Granuloma
   4. Tubercle
      a. 1 only
      b. 3 only
      c. 4 only
      d. 3 and 4 only

3. **The tubercle bacillus is:**
   1. Highly aerobic
   2. Acid-fast
   3. Capable of surviving for months outside of the body
   4. Rod-shaped
      a. 2 only
      b. 4 only
      c. 2 and 3 only
      d. 1, 2, 3, and 4

4. **At which size wheal is a tuberculin skin test considered to be positive?**
   a. Greater than 4 mm
   b. Greater than 6 mm
   c. Greater than 8 mm
   d. Greater than 10 mm

5. **Which of the following is often prescribed as a prophylactic daily dose for 1 year in individuals who have been exposed to tuberculosis bacilli?**
   a. Streptomycin
   b. Ethambutol
   c. Isoniazid
   d. Rifampin

CHAPTER 19 Fungal Diseases of the Lung

Chapter Objectives

After reading this chapter, you will be able to:

- List the anatomic alterations of the lungs associated with fungal disease.
- Describe the causes of fungal disease.
- List the cardiopulmonary clinical manifestations associated with fungal disease.
- Describe the general management of fungal disease.
- Describe the clinical strategies and rationales of the SOAPs presented in the case study.

Key Terms

Acute Symptomatic Pulmonary Histoplasmosis
Allergic Bronchopulmonary Aspergillosis
Amphotericin B
Anidulafungin
Aspergillus
Asymptomatic Primary Histoplasmosis
Azoles
Blastomyces dermatitidis
Blastomycosis
"California Disease"
Candida albicans
Caseous Tubercles
Caspofungin
Cavity Formation
"Chicago Disease"
Chronic Histoplasmosis
Coccidioides immitis
Coccidioidomycosis
Cryptococcus neoformans
"Desert Arthritis"
"Desert Bumps"
"Desert Fever"
"Desert Rheumatism"
Disseminated Histoplasmosis
Echinocandins
Fluconazole
Gilchrist's Disease
Granulomas
Histoplasma capsulatum
Histoplasmin Skin Test
Histoplasmosis
Itraconazole
Ketoconazole
Micafungin
North American Blastomycosis
"Ohio Valley Fever"
"San Joaquin Valley Disease"
Thrush
"Valley Fever"

Chapter Outline

Anatomic Alterations of the Lungs
Etiology and Epidemiology
Primary Pathogens
   Histoplasmosis
   Coccidioidomycosis
   Blastomycosis
   Opportunistic Pathogens
Overview of the Cardiopulmonary Clinical Manifestations
   Associated with Fungal Diseases of the Lungs
General Management of Fungal Disease
   Respiratory Care Treatment Protocols
Case Study: Fungal Disease
Self-Assessment Questions

Anatomic Alterations of the Lungs

When fungal spores are inhaled, they may reach the lungs and germinate. When this happens, the spores produce a frothy, yeast-like substance that leads to an inflammatory response. Polymorphonuclear leukocytes and macrophages move into the infected area and engulf the fungal spores. The pulmonary capillaries dilate, the interstitium fills with fluid, and the alveolar epithelium swells with edema fluid. Regional lymph node involvement commonly occurs during this period. Because of the inflammatory reaction, the alveoli in the infected area eventually become consolidated (Figure 19-1). Airway secretions may also develop at this time.

In severe cases, tissue necrosis, **granulomas,** and cavity formation may be seen. During the healing process, fibrosis and calcification of the lung parenchyma ultimately replace the granulomas. In response to the fibrosis and occasional calcification, the lung tissue retracts and becomes firm. The apical and posterior segments of the upper lobes are most commonly involved. The anatomic changes of the lungs caused by fungal diseases are similar to those seen in tuberculosis.

Fungal diseases of the lung cause a chronic restrictive pulmonary disorder. The major pathologic or structural changes of the lungs associated with fungal diseases of the lungs are as follows:

- Alveolar consolidation
- Alveolar-capillary destruction
- Caseous tubercles or granulomas
- Cavity formation

283

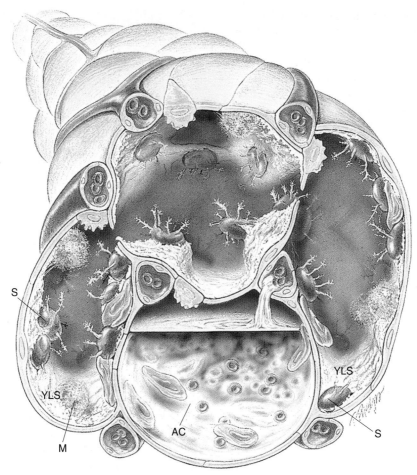

FIGURE 19-1 Fungal disease of the lung. Cross-sectional view of alveoli infected with *Histoplasma capsulatum.* *AC,* Alveolar consolidation; *M,* alveolar macrophage; *S,* fungal spore; *YLS,* yeastlike substance.

- Fibrosis and secondary calcification of the lung parenchyma
- Bronchial secretions

Etiology and Epidemiology

Fungal spores of various types are widely distributed throughout the air, soil, fomites, and animals, and even exist in the normal flora of humans. As many as 300 fungal species may be linked to disease in animals. In plants, fungal disease is the most common cause of death and destruction. In humans, most exposures to fungal pathogens do *not* lead to overt infection because humans have a relatively high resistance to them. Human fungal disease (also called *mycotic disease* or *mycosis*) can be caused by primary or "true" fungal pathogens that exhibit some degree of virulence or by opportunistic or secondary pathogens that take advantage of a weakened immune defense system (e.g., in acquired immunodeficiency syndrome and human immunodeficiency virus [HIV] infection).

Primary Pathogens

Histoplasmosis

Histoplasmosis is the most common fungal infection in the United States. It is caused by the dimorphic fungus *Histoplasma capsulatum*. In the United States, the prevalence of histoplasmosis is especially high along the major river valleys of the Midwest and South (e.g., in Ohio, Michigan, Illinois, Mississippi, Missouri, Kentucky, Tennessee, Georgia, and Arkansas). On the basis of skin test surveys it is estimated that 80% to 90% of the population throughout these areas shows signs of previous infection. Histoplasmosis is often called **Ohio Valley Fever**.

H. capsulatum is commonly found in soils enriched with bird excreta, such as the soil near chicken houses, pigeon lofts, barns, and trees where starlings and blackbirds roost. The birds themselves, however, do not carry the organism, although the *H. capsulatum* spore may be carried by bats. Generally, an individual acquires the infection by inhaling the fungal spores that are released when the soil from an infected area is disturbed (e.g., children playing in dirt).

When the *H. capsulatum* organism reaches the alveoli at body temperature, it converts from its mycelial form (mold) to a parasitic yeast form. The clinical manifestations of histoplasmosis are strikingly similar to those of tuberculosis. The incubation period for the infection is approximately 17 days. Only about 40% of those infected demonstrate symptoms, and only about 10% of these patients are ill enough to consult a physician. Depending on the individual's immune system, the disease may take one of the following forms: **asymptomatic primary histoplasmosis, acute symptomatic pulmonary histoplasmosis, chronic histoplasmosis,** or **disseminated histoplasmosis.**

Asymptomatic histoplasmosis is the most common form of histoplasmosis. Normally it produces no signs or symptoms in otherwise healthy individuals who become infected. The only residual sign of infection may be a small, healed lesion of the lung parenchyma or calcified hilar lymph nodes. The patient will have a positive **histoplasmin skin test** result, much like that for tuberculosis described in Chapter 18.

Acute symptomatic pulmonary histoplasmosis tends to occur in otherwise healthy individuals who have had an intense exposure to *H. capsulatum*. Depending on the number of spores inhaled, the individual signs and symptoms may range from mild to serious illness. Mild signs and symptoms include fever, muscle and joint pain, headache, dry hacking cough, chills, chest pain, weight loss, and sweats. People who have inhaled a large number of spores may develop a severe acute pulmonary syndrome, a potentially life-threatening condition in which the individual becomes extremely short of breath. This is often referred to as *spelunker's lung* because it frequently develops after excessive exposure to bat excrement stirred up by individuals exploring caves. During this phase of the disease, the patient's chest radiograph generally shows single or multiple infection sites resembling those associated with pneumonia.

Chronic pulmonary histoplasmosis is characterized by infiltration and cavity formation in the upper lobes of one or both lungs. This type of histoplasmosis often affects people with an underlying lung disease such as emphysema. It is most commonly seen in middle-aged white men who smoke. Signs and symptoms include fatigue, fever, night sweats, weight loss, productive cough, and hemoptysis—similar to signs and symptoms of tuberculosis. Often the infection is self-limiting. In some patients, however, progressive destruction of lung tissue and dissemination of the infection may occur.

Disseminated histoplasmosis may follow either self-limited histoplasmosis or chronic histoplasmosis. It is most often seen in very young or very old patients with compromised immune systems (e.g., patients with HIV infection). Even though the macrophages can remove the fungi from the bloodstream, they are unable to kill the fungal organisms. As a result, disseminated histoplasmosis can affect nearly any part of the body, including eyes, liver, bone marrow, skin, adrenal glands, and intestinal tract. Depending on which body organs are affected, the patient may develop anemia, pneumonia, pericarditis, meningitis, or adrenal insufficiency and ulcers of the mouth, tongue, or intestinal tract. If untreated, disseminated histoplasmosis is usually fatal.

Screening and Diagnosis

Fungal culture. The fungal culture test is considered the gold standard for detecting histoplasmosis. A small amount of blood, sputum, or tissue from a lymph node, lung, or bone marrow is cultured. The disadvantage of this test is that it takes time for the fungus to grow—4 weeks or longer. For this reason, it is not the test of choice in cases of disseminated histoplasmosis. Treatment delays in patients may prove fatal.

Fungal stain. In the fungal stain test, a tissue sample, which may be obtained from sputum, bone marrow, lungs, or a skin lesion, is stained with dye and examined under a microscope for *H. capsulatum* (Figure 19-2). A positive test

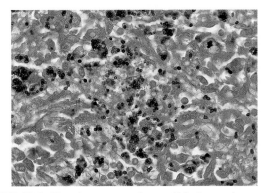

FIGURE 19-2 *Histoplasma capsulatum.* This is a micrograph of tissue infected with *H. capsulatum*, a fungus whose yeast cell stage causes the disease histoplasmosis. (From VanMeter KC, VanMeter WG, Hubert RJ: *Microbiology for the healthcare professional*, St. Louis, 2010, Mosby.)

result is 100% accurate. The disadvantage of this test is that obtaining a sputum sample can be difficult, and obtaining a sample from other sites requires invasive procedures.

Serology. A blood serology test checks blood serum for antigens and antibodies. When an individual is exposed to histoplasmosis spores (antigens), the body's immune system produces antibodies (proteins) to react to the histoplasmosis antigens. Tests that check for histoplasmosis antigen and antibody reactions are relatively fast and fairly accurate. False-negative results, however, may occur in people who have compromised immune systems or who are infected with other types of fungi.

Coccidioidomycosis

Coccidioidomycosis is caused by inhalation of the spores of *Coccidioides immitis*, which are spherical fungi carried by wind-borne dust particles. The disease is endemic in hot, dry regions. In the United States, coccidioidomycosis is especially prevalent in California, Arizona, Nevada, New Mexico, Texas, and Utah. About 80% of the people in the San Joaquin Valley have positive coccidioidin skin-test results. Because the prevalence of coccidioidomycosis is high in these regions, the disease is also known as **"California fever," "Desert rheumatism," "San Joaquin Valley Disease,"** and **"Valley Fever."** The fungus has been isolated in these regions from soils, plants, and a large number of vertebrates (e.g., mammals, birds, reptiles, and amphibians).

When *C. immitis* spores are inhaled, they settle in the lungs, begin to germinate, and form round, thin-walled cells called *spherules*. The spherules, in turn, contain endospores that make more spherules (the spherule-endospore phase). The disease usually takes the form of an acute, primary, self-limiting pulmonary infection with or without systemic involvement. Some cases, however, progress to disseminated disease.

Clinical manifestations are absent in about 60% of the people who have a positive skin-test result. In the remaining 40%, cold-like symptoms such as fever, chest pain, cough, headaches, and malaise are often present. In uncomplicated cases, patients generally recover completely and enjoy lifelong immunity. In approximately 1:200 cases, however, the primary infection does not resolve and progresses with

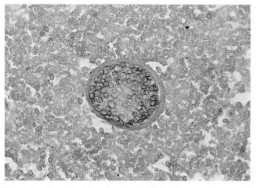

FIGURE 19-3 *Coccidioides immitis.* This is a micrograph of *C. immitis,* a dimorphic fungus that causes coccidioidomycosis. The numerous small spherules are seen within the large, encircling outer capsule. (From VanMeter KC, VanMeter WG, Hubert RJ: *Microbiology for the healthcare professional,* St. Louis, 2010, Mosby.)

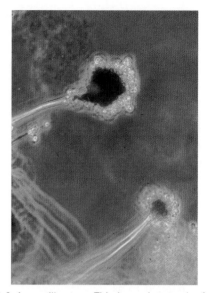

FIGURE 19-4 *Aspergillus* spp. This is a micrograph of *Aspergillus,* an opportunistic fungal pathogen that can cause a variety of diseases collectively called *aspergillosis.* (From VanMeter KC, VanMeter WG, Hubert RJ: *Microbiology for the healthcare professional,* St. Louis, 2010, Mosby.)

varied clinical manifestations. Chronic progressive pulmonary disease is characterized by nodular growths called *fungomas* and cavity formation in the lungs. Disseminated coccidioidomycosis occurs in about 1 : 6000 exposed persons. When this condition exists, the lymph nodes, meninges, spleen, liver, kidney, skin, and adrenals may be involved. The skin lesions (e.g., bumps on the face and chest) are commonly accompanied by arthralgia or arthritis, especially in the ankles and knees. This condition is commonly called **"desert bumps," "desert arthritis,"** or **"desert rheumatism."**

Screening and Diagnosis

The diagnosis of coccidioidomycosis can be made by direct visualization of distinctive spherules in microscopy of the patient's sputum, tissue exudates, biopsies, or spinal fluid (Figure 19-3). The diagnosis can be further supported by blood tests that detect antibodies to the fungus or from a culture of the organism from infected fluid or tissue.

Blastomycosis

Blastomycosis (also called **"Chicago disease," Gilchrist's disease,** and **North American blastomycosis**) is caused by *Blastomyces dermatitidis.* Blastomycosis occurs in people living in the south-central and midwestern United States and in Canada. The infection occurs in 1 to 2 of every 100,000 people in these areas. Cases also have been reported in Central America, South America, Africa, and the Middle East. *B. dermatitidis* inhabits areas high in organic matter, such as forest soil, decaying wood, animal manure, and abandoned buildings. Blastomycosis is most common among pregnant women and middle-aged African-American men. The disease also is found in dogs, cats, and horses.

The primary portal of entry of *B. dermatitidis* is the lungs. The acute clinical manifestations resemble those of acute histoplasmosis, including fever, cough, hoarseness, joint and muscle aches, and, in some cases, pleuritic pain. Unlike in histoplasmosis infection, however, the cough is frequently productive, and the sputum is purulent. Acute pulmonary infections may be self-limiting or progressive. When the condition is progressive, nodules and abscesses develop in the lungs. Extrapulmonary lesions commonly involve the skin,

bones, reproductive tract, spleen, liver, kidney, or prostate gland. The skin lesions may, in fact, be the first signs of the disease. It often begins on the face, hands, wrists, or legs as subcutaneous nodules that erode to the skin surface. Yeast dissemination also may cause arthritis and osteomyelitis, and involvement of the central nervous system causes headache, convulsions, coma, and mental confusion. Standardized serologic testing procedures for blastomycosis are not available, and neither is an accurate blastomycin skin test. The diagnosis of blastomycosis can be made from direct visualization of the yeast in sputum smears, or the fungus can be cultured.

Opportunistic Pathogens

Opportunistic yeast pathogens such as ***Candida albicans, Cryptococcus neoformans,*** and ***Aspergillus*** also are associated with lung infections in certain patients.

C. albicans occurs as normal flora in the oral cavity, genitalia, and large intestine. *C. albicans* infection of the mouth, or **thrush,** is characterized by a white, adherent, patchy infection of the mouth, gums, cheeks, and throat. In patients with HIV infection, *C. albicans* often causes infection of the mouth, pharynx, vagina, skin, and lungs.

C. neoformans proliferates in the high nitrogen content of pigeon droppings and is readily scattered into the air and dust. Today, *Cryptococcus* is most often seen in patients with HIV infection and persons undergoing steroid therapy.

Aspergillus may be the most pervasive of all fungi (Figure 19-4). *Aspergillus* is found in soil, vegetation, leaf detritus, food, and compost heaps. Persons breathing the air of granaries, barns, and silos are at greatest risk. *Aspergillus* infection usually occurs in the lungs where it may present in the form of **allergic bronchopulmonary aspergillosis,** a form of asthma (see Chapter 13). It is almost always an opportunistic infection and poses a serious threat to patients with HIV infection.

OVERVIEW of the Cardiopulmonary Clinical Manifestations Associated with Fungal Diseases of the Lungs

The following clinical manifestations result from the pathophysiologic mechanisms caused (or activated) by **Alveolar Consolidation** (see Figure 9-8) and, in severe cases, with fibrosis. Alveolar Consolidation and increased **Alveolar-Capillary Membrane Thickness** (see Figure 9-9) are the major anatomic alterations of the lungs associated with fungal diseases of the lungs (see Figure 19-1).[1]

CLINICAL DATA OBTAINED AT THE PATIENT'S BEDSIDE

The Physical Examination

Vital Signs

Increased Respiratory Rate (Tachypnea)

Several pathophysiologic mechanisms operating simultaneously may lead to an increased ventilatory rate:

- Stimulation of peripheral chemoreceptors
- Decreased lung compliance–increased ventilatory rate relationship
- Pain, anxiety, fever

Increased Heart Rate (Pulse) and Blood Pressure

Chest Pain, Decreased Chest Expansion
Cyanosis
Digital Clubbing
Peripheral Edema and Venous Distention

Because polycythemia and cor pulmonale are associated with severe fungal disease of the lungs, the following may be seen:

- Distended neck veins
- Pitting edema
- Enlarged and tender liver

Cough, Sputum Production, and Hemoptysis
Chest Assessment Findings

- Increased tactile and vocal fremitus
- Dull percussion note
- Bronchial breath sounds
- Crackles, wheezing
- Pleural friction rub (if process extends to pleural surface)
- Whispered pectoriloquy

CLINICAL DATA OBTAINED FROM LABORATORY TESTS AND SPECIAL PROCEDURES

Pulmonary Function Test Findings
(Moderate to Severe) (Restrictive Lung Pathology)

FORCED EXPIRATORY VOLUME AND FLOW RATE FINDINGS

FVC	FEV_T	FEV_1/FVC ratio	$FEF_{25\%-75\%}$
↓	N or ↓	N or ↑	N or ↓

$FEF_{50\%}$	$FEF_{200-1200}$	PEFR	MVV
N or ↓	N or ↓	N or ↓	N or ↓

LUNG VOLUME AND CAPACITY FINDINGS

V_T	IRV	ERV	RV	
N or ↓	↓	↓	↓	

VC	IC	FRC	TLC	RV/TLC ratio
↓	↓	↓	↓	N

Arterial Blood Gases

MODERATE FUNGAL DISEASE

Acute Alveolar Hyperventilation with Hypoxemia*
(Acute Respiratory Alkalosis)

pH	$PaCO_2$	HCO_3^-	PaO_2	SaO_2 or SpO_2
↑	↓	↓ (but normal)	↓	↓

SEVERE FUNGAL DISEASE WITH PULMONARY FIBROSIS

Chronic Ventilatory Failure with Hypoxemia[†]
(Compensated Respiratory Acidosis)

pH	$PaCO_2$	HCO_3^-	PaO_2	SaO_2 or SpO_2
N	↑	↑ (significantly)	↓	↓

ACUTE VENTILATORY CHANGES SUPERIMPOSED ON CHRONIC VENTILATORY FAILURE[‡]

Because acute ventilatory changes are frequently seen in patients with chronic ventilatory failure, the respiratory therapist must be familiar with—and alert for—the following dangerous arterial blood gas (ABG) findings:

- Acute alveolar hyperventilation superimposed on chronic ventilatory failure—which should further alert the respiratory therapist to record the following important ABG assessment: possible *impending acute ventilatory failure*.
- Acute ventilatory failure (acute hypoventilation) superimposed on chronic ventilatory failure.

Oxygenation Indices[§]
Moderate to Severe Stages

$\dot{Q}_S/\dot{Q}_T$	DO_2[‖]	$\dot{V}O_2$[¶]	$C(a-\bar{v})O_2$[¶]	O_2ER	$S\bar{v}O_2$
↑	↓	N or ↑	N or ↑	↑	↓

---

*See Figure 4-3 and related discussion for the acute pH, $PaCO_2$, and HCO_3^- changes associated with acute alveolar hyperventilation.

[†]See Figure 4-2 and related discussion for the pH, $PaCO_2$, and HCO_3^- changes associated with chronic ventilatory failure.

[‡]See TABLE 4-7 and related discussion for the pH, $PaCO_2$, and HCO_3^- changes associated with Acute Ventilatory Changes Superimpoosed on Chronic Ventilatory Failure.

[§]$C(a-\bar{v})O_2$, Arterial-venous oxygen difference; DO_2, total oxygen delivery; O_2ER, oxygen extraction ratio; $\dot{Q}_S/\dot{Q}_T$, pulmonary shunt fraction; $S\bar{v}O_2$, mixed venous oxygen saturation; $\dot{V}O_2$, oxygen consumption.

[‖]The DO_2 may be normal in patients who have compensated to the decreased oxygenation status with (1) an increased cardiac output, (2) an increased hemoglobin level, or (3) a combination of both. When the DO_2 is normal, the O_2ER is usually normal.

[¶]Increased if febrile.

---

[1]In allergic bronchopulmonary aspergillosis, airway obstruction is the major presenting complaint, with refractory wheezing (see Figure 9-10).

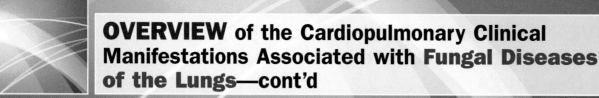
Hemodynamic Indices
Severe Fungal Disease

CVP	RAP	$\overline{PA}$	PCWP	CO	SV
↑	↑	↑	N	N	N

SVI	CI	RVSWI	LVSWI	PVR	SVR
N	N	↑	N	↑	N

ABNORMAL LABORATORY TEST AND PROCEDURE RESULTS

Radiologic Findings
Chest Radiograph

- Increased opacity
- Cavity formation
- Pleural effusion
- Calcification and fibrosis
- Right ventricular enlargement

During the early stages of many pulmonary fungal infections, localized infiltration and consolidation with or without lymph node involvement are commonly seen (Figure 19-5). Single or numerous spherical nodules may be seen (Figure 19-6). During

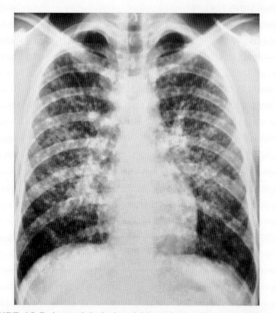

FIGURE 19-5 Acute inhalational histoplasmosis in an otherwise healthy patient. This young man developed fever and cough after tearing down an old barn. The radiograph shows bilateral hilar adenopathy and diffuse nodular opacities. (From Hansell DM, Armstrong P, Lynch DA, McAdams HP, eds: *Imaging of diseases of the chest*, ed 4, Philadelphia, 2005, Elsevier.)

CO, Cardiac output; *CVP*, central venous pressure; *LVSWI*, left ventricular stroke work index; *PA*, mean pulmonary artery pressure; *PCWP*, pulmonary capillary wedge pressure; *PVR*, pulmonary vascular resistance; *RAP*, right atrial pressure; *RVSWI*, right ventricular stroke work index; *SV*, stroke volume; *SVI*, stroke volume index; *SVR*, systemic vascular resistance.

the advanced stages, bilateral cavities in the apical and posterior segments of the upper lobes are often seen (Figure 19-7). In disseminated disease a diffuse bilateral micronodular pattern and pleural effusion may be seen. Fibrosis and calcification of healed lesions can be identified. Finally, because right-sided heart failure may develop as a secondary problem during the advanced stages of fungal disease, an enlarged heart may be seen on the chest radiograph. These radiologic findings are very similar to those seen in pulmonary tuberculosis.

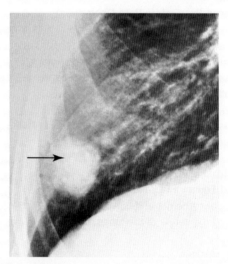

FIGURE 19-6 Histoplasmoma, showing a well-defined spherical nodule. The central portion of the nodule shows calcification. (From Hansell DM, Armstrong P, Lynch DA, McAdams HP, eds: *Imaging of diseases of the chest*, ed 4, Philadelphia, 2005, Elsevier.)

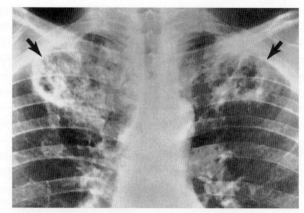

FIGURE 19-7 Chronic cavitary histoplasmosis. Note the striking upper zone predominance of the shadows resembling tuberculosis. Numerous large cavities. (From Hansell DM, Armstrong P, Lynch DA, McAdams HP, eds: *Imaging of diseases of the chest*, ed 4, Philadelphia, 2005, Elsevier.)

General Management of Fungal Disease

Amphotericin B is the treatment of choice for most fungal infections. However, because of the high incidence of nephrotoxicity associated with amphotericin B, the *azole* antifungal agents now serve as an excellent alternative. Although **ketoconazole** was the first agent in this class, it has largely been replaced with fluconazole and **itraconazole**. In addition, a new class of antifungals known as the *echinocandins* is now available. Common antifungal agents, including route and clinical use, are summarized in Table 19-1.

Respiratory Care Treatment Protocols

Oxygen Therapy Protocol

Oxygen therapy is used to treat hypoxemia, decrease the work of breathing, and decrease myocardial work. Because of the hypoxemia associated with the fungal pulmonary condition, supplemental oxygen may be required. Because of the alveolar consolidation produced by a fungal disorder, capillary shunting may be present. Hypoxemia caused by capillary shunting is often refractory to oxygen therapy (see Oxygen Therapy Protocol, Protocol 9-1).

Bronchopulmonary Hygiene Therapy Protocol

Because of the excessive production and accumulation of mucus sometimes associated with fungal disease, a number of bronchial hygiene treatment modalities may be used to enhance the mobilization of bronchial secretions (see Bronchopulmonary Hygiene Therapy Protocol, Protocol 9-2).

Mechanical Ventilation Protocol

Mechanical ventilation may be necessary to provide and support alveolar gas exchange and eventually return the patient to spontaneous breathing. Because acute ventilatory failure is occasionally seen in patients with severe fungal disease, continuous mechanical ventilation may be required. Continuous mechanical ventilation is justified when the acute ventilatory failure is thought to be reversible (see Mechanical Ventilation Protocol, Protocol 10-1, and Mechanical Ventilation Weaning Protocol, Protocol 10-2).

TABLE 19-1 Antifungal Agents

Antifungal Class and Generic Name	Brand Name and Route	Common Uses (Microorganisms)
Polyenes		
Amphotericin B	Fungizone IV, PO*	*Candida* spp., *Aspergillus* spp., *Cryptococcus neoformans, Histoplasma capsulatum, Blastomyces dermatitidis, Coccidioides immitis*
Amphotericin B colloidal dispersion (Amphotec)	Amphotec IV	*Candida* spp., *Aspergillus* spp., mucormycosis, *C. neoformans*
Amphotericin B lipid complex	Abelcet IV	*Candida* spp., *Aspergillus* spp., mucormycosis, *C. neoformans*
Liposomal amphotericin B	AmBisome IV	*Candida* spp., *Aspergillus* spp., mucormycosis, *C. neoformans, leishmaniasis*
Azoles		
Ketoconazole	Nizoral PO	*Candida* spp.[†], *C. neoformans, H. capsulatum, B. dermatitidis*
Fluconazole	Diflucan IV, PO	*Candida* spp.[†], *C. neoformans*
Itraconazole	Sporanox PO	*Candida* spp.[†], *Aspergillus* spp., *C. neoformans, H. capsulatum, B. dermatitidis, C. immitis, Sporothrix schenckii*
Voriconazole	Vfend IV, PO	*Candida* spp.[†], *Aspergillus* spp., *C. neoformans, C. immitis, H. capsulatum, B. dermatitidis, Fusarium* spp., *Scedosporium* spp.
Posaconazole	Noxafil PO	*Candida* spp.[†], *Aspergillus* spp., *C. neoformans, C. immitis, H. capsulatum, B. dermatitidis, Fusarium* spp., *Scedosporium* spp.
Echinocandins		
Caspofungin	Cancidas IV	*Aspergillus* spp., *Candida* spp.
Micafungin	Mycamine IV	*Aspergillus* spp., *Candida* spp.
Anidulafungin	Eraxis IV	*Aspergillus* spp., *Candida* spp.
Other Antifungals		
Flucytosine	Ancobon PO	*Aspergillus* spp., *Candida* spp., *C. neoformans*
Griseofulvin	Fulvicin PO	Tinea corporis, tinea cruris, tinea barbae, tinea capitis, and tinea unguium
Terbinafine	Lamisil PO, TOP	Tinea corporis, tinea pedis, tinea manuum, tinea cruris, tinea imbricata, tinea capitis, and tinea unguium

Modified from Gardenhire DS: *Rau's respiratory care pharmacology*, ed 8, 2012, Elsevier/Mosby.
IV, Intravenous; *PO*, oral; *TOP*, topical.
*The oral form of amphotericin B is not absorbed through the gastrointestinal tract.
[†]*Candida krusei* is intrinsically resistant to all azoles.

Admitting History

A 56-year-old cattle driver was admitted to the arthritis clinic of a small hospital just outside Phoenix, Arizona, because of joint pain. The man stated that the tenderness in his joints prevented him from riding his horse for any extended period. He was born on a cattle ranch in New Mexico and spent most of his adult life working as a cattle driver in Arizona, New Mexico, and Colorado. He had always considered himself an "outdoors" kind of man. He loved the range, wide open spaces, clear air, and beauty of the desert.

In his early 20s he traveled to the East Coast to attend college. While there, he became withdrawn and depressed and felt confined. After 1 year he dropped out of college and returned to New Mexico. Shortly after returning home, his symptoms of depression disappeared. He worked on a large cattle ranch, made several new friends, and was content with the fact that he "belonged on the open range." He never married or settled down in one place he could call home. He often said that the great outdoors was his home. He never owned an automobile; in fact, he often said that the only things of real value he owned were a roan quarter horse and a saddle.

The hospital had no past medical records for the patient. The man reported, however, that although he was rarely ill, he had seen a doctor in Colorado about a year ago for severe "cold" symptoms, which included fever, cough, chest pain, headaches, and a general feeling of fatigue. He was a nonsmoker, although he did chew tobacco for a short time in his teens. The patient verified that he consumed alcohol regularly on Friday and Saturday nights; he estimated that on average he drank between 6 and 10 beers per outing and sometimes more. Despite the patient's somewhat rugged living conditions and alcohol consumption, he was not overweight and was in reasonably good physical condition.

Physical Examination

The patient was a well-developed, well-nourished white man in moderate respiratory distress. He complained of soreness and stiffness in all his joints. He also stated that he thought he had a "bad cold" and that he was short of breath.

The patient's knees and ankle joints were warm, swollen, and tender to the touch. Although his skin appeared weathered and tan, his lips and nail beds were cyanotic. He demonstrated a frequent cough that produced a moderate amount of thick, yellow sputum. Although the cough was strong, he experienced difficulty expectorating sputum during each coughing episode. His vital signs were as follows: blood pressure 160/90, heart rate 90 beats/min, respiratory rate 18 breaths/min, and oral temperature $37.8°C$ ($100°F$). Palpation revealed a few erythematous lesions on his anterior chest, of which he was unaware. In addition, a walnut-sized erythematous lesion was present on the patient's left cheek. Percussion of the chest was not remarkable. Auscultation revealed bilateral coarse crackles in the lung apices.

The patient's chest radiographic film showed scattered infiltrates consistent with fibrosis and calcification and multiple spherical nodules throughout both lungs. In the upper lobes of both lungs, two or three small, 1- to 3-cm cavities were visible. On room air the patient's ABGs were pH 7.51, $PaCO_2$ 29 mm Hg, HCO_3^- 22 mEq/L, PaO_2 64 mm Hg, and SaO_2 94%. The patient was admitted to the hospital, and a respiratory care consultation was requested. On the basis of these clinical data, the following SOAP was documented.

Respiratory Assessment and Plan

S "I feel short of breath, and my joints are swollen and painful."

O Cyanosis; cough: frequent and strong, producing moderate amounts of thick, yellow sputum; vital signs: BP 160/90, HR 90, RR 18, temperature $37.8°C$ ($100°F$); palpation: red lesions on anterior chest and left cheek; auscultation: bilateral coarse crackles in lung apices; chest radiograph: bilateral fibrosis, calcification, and spherical nodules; two to three 1- to 3-cm cavities in both upper lobes; ABGs (room air): pH 7.51, $PaCO_2$ 29, HCO_3^- 22, PaO_2 64, SaO_2 94%.

A • Moderate respiratory distress (cyanosis, vital signs)
   • Large amounts of thick, yellow secretions (sputum, rhonchi)
   • Infection likely (yellow sputum)
   • Pulmonary fibrosis, calcification, and cavities (chest radiograph)
   • Acute alveolar hyperventilation with mild hypoxemia (ABGs)

P Initiate **Oxygen Therapy Protocol** (2 L/min per nasal cannula) and **Bronchopulmonary Hygiene Therapy Protocol** (deep breathing and coughing instruction, PD to both upper lobes each shift for 3 days). Order sputum culture (routine, acid-fast bacillus, and fungal). Encourage fluid intake. Monitor (oximeter, I&O).

5 Days after Admission

After microscopy of the patient's sputum and a spherulin skin test, coccidioidomycosis was diagnosed. The patient had been receiving amphotericin B intravenously for 2 days. A complete pulmonary function study revealed a moderate-to-severe restrictive disorder, with a moderate obstructive component as well.

When the respiratory therapist entered the patient's room, the man was sitting up in bed, appearing cyanotic, short of breath, and fatigued. He stated that he was becoming tired of people in white outfits coming in and out of his room, day and night, with "needles, pills, and bills." He further stated that he still could not get a good breath of air. In fact, he said it was more difficult for him to breathe today than it had been on the day he entered the hospital.

The patient still had a frequent, strong cough productive of moderate amounts of thick, opaque sputum. His vital signs were as follows: blood pressure 165/95, heart rate 96 beats/min, respiratory rate 24 breaths/min, and temperature 37°C (98.6°F). Auscultation revealed persistent bilateral tight wheezes, and bilateral coarse crackles in the apices of both lungs. A current chest x-ray film was not available. His ABGs on 2 L/min cannula were pH 7.54, $PaCO_2$ 27 mm Hg, HCO_3^- 21 mEq/L, PaO_2 55 mm Hg, and SaO_2 92%. At this time, the following SOAP was charted.

Respiratory Assessment and Plan

S "I still can't get a good breath of air."

O Respiratory distress: cyanotic, short of breath; positive spherulin skin test; coccidioidomycosis organisms seen on sputum smear; frequent strong cough: moderate amount of thick, opaque sputum; vital signs: BP 165/95, HR 96, RR 24, temperature normal; bilateral tight wheezes and coarse crackles in the lung apices; ABGs: pH 7.54, $PaCO_2$ 27, HCO_3^- 21, PaO_2 55, SaO_2 92%.

A • Coccidioidomycosis (positive spherulin skin test, sputum smear)
  • Continued respiratory distress (cyanosis, vital signs)
  • Bronchospasm (bilateral tight wheezes)
  • Excessive amounts of thick bronchial secretions (sputum, coarse crackles)
  • Acute alveolar hyperventilation with moderate hypoxemia (worsening ABGs)

P Up-regulate **Oxygen Therapy Protocol** (3 L/min nasal cannula). Add **Aerosolized Medication Protocol and** up-regulate **Bronchopulmonary Hygiene Therapy Protocol** (2 mL 10% acetylcysteine with 0.2 mL albuterol q6h, followed by deep breathing and coughing and PD to both upper lobes). Add supervised use of flutter valve 2 times per shift. Request repeat chest radiograph. Continue to monitor and reevaluate.

10 Days after Admission

On this day, the respiratory therapist found the patient walking up and down the corridor talking to various staff members and patients. The man appeared to be in no respiratory distress. He stated that he was breathing much better and was ready to ride his horse a long distance in any direction away from the hospital.

No spontaneous cough was noted. When asked to generate a cough, the patient produced a strong, nonproductive cough. His vital signs were as follows: blood pressure 135/88, heart rate 80 beats/min, respiratory rate 14 breaths/min, and normal temperature. Auscultation revealed persistent bilateral crackles in the apices of both lungs. A recent chest x-ray film was not available. His ABGs were pH 7.44, $PaCO_2$ 34 mm Hg, HCO_3^- 23 mEq/L, PaO_2 71 mm Hg and SaO_2 95%. On the basis of these clinical data, the following SOAP note was written.

Respiratory Assessment and Plan

S "I'm breathing much better."

O No obvious respiratory distress; no spontaneous cough; strong, nonproductive cough on request; vital signs: BP135/88, HR 80, RR 14, temperature normal; bilateral crackles in the lung apices; ABGs: pH 7.44, $PaCO_2$ 34, HCO_3^- 23, PaO_2 71, SaO_2 95%.

A • Adequate bronchial hygiene status (nonproductive cough, crackles expected in lung fibrosis)
  • Normal acid-base status with mild hypoxemia (ABGs)

P Discontinue Oxygen Therapy Protocol. Recheck SpO_2 on room air ("spot check") in 1 hour. Discontinue Bronchopulmonary Hygiene Therapy Protocol and Aerosolized Medication Protocol.

Discussion

Respiratory therapists who work in the Southwest, where coccidioidomycosis is endemic, would probably anticipate this diagnosis in the patient with bilateral pulmonary infiltrates, swollen tender joints, and the skin rash typical of this lesion. Others could not be blamed if they missed this potential diagnosis until the coccidioidal skin test came back positive and the sputum fungal smear demonstrated the presence of the coccidioidomycosis organism. In this case, the patient demonstrated the clinical manifestations associated with the following two anatomic alterations of the lungs: **Increased Alveolar-Capillary Membrane Thickness** (e.g., bilateral fibrosis and calcification; see Figure 9-9) and **Excessive Bronchial Secretions** (e.g., cough, sputum, and rhonchi; see Figure 9-11).

The first assessment was correct: The patient was hypoxemic despite alveolar hyperventilation and he had alveolar fibrosis and cavity formation. For the hypoxemia, oxygen therapy was appropriately started with a nasal oxygen cannula at 1 to 2 L/min and then regulated with a pulse oximeter. In treating this patient, as with any other patient with pneumonia, the assessing respiratory therapist should quickly obtain sputum for Gram stain, acid-fast bacillus, and fungal testing; this was appropriately done in this case.

In the second assessment, the offending organism had been isolated and appropriate therapy with intravenous amphotericin B was started. The patient was still hypoxemic, and up-regulation of his **Oxygen Therapy** (perhaps to 3 or 4 L/min) was indicated. In addition, if the patient continued to respond poorly to oxygen therapy, refractory hypoxemia and continuous positive airway pressure should have been considered.

Because the patient was still wheezing and coughing up thick, opaque sputum and his dyspnea was not relieved, up-regulation of the **Bronchopulmonary Hygiene Therapy Protocol** and addition of the **Aerosolized Medication Protocol** with a trial of bronchodilator therapy and mucolytic therapy were in order. A repeat chest x-ray also appears to be indicated.

At the last assessment 10 days after the patient's hospital admission, clear improvement was noted. Oximetry revealed good peripheral oxygen saturation, and the blood gases were much improved. This was the time for the treating therapist to reduce the intensity of the patient's respiratory care, and this step is illustrated in the appropriate response for this section of the case study. Follow-up pulmonary function testing 6 to 12 months after the abatement of acute illness would be worthwhile.

SELF-ASSESSMENT QUESTIONS

Answers to questions can be found on Evolve. To access additional student assessment questions visit **http://evolve.elsevier.com/DesJardins/respiratory**.

1. Which of the following is the most common fungal infection in the United States?
   a. Coccidioidomycosis
   b. Histoplasmosis
   c. San Joaquin Valley disease
   d. Blastomycosis

2. Incidence of histoplasmosis is especially high in which of the following area(s)?
   1. Arizona
   2. Mississippi
   3. Nevada
   4. Texas
      a. 2 only
      b. 4 only
      c. 2 and 4 only
      d. 2 and 3 only

3. The condition called "desert bumps," "desert arthritis," or "desert rheumatism" is associated with which fungal disorder?
   a. Histoplasmosis
   b. Blastomycosis
   c. Coccidioidomycosis
   d. Aspergillosis

4. Which of the following is or are used to treat fungal diseases?
   1. Streptomycin
   2. Amphotericin B
   3. Penicillin G
   4. Itraconazole
      a. 1 only
      b. 2 only
      c. 4 only
      d. 2 and 4 only

5. Which of the following forms of histoplasmosis is characterized by healed lesions in the hilar lymph nodes as well as a positive histoplasmin skin test response?
   a. Disseminated infection
   b. Latent asymptomatic disease
   c. Chronic histoplasmosis
   d. Self-limiting primary disease

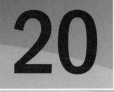

20 Pulmonary Edema

Chapter Objectives

After reading this chapter, you will be able to:
- List the anatomic alterations of the lungs associated with pulmonary edema.
- Describe the causes of pulmonary edema.
- List the cardiopulmonary clinical manifestations associated with cardiogenic and non-cardiogenic pulmonary edema.
- Describe the general management of pulmonary edema.
- Describe the clinical strategies and rationales of the SOAPs presented in the case study.

Key Terms

Afterload Reduction
Albumin
Angiotensin-Converting Enzyme (ACE) Inhibitors
Antidysrhythmic Agents
Brain Natriuretic Peptide (BNP)
Bretylium
Calcium Channel Blockers
Captopril
Cardiogenic Pulmonary Edema
Cardiomegaly
Cephalogenic Pulmonary Edema
Cheyne-Stokes Respiation
Congestive Heart Failure (CHF)
Decompression Pulmonary Edema
Digitalis
Direct-Acting Vasodilators
Dobutamine
Dopamine
Echocardiogram
High Altitude Pulmonary Edema
Hydralazine
Increased Capillary Permeability
Indirect-Acting Vasodilators

Isosorbide
Kerley A and B Lines
Left Ventricular Ejection Fraction (LVEF)
Lisinopril
Mannitol
Mask Continuous Positive Airway Pressure (CPAP)
Metoprolol
Minoxidil
Morphine Sulfate
Nifedipine
Nitroglycerin
Nitroprusside
Noncardiogenic Pulmonary Edema
Oncotic Pressure
Orthopnea
Paroxysmal Nocturnal Dyspnea (PND)
Positive Inotropic Agent
Prazosin
Procainamide
Starling's Equation
Transudate
Trimazosin
Verapamil

Chapter Outline

Anatomic Alterations of the Lungs

Pulmonary edema results from excessive movement of fluid from the pulmonary vascular system to the extravascular system and air spaces of the lungs. Fluid first seeps into the perivascular and peribronchial interstitial spaces; depending on the degree of severity, fluid may progressively move into the alveoli, bronchioles, and bronchi (Figure 20-1).

As a consequence of this fluid movement, the alveolar walls and interstitial spaces swell. As the swelling intensifies, the alveolar surface tension increases and causes alveolar shrinkage and atelectasis. Moreover, much of the fluid that accumulates in the tracheobronchial tree is churned into a frothy white (sometimes blood-tinged or pink) sputum as a result of air moving in and out of the lungs. The abundance of fluid in the interstitial spaces causes the lymphatic vessels to widen and the lymph flow to increase.

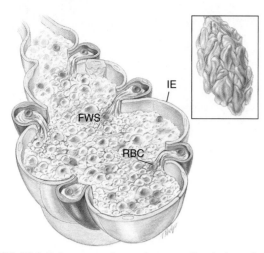

FIGURE 20-1 Pulmonary edema. Cross-sectional view of alveoli and alveolar duct in pulmonary edema. *FWS,* Frothy white secretions; *IE,* interstitial edema; *RBC,* red blood cell. *Inset,* Atelectasis, a common secondary anatomic alteration of the lungs.

Pulmonary edema produces a restrictive pulmonary disorder. The major pathologic or structural changes of the lungs associated with pulmonary edema are as follows:

- Interstitial edema, including fluid engorgement of the perivascular and peribronchial spaces and the alveolar wall interstitium
- Alveolar flooding
- Increased surface tension of alveolar fluids
- Alveolar shrinkage and atelectasis
- Frothy white (or pink) secretions throughout the tracheobronchial tree

Etiology and Epidemiology

The causes of pulmonary edema can be divided into two major categories: *cardiogenic* and *noncardiogenic*.

Cardiogenic Pulmonary Edema

The most common cause of cardiac pulmonary edema is left-sided heart failure—commonly called **congestive heart failure (CHF).** According to the Centers for Disease Control and Prevention (CDC), over 5 million people in the United States have CHF—or about 1.7% of the overall population. About 550,000 new cases of CHF are diagnosed annually. Heart failure is most common in people over age 65 years and is more common in African-Americans. CHF is a leading cause of hospitalization in people over the age of 65 years and is estimated to be a contributing factor to nearly 300,000 deaths annually. As the median age of the U.S. population of "baby boomers" continues to grow older—between the present and 2040—the number of patients diagnosed with CHF will undoubtedly continue to rise. The mortality rate for patients with CHF is about 12% in the first 30 days after admission to the hospital, and 50% within 5 years of diagnosis.

Cardiac pulmonary edema occurs when the left ventricle is unable to pump out a sufficient amount of blood during each ventricular contraction. The ability of the left ventricle to pump blood can be determined by means of the **left ventricular ejection fraction (LVEF)**—a noninvasive, cardiac imaging procedure **Echocardiogram** that reflects the patient's left ventricular *systolic* cardiac contractility. A poor ventricular function may also be caused by an increased ventricular stiffness or impaired myocardial relaxation. This condition is called *diastolic* dysfunction and is currently associated with a relatively normal LVEF. Normal values for the LVEF range between 55% and 70%. An LVEF less than 40% may confirm heart failure; an LVEF less than 35% is life threatening and cardiac arrhythmias are likely.

When the patient's LVEF is low, the blood pressure inside the pulmonary veins and capillaries increases as a result. This action literally causes fluid to be pushed through the capillary walls and into the alveoli in the form of a **transudate.** The basic pathophysiologic mechanism for this action is described in the following sections.

Ordinarily, hydrostatic pressure of about 10 to 15 mm Hg tends to move fluid *out* of the pulmonary capillaries into the interstitial space. This force is normally offset by colloid osmotic forces of about 25 to 30 mm Hg that tend to keep fluid *in* the pulmonary capillaries. The colloid osmotic pressure is referred to as **oncotic pressure** and is produced by the **albumin** and globulin in the blood. The stability of fluid within the pulmonary capillaries is determined by the balance between hydrostatic and oncotic pressure. This relationship also maintains fluid stability in the interstitial compartments of the lung.

Movement of fluid in and out of the capillaries is expressed by **Starling's equation:**

$$J = K(Pc - Pi) - (\pi c - \pi i)$$

where J is the net fluid movement out of the capillary, K is the capillary permeability factor, Pc and Pi are the hydrostatic pressures in the capillary and interstitial space, and πc and πi are the oncotic pressures in the capillary and interstitial space.

Although conceptually valuable, this equation has limited practical use. Of the four pressures, only the oncotic and hydrostatic pressures of blood in the pulmonary capillaries can be measured with any certainty. The oncotic and hydrostatic pressures within the interstitial compartments cannot be readily determined.

When the hydrostatic pressure within the pulmonary capillaries rises to more than 25 to 30 mm Hg, the oncotic pressure loses its holding force over the fluid within the pulmonary capillaries. Consequently, fluid starts to spill into the interstitial and air spaces of the lungs (Figure 20-1).

Clinically, the patient with left ventricular failure often has activity intolerance, weight gain, anxiety, delirium, dyspnea, orthopnea, paroxysmal nocturnal dyspnea, cough, fatigue, cardiac arrhythmias (particularly atrial fibrillation), and adventitious breath sounds. Because of poor peripheral circulation, such patients often have cool skin, diaphoresis, cyanosis of the digits, and peripheral pallor. Major organ failure of the brain and kidney may be the result of hypoperfusion. Increased pulmonary capillary hydrostatic pressure is the most common cause of pulmonary edema. Box 20-1 provides common causes of **cardiogenic pulmonary edema.** Box 20-2 provides common risk factors for coronary heart disease (CHD).

Noncardiogenic Pulmonary Edema

There are numerous noncardiogenic causes of pulmonary edema. In these conditions, fluid can readily flow from the pulmonary capillaries into the alveoli. The more common conditions include those discussed in the following paragraphs.

Increased Capillary Permeability

Pulmonary edema may develop as a result of **increased capillary permeability** stemming from infectious, inflammatory, and other processes. The following are some causes of increased capillary permeability:

- Alveolar hypoxia
- Acute respiratory distress syndrome (ARDS)
- Inhalation of toxic agents such as chlorine, sulfur dioxide, nitrogen dioxides, ammonia, and phosgene
- Pulmonary infections (e.g., pneumonia)
- Therapeutic radiation of the lungs
- Acute head injury (also known as **cephalogenic pulmonary edema**)

Lymphatic Insufficiency

Should the normal lymphatic drainage of the lungs be decreased, intravascular and extravascular fluid begins to pool, and pulmonary edema ensues. Lymphatic drainage may be slowed because of obliteration or distortion of lymphatic vessels. The lymphatic vessels may be obstructed by tumor cells in lymphangitic carcinomatosis. Because the lymphatic vessels empty into systemic veins, increased systemic venous pressure may slow lymphatic drainage. Lymphatic insufficiency also has been observed after lung transplantation.

Decreased Intrapleural Pressure

Reduced intrapleural pressure may cause pulmonary edema. With severe airway obstruction, for example, the negative pressure exerted by the patient during inspiration may create a suction effect on the pulmonary capillaries and cause fluid to move into the alveoli. Furthermore, the increased negative intrapleural pressure promotes filling of the right side of the heart and hinders blood flow in the left side of the heart. This condition may cause pooling of the blood in the lungs and subsequently an elevated hydrostatic pressure and pulmonary edema. A related kind of pulmonary edema is caused by the sudden removal of a pleural effusion. Clinically, this condition is called **decompression pulmonary edema.**

Decreased Oncotic Pressure

Although this condition is rare, if the oncotic pressure is reduced from its normal 25 to 30 mm Hg and falls below the patient's normal hydrostatic pressure of 10 to 15 mm Hg, fluid may begin to seep into the interstitial and air spaces of the lungs. Decreased oncotic pressure may be caused by the following:

- Overtransfusion and/or rapid transfusion of intravenous fluids
- Uremia
- Hypoproteinemia (e.g., severe malnutrition)
- Acute nephritis
- Polyarteritis nodosa

Although the exact mechanisms are not known, Box 20-3 provides other causes of conditions associated with **noncardiogenic pulmonary edema.**

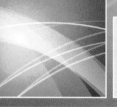

OVERVIEW of the Cardiopulmonary Clinical Manifestations Associated with Pulmonary Edema

The following clinical manifestations result from the pathologic mechanisms caused (or activated) by Atelectasis (see Figure 9-7), Increased Alveolar-Capillary Membrane Thickness (see Figure 9-9), and, in severe cases, Excessive Bronchial Secretions (see Figure 9-11)—the major anatomic alterations of the lungs associated with pulmonary edema (Figure 20-1).

CLINICAL DATA OBTAINED AT THE PATIENT'S BEDSIDE

The Physical Examination

Vital Signs

Increased Respiratory Rate (Tachypnea)

Several pathophysiologic mechanisms operating simultaneously may lead to an increased ventilatory rate:
- Stimulation of peripheral chemoreceptors (hypoxemia)
- Decreased lung compliance–increased ventilatory rate relationship
- Stimulation of J receptors
- Anxiety

Increased Heart Rate (Pulse) and Blood Pressure

Cheyne-Stokes Respiration

Cheyne-Stokes respiration may be seen in patients with severe left-sided heart failure and pulmonary edema. Some authorities have suggested that the cause of Cheyne-Stokes respiration in these patients may be related to the prolonged circulation time between the lungs and the central chemoreceptors. Cheyne-Stokes respiration is a classic clinical manifestation in central sleep apnea (see Chapter 31).

Paroxysmal Nocturnal Dyspnea (PND) and Orthopnea

Patients with pulmonary edema often awaken with severe dyspnea after several hours of sleep. This condition is called **paroxysmal nocturnal dyspnea**. This condition is particularly prevalent in patients with cardiogenic pulmonary edema. While the patient is awake, more time is spent in the erect position and, as a result, excess fluids tend to accumulate in the dependent portions of the body. When the patient lies down, however, the excess fluids from the dependent parts of the body move into the bloodstream and cause an increase in venous return to the lungs. This action raises the pulmonary hydrostatic pressure and promotes pulmonary edema. The pulmonary edema in turn produces pulmonary shunting, venous admixture, and hypoxemia. When the hypoxemia becomes severe, the peripheral chemoreceptors are stimulated and initiate an increased ventilatory rate (see Figure 4-4). The decreased lung compliance, J receptor stimulation, and anxiety may also contribute to the paroxysmal nocturnal dyspnea commonly seen in this disorder at night. A patient is said to have **orthopnea** when dyspnea increases while the patient is in a recumbent position.

Cyanosis

Cough and Sputum (Frothy and Pink in Appearance)

Chest Assessment Findings

- Increased tactile and vocal fremitus
- Crackles and wheezing

CLINICAL DATA OBTAINED FROM LABORATORY TESTS AND SPECIAL PROCEDURES

Pulmonary Function Test Findings
(Moderate to Severe Pulmonary Edema)
(Restrictive Lung Pathology)

FORCED EXPIRATORY VOLUME AND FLOW RATE FINDINGS*

FVC	FEV_T	FEV_1/FVC ratio	$FEF_{25\%-75\%}$
↓	N or ↓	N or ↑	N or ↓

$FEF_{50\%}$	$FEF_{200-1200}$	PEFR	MVV
N or ↓	N or ↓	N or ↓	N or ↓

LUNG VOLUME AND CAPACITY FINDINGS

V_T	IRV	ERV	RV
N or ↓	↓	↓	↓

VC	IC	FRC	TLC	RV/TLC ratio
↓	↓	↓	↓	N

Arterial Blood Gases

MILD TO MODERATE PULMONARY EDEMA

Acute Alveolar Hyperventilation with Hypoxemia[†]
(Acute Respiratory Alkalosis)

pH	$PaCO_2$	HCO_3^-	PaO_2	SaO_2 or SpO_2
↑	↓	↓ (but normal)	↓	↓

SEVERE STAGE PULMONARY EDEMA

Acute Ventilatory Failure with Hypoxemia[†]
(Acute Respiratory Acidosis)

pH[§]	$PaCO_2$	HCO_3^-[§]	PaO_2	SaO_2 or SpO_2
↓	↑	↑ (but normal)	↓	↓

*The decreased forced expiratory volumes and flow rate findings are primarily caused by the low vital capacity associated with the disorder.
[†]See Figure 4-3 and related discussion for the acute pH, $PaCO_2$, and HCO_3^- changes associated with acute alveolar hyperventilation.
[†]See Figure 4-2 and related discussion for the acute pH, $PaCO_2$, and HCO_3^- changes associated with acute ventilatory failure.
[§]When tissue hypoxia is severe enough to produce lactic acid, the pH and HCO_3^-[§] Values will be lower than expected for a particular $PaCO_2$ level.

Oxygenation Indices*

$\dot{Q}s/\dot{Q}T$	DO_2†	$\dot{V}O_2$	$C(a\text{-}\bar{v})O_2$	O_2ER	$S\bar{v}O_2$
↑	↓	N	N	↑	↓

Hemodynamic Indices†
Cardiogenic Pulmonary Edema Moderate to Severe Stages

CVP	RAP	$\overline{PA}$	PCWP	CO	SV
↑	↑	↑	↑	↓	↓

SVI	CI	RVSWI	LVSWI§	PVR	SVR
↓	↓	↑	↓	↑	↑

ABNORMAL LABORATORY TEST AND PROCEDURE RESULTS

- Serum potassium: low
- Serum sodium: low
- Serum chloride: low
- Brain natriuretic peptide (BNP): elevated

Hypokalemia, hyponatremia, and hypochloremia are often seen in patients with left-sided heart failure and may result from diuretic therapy or excessive fluid retention. The **Brain Natriuretic peptide (BNP)**, also known as **B-type natriuretic peptide** or **Ventricular Natriuretic Peptide** (still BNP) is an important biomarker used to help establish the diagnosis of CHF. The BNP hormone is produced by the heart and reflects how well the heart is functioning. Normally, only a low amount of BNP (<100 pg/mL) is found in blood. However, when the heart is working harder than normal over a long period of time, the heart releases more BNP, increasing the blood level of BNP. The following provides various BNP levels and the cardiac status associated with these levels:

- BNP levels below 100 pg/mL indicate no heart failure.
- BNP levels of 100 to 300 pg/mL suggest heart failure is present.
- BNP levels above 300 pg/mL indicate mild heart failure.
- BNP levels above 600 pg/mL indicate moderate heart failure.
- BNP levels above 900 pg/mL indicate severe heart failure.

*$C(a\text{-}\bar{v})O_2$, Arterial-venous oxygen difference; DO_2, total oxygen delivery; O_2ER, oxygen extraction ratio; $\dot{Q}s/\dot{Q}T$, pulmonary shunt fraction; $S\bar{v}O_2$, mixed venous oxygen saturation; $\dot{V}O_2$, oxygen consumption.
†The DO_2 may be normal in patients who have compensated to the decreased oxygenation status with (1) an increased cardiac output, (2) an increased hemoglobin level, or (3) a combination of both. When the DO_2 is normal, the O_2ER is usually normal.
†CO, Cardiac output; CVP, central venous pressure; LVSWI, left ventricular stroke work index; $\overline{PA}$, mean pulmonary artery pressure; PCWP, pulmonary capillary wedge pressure; PVR, pulmonary vascular resistance; RAP, right atrial pressure; RVSWI, right ventricular stroke work index; SV, stroke volume; SVI, stroke volume index; SVR, systemic vascular resistance; LVEF, left ventricular ejection fraction.
§Decreased LVEF when cardiogenic pulmonary edema is present. May be normal in noncardiogenic pulmonary edema.

RADIOLOGIC FINDINGS
Chest Radiograph

- Bilateral fluffy opacities
- Dilated pulmonary arteries
- Left ventricular hypertrophy (cardiomegaly)
- Kerley A and B lines
- Bat's wing or butterfly pattern
- Pleural effusion

CARDIOGENIC PULMONARY EDEMA

The radiographic findings associated with left heart failure are commonly described as follows:

- Mild left-sided heart failure: Pulmonary venous congestion with dilated pulmonary arteries is present.
- Moderate left-sided heart failure: **Cardiomegaly**, engorgement of the pulmonary arteries, and Kerley A and Kerley B lines are present. When cardiomegaly is present, the heart is greater than half the diameter of the thorax in a posterior-anterior chest radiograph (Figure 20-2). Because radiographic densities primarily reflect alveolar filling and not early interstitial edema, by the time abnormal findings are encountered, the pathologic changes associated with pulmonary edema are advanced. Chest x-ray films typically reveal dense, fluffy opacities that spread outward from the hilar areas to the peripheral borders of the lungs (Figures 20-2 and 20-4). **Kerley A lines**, which represent deep interstitial edema, radiate out from the hilum into the central portions of the lungs. Kerley A lines do not reach the pleura and are most prevalent in the middle and upper lung regions. **Kerley B lines** are short, thin, horizontal lines of interstitial edema, usually less than 1 cm in length, that extend inward from the pleural surface. They appear peripherally in contact with the pleura

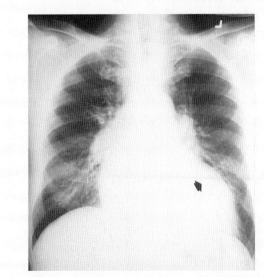

FIGURE 20-2 Cardiomegaly *(arrow)*, hilar prominence, and pulmonary edema in congestive heart failure. Note that the heart diameter is greater than half the diameter of the thorax.

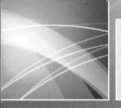
and are parallel to one another at right angles to the pleura. Although they may be seen in any lung region, they are most commonly seen in the lung bases (Figure 20-3).

- Severe left-sided heart failure: During this stage, the patient's chest radiograph shows cardiomegaly; pulmonary artery engorgement; interstitial pulmonary edema; fluffy, patchy areas of alveolar edema; and often the appearance of the **bat's wing pattern** (also called the butterfly pattern)—the peripheral portion of the lungs often remains clear, and this produces what is described as a "butterfly" or "bat's wing" distribution (Figure 20-4). Pleural effusion may also be seen.

NONCARDIOGENIC PULMONARY EDEMA

In noncardiogenic pulmonary edema the chest radiograph commonly shows areas of fluffy densities that are usually more dense near the hilum. The infiltrates may be unilateral or bilateral. Pleural effusion is usually not present and (most important) the cardiac silhouette is not enlarged.

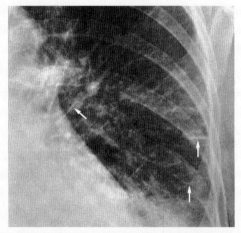

FIGURE 20-3 Kerley lines. Septal lines caused by pulmonary edema. Kerley B lines are short horizontal lines at the lung periphery *(vertical arrows)*. Kerley A lines are lines radiating from the hila *(oblique arrow)*. (From Hansell DM, Armstrong P, Lynch DA, McAdams HP, eds: *Imaging of diseases of the chest*, ed 4, Philadelphia, 2005, Elsevier.)

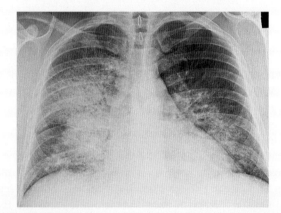

FIGURE 20-4 Bat's wing or butterfly pattern caused by pulmonary edema. This example is typical in that it is bilateral but not symmetrical. The shadowing is maximal in the central (perihilar) portions of the lung, and the outer portions of the lungs are relatively clear. (From Hansell DM, Armstrong P, Lynch DA, McAdams HP, eds: *Imaging of diseases of the chest*, ed 4, Philadelphia, 2005, Elsevier.)

General Management of Pulmonary Edema

The treatment for pulmonary edema is based on (1) the cause—that is, noncardiogenic versus cardiogenic pulmonary edema—and (2) the severity.

The treatment for noncardiogenic pulmonary edema is largely supportive and aimed at ensuring adequate ventilation and oxygenation. Unfortunately, there are no specific treatments to correct an underlying alveolar-capillary membrane permeability problem, or to control the pulmonary inflammatory events that ensue once they are triggered—for example, by inhaled toxic agents or a drug overdose—beyond mechanical ventilation and supportive care. Occasionally, the specific cause of the noncardiogenic pulmonary edema can be identified and treated. For example, noncardiogenic pulmonary edema caused by a severe infection—for example, sepsis—is treated with antibiotics, and **high altitude pulmonary edema** by returning to a lower elevation or by positive pressure ventilation.

For *cardiogenic pulmonary edema*, the initial management is directed at maintaining the patient's airways, oxygenation, and ventilation (see Bronchopulmonary Hygiene, Oxygen Therapy, and Mechanical Ventilation Protocols below). The therapeutic intervention to address the patient's circulatory systems has the following three main goals: (1) reduction of pulmonary venous return (preload reduction); (2) reduction of systemic vascular resistance (afterload reduction); and (3) inotropic support.

Reduction of the preload decreases pulmonary capillary hydrostatic pressure and reduces fluid transudation into the pulmonary interstitium and alveoli. Reduction of afterload increases cardiac output and improves renal perfusion, which in turn allows for diuresis in the patient with fluid overload. Inotropic agents are used to treat hypotension or signs of organ hypoperfusion. While the patient's circulatory problem(s) is/are treated, intubation and mechanical ventilation may be necessary to achieve adequate ventilation, oxygenation, and airway management. Common medications used to treat cardiogenic pulmonary edema are discussed as follows:

Preload Reducers

Reduced pulmonary venous return decreases pulmonary capillary hydrostatic pressure and reduces fluid transudation into the pulmonary interstitium and alveoli. Preload reducers include:

Nitroglycerin (Nitro-Bid, Minitra, Nitrostat)—is a very effective, predictable, and rapid-acting medication for preload.

Loop diuretics (e.g., furosemide)—are considered a cornerstone in the treatment of cardiogenic pulmonary edema. Loop diuretics are presumed to decrease preload through diuresis and direct vasodilation.

Morphine sulfate—may be used in some cases to reduce preload. However, the adverse effects (e.g., nausea and vomiting or respiratory depression) may outweigh the potential benefit, especially with the availability of nitroglycerin, which is a more effective preload reducing agent.

Afterload Reducers

Reduced systemic vascular resistance increases cardiac output and improves renal perfusion, allowing for diuresis. Afterload reducers include:

Captopril—prevents the conversion of angiotensin I to angiotensin II. It is a potent vasodilator. Afterload and cardiac output usually improves in 10 to 15 minutes.

Enalapril (Vasotec)—is a competitive angiotensin-converting enzyme (ACE) inhibitor and reduces angiotensin II levels.

Nitroprusside (Nitropress)—is a potent, direct smooth muscle-relaxing agent that primarily reduces afterload. It can also mildly reduce preload.

Inotropic Agents

These agents produce vasodilation and increase cardiac output. Inotropic agents include:

Dobutamine—is a synthetic catecholamine that mainly has beta$_1$-receptor activity, but also has some beta$_2$-receptor and alpha-receptor activity. Commonly used for patients with mild hypotension (e.g., systolic blood pressure 90 to 100 mm Hg).

Dopamine—is a naturally occurring catecholamine that acts as a precursor to norepinephrine. Dopamine hemodynamic effect is dose dependent. A low dose is associated with dilation in renal and splanchnic vasculature, enhancing diuresis. A moderate dose enhances cardiac contractility and heart rate. A high does increases afterload due to peripheral vasoconstriction. **Dopamine**—is generally reserved for patients with moderate hypotension (e.g., systolic blood pressure 70 to 90 mm Hg).

Norepinephrine (Levophed)—is a naturally occurring catecholamine with potent alpha-receptor and mild beat-receptor activity. It simulates beta$_1$-adrenergic and alpha-adrenergic receptors, increasing myocardial contractility, heart rate, and vasoconstriction. Norepinephrine increases blood pressure and afterload. Norepinephrine is generally reserved for patients with severe hypotension (e.g., systolic blood pressure <70 mm Hg).

Milrinone—is a positive inotropic agent and vasodilator. It reduces afterload and preload and increases cardiac output.

Other Agents

Antidysrhythmic Agents—such as drugs to control bradycardia (e.g., atropine) or tachycardia (e.g., **procainamide, metoprolol,** or **bretylium**) may be administered.

Albumin or mannitol—is sometimes administered to increase the patient's oncotic pressure in an effort to offset the increased hydrostatic forces of cardiogenic pulmonary edema, if the patient's osmotic pressure is extremely low.

Respiratory Care Treatment Protocols

Oxygen Therapy Protocol

Oxygen therapy is used to treat hypoxemia, decrease the work of breathing, and decrease myocardial work. The hypoxemia that develops in pulmonary edema is most commonly caused by the interstitial and alveolar fluid, atelectasis, and capillary shunting associated with the disorder. Hypoxemia caused by capillary shunting is at least partially refractory to oxygen therapy (see Oxygen Therapy Protocol, **Protocol 9-1**).

Bronchopulmonary Hygiene Therapy Protocol

Because of the excessive frothy white secretions associated with pulmonary edema, bronchial hygiene treatment modalities may be used to enhance the mobilization of bronchial secretions (see Bronchopulmonary Hygiene Therapy Protocol, **Protocol 9-2**).

Lung Expansion Therapy Protocol

Lung expansion therapy is commonly used to offset the fluid accumulation and atelectasis associated with cardiogenic pulmonary edema. High-flow mask continuous positive airway pressure (CPAP) has been shown to produce a significant and rapid improvement in oxygenation and ventilatory status in patients with pulmonary edema. **Mask CPAP** improves decreased lung compliance, reduces the work of breathing, enhances gas exchange, and decreases vascular congestion in patients with pulmonary edema. In fact, mask CPAP is prescribed (at least for a trial period) for patients with pulmonary edema who have arterial blood gas (ABG) values that indicate impending ventilatory failure or acute ventilatory failure—the hallmark clinical manifestations for mechanical ventilation. Often, mask CPAP dramatically improves oxygenation and ventilatory status in these patients and eliminates the need for mechanical ventilation (see Lung Expansion Therapy Protocol, **Protocol 9-3**).

Mechanical Ventilation Protocol

Mechanical ventilation may be necessary to provide and support alveolar gas exchange and eventually return the patient to spontaneous breathing. Because acute ventilatory failure is occasionally seen in patients with severe cardiogenic and noncardiogenic pulmonary edema, continuous mechanical ventilation may be required. Continuous mechanical ventilation is justified when the acute ventilatory failure is thought to be reversible (see Mechanical Ventilation Protocol, **Protocol 10-1** and Mechanical Ventilation Weaning Protocol, **Protocol 10-2**).

Aerosolized Medication Protocol

Both sympathomimetic and parasympatholytic agents are commonly used to induce bronchial smooth muscle relaxation (see Aerosolized Medication Protocol, **Protocol 9-4** and Appendix II). In should be noted, however, that aerosolized medications are often not effective in this disorder. In addition, bronchodilator agents must be used with caution, as they may induce cardiac arrhythmias.

Others

Alcohol (Ethanol, Ethyl Alcohol). Because alcohol is a specific surface-active agent, it may be aerosolized into the patient's lungs to lower the surface tension of the frothy secretions. This action enhances the mobilization of secretions. Generally, 5 to 15 mL of 30% to 50% alcohol solution is administered. This therapy is only for cardiogenic pulmonary edema and is rarely used today.

Decreasing Hydrostatic Pressure. In an effort to lower hydrostatic pressure, the physician may order the following:
- Positioning the patient in Fowler's position (sitting up)
- Rotating tourniquets (rarely used)
- Phlebotomy (rarely used)

CASE STUDY Pulmonary Edema

Admitting History and Physical Examination

This 76-year-old man was admitted to the emergency room in obvious respiratory distress. His wife reported that her husband had gone to bed feeling well. He woke up with chest pain at about 2:30 AM, very short of breath. She became concerned and called an ambulance. Neither the patient nor the wife were good historians, but they did report that the patient had been under a physician's care for some time for "heart trouble" and that he was taking "little white pills" on a daily basis. For the previous 3 days, he had not taken any medication.

On admission to the emergency room, the patient was mildly disoriented and slightly cyanotic. He repeatedly tried to take the oxygen mask from his face. He complained of a feeling of suffocation. His neck veins were distended, and the skin of his extremities was mottled. On auscultation, there were coarse crackles in both lower lung fields and some crackles in the middle and upper lung fields.

His cough was productive of pinkish, frothy sputum. His vital signs were as follows: blood pressure 105/50, heart rate 124 beats/min, and respiratory rate 28 breaths/min. He was afebrile. ECG showed evidence of an old infarct, sinus tachycardia, and an occasional premature ventricular contraction. X-ray films taken in the emergency room with the patient in a sitting position revealed bilateral fluffy infiltrates, more marked in the lower lung fields. The heart was enlarged. All other laboratory findings were within normal limits. Blood gases on an FIO_2 of 0.30 were pH 7.11, $PaCO_2$ 72 mm Hg, HCO_3^- 22 mEq/L, PaO_2 56 mm Hg, and SaO_2 75%.

The respiratory therapist working in the emergency room during the night shift recorded the following SOAP note.

Respiratory Assessment and Plan

S Patient states "a feeling of suffocation."
O Cyanosis, disorientation. Distended neck veins and mottled extremities. BP 105/50, HR 124, RR 28. ECG: sinus tachycardia and occasional PVCs. Coarse crackles bilaterally. Frothy pink sputum. CXR: Bilateral fluffy infiltrates and an enlarged heart. ABG: pH 7.11, $PaCO_2$ 72, HCO_3^- 22, PaO_2 56, SaO_2 75% (FIO_2 0.30).

A • Acute pulmonary edema (CXR)
   • Acute ventilatory failure with moderate hypoxemia (ABG)
      • Lactic acidosis likely
   • Large and small airway secretions (coarse crackles)
P **Oxygen Therapy Protocol**: Increase FIO_2 to 0.60 via continuous CPAP mask at 25 cm H_2O per **Lung Expansion Therapy Protocol.** Remain on standby for emergency endotracheal intubation and ventilator support. Continue ECG and oximetry monitoring, and repeat ABG in 30 minutes.

The patient was admitted on the cardiology service with a diagnosis of pulmonary edema–CHF. ECG monitoring and continuous oximetry were followed. Treatment consisted of intravenous furosemide, dopamine, and nitroprusside, as well as mask CPAP at 25 cm H_2O pressure with an FIO_2 of 0.60. A Foley catheter was placed.

Two hours later, the patient's condition was very much improved, and he was no longer cyanotic. Vital signs were as follows: blood pressure 126/70, heart rate 96 beats/min, and respiratory rate 18 breaths/min. ECG revealed mild sinus tachycardia and no ectopic beats. Auscultation showed considerable improvement. There were still some basilar crackles, but the upper lung fields were clear. Cough was much reduced and no longer productive. Repeat chest x-ray examination at the bedside showed considerable improvement. Urine output was in excess of 600 mL/h. The patient was calm and rational, stating that he was less short of breath and had no pain. Repeat ABGs revealed pH 7.35, $PaCO_2$ 46 mm Hg, HCO_3^- 24 mEq/L, PaO_2 120 mm Hg, SaO_2 97% on an FIO_2 of 0.60 and CPAP of 25 cm H_2O. His LVEF was 47%.

The following respiratory therapy SOAP note was made at the time.

Respiratory Assessment and Plan

S Patient states, "I'm less short of breath. No pain."
   Not cyanotic. BP 126/70, HR 96, RR 18. ECG: Mild sinus tachycardia without ectopic beats. Fewer crackles; no sputum production; CXR: Improved. ABG: pH 7.35, $PaCO_2$ 46, HCO_3^- 24, PaO_2 120, SaO_2 97% (FIO_2 0.60 and CPAP of 25 cm H_2O).

A • Decreased pulmonary edema (overall impression from the data)
- No longer in acute ventilatory failure (ABG)
- Acceptable acid-base status with mildly overly corrected hypoxemia (ABG)
- Secretions controlled (no sputum and fewer crackles)
- Congestive heart failure with resolving pulmonary edema

P Reduce O_2 per **Oxygen Therapy Protocol** to 2 L/min by nasal cannula. Discontinue CPAP per **Lung Expansion Therapy Protocol**. Continue ECG and oximetry monitoring. Repeat ABG in 60 minutes.

Discussion

Acute pulmonary edema is a classic finding in severe CHF. Several clinical manifestations associated with **Increased Alveolar-Capillary Membrane Thickness** (see Figure 9-9) were present in this case. For example, the patient's decreased lung compliance was manifested in his tachycardia and tachypnea, whereas his hypoxemia reflected diffusion blockade and intrapulmonary shunting associated with classic pulmonary edema. His lung compliance was so reduced that he had progressed to acute ventilatory failure—that is, the severe stage of pulmonary edema. Frank pulmonary edema due to left ventricular failure typically improves markedly when treated with CPAP. Some **Atelectasis** (see Figure 9-7) was doubtless also present and provided further rationale for CPAP therapy. In addition, the clinical scenario associated with **Excessive Bronchial Secretions** (see Figure 9-11) also was evident initially with frothy blood-tinged sputum and coarse crackles in both lower lung fields. The patient was too ill to allow valid pulmonary function testing, but the suspicion is that a combined obstructive and restrictive pattern may have been present at the time of the first assessment.

The **Aerosolized Medication Protocol** and **Bronchopulmonary Hygiene Therapy Protocol** were not used in this case. Often, the first-line management of pulmonary edema consists only of improving myocardial efficiency, decreasing the cardiovascular afterload, decreasing the hypervolemia, providing CPAP, and improving oxygenation. Furosemide (Lasix) is a potent loop diuretic, dopamine has direct inotropic effects, and nitroprusside is a potent peripheral vasodilator. In this case, the combination of all these therapies resulted in a marked improvement of the patient's condition.

In short, this patient had an acute respiratory problem, but the basic cause was cardiac. After the cardiac condition was treated, the respiratory symptoms rapidly disappeared. CPAP and an increased FIO_2 were adequate, and this patient was spared the trauma and risk associated with intubation and mechanical ventilation. No evidence of acute myocardial infarction was found. He was discharged after 48 hours, his condition much improved. He was instructed to take his cardiac medication and diuretics without fail and to return to his family physician in 3 days.

SELF-ASSESSMENT QUESTIONS

ⓔ Answers to questions can be found on Evolve. To access additional student assessment questions visit **http://evolve.elsevier.com/DesJardins/respiratory**.

1. **Which of the following is an afterload reducer?**
   a. Procainamide
   b. Dopamine
   c. Furosemide
   d. Nitroprusside

2. **What is the normal hydrostatic pressure in the pulmonary capillaries?**
   a. 5 to 10 mm Hg
   b. 10 to 15 mm Hg
   c. 15 to 20 mm Hg
   d. 20 to 25 mm Hg

3. **What is the normal oncotic pressure of the blood?**
   a. 10 to 15 mm Hg
   b. 15 to 20 mm Hg
   c. 20 to 25 mm Hg
   d. 25 to 30 mm Hg

4. **Which of the following are causes of cardiogenic pulmonary edema?**
   1. Excessive fluid administration
   2. Right ventricular failure
   3. Mitral valve disease
   4. Pulmonary embolus
      a. 1 and 2 only
      b. 1, 2, and 3 only
      c. 2, 3, and 4 only
      d. 1, 3, and 4 only

5. **As a result of pulmonary edema, the patient's:**
   1. RV is decreased
   2. FRC is increased
   3. VC is increased
   4. TLC is increased
      a. 1 only
      b. 1 and 4 only
      c. 2 and 3 only
      d. 3 and 4 only

6. **The left ventricular ejection fraction:**
   1. Normally is greater than 75%
   2. Is a good measure of alveolar ventilation
   3. Correlates well with the brain natriuretic peptide values
   4. Provides a noninvasive measurement of cardiac contractility
      a. 1 and 2 only
      b. 2 and 4 only
      c. 3 and 4 only
      d. 2, 3, and 4 only

Chapter Objectives

After reading this chapter, you will be able to:
- List the anatomic alterations of the lungs associated with pulmonary embolism.
- Describe the causes of pulmonary embolism.
- List the cardiopulmonary clinical manifestations associated with pulmonary embolism.
- Describe the general management of pulmonary embolism.
- Define pulmonary hypertension.
- Differentiate the five clinical classifications of pulmonary hypertension.
- Identify the common signs and symptoms associated with pulmonary hypertension.
- Describe the tests and procedures used to diagnose pulmonary hypertension.
- Describe the pulmonary hypertension severity rating.
- Differentiate the signs and symptoms between right-sided heart failure and left-sided heart failure.
- Describe the role of the respiratory therapist in pulmonary vascular disorders.
- Discuss the treatment selections used to manage pulmonary hypertension.
- Describe the clinical strategies and rationales of the SOAPs presented in the case study.

Key Terms

Alteplase
Biventricular Failure
Calcium Channel Blocker
Chronic Thromboembolic Pulmonary Hypertension (CTEPH)
Computed Tomography Pulmonary Angiogram (CTPA)
Coumadin
D-dimer Blood Test
Deep Venous Thrombosis (DVT)
Dihydropyridine
Diltiazem
Echocardiography
Embolus/Embolism
Endothelin Receptor Antagonists
Extremity Venography
High–Molecular-Weight Heparin
Inferior Vena Cava Vein Filter (Greenfield Filter)
Low–Molecular-Weight Heparins
Panwarfarin
Phosphodiesterase-5 Inhibitors
Prostanoids
Pulmonary Angiogram
Pulmonary Thromboembolectomy
Pulmonary Embolism (PE)
Pulmonary Hypertension (PH)
Pulmonary Infarction
Reteplase
Saddle Embolus
Streptokinase
Thrombolytic Agents
Thrombus
Ultrasonography
Urokinase
Ventilation-Perfusion Lung Scan ($\dot{V}/\dot{Q}$ Scan)
Virchow's Triad
Warfarin

Chapter Outline

Anatomic Alterations of the Lungs
Etiology and Epidemiology
    Diagnosis and Screening
Overview of Cardiopulmonary Clinical Manifestations
    Associated with Pulmonary Embolism
General Management of Pulmonary Embolism
    Thrombolytic Agents
    Preventive Measures
    Respiratory Care Treatment Protocols
Pulmonary hypertension
    Diagnosis
    Management of Pulmonary Hypertension
The Role of the Respiratory Therapist in Pulmonary Vascular
    Disorders
Case Study: Pulmonary Embolism
Self-Assessment Questions

PULMONARY EMBOLISM

Anatomic Alterations of the Lungs

A blood clot that forms and remains in a vein is called a **thrombus.** A blood clot that becomes dislodged and travels to another part of the body is called an **embolus (embolism).** In some cases, when the embolus significantly disrupts pulmonary arterial blood flow, **pulmonary infarction** may develop—which, in turn, may cause alveolar atelectasis, consolidation, and tissue necrosis. Bronchial smooth muscle constriction occasionally accompanies pulmonary embolism. Although the precise mechanism is not known, it is believed that the embolism causes the release of cellular mediators such as serotonin, histamine, and prostaglandins from platelets, which in turn leads to bronchoconstriction. Local areas of alveolar hypocapnia and hypoxemia may also contribute to the bronchoconstriction associated with pulmonary embolism.

An embolus may originate from one large thrombus or occur as a shower of small thrombi and may or may not interfere with the right side of the heart's ability to perfuse the lungs adequately. When a large embolus detaches from a thrombus and passes through the right side of the heart, it may lodge in the bifurcation of the pulmonary artery, where it forms what is known as a **saddle embolus.** A large saddle embolus is often quickly fatal, because it can significantly block pulmonary blood from moving to the left ventricle and being pumped out to the systemic circulation (partially shown in Figure 21-1, *A*).

The major pathologic or structural changes of the lungs associated with pulmonary embolism are as follows:
- Blockage of the pulmonary vascular system
- Pulmonary infarction (when severe)
  - Alveolar atelectasis
  - Alveolar consolidation
- Bronchial smooth muscle constriction (bronchospasm)

Etiology and Epidemiology

Deep vein thrombosis (DVT) and **pulmonary embolism (PE)** are often clinically insidious disorders. If the pulmonary embolus is relatively small, the early signs and symptoms of its presence are often vague and nonspecific. By contrast, sudden death is often the first symptom in about 25% of people who have a large pulmonary embolus. A massive pulmonary embolism is one of the most common causes of sudden and unexpected death in all age groups. Many pulmonary emboli are undiagnosed and therefore untreated. In fact, because of the subtle and misleading clinical manifestations associated with a pulmonary embolus, the possibility of a blood clot lodged in the lung is often not considered *until autopsy* in about 70% to 80% of cases.

It is estimated that 300,000 to 600,000 cases of pulmonary embolism are reported each year in the United States. Between 60,000 and 100,000 Americans die annually from the condition. The experienced health-care practitioner actively works to confirm the diagnosis of a pulmonary embolism as *soon as the suspicion arises.* This is especially true when the origin of the signs and symptoms cannot be identified.

Although there are many possible sources of pulmonary emboli (e.g., fat, air, amniotic fluid, bone marrow, tumor fragments), blood clots are by far the most common. Most pulmonary blood clots originate—or break away from—sites of **deep venous thrombosis** in the lower part of the body (i.e., the leg and pelvic veins and the inferior vena cava). When a thrombus or a piece of a thrombus breaks loose in a deep vein, the blood clot (now called an *embolus*) is carried through the venous system to the right atrium and ventricle of the heart and ultimately lodges in the pulmonary arteries or arterioles. There are three primary factors (known as **Virchow's triad**) associated with the formation of DVT. Virchow's triad includes (1) venous stasis (i.e., slowing or stagnation of blood flow through the veins), (2) hypercoagulability (i.e., the increased tendency of blood to form clots), and (3) injury to the endothelial cells that line the vessels.

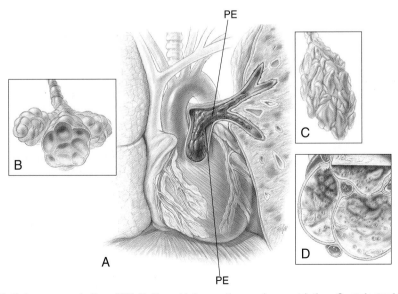

FIGURE 21-1 A, Pulmonary embolism (PE). **B,** Bronchial smooth muscle constriction; **C,** atelectasis; and **D,** alveolar consolidation are common secondary anatomic alterations of the lungs.

Box 21-1 provides common risk factors for pulmonary embolism.

Diagnosis and Screening

The diagnosis of a pulmonary embolism is primarily based on the clinical manifestations that support the possibility of pulmonary embolism—followed by the results of a variety of possible blood tests, venous ultrasonography, and one or more lung imaging techniques to secure a definitive diagnosis.[1] Box 21-2 provides common signs and symptoms associated with a suspected pulmonary embolism. When a pulmonary embolism is possible, the most commonly used tool to predict the clinical probability of a pulmonary embolism is the modified **Wells Scoring System** (Table 21-1). Table 21-2 provides

---

[1]Depending on how much of the lung is involved, the size of the embolism, and the overall health of the patient, the signs and symptoms of a pulmonary embolism can vary greatly.

BOX 21-1 Risk Factors Associated with Pulmonary Embolism

Venous Stasis
- Inactivity
  - Prolonged bed rest and/or immobilization
  - Prolonged sitting (e.g., car or plane travel)
- Congestive heart failure
- Varicose veins
- Thrombophlebitis

Surgical Procedures
- Hip surgery
- Pelvic surgery
- Knee surgery
- Certain obstetric or gynecologic procedures

Trauma
- Bone fractures (especially of the pelvis and the long bones of the lower extremities)
- Extensive injury to soft tissue
- Postoperative or postpartum states
- Extensive hip or abdominal operations
- Phlegmasia alba dolens puerperarum ("milk-leg" of pregnancy)

Hypercoagulation Disorders
- Oral contraceptives
- Polycythemia
- Multiple myeloma

Others
- Obesity
- Pacemakers or venous catheters
- Pregnancy and childbirth
- Supplemental estrogen (estrogen in birth control formulations can increase clotting factors)
- Family history of venous thromboembolism
- Smoking
- Malignant neoplasms
- Burns

---

the **Wells Clinical Prediction Rule for Deep Venous Thrombosis.**

Common Tests for Suspected Pulmonary Embolism

Blood Tests. Once it has been established that there is a likely probability of a pulmonary embolism, an array of blood tests may be performed to exclude important secondary causes of pulmonary embolism—including a full blood count, clotting status, and some screening tests (e.g., erythrocyte sedimentation rate, renal function, liver enzymes, electrolytes). Should any of these tests be abnormal, further investigation is justified.

In individuals who (1) have a family history of blood clots, (2) have had more than one episode of blood clots, or (3) have experienced blood clots for no known reason, the doctor may prescribe a series of blood tests to determine if there are any inherited abnormalities in the blood-clotting system. When genetic abnormalities (e.g., Factor V [Leyden] Deficiency) are found or there is a history of blood clots, the physician may recommend a lifelong therapy of anticoagulants. The doctor may also recommend that other members of the family receive a series of blood tests.

D-dimer Blood Test. The **D-dimer blood test** (also called the *fibrinogen test*) is used to check for an increased level of the protein fibrinogen—an integral component of the blood-clotting process. The test is relatively simple and fast; it

---

BOX 21-2 Signs and Symptoms Commonly Associated with Pulmonary Embolism

- Sudden shortness of breath
- Cardiac arrhythmias
  Sinus tachycardia
  - Atrial arrhythmias
  - Atrial tachycardia
  - Atrial flutter
  - Atrial fibrillation
  - Acute right ventricular strain pattern and right bundle branch block
  - P pulmonale (peaked P waves)
- Weak pulse
- Lightheadedness or fainting
- Anxiety
- Excessive sweating
- Cyanosis
- Cool or clammy skin to the touch
- Chest pain that resembles a heart attack—that is, chest pain that may radiate to the shoulder, arm, neck, or jaw. The pain is often described as sharp, stabbing, aching, or dull. The pain often intensifies when the patient inhales deeply, coughs, eats, or bends over. The pain often intensifies during exertion but will not go away during rest.
- Cough
- Blood-streaked sputum
- Wheezing
- Leg swelling

TABLE 21-1 Wells Clinical Prediction Rule for Pulmonary Embolism

Clinical Feature	Points
Clinical symptoms of DVT	3
Other diagnosis less likely than PE	3
Heart rate greater than 100 beats per minute	1.5
Immobilization or surgery within past 4 weeks	1.5
Previous DVT or PE	1.5
Hemoptysis	1
Malignancy	1
Total points	
Clinical Probability of Pulmonary Embolism	

- High: >6 points
- Moderate: 2 to 6
- Low: <2

DVT, Deep venous thrombosis; *PE*, pulmonary embolism.
PE = pulmonary embolism

TABLE 21-2 Wells Clinical Prediction Rule for Deep Venous Thrombosis

Clinical Feature	Points
Active cancer (treatment within 6 months, or palliation)	1
Paralysis, paresis, or immobilization of lower extremity	1
Bedridden for more than 3 days because of surgery (within 4 weeks)	1
Localized tenderness along distribution of deep veins	1
Entire leg swollen	1
Unilateral calf swelling of greater than 3 cm (below tibial tuberosity)	1
Unilateral pitting edema	1
Collateral superficial veins	1
Alternative diagnosis as likely as or more likely than DVT	−2
Total points	
Clinical Probability of Deep Venous Thrombosis	

- High: >3
- Moderate: 1 to 2
- Low: <1

DVT, Deep venous thrombosis.

entails drawing a blood sample, and the results can be available in less than 1 hour. D-dimer values higher than 500 ng/mL are considered positive—which may suggest the possibility of blood clots. However, it should be emphasized that there are many conditions that can increase an individual's D-dimer level, including recent surgery. Thus, an elevated D-dimer value is usually used to supplement other clinical information. A normal D-dimer level essentially rules out the possibility of blood clots.

Ultrasonography. An **ultrasonography** test uses high-frequency sound waves to detect blood clots in the thigh veins. The test is noninvasive and takes only 30 minutes or less to

perform. A wand-shaped transducer is used to direct the sound waves to the thigh veins being tested. The sound waves are then reflected back to the transducer and converted to a moving image on a computer screen. The test is very accurate for the diagnosis of blood clots behind the knee or thigh. Although it is relatively sensitive in detecting DVT above the knee, it is insensitive in detecting DVT below the knee

Chest x-Ray. Although the chest x-ray is often normal in the patient with a pulmonary embolism, it can be used to rule out conditions that mimic a pulmonary embolism, such as pneumonia and pneumothorax. In addition, infiltrates or atelectasis will be seen in about 50% of pulmonary embolism cases, and an elevated hemidiaphragm occurs in about 40% of cases.

Computed Tomography Pulmonary Angiogram. The spiral (helical) volumetric **computed tomography pulmonary angiogram** (CTPA) (also called a CT pulmonary angiography) with intravenous contrast is fast becoming the first-line test for diagnosing suspected pulmonary embolism. The CTPA is increasingly being preferred to the previous gold standards for diagnosing a pulmonary embolism—ventilation-perfusion scanning or direct pulmonary angiography—because (1) the scan only requires an intravenous line, (2) the image resolution is very good, (3) the volumetric scanning allows the contrast material to be administered more economically and timed more precisely, and (4) the entire chest can be scanned in a single breath hold, or in several successive short breath holds. (See CTPA scan in Radiologic Findings, page 309).

Ventilation-Perfusion Scan. The $\dot{V}/\dot{Q}$ scan is rarely used today to identify a pulmonary embolus. A $\dot{V}/\dot{Q}$ scan is reliable only at the extremes of interpretation (i.e., the test confirms that the lungs are normal or that there is a high probability of a pulmonary embolism). The $\dot{V}/\dot{Q}$ scan often raises more questions than it answers. This test is fast being replaced by more sensitive and rapid tests, such as spiral CTPA scans (see above).

Pulmonary Angiogram. A pulmonary angiogram provides a clear image of the blood flow in the lung's arteries. It is an extremely accurate test for diagnosis of pulmonary embolism. However, because it is invasive (catheter insertion and dye injection) and time consuming (about 1 hour), and requires a high degree of skill to administer, it is usually only performed when other tests have failed to provide a definitive diagnosis. More contrast dye is used in this study than in the pulmonary embolism CTPA scan. (see Pulmonary Angiogram in Radiologic Findings, page 309).

Magnetic Resonance Imaging. A magnetic resonance imaging (MRI) scan of the chest may be used for individuals whose kidneys may be harmed by dyes used in x-ray tests and for women who are pregnant.

Magnetic Resonance Angiography. Magnetic resonance angiography (MRA) may be used to differentiate between blood (usual), thromboemboli, and tumor emboli in patients with malignancy.

The following clinical manifestations result from the pathologic mechanisms caused (or activated) by Atelectasis (see Figure 9-7)—the major anatomic alteration of the lungs associated with a pulmonary embolism (see Figure 21-1). Bronchospasm (see Figure 9-10) may also explain some of the following findings. It occurs rarely and is of little clinical significance compared with atelectasis caused by **pulmonary infarction** and increased physiologic dead space.

CLINICAL DATA OBTAINED AT THE PATIENT'S BEDSIDE
The Physical Examination
Vital Signs
Increased Respiratory Rate (Tachypnea)
Several unique mechanisms probably work simultaneously to increase the rate of breathing in patients with pulmonary embolism.
Stimulation of Peripheral Chemoreceptors (Hypoxemia)
When an embolus lodges in the pulmonary vascular system, blood flow is reduced or completely absent distal to the obstruction. Consequently, the alveolar ventilation beyond the obstruction is wasted, or dead space, ventilation, and no carbon dioxide–oxygen exchange occurs. The ventilation-perfusion ($\dot{V}/\dot{Q}$) ratio distal to the pulmonary embolus is high and may even be infinite if there is no perfusion at all (Figure 21-2).

Although portions of the lungs have a high $\dot{V}/\dot{Q}$ ratio at the onset of a pulmonary embolism, this condition is quickly reversed, and a decrease in the $\dot{V}/\dot{Q}$ ratio occurs. The pathophysiologic mechanisms responsible for the decreased $\dot{V}/\dot{Q}$ ratio are as follows: In some cases of the pulmonary embolus, pulmonary infarction may develop and causes alveolar atelectasis, consolidation, and parenchymal necrosis. In addition, the embolus is believed to

activate the release of humoral agents such as serotonin, histamine, and prostaglandins into the pulmonary circulation, causing bronchial constriction. Collectively, the alveolar atelectasis, consolidation, tissue necrosis, and bronchial constriction lead to decreased alveolar ventilation relative to the alveolar perfusion (decreased $\dot{V}/\dot{Q}$ ratio). As a result of the decreased $\dot{V}/\dot{Q}$ ratio, pulmonary shunting and venous admixture ensue.

The result of the venous admixture is a decrease in the patient's PaO_2 and CaO_2 (Figure 21-3). It should be emphasized that it is not the pulmonary embolism but rather the decreased $\dot{V}/\dot{Q}$ ratio that develops from the pulmonary infarction (atelectasis and consolidation) and bronchial constriction (release of cellular mediators) that actually causes the reduced PaO_2. As this condition intensifies, the patient's oxygen level may decline to a point low enough to stimulate the peripheral chemoreceptors, which in turn initiates an increased ventilatory rate.

Reflexes from the Aortic and Carotid Sinus Baroreceptors
If obstruction of the pulmonary vascular system is severe, left ventricular output will diminish and cause the systemic blood pressure to drop. The decreased systemic blood pressure reduces the tension of the walls of the aorta and carotid artery, which activates the baroreceptors. Activation of the baroreceptors in turn initiates an increased heart and ventilatory rate.

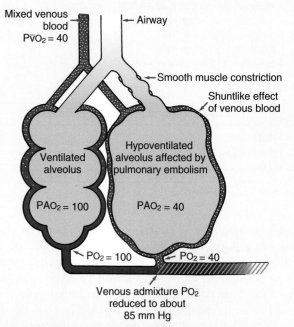

FIGURE 21-3 Venous admixture may develop in pulmonary embolism as a result of bronchial smooth muscle constriction (shuntlike effect). Venous admixture may also occur when an embolus leads to pulmonary infarction and causes alveolar atelectasis and consolidation (true capillary shunt). Alveolar atelectasis and consolidation are not shown in this illustration.

---

*In an uncomplicated pulmonary embolism, none of the clinical scenarios presented in Figures 9-7 through 9-12 are activated. In these patients, "wasted" or increased alveolar dead space ventilation is the primary pathophysiologic mechanism (i.e., the ventilation of embolized [nonperfused] pulmonary subsegments, segments, or lobes).

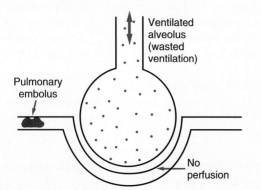

FIGURE 21-2 Dead-space ventilation in pulmonary embolism.

Other pathophysiologic mechanisms that may increase the patient's ventilatory rate include the following:

- Stimulation of the J receptors
- Anxiety, pain

Increased Heart Rate

The two major mechanisms responsible for the increased heart rate associated with pulmonary embolism are (1) reflexes from the aortic and carotid sinus baroreceptors and (2) stimulation of the pulmonary reflex mechanism.

For a discussion of reflexes from the aortic and carotid sinus baroreceptors, see the previous section on increased respiratory rate. The increased heart rate may also reflect an indirect response to hypoxic stimulation of the peripheral chemoreceptors, mainly the carotid bodies. When the carotid bodies are stimulated in this manner, the patient's ventilatory rate increases. As a result of the increased rate of lung inflation, the pulmonary reflex mechanism is activated; this mechanism triggers tachycardia.

Systemic Hypotension (Decreased Blood Pressure)

When significant pulmonary hypertension (PH) develops in pulmonary embolic disease, it is nearly always present because of the decrease in the cross-sectional area of the pulmonary vascular system, which reduces cardiac return and causes a decrease in left ventricular output and systemic hypotension.

Cyanosis

Cough and Hemoptysis

As a result of the PH, the pulmonary hydrostatic pressure, normally about 15 mm Hg, often becomes higher than the pulmonary oncotic pressure (normally about 25 mm Hg). This increase in the hydrostatic pressure permits plasma and red blood cells to move across the alveolar-capillary membrane and into alveolar spaces. If this process continues, the subepithelial mechanoreceptors located in the bronchioles, bronchi, and trachea are stimulated. Such stimulation initiates a cough reflex and the expectoration of blood-tinged sputum.

Peripheral Edema and Venous Distention

- Distended neck veins
- Swollen and tender liver
- Ankle and feet swelling
- Pitting edema

Chest Pain and Decreased Chest Expansion

Chest pain is frequently noted in patients with pulmonary embolism. The origin of the pain is obscure. It may be cardiac or pleural, but it is one of the common early findings in all forms of pulmonary embolism, even in the absence of clinically obvious cor pulmonale or pleural involvement. If the patient has systemic hypotension, perfusion of the coronary arteries decreases, and angina-like chest pain (and electrocardiographic [ECG] findings) may result.

Syncope, Lightheadedness, and Confusion

If the left ventricular output and systemic blood pressure decrease substantially, blood flow to the brain may also diminish significantly. This may cause periods of lightheadedness, confusion, and even syncope.

Abnormal Heart Sounds

- Increased second heart sound (S_2)
- Increased splitting of the second heart sound (S_2)
- Third heart sound (or ventricular gallop) (S_3)

Increased Second Heart Sound (S_2)

As a result of pulmonary embolization, abnormally high blood pressure develops in the pulmonary artery. This condition causes the pulmonic valve to close more forcefully. As a result, the sound produced by the pulmonic valve (P_2) is often louder than the aortic sound (A_2), which causes a louder second heart sound, or S_2. This finding may be noted in the patient's chart as "$P_2>A_2$," which reflects that S_2 is louder when the area over the pulmonic valve, left of the sternal notch, is compared to the intensity of sound to the right of the sternal notch.

Increased Splitting of the Second Heart Sound (S_2)

Two major mechanisms either individually or together may contribute to the increased splitting of S_2 sometimes noted in pulmonary embolism: (1) increased PH and (2) incomplete right bundle branch block.

The incomplete right bundle branch block that sometimes accompanies pulmonary embolism may also contribute to the increased splitting of S_2. In incomplete heart block, the electrical activity through the right side of the heart is delayed; this delayed activity in turn slows right ventricular contraction. The blood pressure in the pulmonic valve area remains higher than normal for a longer time during right ventricular contraction. As a result, the closure of the pulmonic valve is delayed, which may further widen the S_2 split.

Third Heart Sound (Ventricular Gallop)

A third heart sound (S_3), or ventricular gallop, is sometimes heard in patients with pulmonary embolism. It occurs early in diastole, about 0.12 to 0.16 seconds after S_2. Although its precise origin is unknown, S_3 is thought to be created by cardiac wall vibrations during diastole, when the rush of blood into the ventricles is abruptly stopped by ventricular walls that have lost some of their elasticity because of hypertrophy. An S_3 generated in the right ventricle usually is best heard to the right of the cardiac apex, close to the lower sternal border during inspiration.

Other Cardiac Manifestations

Right Ventricular Heave or Lift

As a consequence of the elevated pulmonary blood pressure, right ventricular strain or right ventricular hypertrophy (or both) often develops. When this occurs, a sustained lift of the chest wall can be felt at the lower left side of the sternum during

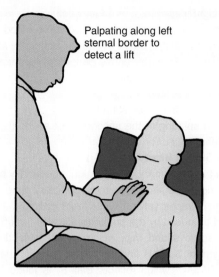

Palpating along left sternal border to detect a lift

FIGURE 21-4 A right ventricular lift can be detected in patients with a pulmonary embolism if significant pulmonary hypertension is present.

systole (Figure 21-4), because the right ventricle lies directly beneath the sternum.

Chest Assessment Findings

- Crackles
- Wheezes
- Pleural friction rub (especially when pulmonary infarction involves the pleura)

CLINICAL DATA OBTAINED FROM LABORATORY TESTS AND SPECIAL PROCEDURES

Arterial Blood Gases

MILD TO MODERATE STAGES

Acute Alveolar Hyperventilation with Hypoxemia[†]
(Acute Respiratory Alkalosis)

pH	$PaCO_2$	HCO_3^-	PaO_2[†]	SaO_2 or SpO_2[†]
↑	↓	↓	↓	↓
		(but normal)		

SEVERE STAGE

Acute Ventilatory Failure with Hypoxemia[§]
(Acute Respiratory Acidosis)

pH[*]	$PaCO_2$	HCO_3^-[*]	PaO_2[†]	SaO_2 or SpO_2[†]
↓	↑	↑	↓	↓
		(but normal)		

[†]See Figure 4-3 and related discussion for the acute pH, $PaCO_2$, and HCO_3^- changes associated with acute alveolar hyperventilation.
[†]Note: a large saddle embolus can cause a sudden and dramatic drop in PaO_2, SaO_2, or SpO_2 values.
[§]See Figure 4-2 and related discussion for the acute pH, $PaCO_2$, and HCO_3^- changes associated with acute ventilatory failure.
[*]When tissue hypoxia is severe enough to produce lactic acid, the pH and HCO_3^- values will be lower than expected for a particular $PaCO_2$ level.

Oxygenation Indices[*]

$\dot{Q}s/\dot{Q}T$	DO_2[†]	$\dot{V}O_2$	$C(a\text{-}\bar{v})O_2$	O_2ER	$S\bar{v}O_2$
↑	↓	N	N	↑	↓

Hemodynamic Indices[†]

EXTENSIVE PULMONARY EMBOLISM

CVP	RAP	$\overline{PA}$	PCWP	CO	SV
↑	↑	↑	↓ or N	↓	↓

SVI	CI	RVSWI	LVSWI	PVR	SVR
↓	↓	↑	↓	↑	N

Normally the pulmonary artery pressure is no greater than 25/10 mm Hg, with a mean pulmonary artery pressure of about 15 mm Hg. Most patients with a pulmonary embolism, however, have a mean pulmonary artery pressure in excess of 20 mm Hg. Three major mechanisms may contribute to PH: (1) decreased cross-sectional area of the pulmonary vascular system because of the embolism, (2) vasoconstriction induced by humoral agents, and (3) vasoconstriction induced by alveolar hypoxia.

Decreased Cross-Sectional Area of the Pulmonary Vascular System Because of the Embolus

The cross-sectional area of the pulmonary vascular system will decrease significantly if a large embolus becomes lodged in a major artery or if many small emboli become lodged in numerous small pulmonary vessels.

Vasoconstriction Induced by Humoral Agents

One of the consequences of pulmonary embolism is the release of certain humoral agents, primarily serotonin and prostaglandin. These agents induce smooth muscle constriction of both the tracheobronchial tree and the pulmonary vascular system. Such smooth muscle vasoconstriction may further reduce the total cross-sectional area of the pulmonary vascular system and cause the pulmonary artery pressure to rise further.

Vasoconstriction Induced by Alveolar Hypoxia

In response to the humoral agents liberated in pulmonary embolism, the smooth muscles of the tracheobronchial tree

[*]$C(a\text{-}\bar{v})O_2$, Arterial-venous oxygen difference; DO_2, total oxygen delivery; O_2ER, oxygen extraction ratio; $\dot{Q}s/\dot{Q}T$, pulmonary shunt fraction; $S\bar{v}O_2$, mixed venous oxygen saturation; $\dot{V}O_2$, oxygen consumption.
[†]The DO_2 may be normal in patients who have compensated to the decreased oxygenation status with (1) an increased cardiac output, (2) an increased hemoglobin level, or (3) a combination of both. When the DO_2 is normal, the O_2ER is usually normal.
[†]CO, Cardiac output; CVP, central venous pressure; LVSWI, left ventricular stroke work index; $\overline{PA}$, mean pulmonary artery pressure; PCWP, pulmonary capillary wedge pressure; PVR, pulmonary vascular resistance; RAP, right atrial pressure; RVSWI, right ventricular stroke work index; SV, stroke volume; SVI, stroke volume index; SVR, systemic vascular resistance.

constrict and cause the $\dot{V}/\dot{Q}$ ratio to decrease and the PaO_2 to decline. Although the precise mechanism is unclear, when the PaO_2 and $PaCO_2$ decrease, pulmonary vasoconstriction routinely ensues. This action appears to be a normal compensatory mechanism that offsets the shunt produced by underventilated alveoli. When the number of hypoxic areas becomes significant, however, generalized pulmonary vasoconstriction may develop and further contribute to the increase in pulmonary blood pressure. When the pulmonary embolism is severe, right-sided heart strain and cor pulmonale may ensue. Cor pulmonale leads to an increased CVP, distended neck veins, and a swollen and tender liver.

ABNORMAL ELECTROCARDIOGRAPHIC PATTERNS

- Sinus tachycardia
- Atrial arrhythmias
  - Atrial tachycardia
  - Atrial flutter
  - Atrial fibrillation
- Acute right ventricular strain pattern and right bundle branch block
- P pulmonale (peaked P waves)

In some cases, the obstruction of pulmonary blood flow produced by pulmonary emboli leads to abnormal ECG patterns. However, there is no single ECG pattern diagnostic of pulmonary embolism. Abnormal patterns merely suggest the possibility of pulmonary embolic disease. Sinus tachycardia is the most common arrhythmia seen. The sinus tachycardia and atrial arrhythmias sometimes noted are also thought to be related to the increased right-sided heart strain and cor pulmonale. In about 15% to 25% of patients with a pulmonary embolism, an $S_1Q_3T_3$ pattern may be seen—which is a large S wave in Lead I, plus a large Q wave and an inverted T wave in Lead III.

RADIOLOGIC FINDINGS

Chest Radiograph

- Increased density (in infarcted areas)
- Hyperradiolucency distal to the embolus (in noninfarcted areas)
- Dilation of the pulmonary arteries
- Pulmonary edema
- Right ventricular cardiomegaly (cor pulmonale)
- Pleural effusion (usually small)

Patients with a pulmonary embolus often demonstrate no radiographic signs. However, a density with an appearance similar to that of pneumonia may be seen if infarction has occurred. Hyperradiolucency may also be apparent distal to the embolus; it is caused by decreased vascularity (Westermark's sign). Dilation of the pulmonary artery on the affected side, pulmonary edema (common after a fat embolus), right ventricular cardiomegaly, and pleural effusions may also be seen.

COMPUTED TOMOGRAPHY PULMONARY ANGIOGRAM (CTPA)

The CTPA scan is fast becoming the first-line diagnostic imaging tool to confirm a pulmonary embolism. As shown in Figure 21-5, a relatively dark area—the thrombus—is clearly outlined by the brighter contrast (blood flow).

VENTILATION-PERFUSION LUNG SCAN FINDINGS

Although the ventilation-perfusion lung scan ($\dot{V}/\dot{Q}$ lung scan) has largely been replaced by the CTPA scan (see above), Figure 21-6 provides a nice example of how one or more pulmonary emboli might appear on the $\dot{V}/\dot{Q}$ lung scan. In this case, Figure 21-6, V shows how the radioactive gas, xenon-133, confirmed normal lung ventilation—that is, a black appearance throughout both lungs. By contrast, Figure 21-6, P shows how the intravenous radiolabeled particles (a gamma-emitting isotope, usually iodine or technetium) confirmed multiple peripheral subsegmental pulmonary emboli—that is, the white areas interspersed throughout the black areas of the lungs.

PULMONARY ANGIOGRAPHY

Because pulmonary angiography is invasive (catheter insertion and dye injection), time consuming (about 1 hour), and requires a high degree of skill to administer, it is rarely performed today. The procedure requires a catheter to be advanced through the right side of the heart and into the pulmonary artery. A radiopaque dye is then rapidly injected into the pulmonary artery while serial roentgenograms are taken. Pulmonary embolism is confirmed by abnormal filling within the artery or a cutoff of the artery. A dark area appears on the angiogram distal to the embolization because the radiopaque material is prevented from flowing past the obstruction (Figure 21-7). The procedure generally poses no risk to the patient unless there is severe PH (mean pulmonary artery pressure >45 mm Hg) or the patient is in shock or is allergic to the contrast medium. Pulmonary angiography has primarily been replaced by the high-resolution CT scan (see above).

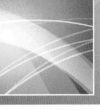
Normal right pulmonary artery | Superior vena cava | **Thrombus in right pulmonary artery**

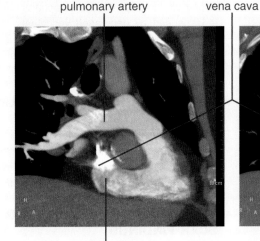 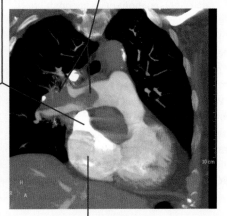 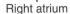

Right atrium | Right atrium

FIGURE 21-5 Oblique coronal projections from a computed tomography pulmonary angiogram (CTPA). Intravenous contrast material is very bright in the visible portions of the superior vena cava and in the superior portion of the right atrium because the contrast material was injected into an antecubital vein. The contrast material mixes in the right atrium with darker blood (without contrast) from the inferior vena cava, resulting in moderate brightness in that chamber, the right ventricle, and the pulmonary artery. The relatively dark area (thrombus) in the right pulmonary artery is clearly outlined by the brighter area (blood flow). CTPA is the best imaging procedure when pulmonary embolus is suspected. (From Vilensky JA, Weber EC, Carmichael SW, Sarosi TE: *Medical imaging of normal and pathologic anatomy*, Philadelphia, 2010, Saunders.)

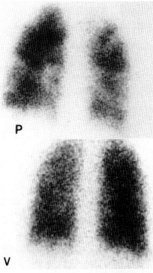

FIGURE 21-6 Fat embolism in a patient with dyspnea and hypoxemia after a recent orthopedic procedure. Perfusion (P) and ventilation (V) radionuclide scans show multiple peripheral subsegmental perfusion defects suggestive of fat embolism. (From Hansell DM, Armstrong P, Lynch DA, McAdams HP, eds: *Imaging of diseases of the chest*, ed 4, Philadelphia, 2005, Elsevier.)

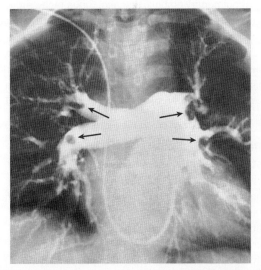

FIGURE 21-7 Pulmonary emboli. Pulmonary angiogram shows numerous filling defects. Trailing ends of the occluding thromboemboli are particularly well shown *(arrows)*. (From Hansell DM, Armstrong P, Lynch DA, McAdams HP, eds: *Imaging of diseases of the chest*, ed 4, Philadelphia, 2005, Elsevier.)

General Management of Pulmonary Embolism

The treatment of pulmonary embolism usually begins with treating the symptoms. Oxygen is administered per the Oxygen Therapy Protocol. The physician provides analgesics for pain, and fluids and cardiovascular agents to correct blood pressure.

Fast-acting anticoagulants, such as heparin, are given (1) to prevent existing blood clots from growing, and (2) to prevent the formation of new ones. Heparin is administered intravenously to achieve a rapid effect. **High–molecular-weight heparin** (unfractionated heparin) has, until recently, been the mainstay of treatment for patients with acute pulmonary embolism. The unfractionated heparin dosing must be governed by frequent monitoring of the activated partial thromboplastin time (APTT). This is because bleeding from unfractionated heparin can develop. Recently, **low–molecular-weight heparins** have become available (e.g., enoxaparin, dalteparin, and tinzaparin) and have been shown to be safer and more effective than unfractionated heparin for prophylaxis of DVT or pulmonary emboli. They are also more cost-effective and do not necessitate APTT monitoring. Doctors strive to achieve a full anticoagulant effect within the first 24 hours of treatment.

This is typically followed by the administration of slow-acting, oral anticoagulant **warfarin (Coumadin, Panwarfarin).** Heparin and warfarin are given together for 5 to 7 days, until blood tests show that the warfarin is effectively preventing clotting. Then the heparin is discontinued. How long anticoagulants are given varies, based on each patient's condition. For example, if the pulmonary embolism is caused by a temporary risk factor, such as surgery, treatment is given for 2 to 3 months. If the cause is from some long-term condition, such as prolonged bed rest, the treatment is usually given for 3 to 6 months. Some patients may need to take anticoagulants indefinitely. For example, patients who have recurrent pulmonary embolism because of a hereditary clotting disorder may need to take anticoagulants for life. Patients taking warfarin need to have their blood tested periodically to determine if the dose needs to be adjusted.

Because many drugs can adversely interact with warfarin, the patient needs to be careful—that is, check with the physician—before taking any other drugs. Drugs that alter the blood's ability to clot include over-the-counter acetaminophens, ibuprofens, herbal preparations, and dietary supplements. In addition, foods that are high in vitamin K (which affects blood clotting), such as broccoli, spinach, and other leafy green vegetables, liver, grapefruit and grapefruit juice, and green tea, may also need to be avoided.

Thrombolytic Agents

Fibrinolytic agents such as **streptokinase** (Streptase), **urokinase** (Abbokinase), **alteplase** (Activase), and **reteplase** (Retavase) actually dissolve blood clots. These agents (commonly referred to as "clot-busters") have proved beneficial in treating acute pulmonary embolism. These **thrombolytic agents** are sometimes used in conjunction with heparin. Their effect in patients with hemodynamic instability may be dramatic. Because of the excessive risk of bleeding, however, the use of fibrinolytic agents in treating pulmonary embolism is somewhat limited.

Preventive Measures

Directions to patients at high risk for thromboembolic disease include the following:

- Walking—If possible, walk frequently. When riding in a car, stop often to walk around or perform a few deep knee bends. When flying in an airplane, move around the cabin every hour or so.
- Exercise while seated—When sitting, flex, extend, and rotate your ankles or press your feet against the seat in front of you. Try rising up and down on your toes. Avoid sitting with your legs crossed.
- Drink fluids—Drink plenty of water to avoid dehydration, which can contribute to the formation of blood clots. Avoid alcohol, which also contributes to fluid loss.
- Graduated compression stockings—Tight-fitting elastic stockings squeeze the patient's legs, helping the veins and leg muscles move blood more efficiently. They provide a safe, simple, and inexpensive way to keep blood from stagnating. Research has shown that compression stockings used in combination with heparin are much more effective than heparin alone.

Inferior Vena Cava Filter

An **inferior vena cava (Greenfield) vein filter** may be surgically placed in the inferior vena cava to prevent clots from being carried into the pulmonary circulation. Their effectiveness and safety of the filter is not well established and, in general, are only recommended in some high-risk patients. Edema distal to the filters is a complicating factor.

Pneumatic Compression

This treatment uses thigh-high cuffs that automatically inflate every few minutes to massage and compress the veins in a patient's legs. Studies show that this procedure can significantly decrease the risk of blood clots, especially in patients who undergo hip replacement surgery.

Pulmonary Embolectomy

Surgical removal of blood clots from the pulmonary circulation (**pulmonary embolectomy**) is generally a last resort in treating pulmonary embolism because of the mortality rate associated with the procedure and because of the availability of fibrinolytic agents to treat pulmonary embolism.

Respiratory Care Treatment Protocols

Oxygen Therapy Protocol

Oxygen therapy is used to treat hypoxemia, decrease the work of breathing, and decrease myocardial work. (See Oxygen Therapy Protocol, Protocol 9-1).

Aerosolized Medication Protocol

Both sympathomimetic and parasympatholytic agents may be used to induce bronchial smooth muscle relaxation when wheezing is present (see Aerosolized Medication Protocol, Protocol 9-4 and Appendix II).

PULMONARY HYPERTENSION

Pulmonary hypertension (PH) is defined as an increase in mean pulmonary artery pressure greater than 25 mm Hg (normal range: 10 to 20 mm Hg) at rest. PH is a frequent complication of chronic pulmonary disease (e.g., chronic obstructive pulmonary disease [COPD] and interstitial lung disease [ILD]), and is more common among women than among men at a ratio of 3:1. The World Health Organization divides PH into five different group classifications based on the cause and treatment options (Box 21-3).

Diagnosis

PH can oftentimes be very insidious. The patient may have mild to moderate PH for years with no remarkable signs or symptoms. Box 21-4 provides signs and symptoms associated with PH. The diagnosis of PH is based on the patient's medical and family histories, physical examination, and the results from a variety of tests and procedures. A number of tests, such as echocardiography, chest x-ray, electrocardiograms, and right heart catheterization, may be used to diagnose PH. Table 21-3 provides an overview of tests and procedures used to diagnose PH. Exercise testing may be used to assess the severity of PH. Table 21-4 shows a PH severity rating scale.

Left-Sided Heart Failure versus Right-Sided Heart Failure

Although there are several clinical conditions that can cause **right-sided heart failure** and cor pulmonale (e.g., COPD, coronary artery disease, pulmonic stenosis, tricuspid stenosis, and tricuspid regurgitation), **left-sided heart failure** (congestive heart failure) is more commonly the cause of PH. Because the respiratory therapist frequently encounters patients in left-sided or right-sided failure—or, a combination of both (**biventricular failure**)—it is important to differentiate and identify the major signs and symptoms (although sometimes overlapping) associated with left-sided and right-sided heart failure. On the basis of the patient's history and physical examination, the common signs and symptoms caused by either left-sided or right-sided heart failure are presented in Box 21-5.

Management of Pulmonary Hypertension

Although PH has no cure, treatment may help reduce the symptoms and slow the progress of the disease. The management of PH includes medicines, procedures, and other therapies. The precise treatment selection depends on what type of PH you have and its severity. Table 21-5 provides an overview of the treatment selections currently used to manage

---

BOX 21-3 Clinical Classification of Pulmonary Hypertension*

Group 1 Pulmonary Arterial Hypertension (PAH)
- PAH includes
  - Idiopathic (IPAH)
  - Heritable (HPAH)
- Drugs or toxins and certain diet medicines induced
- PAH that is caused by conditions such as:
  - Connective tissue diseases
  - Human immunodeficiency virus (HIV) infection
  - Liver disease
  - Congenital heart disease
  - Sickle cell disease
  - Schistosomiasis (parasite infection—one of the most common causes of PAH in many parts of the world)
  - Abnormal vascular conditions of the lungs

Group 2 Pulmonary Hypertension (PH)
- PH due to left heart disease
  - Systolic dysfunction
  - Diastolic dysfunction
  - Valvular disease

Group 3 Pulmonary Hypertension (PH)
- PH due to chronic lung disease and/or chronic hypoxemia

- Chronic obstructive pulmonary disease (COPD)
- Interstitial lung disease (ILD)
- Sleep-related disorders (e.g., sleep apnea)
- Chronic exposure to high altitude

Group 4 Pulmonary Hypertension (PH)
- PH due to **chronic thromboembolic pulmonary hypertension (CTEPH)**

Group 5 Pulmonary Hypertension (PH)
- PH due to unclear multifactorial mechanisms, including:
  - Polycythemia
  - Essential thrombocythemia
  - Sarcoidosis
  - Vasculitis
  - Metabolic disorders:
    - Thyroid disease
    - Glycogen storage disease
  - Other conditions:
    - Tumors that press on the pulmonary arteries
    - Kidney disease

*The World Health Organization first defined the classifications of pulmonary hypertension in 1973 and the classifications have been revised over the years. The classifications of PH were most recently updated in Dana Point, California, in 2008. (Modified from Simonneau G, Robbins IM, Beghetti M et al: Updated clinical classification of pulmonary hypertension, *J Am Coll Cardiol* 5-4:S54, 2009.)

BOX 21-4 Common Signs and Symptoms Associated with Pulmonary Hypertension (PH)

General Findings
- Dyspnea (during routine activity)
- Lightheaded, dizziness, confusion
- Fatigue
- Nonproductive cough
- Hemoptysis
- Hoarseness
- Fainting or syncope
- Chest pain and decreased chest expansion
- A racing heartbeat
- Pain on the upper right side of the abdomen
- Decreased appetite
- Peripheral edema and venous distention
  - Distended neck veins
  - Swollen and tender liver
  - Ankle and feet swelling
  - Pitting edema
- Cyanosis
- Raynaud's phenomenon (blanching of the fingers on exposure to cold)
- Fluid in the abdomen.

Test and Procedure Findings
- Abnormal heart sounds
  - Loud second heart sound (S_2)
- Increased splitting (time delay) of the second heart sound (S_2)
- Third heart sound (or ventricular gallop) (S_3)
- Palpable right ventricular heave or lift
- Abnormal electrocardiographic (ECG) findings
  - Sinus tachycardia
  - Atrial arrhythmias
    - Atrial tachycardia
    - Atrial flutter
    - Atrial fibrillation
  - Acute right ventricular strain pattern and right bundle branch block
  - P pulmonale (peaked P waves)
- Radiologic findings
  - Enlargement of the pulmonary arteries
  - Pulmonary edema
  - Narrowing of the peripheral arteries
  - Enlargement of the right ventricle and atrium (cor pulmonale)
  - Pleural effusion
- Echocardiography
  - Enlarged heart chambers
- Right heart catheterization
  - High pulmonary artery pressure—confirming pulmonary hypertension

TABLE 21-3 Tests and Procedures Used to Diagnose Pulmonary Hypertension

Test or Procedure	Description
Echocardiography	The echocardiogram can be used to show the size and thickness of the right ventricle and right atrium and tricuspid regurgitation. It can also be used to estimate the pressure in the pulmonary arteries (Figure 21-8).
Chest x-ray	A chest x-ray can show whether the pulmonary arteries and right ventricle are enlarged. The chest x-ray can also show signs of an underlying lung disease causing or contributing to pulmonary hypertension (PH).
Electrocardiogram (ECG)	Used to establish whether cardiac rhythm is steady or irregular. ECG findings often reveal right-axis deviation, right ventricular hypertrophy, and strain.
Right heart catheterization (Swan-Ganz Catheter)	Used to confirm the diagnosis of PH and to establish the degree of hemodynamic damage, the presence of vasoreactivity (via a vasoreactivity test), and prognosis (Figure 21-9). A vasoreactivity test is recommended for patients in Group 1 Pulmonary Arterial Hypertension (PAH) (because they are most likely to respond favorably). This involves the administration of a short-acting vasodilator and then the measurement of the hemodynamic response using a right heart catheter. Agents commonly used for vasoreactivity testing include epoprostenol, adenosine, and inhaled nitric oxide. The purpose of vasoreactivity testing is to identify the small minority of patients with a positive test result who may benefit from an oral calcium channel blocker (CCB) with a dihydropyridine or diltiazem. In contrast, patients with a negative vasoreactivity test require advanced therapy with a prostanoid, endothelin receptor antagonist, or phosphodiesterase-5 inhibitor (see Table 21-5).
Chest high-resolution computed tomography (CT) scan	Used to rule out underlying etiologies or condition(s) that may be causing PH.
Chest MRI	Chest magnetic resonance imaging, or chest MRI, can also help detect signs of PH or an underlying condition causing PH. The chest MRI shows how the right ventricle is working and how blood is moving through the lungs.

Continued

TABLE 21-3 Tests and Procedures Used to Diagnose Pulmonary Hypertension—cont'd

Test or Procedure	Description
Pulmonary function tests	Used to rule out the presence of significant restrictive or obstructive pulmonary disease—for example, chronic obstructive pulmonary disease (COPD) versus interstitial lung disease (ILD). Patient with idiopathic pulmonary arterial hypertension (IPAH) commonly have a decreased pulmonary diffusion capacity (D_{LCO}).
Polysomnogram (PSG)	Used to help determine apneas and low oxygen levels during sleep, which are common in PH (see Chapter 31).
Ventilation/perfusion (VQ) scan	Used to help detect blood clots in the lungs.
Blood tests	Used to rule out other diseases, such as HIV, liver disease, and autoimmune diseases (such as rheumatoid arthritis).

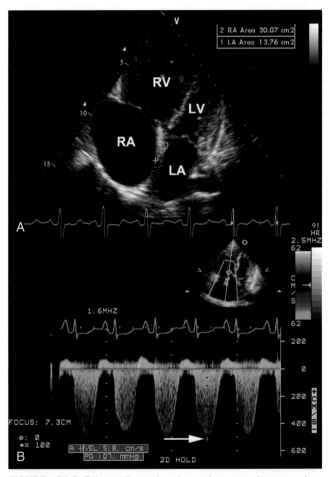

FIGURE 21-8 Echocardiography in pulmonary hypertension. **A,** Apical four-chamber view of the heart reveals enlarged right atrium and ventricle compressing the left cardiac chambers. **B,** Doppler echocardiography shows tricuspid insufficiency jet *(arrow)* used to estimate the right ventricular systolic pressure, in this case 107 mm Hg. *LA,* Left atrium; *LV,* left ventricle; *RA,* right atrium; *RV,* right ventricle. (From Kacmarek RM, Stoller JK, Albert HJ: *Egan's fundamentals of respiratory care,* ed 10, St Louis, 2013, Elsevier.)

TABLE 21-4 Pulmonary Hypertension Severity Rating Based on Exercise Testing*

Class	Description
Class 1	No remarkable limits. The patient performs regular physical activities (e.g., walking or climbing stairs) without causing pulmonary hypertension (PH) symptoms (e.g., tiredness, shortness of breath, or chest pain).
Class 2	Slight or mild limits. The patient is comfortable while resting, but regular physical activity (e.g., walking or climbing stairs) causes PH symptoms.
Class 3	Marked or noticeable limits. Comfortable while resting. However, regular physical activity (e.g., walking or climbing stairs) causes PH symptoms.
Class 4	Severe limits. Patient unable to do any physical activity without discomfort. PH symptoms may be present at rest.

*Exercise testing typically entails either (1) a 6-minute walk test, which measures the distance the patient can quickly walk in 6 minutes, or (2) a cardiopulmonary exercise test, which measures how well the cardiopulmonary system functions while exercising on a treadmill or bicycle.

PH. In addition, several different treatments may be used to manage all types of PH. For example, therapies commonly used to treat all types of PH include the following:

- **Diuretics**—to help decrease fluid buildup—including swelling in ankles and feet.
- **Blood-thinning medications**—to help prevent blood clots from forming or getting larger.
- **Digoxin**—to help the heart to pump stronger or to control the heart rate.
- **Oxygen therapy**—to treat hypoxemia.
- **Physical activity**—to improve exercise tolerance.

The Role of the Respiratory Therapist in Pulmonary Vascular Disorders

In the future, the role of the respiratory therapist will, undoubtedly, expand in the diagnosis and management areas of patients with pulmonary vascular disease. For example, at the patient bedside, the perceptive respiratory therapist may

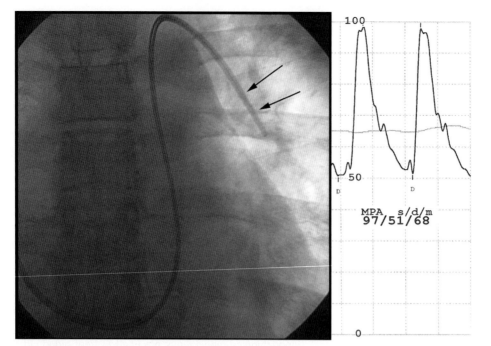

FIGURE 21-9 Right heart catheterization in pulmonary hypertension. In the *left panel*, a pulmonary artery catheter is observed in the left pulmonary artery *(arrows)*. In the *right panel*, the corresponding pulmonary artery pressure tracing is shown, confirming the diagnosis of pulmonary hypertension. In this case, the pulmonary artery systolic, diastolic, and mean pressures were 97 mm Hg, 51 mm Hg, and 68 mm Hg. (From Kacmarek RM, Stoller JK, Albert HJ: *Egan's fundamentals of respiratory care*, ed 10, St Louis, 2013, Elsevier.)

BOX 21-5 Signs and Symptoms: Left-Sided Heart Failure versus Right-Sided Heart Failure

Right-Sided Heart Failure
- Shortness of breath
- Irregular fast heart rate
- Distended neck veins
- Peripheral edema and venous distention
  - Distended neck veins
  - Swollen and tender liver
  - Ankle and feet swelling
  - Pitting edema
- Heart palpitations
- Abdominal distension (bloating)—ascites
- Abdominal pain
- Urinating more frequently at night
- Anorexia
- Nausea
- Fatigue, weakness, faintness
- Weight gain

Left-Sided Heart Failure
- Shortness of breath
- Lightheadedness or fainting
- Frothy, blood-tinged sputum
- Crackles
- Cough and hemoptysis
- Orthopnea
- Paroxysmal nocturnal dyspnea
- Weak pulse
- Hypotension
- Decreased urine production
- Activity intolerance
- Fatigue, weakness, faintness
- Weight gain and fluid retention
- Heart palpitations
- Anxiety
- Excessive sweating
- Cyanosis
- Cool or clammy skin to touch

---

likely be the first to recognize and report important signs and symptoms associated with left-heart sided failure or right-sided heart failure—and, importantly, identify key signs and symptoms of deep venous thrombosis, pulmonary embolism, or PH. Such information-gathering and timely communication may be lifesaving. In addition, the role of the respiratory therapist in the management of pulmonary vascular diseases will further broaden as inhaled gas (e.g., inhaled nitric oxide

[iNO]), and various aerosolized medications (e.g., iloprost and treprostinil), continue to demonstrate long-term therapeutic benefits.[2]

---

[2]See more on the role of the respiratory therapist in administering iNO in treating **persistent pulmonary hypertension of the newborn** (PPHN), Chapter 32.

TABLE 21-5 Treatment Selections Used to Manage Pulmonary Hypertension

Group 1
Pulmonary Arterial Hypertension (PAH)
	Treatments for Group 1 PAH include the following medications and medical procedures:
	Medications
	Positive Vasoreactivity Test
	    Oral calcium channel blocker (CCB) with a dihydropyridine or diltiazem
	Negative Vasoreactivity Test (Advanced Therapy)
	    Prostanoids, (e.g., treprostinil, iloprost, and epoprostenol)
	    Endothelin receptor antagonists (e.g., bosentan and ambrisentan)
	    Phosphodiesterase-5 inhibitors (e.g., sildenafil)
	Surgical Procedures
	    Lung transplant
	    Heart transplant

Group 2 **Pulmonary Hypertension (PH)**	Treating the underlying condition—for example, mitral valve disease in left-side heart failure—can help Group 2 PH. Management includes lifestyle changes, medications, and surgery.
Group 3 **Pulmonary Hypertension (PH)**	Oxygen therapy is the primary treatment selection in Group 3 when the PH is caused by hypoxemia resulting from chronic obstructive pulmonary disease (COPD), chronic interstitial lung disease (ILD), and sleep apnea.
Group 4 **Pulmonary Hypertension (PH)**	Blood-thinning medications are used to treat blood clots in the lungs or blood-clotting disorders associated with Group 4 PH. Potentially curative pulmonary thromboendarterectomy surgery must be considered.
Group 5 **Pulmonary Hypertension (PH)**	Because various different diseases or conditions, such as thyroid disease and sarcoidosis, can cause Group 5 PH, treatment is directed at the cause of the PH.

As many as 25–30% of patients with CTEPH may never have had a diagnosed pulmonary embolism or even a history suggestive of pulmonary embolism, and 45–55% may never have had a history of deep vein thrombus.

CASE STUDY Pulmonary Embolism

Admitting History

A 32-year-old motorcycle enthusiast who smoked one pack of cigarettes per day fell from his bike while riding with a group of Harley "hogs" to the annual Sturgis Rally in North Dakota. Although his motorcycle sustained extensive damage, the man was conscious when the ambulance arrived. Before he was transported to the local hospital, he was treated in the field; splints and an immobilizer were applied. His injuries were thought to include a fractured pelvis, left tibia, and left knee.

En route to the hospital, a non-rebreathing oxygen mask was placed over the man's face. An intravenous infusion was started with 5% glucose solution. The patient was alert and able to answer questions. His vital signs were as follows: blood pressure 150/90, heart rate 105 bpm, and respiratory rate 20/min. Various small lacerations and scrapes on his face and left shoulder were treated. Each time the man was moved slightly or when the ambulance suddenly bounced or turned sharply as it moved over the highway, he complained of abdominal and bilateral chest pain. The emergency medical technician (EMT) crew all believed that his helmet and his youth had saved his life.

In the emergency room, a laboratory technician drew the patient's blood; several x-ray films were taken, and the man was given morphine for the pain. Within an hour the patient was taken to surgery to have the broken bones in his left leg repaired. He was transferred 4 hours later to the intensive care unit (ICU) with his left leg in a cast. Thrombosis and embolism prophylaxis had been started with low-dose heparin. Busy with another surgery, the physician ordered a respiratory care consultation for the patient.

Physical Examination

The respiratory therapist found the patient lying in bed with his left leg suspended about 25 cm (10 inches) above the bed surface. He had a partial rebreathing oxygen mask on his face, and was alert. His wife and twin boys, who were 10 years of age and wearing black motorcycle jackets, were at the man's

bedside. The patient stated that he was feeling much better and that his breathing was "OK."

His vital signs were as follows: blood pressure 115/75, heart rate 75 beats/min and respiratory rate 12 breaths/min. He was afebrile, and his skin color appeared good. No remarkable breathing problems were noted. Palpation revealed mild tenderness over the left shoulder and left anterior chest area. Percussion was unremarkable, and auscultation revealed normal vesicular breath sounds. The chest x-ray taken earlier that morning in the emergency room was normal. His arterial blood gas values (ABGs) on a non-rebreathing oxygen mask were as follows: pH 7.40, $PaCO_2$ 41 mm Hg, HCO_3^- 24 mEq/L, PaO_2 504 mm Hg, and SaO_2 97%. On the basis of these clinical data, the following SOAP was documented.

Respiratory Assessment and Plan

S "My breathing is OK."

O No remarkable respiratory distress noted. Vital signs: BP 115/75, HR 75, RR 12; afebrile; tenderness over left shoulder and left anterior chest area; normal vesicular breath sounds; CXR: normal; ABGs (partial rebreathing mask): pH 7.40, $PaCO_2$ 41, HCO_3^- 24, PaO_2 504 mm Hg, SaO_2 97%.

A • No remarkable respiratory problems
  • Normal acid-base status with overoxygenation

P Reduce FIO_2 per protocol (2 L/min by nasal cannula). Recheck SpO_2.

3 Days after Admission

On the second hospital day, he was transferred out of the ICU. The man's general course of recovery was uneventful until the third day after his admission, when the nurses noticed swelling of the left calf while giving him a bath. Venous ultrasonography revealed a large left femoral vein deep venous thrombosis (DVT). The physician was informed and anticoagulant therapy was started. Five hours later, the patient became short of breath and agitated. A spontaneous cough was noted, with production of a small amount of blood-tinged sputum. Concerned, the nurse called the physician and respiratory care.

When the therapist walked into the patient's room, the man appeared cyanotic, extremely short of breath, and stated that he felt awful. The patient also said that he had precordial chest pain, felt lightheaded, and had a feeling of impending doom. His vital signs were as follows: blood pressure 90/45, heart rate 125 beats/min respiratory rate 30 breaths/min, and oral temperature 37.2 °C (99 °F). Palpation and percussion of the chest were unremarkable. Auscultation revealed faint wheezing throughout both lung fields. A pleural friction rub was audible anteriorly over the right middle lobe. The patient's electrocardiogram (ECG) pattern alternated between a normal sinus rhythm, sinus tachycardia, and atrial flutter.

The chest x-ray showed increased density in the right middle lobe consistent with atelectasis and consolidation. On an FIO_2 of 0.50, the ABGs were as follows: pH 7.53, $PaCO_2$ 26 mm Hg, HCO_3^- 21 mEq/L, PaO_2 53, and SaO_2 91%. Because a pulmonary embolism was suspected, a modified

Wells Scoring System was administered and produced a score of 7—which revealed a high probability that the patient had developed a pulmonary embolism. At this time, the physician started the patient on intravenous streptokinase, ordered a computed tomography pulmonary angiogram (CTPA), and requested that respiratory care see the patient again. On the basis of these clinical data, the following SOAP was documented.

Respiratory Assessment and Plan

S "I feel awful. I'm short of breath and lightheaded."

O Cyanosis; agitation; dyspnea; cough productive of small amount of blood-tinged sputum; vital signs: BP 90/45, HR 125, RR 30, T 37.2 °C (99 °F), slight wheezing throughout both lung fields; pleural friction rub, right mid-lung; ECG: varies among normal sinus rhythm, sinus tachycardia, atrial flutter. CXR: atelectasis and consolidation in the right middle lobe. On FIO_2 = 0.5, ABGs: pH 7.53, $PaCO_2$ 26, HCO_3^- 21, PaO_2 53, SaO_2 91%. Wells Score: 7.

A • High probability of a pulmonary embolism (Wells score of 7)
  • Hypotension (BP)
  • Tachycardia, atrial flutter (ECG)
  • Respiratory distress (cyanosis, heart rate, respiratory rate, ABGs)
  • Pulmonary embolism and infarction likely (history, vital signs, CXR, ECG, blood-tinged sputum, wheezing, pleural friction rub)
  • Bronchospasm, probably secondary to pulmonary embolism or infarction (wheezing)
  • Alveolar atelectasis and consolidation (CXR)
  • Acute alveolar hyperventilation with moderate hypoxemia (ABGs)

P Contact physician and transfer to ICU. Increase **oxygen therapy** per **Protocol.** Begin **Aerosolized Medication Protocol** (med. neb. with 2 mL albuterol premix qid). Monitor and reevaluate in 30 minutes (e.g., ABG). Remain on standby with mechanical ventilator available.

2 Hours Later

The CTPA scan showed no blood flow to the right middle lobe. The patient's eyes were closed, and he no longer was responsive to questions. His skin appeared cyanotic, and his cough was productive of a small amount of blood-tinged sputum. His vital signs were as follows: blood pressure 70/35, heart rate 160 beats/min respiratory rate 25 breaths/min and shallow, and rectal temperature 37.5 °C (99.2 °F). Findings on palpation of the chest were normal. Dull percussion notes were elicited over the right mid-lung. Wheezing was heard throughout both lung fields, and a pleural friction rub was audible over the right middle lobe.

The patient's ECG pattern alternated between a normal sinus rhythm, sinus tachycardia, and atrial flutter. The patient's ABGs on 100% oxygen were as follows: pH 7.25, $PaCO_2$ 69 mm Hg, HCO_3^- 27 mEq/L, PaO_2 37 mm Hg, and SaO_2 59%.

On the basis of these clinical data, the following SOAP was documented.

Respiratory Assessment and Plan

S N/A (patient not responsive)

O CTPA scan: no blood flow to right middle lobe; cyanosis; cough: small amount of blood-tinged sputum; vital signs: BP 70/35, HR 160, RR 25 and shallow, T 37.5°C (99.2°F); palpation negative; dull percussion notes over right middle lobe; wheezing over both lungs; pleural friction rub over right middle lobe; ECG: alternating among normal sinus rhythm, sinus tachycardia, and atrial flutter; ABGs on 100% O_2: pH 7.25, $PaCO_2$ 69, HCO_3^- 27, PaO_2 37, SaO_2 59%.

A • Acute ventilatory failure with severe hypoxemia (ABGs)
   • Pulmonary embolism and infarction (CTPA scan)
   • Bronchospasm (wheezing)

P Contact physician stat. Discuss acute ventilatory failure and need for intubation and **Mechanical Ventilation Protocol.** Manually ventilate until physician arrives. Continue **Oxygen Therapy Protocol** via manual resuscitation at an FIO_2 of 1.0—add continuous positive airway pressure (CPAP) at 10 cm H_2O. Increase **Aerosolized Medication Protocol** (changing med. nebs. to IPPB to assist patient's work of breathing q4 h).

Discussion

Risk factors for development of a fatal pulmonary embolism include pelvis and long bone fractures, immobilization, malignant disease, and a history of thrombotic disease (including venous thrombosis), congestive heart failure, and chronic lung disease. Only about 10% of patients with pulmonary emboli do not have at least one of these risk factors. The symptoms of ultimately fatal pulmonary embolism include dyspnea (in about 60% of patients), syncope (in about 25% of patients), altered mental status, apprehension, nonpleuritic chest pain, sweating, cough, and hemoptysis (in a smaller percentage of patients).

The signs of acute pulmonary embolism and infarction include tachypnea, tachycardia, crackles, low-grade fever, lower extremity edema, hypotension, cyanosis, gallop rhythm, diaphoresis, and clinically evident phlebitis (in a small percentage of patients).

It is interesting to note that in surgical patients, at least half of the deaths caused by pulmonary embolism occur within the first week after the surgical procedure, most commonly on the third to seventh day after the operation. The remainder of the deaths, however, divide equally among the second, third, and fourth postoperative weeks. The current patient certainly had one of the obvious causes for pulmonary embolism—namely, pelvis and long bone fractures and immobilization of the left leg, which was put in a cast after surgery.

At the time of the first assessment, the patient was not in any respiratory distress. His chest physical examination was basically unremarkable, as were the chest x-ray and ABGs. The patient might well have been placed on hyperexpansion therapy, such as incentive spirometry or even mask CPAP therapy, to be proactive in preventing atelectasis. This fact was particularly important for this patient, who was on morphine and might have been prone to hypoventilate because of his left shoulder and left anterior chest pain and tenderness.

By the time of the second assessment, however, things had changed dramatically—the patient demonstrated many of the signs and symptoms associated with a pulmonary embolism and infarction. The assessing therapist should have recognized the seriousness of the situation from the patient's complaints, history, physical findings, Wells score of 7, and ABGs. The patient's wheezing most likely was a result of pulmonary embolism and infarction, as was the atelectasis. However, a trial of aerosolized bronchodilation was not inappropriate given the patient's smoking history. The data were abnormal enough to prompt the therapist to suggest that the patient be transferred to ICU and to prepare for ventilator support because acute ventilatory failure might not have been far off.

Indeed, in the last assessment, things had progressed to the point at which the patient was in severe respiratory acidosis with severe hypoxemia, and mechanical ventilation became necessary. Much more lung tissue than just the right middle lobe must have been embolized, and a repeat CTPA later in the patient's clinical coarse was almost certainly indicated, and might have justified even more aggressive therapy. The treating therapist should recognize that the therapeutic options in such cases are limited by the amount of ventilation "wasted" in these patients because of their embolic disease. High minute volume ventilation may be necessary to improve (even slightly) the ABGs in such patients. Some centers would have considered an attempt at pulmonary embolectomy at this juncture.

One final note: The outlook for this patient was extremely poor. Indeed, he died during the fifth week of his hospitalization. He remained on ventilator support until the time of his death.

SELF-ASSESSMENT QUESTIONS

Ⓔ Answers to questions can be found on Evolve. To access additional student assessment questions visit
http://evolve.elsevier.com/DesJardins/respiratory.

1. Most pulmonary emboli originate from thrombi in the:
   a. Lungs
   b. Right side of the heart
   c. Leg and pelvic veins
   d. Pulmonary veins

2. The aortic and carotid sinus baroreceptors initiate which of the following in response to a decreased systemic blood pressure?
   1. Increased heart rate
   2. Increased ventilatory rate
   3. Decreased heart rate
   4. Decreased ventilatory rate
   5. Ventilatory rate is not affected by the aortic and carotid sinus baroreceptors.
      a. 1 and 5 only
      b. 2 and 3 only
      c. 3 and 4 only
      d. 1 and 2 only

3. What is the upper limit of the normal mean pulmonary artery pressure?
   a. 5 mm Hg
   b. 10 mm Hg
   c. 15 mm Hg
   d. 20 mm Hg

4. Pulmonary hypertension develops in pulmonary embolism because of which of the following?
   1. Increased cross-sectional area of the pulmonary vascular system
   2. Vasoconstriction caused by humoral agent release
   3. Vasoconstriction induced by decreased arterial oxygen pressure (PaO_2)
   4. Vasoconstriction induced by decreased alveolar oxygen pressure (PaO_2)
      a. 1 and 3 only
      b. 2 and 4 only
      c. 1, 2, and 3 only
      d. 2, 3, and 4 only

5. In severe pulmonary embolism, which of the following hemodynamic indices is or are commonly seen?
   1. Decreased pulmonary vascular resistance
   2. Increased mean pulmonary artery pressure
   3. Decreased central venous pressure
   4. Increased pulmonary capillary wedge pressure
      a. 2 only
      b. 3 only
      c. 4 only
      d. 1 and 2 only

6. When humoral agents such as serotonin are released into the pulmonary circulation, which of the following occur?
   1. The bronchial smooth muscles dilate
   2. The ventilation-perfusion ratio decreases
   3. The bronchial smooth muscles constrict
   4. The ventilation-perfusion ratio increases
      a. 1 only
      b. 2 only
      c. 4 only
      d. 2 and 3 only

7. Which of the following is or are thrombolytic agents?
   1. Urokinase
   2. Heparin
   3. Warfarin
   4. Streptokinase
      a. 1 only
      b. 4 only
      c. 2 and 3 only
      d. 1 and 4 only

8. Which of the following is the most prominent source of pulmonary emboli?
   a. Fat
   b. Blood clots
   c. Bone marrow
   d. Air

9. Pulmonary hypertension is defined as an increase in mean pulmonary pressure greater than:
   a. 15 mm Hg
   b. 20 mm Hg
   c. 25 mm Hg
   d. 30 mm Hg

10. An oral calcium channel blocker may be used to help manage some patients who have which of the following classifications of pulmonary hypertension?
    a. Group 1 Pulmonary Arterial Hypertension
    b. Group 3 Pulmonary Hypertension
    c. Group 4 Pulmonary Hypertension
    d. Group 5 Pulmonary Hypertension

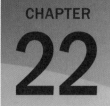

Chapter Objectives

After reading this chapter, you will be able to:

- List the anatomic alterations of the lungs associated with a flail chest.
- Describe the causes of a flail chest.
- Describe the cardiopulmonary clinical manifestations associated with a flail chest.
- Describe the general management of a flail chest.
- Describe the clinical strategies and rationales of the SOAPs presented in the case study.

Key Terms

Double Fractures
Flail
Fractured Ribs

Paradoxical Movement of the Chest Wall
Pendelluft
Positive End-Expiratory Pressure (PEEP)
Pulmonary Contusion
Venous Admixture

Chapter Outline

Anatomic Alterations of the Lungs
Etiology and Epidemiology
Overview of Cardiopulmonary Clinical Manifestations
   Associated with Flail Chest
General Management of Flail Chest
   Respiratory Care Treatment Protocols
Case Study: Flail Chest
Self-Assessment Questions

Anatomic Alterations of the Lungs

A flail chest is the result of **double fractures** of at least three or more adjacent ribs, which causes the thoracic cage to become unstable—to flail, which is defined as to wave, swing, or have abnormal movement (Figure 22-1). The affected ribs cave in (**flail**) during inspiration as a result of the generated subatmospheric intrapleural pressure. This compresses and restricts the underlying lung and promotes a number of pathologies, including atelectasis and lung collapse. In addition, the lung may also be contused (i.e., alveolar hemorrhage and parenchymal damage) under the fractured ribs. Sharp rib fragments may also damage underlying tissue such as the diaphragm, spleen, liver, and large blood vessels.

A flail chest causes a restrictive lung disorder, is often life threatening in severe cases, and requires immediate medical intervention. The major pathologic or structural changes of the lungs that may result from a flail chest are as follows:

- Double fracture of numerous adjacent ribs
- Rib instability
- Lung volume restriction
- Atelectasis
- Lung collapse (pneumothorax)
- Lung contusion (e.g., from trauma)
- Secondary pneumonia (e.g., from weak cough due to pain)

Etiology and Epidemiology

A blunt or crushing injury to the chest is usually the cause of flail chest. Such trauma may result from the following:

- Motor vehicle accidents
- Falls
- Blast injury
- Direct compression by a heavy object
- Occupational and industrial accidents

General Management of Flail Chest

In mild cases, analgesia and routine bronchial hygiene may be the only treatments needed. In more severe cases, however, stabilization of the chest is usually required to allow bone healing and prevent atelectasis. Today, continuous mechanical ventilation, accompanied by **positive end-expiratory pressure** (PEEP), is commonly used to stabilize a flail chest. The use of pharmacological paralytics may be required in severe flail chest for ventilatory control. Generally, mechanical ventilation for 5 to 10 days is adequate for sufficient bone healing to occur.*

---

*Prior to mechanical ventilation with PEEP, external fixation and stabilization was the common treatment for large flail chest injuries.

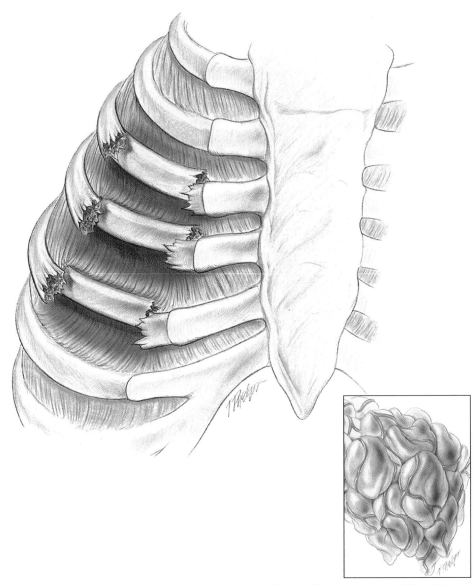

FIGURE 22-1 Flail chest. Double fractures of three or more adjacent ribs produce instability of the chest wall and paradoxic motion of the thorax. *Inset*, Atelectasis, a common secondary anatomic alteration of the lungs.

Respiratory Care Treatment Protocols

Oxygen Therapy Protocol

Oxygen therapy is used to treat hypoxia, decrease the work of breathing, and decrease myocardial work. It should be noted, however, that the hypoxemia that develops in flail chest is most commonly caused by the alveolar atelectasis and capillary shunting associated with the disorder. Hypoxemia caused by capillary shunting is often refractory to oxygen therapy (see Oxygen Therapy Protocol, Protocol 9-1).

Lung Expansion Therapy Protocol

Lung expansion techniques are commonly administered to offset and prevent the alveolar consolidation and atelectasis associated with flail chest (see Lung Expansion Therapy Protocol, Protocol 9-3).

Mechanical Ventilation Protocol

Because acute ventilatory failure is associated with flail chest, continuous mechanical ventilation, often with PEEP, is often required to maintain an adequate ventilatory status (see Mechanical Ventilation Protocol, Protocol 10-1 and Mechanical Ventilation Weaning Protocol, Protocol 10-2).

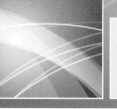

OVERVIEW of the Cardiopulmonary Clinical Manifestations Associated with Flail Chest

The following clinical manifestations result from the pathologic mechanisms caused (or activated) by Atelectasis (see Figure 9-7) and Consolidation (see Figure 9-8)—the major anatomic alterations of the lungs associated with flail chest (see Figure 22-1).

CLINICAL DATA OBTAINED AT THE PATIENT'S BEDSIDE
The Physical Examination
Vital Signs
Increased Respiratory Rate (Tachypnea)

Several pathophysiologic mechanisms operating simultaneously may lead to an increased ventilatory rate. These include the following:

- Stimulation of peripheral chemoreceptors (hypoxemia)
- Paradoxical movement of the chest wall

Paradoxical Movement of the Chest Wall

When double fractures exist in at least three or more adjacent ribs, a **paradoxical movement of the chest wall** is seen. During inspiration the fractured ribs are pushed inward by the atmospheric pressure surrounding the chest and negative intrapleural pressure. During expiration (and particularly during forced exhalation), the flail area bulges outward when the intrapleural pressure becomes greater than the atmospheric pressure.

As a result of the paradoxical movement of the chest wall, the lung area directly beneath the broken ribs is compressed during inspiration and is pushed outward with the flail segment during expiration. This abnormal chest and lung movement causes gas to be shunted from one lung to another during a ventilatory cycle.

When the lung on the affected side is compressed during inspiration, gas moves into the lung on the unaffected side. During expiration, however, gas from the unaffected lung moves into the affected lung. The shunting of gas from one lung to another is known as **pendelluft** (Figure 22-2). As a consequence of the pendelluft, the patient rebreathes dead-space gas and hypoventilates. In addition to the

hypoventilation produced by the pendelluft, alveolar ventilation may also be decreased by the lung compression and atelectasis associated with the unstable chest wall.

As a result of the pendelluft, lung compression, and atelectasis, the $\dot{V}/\dot{Q}$ ratio decreases. This leads to intrapulmonary shunting and venous admixture (Figure 22-3). Because of the venous admixture, the patient's PaO_2 and CaO_2 decrease. As this condition intensifies, the patient's oxygen level may decline to a point low enough to stimulate the peripheral chemoreceptors, which in turn initiate an increased ventilatory rate.

Other Possible Mechanisms

- Decreased lung compliance–increased ventilatory rate relationship
- Activation of the deflation receptors
- Activation of the irritant receptors

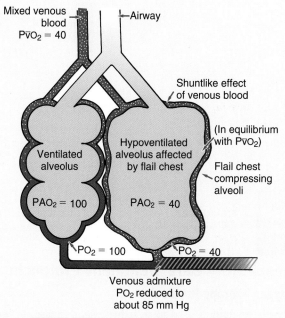

FIGURE 22-3 Venous admixture in flail chest.

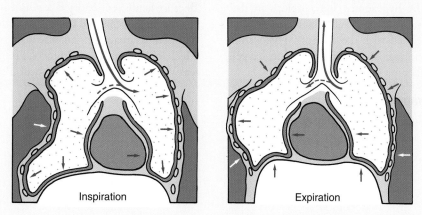

FIGURE 22-2 Lateral flail chest with accompanying pendelluft.

- Stimulation of the J receptors
- Pain, anxiety

Increased Heart Rate (Pulse) and Blood Pressure (e.g., caused by hypoxemia and pain)

Cyanosis

Chest Assessment Findings

- Diminished breath sounds, on both the affected and the unaffected sides

CLINICAL DATA OBTAINED FROM LABORATORY TESTS AND SPECIAL PROCEDURES

Pulmonary Function Test Findings
(Restrictive Lung Pathology)

LUNG VOLUME AND CAPACITY FINDINGS

V_T	IRV	ERV	RV
N or $\downarrow$	$\downarrow$	$\downarrow$	$\downarrow$

VC	IC	FRC	TLC	RV/TLC ratio
$\downarrow$	$\downarrow$	$\downarrow$	$\downarrow$	N

Arterial Blood Gases

MILD TO MODERATE FLAIL CHEST

Acute Alveolar Hyperventilation with Hypoxemia[†]

(Acute Respiratory Alkalosis)

pH	$PaCO_2$	HCO_3^-	PaO_2	SaO_2 or SpO_2
$\uparrow$	$\downarrow$	$\downarrow$ (but normal)	$\downarrow$	$\downarrow$

SEVERE FLAIL CHEST

Acute Ventilatory Failure with Hypoxemia[†]

(Acute Respiratory Acidosis)

pH*	$PaCO_2$	HCO_3^-*	PaO_2	SaO_2 or SpO_2
$\downarrow$	$\uparrow$	$\uparrow$ (but normal)	$\downarrow$	$\downarrow$

[†]See Figure 4-3 and related discussion for the acute pH, $PaCO_2$, and HCO_3^- changes associated with acute alveolar hyperventilation.

[†]See Figure 4-2 and related discussion for the acute pH, $PaCO_2$, and HCO_3^- changes associated with acute ventilatory failure.

*When tissue hypoxia is severe enough to produce lactic acid, the pH and HCO_3^- values will be lower than expected for a particular $PaCO_2$ level.

Oxygenation Indices*

$\dot{Q}_S/\dot{Q}_T$	DO_2[†]	$\dot{V}O_2$	$C(a-\bar{v})O_2$	O_2ER	$S\bar{v}O_2$
$\uparrow$	$\downarrow$	N	$\uparrow$ (severe)	$\uparrow$	$\downarrow$

Hemodynamic Indices[†]
Severe Flail Chest Disorder

CVP	RAP	$\overline{PA}$	PCWP	CO	SV
$\uparrow$	$\uparrow$	$\uparrow$	$\downarrow$	$\downarrow$	$\downarrow$

SVI	CI	RVSWI	LVSWI	PVR	SVR
$\downarrow$	$\downarrow$	$\uparrow$	$\downarrow$	$\uparrow$	$\downarrow$

RADIOLOGIC FINDINGS
Chest Radiograph

- Increased opacity (in atelectatic areas or areas with post-flail pneumonia).
- Rib fractures may need a special radiologic technique (rib series)—to demonstrate.
- Because of the lung compression and atelectasis associated with flail chest, the density of the lung on the affected side increases. The increase in lung density is revealed on the chest radiograph as increased opacity (i.e., whiter in appearance). The chest radiograph may also show the rib fractures (Figure 22-4).

*$C(a-\bar{v})O_2$, Arterial-venous oxygen difference; DO_2, total oxygen delivery; O_2ER, oxygen extraction ratio; $\dot{Q}_S/\dot{Q}_T$, pulmonary shunt fraction; $S\bar{v}O_2$, mixed venous oxygen saturation; $\dot{V}O_2$, oxygen consumption.

[†]The DO_2 may be normal in patients who have compensated to the decreased oxygenation status with (1) an increased cardiac output, (2) an increased hemoglobin level, or (3) a combination of both. When the DO_2 is normal, the O_2ER is usually normal.

[†]CO, Cardiac output; CVP, central venous pressure; LVSWI, left ventricular stroke work index; $\overline{PA}$, mean pulmonary artery pressure; PCWP, pulmonary capillary wedge pressure; PVR, pulmonary vascular resistance; RAP, right atrial pressure; RVSWI, right ventricular stroke work index; SV, stroke volume; SVI, stroke volume index; SVR, systemic vascular resistance.

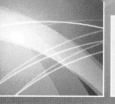

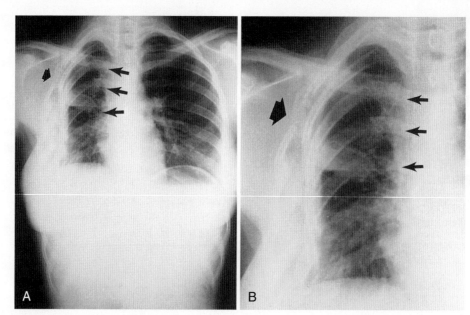

FIGURE 22-4 **A**, Chest x-ray of a 20-year-old woman with a severe right-sided flail chest. **B**, Close-up of the same x-ray film, demonstrating rib fractures *(arrows)*.

CASE STUDY Flail Chest

Admitting History and Physical Examination

A 40-year-old obese male truck driver was involved in a serious four-vehicle accident and was taken to the emergency department of a nearby medical center, where he was found to be markedly agitated and uncooperative. He was conscious and in obvious respiratory distress. His vital signs were as follows: blood pressure 80/62, pulse 90 beats/min, respiration rate 42 breaths/min and shallow. Bilateral **paradoxical movement of the chest wall** was evident.

He had a laceration of the right eyelid and deep lacerations of the right thigh with rupture of the patellar tendon. Pain and tenderness were present on palpation of the right posterolateral chest wall. The ribs moved inward with inspiration. The anteroposterior (AP) diameter of the chest was increased. Breath sounds were decreased bilaterally, and expiration was prolonged.

Chest radiographs revealed double fractures of ribs 2 through 10 on the patient's right posterolateral chest. He had 4+ hematuria, but his other laboratory findings were within normal limits.

The patient was intubated in the emergency department and placed on a mechanical ventilator with 5 cm H_2O PEEP, a V_T of 8 mL/kg, and ventilatory rate of 12. An arterial line was placed, and the patient was taken to the operating room, where surgical repair of the eyelid and thigh was performed. In the operating room, with an FIO_2 of 1.0, the patient's blood gas values were pH 7.48, $PaCO_2$ 30 mm Hg, HCO_3^- 23 mEq/L, PaO_2 360 mm Hg, and SaO_2 98%. His blood pressure was 110/70 and his heart rate was 100 beats/min. The patient was transferred to the surgical intensive care unit, where the respiratory therapist on duty made the following assessment.

Respiratory Assessment and Plan

S N/A—patient is intubated, put on mechanical ventilator, sedated, and pharmacologically paralyzed (vecronium bromide).

O No spontaneous respirations. No paradoxical movement of chest wall on ventilator. BP 110/70, HR 100 regular, RR 12 on vent. On FIO_2 1.0, pH 7.48, $PaCO_2$ 30,

HCO_3^- 23, PaO_2 360, SaO_2 98%. Double fractures of ribs 2 through 10 on the patient's right posterolateral chest: No pneumothorax, no hemothorax.

A • Flail chest (history, paradoxical chest movement, CXR)
  • Acute alveolar hyperventilation with overoxygenation (arterial blood gas, ABG)

P **Mechanical Ventilation Protocol:** Decrease V_T to correct acute alveolar hyperventilation and maintain patient on controlled ventilation and PEEP per protocol until chest wall is stable. Wean oxygen per **Ventilator Protocol** (decreased to FIO_2 0.40). Routine ABG monitoring. Careful chest assessment and auscultation to monitor for secondary pneumothorax and pneumonia.

Over the next 72 hours, the patient was kept intubated and ventilated with an FIO_2 of 0.40 and a mechanical ventilation rate of 12/min. However, his hospital course was stormy. Aggressive fluid volume resuscitation with intravenous fluids at the rate of 100 mL/h was given. His sputum rapidly became thick and yellow. **Lung Expansion Therapy Protocol** was increased to a PEEP of 8 cm H_2O. On the second day, a right pneumothorax was demonstrated and a chest tube was inserted. A persistent air leak was present.

The next day, his pulse increased to 160 breaths/min. His blood pressure was 142/82. His rectal temperature was 99.2 °F. His ventilator rate was 12 breaths/min, with a PEEP of 10 cm H_2O. Auscultation revealed bilateral crackles. On an FIO_2 of 0.70, his ABG values were as follows: pH 7.37, $PaCO_2$ 38 mm Hg, HCO_3^- 23 mEq/L, PaO_2 58 mm Hg, and SaO_2 90%. He was rapidly diuresed, and his cardiac function improved dramatically. Over the next few days, the chest radiograph showed dense infiltrates in both lungs, and it was difficult to maintain adequate oxygenation, even with high inspired oxygen concentrations. His sputum was yellow and thick. At this time, the respiratory assessment was as follows:

Respiratory Assessment and Plan

S N/A—intubated, sedated, and paralyzed.
O Afebrile. HR 160 regular, BP 142/82, RR 12 (on vent). Right chest tube shows air leak. Crackles bilaterally. CXR: Fractures appear in line; bilateral dense infiltrates. ABG on an FIO_2 of 0.70: pH 7.37, $PaCO_2$ 38, HCO_3^- 23, PaO_2 58, and SaO_2 90%. Sputum thick, yellow.
A • Persistent bilateral flail chest (CXR)
  • Bilateral dense infiltrates suggest atelectasis versus pulmonary edema versus acute respiratory distress syndrome (ARDS) versus pneumonia (CXR)
  • Adequate alveolar ventilation with moderate hypoxemia on present ventilator settings; oxygenation continues to worsen (ABG)

• Thick, yellow bronchial secretions (sputum)
• Pneumonia possible (despite normal temperature)
• Bronchopleural fistula on right side (chest tube bubbles)

P **Mechanical Ventilation Protocol** and **Lung Expansion Therapy Protocol**. Increase PEEP to 12 cm H_2O. Oxygen therapy per protocol (maintain FIO_2 of 0.70). Institute **Bronchopulmonary Hygiene Therapy Protocol** and **Aerosolized Medication Protocol** (in-line med. neb. with 3.0 mL premixed albuterol, followed by direct instillation of acetylcysteine q4 h, and suction prn. Obtain sputum for Gram stain and culture). Continue SaO_2 monitoring.

During the patient's first week of hospitalization, his blood urea nitrogen (BUN) increased to 60 mg/dL and his creatinine to 1.9 mg/dL. Liver function values remained within normal limits. The abnormal BUN and creatinine gradually returned to normal during the second week. The patient was slowly but successfully was weaned off the ventilator over the next 2 weeks.

Discussion

This complicated case demonstrates the care of the traumatized patient with multiorgan failure. In this case, the second organ system affected was the cardiovascular system, probably secondary to fluid overload. Initial therapy included chest wall rest and internal stabilization with mechanical ventilation and PEEP. By the time of the second assessment, the more classic clinical manifestations of pulmonary parenchymal change secondary to flail chest had developed. The clinical scenarios of **Atelectasis** (see Figure 9-7) and/or **Alveolar Consolidation** (see Figure 9-8) were well established, with oxygen-refractory pulmonary capillary shunting clearly in evidence.

Later, when what appeared to be acute respiratory distress syndrome (ARDS) supervened, additional PEEP was added, both for its effect on the ARDS and to stabilize the chest wall. Although these problems were dramatic enough, the therapist alertly noted the thick yellow bronchial secretions and added acetylcysteine and vigorous suctioning to deal with this problem. **Aerosolized Bronchodilator Therapy** (in this case albuterol) must always be given before or concurrently with acetylcysteine because the latter agent may cause bronchospasm if given alone. The ordering of a sputum Gram stain and culture was appropriate.

Clearly, a patient this ill should be assessed at least once—possibly more—per shift. Because this patient was hospitalized for 40 days, more than 120 such assessments were found in his chart. As we reviewed his case, this certainly did not seem to be excessive.

SELF-ASSESSMENT QUESTIONS

1. In flail chest, which of the following occur?
   1. Tidal volume (V_T) increases
   2. Atelectasis often occurs
   3. Intrapulmonary shunting occurs
   4. Pneumothorax is rare
      a. 1, 2, and 4 only
      b. 1 and 3 only
      c. 2 and 3 only
      d. 2 and 4 only

2. When a patient has a severe flail chest, which of the following occurs?
   a. Venous return increases
   b. Cardiac output increases
   c. Systemic blood pressure increases
   d. Central venous pressure increases

3. A flail chest consists of a double fracture of at least:
   a. Two adjacent ribs
   b. Three adjacent ribs
   c. Four adjacent ribs
   d. Five adjacent ribs

4. Which of the following respiratory care technique(s) is/are commonly used in the treatment of severe flail chest?
   1. Cough and deep breathe
   2. Intubation with continuous mandatory ventilation
   3. Negative pressure ventilation (cuirass)
   4. Positive end-expiratory pressure/continuous positive airway pressure (PEEP/CPAP)
      a. 1 only
      b. 3 only
      c. 2 and 4 only
      d. 2, 3, and 4 only

5. When mechanical ventilation is used to stabilize a flail chest, how much time generally is needed for adequate bone healing to occur?
   a. 5 to 10 days
   b. 10 to 15 days
   c. 15 to 20 days
   d. 20 to 25 days

Chapter Objectives

After reading this chapter, you will be able to:
- List the anatomic alterations of the lungs associated with a pneumothorax.
- Describe the causes of a pneumothorax.
- List the cardiopulmonary clinical manifestations associated with a pneumothorax.
- Describe the general management of a pneumothorax.
- Describe the clinical strategies and rationales of the SOAPs presented in the case study.

Key Terms

Bleomycin Sulfate Pleurodesis
Chest (Thoracostomy) Tube
Closed Pneumothorax
Iatrogenic Pneumothorax
Open Pneumothorax
Pendelluft
Pleurisy
Pleurodesis
Sclerosant
Spontaneous Pneumothorax
Sucking Chest Wound
Talc Pleurodesis
Tension Pneumothorax
Tetracycline Pleurodesis
Traumatic Pneumothorax

Chapter Outline

Anatomic Alterations of the Lungs
Etiology and Epidemiology
  Traumatic Pneumothorax
  Spontaneous Pneumothorax
  Iatrogenic Pneumothorax
Overview of Cardiopulmonary Clinical Manifestations Associated with Pneumothorax
General Management of Pneumothorax
  Respiratory Care Treatment Protocols
  Pleurodesis
Case Study: Pneumothorax
Self-Assessment Questions

Anatomic Alterations of the Lungs

A pneumothorax exists when gas (sometimes called *free air*) accumulates in the pleural space (Figure 23-1). When gas enters the pleural space, the visceral and parietal pleura separate. This enhances the natural tendency of the lung to recoil, or collapse, and the natural tendency of the chest wall to move outward, or expand. As the lung collapses, the alveoli are compressed and atelectasis ensues. In severe cases, the great veins may be compressed and cause the venous return to the heart to diminish.

A pneumothorax produces a restrictive lung disorder. The major pathologic or structural changes associated with a pneumothorax are as follows:
- Lung collapse
- Atelectasis
- Chest wall expansion (in tension pneumothorax)
- Compression of the great veins and decreased cardiac venous return

Etiology and Epidemiology

Gas can gain entrance to the pleural space in the following three ways:

1. From the lungs through a perforation of the visceral pleura.
2. From the surrounding atmosphere through a perforation of the chest wall and parietal pleura or, rarely, through an esophageal fistula or a perforated abdominal viscus.
3. From gas-forming microorganisms in an empyema in the pleural space (rare).

A pneumothorax may be classified as either closed or open according to the way gas gains entrance to the pleural space. In a **closed pneumothorax,** gas in the pleural space is not in direct contact with the atmosphere. An **open pneumothorax,** however, is a condition in which the pleural space is in direct contact with the atmosphere such that gas can move freely in and out. A pneumothorax in which the intrapleural pressure exceeds the intra-alveolar (or atmospheric) pressure is known as a **tension pneumothorax.** Some forms of pneumothorax are identified on the basis of origin, as follows:
- Traumatic pneumothorax
- Spontaneous pneumothorax
- Iatrogenic pneumothorax

Traumatic Pneumothorax

Penetrating wounds to the chest wall from a knife, a bullet, or an impaling object in an automobile or industrial accident are

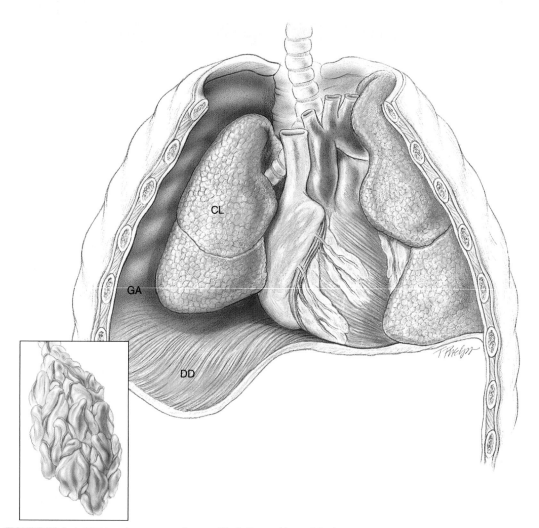

FIGURE 23-1 A right tension pneumothorax. *CL,* Collapsed lung; *DD,* depressed diaphragm; *GA,* gas accumulation in the pleura cavity; *Inset,* Atelectasis, a common secondary anatomic alteration of the lungs.

common causes of traumatic pneumothorax. When this type of trauma occurs, the pleural space is in direct contact with the atmosphere, and gas can move into and out of the pleural cavity. This condition is known as a **sucking chest wound** and is classified as an *open pneumothorax* (Figure 23-2).

A piercing chest wound also may result in a **closed** (valvular) or **tension pneumothorax** through a one-way valve-like action of the ruptured parietal pleura. In this form of pneumothorax, gas enters the pleural space during inspiration but cannot leave during expiration because the parietal pleura (or more infrequently, the chest wall itself) acts as a check valve. This condition may cause the intrapleural pressure to exceed the atmospheric pressure in the affected area. Technically this form of pneumothorax is classified as a *tension pneumothorax* (Figure 23-3). This form of pneumothorax is the most serious of all—since gas continues to accumulate in the intrapleural space and progressively increases the compressing pressures on the lungs and mediastinal structures of the affected area.

When a crushing chest injury occurs, the pleural space may not be in direct contact with the atmosphere, but the sharp end of a fractured rib may pierce or tear the visceral pleura. This may permit gas to leak into the pleural space

from the lungs. Technically, this form of pneumothorax is classified as a *closed pneumothorax.*

Spontaneous Pneumothorax

When a pneumothorax occurs suddenly and without any obvious underlying cause, it is referred to as a *spontaneous pneumothorax.* A spontaneous pneumothorax is secondary to certain underlying pathologic processes such as pneumonia, tuberculosis, and chronic obstructive pulmonary disease (COPD). A spontaneous pneumothorax is sometimes caused by the rupture of a small bleb or bulla on the surface of the lung. This type of pneumothorax often occurs in tall, thin people aged 15 to 35 years. It may result from the high negative intrathoracic pressure and mechanical stresses that take place in the upper zone of the upright lung (Figure 23-4).

A spontaneous pneumothorax also may behave as a tension pneumothorax. Air from the lung parenchyma may enter the pleural space via a tear in the visceral pleura during inspiration but is unable to leave during expiration because the visceral tear functions as a check valve (Figure 23-4). This condition may cause the intrapleural pressure to exceed the intraalveolar pressure. This form of pneumothorax is classified as both a *closed pneumothorax* and a *tension pneumothorax.*

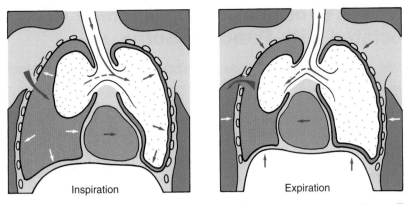

FIGURE 23-2 Sucking chest wound with accompanying pendelluft in an open pneumothorax. The large arrow illustrates the chest wall injury.

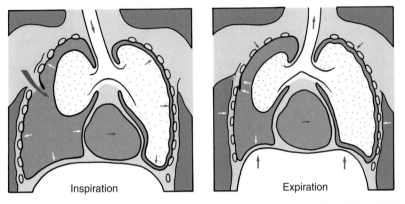

FIGURE 23-3 Closed (tension) pneumothorax produced by a chest wall wound. The large arrow illustrates the chest wall injury. The small arrows indicate the parietal pleural "value."

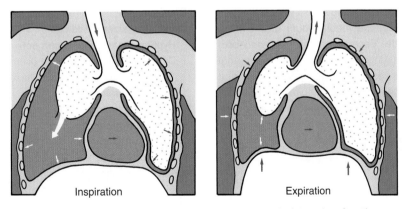

FIGURE 23-4 Right pneumothorax produced by a rupture in the visceral pleura that functions as a check valve. Progressive enlargement of the pneumothorax occurs, producing atelectasis on the affected side.

Iatrogenic Pneumothorax

An *iatrogenic pneumothorax* sometimes occurs during specific diagnostic or therapeutic procedures. For example, a pleural or liver biopsy may cause a pneumothorax, as may a transthoracic needle biopsy of the lung itself. Thoracentesis, intercostal nerve block, cannulation of a subclavian vein, and tracheostomy are other possible causes of an iatrogenic pneumothorax.

An iatrogenic pneumothorax is always a hazard during positive-pressure mechanical ventilation—particularly when high tidal volumes or high system pressures are used. This is particularly common in COPD and in human immunodeficiency virus (HIV)–related acute respiratory distress syndrome (ARDS).

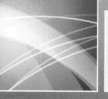
The following clinical manifestations result from the pathologic mechanisms caused (or activated) by Atelectasis (see Figure 9-7)—the major anatomic alteration of the lungs associated with pneumothorax (Figure 23-1).

CLINICAL DATA OBTAINED AT THE PATIENT'S BEDSIDE

The Physical Examination

Vital Signs

Increased Respiratory Rate (Tachypnea)

Several pathophysiologic mechanisms operating simultaneously may lead to an increased ventilatory rate.

Stimulation of Peripheral Chemoreceptors (Hypoxemia)

As gas moves into the pleural space, the visceral and parietal pleura separate and the lung on the affected side begins to collapse. As the lung collapses, atelectasis develops, and alveolar ventilation decreases.

If the patient has a pneumothorax as a result of a sucking chest wound, an additional mechanism may also promote hypoventilation. In other words, when a patient with this type of pneumothorax inhales, the intrapleural pressure on the unaffected side decreases. As a result the mediastinum often moves to the unaffected side, where the pressure is lower, and compresses the normal lung. The intrapleural pressure on the affected side also may decrease, and some air may enter through the chest wound and further shift the mediastinum toward the normal lung. During expiration the intrapleural pressure on the affected side rises above atmospheric pressure, and gas escapes from the pleural space through the chest wound. As gas leaves the pleural space, the mediastinum moves back toward the affected side. Because of this back-and-forth movement of the mediastinum, some gas from the normal lung may enter the collapsed lung during expiration and cause it to expand slightly. During inspiration, however, some of this "rebreathed dead space gas" may move back into the normal lung. This paradoxical movement of gas within the lungs is known as **pendelluft**. As a result of the pendelluft, the patient hypoventilates (Figure 23-2).

Therefore when a patient has a pneumothorax, alveolar ventilation is reduced because of lung collapse and atelectasis. If the pneumothorax is accompanied by a sucking chest wound, alveolar ventilation may be further decreased by pendelluft.

As a result of the reduced alveolar ventilation, the patient's $\dot{V}/\dot{Q}$ ratio decreases. This leads to intrapulmonary shunting and venous admixture (Figure 23-5). Because of the venous admixture, the PaO_2 and CaO_2 decrease. As this condition intensifies, the patient's arterial oxygen level may decline to a point low enough to stimulate the peripheral chemoreceptors. Stimulation of the peripheral chemoreceptors, in turn, initiates an increased ventilatory rate.

Other Possible Mechanisms

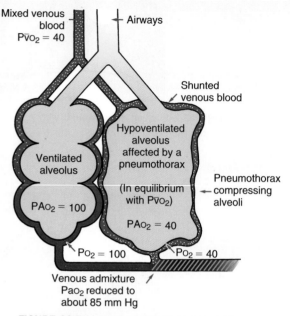

FIGURE 23-5 Venous admixture in pneumothorax.

- Decreased lung compliance–increased ventilatory rate relationship
- Activation of the deflation receptors
- Activation of the irritant receptors
- Stimulation of the J receptors
- Pain, anxiety

Increased Heart Rate (Pulse) and Blood Pressure (Small Pneumothorax)

Cyanosis

Chest Assessment Findings

- Hyperresonant percussion note over the pneumothorax
- Diminished breath sounds over the pneumothorax
- Tracheal shift (away from the affected side in a tension pneumothorax)
- Displaced heart sounds
- Increased thoracic volume on the affected side (particularly in tension pneumothorax)

As gas accumulates in the pleural space, the ratio of air to solid tissue increases. Percussion notes resonate more freely throughout the gas in the pleural space as well as in the air spaces within the lung (Figure 23-6). When this area is auscultated, however, the breath sounds are diminished (Figure 23-7). When intrapleural gas accumulates, and intrathoracic pressure is excessively high, the mediastinum may be forced to the unaffected side. If this is the case, there will be a tracheal shift and the heart sounds will be displaced during auscultation.

Finally, the gas that accumulates in the pleural space enhances not only the natural tendency of the lungs to collapse, but also the natural tendency of the chest wall to expand. Therefore in a large pneumothorax the chest often appears larger on the affected side. This is especially true in patients with a severe tension pneumothorax (Figure 23-8).

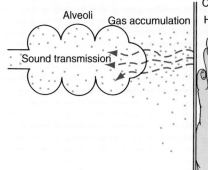

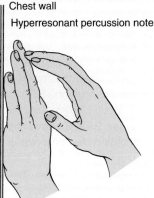

FIGURE 23-6 Because the ratio of extrapulmonary gas to solid tissue increases in a pneumothorax, hyperresonant percussion notes are produced over the affected area.

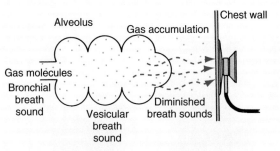

FIGURE 23-7 Breath sounds diminish as gas accumulates in the intrapleural space.

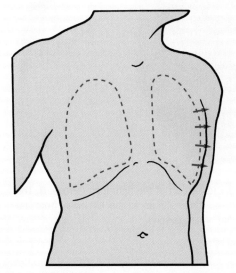

FIGURE 23-8 As gas accumulates in the intrapleural space, the chest diameter increases on the affected side in a tension pneumothorax.

CLINICAL DATA OBTAINED FROM LABORATORY TESTS AND SPECIAL PROCEDURES

Pulmonary Function Test Findings
(Restrictive Lung Pathology)

LUNG VOLUME AND CAPACITY FINDINGS

V_T	IRV	ERV	RV	
N or ↓	↓	↓	↓	

VC	IC	FRC	TLC	RV/TLC ratio
↓	↓	↓	↓	N

Arterial Blood Gases

SMALL PNEUMOTHORAX

Acute Alveolar Hyperventilation with Hypoxemia[†]
(Acute Respiratory Alkalosis)

pH	$PaCO_2$	HCO_3^-	PaO_2	SaO_2 or SpO_2
↑	↓	↓	↓	↓
		(but normal)		

LARGE PNEUMOTHORAX

Acute Ventilatory Failure with Hypoxemia[†]
(Acute Respiratory Acidosis)

pH*	$PaCO_2$	HCO_3^-*	PaO_2	SaO_2 or SpO_2
↓	↑	↑	↓	↓
		(but normal)		

Oxygenation Indices[§]

$\dot{Q}_S/\dot{Q}_T$	DO_2[‖]	$\dot{V}O_2$	$C(a-\bar{v})O_2$	O_2ER	$S\bar{v}O_2$
↑	↓	N	↑	↑	↓
			(severe)		

[†]See Figure 4-3 and related discussion for the acute pH, $PaCO_2$, and HCO_3^- changes associated with acute alveolar hyperventilation.
[†]See Figure 4-2 and related discussion for the acute pH, $PaCO_2$, and HCO_3^- changes associated with acute ventilatory failure.
*When tissue hypoxia is severe enough to produce lactic acid, the pH and HCO_3^- values will be lower than expected for a particular $PaCO_2$ level.
[§]$C(a-\bar{v})O_2$, Arterial-venous oxygen difference; DO_2, total oxygen delivery; O_2ER, oxygen extraction ratio; $\dot{Q}_S/\dot{Q}_T$, pulmonary shunt fraction; $S\bar{v}O_2$, mixed venous oxygen saturation; $\dot{V}O_2$, oxygen consumption.
[‖]The DO_2 may be normal in patients who have compensated to the decreased oxygenation status with (1) an increased cardiac output, (2) an increased hemoglobin level, or (3) a combination of both. When the DO_2 is normal, the O_2ER is usually normal.

Hemodynamic Indices¶
(Large Pneumothorax)

CVP	RAP	$\overline{PA}$	PCWP	CO	SV
↑	↑	↑	↓	↓	↓

SVI	CI	RVSWI	LVSWI	PVR	SVR
↓	↓	↑	↓	↑	↓

RADIOLOGIC FINDINGS
Chest Radiograph

- Increased translucency (darker lung fields) on the side of pneumothorax
- Mediastinal shift to unaffected side in tension pneumothorax
- Depressed diaphragm
- Lung collapse
- Atelectasis

Ordinarily, the presence of a pneumothorax is easily identified on the chest radiograph in the upright posteroanterior view. A small collection of air is often visible if the exposure is made at the end of maximal expiration, because the translucency of the pneumothorax is more obvious when contrasted with the density of a partially deflated lung. The pneumothorax is usually seen in the upper part of the pleural cavity when the film is exposed, while the patient is in the upright position. Severe adhesions, however, may limit the collection of gas to a specific portion of the pleural space. Figure 23-9, *A* shows the development of a tension pneumothorax in the lower part of the right lung. Figure 23-9, *B* shows progression of the same pneumothorax 30 minutes later. Figure 23-10 shows the classic body shape of a 19-year-old man, who is 6 feet 5 inches tall, and who experienced a spontaneous left-sided pneumothorax while playing a round of golf.

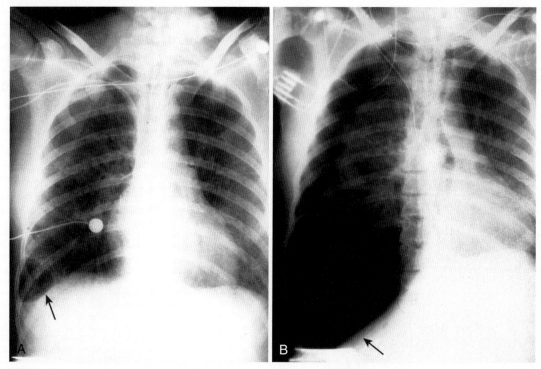

FIGURE 23-9 A, Development of a small tension pneumothorax in the lower part of the right lung *(arrow).* **B,** The same pneumothorax 30 minutes later. Note the shift of the heart and mediastinum to the left away from the tension pneumothorax. Also note the depression of the right hemidiaphragm *(arrow).*

¶*CO,* Cardiac output; *CVP,* central venous pressure; *LVSWI,* left ventricular stroke work index; *$\overline{PA}$,* mean pulmonary artery pressure; *PCWP,* pulmonary capillary wedge pressure; *PVR,* pulmonary vascular resistance; *RAP,* right atrial pressure; *RVSWI,* right ventricular stroke work index; *SV,* stroke volume; *SVI,* stroke volume index; *SVR,* systemic vascular resistance.

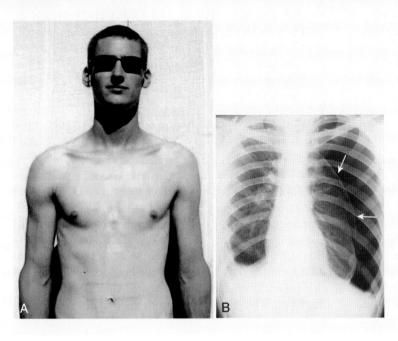

FIGURE 23-10 A, A 19-year-old male patient, 6 feet 5 inches tall, who experienced a sudden spontaneous left-sided pneumothorax while playing a round of golf. A spontaneous pneumothorax is not uncommon in people who are tall and thin. **B**, Chest radiograph of the same patient 45 minutes later in the emergency room. Note the shift of the heart and mediastinum to the right (toward the unaffected side), away from the tension pneumothorax, and the depressed diaphragm on the patient's left side.

General Management of Pneumothorax

The management of pneumothorax depends on the degree of lung collapse. When the pneumothorax is relatively small (15% to 20%), the patient may need only bed rest or limited physical activity. In such cases, reabsorption of intrapleural gas usually occurs within 30 days.

When the pneumothorax is larger than 20%, it should be evacuated. In less severe cases, air may simply be withdrawn from the pleural cavity by needle aspiration. In more serious cases, a **thoracostomy chest tube** attached to an underwater seal is inserted into the patient's pleural cavity. Because air rises, the tube is usually placed anteriorly near the lung's apex, above the rib to avoid injury to the vessels and nerve that run under the ribs in the costal grooves. Typically, a No. 28 to No. 36 French gauge thoracostomy tube is used for adults, with smaller sizes used for children. The tube permits evacuation of air and enhances the reexpansion and pleural adherence of the affected lung. The chest tube may or may not be attached to gentle suction. When suction is used, the negative pressure need not exceed 12 cm H_2O; ~5 cm H_2O is generally all that is needed. After the lung has reexpanded and bubbling from the chest tube has ceased, the tube is clamped and left in place without suction for another 24 to 48 hours.

Respiratory Care Treatment Protocols

Oxygen Therapy Protocol

Oxygen therapy is used to treat hypoxemia, decrease the work of breathing, and decrease myocardial work. It should be noted, however, that the hypoxemia that develops in a pneumothorax is most commonly caused by the alveolar atelectasis and capillary shunting associated with the disorder. Hypoxemia caused by capillary shunting is often refractory to oxygen therapy (see Oxygen Therapy Protocol, Protocol 9-1).

Lung Expansion Therapy Protocol

With caution, lung expansion techniques are commonly administered to offset the atelectasis associated with a pneumothorax (see Lung Expansion Therapy Protocol, Protocol 9-3) in patients with chest tubes.

Mechanical Ventilation Protocol

Because acute ventilatory failure may develop with severe pneumothorax, continuous mechanical ventilation with positive end-expiratory pressure (PEEP) may be required to maintain an adequate ventilatory status (see Mechanical Ventilation Protocol 10-1 and Mechanical Ventilation Weaning Protocol 10-2).

Pleurodesis

On occasion, a thoracentesis may be performed before a procedure called **pleurodesis**. During the pleurodesis procedure a **sclerosant** (**talc, tetracycline,** or **bleomycin sulfate**) is injected into the chest cavity. The chemical substance or medication causes an intense inflammatory reaction over the outer surface of the lung and inside of the chest cavity. This procedure is performed to cause the surface of the lung to adhere to the chest cavity, thus preventing or reducing recurrent pneumothorax or recurrent pleural effusions. An intense pleuritis is produced, which may be quite painful (**pleurisy**).

Admitting History and Physical Examination

This patient was a 20-year-old man, a university student who was in excellent health until 5 hours before admission. He was sitting quietly in his dorm room studying for an examination when he suddenly developed a sharp pain in his left lower thoracic region. It was most acute in the anterior axillary line. The pain was exacerbated by deep inspiration and radiated anteriorly, almost to the midline. It did not radiate into the shoulder or neck. The patient became mildly dyspneic and had episodes of nonproductive cough that seemed to increase the chest pain. These symptoms worsened, and at 1 AM his roommate drove him to the university hospital emergency department.

On examination the patient was a tall, thin, well-nourished young man in moderately acute distress. His trachea was shifted to the right of the midline. His blood pressure was 150/82, pulse 96 beats/min, and respirations 28 breaths/min and shallow. On room air, his SpO_2 was 90%. The left side of the chest was hyperresonant to percussion, and the breath sounds were described as "distant." The patient was not cyanotic. The emergency department physician was momentarily busy with another patient and asked the respiratory therapist on duty to assess the patient's respiratory status.

The respiratory therapist assigned to the emergency room during the night shift made the following assessments and plans.

Respiratory Assessment and Plan

S   Left chest pain worsened by cough; shortness of breath
O   Normal vital signs. Left chest hyperresonant. Trachea shifted to the right. Breath sounds on left "distant." Room air SpO_2 90%.
A   Probable left tension pneumothorax (history and objective indicators)
P   Notify physician (who is in the next room). Request stat CXR and ABG. **Oxygen Therapy Protocol** (partial rebreathing mask). Obtain supplies for tube thoracostomy and place at the patient's bedside.

The patient stated that he was more comfortable on the oxygen mask, but that some left-sided chest pain was still present. His physical findings were unchanged from his initial evaluation. The chest radiograph confirmed the diagnosis of a 50% left-sided pneumothorax, lung collapse, and mediastinal shift to the right. The arterial blood gas values on a partial rebreathing mask were pH 7.53, $PaCO_2$ 29 mm Hg, HCO_3^- 21 mEq/L, PaO_2 56 mm Hg, and SaO_2 92%. The physician was still busy with the patient in the next room.

With this new information, the respiratory therapist charted the following.

Respiratory Assessment and Plan

S   "This oxygen mask helps a little."
O   Persistent symptoms and physical findings as in SOAP-1 above. CXR: 50% left tension pneumothorax. Mediastinum

shifted to right. ABGs: pH 7.53, $PaCO_2$ 29, HCO_3^- 21, PaO_2 56, and SaO_2 92% (on partial rebreathing mask).
A   • 50% left pneumothorax with mediastinal shift—lung collapse and atelectasis (CXR)
    • Acute alveolar hyperventilation with moderate hypoxemia (ABG)
P   Inform physician of previous and current assessment. Up-regulate **Oxygen Therapy Protocol** (Increase FIO_2 via a nonrebreathing mask). Stay at patient's bedside until physician arrives. Assist in placement of chest tube.

Approximately 15 minutes later, the attending physician entered the room and quickly reviewed the clinical data and assessments. Moments later, she performed a needle decompression, followed by the placement of a chest tube. The respiratory therapist placed a CPAP mask on the patient's face at 5 cm H_2O. The FIO_2 on the mask was adjusted to 0.80. Over the next 30 minutes, the lung expanded well and the patient's ventilatory and oxygenation status quickly improved. The chest tube was removed after 48 hours. Follow-up examination after 2 weeks revealed full expansion of the left lung. There was no evidence of blebs or bullae. A tuberculin skin test result was negative, and the cause of the pneumothorax was never found.

Discussion

The spontaneous pneumothorax described in this case study is often seen in tall, thin people between the ages of 15 and 35 years (Figure 23-10). It also can develop in hospitalized patients as a complication of ventilator management, as discussed in Chapter 10. Few respiratory conditions persist with a "crisis" onset, and this is one of them. In short, a spontaneous pneumothorax is an emergency that requires immediate attention—the respiratory therapist should aggressively work to help stabilize the patient's condition as soon as possible! Other instances include foreign body aspiration, pulmonary embolism, anaphylactic shock, and some cases of asthma.

This case nicely demonstrates the signs and symptoms of **Atelectasis** and oxygen-refractory intrapulmonary shunting (see Figure 9-7). The physician and respiratory therapist could not hear crackles, however, presumably because the atelectatic segments were separated (distant) from the chest wall and the examiner's stethoscope.

Although the respiratory care administered in this case (oxygen therapy) was fairly routine and ordinary, the therapist's assistance in the assessment of this patient and his presence at bedside made a great difference in the speed and ease with which the patient was treated. The value of an assessing and treating therapist in this situation cannot be overestimated.

SELF-ASSESSMENT QUESTIONS

Answers to questions can be found on Evolve. To access additional student assessment questions visit **http://evolve.elsevier.com/DesJardins/respiratory**.

1. When gas moves between the pleural space and the atmosphere during a ventilatory cycle, the patient is said to have a(n):
   a. Closed pneumothorax
   b. Iatrogenic pneumothorax
   c. Valvular pneumothorax
   d. Sucking chest wound

2. When gas enters the pleural space during inspiration but is unable to leave during expiration, the patient is said to have a(n):
   1. Iatrogenic pneumothorax
   2. Valvular pneumothorax
   3. Tension pneumothorax
   4. Open pneumothorax
      a. 1 only
      b. 3 only
      c. 2 and 3 only
      d. 3 and 4 only

3. Which of the following may cause a pneumothorax?
   1. Pneumonia
   2. Tuberculosis
   3. Chronic obstructive pulmonary disease
   4. Blebs
      a. 1 and 2 only
      b. 2 and 3 only
      c. 2, 3, and 4 only
      d. 1, 2, 3, and 4

4. When a patient has a pneumothorax because of a sucking chest wound, which of the following occurs?
   1. Intrapleural pressure on the unaffected side increases during inspiration.
   2. The mediastinum often moves to the unaffected side during inspiration.
   3. Intrapleural pressure on the affected side often rises above the atmospheric pressure during expiration.
   4. The mediastinum often moves to the affected side during expiration.
      a. 1 and 4 only
      b. 1 and 3 only
      c. 2 and 3 only
      d. 2, 3, and 4 only

5. The increased ventilatory rate commonly manifested in patients with pneumothorax may result from which of the following?
   1. Stimulation of the J receptors
   2. Increased lung compliance
   3. Increased stimulation of the Hering-Breuer reflex
   4. Stimulation of the irritant reflex
      a. 1 and 4 only
      b. 2 and 3 only
      c. 3 and 4 only
      d. 2, 3, and 4 only

6. The physician usually elects to evacuate the intrathoracic gas when the pneumothorax is greater than:
   a. 5%
   b. 10%
   c. 15%
   d. 20%

7. During treatment of a pneumothorax with a chest tube and suction, the negative (suction) pressure usually need not exceed:
   a. -6 cm H_2O
   b. -8 cm H_2O
   c. -10 cm H_2O
   d. -12 cm H_2O

8. A patient with a severe tension pneumothorax demonstrates which of the following on the affected side?
   1. Diminished breath sounds
   2. Hyperresonant percussion note
   3. Dull percussion notes
   4. Whispered pectoriloquy
      a. 2 only
      b. 1 and 2 only
      c. 3 and 4 only
      d. 1, 2, and 4 only

9. When a patient has a large tension pneumothorax, which of the following occur(s)?
   a. pH increases.
   b. $PaCO_2$ increases.
   c. HCO_3^- decreases.
   d. $PaCO_2$ decreases.

10. When a patient has a large tension pneumothorax, which of the following occur(s)?
    a. PVR decreases.
    b. $\overline{PA}$ increases
    c. CVP decreases.
    d. CO increases.

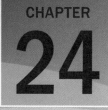

Chapter Objectives

After reading this chapter, you will be able to:

- List the anatomic alterations of the lungs associated with pleural diseases.
- Describe the causes of pleural diseases.
- List the cardiopulmonary clinical manifestations associated with pleural diseases.
- Describe the general management of pleural diseases.
- Describe the clinical strategies and rationales of the SOAPs presented in the case study.

Key Terms

Chylothorax
Empyema
Exudative Pleural Effusion
Fungal Diseases
Hemothorax
Hepatic Hydrothorax
Lateral Decubitus Radiograph
Malignant Mesothelioma
Meniscus Sign
Nephrotic Syndrome
Peritoneal Dialysis
Pleurodesis
Postpneumonic Pleural Effusion
Pulmonary Embolism or Infarction
Reexpansion Pulmonary Edema
Right-Sided Heart Failure
Thoracentesis
Transudative Pleural Effusion
Tuberculosis

Chapter Outline

Anatomic Alterations of the Lungs

A number of pleural diseases can cause fluid to accumulate in the pleural space; this fluid is called a **pleural effusion,** or, if infected, an **empyema** (Figure 24-1). Similar to free air in the pleural space, fluid accumulation separates the visceral and parietal pleura and compresses the lungs. In severe cases, atelectasis will develop, the great veins may be compressed, and cardiac venous return may be diminished. Pleural effusion and empyema produce a restrictive lung disorder.

The major pathologic or structural changes associated with significant pleural effusion are as follows:

- Lung compression
- Atelectasis
- Compression of the great veins and decreased cardiac venous return

Etiology and Epidemiology

Pleural effusion affects approximately 1.3 million people each year in the United States. Early signs and symptoms include pleuritic chest pain, "chest pressure," dyspnea, and cough. Chest *pain* can occur early when there is intense inflammation of the pleural surfaces. Chest pressure does not usually develop until the effusion is in the moderate (500 to 1500 mL) to large (>1500 mL) category. Dyspnea rarely occurs in small effusions unless significant pleurisy is present. A cough is usually directly related to the degree of atelectasis caused by the effusion.

A pleural effusion may be transudative or exudative. A transudate develops when fluid from the pulmonary capillaries moves into the pleural space. The fluid is thin and watery, containing a few blood cells and little protein. The pleural

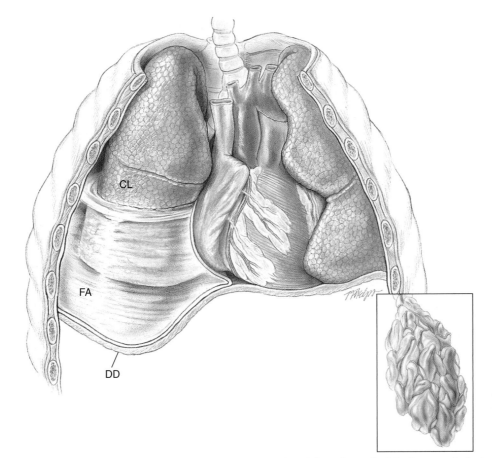

FIGURE 24-1 Right-sided pleural effusion. *CL,* Collapsed lung (partially collapsed); *DD,* depressed diaphragm; *FA,* fluid accumulation. *Inset,* Atelectasis, a common secondary anatomic alteration of the lungs.

surfaces are not involved in producing the transudate. In contrast, an exudate develops when the pleural surfaces are diseased. The fluid has a high protein content and a great deal of cellular debris. Exudate is usually caused by inflammation, infection, or malignancy. **Transudative pleural effusions** and **exudative pleural effusions** are differentiated by comparing the chemistries of the pleural fluid with those of the blood. The pleural effusion is classified as exudative when one or more of the following is found in the pleural fluid:

- Pleural fluid protein >2.9 g/dL (29 g/L)
- Pleural fluid cholesterol >45 mg/dL (1.16 mmol/L)
- Pleural fluid lactate dehydrogenase >60% of upper limit for serum

Common Causes of Transudative Pleural Effusion

Congestive Heart Failure

Congestive heart failure is the most common cause of pleural effusion. Both right- and left-sided heart failure can result in pleural effusion. In general, left-sided heart failure is more likely to produce pleural effusion than right-sided heart failure. In **left-sided heart failure**, an increase in hydrostatic pressure in the pulmonary circulation can (1) decrease the rate of pleural fluid absorption through the visceral pleura and (2) cause fluid movement through the visceral pleura into the pleural space. In **right-sided heart failure** (cor

pulmonale), an increase in the hydrostatic pressure in the systemic circulation can (1) increase the rate of pleural fluid formation and (2) decrease lymphatic drainage from the pleural space because of the elevated systemic venous pressure.

Hepatic Hydrothorax

Hepatic hydrothorax is defined as a pleural effusion, usually >500 mL, in patients with cirrhosis (particularly when ascitic fluid is present in the abdomen) and without primary cardiac, pulmonary, or pleural disease. It develops most likely because of diaphragmatic defects that have been opened by increased peritoneal pressure—thus, allowing the passage of fluid from the peritoneal space to the pleural space. Hepatic hydrothorax is often difficult to manage in end-stage liver failure and often fails to respond to therapy. Because of the location of the liver, the pleural effusion in these patients is generally right-sided.

Peritoneal Dialysis

As in the pleural effusion that occurs as a result of abdominal ascites (see hepatic hydrothorax above), on rare occasions a pleural effusion may develop as a complication of **peritoneal dialysis** in the treatment of severe chronic kidney disease. Peritoneal dialysis uses the patient's peritoneum in the abdomen as a membrane across which fluids and dissolved substances (electrolytes, urea, glucose, albumin and other small molecules) are exchanged with the blood. When the peritoneal dialysis is stopped, the pleural effusion usually disappears rapidly.

Nephrotic Syndrome

Pleural effusion is commonly seen in patients with **nephrotic syndrome.** It is generally bilateral. The effusion is a result of the decreased plasma oncotic pressure that develops in patients with this disorder.

Pulmonary Embolism or Infarction

Between 30% to 50% of patients with pulmonary arterial emboli develop pleural effusion. Two distinct mechanisms are responsible. First, obstruction of the pulmonary vasculature can lead to right-sided heart failure, which in turn can lead to pleural effusion. Second, increased permeability of the capillaries in the visceral pleura develops in response to the ischemic infarction caused by the pulmonary emboli.

Common Causes of Exudative Pleural Effusion

Malignant Pleural Effusions

About two thirds of malignant pleural effusions occur in women. Malignant pleural effusions are highly associated with breast cancer. The pleural effusion is usually caused by a disturbance of the normal Starling forces regulating reabsorption of fluid in the pleural space, secondary to obstruction of mediastinal lymph nodes draining the parietal pleura. Tumors that metastasize frequently to these nodes (e.g., lung cancer, breast cancer, and lymphoma) cause most malignant effusions.

Malignant mesothelioma arises from the mesothelial cells that line the pleural cavities. Individuals who have had chronic exposure to asbestos have a much greater risk for developing mesothelioma. The pleural fluid is exudative and generally contains a mixture of normal mesothelial cells, differentiated and undifferentiated malignant mesothelial cells, and a varying number of lymphocytes and polymorphonuclear leukocytes.

Bacterial Pneumonias

As many as 40% of patients with bacterial pneumonia have an accompanying pleural effusion. Most pleural effusions associated with pneumonia resolve without any specific therapy. Approximately 10%, however, require some sort of therapeutic intervention. If appropriate antibiotic therapy is not instituted, bacteria invade the pleural fluid from the lung parenchyma. Eventually, pus will accumulate in the pleural cavity **(empyema).** Pleural effusion also can be produced by viruses, *Mycoplasma pneumoniae,* and *Rickettsia,* although the pleural effusions are usually small.

Tuberculosis

Pleural effusion may develop from extension of a caseous tubercle into the pleural cavity. It also is possible that the inflammatory reaction that develops in tuberculosis obstructs the lymphatic pores in the parietal pleura. This in turn leads to an accumulation of protein and fluid in the pleural space.

Pleural effusion caused by tuberculosis is generally unilateral and small to moderate in size (see Chapter 17).

Fungal Diseases

Patients with fungal diseases occasionally have secondary pleural effusions. Common fungal diseases that may produce pleural effusions are histoplasmosis, coccidioidomycosis, and blastomycosis (see Chapter 18).

Pleural Effusion Resulting from Diseases of the Gastrointestinal Tract

Pleural effusion is sometimes associated with diseases of the gastrointestinal tract such as pancreatitis, subphrenic abscess, intrahepatic abscess, esophageal perforation, abdominal operations, and diaphragmatic hernia.

Pleural Effusion Resulting from Collagen Vascular Diseases

Pleural effusion occasionally develops as a complication of collagen vascular diseases. Such diseases include rheumatoid pleuritis, systemic lupus erythematosus, Sjögren's syndrome, familial Mediterranean fever, and Wegener's granulomatosis.

Other Pathologic Fluids That Separate the Parietal from the Visceral Pleura

In addition to transudates and exudates, other pathologic fluids can separate the parietal pleura from the visceral pleura.

Empyema

The accumulation of pus in the pleural cavity is called *empyema.* Empyema commonly develops as a result of inflammation. Thoracentesis may confirm the diagnosis and determine the specific causative organism. The pus is usually removed by thoracostomy tube drainage. Open thoracotomy drainage may occasionally be necessary.

Chylothorax

Chylothorax is the presence of chyle in the pleural cavity. Chyle is a milky liquid produced from the food in the small intestine during digestion. It consists mainly of fat particles in a stable emulsion. Chyle normally is taken up by fingerlike intestinal lymphatics called *lacteals* and transported by the thoracic duct to the neck. From the thoracic duct the chyle moves into the venous circulation and mixes with blood. The presence of chyle in the pleural cavity is usually caused by trauma to the neck or thorax or by cancer occluding the thoracic duct.

Hemothorax

The presence of blood in the pleural space is known as a **hemothorax.** Most of these are caused by penetrating or blunt chest trauma. An iatrogenic hemothorax may develop from trauma caused by the insertion of a central venous or pulmonary artery catheter.

Blood can gain entrance into the pleural space from trauma to the chest wall, diaphragm, lung, or mediastinum. A hematocrit of the pleural fluid should always be obtained if the pleural fluid looks like blood. A hemothorax is said to be present only when the hematocrit of the pleural fluid is at least 50%.

OVERVIEW of the Cardiopulmonary Clinical Manifestations Associated with Pleural Effusion and Empyema

The following clinical manifestations result from the pathologic mechanisms caused (or activated) by Atelectasis (see Figure 9-7)—the major anatomic alteration of the lungs associated with pleural effusion (see Figure 24-1).

CLINICAL DATA OBTAINED AT THE PATIENT'S BEDSIDE

The Physical Examination

Vital Signs

Increased Respiratory Rate (Tachypnea)

Several pathophysiologic mechanisms operating simultaneously may lead to an increased ventilatory rate:

- Stimulation of peripheral chemoreceptors (hypoxemia)
- Decreased lung compliance–increased ventilatory rate relationship
- Activation of the deflation receptors
- Activation of the irritant receptors
- Stimulation of J receptors
- Pain, anxiety

Increased Heart Rate (Pulse) and Blood Pressure

Chest Pain (often pleuritic) Decreased Chest Expansion

Cyanosis

Cough (Dry, Nonproductive)

Chest Assessment Findings

- Tracheal shift
- Decreased tactile and vocal fremitus
- Dull percussion note
- Diminished breath sounds
- Displaced heart sounds
- Pleural friction rub (occasionally)

CLINICAL DATA OBTAINED FROM LABORATORY TESTS AND SPECIAL PROCEDURES

Pulmonary Function Test Findings
(Restrictive Lung Pathology)

LUNG VOLUME AND CAPACITY FINDINGS

V_T	IRV	ERV	RV	
N or ↓	↓	↓	↓	

VC	IC	FRC	TLC	RV/TLC ratio
↓	↓	↓	↓	N

Arterial Blood Gases

SMALL PLEURAL EFFUSION

Acute Alveolar Hyperventilation with Hypoxemia[†]
(Acute Respiratory Alkalosis)

pH	$PaCO_2$	HCO_3^-	PaO_2	SaO_2 or SpO_2
↑	↓	↓ (but normal)	↓	↓

LARGE PLEURAL EFFUSION

Acute Ventilatory Failure with Hypoxemia[‡]
(Acute Respiratory Acidosis)

pH*	$PaCO_2$	HCO_3^-*	PaO_2	SaO_2 or SpO_2
↓	↑	↑ (but normal)	↓	↓

Oxygenation Indices[§]
(large pleural effusion)

$\dot{Q}_T/\dot{Q}_S$	$DO_2^{\|}$	$\dot{V}O_2$	$C(a-\bar{v})O_2$	O_2ER	$S\bar{v}O_2$
↑	↓	N	↓ (severe)	↑	↓

Hemodynamic Indices[¶]
(large pleural effusion)

CVP	RAP	$\overline{PA}$	PCWP	CO	SV
↑	↑	↑	↓	↓	↓

SVI	CI	RVSWI	LVSWI	PVR	SVR
↓	↓	↑	↓	↑	↓

RADIOLOGIC FINDINGS

Chest Radiograph

- Blunting of the costophrenic angle
- Fluid level on the affected side (Figure 24-2)
- Depressed diaphragm
- Mediastinal shift (possibly) to unaffected side
- Atelectasis
- "Meniscus sign"

The diagnosis of a pleural effusion is generally based on the chest radiograph. A pleural effusion of <300 mL usually cannot be seen on a chest radiograph in an upright patient. In a moderate pleural effusion (>1000 mL) in the upright position, an increased density usually appears at the costophrenic

---

[†]See Figure 4-3 and related discussion for the acute pH, $PaCO_2$, and HCO_3^- changes associated with acute alveolar hyperventilation.

[‡]See Figure 4-2 and related discussion for the acute pH, $PaCO_2$, and HCO_3^- changes associated with acute ventilatory failure.

*When tissue hypoxia is severe enough to produce lactic acid, the pH and HCO_3^- values will be lower than expected for a particular $PaCO_2$ level.

[§]$C(a-\bar{v})O_2$, Arterial-venous oxygen difference; DO_2, total oxygen delivery; O_2ER, oxygen extraction ratio; $\dot{Q}_S/\dot{Q}_T$, pulmonary shunt fraction; $S\bar{v}O_2$, mixed venous oxygen saturation; $\dot{V}O_2$, oxygen consumption.

[‖]The DO_2 may be normal in patients who have compensated to the decreased oxygenation status with (1) an increased cardiac output, (2) an increased hemoglobin level, or (3) a combination of both. When the DO_2 is normal, the O_2ER is usually normal.

[¶]CO, Cardiac output; CVP, central venous pressure; LVSWI, left ventricular stroke work index; $\overline{PA}$, mean pulmonary artery pressure; PCWP, pulmonary capillary wedge pressure; PVR, pulmonary vascular resistance; RAP, right atrial pressure; RVSWI, right ventricular stroke work index; SV, stroke volume; SVI, stroke volume index; SVR, systemic vascular resistance.

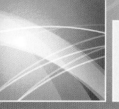
angle. The fluid first accumulates posteriorly in the most dependent part of the thoracic cavity between the inferior surface of the lower lobe and the diaphragm. As the fluid volume increases, it extends upward around the anterior, lateral, and posterior thoracic walls in the so-called "**meniscus sign**" (Figure 24-3). Interlobar fissures are sometimes highlighted as a result of fluid filling.

As nicely illustrated in the chest radiograph of a pleural effusion shown in Figure 24-2, the lateral costophrenic angle is usually obliterated, and the outline of the diaphragm on the affected side is lost. In severe cases the weight of the fluid

may cause the diaphragm to become inverted (concave). Clinically this inversion is seen only in left-sided pleural effusions; the gastric air bubble is pushed downward, and the superior border of the left diaphragmatic leaf is concave. In addition, the mediastinum may be shifted to the unaffected side, and the intercostal spaces may appear widened.

Pleural effusion, atelectasis, and parenchymal infiltrates can obliterate one or both diaphragms. Therefore, when a posteroanterior or lateral chest radiograph suggests pleural effusion, additional radiographic studies are generally necessary to document the presence of pleural fluid or other pathology. The **lateral decubitus radiograph** is recommended because free fluid gravitates to the most dependent part of the pleural space and layers out there (Figure 24-3).

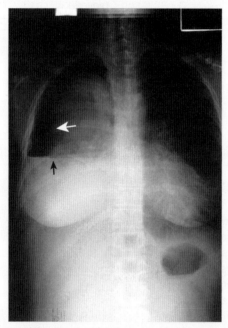

FIGURE 24-2 Right-sided pleural effusion *(small black arrow)* complicated by a pneumothorax *(large white arrow)*. Note that the lateral costophrenic angle on the right side is obliterated, and the outline of the diaphragm on the affected side is lost.

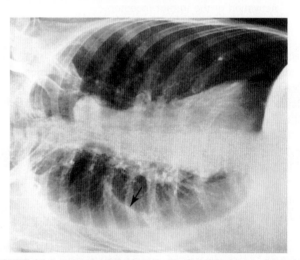

FIGURE 24-3 Subpulmonic pleural effusion. Right lateral decubitus view. Subdiaphragmatic fluid has run up the lateral chest wall, producing a band of soft tissue or water density (meniscus sign). The medial curvilinear shadow *(arrow)* indicates fluid in the major fissure.

General Management of Pleural Effusion

The management of each patient with a pleural effusion must be individualized. Questions to be asked include the following: Should a **thoracentesis** be performed? Can the underlying cause be treated? What is the appropriate antibiotic? Should a chest tube be inserted? When it is determined that a chest tube should be inserted, it is normally placed in the fourth or fifth intercostal space at the midaxillary line. Typically, a No. 28 to No. 36 French gauge thoracostomy tube is used for adults, with a smaller size for children.

The best way to resolve a pleural effusion is to direct the treatment at what is causing it, rather than treating the effusion itself. For example, if the heart failure is reversed or the lung infection is cured by antibiotics, the effusion usually resolves. When the cause of the pleural effusion is not readily evident, microscopic and chemical examination of pleural fluid may determine whether the effusion is a transudate or an exudate. If the fluid is a transudate, treatment is directed to the underlying problem (e.g., congestive heart failure, cirrhosis, nephrosis).

When an exudate is present, a cytologic examination may identify a malignancy. The fluid also may be examined for its biochemical makeup (e.g., protein, sugar, various enzymes) and for the presence of bacteria. Examination of the effusion may reveal blood after trauma or surgery, pus in empyema, or milky fluid in chylothorax. The presence of blood in the pleural fluid in the absence of trauma or surgery suggests malignant disease or pulmonary embolization or infarction.

Respiratory Care Treatment Protocols

Oxygen Therapy Protocol

Oxygen therapy is used to treat hypoxemia, decrease the work of breathing, and decrease myocardial work. The hypoxemia that develops in pleural effusion is mostly caused by the **atelectasis** and pulmonary shunting associated with the disorder. Hypoxemia caused by capillary shunting is often refractory to oxygen therapy (see Oxygen Therapy Protocol, Protocol 9-1).

Lung Expansion Therapy Protocol

Lung expansion techniques are often administered to offset the alveolar atelectasis associated with pleural effusions, and are particularly helpful once the pleural fluid has been removed by thoracentesis or thoracostomy (see Lung Expansion Therapy Protocol, Protocol 9-3).

Mechanical Ventilation Protocol

Because acute ventilatory failure and hypoxemia may be seen in severe pleural effusions, continuous mechanical ventilation may be required to maintain an adequate ventilatory status. Continuous mechanical ventilation is justified when the acute ventilatory failure is thought to be reversible (see Mechanical Ventilation Protocol, Protocol 10-1, and Mechanical Ventilation Weaning Protocol, Protocol 10-2).

Pleurodesis

A **pleurodesis** may be performed to cause irritation and inflammation (pleuritis) between the parietal and visceral layers of the pleural. During the pleurodesis procedure a **sclerosant (talc, tetracycline, or bleomycin sulfate)** is injected into the chest cavity. The chemical substance or medication causes an intense inflammatory reaction over the outer surface of the lung and inside of the chest cavity. This procedure is performed to cause the surface of the lung to adhere to the chest cavity, thus preventing or reducing recurrent pneumothorax or recurrent pleural effusions. An intense pleuritis is produced, which may be quite painful **(pleurisy)**.

CASE STUDY Pleural Disease

Admitting History

A 38 year old woman had discharged herself from the hospital against medical advice 2 months prior to the admission discussed here. She had originally been admitted for severe right lower lobe pneumonia. After 5 days of treatment, she became angry because she was not allowed to smoke. She was a longtime, three-pack-per-day smoker. When a nurse found her smoking in her hospital bed while on a 2 L/min oxygen nasal cannula, the nurse quickly confiscated her cigarettes and matches.

The woman became upset. She told her doctor that this was the last straw and that she was going to leave the hospital on her own. Her doctor wanted her to remain so that a thorough follow-up could be performed for what was described as a "spot" on her lower right lung. The woman promised that she would make an appointment at the doctor's office the next week. She then got dressed and left. However, 2 days later, she felt so much better that she decided the spot on her lung was not an issue for concern. The woman told her friends that smoking one pack of cigarettes made her feel better than 5 days' worth of nurses, doctors, and hospitals.

On the day of the admission discussed here, the woman appeared at her doctor's office without an appointment. She told the receptionist that something was very wrong. She thought that she had the flu and that it had been getting progressively worse over the previous 4 days. At the time of the office visit, she could speak in short sentences only and was unable to inhale deeply. Seeing that the woman was in obvious respiratory distress, the physician was notified. The doctor had the woman transported and admitted to the hospital a few blocks away.

Physical Examination

The woman appeared malnourished, exhibited poor personal hygiene, and had yellow tobacco stains around her fingers. She appeared to be in moderate to severe respiratory distress. Her nails and mucous membranes were cyanotic, and her shirt was wet from perspiration. She demonstrated an occasional hacking, nonproductive cough. She stated that she could not take a deep breath and that maybe the problem stemmed from "that spot" on her lung.

Her vital signs were as follows: blood pressure 130/60, heart rate 112 beats/min, and respiratory rate 36 breaths/min with shallow respirations. She was slightly febrile, with an oral temperature of 37.7° C (99.8° F). Palpation showed that the trachea was shifted slightly to the left. Dull percussion notes were found over the right middle and right lower lobes. Auscultation revealed normal vesicular breath sounds over the left lung fields and upper right lobe. No breath sounds could be heard over the right middle and right lower lobes.

The patient's chest radiograph showed a large, right-sided pleural effusion. The right costophrenic angle demonstrated severe blunting, the right hemidiaphragm was depressed, and the right middle and lower lung lobes were partially collapsed and showed changes consistent with pneumonia. The patient was immediately placed on a nonrebreathing mask and an arterial blood gas (ABG) was drawn. The results were as follows: pH 7.48, $PaCO_2$ 24 mm Hg, HCO_3^- 17 mEq/L, PaO_2 37 mm Hg, and SaO_2 73%. The doctor, assisted by the respiratory therapist, performed a thoracentesis, and slightly more than 2 L of yellow fluid was withdrawn.[1] The patient then was started on intravenous antibiotics. A portable radiograph of the chest was ordered, and a respiratory therapy consultation was requested. On the basis of these clinical data, the following SOAP was documented.

Respiratory Assessment and Plan

S   "I can't take a deep breath."

O   Malnourished appearance with poor personal hygiene; cyanosis with an occasional hacking, nonproductive cough; vital signs: BP 130/60, HR 112, RR 36 and shallow, temperature 37.7° C (99.8° F); trachea slightly shifted to the left; dull percussion notes over the right middle and right lower lobes; normal vesicular breath sounds over the left lung fields and right upper lobe; no breath sounds over the right middle and right lower lobes; chest x-ray (CXR): large, right-sided pleural effusion, right middle and right lower lobes partially collapsed and consolidated; about 2 L of yellow fluid obtained via thoracentesis. ABGs (on 3 L/min O_2 by nasal cannula) before thoracentesis: pH 7.48 , $PaCO_2$ 24, HCO_3^- 17, PaO_2 37, SaO_2 73%

A   • Right-sided pneumonia and pleural effusion (CXR)
    • Partially collapsed right middle and lower lobes (CXR)
    • Respiratory distress (vital signs, ABGs)
    • Acute alveolar hyperventilation with severe hypoxemia (ABGs)
    • Metabolic (lactic) acidosis likely (ABGs compared with PCO_2/ HCO_3^- /pH relationship nomogram)

P   Begin **Lung Expansion Therapy Protocol** (e.g., PEP or continuous positive airway pressure [CPAP] therapy q2h) and **Oxygen Therapy Protocol** (FIO_2 0.50 per venturi mask). Monitor vital signs carefully and reevaluate.

Three Hours after Admission

At this time the patient was sitting up in bed. She stated that although she was feeling better, she did not feel great. She still had an occasional dry-sounding, nonproductive cough. Her skin appeared pale. She was still cyanotic. She was no longer perspiring, as she was when she was first admitted.

Her vital signs were blood pressure 135/85, heart rate 100 beats/min, respiratory rate 24 breaths/min, and temperature normal. Her respiratory efforts, however, no longer appeared shallow. Palpation of the chest was not remarkable. Dull percussion notes were found over the right middle and right lower lobes. Normal vesicular breath sounds were heard over the left lung and upper right lung. Loud bronchial breath sounds were audible over the right middle and right lower lobes.

The patient's chest radiograph showed a small, right-sided pleural effusion. Increased opacity was still present in the right middle and lower lung, consistent with pneumonia. The patient's trachea and mediastinum were in their normal positions. On an FIO_2 of 0.50, her ABGs were as follows: pH 7.52, $PaCO_2$ 29 mm Hg, HCO_3^- 23 mEq/L, PaO_2 57 mm Hg, SaO_2 92%. At this time, the following SOAP was charted.

Respiratory Assessment and Plan

S   "I'm feeling better but not great yet."

O   Cyanotic and pale appearance; occasional dry, nonproductive cough; vital signs: BP 135/85, HR 100, RR 24, temperature normal; dull percussion notes over right middle and right lower lobes; normal vesicular breath sounds over left lung and over right upper lobe; bronchial breath sounds over right middle and lower lobes; CXR: small right-sided pleural effusion; right middle and right lower lobe consolidation; ABGs: pH 7.52, $PaCO_2$ 29, HCO_3^- 23, PaO_2 57; SaO_2 92% on an FIO_2 of 0.50.

A   • Small right-sided pneumonia and pleural effusion, greatly improved (CXR)
    • Atelectasis and consolidation in right middle and lower lung lobes (CXR)
    • Continued respiratory distress, but improving (vital signs, ABGs)
    • Acute alveolar hyperventilation with moderate hypoxemia, improved (ABGs)

P   Up-regulate **Lung Expansion Therapy Protocol** (CPAP mask at 10 cm H_2O q2h for 15 minutes). Up-regulate **Oxygen Therapy Protocol** (FIO_2 0.60 per venturi mask). Monitor and reevaluate.

Five Hours after Admission

The patient was sitting in a semi-Fowler's position. She appeared relaxed and alert. She stated that she had finally caught her breath. Although she still appeared pale, she did not look cyanotic. No spontaneous cough was observed at this time.

Her vital signs were blood pressure 128/79, heart rate 88/min, respiratory rate 16/min, and temperature normal. Palpation of the chest was unremarkable. Dull percussion notes were found over the right middle and right lower lobes. Normal vesicular breath sounds were heard over the left lung and right upper lobe. Bronchial breath sounds were audible over the right middle and right lower lobes. No current chest radiograph was available. The patient's ABG values on an FIO_2 of 0.60 were as follows: pH 7.45, $PaCO_2$ 36 mm Hg, HCO_3^- 24 mEq/L, PaO_2 77 mm Hg, and SaO_2 95%.

---

[1]See **reexpansion pulmonary edema** in discussion section of this case.

On the basis of these clinical data, the following SOAP was documented.

Respiratory Assessment and Plan

S "I've finally caught my breath."

O Relaxed, alert appearance, in semi-Fowler's position; paleness but no cyanosis; no spontaneous cough; vital signs: BP 128/79, HR 88, RR 16, temperature normal; dull percussion notes in right middle and right lower lung lobes; normal vesicular breath sounds over left lung and right upper lobe; bronchial breath sounds over right middle and right lower lobes; ABGs: pH 7.45, $PaCO_2$ 36, HCO_3^- 24, PaO_2 77; SaO_2 95%.

A • Small, right-sided pneumonia and pleural effusion, greatly improved (previous CXR)
  • Atelectasis and consolidation in right middle and right lower lung lobes (previous CXR)
  • Normal acid-base status with mild hypoxemia (ABGs)

P Maintain present level of **Lung Expansion Therapy Protocol** and **Oxygen Therapy Protocols.** Monitor and reevaluate each shift. Provide patient with smoking cessation materials and suggest pulmonary function testing as an outpatient.

Discussion

This case illustrates a patient with postpneumonic pleural effusion, one of the pleural diseases that generally can be improved with appropriate therapy—in this case, the removal of a large amount of yellow fluid via a thoracentesis. This portion of the case study provides a good opportunity to introduce the concept of **reexpansion pulmonary edema.** Reexpansion pulmonary edema is a rare complication resulting from rapid emptying of air or liquid from the pleural cavity performed by either thoracentesis or chest drainage. The condition usually appears unexpectedly—and dramatically—within the first few minutes to an hour after the fluid or air removal. The radiographic evidence of reexpansion pulmonary edema is a unilateral alveolar filling pattern, seen within a few hours of reexpansion of the lung. The edema may progress for 24 to 48 hours and persist for 4 to 5 days.

During the first assessment, the respiratory therapist recognized that the patient had significant respiratory morbidity. Indeed, the patient had an extensive right-sided pneumonia and pleural effusion and partially collapsed right middle and lower lobes. Clearly the patient was in respiratory distress. The patient's acute alveolar hyperventilation and severe hypoxemia were a direct result of the partial collapse of the lung lobes. Because of the extremely low PaO_2 noted on the initial ABG, the presence of lactic acid was very likely. In fact, this was confirmed by the respiratory therapist with the $PCO_2/HCO_3^-/pH$ nomogram. Understanding that **Atelectasis** was the main pathophysiologic mechanism in this case (see Figure 9-7), the therapist correctly assessesed the situation as one that required careful monitoring and began the **Lung Expansion Therapy Protocol** (Protocol 9-3) (e.g., PEP or CPAP therapy) and the **Oxygen Therapy Protocol** (Protocol 9-1) (with a high concentration of oxygen).

Given the patient's history, the respiratory therapist also would be interested in the results of the cytologic studies for malignancy in both the sputum and thoracentesis fluid. Frequently, blood gases do not improve immediately after a thoracentesis, despite the fluid removal, because the atelectasis under the pleural effusion takes some time (hours or days) to dissipate. For this reason, the **Lung Expansion Therapy Protocol,** after thoracentesis, was appropriate.

At the time of the second assessment, the patient was beginning to improve, although she still had signs of right middle and lower lobe **Consolidation** (Figure 9-8). Good breath sounds were heard over the left lung and upper right lung, although bronchial breath sounds reflecting consolidation were still noted on the right. The respiratory therapist was appropriately concerned that atelectasis was still present, and in such a case he or she should increased the **Lung Expansion Therapy Protocol** (Protocol 9-3). In this case, the therapist selected a CPAP mask at 10 cm H_2O every 2 hours for 15 minutes. The therapist could have also intensified use of incentive spirometry, carefully used intermittent positive-pressure breathing, or extended the amount of time the patient was using the CPAP mask.

In the last assessment the patient continued to do fairly well, although she was far from returning to baseline values. The pneumonia, atelectasis, and mild hypoxemia, which persisted despite supplemental oxygen therapy, suggested the need for continued significant (though unchanged) therapy. This case demonstrates that in-place therapy often does not need to be changed at each assessment. Indeed, this guide may apply to as many as 50% to 60% of accurately performed serial assessments. For pedagogic reasons, this option has not been exercised often in this text. However, this third assessment (in a patient with pleural effusion and underlying atelectasis and pneumonia) is a good case in point.

SELF-ASSESSMENT QUESTIONS

Answers to questions can be found on Evolve. To access additional student assessment questions visit
http://evolve.elsevier.com/DesJardins/respiratory.

1. **Which of the following is or are associated with exudative effusion?**
   1. Few blood cells
   2. Inflammation
   3. Thin and watery fluid
   4. Disease of the pleural surfaces
      a. 2 only
      b. 4 only
      c. 1 and 3 only
      d. 2 and 4 only

2. **Which of the following is probably the most common cause of a transudative pleural effusion?**
   a. Pulmonary embolus
   b. Congestive heart failure
   c. Hepatic hydrothorax
   d. Nephrotic syndrome

3. **A hemothorax is said to be present when the hematocrit of the pleural fluid is at least?**
   a. 20%
   b. 30%
   c. 40%
   d. 50%

4. **What percentage of patients with pulmonary emboli develop pleural effusion?**
   a. 0% to 20%
   b. 20% to 30%
   c. 30% to 50%
   d. 50% to 60%

5. **Which of the following is or are associated with pleural effusion?**
   a. Increased RV
   b. Decreased RV/TLC ratio
   c. Increased V_T
   d. Decreased VC

25 Kyphoscoliosis

Chapter Objectives

After reading this chapter, you will be able to:

- List the anatomic alterations of the lungs associated with kyphoscoliosis.
- Describe the causes of kyphoscoliosis.
- List the cardiopulmonary clinical manifestations associated with kyphoscoliosis.
- Describe the general management of kyphoscoliosis.
- Describe the clinical strategies and rationales of the SOAPs presented in the case study.

Key Terms

Adolescent Scoliosis
Boston Brace
Cervicothoracolumbosacral Orthosis [CTLSO])
Charleston Bending Brace
Cobb Angle
Congenital Scoliosis
Cotrel-Dubousset Technique
Harrington Rod
Idiopathic Scoliosis
Infantile Scoliosis
Juvenile Scoliosis
Kyphoscoliosis
Kyphosis
Milwaukee Brace

Neuromuscular Scoliosis
Nonstructural Scoliosis
Rod Instrumentation
Scoliosis
Scheurmann's Disease
Spinal Fusion
Structural Scoliosis
Therapeutic Bronchoscopy
Thoracolumbarsacral Orthosis (TSLO)

Chapter Outline

Anatomic Alterations of the Lungs
Etiology and Epidemiology
Diagnosis of Scoliosis
Overview of Cardiopulmonary Clinical Manifestations Associated with Kyphoscoliosis
General Management of Scoliosis
   Braces
   Surgery
   Other Approaches
Respiratory Care Treatment Protocols
   Oxygen Therapy Protocol
   Bronchopulmonary Hygiene Therapy Protocol
   Lung Expansion Therapy Protocol
Case Study: Kyphoscoliosis
Self-Assessment Questions

Anatomic Alterations of the Lungs

Kyphoscoliosis is a combination of two different thoracic deformities that commonly appear together. In **Kyphosis**, there is a posterior curvature of the spine (humpback or hunchback). In **scoliosis,** the spine is curved to one side, typically appearing as an S or C shape. Its appearance is most obvious in the anterior-posterior plane.

When these two disorders appear together as kyphoscoliosis, the deformity of the thorax can—in severe cases—compress the lungs and restrict alveolar expansion. This condition, in turn, can lead to alveolar hypoventilation and atelectasis. In addition, the patient's ability to cough and mobilize secretions may also be impaired, further causing atelectasis as secretions accumulate throughout the tracheobronchial tree. Because kyphoscoliosis involves both a posterior and a lateral curvature of the spine, the thoracic contents generally twist in such a way as to cause a mediastinal shift in the same direction as the lateral curvature of the spine. Severe kyphoscoliosis causes a chronic restrictive lung disorder that makes it more difficult to clear airway secretions. Figure 25-1 illustrates the lung and chest wall abnormalities in a typical case of kyphoscoliosis.

The major pathologic or structural changes of the lungs associated with kyphoscoliosis are as follows:

- Lung restriction and compression as a result of the thoracic deformity
- Mediastinal shift
- Mucous accumulation throughout the tracheobronchial tree
- Atelectasis

Etiology and Epidemiology

Kyphoscoliosis affects approximately 1% to 2% of people in the United States—mostly young children who are going through a growing spurt. The precise reason why scoliosis and kyphosis often appear together as a combined disorder called kyphoscoliosis is often unclear. However, some of the

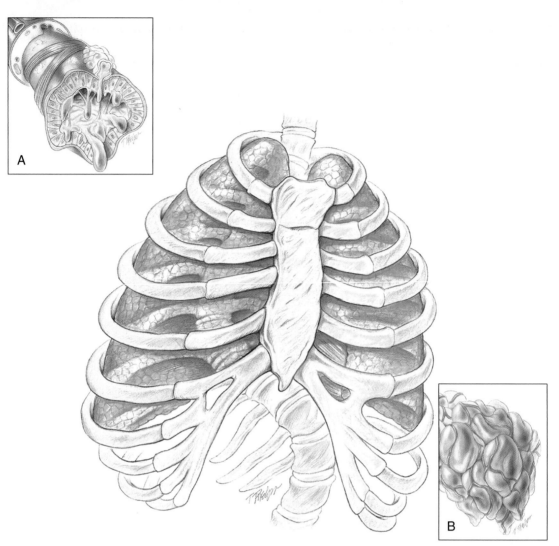

FIGURE 25-1 Kyphoscoliosis. Posterior and lateral curvature of the spine causing lung compression. **A**, Excessive bronchial secretions and **B**, atelectasis are common secondary anatomic alterations of the lungs.

known causes, classifications, and risk factors associated with both scoliosis and kyphosis are as follows:

Scoliosis

In most cases of scoliosis, the cause is unknown. However, in some cases, the scoliosis can be placed in one of the following categories:

Congenital Scoliosis

- A condition resulting from a formation of the spine or fused ribs during fetal development.

Neuromuscular Scoliosis

- A condition caused by poor muscle control, muscle weakness, or paralysis because of diseases such as cerebral palsy, muscular dystrophy, spina bifida, or poliomyelitis.

Idiopathic Scoliosis

- Scoliosis from an unknown cause. It appears in a previously straight spine. When kyphoscoliosis arises without

a known cause (80% to 85% of cases), it is called *idiopathic kyphoscoliosis.*

Other possible causes include hormonal imbalance, trauma, extraspinal contractures, infections involving the vertebrae, metabolic bone disorders (e.g., rickets, osteoporosis, osteogenesis imperfecta), joint disease, and tumors.

Depending on the child's age at the time of onset, idiopathic scoliosis is classified as infantile, juvenile, or adolescent. In **infantile scoliosis** the curvature of the spine develops during the first 3 years of life. In **juvenile scoliosis** the curvature occurs at 4 years of age to the onset of adolescence. In **adolescent scoliosis** the spinal curvature develops after the age of 10 years. Adolescent scoliosis is the most common. Early signs (i.e., appearing when a child is approximately 8 years of age) of scoliosis include uneven shoulder height, prominent shoulder blade(s), uneven waist height, elevated hips, and leaning to one side.

Risk factors include the following:

- **Gender**—Girls are more likely to develop curvature of the spine than boys.

- **Age**—The younger the child is when the diagnosis is first made, the greater the chance of curve progression.
- **Angle of the curve**—The greater the curvature of the spine, the greater the risk that the curve progression will worsen.
- **Location**—Curves in the middle to lower spine are less likely to progress than those in the upper spine.
- **Height**—Taller people have a greater chance of curve progression.
- **Spinal problems at birth**—Children with scoliosis at birth (congenital scoliosis) have a greater risk for worsening of the curve.

Diagnosis of Scoliosis

Scoliosis is diagnosed by means of the patient's medical history, physical examination, x-ray evaluation, and curve measurement. Clinically, scoliosis is commonly defined according to the following factors related to the curvature of the spine:
- Shape (**nonstructural scoliosis** and **structural scoliosis**)—A nonstructural scoliosis is a curve that develops side-to-side as a C- or S-shaped curve. This form of scoliosis results from a cause other than the spine itself (e.g., poor posture, leg length discrepancy, pain). A structural scoliosis is a curvature of the spine associated with vertebral rotation. A structural scoliosis involves the twisting of the spine and appears in three dimensions.

- **Location**—The curve of the spine may develop in the upper back area where the ribs are located (thoracic), the lower back area (lumbar), or in both areas (thoracolumbar).
- **Direction**—Scoliosis can bend the spine left or right.
- **Angle**—A normal spine viewed from the back is zero degrees—a straight line. Scoliosis is defined as a spinal curvature of greater than 10 degrees (i.e., bending toward the ground when in the upright position). The degree of the lateral curvature is expressed by the **Cobb angle,** which is calculated from a radiograph as shown in Figure 25-2.

Kyphosis

Kyphosis can occur at any age, although it is rare at birth. Known causes of kyphosis are (1) degenerative diseases of the spine (such as arthritis or disc degeneration), (2) fractures caused by osteoporosis (osteoporotic compression fractures), and (3) slipping of one vertebra forward on another (spondylolisthesis). Other disorders associated with the cause of kyphosis include certain endocrine diseases, connective tissue disorders, infections (such as tuberculosis), muscular dystrophy, neurofibromatosis, Paget's disease, polio, spina bifida, and tumors. Kyphosis may also be caused by **Scheuermann's disease,** which is the wedging together of several bones of the vertebrae in a row. The precise cause of Scheuermann's disease is unknown.

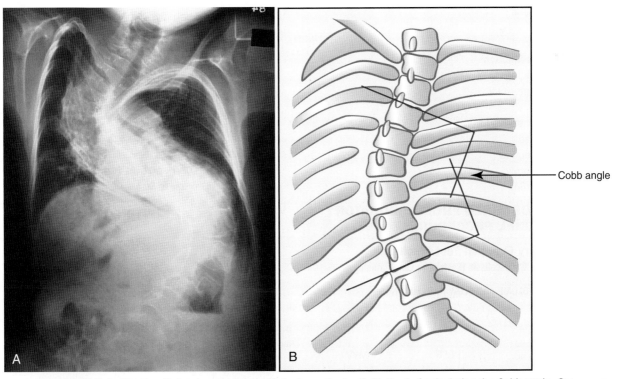

Cobb angle

FIGURE 25-2 A, Chest radiograph on patient with kyphoscoliosis. **B**, Method of calculating the Cobb angle. *Scoliosis* is defined as a spinal curvature of 10 degrees or greater. Because the Cobb angle reflects curvature only in a single plane, it may fail to fully identify the severity of the scoliosis—especially when the patient has vertebral rotation and three-dimensional spinal deformity.

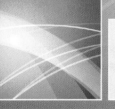

OVERVIEW of the Cardiopulmonary Clinical Manifestations Associated with Kyphoscoliosis[1]

The following clinical manifestations result from the patho-physiologic mechanisms caused (or activated) by Atelectasis (see Figure 9-7) and Excessive Airway Secretions (see Figure 9-11)—the major anatomic alterations of the lungs associated with kyphoscoliosis (Figure 25-1).

CLINICAL DATA OBTAINED AT THE PATIENT'S BEDSIDE
The Physical Examination
Vital Signs
Increased Respiratory Rate (Tachypnea)
Several pathophysiologic mechanisms operating simultane-ously may lead to an increased ventilatory rate:
- Stimulation of peripheral chemoreceptors (hypoxemia)
- Decreased lung compliance–increased ventilatory rate relationship
- Activation of the deflation receptors
- Activation of the irritant receptors
- Stimulation of the J receptors
- Pain, anxiety

Increased Heart Rate (pulse) and Blood Pressure
Cyanosis
Digital Clubbing
Peripheral Edema and Venous Distention
Because polycythemia and cor pulmonale are late findings associated with kyphoscoliosis, the following may be seen:
- Distended neck veins
- Pitting edema
- Enlarged and tender liver

Cough and Sputum Production
Chest Assessment Findings
- Obvious thoracic deformity
- Tracheal shift
- Increased tactile and vocal fremitus
- Dull percussion note
- Bronchial breath sounds
- Whispered pectoriloquy
- Crackles and wheezing

CLINICAL DATA OBTAINED FROM LABORATORY TESTS AND SPECIAL PROCEDURES

Pulmonary Function Test Findings
Moderate to Severe Kyphoscoliosis (Restrictive Lung Pathology)

FORCED EXPIRATORY VOLUME AND FLOW RATE FINDINGS

FVC	FEV_T	FEV_1/FVC ratio	$FEF_{25\%-75\%}$
↓	N or ↓	N or ↑	N or ↓

$FEF_{50\%}$	$FEF_{200-1200}$	PEFR	MVV
N or ↓	N or ↓	N or ↓	N or ↓

LUNG VOLUME AND CAPACITY FINDINGS

V_T	IRV	ERV	RV	
N or ↓	↓	↓	↓	

VC	IC	FRC	TLC	RV/TLC ratio
↓	↓	↓	↓	N

Arterial Blood Gases

MILD TO MODERATE KYPHOSCOLIOSIS
Acute Alveolar Hyperventilation with Hypoxemia*
(Acute Respiratory Alkalosis)

pH	$PaCO_2$	HCO_3^-	PaO_2	SaO_2 or SpO_2
↑	↓	↓	↓	↓
		(but normal)		

SEVERE KYPHOSCOLIOSIS
Chronic Ventilatory Failure with Hypoxemia[†]
(Compensated Respiratory Acidosis)

pH	$PaCO_2$	HCO_3^-	PaO_2	SaO_2 or SpO_2
N	↑	↑	↓	↓
		(significantly)		

ACUTE VENTILATORY CHANGES SUPERIMPOSED ON CHRONIC VENTILATORY FAILURE[‡]
Because acute ventilatory changes are frequently seen in patients with chronic ventilatory failure, the respiratory therapist must be familiar with—and alert for—the follow-ing two dangerous arterial blood gas (ABG) findings:
- Acute alveolar hyperventilation superimposed on chronic ventilatory failure—which should further alert the respira-tory therapist to record the following important ABG assessment: possible *impending acute ventilatory failure*
- Acute ventilatory failure (acute hypoventilation) superim-posed on chronic ventilatory failure

Oxygenation Indices[§]
Moderate to Severe Kyphoscoliosis

$\dot{Q}_S/\dot{Q}_T$	$DO_2^{\parallel}$	$\dot{V}O_2$	$C(a\text{-}\bar{v})O_2$	O_2ER	$S\bar{v}O_2$
↑	↓	N	N	↑	↓

---

*See Figure 4-3 and related discussion for the acute pH, $PaCO_2$, and HCO_3^- changes associated with acute alveolar hyperventilation.
†See Figure 4-2 and related discussion for the pH, $PaCO_2$, and HCO_3^- changes associated with chronic ventilatory failure.
†See TABLE 4-7 and related discussion for the pH, $PaCO_2$, and HCO_3^- changes associated with Acute Ventilatory Changes Superimposed on Chronic Ventilatory Failure
§$C(a\text{-}\bar{v})O_2$, Arterial–venous oxygen difference; DO_2, total oxygen delivery; O_2ER, oxygen extraction ratio; $\dot{Q}_S/\dot{Q}_T$, pulmonary shunt fraction; $S\bar{v}O_2$, mixed venous oxygen saturation; $\dot{V}O_2$, oxygen consumption.
‖The DO_2 may be normal in patients who have compensated to the decreased oxygenation status with (1) an increased cardiac output, (2) an increased hemoglobin level, or (3) a combination of both. When the DO_2 is normal, the O_2ER is usually normal.

---

[1]It is important to note that kyphoscoliosis is a progressive disease and thus changes in the clinical manifestations associated with this disorder will occur over time as the patient ages and the disease progresses.

CVP	RAP	$\overline{PA}$	PCWP	CO	SV
↑	↑	↑	N	N	N

SVI	CI	RVSWI	LVSWI	PVR	SVR
N	N	↑	N	↑	N

Hemodynamic Indices*
Moderate to Severe Kyphoscoliosis

When present, a mediastinal shift is best shown on an antero-posterior chest radiograph. As the alveoli collapse, the density of the lung increases and is revealed on the chest radiograph as increased opacity (Figure 25-3). In severe cases, cor pulmonale may be seen.

LABORATORY FINDINGS

Severe and/or Late Stage Kyphoscoliosis (if the patient is chronically hypoxemic)

- Increased hematocrit and hemoglobin (polycythemia)
- Hypochloremia (Cl⁻)
- Hypernatremia (Na⁺)

RADIOLOGIC FINDINGS

Chest Radiograph
- Thoracic deformity
- Mediastinal shift
- Increased lung opacity
- Atelectasis in areas of compressed (atelectatic) lungs
- Enlarged heart (cor pulmonale)

The extent of the thoracic deformity in kyphoscoliosis is demonstrated in anteroposterior and lateral radiographs.

*CO, Cardiac output; CVP, central venous pressure; LVSWI, left ventricular stroke work index; $\overline{PA}$, mean pulmonary artery pressure; PCWP, pulmonary capillary wedge pressure; PVR, pulmonary vascular resistance; RAP, right atrial pressure; RVSWI, right ventricular stroke work index; SV, stroke volume; SVI, stroke volume index; SVR, systemic vascular resistance.

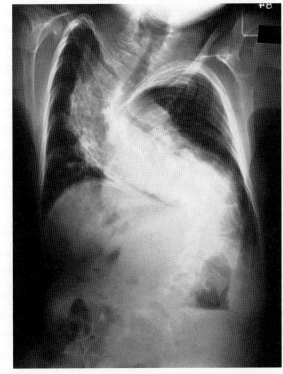

FIGURE 25-3 Severe kyphoscoliosis in a 14-year-old male patient.

General Management of Scoliosis

The treatment of scoliosis largely depends on the cause of the scoliosis, the size and location of the curve, and how much more growing the patient is expected to do. In most cases of scoliosis (less than 20 degrees), the degree of abnormal spine curvature is relatively small and requires only observation to ensure that the curve does not worsen. Observation is usually recommended in patients with a spine curvature of less than 20 degrees. In young children who are still growing, observation checkups are usually scheduled at 3- to 6-month intervals. When the curve is determined to be progressing to a more serious degree (more than 25 to 30 degrees in a child who is still growing), the following treatments options are available:

Braces

A brace device is usually recommended as the first line of defense for growing children who have a spinal curvature of 25 to 45 degrees. Bracing is the primary treatment for adolescent idiopathic scoliosis (AIS). The mechanical objective of the brace is to hyperextend the spine and to limit forward flexion. It does not reverse the curve. Although a brace does not cure scoliosis (or even improve the condition), it has been shown to prevent the curve progression in more than 90% of patients who wear it. Bracing is not effective in congenital or neuromuscular scoliosis. The therapeutic effects of bracing are also less helpful in infantile and juvenile idiopathic scoliosis. Today a number of braces are available, including the **Boston brace, Charleston bending brace,** and **Milwaukee**

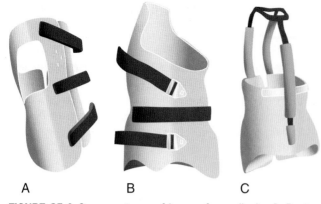

A   B   C

FIGURE 25-4 Common types of braces for scoliosis. **A**, Boston back brace (also called a *thoracolumbosacral orthosis* [TLSO], a *low-profile brace*, or an *underarm brace*). Typically used for curves in the lumbar (low-back) or thoracolumbar sections of the spine. **B**, Charleston bending brace (also known as a *part-time brace*). Commonly used for spinal curves of 20 to 35 degrees, with the apex of the curve below the level of the shoulder blade. **C**, Milwaukee brace (also called cervicothoracolumbosacral orthosis [CTLSO]) is used for high thoracic (mid-back) curves.

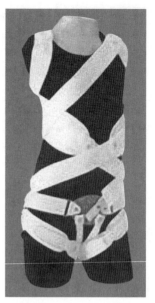

FIGURE 25-5 The SpineCor brace is composed of soft, elastic corrective bands that wrap around the patient's body and resist the body's movement back to the abnormal position.

brace (Figure 25-4). A soft brace, called **SpineCor**, is also available in the United States, Canada, and Europe. The type of brace is selected according to the patient's age, the specific characteristics of the curve, and the willingness of the patient to tolerate a specific brace.

Boston Brace

The Boston brace (also called a **thoracolumbosacral orthosis [TLSO]**, a *low-profile brace,* or an *underarm brace*) is composed of plastic that is custom-molded to fit the patient's body. The Boston brace is the most commonly used brace for AIS. The brace extends from below the breast to the top of the pelvic area in front, and from below the scapula to the coccyx in the back. The Boston brace is typically used for curves in the lumbar (low-back) or thoracolumbar sections of the spine. The Boston brace is worn about 23 hours a day but can be taken off to shower, swim, or engage in sports (Figure 25-4, *A*).

Charleston Bending Brace

The Charleston bending brace (also known as a *part-time brace*) is worn only for 8 to 10 hours at night, when the human growth hormone level is at its highest. The Charleston bending brace is molded to conform to the patient's body when the patient bends toward the convexity—or outward bulge—of the curve. This brace works to overcorrect the curve while the patient is asleep. In order for the Charleston brace to be effective, the patient's curve must be in the 20- to 40-degree range and the apex of the curve needs to be below the level of the scapula. The Charleston bending brace works on the principle that the spine should be bent to grow in the correct direction during the time of day that most growing occurs. Many studies have shown that the Charleston night-time brace is as effective as the braces that need to be worn for 23 hours (Figure 25-4, *B*).

Milwaukee Brace

The Milwaukee brace (also known as a **cervicothoracolumbosacral orthosis [CTLSO]**) is used for high thoracic (mid-back) curves. The Milwaukee brace is a full-torso brace with a neck ring that serves as a rest for the chin and for the back of the head. It extends from the neck to the pelvis. It consists of a specially contoured plastic pelvic girdle and a neck ring that is connected by metal bars in the front and back of the brace. The metal bars work to extend the length of the torso, and the neck ring keeps the head centered over the pelvis. The Milwaukee brace is used less frequently now that more form-fitting plastic braces are available (Figure 25-4, *C*).

SpineCor Brace

The SpineCor brace is a soft and dynamic brace designed to provide a progressive correction of idiopathic scoliosis from 15 degrees Cobb angle and above. It is comfortably worn under clothing. The brace is composed of soft, elastic corrective bands that wrap around the patient's body and resist the body's movement back to the abnormal position (Figure 25-5). The corrective movements of the SpineCor brace is able to put the patient's body through countless repetitions each day—as opposed to the 10 to 50 repetitions that are the typical routine with other rehabilitation techniques. The SpineCor brace is designed to generate a constant correction and relaxation action that gently guides the patient's posture and spinal alignment in an optimal direction. The brace works well to preserve normal body movements, growth, and better allows for normal daily living activities. The brace is usually worn 20 hours a day. The patient should not have it off for more than 2 hours at a time.

Surgery

In general, surgery is performed to correct unacceptable deformity and prevent further curvature. Surgery is usually

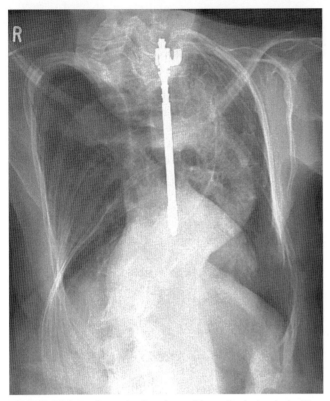

FIGURE 25-6 Radiograph of patient with scoliosis treated with a Harrington rod. (From Albert RK, Spiro SG, Jett JR: *Clinical respiratory medicine*, ed 3, St Louis, 2008, Elsevier.)

recommended in patients who have curvatures of the spine greater than 40 to 50 degrees. As a general rule, even the best surgical techniques do not completely straighten the patient's spine. Also, surgery often does not improve ventilatory function. Surgical procedures include the following:

Spinal Fusion

Spinal fusion is the most widely performed surgery for scoliosis. A spinal fusion, followed by casting, involves placing pieces of bone between two or more vertebrae. The bone sections are taken from the patient's pelvis or rib. Eventually the bone pieces and the vertebrae fuse together. This procedure has now been largely replaced by **rod instrumentation.**

Rod Instrumentation

In 1962, Paul Harrington introduced a metal spinal system that involved the insertion of a metal rod (the **Harrington rod**), hooks, screws, and wires to prevent the curve from moving for 3 to 12 months and to allow the fusion to become solid (Figure 25-6). The system provides disruption to the concave side of the spine and compression to the convex side. This action enhances stabilization, reduces any rotational tendency, and applies force to the spine to correct the curvature. Although the Harrington rod improved up to 50% of the curvature in patients who elected to have the procedure, it is now obsolete. Its major shortcoming was (1) it failed to produce a posture that allowed the skull to be in proper alignment with the pelvis, and (2) it did not address rotational deformity. Currently, the Cotrel-Dubousset system is the most common technique for this procedure. The **Cotrel-Dubousset technique** has been shown to work well in improving pelvic area sagittal imbalance and rotational defects. The Cotrel-Dubousset technique has shown relatively good success (e.g., the rib hump) and low rates of infection. The long-term success of this technique is still being studied.

Other Approaches

Some physicians may try electrical stimulation of muscles, chiropractic manipulation, and exercise to treat scoliosis. There is no evidence that any of these procedures will stop the progression of spine curvature. Exercise, however, may improve the patient's overall health and well-being. Prophylactic deep breathing and coughing (DB&C) exercises are also taught. Their long-term effect is debatable.

Respiratory Care Treatment Protocols

Oxygen Therapy Protocol

Oxygen therapy is used to treat hypoxemia, decrease the work of breathing, and decrease myocardial work. The hypoxemia that develops in kyphoscoliosis is commonly caused by **atelectasis** and pulmonary shunting. Hypoxemia caused by capillary shunting is often refractory to oxygen therapy. (See Oxygen Therapy Protocol, Protocol 9-1).

Bronchopulmonary Hygiene Therapy Protocol

A number of bronchial hygiene treatment modalities may be used to enhance the mobilization of the excessive bronchial secretions associated with kyphoscoliosis (see Bronchopulmonary Hygiene Therapy Protocol, Protocol 9-2).

Lung Expansion Therapy Protocol

Lung expansion therapy is often used to offset atelectasis (see Lung Expansion Therapy Protocol, Protocol 9-3).

Admitting History

A 62-year-old woman began to develop kyphoscoliosis when she was 6 years old. She lived in the mountains of Virginia all her life, first with her parents and later with her two older sisters. Although she wore various types of body braces until she was 17 years old, her disorder was classified as severe by the time she was 15 years old. Her doctors, who were few and far between, always told her that she would have to learn to live with her condition the best she could, and as a general rule she did.

She finished high school with no other remarkable physical or personal problems. She was well liked by her classmates and was actively involved in the school newspaper and art club. After graduation she continued to live with her parents for a few more years. At 21 years of age, she moved in with her two older sisters, who were buying a large farmhouse near a small but popular tourist town. All three sisters made various arts and crafts, which they sold at local tourist shops. The woman's physical disability and general health were relatively stable until she was about 40 years old. At that time, she started to experience frequent episodes of dyspnea, coughing, and sputum production. As the years progressed, her baseline condition was marked by increasingly severe dyspnea.

Because the sisters rarely ventured into the city, the woman's medical resources were poor until she was introduced to a social worker at a nearby church. The church had just become part of an outreach program based in a large city nearby. The social worker was charmed by the woman and fascinated by the beauty of the colorful quilts she made.

The social worker, however, was also concerned by the woman's limited ability to move because of her severe chest deformity. In addition, the social worker thought that the woman's cough sounded serious. She noted that the woman appeared grayish-blue, weak, and ill. The sisters told the social worker that their sibling had had a bad "cold" for about 6 months. After much urging, the social worker persuaded the woman to travel, accompanied by her sisters, to the city to see a doctor at a large hospital associated with the church outreach program. The woman was immediately admitted to the hospital. The sisters stayed in a nearby hotel room provided by the hospital.

Physical Examination

Although the patient appeared to be well nourished, the lateral curvature of her spine was twisted significantly to the left. She also demonstrated anterior bending of the thoracic spine. She appeared older than her stated age, and she was in obvious respiratory distress. The patient stated that she was having trouble breathing. Her skin was cyanotic. She had digital clubbing, and her neck veins were distended, especially on the right side. The woman demonstrated a frequent and strong cough. During each coughing episode she expectorated a moderate amount of thick, yellow sputum.

When the patient generated a strong cough, a large unilateral bulge appeared at the right anterolateral base of her neck, directly posterior to the clavicle. The patient referred to the bulge as her "Dizzy Gillespie pouch*." The doctor thought that the bulge was a result of the severe kyphoscoliosis, which had in turn stretched and weakened the suprapleural membrane that normally restricts and contains the parietal pleura at the apex of the lung. Because of the weakening of the suprapleural membrane, any time the woman performed Valsalva's maneuver for any reason (e.g., for coughing), the increased intrapleural pressure herniated the suprapleural membrane outward. Despite the odd appearance of the bulge, the doctor did not consider it a serious concern.

The patient's vital signs were as follows: blood pressure 160/100, heart rate 90 bpm, respiratory rate 18/min, and oral temperature 36.3 °C (97.4 °F). Palpation revealed a trachea deviated to the right. Dull percussion notes were produced over both lungs; coarse crackles were also heard over them. There was 2+ pitting edema below both knees. A pulmonary function test (PFT) conducted that morning showed vital capacity (VC), functional residual capacity (FRC), and residual volume (RV) of 45% to 50% of predicted values.

Although the patient's electrolyte levels were all normal, her hematocrit was 58%, and her hemoglobin level was 18 g%. A chest radiograph examination revealed a severe thoracic and spinal deformity, a mediastinal shift, an enlarged heart with prominent pulmonary artery segments bilaterally, and bilateral infiltrates in the lung bases consistent with pneumonia and atelectasis. The patient's arterial blood gas values (ABGs) on room air were as follows: pH 7.52, $PaCO_2$ 58 mm Hg, HCO_3^- 46 mEq/L, PaO_2 49 mm Hg, and SaO_2 88%. The physician requested a respiratory care consultation and stated that mechanical ventilation was not an option at this time per the patient's request and his knowledge of the case. On the basis of these clinical data, the following SOAP was documented.

Respiratory Assessment and Plan

S "I'm having trouble breathing."

O Well-nourished appearance; severe anterior and left lateral curvature of the spine; cyanosis, digital clubbing, and distended neck veins—especially on the right side;

---

*The "Dizzy Gillepie pouch" refers to the condition in which the cheeks of the mouth expand greatly with pressure, similar to the famous bebop trumpet player Dizzy Gillespie. Dizzy played his horn incorrectly for some 50 years, letting his cheeks expand when he played, instead of keeping them taut as is considered correct. This was mostly due to his general lack of early musical education. Although Mr. Gillespie was able to create a surprisingly good sound using this form, over time it left his cheeks saggy and loose. A doctor who wanted to use his image in a book named the condition after him. With Gillespie pouches, the cheeks inflate to look almost like balloons. Besides brass players, Gillespie pouches may be found among some balloon artists, who regularly apply great pressure to their cheeks while inflating balloons.

strong cough: frequent, adequate, and productive of moderate amounts of thick yellow sputum; 2+ pitting edema below both knees; vital signs: BP 160/100, HR 90, RR 18, T 36.3 °C (97.4 °F); trachea deviated to the right; both lungs: dull percussion notes, coarse crackles; PFT: VC, FRC, and RV 45% to 50% of predicted; Hct 58%, Hb 18 g%; CXR: severe thoracic and spinous deformity, mediastinal shift, cardiomegaly, and bilateral infiltrates in the lung bases consistent with pneumonia or atelectasis; ABGs (room air): pH 7.52, $PaCO_2$ 58, HCO_3^- 46, PaO_2 49; SaO_2 88%.

A • Severe kyphoscoliosis (history, CXR, physical examination)
  • Increased work of breathing (elevated blood pressure, heart rate, and respiratory rate)
  • Excessive bronchial secretions (sputum, coarse crackles)
  • Infection likely (thick, yellow sputum)
  • Good ability to mobilize secretions (strong cough)
  • Atelectasis and consolidation (CXR)
  • Acute alveolar hyperventilation superimposed on chronic ventilatory failure with moderate hypoxemia (ABGs)
    • Impending ventilatory failure
  • Cor pulmonale (CXR and physical examination)

P Initiate **Oxygen Therapy Protocol** (venturi mask at FIO_2 0.28). **Bronchopulmonary Hygiene Therapy Protocol** (obtain sputum for culture; DB&C instructions and oral suction prn). **Lung Expansion Therapy Protocol** (incentive spirometry qid and prn). Notify physician of admitting ABGs and impending ventilatory failure. Monitor closely.

10 Hours after Admission

The patient's condition had not improved, and she was transferred to an intensive care unit. The physician had trouble titrating the cardiac drugs and decided to insert a pulmonary artery catheter, a central venous catheter, and an arterial line. Because of the woman's cardiac problems, several medical students, respiratory therapists, nurses, and doctors were constantly in and out of her room, performing and assisting in various procedures. As a result, working with the patient for any length of time was difficult, and the intensity of respiratory care was less than desirable. Eventually, the patient's cardiac status stabilized, and the physician requested an update on the woman's pulmonary condition.

The respiratory therapist working on the pulmonary consultation team found the patient in extreme respiratory distress. She was sitting up in bed, appeared frightened, and stated that she was extremely short of breath. Both of her sisters were in the room; one sister was putting cold towels on the patient's face while the other sister was holding the patient's hands. Both sisters were crying softly. The woman's skin appeared cyanotic, and perspiration was visible on her face. Her neck veins were still distended. She demonstrated a weak, spontaneous cough. Although no sputum was noted, she sounded congested when she coughed. Dull percussion notes, and coarse crackles were still present throughout both lungs. Her vital signs were as follows: blood pressure 180/120, heart rate 130 bpm, respiratory rate 26/min, and rectal temperature 37.8 °C (100 °F).

Several of the patient's hemodynamic indices were elevated: CVP, RAP, PA, RVSWI, and PVR.* Her oxygenation indices were as follows: increased $\dot{Q}_S/\dot{Q}_T$ and O_2ER and decreased DO_2 and $S\bar{v}O_2$. Her $\dot{V}O_2$ and $C(a-\bar{v})O_2$ were normal.† No recent chest radiograph was available. Her ABGs on an FIO_2 of 0.28 were as follows: pH 7.57, $PaCO_2$ 49 mm Hg, HCO_3^- 43 mEq/L, PaO_2 43 mm Hg, and SaO_2 87%. On the basis of these clinical data, the following SOAP was documented.

Respiratory Assessment and Plan

S Severe dyspnea; "I'm extremely short of breath."

O Extreme respiratory distress; cyanosis and perspiration; distended neck veins; weak, spontaneous cough; sounds of congestion but no sputum produced; bilateral dull percussion notes, coarse crackles; vital signs: BP 180/120, HR 130, RR 26, T 37.8 °C (100 °F); hemodynamics: increased CVP, RAP, PA, RVSWI, and PVR; oxygenation indices: increased $\dot{Q}_S/\dot{Q}_T$, and O_2ER and decreased DO_2 and $S\bar{v}O_2$; $\dot{V}O_2$ and $C(a-\bar{v})O_2$ normal; ABGs; on FIO_2 0.28: pH 7.57, $PaCO_2$ 49, HCO_3^- 43, PaO_2 43; SaO_2 87%.

A • Severe kyphoscoliosis (history, physical examination, CXR)
  • Increased work of breathing, worsening (increased blood pressure, heart rate, and respiratory rate)
  • Excessive bronchial secretions (coarse crackles, congested cough)
  • Atelectasis and consolidation (previous CXR)
  • Acute alveolar hyperventilation superimposed on chronic ventilatory failure with moderate-to-severe hypoxemia (ABGs and history)
    • Impending ventilatory failure
  • Pulmonary hypertension (hemodynamic indices)
  • Continued critically ill status, but chances of avoiding ventilatory failure improving

P Up-regulate **Oxygen Therapy Protocol** (Venturi oxygen mask at 0.35). Up-regulate **Bronchopulmonary Hygiene Therapy Protocol** (add chest physical therapy [CPT] and postural drainage [PD] qid). Contact physician regarding impending ventilatory failure. Discuss possibility of noninvasive mechanical ventilation and therapeutic bronchoscopy with physician. Monitor and reevaluate in 30 minutes.

24 Hours after Admission

At this time the respiratory therapist found the patient watching the morning news on television with her two sisters. The woman was situated in a semi-Fowler's position eating the last few bites of her breakfast. The patient stated that she felt "so much better" and that "finally I have enough wind to eat some food."

---

*CVP, Central venous pressure; *PA*, mean pulmonary artery pressure; *PVR*, pulmonary vascular resistance; *RAP*, right atrial pressure; *RVSWI*, right ventricular stroke work index.
†*C(a-$\bar{v}$)O₂*, Arterial–venous oxygen difference; *DO₂*, total oxygen delivery; *O₂ER*, oxygen extraction ratio; $\dot{Q}_S/\dot{Q}_T$, pulmonary shunt fraction; $\dot{V}O_2$, mixed venous oxygen saturation; $\dot{V}O_2$, oxygen consumption.

Although her skin still appeared cyanotic, she did not look as ill as she had the day before. On request, she produced a strong cough and expectorated a small amount of white sputum. Her vital signs were as follows: blood pressure 140/85, heart rate 83 bpm, respiratory rate 14/min, and temperature normal. Chest assessment findings demonstrated coarse crackles, and dull percussion notes over both lung fields. The coarse crackles were less intense, however, than they had been the day before.

Although the patient's hemodynamic and oxygenation indices were better than they had been the day before, she still had room for improvement. Her hemodynamic parameters, still abnormal, revealed an elevated CVP, RAP, PA, RVSWI, and PVR. All other hemodynamic indices were normal. Her oxygenation indices still showed an increased $\dot{Q}_S/\dot{Q}_T$ and O_2ER and a decreased DO_2 and $S\bar{v}O_2$. Her $\dot{V}O_2$ and $C(a-\bar{v})O_2$ were normal. The patient's chest radiograph, taken earlier that morning, showed some clearing of the pneumonia and atelectasis described on admission. Her ABGs on an FIO_2 of 0.35 were as follows: pH 7.45, $PaCO_2$ 73 mm Hg, HCO_3^- 49 mEq/L, PaO_2 68 mm Hg, and SaO_2 94%. On the basis of these clinical data, the following SOAP was recorded.

Respiratory Assessment and Plan

S "I feel so much better. I finally have enough wind to eat some food."

O Cyanotic appearance; cough: strong, small amount of white sputum; vital signs: BP 140/85, HR 83, RR 14, T normal; coarse crackles, and dull percussion notes over both lung fields; coarse crackles improving; hemodynamic and oxygenation indices improving, but still an elevated CVP, RAP, PA, RVSWI, and PVR and still an increased $\dot{Q}_S/\dot{Q}_T$ and O_2ER and a decreased DO_2 and $S\bar{v}O_2$; CXR: improvement of the bilateral pneumonia and atelectasis; ABGs: on FIO_2 0.35: pH 7.45, $PaCO_2$ 73, HCO_3^- 49, PaO_2 68; SaO_2 94%.

A • Generally improved respiratory status (history, CXR, hemodynamic and oxygenation indices, ABGs)
  • Significant improvement in problem with excessive bronchial secretions (coarse crackles, cough)
  • Improvement in atelectasis and consolidation (CXR)
  • Chronic ventilatory failure with mild hypoxemia (ABGs)
  • Persistent pulmonary hypertension (hemodynamic indices)
  • Current ABGs are likely close to patient's normal (baseline) ABGs

P Down-regulate **Oxygen Therapy Protocol** and **Bronchopulmonary Hygiene Therapy Protocol**. Continue to monitor and reevaluate (ABGs on reduced FIO_2). Recommend pulmonary rehabilitation and patient and family education (noninvasive positive pressure ventilation [NIPPV] cuirass ventilation, possibly rocking bed, bilevel positive airway pressure [BIPAP], or positive expiratory pressure [PEP]).

Discussion

This case contains an excessive amount of extraneous historical and personal material. This was done to demonstrate, in part, how the respiratory therapist must cut through to the core of the case in the SOAP notes. Care of the patient with symptomatic advanced kyphoscoliosis consists of (1) treatment of the conditions that can complicate it (e.g., bronchitis, pneumonia, atelectasis, pleural effusion) and (2) treatment of the underlying condition itself.

In the first assessment, the SOAP documented excessive bronchial secretions and a likely infection because of the thick yellow sputum and recent history. The patient had a good ability to mobilize the secretions as charted by a strong cough. The chest radiograph confirmed atelectasis and consolidation. Although acute alveolar hyperventilation on top of chronic ventilatory failure was present, the possibility of impending ventilatory failure was real. The therapist's decisions to oxygenate the patient with a low FIO_2 (0.28), administer bronchial hygiene, and be prepared for ventilator support were all appropriate. The patient's secondary polycythemia and cor pulmonale would have been expected to improve as overall oxygenation improved, although this improvement could take some time. The digital clubbing and cor pulmonale itself suggested that the hypoxemia was long-standing.

At the time of the second assessment, the intensity of the patient's respiratory distress was increasing. This was verified by the continued observation of the high pulse and respiratory rate, excessive bronchial secretions, dull percussion notes, acute alveolar hyperventilation on top of chronic ventilatory failure with moderate to severe hypoxemia, atelectasis on the chest x-ray, and poor response to oxygen therapy. Undoubtedly, impending ventilatory failure was more likely.

Atelectasis is often refractory to oxygen therapy, suggesting that **therapeutic bronchoscopy** might have been worthwhile. At that point in time, the up-regulation of the **Oxygen Therapy Protocol** (Protocol 9-1) **and Bronchopulmonary Hygiene Therapy Protocol** (Protocol 9-2) were all justified by the clinical indicators.

In the last assessment, the clinical manifestations associated with the patient's disorder had all improved substantially. The down-regulation of the **Oxygen Therapy Protocol** and **Bronchopulmonary Hygiene Therapy Protocol** was appropriate. The recommendation of pulmonary rehabilitation and family education was appropriately considered.

The ABGs were most likely at the patient's baseline level, because the pH was in the normal range. In fact, according to the pH (normal, but on the alkalotic side of normal) the patient's usual $PaCO_2$ was most likely somewhat higher than the last assessment value. Moreover, this case nicely demonstrates how a patient with a severe restrictive lung disorder—in this case, kyphoscoliosis—can, over time, demonstrate ABGs with very high $PaCO_2$ levels, a normal pH (which has been corrected by an increased HCO_3^- level provided by kidney compensation), and a low PaO_2 level. In other words, the patient with severe kyphoscoliosis may demonstrate ABG findings that reflect chronic ventilatory failure (compensated respiratory acidosis) with hypoxemia—very similar to the patient with severe chronic obstructive pulmonary disease (i.e., emphysema and chronic bronchitis) who displays chronic ventilatory failure ABGs.

Comparison with baseline values (if available) would be appropriate at such a time, and consideration of cuirass ventilation, a rocking bed, or PEP to assist nocturnal ventilation might be in order. Oxygenation can easily be assessed by oximetry at home. This case is an excellent example of the value of hemodynamic monitoring (specifically the normal PCWP) in differentiating left-sided from right-sided cardiac failure.

SELF-ASSESSMENT QUESTIONS

1. **What kind of curvature of the spine is manifested in kyphosis?**
   a. Posterior
   b. Anterior
   c. Lateral
   d. Medial

2. **Kyphoscoliosis affects approximately what percentage of the U.S. population?**
   a. 2%
   b. 5%
   c. 10%
   d. 15%

3. **Which of the following is associated with kyphoscoliosis?**
   a. Decreased RV/TLC ratio
   b. Increased V_T
   c. Decreased RV
   d. Increased TLC

4. **Which of the following are associated with kyphoscoliosis?**
   a. Bronchial breath sounds
   b. Hyperresonant percussion note
   c. Decreased tactile and vocal fremitus
   d. Diminished breath sounds

5. **During the advanced stages of kyphoscoliosis, the patient commonly demonstrates which of the following arterial blood gas values?**
   1. Increased HCO_3^-
   2. Decreased pH
   3. Increased $PaCO_2$
   4. Normal pH
      a. 2 only
      b. 3 and 4 only
      c. 1 and 4 only
      d. 1, 3, and 4 only

PART VII
Environmental Lung Diseases

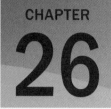

CHAPTER

26

Interstitial Lung Diseases

Chapter Objectives

After reading this chapter, you will be able to:

- List the anatomic alterations of the lungs associated with chronic interstitial lung disease.
- Describe the causes of chronic interstitial lung disease.
- List the cardiopulmonary clinical manifestations associated with chronic interstitial lung disease.
- Describe the general management of chronic interstitial lung disease.
- Describe the clinical strategies and rationales of the SOAPs presented in the case study.

Key Terms

Acute Pneumonitic Phase
Allergic Alveolitis
Asbestos/Asbestosis
Beryllium/Berylliosis
Black Lung
Bronchiolitis Obliterans Organizing Pneumonia (BOOP)
Caplan's Syndrome
Chronic Eosinophilic Pneumonia
Churg-Strauss Syndrome
Coal Miner's Lung
Coal Worker's Pneumoconiosis (CWP)
Connective Tissue (Collagen Vascular) Diseases
Cryptogenic Organizing Pneumonia (COP)
Desquamative Interstitial Pneumonia (DIP)
Extrinsic Allergic Alveolitis
Farmer's Lung
Focal Emphysema
Glomerular Basement Membrane
Goodpasture's Syndrome
Honeycombing
Hypersensitivity Pneumonitis
Idiopathic Pulmonary Fibrosis (IPF)
Idiopathic Pulmonary Hemosiderosis
Interstitial Lung Disease (ILD)
Late Fibrotic Phase
Lymphangioleiomyomatosis (LAM)

Lymphocytic Interstitial Pneumonia (LIP)
Lymphomatoid Granulomatosis
Mononeuritus Multiplex
Plasmapheresis
Pneumoconiosis
Polymyositis-Dermatomyositis
Progressive Massive Fibrosis (PMF)
Progressive Systemic Sclerosis (PSS)
Pulmonary Alveolar Proteinosis
Pulmonary Langerhans Cell Histiocytosis (PLCH)
Pulmonary Vasculitides
Quartz Silicosis (Grinder's Disease)
Rheumatoid Pneumoconiosis
Sarcoidosis
Scleroderma
Silica
Silicosis
Sjögren's Syndrome
Systemic Lupus Erythematosus (SLE)
Usual Interstitial Pneumonia (UIP)
Wegener's Granulomatosis

Chapter Outline

Anatomic Alterations of the Lungs
Etiology and Epidemiology
    Interstitial Lung Diseases of Known Causes or Associations
    Idiopathic Interstitial Pneumonias
    Specific Pathology
    Miscellaneous Diffuse Interstitial Lung Diseases
Overview of Cardiopulmonary Clinical Manifestations Associated with Interstitial Lung Diseases
General Management of Interstitial Lung Disease
    Medications and Procedures Commonly Prescribed by the Physician
    Respiratory Care Treatment Protocols
    Other Treatments
Case Study: Interstitial Lung Disease
Self-Assessment Questions

Introduction

The term **interstitial lung disease (ILD)** (also called *diffuse interstitial lung disease, fibrotic interstitial lung disease, and pulmonary fibrosis*) refers to a broad group of inflammatory lung disorders. More than 180 disease entities are characterized by acute, subacute, or chronic inflammatory infiltration of alveolar walls by cells, fluid, and connective tissue. If left untreated, the inflammatory process can progress to irreversible pulmonary fibrosis. The ILD group consists of a wide range of illnesses with varied causes, treatments, and prognoses. However, because the ILDs all reflect similar anatomic alterations of the lungs and therefore cardiopulmonary clinical manifestations, they are presented as a group in this chapter.

Anatomic Alterations of the Lungs

The anatomic alterations of ILD may involve the bronchi, alveolar walls, and adjacent alveolar spaces. In severe cases the extensive inflammation leads to pulmonary fibrosis, granulomas, **honeycombing,** and cavitation. During the acute stage of any ILD, the general inflammatory condition is characterized by edema and the infiltration of a variety of white blood cells (e.g., neutrophils, eosinophils, basophils, monocytes, macrophages, and lymphocytes) in the alveolar walls and interstitial spaces (Figure 26-1, *A*). Bronchial inflammation and thickening and increasing airway secretions may also be present.

During the chronic stage, the general inflammatory response is also characterized by the infiltration of numerous white blood cells (especially monocytes, macrophages, and lymphocytes), and some fibroblasts may also be present in the alveolar walls and interstitial spaces. This stage may be followed by further interstitial thickening, fibrosis, granulomas, and, in some cases, honeycombing and cavity formation. Pleural effusion may also be present. In the chronic stages the basic pathologic features of interstitial fibrosis are identical in any interstitial lung disorder (so-called *end-stage pulmonary fibrosis*).

As a general rule, the interstitial lung disorders produce restrictive lung disorders. However, because bronchial inflammation and excessive airway secretions can also develop in the small airways, the clinical manifestations associated with an obstructive lung disorder may also be seen. Therefore, the patient with ILD may demonstrate a restrictive disorder, an obstructive disorder, or a combination of both.

The major pathologic or structural changes associated with chronic ILDs are as follows:

- Destruction of the alveoli and adjacent pulmonary capillaries

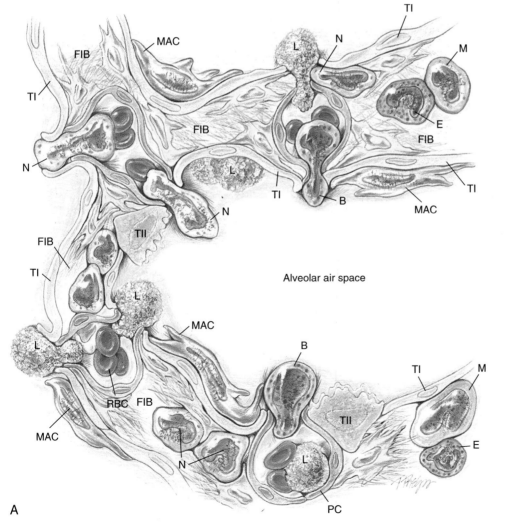

FIGURE 26-1 A, Interstitial lung disease. Cross-sectional microscopic view of alveolar-capillary unit. *B*, Basophil; *E*, eosinophil; *FIB*, fibroblast (fibrosis); *L*, lymphocyte; *M*, monocyte; *MAC*, macrophage; *N*, neutrophil; *PC*, pulmonary capillary; *RBC*, red blood cell; *TI*, type I alveolar cell; *TII*, type II alveolar cell.

Continued

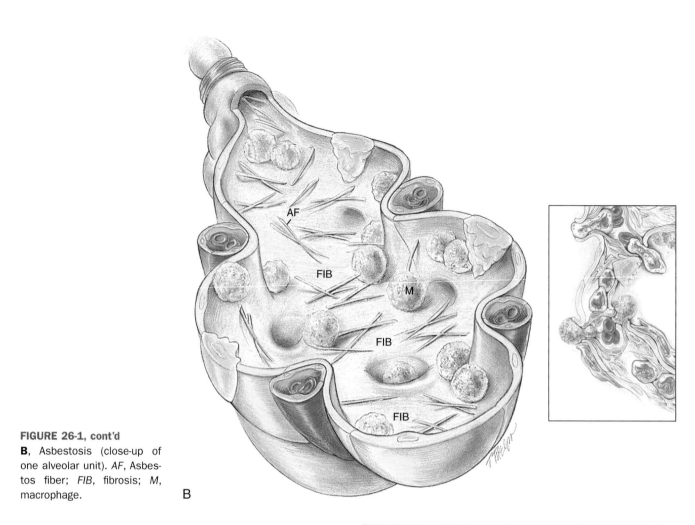

FIGURE 26-1, cont'd
B, Asbestosis (close-up of one alveolar unit). *AF*, Asbestos fiber; *FIB*, fibrosis; *M*, macrophage.

B

- Fibrotic thickening of the respiratory bronchioles, alveolar ducts, and alveoli
- Granulomas
- Honeycombing and cavity formation
- Fibrocalcific pleural plaques (particularly in asbestosis)
- Bronchospasm
- Excessive bronchial secretions (caused by inflammation of airways)

Etiology and Epidemiology

Because there are over 180 different pulmonary disorders classified as ILD, it is helpful to group them according to their occupational or environmental exposure, disease associations, and specific pathology. Table 26-1 provides an overview of common ILD groups. A discussion of the more common ILDs follows.

Interstitial Lung Diseases of Known Causes or Associations (also known as Pneumoconiosis)

Occupational, Environmental, and Therapeutic Exposures

Inorganic Particulate (Dust) Exposure

Asbestos. Exposure to **asbestos** may cause **asbestosis**—a common form of ILD. Asbestos fibers are a mixture of fibrous minerals composed of hydrous silicates of

---

> **BOX 26-1 Common Sources Associates With Asbestos Fibers**
>
> - Acoustic products
> - Automobile undercoating
> - Brake lining
> - Cements
> - Clutch casings
> - Floor tiles
> - Fire-fighting suits
> - Fireproof paints
> - Insulation
> - Roofing materials
> - Ropes
> - Steam pipe material

magnesium, sodium, and iron in various proportions. There are two primary types: the amphiboles (crocidolite, amosite, and anthophyllite) and chrysotile (most commonly used in industry). Asbestos fibers typically range from 50 to 100 μm in length and are about 0.5 μm in diameter. The chrysotiles have the longest and strongest fibers. Box 26-1 lists common sources associated with asbestos fibers.

As shown in Figure 26-1, *B*, asbestos fibers can be seen by microscope within the thickened septa as brown or orange batonlike structures. The fibers characteristically stain for iron with Perls' stain. The pathologic process may affect only

TABLE 26-1 Overview of Interstitial Lung Diseases

Occupational, Environmental, and Therapeutic Exposures	Systemic Diseases	Idiopathic Interstitial Pneumonia	Specific Pathology	Miscellaneous ILDs
Occupation/Environmental	**Connective Tissue Disease**	· Idiopathic pulmonary fibrosis	· Lymphangioleiomyomatosis (LAM)	· Goodpasture's syndrome
Inorganic Exposure	· Scleroderma	· Nonspecific Cryptogenic Organizing Pneumonia (BOOP)	· Pulmonary Langerhans' cell histiocytosis	· Idiopathic pulmonary hemosiderosis
· Asbestosis	· Rheumatoid arthritis	· Lymphocytic interstitial pneumonia (LIP)	· Pulmonary alveolar proteinosis	· Chronic eosinophilic pneumonia
· Coal dust	· Sjögren's syndrome		· The pulmonary vasculitides	
· Silica	· Polymyositis or dermatomyositis		· Wegener's granulomatosis	
· Beryllium	· Systemic lupus erythematosus		· Churg-Strauss Syndrome	
· Aluminum			· Lymphomatoid Granulomatosis	
· Barium	**Sarcoidosis**			
· Clay				
· Iron				
· Certain talcs				
Organic Exposure				
· Hypersensitivity Pneumonitis				
· Moldy hay				
· Silage				
· Moldy sugar cane				
· Mushroom compost				
· Barley				
· Cheese				
· Wood pulp, bark, dust				
· Cork dust				
· Bird droppings				
· Paints				
Medications and Illicit Drugs				
· Antibiotics				
· Anti-inflammatory agents				
· Cardiovascular agents				
· Chemotherapeutic agents				
· Drug-induced systemic lupus erythematosus				
· Illicit drugs				
· Miscellaneous agents				
Radiation Therapy				
Irritant Gases				

one lung, a lobe, or a segment of a lobe. The lower lobes are most commonly affected. Pleural calcification is common and diagnostic in patients with an asbestos exposure history.

Coal Dust. The pulmonary deposition and accumulation of large amounts of coal dust causes what is known as **coal worker's pneumoconiosis (CWP)** (Figure 26-2). CWP is also known as **coal miner's lung and black lung**. Miners who use cutting machines at the coalface have the greatest exposure, but even relatively minor exposures may result in the disease. Indeed, cases have been reported in which coal miners' wives developed the disease, presumably from shaking the dust from their husbands' work clothes.

Simple CWP is characterized by the presence of pinpoint nodules called *coal macules (black spots)* throughout the lungs. The coal macules often develop around the first- and second-generation respiratory bronchioles and cause the adjacent alveoli to retract. This condition is called **focal emphysema.**

Complicated CWP or **progressive massive fibrosis** (PMF) is characterized by areas of fibrotic nodules greater than 1 cm in diameter. The fibrotic nodules generally appear in the peripheral regions of upper lobes and extend toward the hilum with growth. The nodules are composed of dense collagenous tissue with black pigmentation. Coal dust by itself is chemically inert. The fibrotic changes in CWP are usually caused by **silica.**

Silica. Silicosis (also called **grinder's disease** or **quartz silicosis**) is caused by the chronic inhalation of crystalline, free silica, or silicon dioxide particles. Silica is the main component of more than 95% of the rocks of the earth. It is found in sandstone, quartz (beach sand is mostly quartz), flint, granite, many hard rocks, and some clays.

Simple silicosis is characterized by small rounded nodules scattered throughout the lungs. No single nodule is greater than 9 mm in diameter. Patients with simple silicosis are usually symptom-free.

Complicated silicosis is characterized by nodules that coalesce and form large masses of fibrous tissue, usually in the upper lobes and perihilar regions. In severe cases the fibrotic regions may undergo tissue necrosis and cavitate. Box 26-2 lists common occupations associated with silica exposure.

Beryllium. **Beryllium** is a steel-gray, lightweight metal found in certain plastics and ceramics, rocket fuels, and x-ray tubes. As a raw ore, beryllium is not hazardous. When it is processed into the pure metal or one of its salts, however, it may cause a tissue reaction when inhaled or implanted into the skin. The acute inhalation of beryllium fumes or particles may cause a toxic or allergic pneumonitis sometimes accompanied by rhinitis, pharyngitis, and tracheobronchitis. The more complex form of **berylliosis** is characterized by the development of granulomas and a diffuse interstitial inflammatory reaction.

Other Inorganic Causes. Box 26-3 lists other inorganic causes of ILD.

Organic Materials Exposure

Hypersensitivity Pneumonitis. **Hypersensitivity pneumonitis** (also called **allergic alveolitis** or **extrinsic allergic**

BOX 26-2 Common Occupations Associated With Silica Exposure

· Tunneling	· Abrasives work
· Hard-rock mining	· Brick making
· Sandblasting	· Paint making
· Quarrying	· Polishing
· Stonecutting	· Stone drilling
· Foundry work	· Well drilling
· Ceramics work	

BOX 26-3 Additional Inorganic Causes of Interstitial Lung Disease

Aluminium
  · Ammunition workers
Baritosis (barium)
  · Barite millers and miners
  · Ceramic workers
Kalonosis (clay)
  · Brick makers and potters
  · Ceramics workers
Siderosis (iron)
  · Welders
Talcosis (certain talcs)
  · Ceramics workers
  · Papermakers
  · Plastics and rubber workers

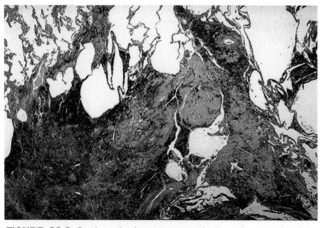

FIGURE 26-2 Coal worker's pneumoconiosis, microscopic view. With massive amounts of inhaled particles (as in "black lung disease" in coal miners), a fibrogenic response can be elicited to produce the coal worker's pneumoconiosis with the coal macule seen here. Progressive massive fibrosis results. (From Klatt E: *Robbins and Cotran atlas of pathology*, ed 2, Philadelphia, 2010, Saunders.)

alveolitis) is a cell-mediated immune response of the lungs caused by the inhalation of a variety of offending agents or antigens. Such antigens include grains, silage, bird droppings or feathers, wood dust (especially redwood and maple), cork dust, animal pelts, coffee beans, fish meal, mushroom compost, and molds that grow on sugar cane, barley, and straw. The immune response to these allergens causes production of antibodies and an inflammatory response. The lung inflammation, or pneumonitis, develops after repeated and prolonged exposure to the allergen. The term *hypersensitivity pneumonitis* (or *allergic alveolitis*) is often renamed according to the type of exposure that caused the lung disorder. For example, the hypersensitivity pneumonitis caused by the inhalation of moldy hay is called **farmer's lung**. Table 26-2 provides common causes, exposure sources, and disease syndromes associated with hypersensitivity pneumonitis.

Medications and Illicit Drugs. As the list of medications and illicit drugs continues to grow, so does the list of possible side effects (Box 26-4). Unfortunately, the lungs are a major target organ affected by these side effects. Although it is impossible to discuss in detail the various lung-related side effects of every drug, it is possible to describe some of the general concerns related to drug-induced lung disease and to list some of the pharmacologic agents that may be responsible.

The chemotherapeutic (anticancer agents) are by far the largest group of agents associated with ILD. Bleomycin, mitomycin, busulfan, cyclophosphamide, methotrexate, and carmustine (BCNU) are the major offenders. Nitrofurantoin (an antibacterial drug used in the treatment of urinary tract infections) is also associated with ILD. Gold and penicillamine for the treatment of **rheumatoid arthritis** have also

TABLE 26-2 Causes of Hypersensitivity Pneumonitis

Antigen	Exposure Source	Disease Syndrome
Bacteria, Thermophilic		
Saccharopolyspora rectivirgula	Moldy hay, silage	Farmer's lung
Thermoactinomyces vulgaris	Moldy sugarcane	Bagassosis
Thermoactinomyces sacchari	Mushroom compost	Mushroom worker's lung
Thermoactinomyces candidus	Heated water reservoirs	Air conditioner lung
Bacteria, Nonthermophilic		
Baccillus subtilis, Bacillus cereus	Water, detergent	Humidifier lung, Washing powder lung
Fungi		
Aspergillus sp.	Moldy hay	Farmer's lung
	Water	Ventilation pneumonitis
Aspergillus clavatus	Barley	Malt worker's lung
Penicillium casiei, P. roqueforti	Cheese	Cheese washer's lung
Alternaria sp.	Wood pulp	Woodworker's lung
Cryptostroma corticale	Wood bark	Maple bark stripper's lung
Graphium, Aureobasidium pullulans	Wood dust	Sequoiosis
Merulius lacrymans	Rotten wood	Dry root lung
Penicillium frequentans	Cork dust	Suberosis
Aureobasidium pullulans	Water	Humidifier lung
Cladosporium sp.	Hot tub mist	Hot tub HP*
Trichosporon cutaneum	Damp wood and mats	Japanese summer-type HP*
Amoebae		
Naegleria gruberi	Contaminated water	Humidifier lung
Acanthamoeba polyphaga	Contaminated water	Humidifier lung
Acanthamoeba castellani	Contaminated water	Humidifier lung
Animal Protein		
Avian proteins	Bird droppings, feathers	Bird-breeder's lung
Urine, serum, pelts	rats, gerbils	Animal handler's lung
Chemicals		
Isocyanates, trimellitic anhydride	Paints, resins, plastics	Chemical worker's lung
Copper sulfate	Bordeaux mixture	Vineyard sprayer's lung
Phthalic anhydride	Heated epoxy resin	Epoxy resin lung
Sodium diazobenzene sulfate	Chromatography reagent	Pauli's reagent alveolitis
Pyrethrum	Pesticide	Pyrethrum HP*

From Selman M: Hypersensitivity pneumonitis. In Schwarz MI, Kin TE, editors: Intersitial Lung Disease, ed 4, Hamilton, 2003, BC Decker.
*HP, Hypersensitivity pneumonitis

BOX 26-4 Medications and Illicit Drugs Associated With the Development of ILD

Antibiotics
- Nitrofurantoin
- Sulfasalazine

Anti-inflammatory agents
- Aspirin
- Gold
- Penicillamine
- Methotrexate
- Etanercept
- Infliximab

Cardiovascular agents
- Amiodarone
- Tocainide

Chemotherapeutic agents
- Bleomycin
- Mitomycin-C
- Busulfan
- Cyclophosphamide
- Chlorambucil
- Melphalan
- Azathioprine
- Cytosine arabinoside
- Methotrexate
- Procarbazine
- Zinostatin
- Etoposide
- Vinblastine
- Imatinib
- Flutamide

Drug-induced systemic lupus erythematosus
- Procainamide
- Isoniazid
- Hydralazine
- Hydantoins
- Penicillamine

Illicit drugs
- Heroin
- Methadone
- Propoxphene
- Talc as an IV contaminant

Miscellaneous agents
- Oxygen
- Drugs inducing pulmonary infiltrates and eosinophilia: L-tryptophan
- Hydrochlorothiazide
- Radiation

From Camus P: Drug-Induced Infiltrative Lung Diseases. In Schwarz MI, King TE, editors: Interstitial Lung Disease, ed 4, Hamilton, 2003, BC Decker.

TABLE 26-3 Common Irritant Gases Associated with ILD

Gas	Industrial Setting
Chlorine	Chemical and plastic industries; water disinfection
Ammonia	Commercial refrigeration; smelting of sulfide ores
Ozone	Welding
Nitrogen dioxide	May be liberated after exposure of nitric acid to air
Phosgene	Used in the production of aniline dyes

interstitial disease may be seen as early as 1 month to as late as several years after exposure to these agents.

The precise cause of drug-induced ILD is not known. Diagnosis is confirmed by an open lung biopsy. When interstitial fibrosis is found with no infectious organisms or known industrial exposure, a drug-induced interstitial process must be suspected.

Radiation Therapy. Radiation therapy in the management of cancer may cause ILD. Radiation-induced lung disease is commonly divided into the following two major phases: the **acute pneumonitic phase** and the **late fibrotic phase**. Acute pneumonitis is rarely seen in patients who receive a total radiation dose of less than 3500 rad. By contrast, doses in excess of 6000 rad over 6 weeks almost always cause ILD in and near the radiated areas. The acute pneumonitic phase develops about 2 to 3 months after exposure. Chronic radiation fibrosis is seen in all patients who develop acute pneumonitis.

The late phase of fibrosis may develop (1) immediately after the development of acute pneumonitis, (2) without an acute pneumonitic period, or (3) after a symptom-free latent period. When fibrosis does develop, it generally does so 6 to 12 months after radiation exposure. Pleural effusion is often associated with the late fibrotic phase.

The precise cause of radiation-induced lung disease is not known. The establishment of a diagnosis is similar to that for drug-induced interstitial disease (i.e., by obtaining a history of recent radiation therapy and confirming the diagnosis with an open lung biopsy).

Irritant Gases. The inhalation of irritant gases may cause an acute chemical pneumonitis and, in severe cases, ILD. Most exposures occur in an industrial setting. Table 26-3 lists some of the more common irritant gases and the industrial settings where they may be found.

Systemic Diseases

Connective Tissue (Collagen Vascular) Diseases

Scleroderma. **Scleroderma** is characterized by chronic hardening and thickening of the skin caused by new collagen formation. It may occur in a localized form or as a systemic disorder (called *systemic sclerosis*). **Progressive systemic sclerosis (PSS)** is a relatively rare autoimmune disorder that

been shown to cause ILD. The excessive long-term administration of oxygen (oxygen toxicity) is also known to cause diffuse pulmonary injury and fibrosis. As a general rule, the risk of these drugs causing an interstitial lung disorder is directly related to the cumulative dosage. However, drug-induced

affects the blood vessels and connective tissue. It causes fibrous degeneration of the connective tissue of the skin, lungs, and internal organs, especially the esophagus, digestive tract, and kidney.

Scleroderma of the lung appears in the form of ILD and fibrosis. Of all the collagen vascular disorders, scleroderma is the one in which pulmonary involvement is most severe and most likely to cause significant scarring of the lung parenchyma. The pulmonary complications include diffuse interstitial fibrosis, severe pulmonary hypertension, pleural disease, and aspiration pneumonitis (secondary to esophageal involvement). Scleroderma may also involve the small pulmonary blood vessels and appears to be independent of the fibrotic process involving the alveolar walls. The disease is most commonly seen in women 30 to 50 years of age.

Rheumatoid Arthritis. Rheumatoid arthritis is primarily an inflammatory joint disease. It may, however, involve the lungs in the form of (1) pleurisy, with or without effusion; (2) interstitial pneumonitis; (3) necrobiotic nodules, with or without cavities; (4) Caplan's syndrome; and (5) pulmonary hypertension secondary to pulmonary vasculitis.

Pleurisy with or without effusion is the most common pulmonary complication associated with rheumatoid arthritis. When present, the effusion is generally unilateral (often on the right side). Men appear to develop rheumatoid pleural complications more often than women. Rheumatoid interstitial pneumonitis is characterized by alveolar wall fibrosis, interstitial and intraalveolar mononuclear cell infiltration, and lymphoid nodules. In severe cases, extensive fibrosing alveolitis and honeycombing may develop. Rheumatoid interstitial pneumonitis is also more common in male patients. Necrobiotic nodules are characterized by the gradual degeneration and swelling of lung tissue.

The pulmonary nodules generally appear as well-circumscribed masses that often progress to cavitation. The nodules usually develop in the periphery of the lungs and are more common in men. Histologically, the pulmonary nodules are identical to the subcutaneous nodules that develop in rheumatoid arthritis.

Caplan's syndrome (also called **rheumatoid pneumoconiosis**) is a progressive pulmonary fibrosis of the lung commonly seen in coal miners. Caplan's syndrome is characterized by rounded densities in the lung periphery that often undergo cavity formation and, in some cases, calcification. Pulmonary hypertension is a common secondary complication caused by the progression of fibrosing alveolitis and pulmonary vasculitis.

Sjögren's Syndrome. **Sjögren's syndrome** is a lymphocytic infiltration that primarily involves the salivary and lacrimal glands and is manifested by dry mucous membranes, usually of the mouth and eyes. Pulmonary involvement also frequently occurs in Sjögren's syndrome and includes (1) pleurisy with or without effusion, (2) interstitial fibrosis that is indistinguishable from that of other collagen vascular disorders, and (3) infiltration of lymphocytes of the tracheobronchial mucous glands, which in turn causes atrophy of the mucous glands, mucous plugging, atelectasis, and secondary

infections. Sjögren's syndrome occurs most often in women (90%) and is commonly associated with rheumatoid arthritis (50% of patients with Sjögren's syndrome).

Polymyositis-Dermatomyositis. *Polymyositis* is a diffuse inflammatory disorder of the striated muscles that primarily weakens the limbs, neck, and pharynx. *Dermatomyositis* is the term used when an erythematous skin rash accompanies the muscle weakness. Pulmonary involvement develops in response to (1) recurrent episodes of aspiration pneumonia caused by esophageal weakness and atrophy, (2) hypostatic pneumonia secondary to a weakened diaphragm, and (3) drug-induced interstitial pneumonitis.

Polymyositis-dermatomyositis is seen more often in women than men, at about a 2:1 ratio. The disease occurs primarily in two age groups: before the age of 10 years and from 40 to 50 years of age. In about 40% of the patients, the pulmonary manifestations are seen 1 to 24 months before the striated muscle or skin shows signs or symptoms.

Systemic lupus erythematosus. **Systemic lupus erythematosus (SLE)** is a multisystem disorder that mainly involves the joints and skin. It may also cause serious problems in numerous other organs, including the kidneys, lungs, nervous system, and heart. Involvement of the lungs appears in about 50% to 70% of cases. Pulmonary manifestations are characterized by (1) pleurisy with or without effusion, (2) atelectasis, (3) diffuse infiltrates and pneumonitis, (4) diffuse ILD, (5) uremic pulmonary edema, (6) diaphragmatic dysfunction, and (7) infections.

Pleurisy with or without effusion is the most common pulmonary complication of SLE. The effusions are usually exudates with high protein concentration and are frequently bilateral. Atelectasis commonly develops in response to the pleurisy, effusion, and diaphragmatic elevation associated with SLE. Diffuse noninfectious pulmonary infiltrates and pneumonitis are common. In severe cases, chronic interstitial pneumonitis may develop. Because SLE frequently impairs the renal system, uremic pulmonary edema may occur. SLE has also been found to be associated with diaphragmatic dysfunction and reduced lung volumes. Some research suggests that a diffuse myopathy affecting the diaphragm is the source of this problem. About 50% of cases have a complicating pulmonary infection.

Sarcoidosis. **Sarcoidosis** is a chronic disorder of unknown origin characterized by the formation of tubercles of nonnecrotizing epithelioid tissue (noncaseating granulomas). Common sites are the eyes, lungs, spleen, liver, skin, mucous membranes, and lacrimal and salivary glands, usually with the involvement of the lymph glands. The lung is the most frequently affected organ, with manifestations generally including ILD, enlargement of the mediastinal lymph nodes, or a combination of both. One of the clinical hallmarks of sarcoidosis is an increase in all three major immunoglobulins (IgM, IgG, and IgA). The disease is more common among African-Americans and appears most frequently in patients 10 to 40 years of age, with the highest incidence at 20 to 30 years of age. Women are affected more often than men, especially among African-Americans.

Idiopathic Interstitial Pneumonias

Some patients with ILD do not have a readily identified specific exposure, a systemic disorder, or an underlying genetic cause. Such instances of ILD are commonly placed in the idiopathic interstitial pneumonia group or the group with specific pathology.

Idiopathic Pulmonary Fibrosis

Idiopathic pulmonary fibrosis (IPF) is a progressive inflammatory disease with varying degrees of fibrosis and, in severe cases, honeycombing. The precise cause is unknown. Although *idiopathic pulmonary fibrosis* is the term most frequently used for this disorder, numerous other names appear in the literature, such as *acute interstitial fibrosis of the lung, cryptogenic fibrosing alveolitis, Hamman–Rich syndrome, honeycomb lung, interstitial fibrosis,* and *interstitial pneumonitis.*

IPF is commonly separated into the following two major disease entities according to the predominant histologic appearance: **desquamative interstitial pneumonia (DIP)** and **usual interstitial pneumonia (UIP)**. In DIP the most prominent features are hyperplasia and desquamation of the alveolar type II cells. The alveolar spaces are packed with macrophages, and there is an even distribution of the interstitial mononuclear infiltrate.

In UIP the most prominent features are interstitial and alveolar wall thickening caused by chronic inflammatory cells and fibrosis. In severe cases, fibrotic connective tissue replaces the alveolar walls, the alveolar architecture becomes distorted, and eventually honeycombing develops. When honeycombing is present, the inflammatory infiltrate is significantly reduced. The prognosis for patients with DIP is significantly better than that for patients with UIP.

Some experts believe that DIP and UIP are two distinct ILD entities. Others, however, believe that DIP and UIP are different stages of the same disease process. IPF is most commonly seen in men 40 to 70 years of age. Diagnosis is generally confirmed by an open lung biopsy. Most patients diagnosed with IPF have a more chronic progressive course, and death usually occurs in 4 to 10 years. Death usually is the result of progressive acute ventilatory failure, complicated by pulmonary infection.

Cryptogenic Organizing Pneumonia

Cryptogenic organizing pneumonia (COP) (also known as **bronchiolitis obliterans organizing pneumonia [BOOP]**) is characterized by connective tissue plugs in the small airways (hence the term *bronchiolitis obliterans*) and mononuclear cell infiltration of the surrounding parenchyma (hence the term *organizing pneumonia*). Although most cases have no identifiable cause and therefore are considered idiopathic, COP has been associated with connective tissue disease, toxic gas inhalation, and infection. The chest radiograph commonly shows patchy infiltrates of alveolar rather than interstitial involvement. Diagnosis may require a surgical biopsy when the clinical and radiographic data are uncertain. COP is one of the ILDs in which both restrictive and obstructive pathologic lesions are present.

Lymphocytic Interstitial Pneumonia

Lymphocytic interstitial pneumonia (LIP) is a diffuse pulmonary disorder characterized by fibrosis and accumulation of lymphocytes in the lungs. It is commonly associated with lymphoma. The diagnosis usually requires a surgical lung biopsy.

Specific Pathology
Lymphangioleiomyomatosis

Lymphangioleiomyomatosis (LAM) is a rare lung disease involving the smooth muscles of the airways and affects women of childbearing age. It is characterized by the proliferation of disorderly smooth muscle proliferation throughout the bronchioles, alveolar septa, perivascular spaces, and lymphatics. LAM causes the obstruction of small airways and lymphatics. Common clinical features associated with LAM are recurrent pneumothorax and chylothorax. The diagnosis of LAM is confirmed with an open lung biopsy. The prognosis is poor; the disease slowly progresses over 2 to 10 years, ending in death resulting from ventilatory failure.

Pulmonary Langerhans Cell Histiocytosis

Pulmonary Langerhans cell histiocytosis (PLCH) is a smoking-related ILD characterized by mid-lung zone star-shaped nodules with adjacent thin-walled cysts. It was once considered a benign condition in adults, but long-term complications such as pulmonary hypertension are becoming increasingly recognized. Diagnosis is confirmed histologically by tissue biopsy.

Pulmonary Alveolar Proteinosis

Pulmonary alveolar proteinosis is a condition of unknown cause in which the alveoli become filled with protein and lipids. The lipoprotein material is similar to the pulmonary surfactant produced by type II cells. In addition, the alveolar macrophages are generally dysfunctional in this disorder. The disease is most commonly seen in adults 20 to 50 years of age. Men are affected twice as often as women. The chest radiograph typically reveals bilateral infiltrates that are most prominent in the perihilar regions (butterfly pattern). It is often indistinguishable from pulmonary edema. Air bronchograms are commonly seen. The diagnosis is confirmed by transbronchial or open lung biopsy, or by analysis of fluid removed during bronchial lavage.

Pulmonary Vasculitides

The **pulmonary vasculitides** (also called *granulomatous vasculitides*) consist of a heterogeneous group of pulmonary disorders characterized by inflammation and destruction of the pulmonary vessels. The major disorders in this category include **Wegener's granulomatosis, Churg-Strauss syndrome,** and **lymphomatoid granulomatosis.**

Wegener's Granulomatosis. Wegener's granulomatosis is a multisystem disorder characterized by (1) a necrotizing, granulomatous vasculitis; (2) focal and segmental glomerulonephritis; and (3) variable degrees of systemic vasculitis of the small veins and arteries. In the lungs, numerous 1- to 9-cm diameter nodules are commonly seen in the upper lobes, and cavity formation is often associated with larger lesions.

Wegener's granulomatosis is considered an aggressive and fatal disorder, although the prognosis has significantly improved with the use of cytotoxic agents (e.g., cyclophosphamide). This disorder is most commonly seen in men older than 50 years of age. Diagnosis is confirmed by an open lung biopsy. Histologic examination reveals lesions with marked central necrosis. The area surrounding the necrotizing lesion consists of inflammatory white blood cells with some fibroblasts. Inflammatory cell infiltrate and necrotizing vasculitis are seen in the adjacent blood vessels.

Churg-Strauss Syndrome. Churg-Strauss syndrome is a necrotizing vasculitis that predominantly involves the small vessels of the lungs. The granulomatous lesions are characterized by a heavy infiltrate of eosinophils, central necrosis, and peripheral eosinophilia. Cavity formation is rare in this disorder. Clinically, symptoms of asthma usually precede the onset of vasculitis. In recent years, rapid tapering of oral steroids with substitution of leukotriene inhibitors such as montelukast (Singulair) and zafirlukast (Accolate) has been associated with deaths from fulminant Churg-Strauss syndrome reactions. Neurologic disorders such as **mononeuritis multiplex**, a simultaneous disease of several peripheral nerves, are frequently associated with this disorder. Diagnosis is usually confirmed with an open lung biopsy, and the disease is often rapidly fatal.

Lymphomatoid Granulomatosis. Lymphomatoid granulomatosis is a rare necrotizing vasculitis that primarily involves the lungs, although neurologic and cutaneous lesions are sometimes seen. The lesions are usually in the lower lobes, and cavities develop in more than one third of cases. Pleural effusion is common.

Although the clinical presentation is similar to that of Wegener's granulomatosis, there are some distinct differences. For example, more mature lymphoreticular cells are involved in the formation of the granulomatous lesions and no glomerulonephritis is seen. Histologically, the lesions simulate malignant lymphoma. This disorder is most commonly seen in men 50 to 70 years of age. Diagnosis is confirmed by open lung biopsy.

Miscellaneous Diffuse Interstitial Lung Diseases

Goodpasture's Syndrome

Goodpasture's syndrome is a disease of unknown cause that involves two organ systems—the lungs and the kidneys. In the lungs there are recurrent episodes of pulmonary hemorrhage and in some cases pulmonary fibrosis, presumably as a consequence of the bleeding episodes. In the kidneys there is a glomerulonephritis characterized by the infiltration of antibodies within the **glomerular basement membrane** (GBM). These circulating antibodies function against the patient's own GBM. They are commonly abbreviated as *anti-GBM antibodies*. It is believed that the anti-GBM antibodies cross-react with the basement membrane of the alveolar wall and that their deposition in the kidneys and lungs is responsible for producing the pathophysiologic processes of the disease.

Goodpasture's syndrome is usually seen in young adults. The average survival period after diagnosis is about 15 weeks. About 50% of patients die from massive pulmonary hemorrhage, and about 50% die from chronic renal failure. An interesting feature of Goodpasture's syndrome is that the patient frequently demonstrates an increased pulmonary diffusion capacity (DLCO), which is in direct contrast to most interstitial lung disorders. The increased carbon monoxide uptake commonly seen in this disorder is thought to be caused by the increased amount of retained hemoglobin in the pulmonary tissue.

Idiopathic Pulmonary Hemosiderosis

Idiopathic pulmonary hemosiderosis is a disease entity of unknown cause that is characterized by recurrent episodes of pulmonary hemorrhage similar to that seen in Goodpasture's syndrome. Histologic examination reveals an alveolar hemorrhage with hemosiderin-laden macrophages and hyperplasia of the alveolar epithelium. Unlike Goodpasture's syndrome, however, there is no evidence of circulating anti-GBM antibodies attacking the alveoli or GBMs, and this disorder is not associated with renal disease.

Idiopathic pulmonary hemosiderosis is most often seen in children. As in Goodpasture's syndrome, patients commonly demonstrate an increased DLCO, which is in direct contrast to most interstitial lung disorders. Again, the increased uptake of carbon monoxide is thought to be caused by the increased amount of hemoglobin retained in the lungs.

Chronic Eosinophilic Pneumonia

Chronic eosinophilic pneumonia is characterized by infiltration of eosinophils and, to a lesser extent, macrophages into the alveolar and interstitial spaces. Clinically, a unique feature of this disorder is often seen on the chest radiograph, consisting of a peripheral distribution of pulmonary infiltrates. This radiographic pattern is commonly referred to as a *photographic negative of pulmonary edema*. This is because of the dense peripheral infiltration, with the sparing of the perihilar areas, seen in chronic eosinophilic pneumonia, compared with the central pulmonary infiltration with the sparing of the lung periphery seen in pulmonary edema. An increased number of eosinophils is also commonly seen in the peripheral blood. Histologic diagnosis is made by means of an open lung biopsy.

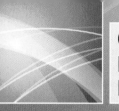

OVERVIEW of the Cardiopulmonary Clinical Manifestations Associated with Chronic Interstitial Lung Diseases

The following clinical manifestations result from the patho-physiologic mechanisms caused (or activated) by an Increased Alveolar-Capillary Membrane Thickness (see Figure 9-9) and Excessive Bronchial Secretions (see Figure 9-11)—the major anatomic alterations of the lungs associated with chronic interstitial lung disease (Figure 26-1).

CLINICAL DATA OBTAINED AT THE PATIENT'S BEDSIDE

The Physical Examination

Vital Signs

Increased Respiratory Rate (Tachypnea)

Several pathophysiologic mechanisms operating simultaneously may lead to an increased ventilatory rate:

- Stimulation of peripheral chemoreceptors (hypoxemia)
- Decreased lung compliance–increased ventilatory rate relationship
- Stimulation of the J receptors
- Pain, anxiety

Increased Heart Rate (Pulse) and Blood Pressure

Cyanosis
Digital Clubbing
Peripheral Edema and Venous Distention

Because polycythemia and cor pulmonale are associated with chronic interstitial lung disease, the following may be seen:

- Distended neck veins
- Pitting edema
- Enlarged and tender liver

Nonproductive Cough
Chest Assessment Findings

- Increased tactile and vocal fremitus
- Dull percussion note
- Bronchial breath sounds
- Crackles
- Pleural friction rub
- Whispered pectoriloquy

CLINICAL DATA OBTAINED FROM LABORATORY TESTS AND SPECIAL PROCEDURES

Pulmonary Function Test Findings
Moderate to Severe Interstitial Lung Disease
(Restrictive Lung Pathology)

FORCED EXPIRATORY VOLUME AND FLOW RATE FINDINGS

FVC	FEV_T	FEV_1/FVC ratio	$FEF_{25\%-75\%}$
↓	N or ↓	N or ↑	N or ↓

$FEF_{50\%}$	$FEF_{200-1200}$	PEFR	MVV
N or ↓	N or ↓	N or ↓	N or ↓

LUNG VOLUME AND CAPACITY FINDINGS

V_T	IRV	ERV	RV
N or ↓	↓	↓	↓

VC	IC	FRC	TLC	RV/TLC ratio
↓	↓	↓	↓	N

DECREASED DIFFUSION CAPACITY

There is an exception to the expected decreased diffusion capacity in the following two interstitial lung diseases: Goodpasture's syndrome and idiopathic pulmonary hemosiderosis. The D_{LCO} is often elevated in response to the increased amount of hemoglobin retained in the alveolar spaces that is associated with these two disorders.

Arterial Blood Gases

MILD TO MODERATE INTERSTITIAL LUNG DISEASE

Acute Alveolar Hyperventilation with Hypoxemia*
(Acute Respiratory Alkalosis)

pH	$PaCO_2$	HCO_3^-	PaO_2	SaO_2 or SpO_2
↑	↓	↓	↓	↓
		(but normal)		

SEVERE CHRONIC INTERSTITIAL LUNG DISEASE

Chronic Ventilatory Failure with Hypoxemia†
(Compensated Respiratory Acidosis)

pH	$PaCO_2$	HCO_3^-	PaO_2	SaO_2 or SpO_2
N	↑	↑	↓	↓
		(significantly)		

ACUTE VENTILATORY CHANGES SUPERIMPOSED ON CHRONIC VENTILATORY FAILURE‡

Because acute ventilatory changes are frequently seen in patients with chronic ventilatory failure, the respiratory therapist must be familiar with—and alert for—the following two dangerous arterial blood gas (ABG) findings:

- Acute alveolar hyperventilation superimposed on chronic ventilatory failure—which should further alert the respiratory therapist to record the following important ABG assessment: possible *impending acute ventilatory failure*
- Acute ventilatory failure (acute hypoventilation) superimposed on chronic ventilatory failure

---

*See Figure 4-3 and related discussion for the acute pH, $PaCO_2$, and HCO_3^- changes associated with acute alveolar hyperventilation.
†See Figure 4-2 and related discussion for the pH, $PaCO_2$, and HCO_3^- changes associated with chronic ventilatory failure.
†See TABLE 4-7 and related discussion for the pH, $PaCO_2$, and HCO_3^- changes associated with Acute Ventilatory Changes Superimposed on Chronic Ventilatory Failure

Oxygenation Indices*
Moderate to Severe Stage Interstitial Lung Disease

$\dot{Q}_S/\dot{Q}_T$	DO_2†	$\dot{V}O_2$	$C(a\text{-}\bar{v})O_2$	O_2ER	$S\bar{v}O_2$
↑	↓	N	N	↑	↓

Hemodynamic Indices†
Severe Interstitial Lung Disease

CVP	RAP	$\overline{PA}$	PCWP	CO	SV
↑	↑	↑	N	N	N

SVI	CI	RVSWI	LVSWI	PVR	SVR
N	N	↑	N	↑	N

LABORATORY FINDINGS

· Increased hematocrit and hemoglobin (polycythemia)

RADIOLOGIC FINDINGS

Radiologic findings vary according to the cause.

Chest Radiograph

· Bilateral reticulonodular pattern
· Irregularly shaped opacities
· Granulomas
· Cavity formation
· Honeycombing
· Pleural effusion (see Chapter 24)

As shown in Figure 26-3, in a patient with severe scleroderma, a bilateral reticulonodular pattern is commonly seen on the radiographs. In patients with asbestosis the opacity is often described as cloudy in appearance or as having a "ground-glass" appearance and is especially apparent in the lower lobes (Figure 26-4). Calcified pleural plaques may be seen on the superior border of the diaphragm or along the chest wall (Figure 26-5). The inflammatory response elicited by the asbestos fibers may also produce a fuzziness and irregularity of the cardiac and diaphragmatic borders.

*$C(a\text{-}\bar{v})O_2$, Arterial–venous oxygen difference; DO_2, total oxygen delivery; O_2ER, oxygen extraction ratio; $\dot{Q}_S/\dot{Q}_T$, pulmonary shunt fraction; $S\bar{v}O_2$, mixed venous oxygen saturation; $\dot{V}O_2$, oxygen consumption.
†The DO_2 may be normal in patients who have compensated to the decreased oxygenation status with (1) an increased cardiac output, (2) an increased hemoglobin level, or (3) a combination of both. When the DO_2 is normal, the O_2ER is usually normal.
†CO, Cardiac output; CVP, central venous pressure; LVSWI, left ventricular stroke work index; $\overline{PA}$, mean pulmonary artery pressure; PCWP, pulmonary capillary wedge pressure; PVR, pulmonary vascular resistance; RAP, right atrial pressure; RVSWI, right ventricular stroke work index; SV, stroke volume; SVI, stroke volume index; SVR, systemic vascular resistance.

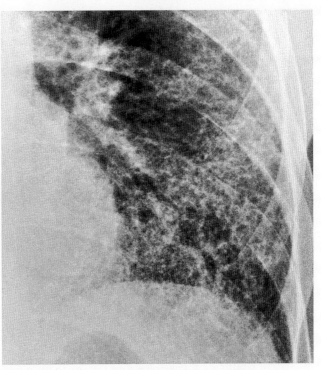

FIGURE 26-3 Reticulonodular pattern of interstitial pulmonary fibrosis in a patient with scleroderma. (From Hansell DM, Armstrong P, Lynch DA, McAdams HP, eds: *Imaging of diseases of the chest,* ed 4, Philadelphia, 2005, Elsevier.)

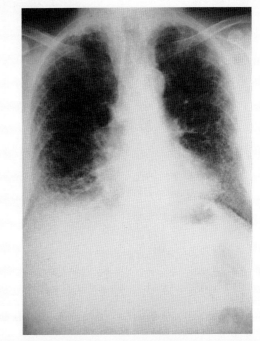

FIGURE 26-4 Chest x-ray film of a patient with asbestosis.

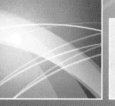
Figure 26-6 shows a diffuse parenchymal ground-glass pattern with some areas of consolidation in a patient with acute farmer's lung. The severity of parenchymal opacification in this case is rare.

In Figure 26-7, the honeycomb appearance is nicely illustrated in a computed tomography (CT) scan of a patient with sarcoidosis. Figure 26-8 shows a patient with Wegener's granulomatosis with numerous nodules with a large cavitary lesion adjacent to the right hilus. Figure 26-9 shows a pleural effusion in a patient with rheumatoid disease.

FIGURE 26-5 Calcified pleural plaques on the superior border of the diaphragm *(arrows)* in a patient with asbestosis. Thickening of the pleural margins is also seen along the lower lateral borders of the chest. **A**, Anteroposterior view. **B**, Lateral view.

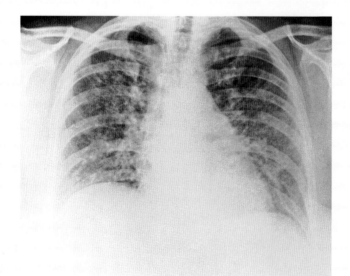

FIGURE 26-6 Acute farmer's lung. Chest radiograph shows diffuse parenchymal ground-glass pattern with some areas of consolidation. The severity of parenchymal opacification in this case is unusual. (From Hansell DM, Armstrong P, Lynch DA, McAdams HP, eds: *Imaging of diseases of the chest,* ed 4, Philadelphia, 2005, Elsevier.)

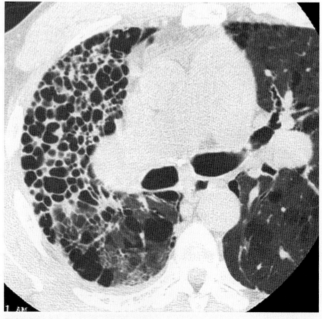

FIGURE 26-7 Honeycomb cysts in sarcoidosis. High-resolution computed tomography (HRCT) through the right mid-lung shows perfuse clustered honeycomb cysts. The cysts are larger than the typical honeycomb cysts seen in usual interstitial pneumonia. Cysts are much less extensive in the left lung. (From Hansell DM, Armstrong P, Lynch DA, McAdams HP, eds: *Imaging of diseases of the chest,* ed 4, Philadelphia, 2005, Elsevier.)

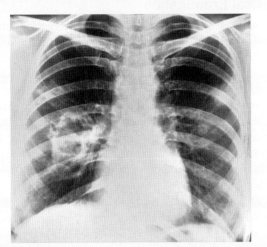

FIGURE 26-8 Wegener's granulomatosis. Numerous nodules with a large (6-cm) cavitary lesion adjacent to the right hilus. Its walls are thick and irregular. (From Hansell DM, Armstrong P, Lynch DA, McAdams HP, eds: *Imaging of diseases of the chest,* ed 4, Philadelphia, 2005, Elsevier.)

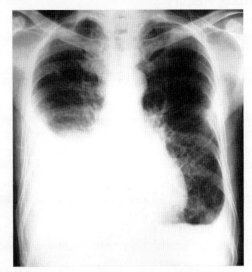

FIGURE 26-9 Pleural effusion in rheumatoid disease. Bilateral pleural effusions are present with mild changes of fibrosing alveolitis. The effusions were painless, and the one on the right had been present, more or less unchanged, for 5 months. Note the bilateral "meniscus signs." (From Hansell DM, Armstrong P, Lynch DA, McAdams HP, eds: *Imaging of diseases of the chest,* ed 4, Philadelphia, 2005, Elsevier.)

General Management of Interstitial Lung Disease

Medications and Procedures Commonly Prescribed by the Physician

The management of interstitial lung disorders is directed at the inflammation associated with the various disorders.

Corticosteroids

Corticosteroids are commonly administered with reasonably good results, but the benefit varies remarkably from one patient and condition (cause) to another (see Appendix II).

Respiratory Care Treatment Protocols

Oxygen Therapy Protocol

Oxygen therapy is used to treat hypoxemia, decrease the work of breathing, and decrease myocardial work. Because of the hypoxemia associated with ILDs, supplemental oxygen is often required. The hypoxemia that develops in an interstitial lung disorder is most commonly caused by **alveolar thickening**, fibrosis, and capillary shunting associated with the disorder (see Oxygen Therapy Protocol, Protocol 9-1).

Mechanical Ventilation Protocol

Mechanical ventilation may be needed to provide and support alveolar gas exchange and eventually return the patient to spontaneous breathing. Because acute ventilatory failure superimposed on chronic ventilatory failure is often seen in patients with severe ILD, continuous mechanical ventilation may be required. Continuous mechanical ventilation is justified when the acute ventilatory failure is thought to be reversible (see Mechanical Ventilation Protocol, Protocol 10-1 and Mechanical Ventilation Weaning Protocol, Protocol 10-2).

Other Treatments

Plasmapheresis

Treatment for Goodpasture's syndrome is directed at reducing the circulating anti-GBM antibodies that attack the patient's GBM. **Plasmapheresis,** which directly removes the anti-GBM antibodies from the circulation, has been of some benefit.

CASE STUDY Interstitial Lung Disease

Admitting History

An 89-year-old man is well known to the treating-hospital staff members, having received care there for more than 12 years. While in the U.S. Navy during World War II, he worked on the East Coast in the ship construction industry. After his discharge in 1945, he returned to his home in Mississippi for about 6 months; he then moved to Detroit, Michigan, and worked for an automobile manufacturer. His primary job for the next 20 years was undercoating automobiles.

In the early 1970s the man was transferred to a nearby automotive plant, where he worked on an assembly line fastening bumpers and chrome trim to cars. He was popular with his fellow workers and considered a hard worker by the management. When he retired in 1980, he was one of four supervisors in charge of the chrome trim assembly line.

Although the man smoked two packs a day for more than 40 years, his health was essentially unremarkable until about 4 years before he retired. At that time he started to experience periods of coughing, dyspnea, and weakness. A complete examination including a chest x-ray provided by the company concluded that the man had moderate interstitial lung disease (ILD).

On the basis of the man's work history, the doctor speculated that the ILD was caused by asbestos fibers. This theory was confirmed later with the finding of asbestos fibers in a Perls' stain of sputum, and the diagnosis of asbestosis was noted in the patient's chart. Just before the man retired, his pulmonary function test results (PFTs) showed a mild-to-moderate combined restrictive and obstructive disorder.

Although the man was able to enjoy a couple of relatively good years of retirement with his wife, his health declined rapidly. His cough and dyspnea quickly became a daily problem. Despite his deteriorating health, the man continued to smoke. When he was 72 years old, he was hospitalized for 8 days for treatment of pneumonia and severe respiratory distress. When he was discharged at that time, his PFTs still showed a moderate-to-severe restrictive disorder. He started using oxygen at home regularly.

Approximately 10 months before the current admission, the man was hospitalized because of congestive heart failure. He was treated aggressively and sent home within 5 days. At the time of discharge, his PFTs showed that he had a worsening restrictive respiratory disorder. His arterial blood gas values (ABGs) on 2 L/min oxygen by nasal cannula were as follows: pH 7.38, PaCO$_2$ 86 mm Hg, HCO$_3^-$ 49 mEq/L, PaO$_2$ 63 mm Hg, and SaO$_2$ 91%.

Approximately 3 hours before the current admission, the man awoke from an afternoon nap extremely short of breath. His wife stated that he coughed almost continuously and had difficulty speaking. She measured his oral temperature, which read 38 °C (100 °F). Concerned, she drove her husband to the hospital emergency room.

Physical Examination

As the man was wheeled into the emergency room, he appeared nervous, weak, and in obvious respiratory distress. He was on 1.5 L/min oxygen by nasal cannula, which was connected to an E-tank that was attached to the wheelchair. His skin felt damp and clammy to the touch. He appeared pale and cyanotic. His neck veins were distended, and his fingers and toes were clubbed. He demonstrated a frequent but weak cough productive of a moderate amount of thick, whitish-yellow secretions. He had 3+ peripheral edema of the ankles and feet. He said this was the worst his breathing had ever been.

The patient's vital signs were as follows: blood pressure 180/96, heart rate 108 beats/min, respiratory rate 32 breaths/min, and oral temperature 38.3 °C (100.8 °F). Palpation of the chest was negative. Percussion produced bilateral dull notes in the lung bases. Coarse crackles were auscultated throughout both lungs. A pleural friction rub could be heard over the right middle lobe between the sixth and seventh ribs, between the anterior axillary line and midaxillary line.

The patient's lower lobes had a diffuse, "ground-glass" appearance on the chest radiograph. Irregularly shaped opacities in the right and left lower pleural spaces were identified by the radiologist as calcified pleural plaques. A possible infiltrate consistent with pneumonia was also visible in the right middle lobe. In addition, the chest x-ray suggested that the right side of the heart was moderately enlarged. His ABGs on a 1.5 L/min oxygen nasal cannula were as follows: pH 7.56, PaCO$_2$ 51 mm Hg, HCO$_3^-$ 43 mEq/L, PaO$_2$ 47 mm Hg, and SaO$_2$ 86%.

The physician started the patient on intravenous furosemide (Lasix) to treat the man's cor pulmonale and began administering an antibiotic to treat suspected pneumonia. A respiratory therapist was called to obtain a sputum culture, perform a respiratory care evaluation, and outline further respiratory therapy. The physician said that she did not want to commit the patient to a ventilator unless absolutely necessary. On the basis of this information, the following SOAP was recorded.

Respiratory Assessment and Plan

S   "This is the worst my breathing has ever been."

O   Vital signs: BP 180/96, HR 108, RR 32, T 38.3 °C (100.8 °F); weak appearance; skin: cyanotic, damp, and clammy; distended neck veins and digital clubbing; cough: frequent, weak, moderate amount of thick, whitish-yellow secretions; peripheral edema 3+ of ankles and feet. Bilateral dull percussion notes in lung bases. Over both lungs: coarse crackles; pleural friction rub over right middle lobe between sixth and seventh ribs, between anterior axillary line and midaxillary line; CXR: ground-glass appearance in lower lobes; calcified pleural plaques in right and left lower pleural spaces; consolidation in right middle lung lobe; right heart enlargement; ABGs

(1.5 L/min O_2 by nasal cannula): pH 7.56, $PaCO_2$ 51, HCO_3^- 43, PaO_2 47, SaO_2 86%.

A • Respiratory distress (general appearance, vital signs, ABGs)
- Pulmonary fibrosis (history, diagnosis of asbestosis, CXR)
- Alveolar consolidation in right middle lobe (CXR)
- Pleurisy (asbestosis or pneumonitis) in area of right middle lobe (pleural friction rub)
- Excessive bronchial secretions (coarse crackles, sputum production)
- Chest infection likely (yellow sputum, fever)
- Acute alveolar hyperventilation superimposed on chronic ventilatory failure with moderate-to-severe hypoxemia (history, ABGs)
- Impending ventilatory failure (ABGs)

P Up-regulate **Oxygen Therapy Protocol** (air entrainment mask at FIO_2 0.35). **Bronchopulmonary Hygiene Therapy Protocol** (DB&C q4 h; obtain sputum for Gram stain and culture). Initiate **Lung Expansion Therapy Protocol** (incentive spirometry followed by C&DB). Monitor with pulse oximeter, set SpO_2 alarm at 85%.

The Next Morning

Throughout the night the patient's condition remained unstable. He continued to cough frequently but could not expectorate secretions adequately on his own. When the therapist assisted the patient during coughing episodes, a moderate amount of thick, white and yellow sputum was produced. Even though he was conscious, alert, and able to follow simple directions, he did not answer any of the respiratory therapist's specific questions about his breathing.

His skin was cold and damp to the touch, and he appeared short of breath. His color was improved, but he still appeared pale and cyanotic. His neck veins were still distended, although not so severely as they had been on admission, and edema of his ankles and feet could still be seen. The patient's vital signs were as follows: blood pressure 192/108, heart rate 113 beats/min, respiratory rate 34 breaths/min, and oral temperature 38 °C (100.4 °F). Palpation of the chest was negative.

Dull percussion notes were elicited over the lung bases. Coarse crackles continued to be auscultated throughout both lungs. A pleural friction rub could still be heard over the right middle lung between the sixth and seventh ribs, between the anterior axillary line and midaxillary line. No recent chest radiograph was available. His ABGs (FIO_2 0.35) were as follows: pH 7.57, $PaCO_2$ 47 mm Hg, HCO_3^- 41 mEq/L, PaO_2 40 mm Hg, and SaO_2 83%.

On the basis of these clinical data, the following SOAP was documented.

Respiratory Assessment and Plan

S N/A (patient too dyspneic to reply)
O Condition unstable; cough: frequent, weak, productive of thick, white and yellow secretions; skin: cyanotic, pale, cool, and damp; distended neck veins and peripheral edema, but improving; vital signs: BP 192/108, HR 113,

RR 34, T 38 °C (100.4 °F); dull percussion notes over both lung bases; coarse crackles throughout both lungs; pleural friction rub over right middle lobe between sixth and seventh ribs, between anterior axillary line and midaxillary line; ABGs (FIO_2 0.35): pH 7.57, $PaCO_2$ 47, HCO_3^- 41, PaO_2 40, SaO_2 83%.

A • Continued respiratory distress (general appearance, vital signs, ABGs)
- Pulmonary fibrosis in lower lobes (history, diagnosis of asbestosis, recent CXR)
- Alveolar consolidation in right middle lobe (CXR, pneumonia)
- Pleurisy or pneumonia that has extended into pleural space over right middle lobe (pleural friction rub)
- Excessive bronchial secretions (coarse crackles, sputum production)
- Infection likely (yellow sputum)
- Acute alveolar hyperventilation superimposed on chronic ventilatory failure with severe hypoxemia, worsening (history, ABGs)
- Impending ventilatory failure (ABGs: increased alveolar hyperventilation and worsening PaO_2)

P Up-regulate **Oxygen Therapy Protocol** (nonrebreather oxygen mask). **Bronchopulmonary Hygiene Therapy Protocol** (adding intensive nasotracheal suctioning q2 h). Start **Aerosolized Medication Protocol** (nebulize 2 mL acetylcysteine mixed with the albuterol dose). Continue **Lung Expansion Therapy Protocol** (continuing to coach and monitor incentive spirometry; if FVC falls below 15 mL/kg, administer CPAP mask at +10 cm H_2O for 20 minutes qid). Continue to monitor closely.

20 Hours Later

At 6:15 AM the alarm on the patient's cardiac monitor sounded. The electrocardiogram (ECG) strip showed frequent premature ventricular contractions followed by ventricular flutter and fibrillation. The head nurse called for a Code Blue. Cardiopulmonary resuscitation was started immediately. Because of the severe hypotension (blood pressure 80/50), epinephrine and dopamine were administered through the patient's intravenous line. Approximately 12 minutes into the code, the patient exhibited a normal sinus rhythm and spontaneous respirations.

The patient was intubated, transferred to the intensive care unit (ICU), and placed on a mechanical ventilator. The initial ventilator settings were as follows: tidal volume 750 mL, 12 breaths per minute, FIO_2 1.0, pressure support 7 cm H_2O, and 5 cm H_2O positive end-expiratory pressure (PEEP). His cardiopulmonary status remained unstable. Premature ventricular contractions were frequently seen on the electrocardiographic monitor. A pulmonary artery catheter and arterial line were inserted.

The patient's skin was pale, cyanotic, and clammy. His neck veins were still distended, and his ankles and feet were swollen. Vital signs were as follows: blood pressure 135/90, heart rate 84 beats/min, and rectal temperature 38.3 °C (100.8 °F). Palpation of the chest wall was negative. Dull percussion notes were noted over the lung bases. Coarse crackles continued to be auscultated throughout both lungs.

Thick, greenish-yellow sputum was frequently suctioned from the patient's endotracheal tube.

A pleural friction rub could still be heard over the right middle lung lobe between the sixth and seventh ribs, between the anterior axillary line and midaxillary line. A chest radiograph had been taken but had not yet been interpreted by the radiologist. His ABGs on FIO_2 1.0 were as follows: pH 7.53, $PaCO_2$ 56 mm Hg, HCO_3^- 45 mEq/L, PaO_2 246 mm Hg, and SaO_2 98%.

At this time, the following SOAP note was charted.

Respiratory Assessment and Plan

S N/A (patient intubated on ventilator)

O Vital signs: BP 135/90 on vasopressors, HR 84, T 38.3 °C (100.8 °F); frequent premature ventricular contractions; skin: pale, cyanotic, and clammy; distended neck veins; peripheral edema of ankles and feet; dull percussion notes over lung bases; coarse crackles throughout both lungs; thick, greenish-yellow sputum frequently suctioned; pleural friction rub over right middle lung lobe between sixth and seventh ribs and between anterior axillary line and midaxillary line; ABGs (FIO_2 1.0): pH 7.53, $PaCO_2$ 56, HCO_3^- 45, PaO_2 246, SaO_2 98%.

A • Pulmonary fibrosis, lower lung lobes (history, diagnosis of asbestosis, recent CXR)

• Alveolar consolidation, right middle lobe (recent CXR showing pneumonia)

• Pneumonia possibly extended into pleural space over right middle lobe (pleural friction rub)

• Excessive bronchial secretions (coarse crackles, sputum production)

• Infection likely (fever, greenish-yellow sputum, possible new organism)

• Acute alveolar hyperventilation superimposed on chronic ventilatory failure and overly corrected hypoxemia (ABGs)

• Alveolar hyperventilation and overoxygenation caused by mechanical ventilator and FIO_2 setting

P Down-regulate **Oxygen Therapy Protocol** (reduce FIO_2 to 0.50). Down-regulate **Mechanical Ventilation Protocol** (e.g., decrease the tidal volume to increase the $PaCO_2$ to patient's baseline—e.g., 80 to 90 mm Hg). Continue **Bronchopulmonary Hygiene Therapy Protocol** and **Aerosolized Medication Protocol**. Continue **Lung Expansion Therapy Protocol** (10 cm H_2O PEEP, but monitor mean airway pressure). Continue to closely monitor and reevaluate.

Discussion

The admitting history revealed that the patient had been diagnosed with moderate pneumoconiosis (probable asbestosis). Not surprisingly, pulmonary function tests in the past had shown mild-to-moderate restrictive pulmonary disorders.

Significant new findings were the recent history suggesting congestive heart failure and the arterial blood gas values on his discharge from the hospital 10 months before the admission under discussion, which demonstrated chronic ventilatory failure. The patient's recent fever and cough before his emergency room admission suggested an infectious cause for his symptoms. His cyanosis, neck-vein distention, and digital clubbing suggested chronic hypoxemia. The sputum purulence confirmed that infection may indeed have been present and that the assessing therapist's desire to obtain a sputum culture was appropriate. The pleural rub demonstrated by this patient could have been related to his asbestosis or to a pneumonic infiltrate extending to the pleural surface.

In the initial assessment the patient's severe hypertension and his fever were noted. Both deserved vigorous therapy if his pulmonary function were to improve at all. The patient's severe hypoxemia reflected common clinical indicators caused by **Alveolar-Capillary Membrane Thickening** (see Figure 9-9) and **Excessive Bronchial Secretions** (see Figure 9-11). Although there is no therapy available to reverse the increased alveolar membrane thickening, the excessive bronchial secretions can be effectively treated in most cases.

The patient was hyperventilating with respect to his earlier outpatient blood gases. During such an assessment the patient's underlying pulmonary conditions (chronic pulmonary fibrosis, bronchitis, and congestive heart failure) should be recorded, but the assessment should really zero in on the treatable issues, specifically in this case the pulmonary infection, as suggested by the patient's fever, sputum purulence, and chest radiograph.

At the time of the second evaluation, the patient's hypoxemia had worsened despite oxygen therapy. If not already being used, Venturi oxygen mask therapy was indicated there, and aggressive endotracheal suctioning could also be indicated. A trial of **Lung Expansion Therapy Protocol** (Protocol 9-3) was appropriate to attempt to offset the pathologic effects of the alveolar consolidation and, possibly, atelectasis. The physician may have ordered a trial of diuretic therapy to reduce the fluid retention and also a course of antibiotic therapy.

The last assessment revealed ventricular arrhythmias. The change in the patient's sputum from thick and white to greenish-yellow suggests superinfection with another organism, and reculture of the sputum was appropriate. The respiratory therapist responded quickly, and appropriately, to readjust the mechanical ventilator. The FIO_2 was decreased to 0.50 to correct the patient's overoxygenation (PaO_2: 246), and the tidal volume was reduced to increase the $PaCO_2$ to the baseline—80 to 90 mm Hg, according to the ABG history. Ventilator parameters should be adjusted to provide good pulmonary expansion while avoiding high mean airway pressures. A cautious trial of PEEP would have been in order.

Despite all that was done for this patient, he died 4 days later as a result of left-sided congestive heart failure and pneumonia complicating his pulmonary asbestosis.

SELF-ASSESSMENT QUESTIONS

Answers to questions can be found on Evolve. To access additional student assessment questions visit **http://evolve.elsevier.com/DesJardins/respiratory**.

1. **Which of the following is another name for hypersensitivity pneumonitis?**
   a. Sarcoidosis
   b. Extrinsic allergic alveolitis
   c. Alveolar proteinosis
   d. Idiopathic pulmonary hemosiderosis

2. **Which of the following is or are considered pulmonary vasculitides?**
   1. Rheumatoid arthritis
   2. Wegener's granulomatosis
   3. Lymphomatoid granulomatosis
   4. Churg-Strauss syndrome
      a. 1 only
      b. 3 only
      c. 2, 3, and 4 only
      d. 1, 2, and 3 only

3. **Which of the following disorders is associated with desquamative interstitial pneumonia and usual interstitial pneumonia?**
   a. Idiopathic pulmonary fibrosis
   b. Eosinophilic granuloma
   c. Rheumatoid arthritis
   d. Sarcoidosis

4. **Which of the following is/are systemic connective tissue diseases?**
   1. Pulmonary Langerhans cell histiocytosis
   2. Rheumatoid arthritis
   3. Sjögren's syndrome
   4. Alveolar proteinosis
      a. 3 only
      b. 2 and 4 only
      c. 1 and 4 only
      d. 2 and 3 only

5. **Which of the following pulmonary function study findings is or are associated with chronic interstitial lung disease?**
   1. Increased FRC
   2. Decreased FEVT
   3. Increased RV
   4. Decreased FVC
      a. 1 only
      b. 3 only
      c. 2 and 4 only
      d. 3 and 4 only

6. **Which of the following hemodynamic indices is or are associated with advanced or severe interstitial lung disease?**
   1. Increased CVP
   2. Decreased PCWP
   3. Increased $\overline{PA}$
   4. Decreased RAP
      a. 1 only
      b. 4 only
      c. 1 and 3 only
      d. 2 and 4 only

7. **Which of the following chest assessment findings is associated with interstitial lung disease?**
   a. Diminished breath sounds
   b. Hyperresonant percussion note
   c. Decreased tactile fremitus
   d. Bronchial breath sounds

8. **Which of the following oxygenation indices is or are associated with the pneumoconioses?**
   1. Decreased $C(a-\overline{v})O_2$
   2. Increased O_2ER
   3. Decreased $S\overline{v}O_2$
   4. Increased $S\overline{v}O_2$
      a. 1 only
      b. 3 only
      c. 2 and 3 only
      d. 1 and 4 only

9. **The fibrotic changes that develop in coal worker's pneumoconiosis usually result from which of the following?**
   a. Barium
   b. Silica
   c. Iron
   d. Coal dust

10. **Which of the following are associated with interstitial lung disease?**
    1. Pleural friction rub
    2. Dull percussion note
    3. Cor pulmonale
    4. Elevated $\overline{PA}$
       a. 2 and 4 only
       b. 3 and 4 only
       c. 2, 3, and 4 only
       d. 1, 2, 3, and 4

CHAPTER

27 Cancer of the Lung

Chapter Objectives

After reading this chapter, you will be able to:

- List the anatomic alterations of the lungs associated with lung cancer.
- Describe the causes of lung cancer.
- List the cardiopulmonary clinical manifestations associated with lung cancer.
- Describe the general management of lung cancer.
- Describe the clinical strategies and rationales of the SOAPs presented in the case study.

Key Terms

Adenocarcinoma
Aerosolized Morphine
Benign Tumors
Brachytherapy
Bronchogenic Carcinoma
Chemotherapy
Coin Lesion
Endobronchial Ultrasound (EBUS)
Environmental Tobacco Smoke (ETS)
External Beam Radiation Therapy (EBRT)
Large Cell Carcinoma (Undifferentiated)
Lobectomy
Malignant Tumors
Mediastinoscopy
Neoplasm
Non–Small Cell Lung Carcinoma (NSCLC)
PET/CT Imaging
Photodynamic Therapy (PDT)
Pneumonectomy

Positron Emission Tomography (PET) Lung Scan
Radiation Therapy
Radiofrequency Ablation (RFA)
Segmentectomy
Small Cell (Oat Cell) Carcinoma
Small Cell Lung Carcinoma (SCLC)
Squamous Cell Carcinoma
Staging of Lung Cancer
Stereotactic Body Radiation Therapy (SBRT)
Stereotactic Radiosurgery (SRS)
Video-Assisted Thoracoscopy Surgery (VATS)
Wedge Resection

Chapter Outline

Anatomic Alterations of the Lungs
Etiology and Epidemiology
    Types of Cancers
    Non–Small Cell Lung Carcinoma
    Small Cell Lung Carcinoma
Screening and Diagnosis
    Staging of Non–Small Cell Lung Carcinoma (NSCLC)
    Staging of Small Cell Lung Carcinoma (SCLC)
Overview of Cardiopulmonary Clinical Manifestations
    Associated with Cancer of the Lung
General Management of Lung Cancer
    Treatment Options for Non–Small Cell Lung Cancer (NSCLC)
    Treatment Options for Small Cell Lung Cancer (SCLC)
Case Study: Cancer of the Lung
Self-Assessment Questions

Anatomic Alterations of the Lungs

Cancer is a general term that refers to abnormal new tissue growth characterized by the progressive, uncontrolled multiplication of cells. This abnormal growth of new cells is called a **neoplasm** or *tumor*. A tumor may be localized or invasive, benign or malignant.

Benign tumors do not endanger life unless they interfere with the normal functions of other organs or affect a vital organ. They grow slowly and push aside normal tissue but do not invade it. They are usually encapsulated, well-demarcated growths. They are not invasive or metastatic; that is, tumor cells do not travel by way of the bloodstream or lymphatics and invade or form secondary tumors in other organs.

Malignant tumors are composed of embryonic, primitive, or poorly differentiated cells. They grow in a disorganized manner and so rapidly that nutrition of the cells becomes a problem. For this reason, necrosis, ulceration, and cavity formation are commonly associated with malignant tumors. They also invade surrounding tissues and may be metastatic. Although malignant changes may develop in any portion of the lung, they most commonly originate in the epithelium of the tracheobronchial tree.

A tumor that originates in the bronchial mucosa is called **bronchogenic carcinoma**. The terms *lung cancer* and *bronchogenic carcinoma* are used interchangeably. As a tumor enlarges, the surrounding bronchial airways and alveoli become irritated, inflamed, and swollen. The adjacent alveoli may fill with fluid or become consolidated or collapse. In addition, as the tumor protrudes into the tracheobronchial tree, excessive mucous production and airway obstruction develop. As the surrounding blood vessels erode, blood enters the tracheobronchial tree. Peripheral tumors may also invade the pleural space and impinge on the mediastinum, chest wall, ribs, or diaphragm. A secondary pleural effusion is often seen in lung cancer. A pleural effusion further compresses the lung and causes atelectasis.

The major pathologic or structural changes associated with bronchogenic carcinoma are as follows:

- Inflammation, swelling, and destruction of the bronchial airways and alveoli
- Excessive mucous production
- Tracheobronchial mucous accumulation and plugging
- Airway obstruction (either from blood, from mucous accumulation, or from a tumor projecting into a bronchus)
- Atelectasis
- Alveolar consolidation
- Cavity formation
- Pleural effusion (when a tumor invades the parietal pleura and mediastinum)

Etiology and Epidemiology

In 2013 in the United States, the American Cancer Society estimated that there were 228,190 new cases of lung cancer (118,080 in men and 110,110 in women), with an estimated 159,480 deaths (87,260 in men and 72,220 among women), which accounted for about 27% of all cancer deaths. Each year, there are more deaths caused by lung cancer than colon, breast, and prostate cancers combined. About 2 out of 3 people diagnosed with lung cancer are 65 years or older; fewer than 2% of all cases are found in people younger than 45 years. The average age at the time of diagnosis is about 70 years. Black men are about 20% more likely to develop lung cancer than white men. The rate is about 10% lower in black women than in white women. More than 380,000 people alive today have been diagnosed with lung cancer.

Cigarette smoking[1] is the most common cause of lung cancer. Although various studies and professional organizations report slightly different numbers, all figures are

---

[1]The role of the respiratory therapist as a patient educator is becoming increasingly important, and nowhere more so than in the field of smoking cessation education. This function occurs best in the outpatient and inpatient settings as part of well-organized pulmonary rehabilitation programs, in the public domain (e.g., lectures to high school students), and on an individual basis with patients. The role of smoking cessation education has been discussed elsewhere (see Chapter 12) as part of evidenced-based practice in chronic obstructive pulmonary disease (COPD). Documentation of efforts and patient adherence and compliance to smoking cessation efforts has become increasingly complex, and important for reimbursement purposes. The effect of smoking cessation of established lung cancer is, unfortunately, not particularly successful.

grim. For example, according to the Centers for Disease Control and Prevention (CDC) and the Surgeon General's report, male smokers are 22 times more likely to develop lung cancer than nonsmokers, whereas female smokers are 12 times more likely than female nonsmokers to develop lung cancer. Heavy smokers are 64 times more likely to develop lung cancer. It is estimated that cigarette smoke contains more than 4000 different chemicals, many of which have proved to be carcinogens. Exposure to secondhand smoke or **environmental tobacco smoke (ETS)** is associated with as much as a 30% increase in the risk for lung cancer. A genetic predisposition toward developing lung cancer also plays a role in the incidence of lung cancer.

Environmental or occupational risk factors for lung cancer include the following:

- Benzopyrene and radon particles associated with uranium mining
- Radiation and nuclear fallout
- Polycyclic aromatic hydrocarbons and arsenicals
- Asbestos fibers
- Diesel exhaust
- Nitrogen mustard gases
- Nickel
- Silica
- Vinyl chloride
- Chloromethyl methyl ether
- Air pollution
- Coal and iron mining

Types of Cancers

As shown in Figure 27-1, bronchogenic carcinomas can be divided into the following two major categories: **Non–small Cell Lung Carcinoma (NSCLC)** and **Small Cell Lung Carcinoma (SCLC)**. The NSCLC category is further subdivided into the following three types of lung cancer: (1) **squamous (epidermoid) cell carcinoma**, (2) **adenocarcinoma** (including bronchial alveolar cell carcinoma), and (3) **large cell carcinoma**. Under the SCLC category is **small cell carcinoma** (also called **oat cell carcinoma**), or **combined small cell carcinoma**, or a **mixture of small cell** and **non–small cell carcinoma**.

Each type of lung cancer grows and spreads in a different way. For example, SCLC spreads aggressively and responds best to **chemotherapy** and **radiation therapy**. SCLC occurs almost exclusively in smokers, and accounts for 15% to 20% of all lung cancers in the United States. NSCLCs are more common and account for 75% to 85% of all lung cancers in the United States. When confined to a small area and identified early, NSCLCs can often be removed surgically. Table 27-1 provides general characteristics of these cancer cell types, including growth rates, metastasis, and means of diagnosis. A more in-depth description of each cancer cell type follows.

Non–Small Cell Lung Carcinoma
Squamous Cell Carcinoma

Squamous cell carcinoma constitutes about 30% of the bronchogenic carcinomas. The incidence of this type of cancer has sharply declined over the past two decades. This type of

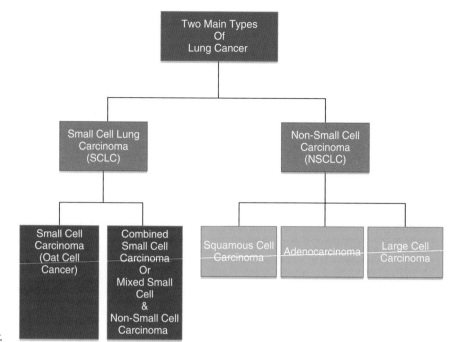

FIGURE 27-1 Types of lung cancer.

Tumor Type	Growth Rate	Metastasis	Means of Diagnosis	Clinical Manifestations and Treatment
Non–Small Cell Lung Carcinoma (NSCLC)				
Squamous cell carcinoma	Slow	Late; mostly to hilar lymph nodes	Biopsy, sputum analysis, bronchoscopy, electron microscopy, immunohistochemistry	Cough, sputum production, airway obstruction; treated surgically, chemotherapy adjunctive
Adenocarcinoma	Moderate	Early	Radiography, fiberoptic bronchoscopy, electron microscopy	Pleural effusion; treated surgically, chemotherapy adjunctive
Large cell carcinoma	Rapid	Early and widespread	Sputum analysis, bronchoscopy, electron microscopy (by exclusion of other cell types)	Chest wall pain, pleural effusion, cough, sputum production, hemoptysis, airway obstruction resulting in pneumonia (if airways involved); treated surgically
Small Cell Lung Carcinoma (SCLC)				
Small cell (oat cell) carcinoma	Very rapid	Very early; to mediastinum or distally in lung	Radiography, sputum analysis, bronchoscopy, electron microscopy, immunohistochemistry, and clinical manifestations (cough, chest pain, dyspnea, hemoptysis, localized wheezing)	Airway obstruction, signs and symptoms of excessive hormone secretion; treated by chemotherapy and ionizing radiation to thorax and central nervous system

TABLE 27-1 Characteristics of Lung Cancers

Modified from McCance KL, Huether SE: *Pathophysiology: the biologic basis for disease in adults and children*, ed 6, St Louis, 2010, Mosby/Elsevier.

tumor is commonly located near a central bronchus or hilus and projects into the large bronchi. Squamous cell tumors are often seen projecting into the bronchi during bronchoscopy. The tumor originates from the basal cells of the bronchial epithelium and grows through the epithelium before invading the surrounding tissues.

The tumor has a slow growth rate and a late metastatic tendency (mostly to hilar lymph nodes). These tumors generally remain fairly well localized and tend not to metastasize until late in the course of lung cancer. Cavitation and necrosis within the center of the cancer is a common finding. Surgical resection is the preferred treatment if metastasis has

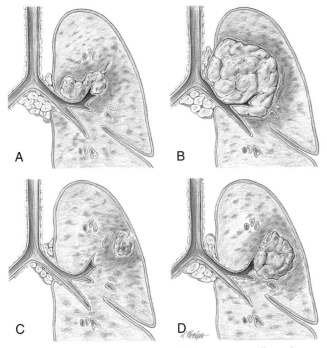

FIGURE 27-2 Cancer of the lung. **A**, Squamous cell carcinoma. **B**, Adenocarcinoma. **C**, Large cell carcinoma. **D**, Small cell (oat cell) carcinoma.

not taken place. Chemotherapy has limited effectiveness. In about one third of cases, squamous cell carcinoma originates in the periphery. Because of the location in the central bronchi, obstructive manifestations are generally nonspecific and include a nonproductive cough and hemoptysis. Pneumonia and atelectasis are often secondary complications of squamous cell carcinoma. Cavity formation with or without an air-fluid interface is seen in 10% to 20% of cases (Figure 27-2, *A*).

Adenocarcinoma

Adenocarcinoma arises from the mucous glands of the tracheobronchial tree. In fact, the glandular configuration and the mucous production caused by this type of cancer are the pathologic features that distinguish adenocarcinoma from the other types of bronchogenic carcinoma. It accounts for 35% to 40% of all bronchogenic carcinomas. Adenocarcinoma has the weakest association with smoking. Among people who have never smoked, adenocarcinoma is the most common form of lung cancer. Adenocarcinoma tumors are usually smaller than 4 cm and are most commonly found in the peripheral regions of the lung parenchyma. The growth rate is moderate and the metastatic tendency is early. Secondary cavity formation and pleural effusion are common (Figure 27-2, *B*). When the cancer is discovered early, surgical resection is possible in a high percentage of cases.

Bronchial alveolar cell carcinoma is included under the category of adenocarcinoma. These tumors typically arise from the terminal bronchioles and alveoli. They have a slow growth rate, and their metastasis pattern is unpredictable.

Large Cell Carcinoma (Undifferentiated)

Large cell carcinoma accounts for about 10% to 15% of all bronchogenic carcinoma cases. Because this tumor has lost

all evidence of differentiation, it is commonly referred to as *undifferentiated large cell anaplastic cancer.* Although these tumors commonly arise peripherally, they may also be found centrally—often distorting the trachea and large airways. Large cell carcinoma has a rapid growth rate and early and widespread metastasis. Common secondary complications include chest wall pain, pleural effusion, pneumonia, hemoptysis, and cavity formation (Figure 27-2, *C*).

Small Cell Lung Carcinoma

Small cell carcinoma accounts for about 14% of all bronchogenic carcinomas. Most of these tumors arise centrally near the hilar region. They tend to arise in the larger airways (primary and secondary bronchi). Cell size ranges from 6 to 8 μm. The tumor grows very rapidly, becoming very large, and metastasizes early. Because the tumor cells are often compressed into an oval shape, this form of cancer is commonly referred to as oat cell carcinoma. Staging for small cell carcinoma is divided into only two categories: limited disease (20% to 30%) or extensive disease (70% to 80%). Small cell carcinoma has the poorest prognosis. The average survival time for untreated small cell carcinoma is about 1 to 3 months. About 90% of patients respond to treatment (e.g., chemotherapy, radiation, or both), but nearly all relapse within 24 months. Small cell carcinoma has the strongest correlation with cigarette smoking and is associated with the worst prognosis (Figure 27-2, *D*).

Screening and Diagnosis

Unfortunately, most lung cancers are not diagnosed until after the patient presents with symptoms that suggest lung cancer. Symptoms associated with lung cancer include: (1) a progressively worsening cough—often includes blood or rust-colored sputum; (2) chest pain—especially with deep breathing, coughing, or laughing; (3) hoarse voice; (4) poor appetite and weight loss; (5) dyspnea; (6) fatigue; (7) frequent bronchial infection or pneumonia episodes; and (8) the sudden onset of wheezing.

When lung cancer spreads to other parts of the body, the patient may have other symptoms of cancer that include bone pain (e.g., back or hips), neurologic problems (e.g., headache, arm and leg weakness or numbness, dizziness or balance problems, seizures, jaundice), and enlarged lymph nodes (e.g., neck or under the arms). In addition, the patient may demonstrate a group of very specific syndromes associated with lung cancer, such as:

- Horner's syndrome—is caused by a tumor near the top of the lung that damages the nerve that passes from the upper chest to the neck; causing drooping or weakness of one eyelid, small pupil in the same eye, and reduced or no perspiration on the same side of the face.
- Superior vena cava syndrome—is caused by a tumor near the upper portion of the right lung that compresses the superior vena cava and restricts blood flow. This condition causes headaches, dizziness, and swelling in the face, neck, arms, and upper chest—sometimes with a bluish-red skin color.

- Paraneoplastic syndromes—are the indirect effects of a tumor that occur distant to the tumor or metastatic site. The tumor produces active proteins, polypeptides, or hormonelike substances that enter the bloodstream and cause problems distant from the tumor. Common paraneoplastic syndromes caused by non–small cell lung cancer include (1) high blood calcium levels (hypercalcemia), (2) excess growth of certain bones (e.g., fingertips), and (3) blood clots.

When symptoms are present that suggest lung cancer, a full medical history and physical examination—along with a check for risk factors—are ordered. When the results of these activities further support the possibility of lung cancer, additional diagnostic tests are ordered—for example, imaging tests and tissue sampling techniques. Table 27-2 provides an overview of the common screening and diagnostic tests for lung cancer. The primary goal of these diagnostic procedures is (1) confirm the presence of a lung carcinoma, (2) establish the cancer cell type, and (3) confirm the stage of the cancer. The definitive diagnosis of lung cancer is made by a microscopic examination of a tissue sample (biopsy). The treatment and prognosis of any cancer depends, to a large extent, on the stage of the cancer. The **staging of lung** cancer is discussed in more detail as follows.

Staging of Non–Small Cell Lung Carcinoma (NSCLC)

The Tumor Node Metastasis (TMN) Staging System

The staging of lung cancer confirms the cell type, the size of the tumor, and the level of lymph node involvement, and the extent to which the cancer has spread. The prognosis and treatment of the patient depend, to a large extent, on the staging results. The staging of NSCLC uses the **American Joint Committee on Cancer TMN staging system** (Table 27-3). The stage of a patient's cancer is determined by a combination of all of the following factors:
- **T**—represents the size and location of the primary tumor
- **N**—denotes the regional lymph node involvement
- **M**—signifies the extent of metastasis (e.g., common sites are the brain, bones, adrenal glands, liver, kidneys, and other lung)

The numbers and letters after the T, N, and M provide more information about each of these factors. The numbers 0 through 4 represent increasing severity.

Stage Grouping for Lung Cancer

Once the T, N, and M categories have been established, the information is grouped together to determine the overall stage of the lung cancer. Stages 0, I, II, III, and IV are used to identify the overall stage of the lung cancer—with Stage 0 and Stage I being the least advanced and Stage IV the most advanced. Table 27-4 provides an overview of the stage grouping for lung cancer.

Staging of Small Cell Lung Carcinoma (SCLC)

SCLC is staged differently than non–small cell cancer. For treatment reasons, SCLC is usually classified as a limited stage, or an extensive stage:
- **Limited Stage**—means the cancer is confined to only one lung and to its neighboring lymph nodes. It can be treated with a single radiation field. In some cases, the lymph nodes at the center of the chest (mediastinal lymph nodes) may be included, even when the cancer is close to the other lung. Between 20% and 30% of the patients with small cell lung cancer have limited stage SCLC.
- **Extensive Stage**—means the cancer has spread beyond one lung and nearby lymph nodes. It may have invaded lungs, more remote lymph nodes, and other distant organs (including bone marrow). Between 70% and 80% of the patients with small cell lung cancer have extensive stage SCLC.

SCLC is commonly staged this way to help identify which patients might benefit more from aggressive treatments—for example, chemotherapy combined with radiation therapy is commonly used to treat limited stage SCLC—as compared to treating the patient with only chemotherapy, which would be the better option for extensive stage SCLC.

5-Year Survival Rate

The average percentage of people who are still alive 5 years after the cancer has been discovered depends on the type and stage of the lung cancer. NSCLC generally grows and spreads more slowly than SCLC. The survival rates decrease when the stage of cancer involves the patient's lymph nodes or other body organs. According to the American Cancer Society, the general 5-year survival rates for NSCLC are shown in Table 27-5. Although SCLC is less common than NSCLC, it generally grows very fast and is more likely to spread to other organs. Table 27-6 provides a general overview of the 5-year survival rates for SCLC.

Text continued on p. 384

TABLE 27-2 Screening and Diagnostic Tests for Lung Cancer

Technique	Description
Imaging for Lung Cancer Imaging is performed to (1) identify suspicious areas of the lungs that might be cancerous, (2) determine if and where the cancer may have spread, (3) evaluate the effectiveness of treatment, and (4) assess signs that a cancer has returned after a treatment program.	
Chest radiograph	The chest x-ray is often the first test used to determine if there are any masses or spots on the lungs. If any suspicious areas are identified, one or more of the following imaging methods are ordered.
Computed tomography (CT) scan	The CT scan better identifies a lung tumor than a routine chest x-ray. It also provides excellent information about the size, shape, and location of the tumor. It can also help identify enlarged lymph nodes that might contain cancer cells.
Positron emission tomography (PET) scan	The PET scan is used to help determine if an abnormal area on the chest x-ray or CT scan might be cancer. It helps to assess if the cancer has spread to nearby lymph nodes or other areas of the body, which helps to determine if surgery is an option.
Magnetic resonance imaging (MRI) scan	The MRI scan may be used to determine if the cancer cells have spread from the lungs to the brain or spinal cord.
Bone scan	The bone scan can also help to determine if the cancer has spread to the bones. Because the PET scan can usually identify if cancer has spread to the bones, the bone scan is now primarily only ordered when the patient has bone pain symptoms.
Diagnostic Tests for Lung Cancer Identifying cancer cells under a microscope makes the actual diagnosis of lung cancer. The cells can be obtained from sputum samples, taken from a suspicious area (biopsy), or removed from pleural (thoracentesis).	
Sputum cytology	A sputum sample is obtained and viewed under the microscope to determine if it has any cancer cells.
Bronchoscopy • Needle biopsy • Bronchial brushing • Bronchial washing	A bronchoscope is commonly used to visually evaluate the tracheobronchial tree of the patient. In addition, small instruments can easily be passed down the bronchoscope to obtain tissue biopsies via needle aspiration, bronchial brushing, or bronchial washing. The tissue and cell samples are then evaluated under a microscope.
Endobronchial ultrasound (EBUS)	EBUS may be performed during a bronchoscopy to view lymph nodes and other structures in the mediastinum area. EBUS may also be used for a needle biopsy. Tissue samples are viewed under the microscope. EBUS may provide sufficient information to stage a cancer without other more invasive procedures, such as mediastinoscopy, thoracoscopy, or thoracotomy.
Endoscopic esophageal ultrasound	Similar to EBUS, the endoscopic esophageal ultrasound can be passed into the esophagus and directed to view lymph nodes and other structures in the chest that appear suspicious for cancer. When enlarged lymph nodes are identified, a hollow needle can pass through the endoscope to obtain a tissue sample.
Mediastinoscopy and mediastinotomy	These procedures are performed to view a suspicious area more directly and to obtain a tissue sample. They are performed in the operating room while the patient is under general anesthesia. The *mediastinoscopy* entails a small incision in the front of the neck, which allows a thin, hollow, lighted tube to be inserted behind the sternum and in front of the trachea. Tissue samples can be obtained from the lymph nodes along the trachea and major bronchi. A mediastinotomy entails a slightly larger incision (about 2 inches long) between the left second and third ribs adjacent to the sternum. This permits the surgeon to reach some lymph nodes that cannot be reached by mediastinoscopy.
Thoracentesis	Thoracentesis is used to obtain fluid that accumulates (pleural effusion) between the chest wall and the lungs. Thoracentesis entails the insertion of a hollow needle between the ribs to aspirate the fluid (and possible cancer cells) for microscopic study.
Video-assisted thoracoscopy surgery (VATS)	VATS may be performed to determine if the cancer has spread to the intrapleural space. It can also be used to obtain tissue biopsies on the outer parts of the lungs, nearby lymph nodes, and fluid. It may also help to assess if a tumor is growing into nearby organs or tissues. Because VATS is performed in the operating room under general anesthesia, it is not often done just to diagnose cancer unless other procedures have been unsuccessful in obtaining a tissue sample.
Lab Tests of Biopsy The tissue samples obtained from one of the above procedures may be used for additional tests to help better classify the cancer.	
Immunohistochemistry	This test entails treating the tissue sample with certain antibodies designed to attach only to specific substances found in certain cancer cells.

Continued

TABLE 27-2 Screening and Diagnostic Tests for Lung Cancer—cont'd

Technique	Description
Molecular tests	In some cases, the identification of specific gene changes in the cancer cells may help pinpoint certain targeted drugs that might be effective in treating the cancer.
Complete blood count (CBC)	Although blood tests are not used to diagnose lung cancer, they are useful in assessing the overall health of the patient and, in some cases, to determine if the patient is healthy enough for surgery. In addition, a CBC is repeated regularly in patients being treated with chemotherapy—which often affect blood-forming cells of the bone marrow. Also, when a cancer has spread to the liver and bones, it may cause abnormal levels of certain chemicals in the blood—e.g., higher than normal level of lactate dehydrogenase (LDH).

Adapted from the American Cancer Society, http://www.cancer.org (Last Medical Review: 05/22/2013) (Last Revised: 07/12/2013).

TABLE 27-3 The American Joint Committee on Cancer (AJCC) Tumor Node Metastasis (TNM) Staging System for Lung Cancer

TNM Category	Description
	Primary Tumor (T)
TX	The main (primary) tumor cannot be assessed, or cancer cells were seen on sputum cytology or bronchial washing but no tumor can be found.
T0	There is no evidence of a primary tumor.
Tis	The cancer is found only in the top layers of cells lining the air passages. It has not invaded into deeper lung tissues. This is also known as *carcinoma in situ*.
T1	The tumor is no larger than 3 cm—slightly less than 1.25 inches—across, has not reached the membranes that surround the lungs (visceral pleura), and does not affect the main branches of the bronchi. If the tumor is 2 cm (about 0.8 of an inch) or less across, it is called **T1a**. If the tumor is larger than 2 cm but not larger than 3 cm across, it is called **T1b**.
T2	The tumor has one or more of the following features: • It is larger than 3 cm across but not larger than 7 cm. • It involves a main bronchus, but is not closer than 2 cm (about 0.75 of an inch) to the carina (the point where the windpipe splits into the left and right main bronchi). • It has grown into the membranes that surround the lungs (visceral pleura). • The tumor partially clogs the airways, but this has not caused the entire lung to collapse or develop pneumonia.
T2a	Tumor >3 cm but ≤5 cm
T2b	Tumor >5 cm but ≤7 cm
T3	The tumor has one or more of the following features: • It is larger than 7 cm across. • It has grown into the chest wall, the breathing muscle that separates the chest from the abdomen (diaphragm), the membranes surrounding the space between the two lungs (mediastinal pleura), or membranes of the sac surrounding the heart (parietal pericardium). • It invades a main bronchus and is closer than 2 cm (about 0.75 of an inch) to the carina, but it does not involve the carina itself. • It has grown into the airways enough to cause an entire lung to collapse or to cause pneumonia in the entire lung. • Two or more separate tumor nodules are present in the same lobe of a lung.
T4	The cancer has one or more of the following features: • A tumor of any size has grown into the space between the lungs (mediastinum), the heart, the large blood vessels near the heart (such as the aorta), the windpipe (trachea), the tube connecting the throat to the stomach (esophagus), the spine, or the carina. • Two or more separate tumor nodules are present in different lobes of the same lung.
	Regional Lymph Nodes (N)
NX	Nearby lymph nodes cannot be assessed.
N0	There is no spread to nearby lymph nodes.
N1	The cancer has spread to lymph nodes within the lung and/or around the area where the bronchus enters the lung (hilar lymph nodes). Affected lymph nodes are on the same side as the primary tumor.

TABLE 27-3 The American Joint Committee on Cancer (AJCC) Tumor Node Metastasis (TNM) Staging System for Lung Cancer—cont'd

TNM Category	Description
Regional Lymph Nodes (N)	
N2	The cancer has spread to lymph nodes around the carina (the point where the windpipe splits into the left and right bronchi) or in the space between the lungs (mediastinum). Affected lymph nodes are on the same side as the primary tumor.
N3	The cancer has spread to lymph nodes near the clavicle on either side, and/or spread to hilar or mediastinal lymph nodes on the side opposite the primary tumor.
Distant Metastasis (M)	
M0	No spread to distant organs or areas. This includes the other lung, lymph nodes further away than those mentioned in the N stages above, and other organs or tissues such as the liver, bones, or brain.
M1a	Any of the following: • The cancer has spread to the other lung. • Cancer cells are found in the pleural fluid (called a *malignant pleural effusion*). • Cancer cells are found in the fluid around the heart (called a *malignant pericardial effusion*).
M1b	The cancer has spread to distant lymph nodes or to other organs such as the liver, bones, or brain.

Adapted from the American Cancer Society, http://www.cancer.org (Last Medical Review: 05/22/2013) (Last Revised: 07/12/2013).

TABLE 27-4 Stage Groupings—Tumor Node Metastasis (TNM) Subsets

After the T, N, and M Categories Have Been Established, the Information is Merged Together to Assign an Overall Stage of 0, I, II, III, or IV.

Stage Grouping	TMN subsets	Description
Occult (hidden) cancer	TX, N0, M0	Cancer cells are found in sputum or other lung fluids, but the cancer is not identified in other tests—thus, the location cannot be established.
Stage 0	Tis, N0, M0	Cancer found only in the top layers of cells lining the airways. It has not invaded deeper into other lung tissue and has not spread to lymph nodes or distant sites.
Stage IA	T1a-T1b, N0, M0	The cancer is no larger than 3 cm across, has not reached the membranes that surround the lungs, and does not affect the main branches of the bronchi. It has not spread to lymph nodes or distant sites.
Stage IB	T2a, N0, M0	The cancer has one or more of the following features: • The main tumor is larger than 3 cm across but not larger than 5 cm. • The tumor has grown into a main bronchus, but is not within 2 cm of the carina (and it is not larger than 5 cm). • The tumor has grown into the visceral pleura (the membranes surrounding the lungs) and is not larger than 5 cm. • The tumor is partially obstructing the airways (and is not larger than 5 cm). The cancer has not spread to lymph nodes or distant sites.
Stage IIA (There are three main combinations of categories that make up this stage)	T1a/T1b, N1, M0	The cancer is no larger than 3 cm across, has not grown into the membranes that surround the lungs, and does not affect the main branches of the bronchi. It has spread to lymph nodes within the lung and/or around the area where the bronchus enters the lung (hilar lymph nodes). These lymph nodes are on the same side as the cancer. It has not spread to distant sites.
	T2a, N1, M0	The cancer has one or more of the following features: • The main tumor is larger than 3 cm across but not larger than 5 cm. • The tumor has grown into a main bronchus, but is not within 2 cm of the carina (and it is not larger than 5 cm). • The tumor has grown into the visceral pleura (the membranes surrounding the lungs) and is not larger than 5 cm. • The tumor is partially obstructing the airways (and is not larger than 5 cm). The cancer has also spread to lymph nodes within the lung and/or around the area where the bronchus enters the lung (hilar lymph nodes). These lymph nodes are on the same side as the cancer. It has not spread to distant sites.

Continued

TABLE 27-4 Stage Groupings—Tumor Node Metastasis (TNM) Subsets—cont'd

After the T, N, and M Categories Have Been Established, the Information is Merged Together to Assign an Overall Stage of 0, I, II, III, or IV.

Stage Grouping	TMN subsets	Description
	T2b, N0, M0	The cancer has one or more of the following features: • The main tumor is larger than 5 cm across but not larger than 7 cm. • The tumor has grown into a main bronchus, but is not within 2 cm of the carina (and it is between 5 and 7 cm across). • The tumor has grown into the visceral pleura (the membranes surrounding the lungs) and is between 5 and 7 cm across. • The tumor is partially obstructing the airways (and is between 5 and 7 cm across). The cancer has not spread to lymph nodes or distant sites.
Stage IIB Two combinations of categories make up this stage.	**T2b, N1, M0**	The cancer has one or more of the following features: • The main tumor is larger than 5 cm across but not larger than 7 cm. • The tumor has grown into a main bronchus, but is not within 2 cm of the carina (and it is between 5 and 7 cm across). • The tumor has grown into the visceral pleura (the membranes surrounding the lungs) and is between 5 and 7 cm across. • The cancer is partially obstructing the airways (and is between 5 and 7 cm across). It has also spread to lymph nodes within the lung and/or around the area where the bronchus enters the lung (hilar lymph nodes). These lymph nodes are on the same side as the cancer. It has not spread to distant sites.
	T3, N0, M0	The main tumor has one or more of the following features: • It is larger than 7 cm across. • It has grown into the chest wall, the breathing muscle that separates the chest from the abdomen (diaphragm), the membranes surrounding the space between the lungs (mediastinal pleura), or membranes of the sac surrounding the heart (parietal pericardium). • It invades a main bronchus and is closer than 2 cm (about 0.75 of an inch) to the carina, but it does not involve the carina itself. • It has grown into the airways enough to cause an entire lung to collapse or to cause pneumonia in the entire lung. • Two or more separate tumor nodules are present in the same lobe of a lung. The cancer has not spread to lymph nodes or distant sites.
Stage IIIA Three main combinations of categories make up this stage.	T1 to T3, N2, M0	The main tumor can be any size. It has not grown into the space between the lungs (mediastinum), the heart, the large blood vessels near the heart (such as the aorta), the windpipe (trachea), the tube connecting the throat to the stomach (esophagus), the spine, or the carina. It has not spread to different lobes of the same lung. The cancer has spread to lymph nodes around the carina (the point where the windpipe splits into the left and right bronchi) or in the space between the lungs (mediastinum). These lymph nodes are on the same side as the main lung tumor. The cancer has not spread to distant sites.
	T3, N1, M0	The cancer has one or more of the following features: • It is larger than 7 cm across. • It has grown into the chest wall, the diaphragm, the membranes surrounding the space between the lungs (mediastinal pleura), or membranes of the sac surrounding the heart (parietal pericardium). • It invades a main bronchus and is closer than 2 cm to the carina, but it does not involve the carina itself. • Two or more separate tumor nodules are present in the same lobe. • It has grown into the airways enough to cause an entire lung to collapse or to cause pneumonia in the entire lung. It has also spread to lymph nodes within the lung and/or around the area where the bronchus enters the lung (hilar lymph nodes). These lymph nodes are on the same side as the cancer. It has not spread to distant sites.

TABLE 27-4 Stage Groupings—Tumor Node Metastasis (TNM) Subsets—cont'd

After the T, N, and M Categories Have Been Established, the Information is Merged Together to Assign an Overall Stage of 0, I, II, III, or IV.

Stage Grouping	TMN subsets	Description
	T4, N0 or N1, M0	The cancer has one or more of the following features: • A tumor of any size has grown into the space between the lungs (mediastinum), the heart, the large blood vessels near the heart (such as the aorta), the trachea, the tube connecting the throat to the stomach (esophagus), the spine, or the carina. • Two or more separate tumor nodules are present in different lobes of the same lung. It may or may not have spread to lymph nodes within the lung and/or around the area where the bronchus enters the lung (hilar lymph nodes). Any affected lymph nodes are on the same side as the cancer. It has not spread to distant sites.
Stage IIIB Two combinations of categories make up this stage.	Any T, N3, M0	The cancer can be of any size. It may or may not have grown into nearby structures or caused pneumonia or lung collapse. It has spread to lymph nodes near the clavicle on either side, and/or has spread to hilar or mediastinal lymph nodes on the side opposite the primary tumor. The cancer has not spread to distant sites.
	T4, N2, M0	The cancer has one or more of the following features: • A tumor of any size has grown into the space between the lungs (mediastinum), the heart, the large blood vessels near the heart (such as the aorta), the trachea, the tube connecting the throat to the stomach (esophagus), the backbone, or the carina. • Two or more separate tumor nodules are present in different lobes of the same lung. The cancer has also spread to lymph nodes around the carina (the point where the windpipe splits into the left and right bronchi) or in the space between the lungs (mediastinum). Affected lymph nodes are on the same side as the main lung tumor. It has not spread to distant sites.
Stage IV Two combinations of categories make up this stage.	Any T, any N, M1a	The cancer can be any size and may or may not have grown into nearby structures or reached nearby lymph nodes. In addition, any of the following is true: • The cancer has spread to the other lung. • Cancer cells are found in the pleural fluid (called a *malignant pleural effusion*). Cancer cells are found in the fluid around the heart (called a *malignant pericardial effusion*).
	Any T, any N, M1b	The cancer can be any size and may or may not have grown into nearby structures or reached nearby lymph nodes. It has spread to distant lymph nodes or to other organs such as the liver, bones, or brain.

Adapted from the American Cancer Society, http://www.cancer.org (Last Medical Review: 05/22/2013) (Last Revised: 07/12/2013).

TABLE 27-5 5-Year Survival Rate for Non–Small Cell Lung Carcinoma (NSCLC)

Stage	Average Percent Survival
I	<50%
II	<30%
III	<15%
IV	<1%

TABLE 27-6 5-Year Survival Rate for Small Cell Lung Carcinoma (SCLC)

Stage	Average Percent Survival
I	<30%
II	<20%
III	<10%
IV	<2%

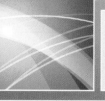

OVERVIEW of the Cardiopulmonary Clinical Manifestations Associated with Cancer of the Lung

The following clinical manifestations result from the pathologic mechanisms caused (or activated) by Atelectasis (see Figure 9-7), Alveolar Consolidation (see Figure 9-8), and Excessive Bronchial Secretions (see Figure 9-11)—the major anatomic alterations of the lungs associated with cancer of the lung (Figure 27-2).

CLINICAL DATA OBTAINED AT THE PATIENT'S BEDSIDE
The Physical Examination
Vital Signs
Increased Respiratory Rate (Tachypnea)
Several pathophysiologic mechanisms operating simultaneously may lead to an increased ventilatory rate:
- Stimulation of peripheral chemoreceptors (hypoxemia)
- Decreased lung compliance–increased ventilatory rate relationship
- Stimulation of J receptors
- Pain, anxiety

Increased Heart Rate (Pulse) and Blood Pressure
Cyanosis
Cough, Sputum Production, and Hemoptysis
Chest Assessment Findings
- Crackles and wheezing

CLINICAL DATA OBTAINED FROM LABORATORY TESTS AND SPECIAL PROCEDURES

Pulmonary Function Test (PFT) Findings

Dependent on where the malignancy originates, the PFT results may show either obstructive or restrictive values. For example, when the malignancy obstructs major airways, the PFT values may show obstructive pathology—especially when chronic obstructive pulmonary disease (COPD) is present. However, when large amounts of pulmonary tissue, chest wall, and/or diaphragm are involved (extensive bronchioloalveolar carcinoma), then the pathology may show restrictive PFT values.

Arterial Blood Gases (ABGs)

LOCALIZED (E.G., LOBAR) LUNG CANCER
Acute Alveolar Hyperventilation with Hypoxemia[†]
(Acute Respiratory Alkalosis)

pH	$PaCO_2$	HCO_3^-	PaO_2	SaO_2 or SpO_2
↑	↓	↓ (but normal)	↓	↓

EXTENSIVE OR WIDESPREAD LUNG CANCER
Acute Ventilatory Failure with Hypoxemia[†]
(Acute Respiratory Acidosis)

pH*	$PaCO_2$	HCO_3^-*	PaO_2	SaO_2 or SpO_2
↓	↑	↑ (but normal)	↓	↓

Oxygenation Indices[§]

$\dot{Q}_s/\dot{Q}_T$	DO_2[‖]	$\dot{V}O_2$	$C(a-\bar{v})O_2$	O_2ER	$S\bar{v}O_2$
↑	↓	N	N	↑	↓

Hemodynamic Indices[¶]

When hypoxemia and acidemia are present, or when a tumor invades the mediastinum and compresses the superior vena cava, the following may be expected.

CVP	RAP	$\overline{PA}$	PCWP	CO	SV
↑	↑	↓	↓ or N	↓ or N	↓ or N

SVI	CI	RVSWI	LVSWI	PVR	SVR
↓ or N	↓ or N	↑	↓ or N	↑	N

RADIOLOGIC FINDINGS
Chest Radiograph
- Small oval or coin lesion
- Large irregular mass
- Alveolar consolidation
- Atelectasis
- Pleural effusion (see Chapter 24)
- Involvement of the mediastinum or diaphragm

[†]See Figure 4-3 and related discussion for the acute pH, $PaCO_2$, and HCO_3^- changes associated with acute alveolar hyperventilation.
[†]See Figure 4-2 and related discussion for the acute pH, $PaCO_2$, and HCO_3^- changes associated with acute ventilatory failure.
*When tissue hypoxia is severe enough to produce lactic acid, the pH and HCO_3^- values will be lower than expected for a particular $PaCO_2$ level.
[§]$C(a-\bar{v})O_2$, Arterial–venous oxygen difference; DO_2, total oxygen delivery; O_2ER, oxygen extraction ratio; $\dot{Q}_s/\dot{Q}_T$, pulmonary shunt fraction; $S\bar{v}O_2$, mixed venous oxygen saturation; $\dot{V}O_2$, oxygen consumption.
[‖]The DO_2 may be normal in patients who have compensated to the decreased oxygenation status with (1) an increased cardiac output, (2) an increased hemoglobin level, or (3) a combination of both. When the DO_2 is normal, the O_2ER is usually normal.
[¶]CO, Cardiac output; CVP, central venous pressure; LVSWI, left ventricular stroke work index; $\overline{PA}$, mean pulmonary artery pressure; PCWP, pulmonary capillary wedge pressure; PVR, pulmonary vascular resistance; RAP, right atrial pressure; RVSWI, right ventricular stroke work index; SV, stroke volume; SVI, stroke volume index; SVR, systemic vascular resistance.

A routine chest radiograph often provides the first indication or suspicion of lung cancer. Depending on how long the tumor has been growing, the chest radiograph may show a small radiodense nodule (called a **coin lesion**) or a large irregular radiodense mass. Unfortunately, by the time a tumor is identified radiographically, regardless of its size, it is usually in the invasive stage and thus difficult to treat. Another common radiograph presentation of lung cancer is that of volume loss involving a single lobe or an individual segment within a lobe.

Because there are four major forms of lung cancer, chest radiograph findings are variable. In general, squamous cell and small cell carcinoma usually appear as a white mass near the hilar region; adenocarcinoma appears in the peripheral portions of the lung; and large cell carcinoma may appear in either the peripheral or the central portion of the lung. Figure 27-3 is a representative example of a large bronchogenic carcinoma in the right lung. Common secondary chest radiograph findings caused by bronchial obstruction include alveolar consolidation, atelectasis, pleural effusion, and mediastinal or diaphragmatic involvement. The radiograph appearance of cavity formation within a bronchogenic carcinoma is similar regardless of the type of cancer.

Clinically, a **positron emission tomography (PET) scan** is an excellent test to rule out a possible cancerous area identified on either a chest radiograph or a computed tomography (CT) scan. For example, Figure 27-4 shows a chest radiograph that

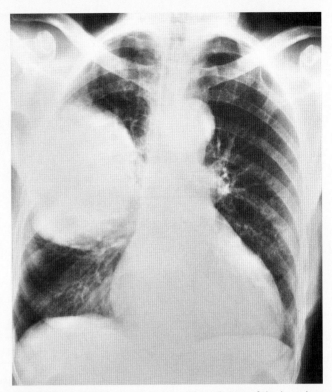

FIGURE 27-3 Right lung squamous cell carcinoma of the bronchus illustrating the huge size these tumors may attain before discovery. (From Hansell DM, Armstrong P, Lynch DA, McAdams HP, eds: *Imaging of diseases of the chest*, ed 4, Philadelphia, 2005, Elsevier.)

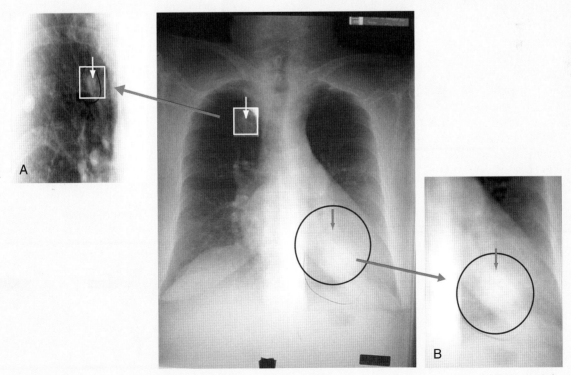

FIGURE 27-4 Chest radiograph identifying two suspicious findings: **A**, in the right upper lobe and **B**, in the left lower lobe, just behind the heart (*white arrows*).

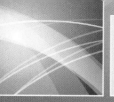

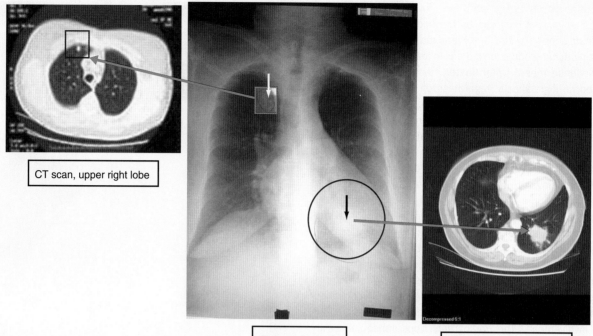

CT scan, upper right lobe

Chest radiograph

CT scan, lower left lobe

FIGURE 27-5 Same chest radiograph as shown in Figure 26-5. Note that the computed tomography (CT) scan also identifies the suspicious nodules and their precise location.

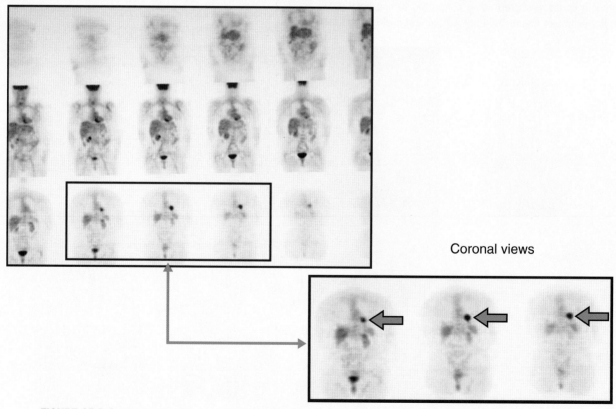

Coronal views

FIGURE 27-6 Positron emission tomography (PET) scan: coronal views. Scans show a hot spot in the left lower lobe.

identifies two suspicious findings—one small nodule in the right upper lung lobe and a larger density in the left lower lung lobe, just behind the heart. Figure 27-5 shows two CT scans that also identify the two suspicious findings and their precise location. Figures 27-6, 27-7, and 27-8 show PET scans that all confirm a "hot spot" (likely cancer) in the lower left lobe. However, the PET scan shown in Figure 27-9 confirms that the nodule in the right upper lobe is benign (i.e., no hot spot is noted).

Finally, the **PET/CT image** provides an image of excellent quality and high sensitivity and specificity in detecting malignant lesions in the chest. Figure 27-10 shows a CT/PET scan

alongside a CT scan and a PET scan; all the images show the same malignant nodule in the right upper lobe.

Bronchoscopy Findings

• Bronchial tumor or mass lesion

The fiberoptic bronchoscope may permit direct visualization of a bronchial tumor for further inspection, biopsy, and assessment of the extent of the disease (Figure 27-11, A and Figure 8-1).

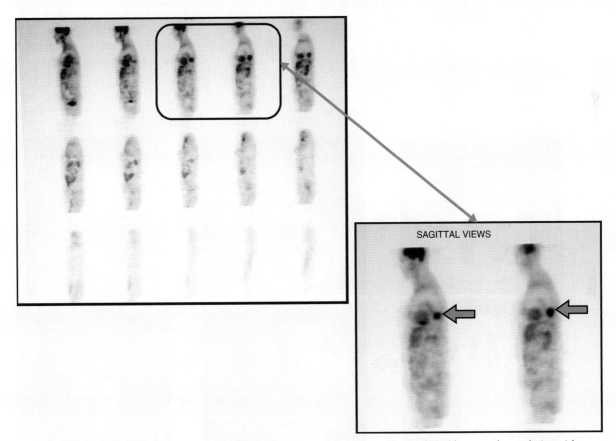

SAGITTAL VIEWS

FIGURE 27-7 Positron emission tomography (PET) scan: sagittal views. The encircled images show a hot spot in the lower left lobe.

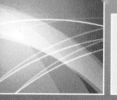

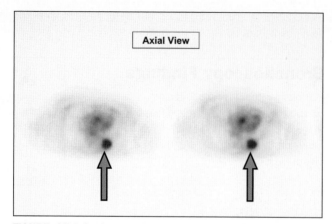

FIGURE 27-8 Positron emission tomography (PET) scan: axial view. A hot spot is further confirmed in left lower lobe.

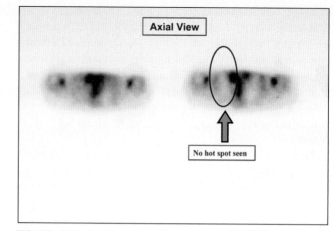

FIGURE 27-9 Positron emission tomography (PET) scan: axial view. This image confirms that the small nodule identified in the upper right lobe in the chest radiograph and computed tomography (CT) scan is benign (i.e., no hot spot is evident).

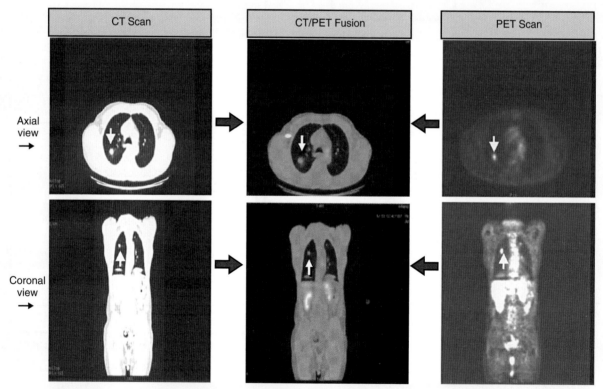

FIGURE 27-10 Computed tomography/positron emission tomography (CT/PET) scan (*center*). CT scan, CT/PET fusion, and PET scan, all showing the same malignant nodule in right upper lobe (*white arrow*). Note: CT/PET fusion is normally presented in color (e.g., red, blue, yellow).

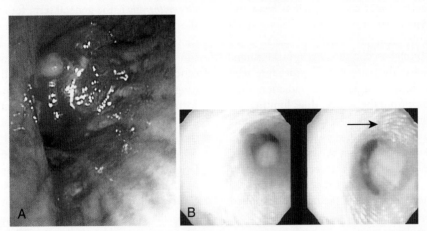

FIGURE 27-11 A, Bronchoscopic view of a small cell carcinoma tumor protruding into the right main stem bronchus. **B**, A wire stent is in place to help hold the airway open (*black arrow*).

General Management of Lung Cancer[2]

Treatment Options for Non–small Cell Lung Cancer (NSCLC)

Depending on the stage of the lung cancer and other factors (e.g., the patient's general health conditions), treatment options for NSCLC include the following.

Surgery

Surgery may be an option for early stage NSCLC. Surgery provides the best chance to cure NSCLC. Surgery is usually an option only for patients who have NSCLC in only one lung, up to Stage IIIA. This is usually confirmed with a CT scan and PET scan. In addition, an adequate respiratory reserve must be present to allow good lung function after the lung tissue has been removed. Common surgical procedures include the following:

- **Pneumonectomy**—the entire lung is removed in this surgery.
- **Lobectomy**—an entire section (lobe) of a lung is removed in this surgery.
- **Segmentectomy or wedge resection**—a part of a lobe is removed in this surgery.
- **Sleeve resection**—entails removal of some tumors in the large airways. The airway is completely cut above and below the tumor and the shortened airway is reattached.

Radiation Therapy

Radiation therapy uses high-intensity rays (such as x-rays) to kill cancer cells. The two primary types of radiation therapy are (1) external beam radiation therapy, and (2) brachytherapy (internal radiation therapy).

- **External beam radiation therapy (EBRT)**—directs radiation from outside the body to the cancer cells. EBRT is the most common form of radiation used to treat primary lung cancer or its spread to other organs. As a general rule, EBRT to the lungs is administered 5 days a week for 5 to 7 weeks. Newer EBRT techniques—which treat the lung cancer more accurately while lowering the radiation exposure offer better success rates and fewer side effects—including the following:
  - **Three-dimensional conformal radiation therapy (3D-CRT)**—uses special computers to precisely map the location of the tumor(s). Radiation beams are directed at the tumor(s) from several directions. This technique is less likely to damage surrounding normal tissues.
  - **Intensity modulated radiation therapy (IMRT)**—is a more advanced type of 3D therapy. IMRT uses a computer-driven machine that moves around the patient while it delivers radiation beams. In addition, the intensity (strength) of the beams can be adjusted to limit the dose reaching the most sensitive normal tissues. IMRT is most commonly used to treat tumors near important structures such as the spinal cord.
  - **Stereotactic body radiation therapy (SBRT)**, also known as stereotactic ablative radiotherapy (SABR)—can be used to treat very early stage lung cancers when surgery is not an option (e.g., because of issues with the patient's health or in patients who do not want surgery). SBRT applies very focused beams of high-dose radiation in fewer (1 to 5) treatments. The success rate for smaller tumors has been very promising and appears to have a low risk of complications.

[2]Adapted from the American Cancer Society, http://www.cancer.org (Last Medical Review: 05/22/2013) (Last Revised: 07/12/2013).

- **Stereotactic radiosurgery (SRS)**—is another form of stereotactic radiation therapy that is given in only one session. These treatments can be repeated if needed.
- **Brachytherapy (internal radiation therapy)**—may be used to shrink tumors in the airways to reduce symptoms. It is used more often for other cancers such as head and neck cancer. This type of treatment entails placing small amounts of radioactive material (usually in the form of small pellets) via a bronchoscope directly into the tumor or into the airway near the cancer. This procedure may also be performed during surgery. The radiation only travels a short distance from the source; thus, limiting the adverse effects on surrounding healthy tissue. After a short period of time, the radiation source is usually removed. Occasionally, small radioactive "seeds" are left in place permanently. The radiation from the seeds gets weaker over several weeks.

Common side effects depend on where the radiation is aimed and can include:

- Sunburnlike skin problems
- Hair loss where the radiation enters the body
- Fatigue
- Nausea and vomiting
- Loss of appetite and weight loss

Other Local Treatments

- In some cases, some treatments other than surgery and radiation may be used to treat lung tumors in specific locations. Such treatments include:
- **Radiofrequency ablation (RFA)**—may be used for some small lung tumors near the outer edge of the lungs. RFA entails the use of high-energy radio waves to heat the tumor. A thin, needlelike probe is inserted into the tumor and, once in place, an electric current is passed through the probe, which heats the tumor and destroys the cancer cell.
- **Photodynamic therapy (PDT)**—may be used to treat early stage lung cancer that is still confined to the outer edge of the lung. PDT may also be used to help open up airways obstructed by a tumor. PDT entails the injection of a light-activated drug called porfimer sodium into a vein. This drug is designed to settle in cancer cells. After a period of time (to allow the drug to build up in the cancer cells), a bronchoscope with a special laser light is directed at the tumor. The laser light activates the drug and causes the cancer cells to die. It should be noted that this drug can also settle in normal cells and make the patient very sensitive to sunlight or strong indoor lights (causing a sunburnlike reaction). It is recommended that the patient stay out of any strong light for 4 to 6 weeks after the injection.
- **Laser therapy**—may be used to treat very small lung cancers along the lining of the airways. It can also be used to help open up airways blocked by tumors. The laser, which is on the end of a bronchoscope, is aimed at the cancer cells.
- **Stent placement**—may be used to help keep the airway open. The stent, which is composed of hard silicone or metal, may be placed in the airway with a bronchoscope.

The stent helps to keep the tumor from moving into the bronchus—which can result in a partial or complete obstruction of the bronchus (Figure 27-11, *B*).

Chemotherapy

Chemotherapy is the general term for any treatment involving the use of chemical agents or drugs that are selectively destructive to malignant cancer cells. Because chemotherapy can eliminate cancer cells at sites away from the original cancer, it is considered a systemic treatment. Because the drugs used in chemotherapy can damage healthy cells along with cancer cells, serious side effects are common. Fast-growing cells are especially likely to be affected (e.g., cells in the digestive tract, bone marrow, and hair). In addition, the patient may experience nausea and vomiting, dizziness, fatigue, and increased risk of infection.

Chemotherapy is usually administered in cycles, which consist of 1 to 3 days of therapy followed by a rest period to allow the body time to recover. Chemotherapy cycles generally last about 3 to 4 weeks. Box 27-1 provides current drugs used to treat NSCLC. The treatment for NSCLC typically uses a combination of two different chemotherapy drugs—for example, cisplatin or carboplatin plus one other drug. The side effects of chemotherapy depend on the type and dose of drugs given and the length of time they are taken. Common side effects include:

- Hair loss
- Mouth sores
- Loss of appetite
- Nausea and vomiting
- Diarrhea or constipation
- Increased chance of infections (from having too few white blood cells)
- Easy bruising or bleeding (from having too few blood platelets)
- Fatigue (from having too few red blood cells)

These side effects are generally short-lived and resolve after treatment is finished.

Targeted Therapies

Researchers have had some success with newer drugs that specifically target certain portions of the cancer cell that help

---

BOX 27-1 Current Drugs Used To Treat Non–Small Cell Lung Carcinoma (NSCLC)

cisplatin
carboplatin
paclitaxel (Taxol)
albumin-bound paclitaxel (nab-paclitaxel, Abraxane)
docetaxel (Taxotere)
gemcitabine (Gemzar)
vinorelbine (Navelbine)
irinotecan (Camptosar)
etoposide (VP-16)
vinblastine
pemetrexed (Alimta)

---

them grow. For example, the drug bevacizumab (Avastin) works to target and block new tumor blood vessels—thus, blocking the nutritional routes to the cancer cells. Other agents, such as erlotinib (Tarceva), cetuximab (Erbitux), and afatinib (Gilotrif), work to block the *epidermal growth factor receptor* (EGFR), which causes cancer cells to grow faster. In about 5% of NSCLC cases, a rearrangement of a gene called anaplastic lymphoma kinase (*ALK*) has been found— especially in nonsmokers who have the adenocarcinoma subtype of NSCLC. This *ALK* gene produces an abnormal protein that causes the cells to grow and spread. Crizotinib (Xalkori) is a drug that blocks the abnormal ALK protein. The drug has shown success in shrinking tumors in more than 50% of patients that have this abnormal *ALK* gene change. It is often the first drug used (instead of chemotherapy) in patients with the *ALK* gene rearrangement.

Treatment Options for Small Cell Lung Cancer (SCLC)

Depending on the stage of the lung cancer and other factors (e.g., the patient's general health conditions), treatment options for SCLC include the following.

Surgery

Surgery is rarely a treatment option for SCLC. Occasionally, surgery may be an option for early stage cancers when a single lung tumor is found, with no lymph node or other organ involvement. Surgery is usually followed by chemotherapy and radiation therapy. Although the types of surgery options are the same as NSCLC, a lobectomy is generally the preferred choice for SCLC if it can be done. This is because a lobectomy offers a better chance of removing all the cancer as compared to a segmentectomy or wedge resection.

Radiation Therapy

Similar to NSCLC, EBRT and the newer radiation techniques, 3D-CRT and IMRT, may be used to treat SCLC (see a description of these techniques above).

Chemotherapy

Chemotherapy for SCLC is usually started as a combination of drugs. Common drug combinations include the following:

- Cisplatin and etoposide
- Carboplatin and etoposide
- Cisplatin and irinotecan
- Carboplatin and irinotecan

Other drugs may be tried if the cancer worsens or returns after treatment is completed.

Respiratory Care Treatment Protocols

Oxygen Therapy Protocol. Oxygen therapy is used to treat hypoxemia, decrease the work of breathing, and decrease myocardial work. Because hypoxemia is associated with lung cancer, supplemental oxygen may be required. However, capillary shunting is common because of the alveolar compression and consolidation often produced by lung cancer. Hypoxemia caused by capillary shunting is often refractory to oxygen therapy (Oxygen Therapy Protocol, Protocol 9-1).

Bronchopulmonary Hygiene Therapy Protocol. Because of the excessive mucous production and accumulation associated with lung cancer, and some of its treatments, a number of bronchial hygiene treatment modalities may be used to enhance the mobilization of bronchial secretions (Bronchopulmonary Hygiene Therapy Protocol, Protocol 9-2).

Lung Expansion Therapy Protocol. Lung expansion techniques are used to offset (at least temporarily) the alveolar compression and consolidation associated with lung cancer (Lung Expansion Therapy Protocol, Protocol 9-3).

Aerosolized Medication Protocol. Aerosolized bronchodilators and occasionally mucolytics are often indicated, particularly when COPD coexists (Aerosolized Medication Protocol, Protocol 9-4).

CASE STUDY Cancer of the Lung

Admitting History

A 66-year-old retired man lives with his wife in a small, two-bedroom ranch house in Peoria, Illinois, during the summer months. During the rest of the year, they live in a 22-foot trailer in a retirement park just outside Las Vegas, Nevada. The trailer park is located conveniently on the casinos' shuttle-bus route; a bus comes by at the top of every hour.

Both the man and his wife are described by their children as addicted gamblers. They gamble almost every day of the year. During the summer months, they play keno and blackjack on the Par-A-Dice Riverboat Casino, which is docked along the shores of the Illinois River in downtown East Peoria. While in Las Vegas, they play bingo, blackjack, and the slot machines at several different casinos. They dress in matching warm-up suits, ride the bus to one of the casinos, and gamble until 10:00 or 11:00 PM every day.

Their children, adults with their own families, homes, and jobs in the Peoria area, have been very concerned about their parents' gambling. They have tried to no avail to get their parents to see a compulsive-gambling therapist, who actually is provided by the Par-A-Dice Riverboat Casino. Their children's concern is justified. Their parents are always gambling on a shoestring budget. Although they still own their trailer and small home in Peoria, within the last 2 years they have gambled away most of their life savings, which included stocks, bonds, and mutual funds. Because they let their health insurance premium lapse, their policy was recently cancelled. They still receive a small monthly pension check, and some Social Security income.

Before he retired, the man worked for 17 years as a boiler tender for Methodist Hospital in Peoria. He also was a part-time firefighter. For more than 52 years, he smoked two and a half to three packs of unfiltered cigarettes daily. While in Las Vegas, the man began experiencing periods of dyspnea, coughing, and weakness. His cough was productive of small amounts of clear secretions. Also around this time, his wife first noticed that his voice sounded hoarse.

Although he missed several days of gambling and remained in bed because of weakness, he did not seek medical attention. He hated doctors and thought that he merely had a bad cold and the flu. When he returned to Peoria for the summer, however, the children became concerned and insisted that he see a doctor. Despite the man's lack of health insurance, two medical students from the University of Illinois, who were working in the office as a team, ordered a full diagnostic workup.

A pulmonary function test showed that the man had a combined restrictive and obstructive pulmonary disorder. CT scanning revealed several masses, ranging from 2 to 5 cm in diameter, in the right and left mediastinum at the level of the hilar region. The masses, especially on the right side, could also be seen clearly on the posteroanterior chest radiograph. Both the CT scan and the chest x-ray showed increased opacity consistent with atelectasis of the medial basal segments of the left lower lobe as well.

A bronchoscopic examination was conducted by the pulmonary physician, with the assistance of a respiratory care practitioner trained in special procedures. It showed several large, protruding bronchial masses in the second- and third-generation bronchi of the right lung; and in the second-, third-, and fourth-generation bronchi of the left lung. During the bronchoscopy, several mucous plugs were suctioned. Biopsy of three of the larger tumors was positive for squamous cell bronchogenic carcinoma, and the man was admitted to the hospital.

The physician told the patient that he had cancer and that his prognosis was poor. Treatment, at best, would be palliative. The patient asked what the odds were on his life expectancy. The physician stated that the patient had only about a 50% chance of living longer than 6 to 8 weeks. Surgery was out of the question. In the interim, however, the physician promised to do what was possible to make the man comfortable. The physician outlined a treatment plan of radiation therapy and chemotherapy and requested a respiratory care consultation.

Physical Examination

The respiratory care practitioner reviewed the admitting history information in the patient's chart and found the man sitting up in bed in obvious respiratory distress. He appeared weak. His skin was cyanotic, and his face, arms, and chest were damp with perspiration. Wheezing was audible without the aid of a stethoscope. He stated in a hoarse voice that he had coughed up a cup of sputum since breakfast 2 hours earlier. He demonstrated a weak cough every few minutes or so. His cough was productive of large amounts of blood-streaked sputum. The viscosity of the sputum was thin. After each coughing episode, he stated that he wanted a cigarette and then laughed.

His vital signs were as follows: blood pressure 155/85, heart rate 90 beats/min, respiratory rate 22 breaths/min, and temperature normal. Palpation was unremarkable. Percussion produced dull notes over the left lower lobe. On auscultation, wheezing and coarse crackles could be heard throughout both lung fields. His arterial blood gas values on a 2 L/min oxygen nasal cannula were as follows: pH 7.51, $PaCO_2$ 29 mm Hg, HCO_3^- 23 mEq/L, PaO_2 66 mm Hg, and SaO_2 94%. On the basis of these clinical data, the following SOAP was documented.

Respiratory Assessment and Plan

S "I've coughed up a cup of sputum since breakfast."

O Vital signs: BP 155/85, HR 90, RR 22, T normal; perspiring and weak and cyanotic appearance; voice hoarse-sounding; weak cough; large amounts of blood-streaked sputum; dull percussion notes over left lower lobe; wheezing and coarse crackles throughout both lung fields; recent PFTs: restrictive and obstructive pulmonary disorder; CT scan and CXR: 2- to 5-cm masses in right and left mediastinum in hilar regions and atelectasis of left lower lobe. Bronchoscopy: protruding tumors in both left and right large airways, mucous plugging. Biopsy: squamous cell bronchogenic carcinoma. ABGs (2 L/min O_2 by nasal cannula): pH 7.51, $PaCO_2$ 29, HCO_3^- 23, PaO_2 66, SaO_2 94%.

A
- Bronchogenic carcinoma (CT scan and biopsy)
- Respiratory distress (vital signs, ABGs)
- Bronchospasm (wheezing)
- Excessive bloody bronchial secretions (sputum, coarse crackles)
- Mucous plugging (bronchoscopy)
- Poor ability to mobilize secretions (weak cough)
- Atelectasis of left lower lobe (CXR)
- Acute alveolar hyperventilation with mild hypoxemia (ABGs)

P Up-regulate **Oxygen Therapy Protocol** (4 L nasal cannula and titration by oximetry). Also begin **Aerosolized Medication Protocol** (0.5 mL albuterol in 2 mL NS q6 h), followed by **Bronchopulmonary Hygiene Therapy Protocol** (DB&C). Begin **Lung Expansion Therapy Protocol** (incentive spirometry q2 h and prn). Closely monitor and reevaluate.

3 Days after Admission

A respiratory therapist evaluated the patient during morning rounds. After reviewing the patient's chart, the practitioner went to the patient's bedside and discovered that the man was not tolerating the chemotherapy well. He had been vomiting intermittently for the past 10 hours and was still in obvious respiratory distress. He appeared cyanotic and tired, and his hospital gown was wet from perspiration. His cough was still weak and productive of large amounts of moderately thick, clear, and white sputum. He stated in a hoarse voice that he was still not breathing very well.

His vital signs were as follows: blood pressure 166/90, heart rate 95 beats/min, respiratory rate 28 breaths/min, and temperature normal. Dull percussion notes were elicited over both the right and left lower lobes. Wheezing and coarse crackles were auscultated throughout both lung fields. His ABG values on a 4 L cannula were as follows: pH 7.55, $PaCO_2$ 25 mm Hg, HCO_3^- 21 mEq/L, PaO_2 53 mm Hg, and SaO_2 92%. On the basis of these clinical data, the following SOAP was documented.

Respiratory Assessment and Plan

S "I'm still not breathing very well."

O Vital signs: BP 166/90, HR 95, RR 28, T normal; vomiting over past 10 hours; cyanosis, tiredness, and dampness from perspiration; cough: weak and productive of moderately thick, clear, and white sputum; dull percussion notes over both right and left lower lobes; wheezing and coarse crackles over both lung fields; ABGs on a 4 L cannula pH 7.55, $PaCO_2$ 25, HCO_3^- 21, PaO_2 53, SaO_2 92%.

A • Bronchogenic carcinoma (previous CT scan and biopsy)
  • Trouble tolerating chemotherapy well (excessive vomiting)
  • Continued respiratory distress
  • Bronchospasm (wheezing)
  • Excessive bronchial secretions (sputum, coarse crackles)
  • Mucous plugging still likely (previous bronchoscopy, secretions becoming thicker)
  • Poor ability to mobilize secretions (weak cough)
  • Atelectasis of left lower lobes; atelectasis likely in right lower lobe now (CXR, dull percussion notes)
  • Acute alveolar hyperventilation with moderate hypoxemia, worsening (ABGs)
    • Possible impending ventilatory failure (ABGs, weak cough, worsening vital signs)

P Up-regulate **Oxygen Therapy Protocol** (simple oxygen mask). Up-regulate **Aerosolized Medication Protocol** (increasing treatment frequency to q3 h; consider adding acetylcysteine q6 h). Up-regulate **Bronchopulmonary Hygiene Therapy Protocol** (CPT and PD q3 h). Up-regulate **Lung Expansion Therapy Protocol** (change incentive spirometry to +5 to +10 cm H_2O CPAP mask, qid). Contact physician about possible ventilatory failure. Discuss therapeutic bronchoscopy. Closely monitor and reevaluate.

16 Days after Admission

Although the physician's original intention and hope were to discharge the patient soon, stabilizing the man for any length of time proved difficult. Over the next 2 weeks, the patient had continued to be nauseated on a daily basis. He did,

however, have occasional periods of relief during which he could breathe easier, but he generally was in respiratory distress. On Day 16 the respiratory therapist observed and collected the following clinical data.

The patient was lying in bed in the supine position. His eyes were closed, and he was unresponsive to the therapist's questions. The patient was in obvious respiratory distress. He appeared pale, cyanotic, and diaphoretic. No cough was observed at this time, but coarse crackles could easily be heard from across the patient's room. The nurse in the patient's room stated that the doctor had called the coarse crackles a "death rattle." The patient's vital signs were as follows: blood pressure 170/105, heart rate 110 beats/min, respiratory rate 12 breaths/min and shallow, and rectal temperature normal. Percussion was not performed. Wheezing and coarse crackles were heard throughout both lung fields. On an FIO_2 of 0.60, his ABG values were as follows: pH 7.28, $PaCO_2$ 63 mm Hg, HCO_3^- 28 mEq/L, PaO_2 66 mm Hg, and SaO_2 89%.

At that time, the following SOAP was recorded.

Respiratory Assessment and Plan

S N/A (patient comatose)

O Unresponsive; pale, cyanotic, and perspiring appearance; no cough noted; coarse crackles heard without stethoscope; vital signs: BP 170/105, HR 110, RR 12 and shallow, T normal; wheezing and coarse crackles over both lung fields; ABGs: pH 7.28, $PaCO_2$ 63, HCO_3^- 28, PaO_2 66, SaO_2 89%.

A • Bronchogenic carcinoma (previous CT scan and biopsy)
  • Bronchospasm (wheezing)
  • Excessive bronchial secretions (coarse crackles)
  • Mucous plugging still likely (previous bronchoscopy, coarse crackles)
  • Poor ability to mobilize secretions (no cough)
  • Atelectasis (CXR)
  • Acute ventilatory failure with moderate hypoxemia (ABGs)

P Contact physician about acute ventilatory failure, and discuss code status. Up-regulate **Oxygen Therapy Protocol**, **Bronchopulmonary Hygiene Therapy Protocol**, and **Aerosolized Medication Therapy Protocol**. Monitor and reevaluate.

Discussion

This case demonstrates the few specific treatments that a respiratory therapist can bring to the care of patients with lung cancer. Specifically, it illustrates that most of the patients that have concomitant obstructive pulmonary disease have a need for good **Bronchopulmonary Hygiene Therapy** (Protocol 9-2). Comfort of the patient must be kept in mind at all times.

The first assessment was performed soon after bronchoscopy and diagnosis. The patient's blood-stained sputum could have reflected the primary tumor or, as likely, bleeding from the bronchoscopy sites. In such cases the practitioner must monitor this sputum as the days go along. No improvement in the patient's wheezing can be expected if a bronchial tumor is the cause, but it may improve if bronchospasm (from cigarette smoking) is the causative factor.

The wheezing and coarse crackles indicated the need for vigorous bronchial hygiene therapy. The atelectasis in the left lower lobe suggested that a trial of careful **Lung Expansion Therapy Protocol** (Protocol 9-3) and **Aerosolized Medication Therapy Protocol** (Protocol 9-4) were in order. The ABG values assessed with the patient on 2 L/min O_2 showed acute alveolar hyperventilation with moderate hypoxemia. At this time, the patient's oxygen therapy was up-regulated to a 4-L nasal cannula. Certainly, a trial of oxygen therapy via an air-entrainment mask (or nonrebreathing mask) would also have been appropriate. Patient anxiety may be alleviated with appropriate treatment of the hypoxemia.

The second assessment revealed that the patient may have developed atelectasis in both the right and left lower lobes (where the tumor masses had been noted previously). This case may present a setting in which therapeutic bronchoscopy or laser-assisted endobronchial resection of the tumor masses may be helpful. The patient continued to be hypoxemic, despite alveolar hyperventilation. A higher FIO_2 (e.g.,

through a Venturi oxygen mask) was indicated. Vigorous suctioning was appropriate. Because of the impending ventilatory failure, ordering at least one cycle of ventilator support, perhaps in the form of noninvasive positive pressure ventilation (see Chapter 10), for such a patient would not be surprising; given that the patient had just recently received radiation and chemotherapy. The patient's wishes in this respect should have been checked against his living will or durable power of attorney for health care, if such a document existed.

The last assessment indicates that the patient did not elect aggressive therapy and that he had slipped into acute ventilatory failure. All health-care personnel had agreed that the patient was close to death. The practitioner may be excused for not suggesting the use of chest physical therapy and postural drainage at this time, because of the patient's wishes. **Aerosolized morphine** is now being used to relieve dyspnea in terminally ill cancer patients. If, however, aggressive therapy were still in order, formal evaluation and treatment of superimposed atelectasis or pneumonia, or both, would be in order.

SELF-ASSESSMENT QUESTIONS

Answers to questions can be found on Evolve. To access additional student assessment questions visit **http://evolve.elsevier.com/DesJardins/respiratory**.

1. Which of the following is commonly located near a central bronchus or hilus and projects into the large bronchi?
   a. Squamous cell carcinoma
   b. Oat cell carcinoma
   c. Large cell carcinoma
   d. Adenocarcinoma

2. Which of the following arises from the mucous glands of the tracheobronchial tree?
   a. Small cell carcinoma
   b. Adenocarcinoma
   c. Squamous cell carcinoma
   d. Oat cell carcinoma

3. Which of the following carcinomas has the strongest correlation with cigarette smoking?
   a. Adenocarcinoma
   b. Small cell carcinoma
   c. Large cell carcinoma
   d. Squamous cell carcinoma

4. Which of the following has the fastest growth (doubling) rate?
   a. Large cell carcinoma
   b. Small cell carcinoma
   c. Adenocarcinoma
   d. Squamous cell carcinoma

5. Which of the following is or are associated with bronchogenic carcinoma?
   1. Alveolar consolidation
   2. Pleural effusion
   3. Alveolar hyperinflation
   4. Atelectasis
      a. 2 and 3 only
      b. 1 and 4 only
      c. 2 and 3 only
      d. 1, 2, and 4 only

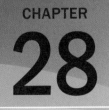

CHAPTER 28

Acute Respiratory Distress Syndrome

Chapter Objectives

After reading this chapter, you will be able to:

- List the anatomic alterations of the lungs associated with acute respiratory distress syndrome.
- Describe the causes of acute respiratory distress syndrome.
- List the cardiopulmonary clinical manifestations associated with acute respiratory distress syndrome.
- Describe the general management of acute respiratory distress syndrome.
- Describe the clinical strategies and rationales of the SOAPs presented in the case study.

Key Terms

ARDSnet Ventilation Protocol
Barotrauma
Berlin Definition of ARDS
Ground Glass Appearance
Hyaline Membrane
Low Tidal Volume Ventilation (LTVV)
Oxygen Toxicity
Permissive Hypercapnia
Volutrauma

Chapter Outline

Anatomic Alterations of the Lungs
Etiology and Epidemiology
Overview of Cardiopulmonary Clinical Manifestations
   Associated with Acute Respiratory Distress Syndrome
General Management of Acute Respiratory Distress
   Syndrome
   Respiratory Care Treatment Protocols
   Ventilation Strategy for Adult Respiratory Distress
      Syndrome
Case Study: Acute Respiratory Distress Syndrome
Self-Assessment Questions

Anatomic Alterations of the Lungs

The lungs of patients affected by acute respiratory distress syndrome (ARDS) undergo similar anatomic changes, regardless of the cause of the disease. In response to injury, the pulmonary capillaries become engorged and the permeability of the alveolar-capillary membrane increases. Interstitial and intraalveolar edema and hemorrhage ensue, as well as scattered areas of hemorrhagic alveolar consolidation. These processes result in a decrease in alveolar surfactant and in alveolar collapse, or atelectasis.

As the disease progresses, the intraalveolar walls become lined with a thick, rippled **hyaline membrane** identical to the hyaline membrane seen in newborns with respiratory distress syndrome (hyaline membrane disease) (see Chapter 35). The membrane contains fibrin and cellular debris. In prolonged cases there is hyperplasia and swelling of the type II cells. Fibrin and exudate develop and lead to intraalveolar fibrosis.

In gross appearance the lungs of patients with ARDS are heavy and "red," "beefy," or "liverlike." The anatomic alterations that develop in ARDS create a restrictive lung disorder (Figure 28-1).

The major pathologic or structural changes associated with ARDS are as follows:

- Interstitial and intraalveolar edema and hemorrhage
- Alveolar consolidation
- Intraalveolar hyaline membrane formation
- Pulmonary surfactant deficiency or abnormality
- Atelectasis

Historically, ARDS was first referred to as the "shock lung syndrome" when the disease was first identified in combat casualties during World War II. Since that time, the disease has appeared in the medical literature under many different names, all based on the conditions believed to be responsible for the disease. In 1967, the disease was first described as a specific entity, and the term *acute respiratory distress syndrome* was suggested. This term is predominantly used today. Box 28-1 provides some of the other names that have appeared in the medical journals to identify ARDS.

Etiology and Epidemiology

A multitude of causative factors may produce ARDS. Although more than 60 possible pulmonary insults have been identified to cause ARDS, only a few common causes account

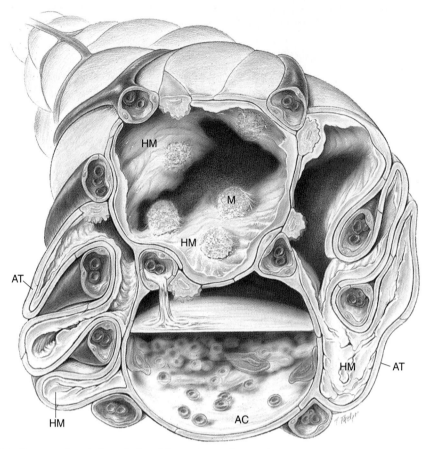

FIGURE 28-1 Cross-sectional view of alveoli in acute respiratory distress syndrome. *AC,* Alveolar consolidation; *AT,* atelectasis; *HM,* hyaline membrane; *M,* macrophage.

BOX 28-1 Previous Names for Acute Respiratory Distress Syndrome (ARDS)

- Adult hyaline membrane disease
- Adult respiratory distress syndrome
- Capillary leak syndrome
- Congestion atelectasis
- Da Nang lung (because of the high incidence of ARDS in the Vietnam War)
- Hemorrhagic pulmonary edema
- Noncardiac pulmonary edema
- Oxygen pneumonitis
- Oxygen toxicity
- Postnontraumatic pulmonary insufficiency
- Postperfusion lung
- Postpump lung
- Posttraumatic pulmonary insufficiency
- Shock lung syndrome
- Stiff lung syndrome
- Wet lung
- White lung syndrome

---

for most cases of ARDS. Box 28-2 provides some of the better-known causes. The clinical manifestations associated with ARDS usually appear within 6 to 72 hours of an inciting event, and worsen rapidly. The patient typically presents with dyspnea, cyanosis, bilateral crackles, tachypnea, tachycardia,

diaphoresis, and use of accessory muscles of inspiration. A cough and chest pain may also be present. The general clinical course is characterized by several days of hypoxemia that requires moderate to high concentrations of inspired oxygen. The bilateral alveolar infiltrates and diffuse crackles are persistent during this period, and the patient's overall health status is often fragile as a result of severe hypoxemia. Most patients who survive this initial clinical course begin to show oxygenation improvements and decreasing alveolar infiltrates over the next several days.

Diagnostic Criteria for ARDS

As shown in Box 28-3, the **Berlin Definition of ARDS** is used as the diagnostic criteria for ARDS. Note that the Berlin Definition of ARDS requires that all the elements listed—in Box 28-3—must be present in order to diagnose ARDS. For the most part, ARDS is a diagnosis of exclusion—that is, excluding other possible causes of acute hypoxemic respiratory failure with bilateral alveolar infiltrates. *Cardiogenic pulmonary edema is the primary alternative that needs to be ruled out.* Other possible alternative causes of acute hypoxemic respiratory failure with bilateral alveolar infiltrates include diffuse alveolar hemorrhage, idiopathic acute exacerbation of pre-existing interstitial lung disease, acute eosinophilic pneumonia, cryptogenic organizing pneumonia, acute interstitial pneumonia, and rapidly disseminating cancer.

BOX 28-2 Causes of Acute Respiratory Distress Syndrome

Most Common

- **Sepsis**—Is the most common cause of ARDS. It should be the first etiology considered whenever ARDS develops in an adult patient.
  - The risk factors are especially high in patients with sepsis who also have a history of alcoholism.
- **Aspiration** (e.g., of gastric contents, or water in near-drowning episodes). ARDS occurs in about one third of patients who have a recognized episode of aspiration of gastric contents.
- **Pneumonia**—Community acquired pneumonia is one of the most common causes of ARDS that develops outside of the hospital. Common pathogens include *Streptococcus pneumonia*, *Legionella pneumophila*, *Pneumocystis jirovecii* (formerly called *Pneumocystis carinii*), *Staphylococcus aureus*, enteric gram-negative organisms, and a variety of respiratory viruses.
- **Severe trauma**—ARDS is a common complication of severe trauma. Such trauma often includes the following:
  - Bilateral lung contusion caused by blunt trauma (e.g., steering wheel smashed into the chest during a car accident).
  - Fat embolism from a long bone fracture (ARDS symptoms typically appear 12 to 48 hours after the trauma).
  - Sepsis—Perhaps the most common cause of ARDS that develops several days after severe trauma.
- Massive traumatic tissue injury—Predisposes the patient to ARDS.
- **Massive blood transfusion** (in stored blood the quantity of aggregated white blood cells [WBCs], red blood cells [RBCs], platelets, and fibrin increases; these blood components may in turn occlude or damage small blood vessels).
- **Lung and hematopoietic stem cell transplantation**—Patients are at risk for ARDS resulting from a variety of infectious and noninfection causes.
- **Drug abuse** (e.g., heroin, barbiturates, morphine, methadone).

Other Causes

- **Central nervous system** (CNS) disease (particularly when complicated by increased intracranial pressure).
- **Cardiopulmonary bypass** (especially when the bypass is prolonged).
- **Disseminated intravascular coagulation** (seen in patients with shock; it is a condition of paradoxic simultaneous clotting and bleeding that produces microthrombi in the lungs).
- **Inhalation of toxins and irritants** (e.g., chlorine gas, nitrogen dioxide, smoke, ozone; oxygen may also be included in this category of irritants).
- **Immunologic reactions** (e.g., allergic alveolar reaction to inhaled material or Goodpasture's syndrome).
- **Oxygen toxicity** (e.g., prolonged exposure to FIO_2 >0.60).

BOX 28-3 The Berlin Definition of ARDS: The Diagnostic Criteria for ARDS

- Respiratory symptoms associated with ARDS have manifested within 1 week of a known clinical event—or, new or worsening symptoms over the past 7 days.
- Bilateral opacities similar to pulmonary edema appear on the chest radiograph or computed tomography scan. The opacities cannot be fully explained by pleural effusion, lobar or lung collapse, or pulmonary nodules.
- The patient's respiratory failure cannot be fully explained by heart failure or fluid overload. An objective assessment to rule out hydrostatic pulmonary edema is required if risk factors are not present for ARDS (e.g., echocardiography).
- A moderate to severe impairment of oxygenation must be present, as defined by the ratio of arterial oxygen tension to fraction of inspired oxygen ratio (PaO_2/FIO_2 ratio). The severity of the hypoxemia defines the severity of the ARDS:*
- **Mild ARDS**: The PaO_2/FIO_2 is >200 mm Hg, but ≤300 mm Hg, on ventilator settings that include positive end-expiratory pressure (PEEP) or continuous positive airway pressure (CPAP) ≥5 cm H_2O.
- **Moderate ARDS**: The PaO_2/FIO_2 is >100 mm Hg, but ≤200 mm Hg, on ventilator settings that include PEEP ≥5 cm H_2O.
- **Severe ARDS**: The PaO_2/FIO_2 is ≤100 mm Hg on ventilator settings that include PEEP ≥5 cm H_2O.

Modified from ARDS Definition Task Force, Ranieri VM, Rubenfeld GD, Thompson BT, Ferguson ND, Caldwell E, Fan E, Camporota L, Slutsky AS: Acute respiratory distress syndrome: the Berlin Definition, *JAMA* 307:2526-2533, 2012.
*To determine the PaO_2/FIO_2 ratio, the PaO_2 is measured in mm Hg and the FIO_2 is expressed as a decimal fraction between 0.21 and 1. For example, if a patient has a PaO_2 of 60 mm Hg while receiving 85% oxygen, then the PaO_2/FIO_2 is 60/0.85 = 70 mm Hg. The normal PaO_2/FIO_2 ratio is between 350 and 450 mm Hg.

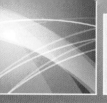

The following clinical manifestations result from the pathologic mechanisms caused (or activated) by Atelectasis (see Figure 9-7), Alveolar Consolidation (see Figure 9-8), and Increased Alveolar-Capillary Membrane Thickness (see Figure 9-9)—the major anatomic alterations of the lungs associated with ARDS (Figure 28-1).

CLINICAL DATA OBTAINED AT THE PATIENT'S BEDSIDE

The Physical Examination

Vital Signs

Increased Respiratory Rate (Tachypnea)

Several pathophysiologic mechanisms operating simultaneously may lead to an increased ventilatory rate:

- Stimulation of peripheral chemoreceptors (hypoxemia)
- Decreased lung compliance–increased ventilatory rate relationship
- Stimulation of J receptors
- Anxiety

Increased Heart Rate (Pulse) and Blood Pressure

Substernal or Intercostal Retractions

Cyanosis

Chest Assessment Findings

- Dull percussion note
- Bronchial breath sounds
- Crackles

CLINICAL DATA OBTAINED FROM LABORATORY TESTS AND SPECIAL PROCEDURES

Pulmonary Function Test Findings
(Restrictive Lung Pathophysiology)

FORCED EXPIRATORY VOLUME AND FLOW RATE FINDINGS

FVC	FEV_T	FEV_1/FVC ratio	$FEF_{25\%-75\%}$
↓	N or ↓	N or ↑	N or ↓

$FEF_{50\%}$	$FEF_{200-1200}$	PEFR	MVV
N or ↓	N or ↓	N or ↓	N or ↓

LUNG VOLUME AND CAPACITY FINDINGS

V_T	IRV	ERV	RV
N or ↓	↓	↓	↓

VC	IC	FRC	TLC	RV/TLC ratio
↓	↓	↓	↓	N

DECREASED DIFFUSION CAPACITY (D_{LCO})

Arterial Blood Gases

MILD TO MODERATE ACUTE RESPIRATORY DISTRESS SYNDROME

Acute Alveolar Hyperventilation with Hypoxemia[†]
(Acute Respiratory Alkalosis)

pH	$PaCO_2$	HCO_3^-	PaO_2	SaO_2 or SpO_2
↑	↓	↓ (but normal)	↓	↓

SEVERE ACUTE RESPIRATORY DISTRESS SYNDROME

Acute Ventilatory Failure with Hypoxemia[‡]
(Acute Respiratory Acidosis)

pH*	$PaCO_2$	HCO_3^- *	PaO_2	SaO_2 or SpO_2
↓	↑	↑ (but normal)	↓	↓

Oxygenation Indices[§]

$\dot{Q}_S/\dot{Q}_T$	DO_2[∥]	$\dot{V}O_2$	$C(a-\bar{v})O_2$	O_2ER	$S\bar{v}O_2$
↑	↓	N	N	↑	↓

Hemodynamic Indices[¶]
Severe

CVP	RAP	$\overline{PA}$	PCWP	CO	SV
↑	↑	↑	N[#] or ↓	N or ↑[¶]	N or ↑[¶]

SVI	CI	RVSWI	LVSWI	PVR	SVR
N or ↑[¶]	N or ↑[¶]	↑	↓	↑	N or ↓[¶]

[†]See Figure 4-3 and related discussion for the acute pH, $PaCO_2$, and HCO_3^- changes associated with acute alveolar hyperventilation.

[‡]See Figure 4-2 and related discussion for the acute pH, $PaCO_2$, and HCO_3^- changes associated with acute ventilatory failure.

*When tissue hypoxia is severe enough to produce lactic acid, the pH and HCO_3^- values will be lower than expected for a particular $PaCO_2$ level.

[§]$C(a-\bar{v})O_2$, Arterial–venous oxygen difference; DO_2, total oxygen delivery; O_2ER, oxygen extraction ratio; $\dot{Q}_S/\dot{Q}_T$, pulmonary shunt fraction; $S\bar{v}O_2$, mixed venous oxygen saturation; $\dot{V}O_2$, oxygen consumption.

[∥]The DO_2 may be normal in patients who have compensated to the decreased oxygenation status with (1) an increased cardiac output, (2) an increased hemoglobin level, or (3) a combination of both. When the DO_2 is normal, the O_2ER is usually normal.

[¶]CO, Cardiac output; CVP, central venous pressure; LVSWI, left ventricular stroke work index; $\overline{PA}$, mean pulmonary artery pressure; PCWP, pulmonary capillary wedge pressure; PVR, pulmonary vascular resistance; RAP, right atrial pressure; RVSWI, right ventricular stroke work index; SV, stroke volume; SVI, stroke volume index; SVR, systemic vascular resistance.

[#]A normal PCWP (<18 mm Hg) is the hallmark of ARDS, distinguishing it from cardiogenic pulmonary edema, in which the PCWP is elevated .

[¶]If sepsis with systemic hypotension is present.

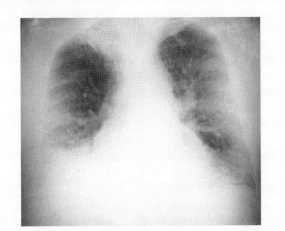

FIGURE 28-2 Chest radiograph of a patient with moderately severe acute respiratory distress syndrome.

RADIOLOGIC FINDINGS

Chest Radiograph

• Increased opacity, diffusely throughout lungs

Because of the bilateral alveolar infiltrates that develop in ARDS, an increased radiodensity is seen on the chest radiograph. The increased lung density resists x-ray penetration and is revealed on the radiograph as increased opacity. Therefore, the more severe the ARDS, the denser the lungs become and the "whiter" the radiograph (Figure 28-2). Ultimately, the lungs may have a **"ground-glass" appearance**.

OTHER CLINICAL MANIFESTATIONS ASSOCIATED WITH ARDS COMPLICATIONS

Patients with ARDS are at high risk for complications. Some of the complications are related to the patient that requires mechanical ventilation (e.g., pulmonary barotrauma and hospital-acquired pneumonia), whereas others are associated

with the patient's critical illness and being in intensive care (e.g., delirium, deep venous thrombosis, gastrointestinal bleeding caused by stress ulceration, and catheter-related infections). Common complications include:

Barotrauma—The patient with ARDS is often susceptible to pulmonary barotrauma resulting from the physical tension of high positive-pressure mechanical ventilation (plateau airway pressure >30 cm H_2O) on acutely damaged alveoli. It is most likely that the areas of the lungs affected by barotrauma are, in fact, the healthy alveoli—which are interspersed with the pathologically altered alveoli. This is because the relatively high pressures required to manage patients with ARDS not only help to recruit collapsed alveoli but may also work to overdistend the healthier alveoli—thus, resulting in the overexpansion of the alveolar, tearing ("popping"), and collapse (called **volutrauma** and/or barotrauma).

This complication is less common now that the low tidal volume ventilation and high respiratory rate strategy for providing ventilator support for ARDS has become widespread (see Mechanical Ventilation Protocol, Protocol 10-1 and Protocol 10-2). This ventilator strategy works to reduce the overall plateau airway pressure (<30 cm H_2O).

Delirium—ARDS, as well as other forms of acute ventilatory failure, is often complicated by delirium. Deep sedation and neuromuscular blocking agents are commonly used to treat agitated delirium.

Deep venous thrombosis—Prolonged bed rest and/or immobilization is commonly associated with a deep venous thrombosis.

Gastrointestinal bleeding attributable to stress ulceration—The incidence of overt gastrointestinal bleeding caused by stress ulceration ranges from 1.5% to 8.5% among all patients in the intensive care unit.

General Management of Acute Respiratory Distress Syndrome

Respiratory Care Treatment Protocols

Oxygen Therapy Protocol

Oxygen therapy is used to treat hypoxemia, decrease the work of breathing, and decrease myocardial work. Because of the hypoxemia associated with ARDS, supplemental oxygen is often required. The hypoxemia that develops in ARDS is most commonly caused by widespread **alveolar consolidation, atelectasis**, and **increased alveolar capillary thickening**. Hypoxemia caused by capillary shunting is often refractory to oxygen therapy (see Oxygen Therapy Protocol, Protocol 9-1).

Lung Expansion Therapy Protocol

Lung expansion measures (e.g., **positive end-expiratory pressure [PEEP]** or **continuous positive airway pressure [CPAP]**) are key to attempt to offset the alveolar consolidation and atelectasis associated with ARDS (see Lung Expansion Protocol, Protocol 9-3).

Mechanical Ventilation Protocol

Mechanical ventilation is usually needed to provide and support alveolar gas exchange and eventually return the patient to spontaneous breathing. Continuous mechanical ventilation is justified when the acute ventilatory failure is thought to be reversible (see Mechanical Ventilation Protocol, Protocol 10-1 and Mechanical Ventilation Weaning Protocol, Protocol 10-2).

Ventilation Strategy for Adult Respiratory Distress Syndrome

For most patients in acute ventilatory failure caused by ARDS, it is recommended that the patient be immediately placed on invasive mechanical ventilation, rather than doing an initial trial of noninvasive positive pressure ventilation. In addition, a full support mode of mechanical ventilation is recommended, rather than a partially supported mode of ventilation. Either volume-limited or pressure-limited modes of ventilation are acceptable.

The recommended ventilatory strategy for ARDS is **low tidal volume ventilation** (LTVV) and **high respiratory rates**. The initial tidal volume is usually set at 8 mL/kg (with the ability to drop down to 6 mL/kg IBW if needed to maintain a low plateau pressure [Pplat] over the next 2 to 4 hours), and the respiratory rate is set at 20 to 25 breaths/min. Ideally, the Pplat should be maintained between 25 and 30 cm H_2O.

If the Pplat drops below 25 cm H_2O, the most common protocol is to increase the tidal volume (V_T) per the following **ARDSnet Protocol**:[1]

Increase V_T by 1 mL/kg until the Pplat is >25 cm H_2O, or the V_T = 6 mL/kg

Ventilatory rates as high as 35 breaths/min may be needed to maintain an adequate minute volume. In the patient with ARDS, a strategy of high PEEP is recommended when the PaO_2/FIO_2 is less than 200 mm Hg. For these patients, it is felt that the benefits of a high PEEP strategy (e.g., opens collapsed alveoli) outweighs the possible negatives (e.g.,

pulmonary barotrauma). However, the optimal level of high PEEP has not been established.

The patient's $PaCO_2$ is often allowed to increase (**permissive hypercapnia**) as a tradeoff to protect the lungs from high airway pressures. In most cases, an increased ventilatory rate adequately offsets the decreased tidal volume used in the management of ARDS. The $PaCO_2$, however, should not be permitted to increase to the point of severe acidosis (e.g., a pH below 7.2).*

The therapeutic goals are to (1) maintain the plateau airway pressures (Pplat) between 25 and 30 cm H_2O, (2) reduce overdistention of the lungs, (3) decrease barotrauma, and to (4) adequately oxygenate the patient. (see Mechanical Ventilation Protocol, Protocol 10-1 and Mechanical Ventilation Weaning Protocol, Protocol 10-2).

Permissive Hypercapnia defined: Mechanical ventilation was traditionally applied with the goal of normalizing arterial blood gas values, particularly the arterial carbon dioxide tension ($PaCO_2$). However, this is no longer the primary objective of mechanical ventilation. Today, the emphasis is on maintaining adequate gas exchange while—and, importantly—minimizing the risks of mechanical ventilation. Common strategies used to reduce the complications of mechanical ventilation include (1) low tidal volume ventilation—to protect the lung from ventilator-associated lung injury in patients with acute lung injury (e.g., ARDS)—and (2) reduction of the tidal volume, respiratory rate, or both—to minimize intrinsic positive end-expiratory pressure (i.e., auto-PEEP) in patients with obstructive lung disease (e.g., COPD).

Although these mechanical ventilation strategies may result in an increased $PaCO_2$ level (hypercapnia), they do help to protect the lung from barotauma (i.e., physical damage to lung tissues caused by excessive gas pressures). The lenient acceptance of the hypercapnia is called **permissive hypercapnia**. In most cases, the patient's $PaCO_2$ is adequately maintained by an increased ventilatory rate that offsets the decreased tidal volume. The $PaCO_2$, however, should not be permitted to increase to the point of severe acidosis. The most current consensus suggests it is safe to allow pH to fall to at least 7.20 (www.ARDSNet).

---

[1]http://www.ardsnet.org/system/files/Ventilator%20Protocol%20Card.pdf

---

CASE STUDY Acute Respiratory Distress Syndrome (ARDS)

Admitting History and Physical Examination

This comatose 47-year-old woman was admitted to the emergency department of a small community hospital. Her husband found her lying in bed with an empty bottle of "sleeping pills" and a "goodbye note" on the bedside table. She had a long history of depression.

In the emergency department she was found to be in a moderately deep coma, responding to deep painful stimulation, but otherwise nonresponsive. She was of average size and, according to the husband, had previously been in good physical health. She did not smoke or drink and was taking no other medication. Her blood pressure and pulse were within normal limits, but her respirations were shallow and noisy. The emergency department physician attempted to

lavage her stomach. During the introduction of the nasogastric tube, the patient vomited and aspirated liquid gastric contents. At this time it was decided to transfer her by ambulance to a tertiary care medical center about 30 miles away. The pH of the gastric contents was not determined.

On arrival at the medical center, the patient was comatose but responsive to mild painful stimulation. Her weight was 50 kg and her rectal temperature was 101.5 °F. Her blood pressure was 100/60, heart rate 114 beats/min, and respirations 10 breaths/min and shallow. On auscultation, there were fine crackles over the left lung, and coarse crackles over the right side. A chest radiograph showed bilateral moderate fluffy infiltrates, mostly on the right side. Blood gases on a nonrebreather oxygen mask were pH 7.29, $PaCO_2$

56 mm Hg, HCO_3^- 26 mEq/L, PaO_2 52 mm Hg, and SaO_2 80%.

At the time the respiratory therapist recorded the following SOAP note:

Respiratory Assessment and Plan

S N/A

O Patient is comatose. BP 100/60; HR 114; RR 28; T 101.5 °F. Auscultation: fine crackles over the left lung, and course crackles over the right side. CXR: bilateral infiltrates, worse on right side. Arterial blood gas values (ABGs) on nonrebreather oxygen mask were pH 7.29, $PaCO_2$ 56, HCO_3^- 26, PaO_2 52, and SaO_2 80%.

A • Sedative drug overdose with coma (history)
   • Aspiration pneumonitis without previous history of pulmonary disease (Aspiration observed)
   • Possible early stages of ARDS (history and x-ray)
   • Acute ventilatory failure with moderate hypoxemia (ABGs)

P Contact physician stat regarding acute ventilatory failure. Manually ventilate and oxygenate patient until the physician's orders are completed. Repeat ABG 1 hour after intubation and prn.

Over the next 30 minutes, the patient was transferred to the intensive care unit, intubated, and mechanically ventilated for possible early stages of mild ARDS. The initial ventilator settings were as follows: V_T 400 mL (8 mL × 50 kg), rate 15 breaths/min, FIO_2 0.50, and 10 cm H_2O of PEEP. The Pplat was 26 cm H_2O. An arterial line was placed in her left radial artery, and an intravenous infusion was started with lactated Ringer's solution.

Over the next 15 hours, the patient's oxygenation status continued to deteriorate—in spite of a progressive increase in the delivered FIO_2, PEEP, and pressure-controlled mechanical ventilation. When the arterial oxygen tension did not improve appreciably on an FIO_2 of 1.0 and a PEEP of 20 cm H_2O, a Swan-Ganz catheter was placed in the pulmonary artery. In view of the PEEP, the pressure readings were difficult to interpret. A mean pulmonary artery pressure of 27 mm Hg, however, did suggest increased pulmonary vascular resistance.

A chest radiograph revealed ARDS with bilateral diffuse infiltrates and atelectasis. The heart was not enlarged. At this time, the physician charted "severe ARDS" in the patient's progress notes. At this time, the respiratory therapist immediately decreased the tidal volume on the ventilator to 300 mL (6 mL × 50 kg) and increased the rate to 20 breaths/min. The FIO_2 remained at 1.0, and the PEEP was increased to 22 cm H_2O. Twenty minutes later the patient's ABGs were pH 7.31, $PaCO_2$ 49 mm Hg, HCO_3^- 24 mEq/L, PaO_2 38 mm Hg, and SaO_2 65%. Her PaO_2/FIO_2 ratio was 38 (38 ÷ 1.0 = 38). She had coarse crackles and bronchial breath sounds throughout all lung fields. Moderate to large amounts of purulent sputum were frequently suctioned from the endotracheal tube. Her blood pressure was 90/60, and her heart rate was 130 beats/min. Her temperature was 100.2 °F.

At this time, the respiratory therapist charted the following SOAP note:

Respiratory Assessment and Plan

S N/A (patient comatose)

O Patient remains comatose. BP 90/60, HR 130, T 100.2 °F. Bilateral coarse crackles and bronchial breath sounds. ABGs on decreased V_T of 300 mL, rate 20, FIO_2 1.0, and +22 PEEP: pH 7.31, $PaCO_2$ 49, HCO_3^- 24, PaO_2 38, and SaO_2 65%. PaO_2/FIO_2 ratio: 38. CXR: ARDS with bilateral diffuse infiltrates and atelectasis, worse on the right side. Purulent sputum. PA pressure (mean) 27 mm Hg.

A • Severe ARDS (symptoms associated with ARDS <1 week, bilateral infiltrates on CXR, PaO_2/FIO_2 ratio <100 [38] on ventilator setting that include PEEP >20 cm H_2O).
   • Persistent coma (physical exam)
   • Aspiration pneumonitis—progressing to ARDS with bilateral infiltrates and atelectasis (CXR, bronchial breath sounds)
   • Increasing airway secretions with infection (fever, coarse crackles, and purulent sputum)
   • Acute ventilatory failure on present ventilator settings (but acceptable hypercapnia in this case)
   • Severe hypoxemia (ABGs, extremely low PaO_2/FIO_2 ratio: 38)

P Call physician to discuss worsening PaO_2 and to confirm an acceptable hypercapnia level and PEEP upper limit. **Bronchopulmonary Hygiene Therapy Protocol** (suction prn). Adjust **Mechanical Ventilation Protocol** (titrate tidal volume and rate to raise $PaCO_2$ to permissive hypercapnia range). Repeat Gram stain and culture sputum. Closely monitor and reevaluate.

After 3 hours it was apparent that current management would not be successful; the physician decided to alert the extracorporeal membrane oxygenation (ECMO) team and place the patient on extracorporeal membrane oxygenation. This was done, and the patient was maintained on ECMO for 13 hours, when she developed ventricular tachycardia followed by ventricular fibrillation. Attempts to reestablish normal cardiac function were not successful, and the patient was pronounced dead 45 minutes later.

Discussion

This was possibly a preventable death. Gastric lavage should *never* be performed on an unconscious patient unless the airway is first protected with a cuffed endotracheal tube. This is one of the very few categoric imperatives in pulmonary medicine. The following three causative factors known to produce ARDS may have been operative in this patient: (1) drug overdose, (2) aspiration of gastric contents, and (3) breathing an excessive FIO_2 for a long period. As time progressed, the patient's lungs became stiffer and physiologically nonfunctional as a result of the anatomic alterations associated with ARDS. The PaO_2/FIO_2 ratio helped to detect this, and raises the point that an initial (or very early) ABG at a known FIO_2 should be established in patients who are acutely ill.

As documented in the first assessment, her crackles, refractory hypoxemia, and radiograph findings all reflected the pathophysiologic changes seen in patients with **Atelectasis** (see Figure 9-7) and/or **Increased Alveolar-Capillary Membrane Thickening** (see Figure 9-9). Aggressive **Lung Expansion Therapy** (Protocol 9-3), in the form of PEEP, was used with mechanical ventilation right from the start. Unfortunately, severe ARDS was confirmed 15 hours later—that is, when the respiratory symptoms associated with ARDS were present in less than 1 week, bilateral infiltrates were seen on the chest radiograph, and the PaO_2/FIO_2 ratio was only 38 mm Hg on ventilator settings that include PEEP >20 cm H_2O (see Box 28-3, The Berlin Definition of ARDS). The respiratory therapist's immediate reduction in the tidal volume of the patient to 300 mL, increase in respiratory rate to 20 breaths/min, and permissive hypercapnia were all clearly indicated and appropriate.

Unfortunately, these therapeutic techniques and use of ECMO to manage the condition were not enough in the final analysis.

SELF-ASSESSMENT QUESTIONS

Answers to questions can be found on Evolve. To access additional student assessment questions visit **http://evolve.elsevier.com/DesJardins/respiratory**.

1. **In response to injury, the lungs of a patient with ARDS undergo which of the following changes?**
   1. Atelectasis
   2. Decreased alveolar-capillary membrane permeability
   3. Interstitial and intraalveolar edema
   4. Hemorrhagic alveolar consolidation
      a. 1 and 3 only
      b. 2 and 4 only
      c. 1, 2, and 4 only
      d. 1, 3, and 4 only

2. **Which of the following is/are recommended ventilation strategies for most patients with ARDS?**
   1. High tidal volumes
   2. Low respiratory rates
   3. High respiratory rates
   4. Low tidal volumes
      a. 1 only
      b. 3 and 4 only
      c. 1 and 3 only
      d. 2 and 4 only

3. **Common chest assessment findings in ARDS include the following:**
   1. Diminished breath sounds
   2. Dull percussion note
   3. Bronchial breath sounds
   4. Crackles
      a. 1 only
      b. 3 only
      c. 2 and 3 only
      d. 2, 3, and 4 only

4. **During the early stages of ARDS, the patient commonly demonstrates which one of the following arterial blood gas values?**
   a. Decreased pH
   b. Decreased $PaCO_2$
   c. Increased HCO_3^-
   d. Normal PaO_2

5. **Which of the following oxygenation indices is/are associated with ARDS?**
   a. Increased $\dot{V}O_2$
   b. Decreased DO_2
   c. Increased $S\overline{v}O_2$
   d. Decreased $\dot{Q}_S/\dot{Q}_T$

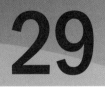

CHAPTER

29 Guillain-Barré Syndrome

Chapter Objectives

After reading this chapter, you will be able to:

- List the anatomic alterations of the lungs associated with Guillain-Barré syndrome.
- Describe the etiology and epidemiology of Guillain-Barré syndrome.
- List the cardiopulmonary clinical manifestations associated with Guillain-Barré syndrome.
- Describe the general management of Guillain-Barré syndrome.
- Describe the clinical strategies and rationales of the SOAPs presented in the case study.

Key Terms

Acute Inflammatory Demyelinating Polyradiculopathy (AIDP)
Acute Motor and Sensory Axonal Neuropathy (AMSAN)
Acute Motor Axonal Neuropathy (AMAN)
Acute Pandysautonomic Neuropathy (APN)
Albuminocytologic Dissociation (Spinal Fluid)
Areflexia
Ascending Paralysis
Autonomic Dysfunction
Axoplasm
Bickerstaff's Brainstem Encephalitis (BBE)
Campylobacter Jejuni
Cytomegalovirus (CMV)
Demyelination
Dysautonomia
Electromyography (EMG)

Hydrotherapy (Whirlpool Therapy)
Hyporeflexia
Intravenous Immune Globulin (IVIG)
Landry's Paralysis
Maximum Inspiratory Pressure (MIP)
Miller Fisher Syndrome (MFS)
Nerve Conduction Studies (NCS)
Non-Steroidal Anti-Inflammatory Drugs (NSAIDs)
Paresthesia or Dysesthesias
Pharyngeal-Cervical-Brachial (PCB)
Plasma Exchange
Plasmapheresis
Stryker Frame

Chapter Outline

Anatomic Alterations of the Lungs Associated with Guillain-Barré Syndrome[1]

Guillain-Barré syndrome (GBS) is an autoimmune disease that causes an acute peripheral nervous system disorder (called polyneuropathy) that results in a flaccid paralysis of the skeletal muscles and loss of muscle reflexes. Box 29-1 lists other names in the literature for GBS. In severe cases, paralysis of the diaphragm and ventilatory failure can develop.

Clinically, this is a medical emergency. In these cases, mechanical ventilation is required. If the patient is not properly managed (e.g., via the Bronchopulmonary Hygiene Therapy Protocol, Protocol 9-2 and Mechanical Ventilation Protocols, Protocol 10-1 and Protocol 10-2), **mucous accumulation with airway obstruction, alveolar consolidation, and atelectasis** may develop.

The major pathologic or structural changes of the lungs associated with poorly managed GBS are as follows:

- Mucous accumulation
- Airway obstruction
- Alveolar consolidation
- Atelectasis

---

[1]The Guillain-Barré syndrome is named after the French physicians Georges Guillain and Jean Alexandre Barré, who described it in 1916.

Etiology and Epidemiology

GBS occurs worldwide with an overall incidence of 1 per 100,000 people. The incidence GBS is **equal** among males and females. The incidence is greater in people over 50 years of age. GBS is 50% to 60% more common in whites than blacks. There is no obvious seasonal clustering of cases. As shown in Table 29-1, there are several different subtypes of GBS.

Although the precise cause of GBS is not fully understood, it is known that all forms of GBS are autoimmune

---

BOX 29-1 Other Names Found in the Literature for Guillain-Barré Syndrome

- Landry-Guillain-Barré-Strohl syndrome
- Acute idiopathic polyneuritis
- Postinfectious polyneuritis
- **Landry's paralysis**
- Acute postinfectious polyneuropathy
- Acute polyradiculitis
- Polyradiculoneuropathy

---

diseases that develop from an immune response to foreign antigens (e.g., an infectious agent) that attack the nerve tissues. For example, **acute inflammatory demyelinating polyradiculopathy (AIDP)** is thought to be caused by an immunologic attack that results in peripheral nerve demyelination and inflammation. Lymphocytes and macrophages appear to attack and strip off the myelin sheath of the peripheral nerves and leave swelling and fragmentation of the neural axon. It is believed that the myelin sheath covering the peripheral nerves (or the myelin-producing Schwann cell) is the actual target of the immune attack. Microscopically, the nerves show **demyelination,** inflammation, lymphocytes, macrophages, and edema. As the anatomic alterations of the peripheral nerves intensify, the ability of the neurons to transmit impulses to the muscles decreases, and eventually paralysis ensues (Figure 29-1).

The onset of GBS often occurs 1 to 4 weeks after a febrile episode caused by a mild respiratory or gastrointestinal viral or bacterial infection. In most cases, *Campylobacter jejuni* or **cytomegalovirus (CMV)** is identified as the cause of the preceding infection. Other precipitating factors include infectious mononucleosis, parainfluenza 2, vaccinia, variola, measles, mumps, hepatitis A and B viruses, *Mycoplasma*

TABLE 29-1 Subtypes of Guillain-Barré Syndrome (GBS)

Acute inflammatory demyelinating polyneuropathy (AIDP)	AIDP is the most common form of GBS in the United States and Europe—representing about 85% to 90% of cases. The typical clinical features are a progressive, fairly symmetric muscle weakness accompanied by absent or depressed deep tendon reflexes. AIDP is caused by an autoimmune response that targets the peripheral nerve myelin—the Schwann cell membranes.
Miller Fisher syndrome (MFS)	MFS is characterized by ophthalmoplegia (paralysis or weakness of one or more of the muscles that control eye movement), ataxia (lack of muscle coordination), and areflexia (absence of a reflex). Antibodies against GQ1b (a ganglioside component of nerve tissue) are present in 85% to 90% of MFS cases. MFS occurs in 5% of cases in the United States, and 25% of cases in Japan
Acute motor axonal neuropathy (AMAN) AMAN is similar to AMSAN (see below)	AMAN attacks motor nodes of Ranvier (i.e., the constrictions in the myelin sheath that surrounds the axons of nerve cells, or neurons). AMAN is primarily an axonal form of GBS. Sensory nerves are not affected. AMAN is probably attributable to an autoimmune response directed against the **axoplasm** of peripheral nerves. Most cases are preceded by *Campylobacter jejuni* infection. AMAN is most prevalent in China and Japan (particularly in the young), but when combined with the AMSAN form of GBS (discussed below), comprises about 5% to 10% of GBS cases in the United States.
Acute motor and sensory axonal neuropathy (AMSAN) AMSAN is similar to AMAN (see above)	AMSAN is a more severe form of AMAN—It affects both sensory and motor fibers with marked axonal degeneration, causing delayed and incomplete recovery. Clinically, AMSAN resembles AMAN, but has more sensory symptoms. Similar to AMAN, it is most prevalent in China and Japan (particularly in the young), but when combined with the AMSAN form of GBS, represents about 5% to 10% of GBS cases in the United States.
Acute pandysautonomic neuropathy (APN)	APN is very rare. Symptoms include diarrhea, vomiting, dizziness, abdominal pain, ileus, orthostatic hypotension, urinary retention, pupillary abnormalities, an unaltered heart rate, decreased sweating, salivation, and lacrimation. Reflexes are absent or diminished and sensory symptoms may be present. APN may respond to intravenous immune globulin.
Bickerstaff's brainstem encephalitis (BBE)	BBE is a brainstem encephalitis with features similar to the MFS form of GBS such as ophthalmoplegia and ataxia, but with an encephalopathy and hyperreflexia. BBE is also associated with anti-GQ1b antibodies and can respond to intravenous immune globulin and plasma exchange.
Pharyngeal-cervical-brachial (PCB)	This subtype is characterized by acute arm weakness and swallowing dysfunction. Facial weakness may also be present. Leg strength and leg reflexes are usually preserved.

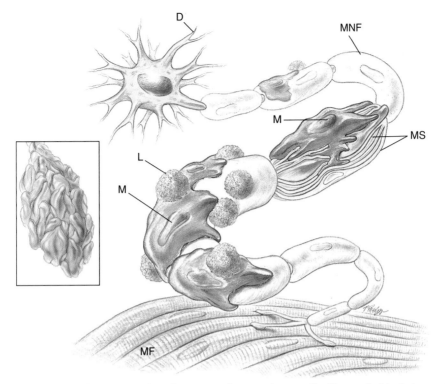

FIGURE 29-1 Guillain-Barré syndrome. Lymphocytes and macrophages attacking and stripping away the myelin sheath of a peripheral nerve. *D*, Dendrite; *L*, lymphocyte; *M*, macrophage; *MF*, muscle fiber; *MNF*, myelinated nerve fiber; *MS*, myelin sheath (cross-sectional view; note the macrophage attacking the myelin sheath). *Inset*, Atelectasis, a common secondary anatomic alteration of the lungs.

pneumoniae, Salmonella typhi, and *Chlamydia psittaci.* Although the significance of the association is controversial, during the nationwide immunization campaign in the United States in 1976, more than 40 million adults were vaccinated with swine influenza vaccine, and more than 500 new cases of GBS were reported among the vaccinated individuals, with 25 deaths. Today, about 2% to 3% of patients with GBS die.

Clinical Presentation

The general clinical history of patients with GBS is (1) symmetric muscle weakness in the distal extremities accompanied by **paresthesia** (tingling, burning, shocklike sensations) **or dysesthesias** (unpleasant, abnormal sense of touch), (2) pain (throbbing, aching, especially in the lower back, buttocks, and leg), and (3) numbness. The muscle paralysis then spreads upward **(ascending paralysis)** to the arms, trunk, and face. The muscle weakness and paralysis may develop within a single day or over several days. The muscle paralysis generally peaks in about 2 weeks. Deep tendon reflexes are commonly absent. More than one half of patients experience severe pain, and about two thirds have autonomic symptoms.

The patient often drools and has difficulty chewing, swallowing, and speaking. The management of oral secretions may be a problem. Oculomotor weakness occurs in about 15% of cases. In 10% to 30% of cases, respiratory muscle paralysis—followed by acute ventilatory failure (hypercapnic respiratory failure)—develops. Although GBS is typically an ascending paralysis—that is, moving from the lower portions

of the legs and body upward—in about 10% of cases, muscle paralysis affects the facial and arm muscles first and then moves downward.

Although the weakness is commonly symmetric, a single arm or leg may be involved before paralysis spreads. The paralysis may also affect all four limbs simultaneously. Progression of the paralysis may stop at any point. After the paralysis reaches its maximum, it usually remains unchanged for a few days or weeks. Improvement generally begins spontaneously and continues for weeks or, in rare cases, months. Between 10% and 20% of patients have permanent residual neurologic deficits. About 90% of patients make a full recovery, but the recovery time may be as long as 3 years.

Diagnosis

If diagnosed early, patients with GBS have an excellent prognosis. The diagnosis is typically based on the patient's clinical history (e.g., sudden ascending paralysis), cerebrospinal fluid (CSF) findings, and abnormal **electromyography (EMG)** and **nerve conduction studies (NCS)** results. In 80% to 90% of cases, the typical CSF finding is an elevated protein level (100 to 1000 mg/dL) with a normal white blood cell (WBC) count. This is called **albuminocytologic dissociation of the spinal fluid.** The EMG and NCS results typically show evidence of an acute polyneuropathy with demyelinating characteristics in *acute inflammatory demyelinating polyneuropathy* (AIDP), whereas the features are predominantly axonal in acute motor axonal neuropathy **(AMAN)** *and acute sensorimotor axonal neuropathy* (AMSAN). Glycolipid antibodies may be associated with some GBS subtypes. For

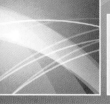

OVERVIEW of the Cardiopulmonary Clinical Manifestations Associated with Guillain-Barré Syndrome

The following clinical manifestations result from the pathologic mechanisms caused (or activated) by Atelectasis (see Figure 9-7), Alveolar Consolidation (see Figure 9-8), and Excessive Bronchial Secretions (see Figure 9-11)—the major anatomic alterations of the lungs associated with GBS, which may occur when the patient is not properly managed via the Bronchopulmonary Hygiene Therapy Protocol, Protocol 9-2 and Mechanical Ventilation Protocols, Protocol 10-1 and Protocol 10-2 (Figure 29-1).[2]

CLINICAL DATA OBTAINED AT THE PATIENT'S BEDSIDE
The Physical Examination
Respiratory Rate
- Varies with the degree of respiratory muscle paralysis
- Apnea (in severe cases)
- Anxiety
Cyanosis
Chest Assessment Findings
- Diminished breath sounds
- Crackles

CLINICAL DATA OBTAINED FROM LABORATORY TESTS AND SPECIAL PROCEDURES

Pulmonary Function Test Findings*
(Restrictive Lung Pathology)

FORCED EXPIRATORY VOLUME AND FLOW RATE FINDINGS

FVC	FEV_T	FEV_1/FVC ratio	$FEF_{25\%-75\%}$
↓	N or ↓	N or ↑	N or ↓

$FEF_{50\%}$	$FEF_{200-1200}$	PEFR	MVV
N or ↓	N or ↓	N or ↓	N or ↓

*Progressive worsening of these values is key to anticipating the onset of ventilatory failure.

LUNG VOLUME AND CAPACITY FINDINGS

V_T	IRV	ERV	RV
↓	↓	↓	↓

VC	IC	FRC	TLC	RV/TLC ratio
↓	↓	↓	↓	N

MAXIMUM INSPIRATORY PRESSURE (MIP) ↓

Arterial Blood Gases
Moderate to Severe Guillain-Barré Syndrome

Acute Ventilatory Failure with Hypoxemia[†]
(Acute Respiratory Acidosis)

pH*	$PaCO_2$	HCO_3*	PaO_2	SaO_2 or SpO_2
↓	↑	↑ (but normal)	↓	↓

Oxygenation Indices[†]

$\dot{Q}s/\dot{Q}T$	DO_2[§]	$\dot{V}O_2$	$C(a-\bar{v})O_2$	O_2ER	$S\bar{v}O_2$
↑	↓	N	N	↑	↓

RADIOLOGIC FINDINGS
Chest Radiograph
- Normal, or
- Increased opacity (when atelectasis or consolidation are present)

If the ventilatory failure associated with GBS is properly managed (e.g., via the Bronchopulmonary Hygiene Therapy and Mechanical Ventilation Protocols, Protocol 9-2, Protocol 10-1, and Protocol 10-2), the chest radiograph should appear normal. However, if the patient is not properly managed, mucous accumulation, alveolar consolidation, and atelectasis may develop. In these cases, the chest radiograph will show an increased density of the lung segments affected.

AUTONOMIC NERVOUS SYSTEM DYSFUNCTIONS
Dysautonomia (autonomic dysfunction) occurs in about 70% of cases. Symptoms include:
- Cardiac arrhythmias
  - Tachycardia (the most common)
  - Bradycardia, ventricular tachycardia, atrial flutter, atrial fibrillation, and asystole
- Urinary retention
- Hypertension alternating with hypotension
- Orthostatic hypotension
- Obstruction of the intestines (ileus)
- Loss of sweating

---

*When tissue hypoxia is severe enough to produce lactic acid, the pH and HCO_3^- values will be lower than expected for a particular $PaCO_2$ level.
[†]See Figure 4-2 and related discussion for the acute pH, $PaCO_2$, and HCO_3^- changes associated with acute ventilatory failure.
[†]$C(a-\bar{v})O_2$, Arterial–venous oxygen difference; DO_2, total oxygen delivery; O_2ER, oxygen extraction ratio; $\dot{Q}s/\dot{Q}T$, pulmonary shunt fraction; $S\bar{v}O_2$, mixed venous oxygen saturation; $\dot{V}O_2$, oxygen consumption.
[§]The DO_2 may be normal in patients who have compensated to the decreased oxygenation status with (1) an increased cardiac output, (2) an increased hemoglobin level, or (3) a combination of both. When the DO_2 is normal, the O_2ER is usually normal.

---

[2]It should be noted that the clinical manifestations associated with Guillain-Barré may occur over hours or days, depending on how quickly the paralysis progresses.

example, antibodies against GQ1b (a ganglioside component of nerve) are found in 85% to 90% of patients with the Miller Fisher syndrome. Antibodies to GM1, GD1a, GalNac-GD1a, and GD1b are mostly associated with axonal subtypes of GBS.

Box 29-2 provides the diagnostic criteria for GBS developed by the National Institute of Neurological Disorders and Stroke (NINDS). These criteria are based on expert consensus and are widely used today in clinical practice.[3]

General Management of Guillain-Barré Syndrome[4]

GBS is a potential medical emergency, and patients must be monitored closely after the diagnosis has been made. About 30% of cases develop acute ventilatory failure and require mechanical ventilation. The primary treatment should be directed at stabilization of vital signs and supportive care for the patient. Close respiratory monitoring with frequent measurements of the patient's forced vital capacity (FVC),

---

[3]These diagnostic criteria have been used for years in research studies and are applicable to about 80% or 90% of patients with GBS in North America and Europe, particularly those with the AIDP form of GBS.

[4]About 80% of GBS cases have a complete recovery within a few months. Even with treatment, about 5% to 10% of cases have a prolonged course with very prolonged and incomplete recovery. About 2% to 3% die despite intensive care. In addition, relapse occurs in up to 10% of patients.

---

maximum inspiratory pressure (MIP), maximum expiratory pressure (MEP), blood pressure, oxygenation saturation, and, when indicated, arterial blood gases (ABGs) should be performed. Mechanical ventilation should be initiated when the clinical data demonstrate impending or acute ventilatory failure.

Good clinical indicators of impending acute ventilatory failure include the following:
- FVC < 20 mL/kg
- MIP < −30 cm H_2O—In other words, the patient is unable to generate a maximum inspiratory pressure of −30 cm H_2O or more. For example, an MIP of only −15 cm H_2O would confirm severe muscle weakness and, importantly, that acute ventilatory failure is likely.
- MEP < 40 cm H_2O
- $PaCO_2$ > 45 mm Hg
- pH < 7.35

The primary treatment modalities for GBS are (1) **plasmapheresis** (also called **plasma exchange**), and (2) **intravenous immune globulin (IVIG)**. These two treatments have been shown to be equally effective. Plasmapheresis, or plasma exchange (PE), has been shown to be effective in decreasing the morbidity and shortening the clinical course of GBS. Plasmapheresis entails the removal of damaged antibodies from the patient's blood plasma, followed by the transfusion of new blood cells. It is believed that plasmapheresis removes the antibodies from the plasma that contribute to the immune system attack on the peripheral nerves. This procedure has been shown to reduce circulating antibody titers during the early stages of the disorder. High-dose IVIG has demonstrated to be at least as effective, and possibly more, than plasmapheresis. IVIG is a blood product that contains the pooled immunoglobulins (IgG) from thousands of donors. The effects of IVIG last between 2 weeks and 3 months. IVIG products are used to treat multiple conditions, including GBS. Glucocorticoids are not recommended.

As in any patient who is paralyzed or immobilized for prolonged periods, the risk of thromboembolism increases. Because of this danger, the patient commonly receives anticoagulants, elastic stockings, and passive range-of-motion exercises (every 3 to 4 hours) for all extremities. To prevent skin breakdown, the patient should be turned frequently. **Nonsteroidal anti-inflammatory agents (NSAIDs)** are helpful for pain control. A rotary bed or **Stryker frame** may be required. Blood pressure disturbances and cardiac arrhythmias require immediate attention. For example, episodes of bradycardia are commonly treated with atropine.

Respiratory Care Treatment Protocols

Oxygen Therapy Protocol

Oxygen therapy is used to treat hypoxemia, decrease the work of breathing, and decrease myocardial work. Because of the hypoxemia that may develop in GBS, supplemental oxygen may be required. However, because of the alveolar consolidation and atelectasis associated with GBS, capillary shunting may be present. Hypoxemia caused by capillary shunting or alveolar hypoventilation is refractory to oxygen therapy (see Oxygen Therapy Protocol, Protocol 9-1).

Bronchopulmonary Hygiene Therapy Protocol

Because of the excessive mucous accumulation, airway obstruction, alveolar consolidation, and atelectasis associated with GBS, a number of bronchopulmonary hygiene modalities may be used to enhance the mobilization of bronchial secretions (see Bronchopulmonary Hygiene Therapy Protocol, Protocol 9-2).

Lung Expansion Therapy Protocol

Lung expansion measures are commonly administered to offset the alveolar consolidation and atelectasis associated with GBS (see Lung Expansion Therapy Protocol, Protocol 9-3).

Mechanical Ventilation Protocol

Mechanical ventilation may be necessary to provide and support alveolar gas exchange and eventually return the patient to spontaneous breathing. Because acute ventilatory failure is seen in patients with severe GBS, continuous mechanical ventilation is often required. Continuous mechanical ventilation is justified because the acute ventilatory failure is thought to be reversible. Noninvasive positive-pressure ventilation (NIPPV) may be helpful if carefully monitored (see Mechanical Ventilation Protocol, Protocol 10-1 and Mechanical Ventilation Weaning Protocol, Protocol 10-2).

Physical Therapy and Rehabilitation

Physical therapy usually begins long before the patient recovers from the effects of GBS—often while the patient is still being mechanically ventilated. In long-term cases, for example, the arms and legs of the patient will be manually moved on a regular basis to keep the muscles flexible. After recovery, the patient frequently requires physical therapy to regain full strength and normal mobility. **Hydrotherapy (whirlpool therapy)** is commonly used to relieve pain and facilitate limb movement. Full recovery may occur in as little as a few weeks or as long as 3 years.

CASE STUDY Guillain-Barré Syndrome

Admitting History and Physical Examination

A 48-year-old career U.S. Navy physician visited the base hospital clinic because of the acute onset of severe muscle weakness. He had joined the Navy immediately after medical school. Throughout his time in the service, he had the opportunity to pursue his passion—competitive water-ski jumping. For many years he was the first-place winner at most tournaments, including the nationals held yearly. For almost 25 years, he progressed through the age divisions, always remaining the top seed, always capturing the highest title.

The man was in outstanding physical condition. He was an avid runner and weightlifter, and during the off-season he often traveled to a warm climate to practice his water-ski jumping. He had never smoked and had never been hospitalized. He had an occasional "cold." About 2 years previously, he had begun to focus all his attention on his 19-year-old son, who was quickly following in his father's footsteps, having just captured the Men's Division I championship in collegiate ice hockey.

The man stated that he had felt good until 3 weeks before his admission, at which time he experienced a flulike syndrome for 3 days. About 10 days after returning to work, he noticed a tingling and burning sensation in his feet during his morning patient rounds. By dinner time that same day, the tingling and burning had radiated from his feet to about the level of his knees. Thinking that he was just tired from being on his feet all day, he went to bed early that evening. The next morning, however, his legs were completely numb, although he could still move them. Alarmed, he asked his son to drive him to the clinic. After examining him, his doctor (a personal friend) admitted him for a diagnostic workup and observation.

Over the next 3 days, the laboratory results showed that the patient's cerebrospinal fluid had an elevated protein concentration with a normal cell count. The electrodiagnostic studies showed a progressive ascending paralysis of the man's legs and arms. He began to have difficulty eating and swallowing his food. The respiratory therapist, who was monitoring his forced vital capacity (FVC), maximum inspiratory pressure (MIP), pulse oximetry, and arterial blood gas values (ABGs), reported a progressive deterioration in all the values. A diagnosis of Guillain-Barré syndrome was recorded in the patient's chart.

When the man's ABGs showed pH 7.29, $PaCO_2$ 53 mm Hg, HCO_3^- 23 mEq/L, PaO_2 86 mm Hg, and SaO_2 96% (on a 2 L/min oxygen nasal cannula), the respiratory therapist called the attending physician and reported his assessment of acute ventilatory failure. The doctor transferred the patient to the intensive care unit (ICU), intubated him, and placed him on a mechanical ventilator. The initial ventilator settings were as follows: synchronized intermittent mandatory ventilation (SIMV) mode, 12 breaths/min, tidal volume 750 mL, and FIO_2 0.50.

About 15 minutes after the patient was committed to the ventilator, he appeared comfortable. No spontaneous breaths were noted between the 12 set breaths per minute. His vital signs were as follows: blood pressure 126/82 and heart rate 68 beats/min. He was afebrile. A portable chest radiograph confirmed that the endotracheal (ET) tube was in a good position and the lungs were adequately aerated. Normal vesicular breath sounds were auscultated over both lung fields. His ABGs were as follows: pH 7.51, $PaCO_2$ 29 mm Hg, HCO_3^- 22 mEq/L, PaO_2 204 mm Hg, and SaO_2 98%. On the basis of these clinical data, the following SOAP was documented.

Respiratory Assessment and Plan

S N/A (intubated on ventilator)

O Vital signs: BP 126/82, HR 68, RR 12 (SIMV); afebrile; no spontaneous breaths; CXR: normal; normal breath sounds; ABGs (on FIO_2 0.50): pH 7.51, $PaCO_2$ 29, HCO_3^- 22, PaO_2 204, SaO_2 98%

A • Acute alveolar hyperventilation with excessive oxygenation (ABGs)
   • Excessive alveolar ventilation (increased pH and decreased $PaCO_2$)
   • FIO_2 too high (ABGs)

P Adjust mechanical ventilator settings (decrease tidal volume to 650 mL and FIO_2 to 0.40) according to **Mechanical Ventilation Protocol** and **Oxygen Therapy Protocol**. Monitor closely and reevaluate.

3 Days after Admission

The patient's cardiopulmonary status had been unremarkable. No improvement was seen in his muscular paralysis. No changes had been made in his ventilator settings over the previous 48 hours. His skin color appeared good. Palpation and percussion of the chest were unremarkable. On auscultation, however, coarse crackles could be heard over both lung fields.

Moderate amounts of thick, whitish, clear secretions were being suctioned from the patient's endotracheal tube regularly. His vital signs were as follows: blood pressure 124/83, heart rate 74 beats/min, and rectal temperature 37.7 °C (99.8 °F). A recent portable chest radiograph revealed no significant pathologic process. His ABGs on an FIO_2 of 0.40, a respiratory rate of 12 breaths/min, and tidal volume of 650 were as follows: pH 7.44, $PaCO_2$ 35 mm Hg, HCO_3^- 24 mEq/L, PaO_2 98 mm Hg, and SaO_2 97%. On the basis of these clinical data, the following SOAP was documented.

Respiratory Assessment and Plan

S N/A

O Skin color good; coarse crackles over both lung fields; moderate amount of whitish, clear secretions being suctioned regularly; vital signs: BP 124/83, HR 74, T 37.7 °C (99.8 °F); CXR: unremarkable; ABGs (FIO_2 0.4): pH 7.44, $PaCO_2$ 35, HCO_3^- 24, PaO_2 98, SaO_2 97%

A • Normal acid-base and oxygenation status on present ventilator settings (ABGs)
   • Excessive sputum accumulation; possible progression to mucous plugging and atelectasis (coarse crackles, whitish and clear secretions)

P Begin **Bronchopulmonary Hygiene Therapy Protocol** (vigorous tracheal suctioning and obtain sputum stain and culture). Begin **Lung Expansion Therapy Protocol** (+10 cm H_2O positive end-expiratory pressure [PEEP] to offset any early development of atelectasis). Monitor and reevaluate (4 × per shift). Continue Mechanical Ventilation Protocol and Oxygen Therapy Protocol.

5 Days after Admission

The patient remained alert and comfortable, except for the presence of the ET tube. His muscular paralysis remained unchanged. His skin color appeared good, and no abnormalities were noted during palpation and percussion of the chest. Although coarse crackles could still be heard over both lung fields, they were not as intense as they had been 48 hours earlier. A small amount of clear secretions was suctioned from the patient's ET tube. His vital signs were as follows: blood pressure 118/79, heart rate 68 beats/min, and temperature normal. Results of a recent portable chest radiograph appeared normal. His ABGs on an FIO_2 of 0.40, a respiratory rate of 12 breaths/min, a tidal volume of 650, and PEEP of +10 cm H_2O were as follows: pH 7.42, $PaCO_2$ 37 mm Hg, HCO_3^- 24 mEq/L, PaO_2 97 mm Hg, SaO_2 97%. The sputum culture was unremarkable. On the basis of these clinical data, the following SOAP note was recorded.

Respiratory Assessment and Plan

S N/A

O Skin color good; coarse crackles over both lung fields improving; small amount of clear secretions suctioned; vital signs: BP 118/79, HR 68, T normal; no spontaneous respirations; CXR: normal; ABGs (FIO_2 0.4): pH 7.42, $PaCO_2$ 37, HCO_3^- 24, PaO_2 97, SaO_2 97%

A • Normal acid-base and oxygenation status on present ventilator settings (ABGs)
   • Respiratory insufficiency (no spontaneous respirations)
   • Secretion control improving (coarse crackles, clear secretions)

P Continue **Mechanical Ventilation Protocol**. Continue **Bronchopulmonary Hygiene Therapy Protocol**. Continue **Lung Expansion Therapy Protocol**. Monitor and reevaluate (SpO_2, maximum inspiratory pressure (MIP), and forced vital capacity (FVC) 2 × per shift).

Discussion

Guillain-Barré syndrome is a neuromuscular paralysis that ensues after infection with a neurotropic virus. This patient had a classic history of ascending paralysis and paresthesia and the diagnostic finding of elevated protein concentration in the spinal fluid. In this setting, serial measurements of the patient's forced vital capacity (FVC), maximum inspiratory pressure (MIP), blood pressure, oxygen saturation, and arterial blood gases (ABGs) must be measured and charted. Once respiratory failure supervened, intubation and respiratory support on a ventilator became necessary. As discussed in this chapter, good clinical indicators of acute ventilatory failure include the following: FVC < 20 mL/kg, MIP < −30 cm H_2O, pH < 7.35, and $PaCO_2$ > 45 mm Hg. As noted by the respiratory therapist, a progressive deterioration was observed in all of these clinical indicators over a 3-day period.

As shown during the first assessment, when acute ventilatory failure developed, the patient was transferred to the ICU, intubated, and placed on a mechanical ventilator. Shortly after the patient was placed on the ventilator, his arterial blood gas values showed hyperoxia and acute alveolar hyperventilation—both of which were caused by the ventilator settings. The appropriate response was to immediately adjust the ventilator settings by reducing the tidal volume or frequency (or both) and the FIO_2. At the time of the assessment, the patient exhibited no evidence of airway obstruction or secretions. Therefore, the **Bronchial Hygiene Therapy Protocol** (Protocol 9-2) was not indicated. Indeed, all that needed to be done at that time was to ensure adequate ventilation and oxygenation on the ventilator.

However, 3 days later, at the time of the second assessment, coarse crackles were heard over all lung fields. There was no indication of fluid overload. Clearly the time had come to initiate the **Bronchial Hygiene Therapy Protocol (Protocol 9-2)**. Because of the risk of atelectasis, the **Lung Expansion Therapy Protocol** (Protocol 9-3), in the form of PEEP on the ventilator, was indicated. In such a case the sputum should be cultured to see whether any infectious organisms were present.

At the time of the final assessment (2 days later), the clinical indicators for airway secretions had decreased—the crackles could no longer be heard over the lung fields, and the small amount of sputum suctioned appeared clear. At that point down-regulation of the **Bronchial Hygiene Therapy Protocol** (Protocol 9-2) was indicated.

Serial SpO_2, FVC, or MIP measurements would continue to be made until the patient was ready to be extubated and thereafter for at least several days. Indeed, extubation occurred about 3 weeks after the initiation of mechanical ventilation. The patient recovered without incident and returned to his active lifestyle within a year.

SELF-ASSESSMENT QUESTIONS

Answers to questions can be found on Evolve. To access additional student assessment questions visit http://evolve.elsevier.com/DesJardins/respiratory.

1. In Guillain-Barré syndrome, which of the following pathologic changes develop in the peripheral nerves?
   1. Inflammation
   2. Increased ability to transmit nerve impulses
   3. Demyelination
   4. Edema
      a. 2 and 3 only
      b. 3 and 4 only
      c. 2, 3, and 4 only
      d. 1, 3, and 4 only

2. Which of the following is associated with Guillain-Barré syndrome?
   1. Alveolar consolidation
   2. Mucous accumulation
   3. Alveolar hyperinflation
   4. Atelectasis
      a. 1 and 2 only
      b. 3 and 4 only
      c. 1, 2, and 4 only
      d. 2, 3, and 4 only

3. Guillain-Barré syndrome is more common in:
   1. People older than 50 years of age
   2. Blacks
   3. Whites than in females
   4. Early childhood
      a. 1 only
      b. 4 only
      c. 1 and 3 only
      d. 3 and 4 only

4. Which of the following are possible precursors to Guillain-Barré syndrome?
   1. Mumps
   2. Swine influenza vaccine
   3. Infectious mononucleosis
   4. Measles
      a. 2 and 4 only
      b. 3 and 4 only
      c. 2, 3, and 4 only
      d. 1, 2, 3, and 4

5. Full recovery from Guillain-Barré syndrome is expected in approximately what percentage of cases?
   a. 30%
   b. 40%
   c. 50%
   d. 90%

6. Which of the following are indicators for intubation and mechanical ventilation in patients with Guillain-Barré syndrome?
   1. pH > 7.40
   2. $PaCO_2 > 45$
   3. FVC < 20 mL/kg
   4. MIP < –30 cm H_2O
      a. 1 and 2 only
      b. 3 and 4 only
      c. 2, 3, and 4 only
      d. 1, 2, and 3 only

Chapter Objectives

After reading this chapter, you will be able to:

- List the anatomic alterations of the lungs associated with myasthenia gravis.
- Describe the etiology and epidemiology of myasthenia gravis.
- Discuss the screening for and diagnosis of myasthenia gravis.
- List the cardiopulmonary clinical manifestations associated with myasthenia gravis.
- Describe the general management of myasthenia gravis.
- Describe the clinical strategies and rationales of the SOAPs presented in the case study.

Key Terms

Acetylcholine (ACh)
Anticholinesterase Inhibitors
Binding AChR Antibodies Test
CMAP Amplitude
Decremental Response
Diplopia
Edrophonium (Tensilon) Test
Electromyography
Generalized Myasthenia Gravis
Ice Pack Test
IgG Antibodies
Inadvertent Right Main Stem Bronchial Intubation
Intravenous Immune Globulin (IVIG)
Lactic Acidosis
MuSK
Myasthenic Crisis
Mycophenolate Mofetil
Neuromuscular Junction
Ocular Myasthenia Gravis

Ophthalmoparesis
Ophthalmoplegia
Plasmapheresis
Ptosis
Pyridostigmine (Mestinon)
Repetitive Nerve Stimulation (RNS)
Seronegative Myasthenia Gravis
Seropositive Myasthenia Gravis
Single-Fiber Electromyography (SFEMG)
Thymectomy
Thymoma

Chapter Outline

Anatomic Alterations of the Lungs Associated with Myasthenia Gravis
Etiology and Epidemiology
Screening and Diagnosis
   Clinical Presentation and History
   Diagnostic (Bedside Diagnostic Tests)
   Immunologic Studies
   Electrodiagnostic Studies
   Evaluation of Conditions Associated with Myasthenia Gravis
Overview of Cardiopulmonary Clinical Manifestations Associated with Myasthenia Gravis
General Management of Myasthenia Gravis
   Acetylcholinesterase Inhibitors
   Immunotherapy
   Rapid Immunotherapies
   Thymectomy
   Respiratory Care Treatment Protocols
Case Study: Myasthenia Gravis
Self-Assessment Questions

Anatomic Alterations of the Lungs Associated with Myasthenia Gravis

Myasthenia gravis is the most common chronic disorder of the **neuromuscular junction**. The disorder interferes with the chemical transmission of **acetylcholine (ACh)** between the axonal terminal and the receptor sites of voluntary muscles (Figure 30-1). The hallmark clinical feature of myasthenia gravis is fluctuating skeletal muscle weakness, often with true muscle fatigue. The fatigue and weakness usually improves following rest. There are two clinical types of myasthenia gravis: *ocular* and *generalized*. In **ocular myasthenia gravis**, the muscle weakness is limited to the eyelids and extraocular muscles. In **generalized myasthenia gravis**, the muscle weakness involves a variable combination of (1) muscles of the mouth and throat responsible for speech and swallowing (called bulbar muscles), (2) limbs, and (3) respiratory muscles. Neck extensor and flexor muscles are commonly affected, producing what is called a "dropped head syndrome." The facial muscles are often involved, causing the patient to appear expressionless. Generalized myasthenia gravis may, or may not, involve the ocular muscle. Because the disorder affects only the myoneural (motor) junction, sensory function is not lost.

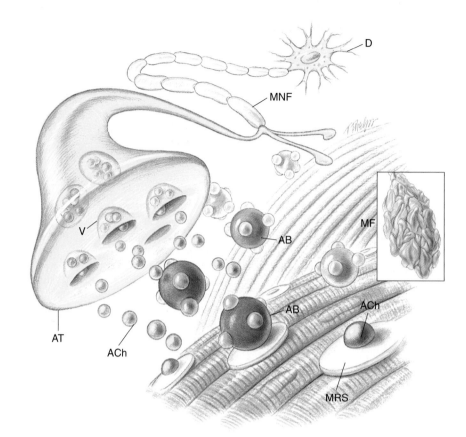

FIGURE 30-1 Myasthenia gravis, a disorder of the neuromuscular junction that interferes with the chemical transmission of acetylcholine. *AB,* Antibody; *ACh,* acetylcholine; *AT,* axonal terminal; *D,* dendrite; *MF,* muscle fiber; *MNF,* myelinated nerve fiber; *MRS,* muscle receptor site; *V,* vesicle. Note that the antibodies have a physical structure similar to that of ACh, which permits them to connect to (and block ACh from) the muscle receptor sites. *Inset:* Atelectasis, a common secondary anatomic alteration of the lungs.

The abnormal weakness may be confined to an isolated group of muscles (e.g., the drooping of one or both eyelids), or it may manifest as a generalized weakness that in severe cases includes the diaphragm. When the diaphragm is involved, ventilatory failure can develop—producing what is called a "**myasthenic crisis.**" In these cases, mechanical ventilation is required. If the patient is not properly managed (e.g., via the Bronchopulmonary Hygiene Therapy Protocol, Protocol 9-2 and Mechanical Ventilation Protocols, Protocol 10-1 and Protocol 10-2), **mucous accumulation with airway obstruction, alveolar consolidation,** and **atelectasis** may develop.

The major pathologic or structural changes of the lungs associated with a poorly managed myasthenic crisis are as follows:

- Mucous accumulation
- Airway obstruction
- Alveolar consolidation
- Atelectasis

Etiology and Epidemiology

The cause of myasthenia gravis appears to be related to ACh receptor (AChR) antibodies (**IgG antibodies**) that block the nerve impulse transmissions at the neuromuscular junction.

Patients who have detectable antibodies to the AChR, or to the muscle-specific receptor tyrosine kinase (**MuSK**), are said to have **seropositive myasthenia gravis,** whereas those lacking both AChR and MuSK antibodies on standard assays are said to have **seronegative myasthenia gravis.** About 50% of patients with only ocular myasthenia gravis are seropositive. About 90% of generalized cases of myasthenia gravis are seropositive.

It is believed that the IgG antibodies disrupt the chemical transmission of ACh at the neuromuscular junction by (1) blocking the ACh from the receptor sites of the muscular cell, (2) accelerating the breakdown of ACh, and (3) destroying the receptor sites (Figure 30-1). Receptor-binding antibodies are present in 85% to 90% of persons with myasthenia gravis. Although the specific events that activate the formation of the antibodies remain unclear, the thymus gland is often abnormal; it is generally presumed that the antibodies arise within the thymus or in related tissue.

According to the Myasthenia Gravis Foundation of America, there are about 36,000 to 60,000 cases of myasthenia gravis in the United States (20 per 100,000 population). The disease usually has a peak age of onset in females of 15 to 35 years, compared with 40 to 70 years in males. The clinical manifestations associated with myasthenia gravis are often provoked by emotional upset, physical stress, exposure to extreme temperature changes, febrile illness, and pregnancy. Death caused by myasthenia gravis is possible, especially during the first few years after onset.

Screening and Diagnosis

Screening methods and tests used to diagnose myasthenia gravis include (1) clinical presentation and history, (2) bedside tests, (3) immunologic studies, (4) electrodiagnostic studies, and (5) evaluation of conditions associated with myasthenia gravis.

Clinical Presentation and History

The hallmark of myasthenia gravis is chronic muscle fatigue. The muscles become progressively weaker during periods of activity and improve after periods of rest. Signs and symptoms include facial muscle weakness; **ptosis** (drooping of one or both eyelids); **diplopia** (double vision); **ophthalmoplegia** (paralysis or weakness of one or more of the muscles that control eye movement); difficulty in breathing, speaking, chewing, and swallowing; unstable gait; and weakness in arms, hands, fingers, legs, and neck brought on by repetitive motions. The muscles that control the eyes, eyelids, face, and throat are especially susceptible and are usually affected first. The respiratory muscles of the diaphragm and chest wall can become weak and impair the patient's ventilation. Impairment in deep breathing and coughing predispose the patient to excessive bronchial secretions, atelectasis, and pneumonia.

The signs and symptoms of myasthenia gravis during the early stages are often elusive. The onset can be subtle, intermittent, or sudden and rapid. The patient may (1) demonstrate normal health for weeks or months at a time, (2) show signs of weakness only late in the day or evening, or (3) develop a sudden and transient generalized weakness that includes the diaphragm. Because of this last characteristic, ventilatory failure is always a sinister possibility. In most cases, the first noticeable symptom is weakness of the eye muscles (droopy eyelids) and a change in the patient's facial expressions. As the disorder becomes more generalized, weakness develops in the arms and legs. The muscle weakness is usually more pronounced in the proximal parts of the extremities. The patient has difficulty in climbing stairs, lifting objects, maintaining balance, and walking. In severe cases, the weakness of the upper limbs may be such that the hand cannot be lifted to the mouth. Muscle atrophy or pain is rare. Tendon reflexes almost always remain intact.

Bedside Diagnostic Tests

Ice Pack Test

The **ice pack test** is a very simple, safe, and reliable procedure for diagnosing myasthenia gravis in patients who have ptosis (droopy eye). In addition, the ice pack test does not require special medications or expensive equipment and is free of adverse effects. The test consists of the application of an ice pack to the patient's symptomatic eye for 3 to 5 minutes (Figure 30-2). The test is considered positive for myasthenia gravis when there is improvement of the ptosis (an increase of at least 2 mm in the palpebral fissure from before to after the test).

A major disadvantage of the ice pack test is that it is useful only when ptosis is present. Even though the symptoms associated with diplopia (double vision) may also improve with the ice pack test, the reliability of the ice pack test in patients with diplopia without ptosis is usually questionable because the patient's personal impression of the diplopia is subjective. Therefore, caution should be exercised in patients with isolated diplopia without ptosis. The ice pack test may be especially useful in patients in whom the edrophonium test is contraindicated by either cardiac status or age.

Edrophonium (Tensilon) Test

The **edrophonium (Tensilon) test** is used in patients with obvious ptosis or **ophthalmoparesis**. Edrophonium, a short-acting drug, blocks cholinesterase from breaking down ACh after it has been released from the terminal axon. This action increases the myoneural concentration of ACh, which in turn offsets the influx of antibodies at the neuromuscular junction. When muscular weakness is caused by myasthenia gravis, a dramatic transitory improvement in muscle function (lasting about 10 minutes) is seen after the administration of edrophonium. A disadvantage of the edrophonium test is that it can be complicated by cholinergic side effects that include cardiac arrhythmias and cardiopulmonary arrest. Cardiac monitoring, or avoiding this test altogether, is suggested in the elderly or those with a history of arrhythmia or heart disease. Although the sensitivity of the Tensilon test for the diagnosis of myasthenia gravis is in the 80% to 90% range, it is associated with many false-negative and false-positive results.

Immunologic Studies

Serologic tests to detect the presence of circulating acetylcholine receptor antibodies (AChR-Abs) is the first step in

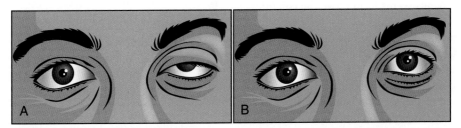

FIGURE 30-2 Ice pack test. **A**, Myasthenia gravis in a patient who has ptosis (droopy left eye). **B**, Same patient after 5-minute application of an ice pack. Note the patient's left eye lid is no longer droopy.

the laboratory confirmation of myasthenia. There are three AChR-Ab assays: binding, blocking, and modulating. The **binding AChR antibodies test** is highly specific for myasthenia gravis (80% to 90%). Most experts use the term AChR-Abs as synonymous with the binding antibodies. In some patients, assays for blocking and modulating antibodies may also be helpful. Blocking AChR-Abs are found in about 50% of patients with generalized myasthenia gravis. Assays for modulating AChR-Abs increase the diagnostic sensitivity by about 5% when combined with the binding studies. When AChR-Abs are negative, an assay for the antibodies to MuSK proteins should be performed.

Electrodiagnostic Studies

The **repetitive nerve stimulation (RNS)** and **single-fiber electromyography (SFEMG)** tests are important diagnostic supplements to the immunologic studies. The RNS study is the most frequently used electrodiagnostic test for myasthenia gravis. The RNS study is performed by electrically stimulating the motor nerve of selected muscles 6 to 10 times at low rates (2 or 3 Hz). In the normal muscle, there is no change in the compound muscle action potential (CMAP) amplitude. In patients with myasthenia gravis, there may be a progressive decline in the **CMAP amplitude** within the first four to five stimuli—called a **decremental response**. The RNS is considered positive when the decrement is greater than 10%.

The SFEMG is the most sensitive diagnostic test for myasthenia gravis, although it is technically more difficult. A specialized needle electrode allows simultaneous recording of the action potential of two muscle fibers innervated by the same motor axon. The variability in time between the two action potentials is called "jitter." In patients with myasthenia gravis, the jitter is increased. The SFEMG is positive in more than 95% of patients with generalized myasthenia gravis. The sensitivity of the SFEMG ranges between 85% and 95% in ocular myasthenia gravis.

Evaluation of Conditions Associated with Myasthenia Gravis

Thymic Tumors and Other Malignancies—Thymic abnormalities are often seen in patients with myasthenia gravis. Computed tomography (CT) or magnetic resonance imaging (MRI) scans may be used to identify an abnormal thymus gland or the presence of a **thymoma** (a usually benign tumor of the thymus gland that may be associated with myasthenia gravis). A **thymectomy** has been shown to reduce symptoms of myasthenia gravis. In fact, a thymectomy may be recommended even when there is no tumor. The removal of the thymus seems to improve the condition in many patients.

Differential diagnosis—Studies to rule out other disease in the differential diagnosis of myasthenia gravis are indicated in some patients. For example, in cases with ocular or bulbar symptoms, an MRI of the brain is indicated. CT scanning or ultrasound of the orbits is helpful in the differential diagnosis of ocular myasthenia and thyroid ophthalmopathy. A lumbar puncture may be helpful in ruling out lymphomatous or carcinomatous meningitis is some cases.

Blood tests should include thyroid function tests. In patients who have symptoms associated with a rheumatologic disorder, assays for antinuclear antibodies and rheumatoid factor should be performed.

Pulmonary Function Testing—May be performed to help evaluate the patient's ventilatory status and the possibility of ventilatory failure—that is, a myasthenic crisis.

Box 30-1 provides a widely accepted clinical classification system of myasthenia gravis, which was developed by the Myasthenia Gravis Foundation of America.

BOX 30-1 Clinical Classifications of Myasthenia Gravis	
Class I	Any ocular muscle weakness; may have weakness of eye closure; all other muscle strength is normal
Class II	Mild weakness affecting other ocular muscles; may also have ocular muscle weakness of any severity
Class IIa	Predominantly affecting limb, axial muscles, or both; may also have lesser involvement of oropharyngeal muscles
Class IIb	Predominantly affecting oropharyngeal, respiratory muscles, or both; may also have lesser or equal involvement of limb, axial muscles, or both
Class III	Moderate weakness affecting other ocular muscles; may also have ocular muscle weakness of any severity
Class IIIa	Predominantly affecting limb, axial muscles, or both; may also have lesser involvement of oropharyngeal muscles
Class IIIb	Predominantly affecting oropharyngeal, respiratory muscles, or both; may also have lesser or equal involvement of limb, axial muscles, or both
Class IV	Severe weakness affecting other ocular muscles; may also have ocular muscle weakness of any severity
Class Iva	Predominantly affecting limb, axial muscles, or both; may also have lesser involvement of oropharyngeal muscles
Class IVb	Predominantly affecting oropharyngeal, respiratory muscles, or both; may also have lesser or equal involvement of limb, axial muscles, or both; use of a feeding tube without intubation
Class V	Defined by the need for intubation, with or without mechanical ventilation, except when used during routine postoperative management

Adapted from Jaretzki A 3rd, Barohn RJ, Ernstoff RM, et al: Myasthenia gravis: recommendations for clinical research standards. Task Force of the Medical Scientific Advisory Board of the Myasthenia Gravis Foundation of America, *Neurology* 55:16–23, 2000.

The following clinical manifestations result from the pathologic mechanisms caused (or activated) by Atelectasis (see Figure 9-7), Alveolar Consolidation (see Figure 9-8), and Excessive Bronchial Secretions (see Figure 9-11)—the major anatomic alterations of the lungs associated with myasthenia gravis, which may occur when the patient is not properly managed via the Bronchopulmonary Hygiene Therapy Protocol, Protocol 9-2 and Mechanical Ventilation Protocols, Protocol 10-1 and Protocol 10-2 (Figure 30-1).[1]

CLINICAL DATA OBTAINED AT THE PATIENT'S BEDSIDE

The Physical Examination

Respiratory Rate
- Varies with the degree of respiratory muscle paralysis
- Apnea (in severe cases)

Cyanosis (in Severe Cases)

Chest Assessment Findings
- Diminished breath sounds
- Crackles

CLINICAL DATA OBTAINED FROM LABORATORY TESTS AND SPECIAL PROCEDURES

Pulmonary Function Test Findings*
(Restrictive Lung Pathology)

FORCED EXPIRATORY VOLUME AND FLOW RATE FINDINGS

FVC	FEV_T	FEV_1/FVC ratio	$FEF_{25\%-75\%}$
↓	N or ↓	N or ↑	N or ↓

$FEF_{50\%}$	$FEF_{200-1200}$	PEFR	MVV
N or ↓	N or ↓	N or ↓	N or ↓

*Progressive worsening of these values is key to anticipating the onset of ventilatory failure.

LUNG VOLUME AND CAPACITY FINDINGS

V_T	IRV	ERV	RV
↓	↓	↓	↓

VC	IC	FRC	TLC	RV/TLC ratio
↓	↓	↓	↓	N

MAXIMUM INSPIRATORY PRESSURE (MIP) ↓

---

[1]It should be noted that the clinical manifestations associated with myasthenia gravis may occur over hours or days, depending on how quickly the paralysis progresses.

Arterial Blood Gases
Moderate to Severe Myasthenia Gravis

Acute Ventilatory Failure with Hypoxemia[†]
(Acute Respiratory Acidosis)

pH*	$PaCO_2$	HCO_3^-*	PaO_2	SaO_2 or SpO_2
↓	↑	↑	↓	↓
		(but normal)		

Oxygenation Indices[†]

$\dot{Q}s/\dot{Q}T$	DO_2[§]	$\dot{V}O_2$	$C(a\text{-}\bar{v})O_2$	O_2ER	$S\bar{v}O_2$
↑	↓	N	N	↑	↓

RADIOLOGIC FINDINGS

Chest Radiograph
- Normal, or
- Increased opacity (when atelectasis or consolidation are present)

If the ventilatory failure associated with myasthenia gravis is properly managed (e.g., via the Bronchopulmonary Hygiene Therapy and Mechanical Ventilation Protocols, Protocol 9-2, Protocol 10-1, and Protocol 10-2), the chest radiograph should appear normal. However, if the patient is not properly managed, mucous accumulation, alveolar consolidation, and atelectasis may develop. In these cases, the chest radiograph will show an increased density of the lung segments affected.

---

*When tissue hypoxia is severe enough to produce lactic acid, the pH and HCO_3^- values will be lower than expected for a particular $PaCO_2$ level.
[†]See Figure 4-2 and related discussion for the acute pH, $PaCO_2$, and HCO_3^- changes associated with acute ventilatory failure.
[‡]$C(a\text{-}\bar{v})O_2$, Arterial–venous oxygen difference; DO_2, total oxygen delivery; O_2ER, oxygen extraction ratio; $\dot{Q}s/\dot{Q}T$, pulmonary shunt fraction; $S\bar{v}O_2$, mixed venous oxygen saturation; $\dot{V}O_2$, oxygen consumption.
[§]The DO_2 may be normal in patients who have compensated to the decreased oxygenation status with (1) an increased cardiac output, (2) an increased hemoglobin level, or (3) a combination of both. When the DO_2 is normal, the O_2ER is usually normal.

General Management of Myasthenia Gravis

In the past, many patients with myasthenia gravis died within the first few years of diagnosis of the disease. Today, a number of therapeutic measures provide most patients with marked relief of symptoms and allow them to live a normal life. Close respiratory monitoring with frequent measurements of the patient's forced vital capacity (FVC), maximum inspiratory pressure (MIP), maximum expiratory pressure (MEP), blood pressure, oxygen saturation, and, when indicated, arterial blood gases (ABGs) should be performed. Mechanical ventilation should be initiated when the clinical data demonstrate impending or acute ventilatory failure.

Good clinical indicators of impending acute ventilatory failure include the following:

- FVC < 20 mL/kg
- MIP < −30 cm H_2O—In other words, the patient is unable to generate a maximum inspiratory pressure of −30 cm H_2O or more. For example, an MIP of only −15 cm H_2O would confirm severe muscle weakness and, importantly, that acute ventilatory failure is likely.
- MEP < 40 cm H_2O
- $PaCO_2$ > 45 mm Hg
- pH < 7.35

The basic therapy modalities for myasthenia gravis include (1) acetylcholinesterase inhibitors, (2) immunotherapy (e.g., glucocorticoids and other immunosuppressive drugs), (3) rapid immunotherapies (plasma exchange and intravenous immune globulins [IVIG]), (4) thymectomy, and (5) the avoidance of drugs that may exacerbate myasthenia.

Acetylcholinesterase Inhibitors

Acetylcholinesterase inhibitors are recommended as the first line of treatment for symptomatic myasthenia gravis. **Pyridostigmine (Mestinon)** is usually the first choice. Pyridostigmine inhibits the function of acetylcholinesterase. This action increases the concentration of ACh to compete with the circulating anti-ACh antibodies, which interfere with the ability of ACh to stimulate the muscle receptors. Although the **anticholinesterase inhibitors** are effective in mild cases of myasthenia gravis, they are not completely effective in severe cases.

Immunotherapy

Most patients with myasthenia gravis need some form of immunotherapy; in addition to an acetylcholinesterase inhibitor (see above). It is recommended that immunotherapy be administered to patients who (1) are significantly symptomatic while on an acetylcholinesterase inhibitor, or (2) who become symptomatic after a temporary response to an acetylcholinesterase inhibitor. Widely used agents include azathioprine, **mycophenolate mofetil**, and cyclosporine. Immunotherapy agents are usually used for more severe cases. The patient's strength often improves strikingly with steroids. Patients receiving long-term steroid therapy, however, may develop serious complications such as diabetes, cataracts, steroid myopathy, gastrointestinal bleeding, infections, aseptic necrosis of the bone, osteoporosis, and psychoses.

Rapid Immunotherapies

Rapid immunotherapy modalities are used most often for (1) myasthenic crisis, (2) preoperatively before thymectomy or other surgery, (3) as a bridge to slower acting immunotherapies, and (4) to help maintain remission in hard-to-control patients. Rapid immunotherapy modalities include plasmapheresis and IVIG therapy.

Plasmapheresis (plasma exchange) directly removes the AChR antibodies from the patient's blood. The beneficial effects of plasmapheresis basically correlate to the decrease in the AChR antibodies. Immunotherapy (e.g., glucocorticoids) is typically administered concurrently to offset an AChR antibody level rebound. Plasmapheresis is a well-established treatment selection for seriously ill patients in a myasthenic crisis. Plasmapheresis can be a life-saving intervention in the treatment of myasthenia gravis. However, it is time-consuming and is associated with many side effects, such as low blood pressure, infection, and blood clots.

Intravenous immune globulin (IVIG) entails the administration of pooled immunoglobulins (IgG) from multiple donors. Although the precise mechanism of IVIG therapy is uncertain, the benefits are typically seen in less than a week and can last for 3 to 6 weeks. Similar to plasmapheresis, IVIG therapy is used to quickly reverse an exacerbation of myasthenia gravis. IVIG therapy also provides an alternative to plasmapheresis or immunosuppressive agents in certain patients with refractory myasthenia gravis, or as a preoperative treatment before a thymectomy, or as a "bridge" to slower acting immunotherapy agents. Transfusion reactions to rapid administrations of IVIG are not uncommon.

Thymectomy

Although controversial, a thymectomy may be recommended for some patients with generalized myasthenia gravis, who are less than 60 years of age and without thymoma. The thymus is the source of the anti-ACh receptor antibodies. Although a thymectomy may improve muscle strength in some patients, the full benefits of this procedure usually take several years to accumulate.

Respiratory Care Treatment Protocols

Oxygen Therapy Protocol

Oxygen therapy is used to treat hypoxemia, decrease the work of breathing, and decrease myocardial work. Because of the hypoxemia that may develop in myasthenia gravis, supplemental oxygen may be required. However, because of the alveolar consolidation and atelectasis associated with myasthenia gravis, capillary shunting may be present. Hypoxemia caused by capillary shunting is refractory to oxygen therapy (see Oxygen Therapy Protocol, Protocol 9-1).

Bronchopulmonary Hygiene Therapy Protocol

Because of the excessive mucous production and accumulation associated with myasthenia gravis, a number of bronchial hygiene treatment modalities may be used to enhance the mobilization of bronchial secretions (see Bronchopulmonary Hygiene Therapy Protocol, Protocol 9-2).

Lung Expansion Therapy Protocol

Lung expansion measures are commonly administered to prevent or offset the alveolar consolidation and atelectasis associated with myasthenia gravis (see Lung Expansion Therapy Protocol, Protocol 9-3).

Mechanical Ventilation Protocol

Mechanical ventilation may be needed to provide and support alveolar gas exchange and eventually return the patient to spontaneous breathing. Because acute ventilatory failure is often seen in patients with severe myasthenia gravis, continuous mechanical ventilation may be required. Continuous mechanical ventilation is justified when the acute ventilatory failure is thought to be reversible. Noninvasive positive-pressure ventilation (NIPPV) may be helpful if carefully monitored (see Mechanical Ventilation Protocol, Protocol 10-1 and Mechanical Ventilation Weaning Protocol, Protocol 10-2).

CASE STUDY Myasthenia Gravis

Admitting History

A 35-year-old Spanish-American woman was a schoolteacher with a 3-year-old son and an unemployed husband who was still "finding his real place in life." The woman was a high achiever. She had recently received her doctoral degree in education, but she continued to work in the classroom with the grade-school children she loved so much. She was named Teacher of the Year in the large city where she lived. Her colleagues at school considered her a nonstop worker. She had never smoked.

At home, she was always on the move. She had just finished remodeling her kitchen and two bathrooms. She also did her own backyard landscaping on the weekends, a job she particularly enjoyed. She read and played with her son whenever they had time together. Although she enjoyed cooking (a skill she learned from her mother), she did not like to shop for groceries. Fortunately, this was a chore that her husband enjoyed.

Three weeks before the current admission, the woman noticed that her eyes "felt tired." She began to experience slight double vision. Thinking that she was working too hard, she slowed down a bit and went to bed earlier for about a week. However, she progressively felt weaker. Her legs quickly became tired, and she began having trouble chewing her food. Concerned, the woman finally went to see her doctor. After reviewing the woman's recent history and performing a careful physical examination, the physician admitted her to the hospital for further evaluation and treatment.

Over the next 48 hours, the woman's physical status declined progressively. At the patient's bedside, an ice pack test was positive for myasthenia gravis when her ptosis improved by 5 mm. She also indicated that her diplopia was better for about 10 minutes after the test. After the administration of edrophonium, her muscle strength increased significantly for about 10 minutes. **Electromyography** disclosed extensive muscle involvement and a high degree of fatigability in all the affected muscles. A diagnosis of myasthenia gravis was recorded in the patient's chart.

The woman began to choke and aspirate food during meals, and a nasogastric feeding tube was inserted. Her speech became more and more slurred. Both her upper eyelids drooped, and she was unable to hold her head off her pillow on request. The respiratory therapists who monitored her forced vital capacity, maximum inspiratory pressure, pulse oximetry, and arterial blood gas values (ABGs) reported a progressive worsening in all parameters.

When the woman's ABGs were pH 7.32, $PaCO_2$ 51 mm Hg, HCO_3^- 23 mEq/L, PaO_2 59 mm Hg, and SaO_2 88% (on room air), the respiratory therapist called the physician and reported an assessment of acute ventilatory failure. The doctor had the patient transferred to the intensive care unit, intubated (No. 7 endotracheal tube with a tube length charted at 23 cm at the lip), and placed on a mechanical ventilator. The initial ventilator settings were as follows: synchronized intermittent mechanical ventilation (SIMV) mode, frequency 10 breaths/min, tidal volume 600 mL, FIO_2 0.50, and positive end-expiratory pressure (PEEP) of +5 cm H_2O.

On these ventilator settings, her ABG values were as follows: pH 7.28, $PaCO_2$ 64 mm Hg, HCO_3^- 29 mEq/L, PaO_2 52 mm Hg, and SaO_2 81%. About 45 minutes after the patient was placed on the ventilator, she appeared agitated. No spontaneous ventilations were seen. Her vital signs were as follows: blood pressure 132/86, heart rate 90 beats/min, and rectal temperature 38 °C (100.5 °F). A portable chest radiograph had been taken, but the image was still being processed. Normal vesicular breath sounds were auscultated over the right lung, and diminished-to-absent breath sounds were auscultated over the left lung. On the basis of these clinical data, the following SOAP was recorded.

Respiratory Assessment and Plan

S N/A (patient intubated)

O No spontaneous ventilations; vital signs: BP 132/86, HR 90, RR 10 (controlled), T 38 °C (100.5 °F); normal breath sounds over right lung; diminished-to-absent breath sounds over left lung; ABGs (on FIO_2 0.50): pH 7.28, $PaCO_2$ 64, HCO_3^- 29, PaO_2 52, SaO_2 81%

A • Endotracheal tube possibly placed in right main stem bronchi (diminished-to-absent breath sounds over left lung, ABGs)
  • Acute ventilatory failure with moderate hypoxemia—on present ventilatory settings (ABGs)
  • Worsening condition likely caused by misplacement of endotracheal tube

P Notify physician stat. Check CXR. Pull endotracheal tube back until breath sounds can be auscultated over both lungs. Confirm initial placement of the endotracheal tube when radiograph is available. **Mechanical Ventilation Protocol** (increase tidal volume to 750 mL and increase FIO_2 to 1.0). Monitor and reevaluate immediately.

45 Minutes Later

After the patient's endotracheal tube was pulled back 3 cm to 20 cm at the lip, normal vesicular breath sounds could be auscultated over both lungs. The first chest radiograph examination confirmed that the endotracheal tube had indeed been inserted too far into the patient's right main stem bronchus. A follow-up chest radiograph examination confirmed that the endotracheal tube was now appropriately positioned about 2 cm above the carina. Her vital signs were as follows: blood pressure 123/75, heart rate 74 beats/min, and temperature normal. On the new ventilatory settings per the last SOAP (see above), the ABGs were as follows: pH 7.53, $PaCO_2$ 27 mm Hg, HCO_3^- 22 mEq/L, PaO_2 376 mm Hg, and SaO_2 98%. On the basis of these clinical data, the following SOAP was written.

Respiratory Assessment and Plan

S N/A (patient intubated on ventilator)
O Vital signs: BP 123/75, HR 74, T normal; normal bronchovesicular breath sounds over both lung fields; CXR: No. 7 endotracheal tube in good position (20 cm at lip); lungs adequately ventilated; ABGs: pH 7.53, $PaCO_2$ 27, HCO_3^- 22, PaO_2 376, SaO_2 98%
A • Acute ventilator-induced alveolar hyperventilation (respiratory alkalosis), with overly corrected hypoxemia (ABGs)

P Adjust present settings per **Mechanical Ventilation Protocol** (decrease tidal volume to 650 mL). Down-regulate **Oxygen Therapy Per Protocol** (decrease FIO_2 to 0.30). Monitor and reevaluate (e.g., SpO_2, maximum inspiratory pressure [MIP], and forcedvital capacity (FVC) 2 × per shift).

3 Days Later

No changes in the patient's ventilator settings were made since the SOAP shown above. No remarkable information was noted during the last 72 hours. However, on this day the woman appeared pale, and her vital signs were as follows: blood pressure 146/88, heart rate 92 beats/min, and temperature 37.9 °C (100.2 °F). Large amounts of thick, yellowish sputum were being suctioned from her endotracheal tube

about every 30 minutes. No improvement was seen in her muscular paralysis.

Coarse crackles were auscultated over both lung fields. A sputum sample was obtained and sent to the laboratory to be cultured. A portable chest radiograph revealed a new infiltrate in the right lower lobe consistent with pneumonia or atelectasis. The ABGs (on FIO_2 0.30, tidal volume 650 mL, respiratory rate of 10, and PEEP of +5) were as follows: pH 7.28, $PaCO_2$ 36 mm Hg, HCO_3^- 16 mEq/L, PaO_2 41 mm Hg, and SaO_2 69%. On the basis of these clinical data, the following SOAP was recorded.

Respiratory Assessment and Plan

S N/A
O No improvement seen in muscular paralysis; skin: pale; vital signs: BP 146/88, HR 92, T 37.9 °C (100.2 °F); large amounts of thick, yellowish sputum; coarse crackles over both lung fields; CXR: pneumonia and atelectasis in right lower lobe; ABGs: pH 7.28, $PaCO_2$ 36, HCO_3^- 16, PaO_2 41, SaO_2 69%
A • Excessive bronchial secretions (coarse crackles, sputum)
  • Infection likely (yellow sputum, fever, CXR: pneumonia)
  • Metabolic acidosis with moderate-to-severe hypoxemia (ABGs)
  • Acidosis likely caused by lactic acid (ABGs)

P Up-regulate **Bronchopulmonary Hygiene Therapy Protocol** (med. neb. with 0.5 mL albuterol in 2 mL 10% acetylcysteine q4 h; therapist to suction patient frequently; sputum culture check in 24 and 48 hours). Up-regulate **Lung Expansion Therapy Protocol** (+10 cm H_2O PEEP). Up-regulate **Oxygen Therapy Protocol** (increase FIO_2 to 0.60). Monitor closely and reevaluate (check ABGs in 30 minutes).

Discussion

As with the patient with Guillain-Barré syndrome, this case of myasthenia gravis provides another chance to discuss ventilatory failure secondary to neuromuscular disease. The presentation of this patient with double vision (diplopia), difficulty in swallowing (dysphagia), and progressive muscle weakness is classic for this condition. The positive edrophonium test noted in the history was necessary for a final diagnosis. Also important to note is that **aspiration of gastric contents** is not uncommon in such cases.

In the first assessment the therapist should have recognized that this case was more than simple respiratory failure. The reader sees that the patient was intubated and that breath sounds no longer were present in the entire left lung (**inadvertent right main stem bronchus intubation**). The therapist appropriately responded quickly and pulled the endotracheal tube back until breath sounds could be auscultated over both lung fields. The inappropriate positioning of the tube was confirmed 45 minutes later in the patient's chest radiograph. The patient's respiratory status could have been seriously compromised if the therapist had waited a full 45 minutes before pulling the tube above the carina. This event further demonstrates the importance of good bedside assessment skills. In addition, because lactic acidosis was probably present at this time, oxygenating the patient was of primary importance. In fact, increasing the FIO$_2$ to 1.0 would have been appropriate in this case.

The second assessment reflected that the patient was improving and was now hyperventilated and hyperoxygenated on the current ventilator settings. The therapist adjusted the ventilator settings accordingly and began the process of longitudinal evaluation of forced vital capacity and maximum inspiratory pressure so that the Mechanical Ventilation Protocol was appropriate for this condition.

The final assessment suggested that the patient had taken another turn for the worse. The sputum was now purulent, coarse crackles were heard over both lung fields, and a right lower lobe pneumonia or atelectasis had developed. The patient had an uncompensated metabolic acidemia that required evaluation. The fact that the patient's PaO$_2$ was only 41 provided a significant clinical indicator that the cause of the metabolic acidosis was probably lactic acid generated from a low tissue oxygen level. It was clearly appropriate for the respiratory therapist to focus on the patient's oxygenation status. This was done by up-regulating the **Oxygen Therapy Protocol** (Protocol 9-1) (increasing the FIO$_2$ to 0.60) and starting the **Lung Expansion Therapy Protocol** (Protocol 9-3) (the addition of 10 cm H$_2$O PEEP to ventilator settings).

The therapist should have anticipated this development, obtained appropriate cultures, and, if not done before, prophylactically started the **Bronchopulmonary Hygiene Therapy Protocol** (Protocol 9-2) and **Aerosolized Medication Therapy Protocol** (Protocol 9-4)—with frequent suctioning, percussion, postural drainage, and possibly mucolytics. Finally, for a better understanding of **lactic acidosis**, the reader may wish to review other possible causes of metabolic acidemia at this time (e.g., diabetic ketoacidosis, renal failure) (see Chapter 4).

Unfortunately the patient's pulmonary condition progressively deteriorated, and she died 3 weeks later.

SELF-ASSESSMENT QUESTIONS

Answers to questions can be found on Evolve. To access additional student assessment questions visit **http://evolve.elsevier.com/DesJardins/respiratory**.

1. The onset of the signs and symptoms of myasthenia gravis is/are:
   1. Slow and insidious
   2. Sudden and rapid
   3. Intermittent
   4. Often elusive
      a. 1 only
      b. 2 only
      c. 2 and 4 only
      d. 1, 2, 3, and 4

2. Myasthenia gravis
   1. Is more common in young men
   2. Has a peak age of onset in females of 15 to 35 years
   3. Is often provoked by emotional upset and physical stress
   4. Is associated with receptor-binding antibodies
      a. 1 only
      b. 2 and 4 only
      c. 2, 3, and 4 only
      d. 1, 2, 3, and 4

3. Which of the following is associated with myasthenia gravis?
   1. Bronchospasm
   2. Mucous accumulation
   3. Alveolar hyperinflation
   4. Atelectasis
      a. 1 and 2 only
      b. 2 and 4 only
      c. 1, 2, and 4 only
      d. 2, 3, and 4 only

4. When monitoring the patient with myasthenia gravis, ALL of the following are indicators of acute ventilatory failure EXCEPT:
   a. pH: 7.31
   b. PaCO$_2$: 55 mm Hg
   c. FVC: 25 mL/kg
   d. MIP: –15 cm H$_2$O

5. Which of the following antibodies is believed to block the nerve impulse transmissions at the neuromuscular junction in myasthenia gravis?
   a. IgG
   b. IgE
   c. IgA
   d. IgM

Sleep-Related Breathing Disorders—Sleep Apnea

Chapter Objectives

After reading this chapter, you will be able to:

- List the major classifications of sleep disorders.
- Define the commonly used terms and phrases associated with sleep-related disorders.
- Describe the derived measurements used to calculate the frequency of respiratory disturbances during sleep.
- Differentiate between obstructive sleep apnea, central sleep apnea, and mixed sleep apnea.
- Describe the anatomic alterations of the lungs associated with sleep apnea.
- Explain the signs and symptoms associated with obstructive sleep apnea.
- List the common risk factors associated with obstructive sleep apnea.
- Differentiate between hyperventilation-related central sleep apnea and hypoventilation-related sleep apnea.
- Differentiate between the advantages and disadvantages of polysomnography and in-home portable monitoring in the diagnosis of sleep apnea.
- Explain the diagnostic criteria for obstructive and sleep apnea.
- Differentiate between the criteria for mild, moderate, and severe obstructive sleep apnea.
- List the cardiopulmonary clinical manifestations associated with sleep apnea.
- Describe the management of obstructive sleep apnea.
- Describe the management of central sleep apnea.
- Describe the clinical strategies and rationales of the SOAPs presented in the case study.

Key Terms

Adaptive Servo-Ventilation (ASV)
Alpha Wave
Apnea-Hypopnea Index (AHI)
Autotitrating Positive Airway Pressure (APAP)
Basal Metabolic Index
Beta Waves
Bilevel Positive Airway Pressure (BPAP)
Blood Pressure "Dippers" vs "Nondippers"
Brady-Tachy Syndrome
Cardiopulmonary Complications of Sleep Apnea
Central Sleep Apnea (CSA)
Cheyne-Stokes Breathing Pattern
COHb-corrected Oxymetry O_2 Saturation
Confusional Arousals
Continuous Positive Airway Pressure (CPAP)
CPAP Compliance/Adherence
CPAP Titration Polysomnogram
"Crossover Syndrome" (COPD)
Delta Waves

Drug-Induced Sleep Endoscopy (DISE)
Electroencephalogram (EEG)
Electromyogram (EMG)
Electrooculogram (EOG)
Epoch
Epworth Sleepiness Scale
Home Sleep Test (HST)
Hyperventilation-related CSA
Hypopneas
Hypoventilation-related CSA
Implantable Upper-Airway Stimulator
K Complexes
Laser-Assisted Uvulopalatoplasty
Mallampati Classification
Mixed Sleep Apnea
Nocturnal Low-Flow Oxygen Therapy
Non-Rapid Eye Movement (Non-REM) Sleep
Obstructive Apneas
Obstructive Sleep Apnea (OSA)
Oxygen Desaturation Index
Pickwickian Syndrome
Polysomnogram (PSG)
Polysomnography
Positive End-Expiratory Pressure (PEEP)
Primary Central Sleep Apnea
Pulmonary Hypertension
Radiofrequency Ablation
Rapid Eye Movement (REM) Sleep
Respiratory Disturbance Index (RDI)
Respiratory Effort-Related Arousals (RERAs)
Sawtoothed Waves
Secondary Central Sleep Apnea
Sleep Apnea Screening Programs
Sleep Spindles
Sleep Stages
Slow Wave Sleep
Split-Night Polysomnogram
Theta Waves
Total Recording Time (TRT)
Total sleep time (TST)
Tonsilar Hypertophy
Uvulopalatopharyngoplasty (UPPP)
Variable Positive Airway Pressure (VPAP)
Vertex Waves

Chapter Outline

Obstructive Sleep Apnea
Central Sleep Apnea
Mixed Sleep Apnea
Sleep-Related Hypoventilation/Hypoxemia Syndromes

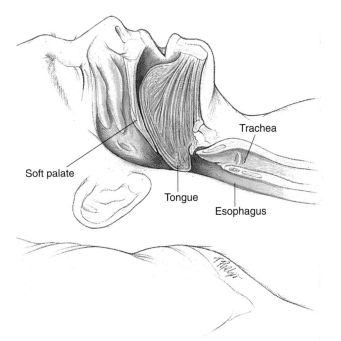

FIGURE 31-1 Obstructive sleep apnea. When the genioglossus muscle fails to oppose the forces that tend to collapse the airway passage during inspiration, the tongue moves into the oropharyngeal area and obstructs the airway.

BOX 31-1 Sleep Disorder Categories

Sleep related breathing disorders
Insomnia
Hypersomnias of central origin
Circadian rhythm sleep disorders
Parasomnias
Sleep related movement disorders
Isolated symptoms and normal variants
Other sleep disorders

Modified from American Academy of Sleep Medicine. *International classification of sleep disorders, 3rd ed: diagnostic and coding manual*, Darien, Illinois, 2014, American Academy of Sleep Medicine.

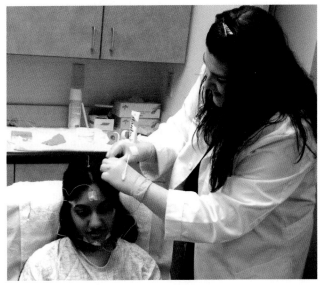

FIGURE 31-2 A sleep disorder specialist (SDS) setting up scalp electrodes on a patient to be studied. While the patient sleeps, the SDS (1) monitors brain waves, eye movements, muscle activity, multiple breathing patterns, and blood oxygen levels using specialized recording equipment, (2) interprets the recordings as they happen and responds appropriately to any emergencies, (3) instructs the patient in recording and maintaining a sleep diary of wake/sleep cycles, and (4) provides support services related to the treatment of sleep-related problems—including helping the patient use various treatment devices for breathing problems during sleep. (Courtesy of George G. Burton, MD, Sleep Disorders Center, Kettering Medical Center, Dayton, Ohio.)

Sleep-related breathing disorders are characterized by abnormal breathing patterns during sleep, and include (1) obstructive sleep apnea (OSA) syndrome (Figure 31-1), (2) central sleep apnea syndrome, (3) mixed sleep apnea, and (4) sleep-related hypoventilation/hypoxemia syndromes. According to the **American Academy of Sleep Medicine (AASM)**,[1] sleep disorders can be classified into eight major groups (Box 31-1). Of particular interest to the respiratory therapist is the category of **sleep-related breathing disorders** and, importantly, the ability to pursue additional education, training, and finally, certification through **the National Board for Respiratory Care**, or the **Board Registered Polysomnographic Technologist (RPSGT)**[2] as a **sleep disorder specialist (SDS)** (Figure 31-2). Table 31-1 provides commonly used terms and phrases associated with sleep-related breathing disorders.

[1]American Academy of Sleep Medicine (AASM) (http://www.aasmnet.org).
[2]National Board for Respiratory Care Inc. (http://www.nbrc.org). Board Registered Polysomnographic Technologist (http://www.brpt.org/).

TABLE 31-1 Common Terms and Phrases Associated with Sleep-Related Breathing Disorders (Sleep Events)

Term and/or Phrase	Definition
Apnea	The cessation, or near cessation, of airflow. Apnea exists when airflow is less than 10% of pre-event baseline for at least 10 seconds in adults. Apneas can be associated with arousals from sleep, increased arterial carbon dioxide, and decreased oxygen levels.
Obstructive apnea	Airflow is absent or nearly absent, but ventilatory effort persists. It is caused by complete, or near complete, upper airway obstruction.
Central apnea	The absence of both airflow and ventilatory efforts (i.e., diaphragmatic contraction as measured by electromyography and esophageal manometry).
Mixed apnea	A period of time during which there is no ventilatory effort (i.e., central apnea pattern) followed by a period of time during which there are obstructed respiratory efforts (obstructive apnea pattern).
Hypopnea	Is present when the following three criteria are present: • Airflow decreased ≥30% from preevent baseline • The decreased airflow lasts ≥10 seconds • The decreased airflow is accompanied by ≥3% SpO_2 desaturation from preevent baseline or an arousal.*
Obstructive hypopnea	Is present when any of the following occur: • Snoring during the event • Increased inspiratory flattening of the nasal pressure waveform or airflow compared to baseline • An associated thoracoabdominal paradox during the event but not during preevent breathing.
Central hypopnea	The hypopnea is called central when none of the three criteria for obstructive hypopnea (snoring, increased inspiratory flattening of nasal pressure waveform, or thoracoabdominal paradox) is present during the event.
Arousals	Arousals range from full awakenings to 3-second transient electroencephalography shifts to a lighter stage of sleep (alpha, theta, and/or frequencies >16 Hz (but not sleep spindles) with at least 10 seconds of stable sleep preceding the change.
Respiratory Effort Related Arousal (RERAs)	Said to be present when: 1. There are a series of ventilatory patterns that have a duration of ≥10 seconds 2. The ventilatory pattern is characterized by increasing ventilatory effort or flattening of the nasal pressure waveform, followed by an arousal from sleep, and 3. The ventilatory patterns do not meet the criteria for an apnea or hypopnea. 4. RERAs are often associated with a terminal snort or an abrupt change in ventilatory measures.
Hypoventilation	An increase in the arterial carbon dioxide ($PaCO_2$) to a value >55 mm Hg for at least 10 minutes, or a ≥10 mm Hg rise in the $PaCO_2$ during sleep (compared with awake supine level) above the patient's normal $PaCO_2$ level, exceeding 50 mm Hg for at least 10 minutes.
Cheynes-Stokes breathing	At least three consecutive central apneas and/or central hypopneas, followed by crescendo-decrescendo breathing—with a cycle length (i.e., time from the beginning of a central apnea, or hypopnea to the beginning of the next apnea or hypopnea) of at least 40 seconds. In addition, there must be at least five apneas or hypopneas per hour associated with the crescendo-decrescendo breathing pattern.

*Previous definitions endorsed by the American Academy of Sleep Medicine (AASM), and still used by the Centers for Medicare and Medicaid Services, use a 4% cutoff for SpO_2 desaturation.

Table 31-2 shows derived measurements used to determine the frequency of respiratory disturbances during sleep. Based on the type and frequency of the respiratory events, the following syndromes of sleep-related breathing disorders can be established:

Obstructive Sleep Apnea

OSA is a common sleep disorder that often requires lifelong care. Cardinal features include **obstructive apneas,** **hypopneas,** and **respiratory effort-related arousals (RERAs)**, which are caused by recurring collapse of the upper airway during sleep (see Figure 31-1). During periods of airway obstruction, patients commonly appear quiet and still, as though they are holding their breath, followed by increasingly desperate efforts to inhale. Often the apneic episode ends only after an intense struggle. A snorting sound called "fricative breathing" may be heard at the end of the apneic periods. In severe cases, the patient may suddenly awaken, sit upright in bed, and gasp for air. Patients with

TABLE 31-2 Derived Measurements Used to Calculate The Frequency of Respiratory Disturbances during Sleep

Measures	Definition
Apnea index (AI)	The total number of apneas per hour of sleep.
Apnea Hypopnea Index (AHI)	The total number of apneas and hypopneas calculated per hour of total sleep. The AHI may also be calculated per hour of non- rapid eye movement (REM) sleep, per hour of REM sleep, or per hour of sleep in a certain position. The AHI may provide information regarding the sleep stage dependency, or sleep position dependency, of the sleep-related breathing disorder.
Respiratory Disturbance Index (RDI)	The total number of events (e.g., apneas, hypopneas, and RERAs) per hour of sleep. The RDI is usually greater than the AHI. This is because the RDI includes the frequency of RERAs; the AHI does not.
Oxygen desaturation (SpO$_2$)	The drop in hemoglobin oxygenation caused by periods of apnea and hypopnea. Serial measurements are normally used to quantify the severity of the desaturation and should be included on the polysomnogram report.
Oxygen Desaturation Index (ODI)	The total time that the oxygen saturation falls by more than 3 percentage points per hour of sleep, or of total recording time.
Arousal index (ArI)	The total number of arousals per hour of sleep.
Total sleep time (TST)	The total duration of light sleep (stages N1 and N2), deep sleep (stage N3), and REM sleep.
Total recording time (TRT)	The total duration of recording time only.
Sleep efficiency (SE)	The TST divided by the total recording time (i.e., time in bed).
Sleep stage percentage (SSP)	The duration of a particular stage divided by the TST.
Sleep stage latency	The duration from the onset of sleep to the initiation of any stage of sleep.

OSA usually demonstrate perfectly normal and regular breathing patterns when awake.

In fact, a large number of patients with OSA demonstrate what is commonly called the **Pickwickian syndrome** (named after a character in Charles Dickens' *The Posthumous Papers of the Pickwick Club*, published in 1837). Dickens' description of Joe, "the fat boy" who snored and had excessive daytime sleepiness, included many of the classic features of what is now recognized as sleep apnea syndrome with hypercapnia, or the obesity hypoventilation syndrome. It should be noted, however, that many patients with sleep apnea are not obese, and therefore clinical suspicion should not be limited to this group. Box 31-2 provides common signs and symptoms associated with OSA. Table 31-3 provides the more common risk factors associated with OSA.

Central Sleep Apnea

Central sleep apnea (CSA) is a disorder characterized by the repetitive stopping or reduction of both airflow and ventilatory effort during sleep. CSA can be classified as **primary CSA** (idiopathic or unknown cause) or **secondary CSA**. Examples of conditions associated with secondary CSA include Cheyne-Stokes breathing (congestive heart failure), medical conditions (e.g., encephalitis, brain stem neoplasm, brain stem infarction, spinal surgery, hypothyroidism, drug or substance abuse), and high-altitude periodic breathing. CSA is further categorized as either (1) **hyperventilation-related CSA** or (2) **hypoventilation-related CSA**.

BOX 31-2 Signs and Symptoms Associated with Obstructive Sleep Apnea

Loud snoring
Observed episodes of breathing cessation during sleep
Abrupt awakenings accompanied by shortness of breath
Difficulty staying asleep (insomnia)
Moodiness or irritability
Lack of concentration
Memory impairment
Awakening with a dry mouth or sore throat
Morning headache
Nausea
Excessive daytime sleepiness (hypersomnia)
Intellectual and personality changes
Depression
Nocturnal enuresis
Sexual impotence
Night sweats

Hyperventilation-related CSA is the most common. It includes primary CSA and CSA associated with **Cheyne-Stokes breathing** (see Table 2-4), medical conditions such as congestive heart failure, or high-altitude periodic breathing. Patients with hyperventilation-related CSA develop alternating cycles of apnea—or hypopneas—with hyperpnea (i.e., increased rate and depth of breathing) during sleep. As a result, this condition produces a sequence of abnormal

TABLE 31-3 Risk Factors Associated with Obstructive Sleep Apnea

Excess weight	More than 50% of patients diagnosed with obstructive sleep apnea (OSA) are overweight. Fat deposits around the upper airway may obstruct breathing.
Neck size	OSA is often seen in patients with a large neck size. A neck circumference >17 inches in males and >16 inches in females increases the risk for OSA.
Hypertension	OSA is commonly seen in patients with high blood pressure.
Anatomic narrowing of upper airway	Common causes of anatomic narrowing of the upper airway include excessive pharyngeal tissue, **tonsilar hypertrophy** or adenoids, deviated nasal septum, laryngeal stenosis, vocal cord dysfunction, and a Mallampati classification score of 3 or 4 (see Figure 31-4).
Chronic nasal congestion	OSA occurs twice as often in patients with chronic nasal congestion from any cause.
Diabetes	Patients with diabetes are three times more likely to have OSA than persons who do not have diabetes.
Male sex	Men are twice as likely to have OSA as women.
Age older than 65 years	OSA is two to three times greater in people older than 65 years.
Age under 35 years, and black, Hispanic, or Pacific Islander heritage	Among individuals under the age of 35, the incidence of OSA is greater in blacks, Hispanics, and Pacific Islanders.
Menopause	The risk of OSA is greater after menopause.
Family history of sleep apnea	Individuals who have one or more family members with OSA are also at greater risk for developing it.
Alcohol, sedatives, or tranquilizers	Depressive agents relax the muscles of the upper airway.
Smoking	Smokers are almost three times more likely to develop OSA.

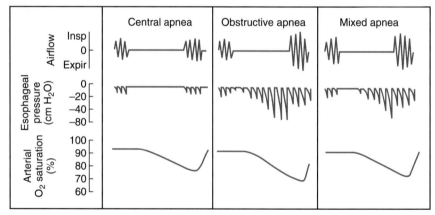

FIGURE 31-3 Patterns of airflow, respiratory efforts (reflected through the esophageal pressure), and arterial oxygen saturation produced by central, obstructive, and mixed apneas.

respiratory events—including periods of ventilatory overshoot, hypocapnia, central apnea, hypercapnia, and recurrent hyperpnea.

Hypoventilation-related CSA is usually a secondary problem related to an underlying condition, such as a central nervous system disease, central nervous system-suppressing drugs or substances (e.g., alcohol, opiates, barbiturates, benzodiazepines, and various tranquilizers), neuromuscular disease (e.g., Guillain-Barré syndrome or myasthenia gravis), or severe disorders of pulmonary mechanics (e.g., chronic obstructive pulmonary disease [COPD], pulmonary fibrosis). During sleep, the patient no longer has the wakefulness stimulus to breathe and, as a result, alveolar hypoventilation and central apnea occur. The patient's breathing is restored

during arousal from sleep, but again decreases when sleep resumes—resulting in cyclic periods of normal ventilation, hypoventilation, and apnea. The choice of therapy is based on whether the patient's central apneas are hyperventilation- or hypoventilation-related (see Management of Sleep Apnea, page 432).

Mixed Sleep Apnea

Mixed sleep apnea is a combination of OSA and CSA. It usually *begins* as central apnea followed by the onset of ventilatory effort without airflow (obstructive apnea). Clinically, patients with predominantly mixed apnea are classified (and treated) as having OSA. Figure 31-3 illustrates the patterns of airflow, respiratory effort (reflected in this illustration through the esophageal pressure tracing), and arterial oxygen saturation in central, obstructive, and mixed apneas. Respiratory effort is classically measured from "effort detections" around the thorax and/or abdomen. *It is essential that the respiratory therapist recognize the differences among these three entities.*

Sleep-Related Hypoventilation/ Hypoxemia Syndromes

Sleep-related hypoventilation/hypoxemia syndromes (SRHHSs) include a broad range of sleep disorders. Some are quite common, such as obesity hypoventilation syndrome (also known as **Pickwickian syndrome**) or co-existing with COPD, the so-called "**crossover syndrome.**" Others are rather rare, such as congenital central hypoventilation syndrome and neuromuscular and chest wall disorders. However, all share the characteristic of abnormal gas exchange that worsens, or may only be present during sleep or sedation. Such abnormalities are usually caused by hypoventilation and result in hypercapnia and hypoxemia. Pulmonary disorders, such as chronic bronchitis or emphysema, are not considered "stand-alone" sleep-related breathing disorders. However, they are known to cause hypoventilation—and hypercapnia and hypoxemia—during sleep. In these cases, the diagnosis of sleep-related hypoventilation/hypoxemia should be considered. Unfortunately, the diagnosis of the crossover syndrome is often missed in critically ill, hospitalized patients.

Diagnosis

The diagnosis of sleep apnea begins with a comprehensive sleep evaluation, which includes a history from the patient and/or the patient's bed partner, especially noting the presence of snoring, sleep fragmentation, periods of apnea during sleep, nonrefreshing sleep, and persistent daytime sleepiness. The **Epworth Sleepiness scale** is routinely used as a validated measure of daytime sleepiness. Sleepiness must be differentiated from fatigue, which can be semi-quantitated with the use of the Fatigue Severity Scale (FSS) or the Visual Analogue Fatigue Scale (VAFS). This is followed by a careful examination of the upper airway and perhaps by pulmonary function studies (especially by analysis of the flow-volume loop) to determine whether upper airway obstruction is present. Abnormalities in the posterior pharynx include a large uvula, enlarged tonsils, a long soft palate, redundant lateral pharyngeal walls, macroglossia (enlarged tongue), and the presence of an overbite of the upper teeth with a posterior placement of the mandible. The **Mallampati classification** score is frequently used in physician notes to describe abnormalities of the soft palate and uvula (Figure 31-4).

The patient's blood may be evaluated for the presence of polycythemia, reduced thyroid function, and bicarbonate retention. Arterial blood gas (ABG) values may be obtained to determine resting, wakeful oxygenation, and acid-base status. When possible, a carboxyhemoglobin level should be obtained. It should be noted that the pulse oximeter used routinely in polysomnography assumes that the patient

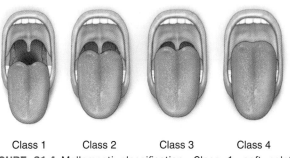

| Class 1 | Class 2 | Class 3 | Class 4 |

FIGURE 31-4 Mallampati classification. Class 1, soft palate, fauces, uvula, pillars are easily seen. Class 2, soft palate, fauces, portion of uvula are seen. Class 3, soft palate, only the base of uvula are seen. Class 4, only the hard palate is seen.

has normal hemoglobin, PaO_2, and SpO_2 relationships. If carboxyhemoglobin is present, it should be subtracted from the pulse oximeter reading. For example, if the pulse oximeter gives an SpO_2 of 90% and the patient has 7% carboxyhemoglobin, the true **COHb-corrected oximetry** O_2 saturation would be 83% (90% − 7% = 83%). A chest x-ray, electrocardiogram (ECG), and echocardiogram are helpful in evaluating the presence of pulmonary hypertension, the state of right and left ventricular compensation, cardiac arrhythmias, and the presence of any other cardiopulmonary disease.

Finally, in patients suspected of having sleep apnea, the diagnosis and type of sleep apnea are confirmed by one of the following methods:

- Polysomnography
- In-home portable monitoring

These diagnostic methods are discussed in more detail below.

Polysomnography

Polysomnography (PSG) is a specialized sleep test that monitors and records a number of physiologic parameters that occur during sleep. The test result is called a polysomnogram (which is also abbreviated PSG). The **PSG** may be administered as either (1) a **full-night, attended, in-laboratory polysomnograph** or (2) a **split-night, attended, in-laboratory polysomnograph**. The *full-night, attended, in-laboratory PSG* is considered the gold-standard diagnostic test for OSA. It is performed on selected patients overnight in a sleep laboratory with a technologist (i.e., SDS) in attendance.

In a *split-night, attended, in-laboratory PSG*, the diagnosis of OSA is established during the first portion of the study, followed by a form of positive airway pressure (CPAP, BPAP, VPAP) treatment—called a CPAP (or BPAP or VPAP) **titration polysomnogram**. The positive airway pressure is applied to prevent upper airway obstruction or central apneas during sleep for the remaining time. This test is both diagnostic and therapeutic. Because of the perceived cost-effectiveness, there is a growing trend to perform split-night studies, if the patient's total sleep time allows.

Table 31-4 provides the physiologic variables that are *required*, and recommended, by the AASM during a PSG. Table 31-5 illustrates the stages of sleep recorded during a PSG. Each sleep stage is associated with characteristic EEG, electrooculogram, electromyogram, behavioral, and breathing patterns. Figure 31-5 provides a representative period of a

TABLE 31-4 Required and Recommended Physiologic Variables to be Measured by Polysomnography (According to the American Academy of Sleep Medicine)

Required Physiologic Variable	Description
Sleep stages	Measured and recorded via (1) an **electroencephalogram (EEG)**, which measures the electrophysiologic changes in the brain; (2) an **electrooculogram (EOG)**, which records the movements of the eyes; (3) an **electromyogram (EMG)**, which monitors muscle activity (see Table 31-5).
Respiratory efforts	Although an esophageal manometry is considered the gold standard for assessing respiratory effort, it not routinely used because placement of the esophageal manometer is invasive. The American Academy of Sleep Medicine recommends the noninvasive method of *respiratory inductive plethysmography* and *electromyography*. Strain gauges, piezo electrodes, or impedance devices spread across the chest wall and abdomen are also acceptable options.
Airflow	Measured via nasal prongs connected to a pressure transducer that detects inspiratory flow. Because the pressure transducer is unable to sense airflow through the mouth, a thermistor is added to detect airflow at the mouth by sensing alterations in heat exchange. Thus the nasal pressure transducer is able to identify hypopneas (decreased airflow), and the thermistor can diagnose apneas.
Snoring	Measured via a microphone placed at the neck to detect the presence or absence of snoring.
Pulse oximetry (SpO$_2$)	Measures the oxyhemoglobin saturation continuously during the polysomnogram.
Electrocardiogram	Detects arrhythmias during sleep. Lead II alone is preferred.
Recommended Physiologic Variable	
Body position	In some patients, the body position can cause abnormal breathing patterns. Thus the monitoring of the patient's body position (supine, left lateral, right lateral, and prone) with a position sensor and/or video monitor may be helpful.
Limb movements	An electromyogram of the anterior tibialis of both legs and arms may be monitored to detect leg movements.

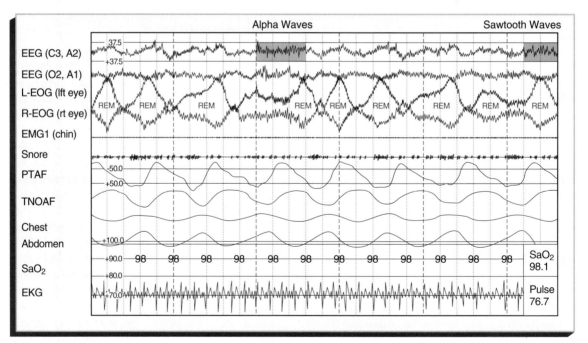

FIGURE 31-5 A 30-second epoch of rapid eye movement (REM) sleep (each vertical line equals 1 second), resembling the eyes open-wake epoch. The electroencephalogram records low-voltage, mixed electroencephalographic activity and frequent saw-toothed waves (*brown bar*). Alpha waves may be present (*purple bar*). The electrooculogram (EOG) records REM. The electromyogram (EMG) records low electrical activity and documents a temporary paralysis of most of the skeletal muscles (e.g., arms, legs). The breathing rate increases and decreases irregularly. During REM sleep, the heart rate becomes inconsistent, with episodes of increased and decreased rates. Snoring may or may not be present. REM is not as restful as non-REM sleep. REM is also known as *paradoxical sleep*. Most dreams occur during REM sleep. *PTAF*, Pneumotachograph air flow; *TNOAF*, thermistor nasal/oral air flow; SaO$_2$, oximetry.

TABLE 31-5 Stages of Sleep and Electroencephalogram Waveforms

Stage	Electroencephalogram (EEG)	Characteristics
Eyes open-wake (Stage W)		The EEG shows **beta waves** and high-frequency, low-amplitude activity. The electrooculogram looks very similar to rapid eye movement (REM) sleep waves—low-amplitude, mixed-frequency, and sawtoothed waves. Electromyogram activity is relatively high.
Eyes closed-wake (drowsy)		The EEG is characterized by prominent **alpha waves** (>50%). The electrooculogram shows slow, rolling eye movements, and electromyogram activity is relatively high.
Non-REM Sleep Stage N1 (light sleep)	Vertex Waves	The EEG shows low-voltage, mixed-frequency activity, **alpha waves** (8-12 Hz <50%), and **theta waves**. Some **beta waves** (>13 Hz) may also appear. Vertex waves commonly appear toward the end of Stage N1. The **electrooculogram** shows slow, rolling eye movements. The electromyogram reveals decreased activity and muscle relaxation. Respirations become regular, and heart rate and blood pressure decrease slightly. Snoring may occur. If awakened, the person may state that he or she was not asleep.
Stage N2 (light sleep)	K Complex	The EEG becomes more irregular and is composed predominantly of **theta waves** (4-7 Hz), intermixed with sudden bursts *of sleep spindles* (12-18 Hz), and one or more **K complexes**. **Vertex waves** may also be seen during this stage. The electrooculogram shows either slow eye movements or absence of slow eye movements. The electromyogram has low electrical activity. The heart rate, blood pressure, respiratory rate, and temperature decrease slightly. Snoring may occur. If awakened, the person may say he or she was thinking or daydreaming.
Stage N3 (**slow wave sleep**)	Medium Sleep	EEG shows 20% to 50% **delta waves**. Both **sleep spindles** and **K complexes** may be present. The electrooculogram shows little or no eye movement, and the electromyogram activity is low. Heart rate, blood pressure, respiratory rate, body temperature, and oxygen consumption continue to decrease. Snoring may occur. Dreaming may occur, and the sleeper becomes more difficult to arouse.
Stage N3 (Deep sleep)		EEG shows more than 50% **delta waves**. The electrooculogram shows no eye movements, and the electromyogram has little or no electrical activity. The sleeper is very relaxed and seldom moves. The vital signs reach their lowest, normal level. Oxygen consumption is low. The patient is very difficult to awaken. Bed-wetting, night terrors, and sleepwalking may occur.
REM Sleep	Saw-Tooth Waves	About 90 minutes into the sleep cycle, there is an abrupt EEG pattern change. The EEG pattern resembles the wakeful state with low-amplitude, mixed frequency EEG activity. **Sawtoothed waves** are frequent and **alpha waves** may be seen. The respiratory rate increases, and respiration is irregular and shallow. The heart rate and blood pressure increase. REM occurs, and there is paralysis of most skeletal muscles. Most dreams occur during REM sleep.

sleep study **PSG** (called an **epoch**) of REM sleep. Box 31-3 shows the diagnostic criteria for OSA. Box 31-4 provides the criteria for mild, moderate, and severe OSA.

Diagnosis of CSA

CSA is diagnosed when the majority of the respiratory events are central apnea or hypopneas. On the PSG, there is an absence of nasal or oral airflow *and* thoracoabdominal movements. Patients diagnosed with CSA are evaluated carefully for the presence of cardiac disease and lesions involving the cerebral cortex and the brain stem. Atrial fibrillation is also associated with CSA. The treatment for CSA depends on its specific cause.

In-home, Unattended, Portable Monitoring

The AASM endorses *in-home, unattended, portable monitoring* —commonly called a **home sleep test (HST)**—as a reasonable alternative for patients who have a high likelihood of either moderate or severe OSA. According to their guidelines, an HST for the diagnosis of OSA should only be performed in conjunction with a comprehensive clinical sleep evaluation —supervised by a practitioner with board certification in sleep medicine or eligible for the sleep medicine certification examination. Box 31-5 reviews the advantages and disadvantages of in-home, unattended, portable monitoring.

Over the past several years, the effectiveness of the in-laboratory PSG vs the HST has stimulated much debate. Some have argued that many of the advantages of HST— such as that it can be performed in the comfort of the patient's home, it can diagnose moderate or severe OSA, and it is more cost-effective—justify its use. Others counter that the quality of the HST can often be compromised—resulting in erroneous, misleading, or completely missed diagnostic information.

For example, in some cases the HST monitors consist of electrodes that are actually placed on the patient in the sleep laboratory by a polysomnographic technician, and then the patient is sent home; in other cases the electrodes are shipped to the patient's home, with instructions on how to attach them to the body—a process that can often be problematic. In addition, the standard HST only records the snoring noise, nasal airflow, pulse rate, chest or abdominal effort, and oximetry. Because of these limitations, there are many significant sleep disorders that can easily be missed. Box 31-6 lists sleep disorders not readily diagnosed with HST devices.

Another significant limitation of HST devices is that an EEG is not recorded—thus sleep staging and scoring are not possible. The HST surrogate for **total sleep time (TST)** is the **total recording time (TRT)**. Thus in the HST the SDS must calculate a **respiratory disturbance index (RDI)** instead of an **apnea-hypopnea index (AHI)** as shown below:

BOX 31-5 In-Home Portable Monitoring

Advantages

It can be done in the patient's home and/or in areas without ready access to sleep centers

Convenience

Patient acceptance

Easily can be performed over multiple nights

Decreased cost

Disadvantages

Absence of a trained technologist to correct and clarify recording artifacts, and to make ongoing equipment adjustments

Inability to intervene in medically unstable patients

Possible data loss or distortion

The potential for interpretation errors due to limited data

Inability to perform subsequent multiple sleep latency testing according to standard protocol

Varied sensor technology

No published standards for scoring or interpretation

Physiologic Measurement Limitations of the Portable Monitor Compared to Polysomnogram (PSG):

PSG (type I) (in-lab studies) has

- Electroencephalogram, measures arousals and true sleep
- Electrooculogram
- Electromyogram (chin and limbs)
- Electrocardiogram—rate, rhythm, and morphology
- Respiratory effort at thorax and abdomen
- Airflow from nasal cannula thermistor or CO_2 detector
- Pulse oximetry
- Addition channels for continuous positive airway pressure /bilevel positive airway pressure levels, CO_2, etc.

Portable monitoring (home sleep test) (type III)

- Respiratory movement
- Airflow (and snoring)
- Electrocardiogram (rate only)
- Pulse oximetry

BOX 31-6 Sleep Disorders That Cannot Be Diagnosed with Home (Portable) Sleep Testing Devices

- Type of sleep apnea (obstructive vs central vs mixed)
- Insomnia (approximately 30% to 35% of insomnia patients may need polysomnogram)
- Nocturnal seizure disorders
- Narcolepsy/hypersomnia
- Periodic limb movement disorder
- Nocturnal cardiac arrhythmias (home sleep test only measures heart rate)
- Rapid eye movement (REM) and position-dependent sleep apnea syndrome
- REM behavior disorder
- Other parasomnias, such as sleep walking, sleep talking, and **confusional arousals**

For the in-lab sleep study, the calculation is:

$$AHI = \frac{\text{number of apneas and hypopneas}}{\text{TST (hours)}}$$

Example: If there are 100 apneas and hypopneas in a measured total sleep time of 8.0 hours, the AHI would be 12.5/hour (100 ÷ 8.0 = 12.5)

Whereas in the HST, the calculation is:

$$RDI = \frac{\text{number of apneas and hypopneas}}{\text{TST (hours)}}$$

A true measure of sleep time is not available in the HST. The patient may sleep for a very short time, but be recorded for a long time. As a result, the patient's RDI can often be falsely low. Thus the HST can lead to miscalculations in estimating the severity of the patient's sleep-disordered breathing problems. It should not be used in patients with comorbidities such as cardiopulmonary disease, seizure disorders, etc.[3]

---

[3]The HST device was originally proposed for use in remote, medically underserved areas and as a screening device for hospitalized, critically ill patients, such as those with COPD and congestive heart failure. Much of the insurance industry, in the meantime, has seized on HST as the new gold standard for sleep diagnostic testing, which has paradoxically reduced access to sleep medicine services in many locations—because, in short, the insurance industry has made "prior authorization" for PSGs extremely time-consuming and tedious. Despite all this, HST has indeed become the "preferred" diagnostic sleep study—at least by the insurance industry—in patients with a high probability of moderate or severe OSA.

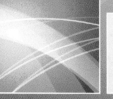

OVERVIEW of the Cardiopulmonary Clinical Manifestations Associated with Sleep Apnea

CLINICAL DATA OBTAINED AT THE PATIENT'S BEDSIDE

The Physical Examination (also see Box 31-2 and Table 31-3)

Apnea or Hypopnea

Cyanosis

CLINICAL DATA OBTAINED FROM LABORATORY TESTS AND SPECIAL PROCEDURES

Pulmonary Function Test Findings

The following findings are expected in patients who are obese or who have congestive heart failure—that is, restrictive pathophysiology.

LUNG VOLUME AND CAPACITY FINDINGS

V_T	IRV	ERV*	RV	
N or ↓	↓	↓	↓	

VC	IC	FRC	TLC	RV/TLC ratio
↓	↓	↓	↓	N

Obviously, pulmonary function cannot easily be studied during sleep. However, patients with OSA may demonstrate a sawtooth pattern on maximal inspiratory and expiratory flow-volume loops (Figure 31-6). Also characteristic of OSA is a ratio of expiratory-to-inspiratory flow rates at 50% of the vital capacity ($FEF_{50\%}/FIF_{50\%}$) that exceeds 1.0 in the absence of obstructive pulmonary disease.

In addition, because the muscle tone of the intercostal muscles is low during periods of rapid eye movement (REM)-related apneas, the large swings in intrapleural pressure generated by the diaphragm often cause a magnified paradoxical motion of the rib cage—that is, during inspiration the tissues between the ribs move inward, and during expiration they bulge outward. This paradoxical motion of the rib cage may cause the vital capacity (VC), expiratory reserve volume (ERV), functional residual capacity (FRC), and total lung capacity (TLC) to decrease further; i.e., toward restrictive pulmonary function pathophysiology as described above. Along with obesity-related atelectasis, this further contributes to the nocturnal hypoxemia seen in patients with sleep apnea syndrome.

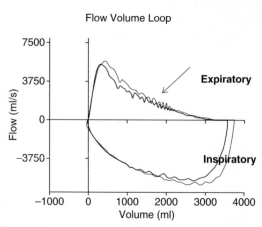

Flow Volume Loop

FIGURE 31-6 Sawtooth pattern. The expiratory limb of the flow volume loop shows fluttering in the midflow portion. This vibratory motion (fluttering) of the soft palate is known as the "sawtooth" sign (see red arrow). The sawtooth pattern may be seen during obstructive sleep apnea (OSA). The arrow highlights the airway fluttering during exhalation. Note similar but less pronounced inspiratory fluttering. Contemporary pulmonary function testing equipment tends to "smooth" the expiratory fluttering that is characteristic of the phenomenon. The absence of sawtoothing does not exclude sleep apnea and neither does its presence rule it in; if present, sawtoothing should prompt a clinician to consider OSA and consider further testing. (From: http://thoracic.org/clinical/sleep/sleep-fragment/pages/fluttering-on-a-flow-volume-loop.php. Charles Atwood, MD, VA Pittsburgh Healthcare System and University of Pittsburgh Medical Center, Pittsburg, Pa.).

Arterial Blood Gases

SEVERE OBSTRUCTIVE SLEEP APNEA

Chronic Ventilatory Failure with Hypoxemia*
(Compensated Respiratory Acidosis)

pH	PaCO₂	HCO₃⁻	PaO₂	SaO₂ or SpO₂
N	↑	↑	↓	↓
	(significantly)			

Acute Ventilatory Changes Superimposed on Chronic Ventilatory Failure†

Because acute ventilatory changes are frequently seen in patients with chronic ventilatory failure, the respiratory therapist must be familiar with—and alert for—the following dangerous ABG findings:

- Acute alveolar hyperventilation superimposed on chronic ventilatory failure—which should further alert the respiratory therapist to record the following important ABG assessment: possible *impending acute ventilatory failure.*

- Acute ventilatory failure (acute hypoventilation) superimposed on chronic ventilatory failure.

*See Figure 4-2 and related discussion for the pH, PaCO₂, and HCO₃⁻ changes associated with chronic ventilatory failure.

†See TABLE 4-7 and related discussion for the pH, PaCO₂, and HCO₃⁻ changes associated with Acute Ventilatory Changes Superimposed on Chronic Ventilatory Failure.

*A decreased ERV is the hallmark of centripetal obesity.

Oxygenation Indices*†
Severe Stage OSA

$\dot{Q}_S/\dot{Q}_T$	DO_2†	$\dot{V}O_2$	$C(a\text{-}\bar{v})O_2$	O_2ER	$S\bar{v}O_2$
↑	↓	N	N	↑	↓

Hemodynamic Indices§
Severe Obstructive Sleep Apnea (with cor pulmonale)

CVP	RAP	$\overline{PA}$	PCWP	CO	SV
↑	↑	↑	N or ↓	N or ↑	N or ↓

SVI	CI	RVSWI	LVSWI	PVR	SVR
↓	↓	↑	↑	↑	↑

Brady-Tachy Syndrome

The presence of upper airway obstruction during apneic episodes often is accompanied by bradycardia and temporary reduction in cardiac output. This is unusual, as hypoxemia usually causes tachycardia. In sleep apnea, oxygen transport ($\dot{Q}_T \times CaO_2 \times 10$) falls, and results in electrocardiographic "brady-tachy syndrome" episodes and swings in heart rate and blood pressure secondary to surges of adrenaline in an attempt to compensate for tissue hypoxia.

The carotid body peripheral chemoreceptors are probably responsible for this response—that is, when ventilation is kept constant or is absent (e.g., during an apneic episode), hypoxic stimulation of the carotid body peripheral chemoreceptors slows the cardiac rate. Therefore it follows that when the lungs are unable to expand (e.g., during periods of obstructive apnea), the depressive effect of the carotid bodies on the heart rate predominates. The increased heart rate noted when ventilation resumes is activated by the excitation of the pulmonary stretch receptors.

Although changes in cardiac output during periods of apnea have been difficult to study, several studies have reported a reduction in cardiac output (about 30%) during periods of

---

*$C(a\text{-}\bar{v})O_2$, Arterial-venous oxygen difference; DO_2, total oxygen delivery; O_2ER, oxygen extraction ratio; $\dot{Q}_S/\dot{Q}_T$, pulmonary shunt fraction; $S\bar{v}O_2$, mixed venous oxygen saturation; $\dot{V}O_2$, oxygen consumption.

†The abnormal oxygenation indices may develop as a result of hypoventilation and/or atelectasis.

†The DO_2 may be normal in patients who have compensated to the decreased oxygenation status with (1) an increased cardiac output, (2) an increased hemoglobin level, or (3) a combination of both. When the DO_2 is normal, the O_2ER is usually normal.

§CO, Cardiac output; CVP, central venous pressure; LVSWI, left ventricular stroke work index; $\overline{PA}$, mean pulmonary artery pressure; PCWP, pulmonary capillary wedge pressure; PVR, pulmonary vascular resistance; RAP, right atrial pressure; RVSWI, right ventricular stroke work index; SV, stroke volume; SVI, stroke volume index; SVR, systemic vascular resistance.

---

apnea, followed by an increase (10% to 15% above controls) after termination of apnea. *Both pulmonary and systemic arterial blood pressures increase in response to the nocturnal oxygen desaturation that develops during periods of sleep apnea.* The magnitude of the *pulmonary hypertension* is related to the severity of the alveolar hypoxia and hypercapnic acidosis. Repetition of these transient episodes of pulmonary hypertension many times a night every night for years may contribute to the development of the right ventricular hypertrophy, cor pulmonale, and eventual cardiac decompensation seen in such patients.

Episodic systemic vasoconstriction secondary to sympathetic adrenergic neural activity is believed to be responsible for the *elevation in systemic blood pressure* that is commonly seen during apneas. In normal individuals, blood pressures drop during sleep, a phenomenon known as **blood pressure dipping**. This often fails to occur in patients with sleep apnea, who are termed **nondippers**. Sleep apnea is now recognized as one of the most frequent and correctable causes of systemic hypertension.

RADIOLOGIC FINDINGS
Chest Radiograph
· Often normal
· Right- or left-sided heart failure

Because of the pulmonary hypertension and polycythemia associated with persistent periods of apnea, right- and/or left-sided heart failure may develop. This condition may be identified as an enlargement of the heart on a chest x-ray or an echocardiogram and may help in diagnosis.

CARDIAC ARRHYTHMIAS
· **Brady-tachy syndrome**
· Sinus arrhythmia
· Sinus bradycardia
· Sinus pauses
· Atrioventricular block (second-degree)
· Premature ventricular contractions
· Supraventricular tachycardia
· Ventricular tachycardia
· Atrial fibrillation
· "Sick sinus" syndrome

In severe cases of sleep apnea, sudden arrhythmia-related death is always possible. Periods of apnea commonly are associated with sinus arrhythmia, sinus bradycardia, and sinus pauses (>2 seconds). The extent of sinus bradycardia is directly related to the severity of the oxygen desaturation. Obstructive apneas usually are associated with the greatest degrees of cardiac slowing. To a lesser extent, atrioventricular heart block (second-degree), premature ventricular contractions, and ventricular tachycardia are also seen. Apnea-related ventricular tachycardia is viewed as a life-threatening event. Atrial fibrillation is extremely common in central sleep apnea.

General Management of Obstructive Sleep Apnea

Once the diagnosis of OSA is confirmed and its severity determined, the patient should be educated about the risk factors, natural history, and long-term consequences of OSA. Importantly, the patient should be warned about the potential danger and consequences of driving or operating other equipment or tools while sleepy. The types of therapy for OSA include the following:

Behavior Modification

Behavior Modification is indicated for all patients who have OSA and modifiable risk factors. Helpful behavior modification areas include weight loss (if overweight or obese), exercise, changing sleep position (e.g., OSA often worsens in the supine position), abstaining from alcohol, and avoidance of certain medications when possible (e.g., medications that inhibit the central nervous system, such as benzodiazepines, benzodiazepine receptor agonists, and barbiturates).

Positive Airway Pressure

Positive airway pressure therapy is considered the first-line therapy for OSA. As discussed earlier, the cause of many cases of OSA is related to (1) an anatomic malconfiguration of the pharynx and (2) the decreased muscle tone that normally develops in the pharynx during REM sleep. When the patient with OSA inhales, the pharyngeal muscles (and surrounding tissues) are sucked inward as a result of the negative airway pressure generated by the contracting diaphragm. Positive airway pressure is useful in preventing the collapse of the hypotonic and obstructed airway and is the standard treatment for most cases of OSA. Positive airway pressure can be delivered as **continuous positive airway pressure (CPAP), bilevel positive airway pressure (BPAP), autotitrating positive airway pressure (APAP),** or **positive endexpiratory pressure (PEEP):**

CPAP—is the most common—and arguably the most effective—treatment for OSA. A CPAP device provides a positive airway pressure at a level that remains constant throughout the ventilatory cycle in a spontaneously breathing patient (Figure 31-7). Figure 31-8 provides a useful protocol algorithm to help improve CPAP adherence in patients with sleep apnea/hypopnea syndrome.[4]

BPAP[5]—with a backup respiratory rate, is often very beneficial in patients with OSA who have frequent apneas and hypopneas during sleep. The backup respiratory rate works to prevent sudden changes in the patient's PaO_2, $PaCO_2$, and pH values (i.e., during periods of apneas or hypopneas, the PaO_2 decreases, the PCO_2 increases, and the pH decreases). The BPAP provides both an adjustable inspiratory positive airway pressure (IPAP) setting and an

---

[4]**CPAP Adherence.** It is estimated that between 30% and 80% of sleep apnea patients are nonadherent to CPAP therapy, when nonadherence is defined as a mean of ≤4 hours of use per night. The mean duration of use is only 3 hours per night—on those nights when it is used—among patients who are nonadherent. The AASM recommends 5 hours per night, every night, for optimal **CPAP compliance.** Even one night without CPAP can diminish the benefits of therapy—which include the number of apneas and hypopneas, and daytime mood and concentration. In short, the patient's use of the CPAP device is both therapeutically critical and problematic. Today, many CPAP devices have downloadable compliance features that provide periodic updates of patient compliance. Objective documentation of the patient's CPAP compliance is increasingly being required by third-party insurance agencies if payment for the CPAP device is to be made. New, evidence-based definitions of compliance and adherence are being evaluated.

[5]BPAP should not be confused with BiPAP®, which is the brand name of a single manufacturer, and is just one of many devices that can be used for BPAP.

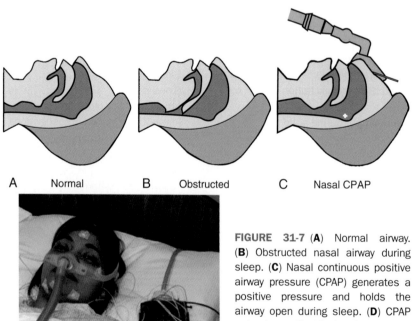

A Normal   B Obstructed   C Nasal CPAP

D

FIGURE 31-7 (A) Normal airway. **(B)** Obstructed nasal airway during sleep. **(C)** Nasal continuous positive airway pressure (CPAP) generates a positive pressure and holds the airway open during sleep. **(D)** CPAP setup in a patient in the sleep center. (Courtesy of George G. Burton, MD, Sleep Disorders Center, Kettering Medical Center, Dayton, Ohio.)

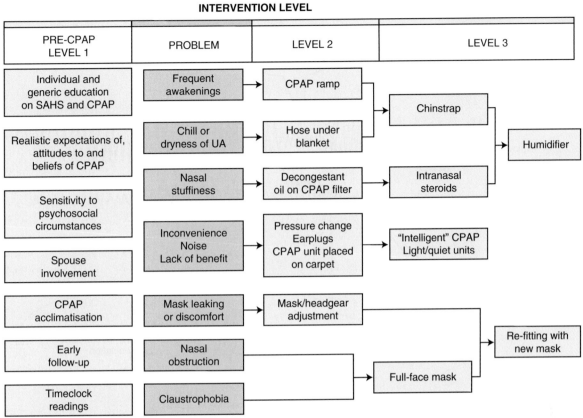

INTERVENTION LEVEL

PRE-CPAP LEVEL 1	PROBLEM	LEVEL 2	LEVEL 3
Individual and generic education on SAHS and CPAP	Frequent awakenings	CPAP ramp	Chinstrap
Realistic expectations of, attitudes to and beliefs of CPAP	Chill or dryness of UA	Hose under blanket	Humidifier
Sensitivity to psychosocial circumstances	Nasal stuffiness	Decongestant oil on CPAP filter	Intranasal steroids
Spouse involvement	Inconvenience Noise Lack of benefit	Pressure change Earplugs CPAP unit placed on carpet	"Intelligent" CPAP Light/quiet units
CPAP acclimatisation	Mask leaking or discomfort	Mask/headgear adjustment	Re-fitting with new mask
Early follow-up	Nasal obstruction		Full-face mask
Timeclock readings	Claustrophobia		

FIGURE 31-8 Protocol algorithm to help improve continuous positive airway pressure adherence. (Modified from Engleman HM, Wild MR. Improving CPAP use by patients with the sleep apnoea/hypopnoea syndrome (SAHS). *Sleep Med Rev* 2003;7:81. Copyright 2003 Elsevier.)

adjustable expiratory positive pressure airway pressure (EPAP) setting. The EPAP portion of BPAP actually functions as a PEEP. BPAP is particularly effective in obese OSA patients who demonstrate CO_2 retention.

APAP—(also called autoPAP) increases or decreases the level of positive airway pressure in response to a change in airflow, a change in circuit pressure, or a vibratory snore. Although APAP has not proven to be more effective than CPAP, patients often prefer it more. The use of APAP is indicated while a formal polysomnographic diagnosis of the precise type of sleep apnea is being made, and thus is of use in hospitalized, not yet fully-diagnosed, patients with sleep apnea.

PEEP—is defined as positive pressure at the end of expiration during either spontaneous breathing or mechanical ventilation. In most cases, however, the term implies that the patient is also receiving mandatory breaths from a ventilator. When PEEP is used for treating OSA, it can be achieved via a disposable nasal device that permits unimpeded inspiration, but provides increased resistance on expiration.

Oral Appliances

Most oral appliances fall under one of the following two categories: a mandibular-repositioning device or a tongue-retaining device. The mandibular-repositioning devices are the most popular. They are designed to reposition the mandible forward and down slightly. The tongue-retaining devices hold the tongue in a more anterior position. Either design works to position the soft tissues of the oropharynx away from the posterior pharyngeal wall.

Surgery

Surgery is most effective in nonobese patients who have OSA due to a severe, surgically correctable, obstructing lesion. For example, tonsillectomy is a reasonable approach in a patient with OSA caused by tonsillar hypertrophy, particularly in children but occasionally in adults. In patients without a strictly defined anatomic lesion, **uvulopalatopharyngoplasty (UPPP)** is one of the most common surgical procedures used to treat snoring and sleep apnea. The posterior third of the soft palate and the uvula are removed. The pillars of the palatoglossal arch and the palatopharyngeal arch are tied together, and the tonsils are removed if present. As much excess lateral posterior wall tissue is removed as possible. The success rate of this type of surgery is 30% to 50%. **Laser-assisted uvulopalatoplasty** and **radiofrequency ablation** are less invasive alternatives to UPPP. Other possible surgical procedures for OSA include septoplasty, rhinoplasty, nasal turbinate reduction, nasal polypectomy, palatal advancement pharyngoplasty, adenoidectomy, palatal implants, tongue reduction (partial glossectomy, lingual tonsillectomy), genioglossus advancement, and maxillomandibular advancement.

Implantable Upper-Airway Stimulator

Recently, studies have shown the effectiveness of an implantable device that stimulates the hypoglossal nerve (XII), which in turn activates the genioglossal muscle (the tongue) to

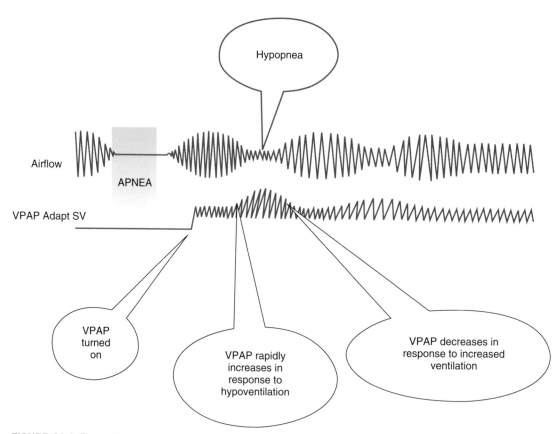

FIGURE 31-9 The variable positive airway pressure (VPAP) adaptive servo-venti responds to apnea by increasing pressure support. Note the progressive dampening of the Cheyne-Stokes cycles with the continued administration of VPAP.

contract and increase the patency of the upper airway. In selected patients who are refractory to CPAP therapy, and in whom complete concentric collapse of the retroplalatal airway can be demonstrated during **Drug-Induced Sleep Endoscopy (DISE)**, this technique shows promise.

General Management of Central Sleep Apnea

For all patients diagnosed with CSA, the initial treatment is directed at the conditions that may be causing the sleep apnea (e.g., congestive heart failure, encephalitis, or brain stem neoplasm). If the CSA continues after such therapy, management is then based on whether the patient has **hyperventilation-related CSA** or **hypoventilation-related CSA**.

Management of Hyperventilation-Related CSA (the most common)

Positive Airway Pressure Therapy

Similar to OSA, CPAP has customarily been the first-line therapy for patients with hyperventilation-related CSA.

Patients who do not respond well to CPAP should receive a trial of **adaptive servo-ventilation (ASV)** with the **variable positive airway pressure adapt (VPAP Adapt)**.[6] ASV provides ventilator support to treat all forms of CSA, mixed

apnea, and periodic breathing (Cheyne-Stokes respiration). The VPAP Adapt responds by increasing pressure support during a central event when the patient's minute ventilation falls below his or her target ventilation (which is 90% of the patient's minute ventilation). To determine the degree of pressure support, the ASV algorithm continuously calculates target ventilation. The algorithm uses the following three factors to achieve synchronization between the needed pressure support and the patient's breathing pattern:

1. The patient's recent average respiratory rate, including the inspiratory-expiratory ratio (I:E) and the time of any expiratory pause.
2. The instantaneous direction of airflow, magnitude, and rate of change of airflow that are measured at specific points during each breath.
3. A backup respiratory rate of 15 breaths/min.

The ASV ensures that ventilator support is synchronized with the patient's ventilatory efforts by means of numbers 1 and 2 above. When the patient experiences an episode of central apnea or hypopnea, the pressure support initially works to reflect the patient's recent pattern. However, if the apnea or hypopnea persists, the ASV increases the backup respiratory rate (number 3 above). Figure 31-9 illustrates this. ASV is often the preferred therapy for patients with hyperventilation-related CSA.

For patients who do not tolerate CPAP or ASV, a trial period of BPAP with a backup ventilator rate is suggested before abandoning positive airway pressure therapy. The use of BPAP is only recommended for patients with

[6]From ResMed Corporation; www.resmed.com.

hyperventilation-related CSA after CPAP and ASV has failed. BPAP in these patients should only be used with a backup respiratory rate. This is because BPAP, with a set rate, may overventilate the patient during periods of normal breathing or hyperpnea, causing discomfort and arousals. It can even cause more CSA events.

Management of Hypoventilation-Related CSA

BPAP, with a backup respiratory rate, is the first-line therapy for patients with hypoventilation-related CSA. Most patients with ventilatory failure tolerate BPAP well.

Other Treatments for Sleep Apnea

Oxygen Therapy

Because of the hypoxemia-related **cardiopulmonary complications of sleep apnea** (arrhythmias and pulmonary hypertension), **nocturnal low-flow oxygen therapy** is sometimes used alone to offset or minimize the oxygen desaturation (see Oxygen Therapy Protocol, Protocol 9-1). The reasoning behind the use of nasal oxygen therapy's effectiveness is that the airway is continually "flooded" with oxygen, which will be inspired during the nonapneic episodes—in effect, "pre-oxygenating" the patient in anticipation of the apnea events. Usually, no improvement in sleep fragmentation or hypersomnolence occurs with the use of supplemental oxygen.

All of the positive airway pressure devices listed in the forgoing section generally use room air as the airway-distending gas. Supplemental oxygen can be "bled" into any of them, if device-related manipulations of inspiratory and expiratory pressure and backup rate fail to adequately oxygenate the patient.

Pharmacologic Therapy

In any patient who does not tolerate or benefit from positive airway pressure or supplemental oxygen during sleep, a respiratory stimulant such as acetazolamide or theophylline may be tried, though the results are extremely variable.

CASE STUDY Obstructive Sleep Apnea

Admitting History

A 55-year-old white man with a history of moderate-to-severe COPD had been in the US Marine Corps for more than 25 years when he retired with honors at 46 years of age with the rank of sergeant. He had completed tours in Vietnam, Grenada, and Beirut. His last assignment had been in Iraq and Kuwait during Operation Desert Storm. During his military career he had received several medals, including a Purple Heart for a leg wound that he incurred in Vietnam when he pulled a fellow Marine to safety. During his last 3 years in the service, he had been assigned to a desk job, working with new recruits as they progressed through boot camp.

Although retirement was not mandatory, he felt that "it was time." He had gained a great deal of weight over the years, and his ability to meet the physical challenge of being a Marine had become progressively more difficult. In addition, when he was doing paperwork at his office, he had become aware that he was "catnapping" while on the job. He knew that if he had observed a fellow Marine doing the same, he would have been quick to issue a severe reprimand. In view of these developments, he regretfully retired from the service.

For a few years after he retired, he continued to work for the Marines as a volunteer at a local recruitment office. At first he had enjoyed this job a great deal. He often found that his military experiences enhanced his ability to talk in a meaningful way to new recruits. Over the past few years, however, working had become progressively more difficult for him, and his attendance had become increasingly sporadic.

He was often tardy. He told the other recruitment volunteers that he was always tired and was experiencing severe morning headaches. His coworkers frequently found him irritable and quick to anger.

The man was having trouble at home, too. Several months before the admission under discussion, his wife had begun sleeping in a room vacated by their daughter. His wife said that she no longer could sleep with her husband because of his loud snoring and constant thrashing in bed. At about this time, he became clinically depressed and sexually impotent. Despite much discussion with and encouragement from his wife, he did not seek medical advice until a few hours before the admission under discussion, when he became extremely short of breath.

Physical Examination

On observation in the Emergency Room, the man appeared to be in severe respiratory distress. He was 5 feet 11 inches tall. He was obese, weighing more than 160 kg (355 lb), and perspiring profusely. His **Basal Metabolic Index** (weight [kg]/height [m²]) was 50. His skin appeared cyanotic, and his neck veins were distended. He had +4 edema of his feet and legs, extending to midcalf. His blood pressure was 164/100, heart rate was 78 beats/min, respiratory rate was 22 breaths/min, and temperature was normal. Although the man was in obvious discomfort, he stated that he was breathing "OK." His wife quickly piped up, "There's that damn Marine coming out again!"

The patient had diminished breath sounds, which were believed to result primarily from his obesity. Palpation of the chest was unremarkable, and percussion was unreliable because of the obesity. A chest radiograph showed cardiomegaly; the lungs appeared unremarkable. To treat the presumed cor pulmonale, the treating physician immediately started the patient on diuretics. His awake ABG values on room air were pH 7.54, $PaCO_2$ 58 mm Hg, HCO_3^- 48 mEq/L, PaO_2 52 mm Hg, and SaO_2 91%.

Because of the patient's history and present clinical manifestations, the emergency room physician diagnosed OSA and requested a full-night, attended, in-laboratory, polysomnographic split study. The physician asked the respiratory therapist to document her assessment.

The following SOAP was charted.

Respiratory Assessment and Plan

S "I'm breathing OK."

O Weight: 160 kg (355 lb); skin: flushed and cyanotic; distended neck veins and edema of feet and legs (4+) to midcalf; vital signs: BP 164/100, HR 78, RR 22, T normal; oropharyngeal examination typical for obstructive sleep apnea; diminished breath sounds, likely because of obesity; chest radiograph: cor pulmonale; lungs appear normal; ABGs (on room air): pH 7.54, $PaCO_2$ 58, HCO_3^- 48, PaO_2 52, SaO_2 91%.

A Obstructive sleep apnea likely (history, cor pulmonale, ABGs, physical appearance).

Acute alveolar hyperventilation superimposed on chronic ventilatory failure with moderate hypoxemia (ABGs and history):
- Impending ventilatory failure

P Place patient on alarming oximeter, set to alarm at 85%. Initiate **Oxygen Therapy Protocol** (venturi oxygen mask at FIO_2 0.24). Monitor and reevaluate (vital signs, ECG, ABGs, and SpO_2 q4h).

Over the Next 72 Hours

A clinical diagnosis of severe OSA was quickly established with a split-night-study PSG the following night. Along with the patient's classic history of OSA, the polysomnogram documented more than 325 periods of obstructive apnea or hypopnea during the study night. His AHI was 64. The CPAP titration polysomnogram indicated that 12 cm H_2O CPAP was required to effectively treat the apneic syndrome. In addition to the patient's short muscular neck and extreme obesity, an oropharyngeal examination revealed a small mouth and large tongue for his body size. The free margin of the soft palate hung low in the oropharynx, nearly obliterating the view behind it (Mallampati class 3). The uvula was widened (4+) and elongated; the tonsillar pillars were widened (3+). Air entry through the nares was reduced bilaterally. The patient's hematocrit was 51%, and hemoglobin level was 17 g/dL.

Results of a complete pulmonary function test showed severe restrictive pulmonary disorder. In addition, a sawtoothed pattern was seen in the maximal inspiratory and expiratory flow-volume loops. A chest x-ray obtained on the patient's second day of hospitalization showed reduced heart size and clear lungs. A brisk diuresis was in process. The patient stated that he was breathing much better.

On inspection the patient no longer appeared short of breath. Although he still appeared flushed, he did not look as cyanotic as he had on admission. His neck veins were no longer distended, and the peripheral edema of his legs and feet had improved. His breath sounds were clear but diminished. His ABGs on an FIO_2 of 0.24 were pH 7.36, $PaCO_2$ 82 mm Hg, HCO_3^- 45 mEq/L, PaO_2 66 mm Hg, and SaO_2 92%. The physician again called for a respiratory care evaluation. On the basis of these clinical data, the following SOAP was recorded.

Respiratory Assessment and Plan

S "I'm breathing much better."

O Recent diagnosis: OSA—more than 325 periods of obstructive apnea or hypopnea documented during baseline sleep study (AHI: 64); short muscular neck; narrow upper airway; obesity; Hct 51%; Hb 17 g/dL; pulmonary function tests: severe restrictive disorder; sawtooth pattern on maximal inspiratory and expiratory flow-volume loops; no longer appearing short of breath; cyanotic appearance improved; clear but diminished breath sounds; ABGs (on room air): pH 7.36, $PaCO_2$ 82, HCO_3^- 45, PaO_2 66, SaO_2 92%.

A Severe OSA confirmed (history, polysomnographic study, ABGs)

Chronic ventilatory failure with mild hypoxemia

Cor pulmonale improved

P Continue **Oxygen Therapy Protocol** (via venturi oxygen at FIO_2 0.24). Start **Continuous Positive Airway Pressure** (12 cm H_2O via mask) at bedtime. Ensure that patient sleeps in the head-up position and refrains from sleeping on his back. Start process to have CPAP device set up at patient's home. Monitor and re-evaluate.

Discussion

Although the diagnosis of OSA is made most frequently in the outpatient setting, it often may be diagnosed in the course of an acute hospitalization. A recent study showed that 78% of over 1000 patients admitted with acute decompensated heart failure (left ventricular ejection fraction <45%) had either OSA or CSA, *and they had never been diagnosed with sleep-disordered breathing.* CSA was an independent predictor of cardiac readmission at 1, 3, and 6 months. In the case under discussion, although the patient was first seen in the emergency room, it soon became clear that he was ill enough to be admitted, and his workup proceeded from there.

In the first assessment the therapist needed to perform and record a more careful examination of the patient's nasopharynx and oropharynx, as well as his chest. The typical upper airway anatomy of OSA was visible and should have been described in more detail—e.g., tongue size? Overbite? Tonsillar enlargement? Uvular enlargement? Mallampati classification score? While the patient's polysomnogram and CPAP titration study were in progress, the therapist appropriately ensured the patient's oxygenation (FIO_2 0.24 venturi oxygen mask) while attempting to prevent alveolar hypoventilation. In as classic a case as this, a **split-night study** (half standard PSG, half CPAP titration) was certainly in order.

The patient's neck vein distention, polycythemia, cardiomegaly, and peripheral edema all suggested cor pulmonale. This condition would improve once the patient's overall hypoventilation and oxygenation were treated. Many physicians would go ahead and give the patient a bicarbonate-losing diuretic, watching for metabolic acidosis while this was being done. The therapist (in the first assessment) correctly analyzed the situation as being potentially hazardous and noted impending ventilatory failure, which was a real possibility.

After the second assessment the diagnosis was made. Pulmonary function tests showed upper airway obstruction and a restrictive disorder. Based on the pH value of 7.36, the patient's $PaCO_2$ appeared to be at its normal baseline level. It is not uncommon for patients with severe OSA to have chronic ventilatory failure (compensated respiratory acidosis). The therapist elected to have the patient refrain from sleeping on his back and to sleep in the head-up position instead. In addition, the physician would likely ask for a nutrition consultation at that time because the patient needed to begin a drastic weight-loss program.

At the end of the assessment and treatment period, the patient's condition still was not markedly improved, and he awaited the long-term benefits of CPAP therapy and weight loss. Indeed, the CPAP therapy was eventually helpful. The patient had a 9-kg (20-lb) diuresis during the first week of combined CPAP and diuretic use, and good oxygenation was achieved with 10 cm H_2O CPAP pressure.

A diagnosis of OSA often can complicate other primary respiratory disorders, such as COPD (the so-called **crossover syndrome**), pneumonia, atelectasis, or chest wall deformity. In these settings, care is more complicated and, if anything, should be even more data-driven, with careful examination of all subjective and objective findings.

Patients with OSA have a significant risk of cardiovascular and central nervous system morbidity and mortality (myocardial infarctions, arrhythmias, hypertension, and cerebrovascular accidents). Psychiatric effects such as depression, sleep-related job malperformance, and daytime motor vehicle accidents also are seen. Current evidence suggests that such patients need not experience these effects if the sleep disorder–related breathing problems are diagnosed early and treated effectively. Most good respiratory care departments now have **sleep apnea screening programs** in place for all hospitalized patients. Compliance with CPAP therapy is important but difficult to achieve. Close clinical monitoring is important if good therapeutic outcomes are to be achieved consistently. One clear function of postdischarge transitional care programs for pneumonia, congestive heart failure, and COPD will be to arrange for further sleep apnea screening and treatment adherence evaluations were indicated.

SELF-ASSESSMENT QUESTIONS

Answers to questions can be found on Evolve. To access additional student assessment questions visit **http://evolve.elsevier.com/DesJardins/respiratory.**

1. **What is or are another name(s) for non–rapid eye movement (non-REM) sleep?**
   1. Slow-wave sleep
   2. Active sleep
   3. Dreaming sleep
   4. Quiet sleep
      a. 1 only
      b. 3 only
      c. 4 only
      d. 1 and 4 only

2. **During non-REM sleep, ventilation becomes slow and regular during which stage?**
   a. Eyes open wake
   b. Stage N1
   c. Stage N2
   d. Stage N3

3. **Moderate sleep apnea is said to be present when the apnea-hypopnea index (AHI) is:**
   a. 3 to 5 episodes/h
   b. 3 to 10 episodes/h
   c. 15 to 30 episodes/h
   d. 30 to 60 episodes/h

4. **During periods of apnea, the patient commonly demonstrates which of the following?**
   1. Systemic hypotension
   2. Decreased cardiac output
   3. Increased heart rate
   4. Transient pulmonary hypertension
      a. 1 and 3 only
      b. 2 and 4 only
      c. 3 and 4 only
      d. 1, 2, and 3 only

5. **Periods of severe sleep apnea are commonly associated with which of the following?**
   1. Ventricular tachycardia
   2. Sinus bradycardia
   3. Premature ventricular contraction
   4. Sinus arrhythmia
      a. 2 and 3 only
      b. 3 and 4 only
      c. 2, 3, and 4 only
      d. 1, 2, 3, and 4

6. During REM sleep, there is paralysis of the:
   1. Arm muscles
   2. Upper airway muscles
   3. Leg muscles
   4. Intercostal muscles
   5. Diaphragm
      a. 4 only
      b. 5 only
      c. 4 and 5 only
      d. 1, 2, 3, and 4 only

7. Normally, REM sleep constitutes about what percentage of the total sleep time?
   a. 5% to 10%
   b. 10% to 20%
   c. 20% to 25%
   d. 25% to 30%

8. Which of the following therapy modalities is or are therapeutic for obstructive sleep apnea?
   1. Phrenic pacemaker
   2. CPAP
   3. Theophylline
   4. Negative-pressure ventilation
      a. 1 only
      b. 2 only
      c. 3 and 4 only
      d. 1 and 4 only

9. Which of the following therapy modalities is or are therapeutic for central sleep apnea?
   a. Negative-pressure ventilation
   b. CPAP
   c. VPAP
   d. Tracheostomy

10. How long do normal periods of apnea during REM sleep last?
    a. 0 to 5 seconds
    b. 5 to 10 seconds
    c. 10 to 15 seconds
    d. 15 to 20 seconds

11. While a formal polysomnographic diagnosis of the precise type and severity of sleep apnea is being made (i.e., obstructive, central, or mixed sleep apnea), which of the following respiratory care modalities would be most safely used?
    a. VPAP
    b. Low-flow nasal oxygen therapy
    c. CPAP
    d. APAP

CHAPTER

32

Newborn and Early Childhood Cardiopulmonary Disorders

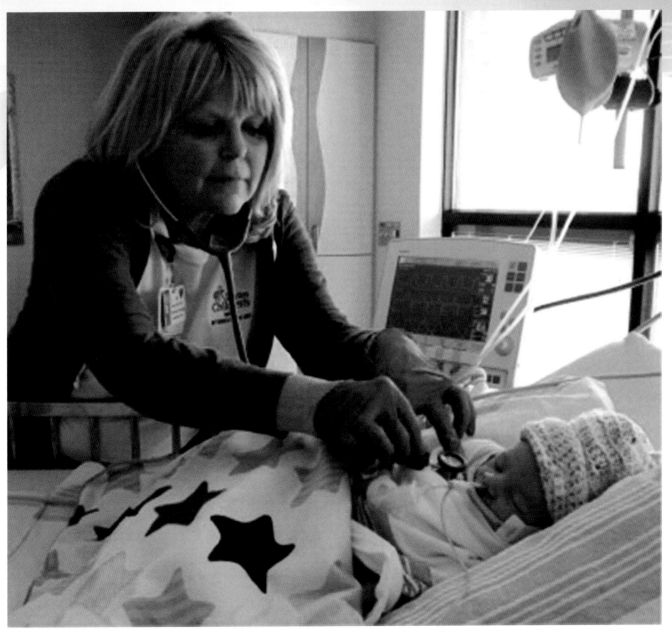

Courtesy of Dayton Children's Hospital, Dayton, Ohio.

Chapter Objectives

After reading this chapter, you will be able to:

- Describe the flow routing and major components of the fetal circulation in utero.
- Discuss the flow routing and major anatomic changes of the fetal circulation at birth.
- Describe persistent pulmonary hypertension of the newborn.
- List the clinical manifestations common in newborn and early childhood respiratory disorders.
- Describe the meaning of "apnea of prematurity."
- List factors that trigger apnea in the premature infant.
- Describe the arterial blood gas values commonly associated with newborn respiratory disorders.
- Discuss the objective data, assessments, and treatment plans commonly associated with the care of newborn respiratory disorders.
- Describe the major components of the Apgar score.
- Describe the respiratory protocols commonly used to treat the newborn and pediatric patient.

Key Terms

Apgar Score
Apnea of Prematurity
Arterial Blood Gases (ABGs)
Auto-PEEP
Capillary Blood Gases (CBGs)
"Chest Wiggle"
Ductus Arteriosus
Ductus Venosus
Echocardiography, use of, in PPHN
Endothelin-1
End-tidal Carbon Dioxide (ETCO2)
Expiratory Grunting
Extracorporeal Membrane Oxygenation (ECMO) in PPHN
Flaring Nostrils (or Nasal Flaring)
Foramen Ovale
Fossa Ovalis
Head Bobbing
High Frequency Jet Ventilation (HFJV)
High Frequency Oscillatory Ventilation (HFOV)
High Frequency Ventilation (HFV)
Inferior Vena Cava
Inhaled Nitric Oxide (iNO) Treatment in PPHN
Intercostal Retractions
Lateral Umbilical Ligaments
Ligamentum Arteriosus
Ligamentum Venosum
Maladaptation Abnormalities (pulmonary vasoconstriction)
Maldevelopment Abnormalities (idiopathic pulmonary hypertension)
Meconium Aspiration Syndrome (MAS)

Meconium Staining
Nasal Flaring
Neurally Activated Ventilatory Assistance (NAVA)
Oxygenation Index
Periodic Breathing
Persistent Pulmonary Hypertension of the Newborn (PPHN)
Placenta
Preductal Pulse Oximetry (SpO$_2$)
Postductal Pulse Oximetry (SpO$_2$)
Prostaglandins
Pulmonary Vascular Resistance (PVR)
Pulmonary/Systemic Vascular Resistance Ratio (PVR/SVR ratio)
Round Ligament (Ligamentum Teres)
Seesaw
Superior Vena Cava
Systemic Vascular Resistance (SVR)
Transcutaneous Gas Monitoring
Umbilical Arteries
Umbilical Artery Catheter
Umbilical Vein
Underdevelopment Abnormalities
Volumetric CO$_2$ Monitoring

Chapter Outline

Normal Fetal Circulation
Normal Circulatory Changes at Birth
Persistent Pulmonary Hypertension of the Newborn
  Etiology and Epidemiology
  Diagnosis
  Clinical Manifestations
Management
Clinical Manifestations Common in Newborn and Early Childhood Respiratory Disorders
  Clinical Manifestations Associated with Increased Negative Intrapleural Pressures during Inspiration
  Flaring Nostrils (or Nasal Flaring)
  Expiratory Grunting
  Head Bobbing
  Apnea of Prematurity
Arterial Blood Gases in Newborns and Infants
Assessment of the Newborn
Apgar Score
Newborn and Pediatric Treatment Protocols
  Oxygen Therapy Protocol
  Bronchopulmonary Hygiene Therapy Protocol
  Lung Expansion Therapy Protocol
  Aerosolized Medication
  Mechanical Ventilation and Ventilator Weaning
  Surfactant Administration Protocol
Self-Assessment Questions

To fully appreciate the common respiratory disorders and congenital heart defects that are associated with the newborn, the respiratory therapist must first have a good understanding of (1) the normal fetal circulation, (2) the normal circulatory changes that occur at birth, and (3) **persistent pulmonary hypertension of the newborn (PPHN)**. The following provides a brief review of the essential components of these important newborn topics.

Normal Fetal Circulation

Fetal circulation differs from circulation after birth for the following main reason: fetal blood must exchange oxygen and carbon dioxide and obtain nutrients from the maternal blood instead of from fetal lungs and digestive organs. Structures outside the fetus that accomplish these functions are the two **umbilical arteries**, the **umbilical vein**, and the

placenta (Figure 32-1). In addition, the following structures located within the body of the fetus play an important part in the plan of the fetal circulation: the **ductus venosus**, **foramen ovale**, and **ductus arteriosus** (Figure 32-2). A brief description of each of these six structures required for life-sustaining fetal circulation follows.

- The two fetal **umbilical arteries** are branches of the internal iliac (hypogastric) arteries. They return deoxygenated blood from the fetus to the placenta. Normally, the PO_2 in the umbilical arteries is about 20 torr and the PCO_2 is about 55 torr. The umbilical arteries wrap around the umbilical vein (see Figure 32-1).

- The **placenta** is attached to the (maternal) uterine wall. Throughout fetal life, the placenta transfers maternal oxygen and nutrients to the fetus and moves waste products from the fetal circulation. No mixing of maternal and fetal blood occurs (see Figure 32-1).

- The **umbilical vein** returns oxygenated blood and nutrients from the placenta to the fetus (see Figure 32-2). Normally, the PO_2 in the umbilical vein is about 30 to 35 torr and the PCO_2 is close to maternal—low 30s torr during the last trimester of pregnancy. The umbilical vein enters the navel of the fetus and ascends anteriorly to the liver. The two umbilical arteries and the umbilical vein together constitute the umbilical cord.

- About half of the blood enters the liver, and the rest flows through the **ductus venosus** and enters the fetal **inferior vena cava** (see Figure 32-2). This results in oxygenated blood (from the placenta) mixing with deoxygenated blood from the lower parts of the fetal body. The newly mixed blood then travels up the inferior vena cava and enters the right atrium of the heart—where it again mixes with deoxygenated blood from the **superior vena cava**.

- Once in the *right atrium*, a portion of the blood moves directly into the *left atrium* through the **foramen ovale.** While in the left atrium, the fetal blood mingles with a small about of deoxygenated blood from the pulmonary veins (see Figure 32-2).

- The remaining blood in the right atrium moves into the right ventricle, where it is then pumped into the pulmonary artery. Once in the pulmonary artery, a small amount of blood (about 15%) in the pulmonary artery flows through the fetal lungs and returns to the left atrium via the pulmonary veins. Most of the blood in the pulmonary artery moves through the **ductus arteriosus** and empties directly into the descending aorta (see Figure 32-2). At this point, the PO_2 is about 20 torr as it moves downstream toward the common iliac arteries, which branch into the external and internal iliacs. The blood in the internal iliac branch moves into the umbilical arteries and back to the placenta.

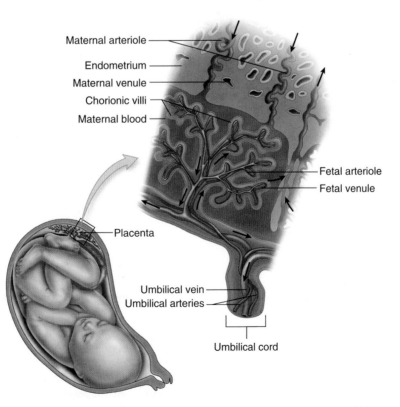

Maternal arteriole
Endometrium
Maternal venule
Chorionic villi
Maternal blood
Fetal arteriole
Fetal venule
Placenta
Umbilical vein
Umbilical arteries
Umbilical cord

FIGURE 32-1 Placental circulation. The placenta is an organ that permits exchange of blood gases (O_2 and CO_2), nutrients, and waste between fetal blood and maternal blood. Note that fetal and maternal blood are separated by a membranous barrier. Other special features of fetal circulation are shown in Figure 32-2 and Figure 32-3. (From Patton KT, Thibodeau GA: *Anatomy & physiology*, ed 8, 2013, Mosby/Elsevier.)

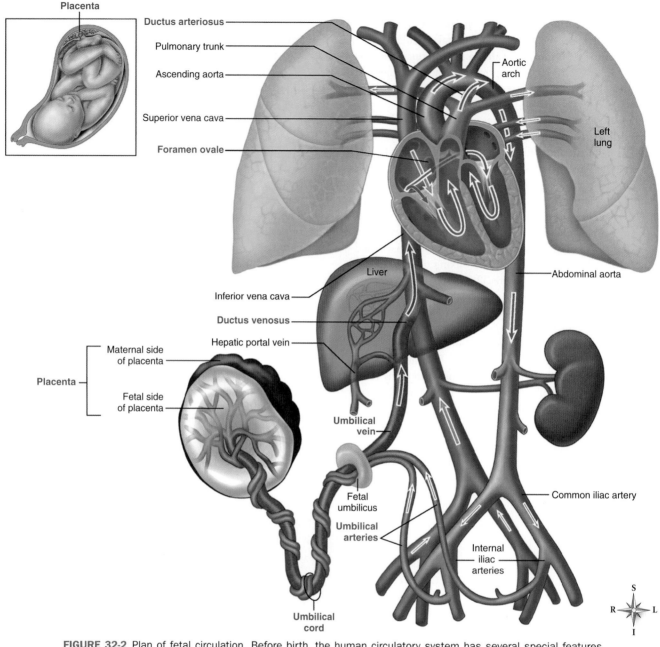

FIGURE 32-2 Plan of fetal circulation. Before birth, the human circulatory system has several special features that adapt the body to life in the womb. These features *(in red)* include two umbilical arteries, one umbilical vein, ductus venosus, foramen ovale, ductus arteriosus, and umbilical cord. The placenta, another essential feature of the fetal circulatory plan, is shown in Figure 32-1. (From Patton KT, Thibodeau GA: *Anatomy & physiology*, ed 8, 2013, Mosby/Elsevier.)

Normal Circulatory Changes at Birth

Shortly after birth—and after the normal extrauterine cardiopulmonary, renal, digestive, and liver functions are established—the six structures that serve fetal circulation are no longer needed (Figure 32-3). These structural changes are briefly described below:

- As soon as the umbilical cord is cut, the mother sheds the umbilical arteries, umbilical vein, and placenta as the *afterbirth*. The sections of these vessels that remain in the infant's body eventually become fibrous cords and remain throughout life. The two *umbilical arteries* atrophy and become the **lateral umbilical ligaments.** The *umbilical vein* becomes the **round ligament** (*ligamentum teres*) of the liver.

- The *ductus venosus* becomes the **ligamentum venosum,** which is a fibrous cord in the liver.

- The flap on the *foramen ovale* functionally closes (as a result of increased left atrial blood pressure [BP]) soon after the newborn takes the first breath and full circulation through the lungs becomes established. The closed foramen ovale becomes a depression—called the **fossa ovalis**—in the interatrial septum.

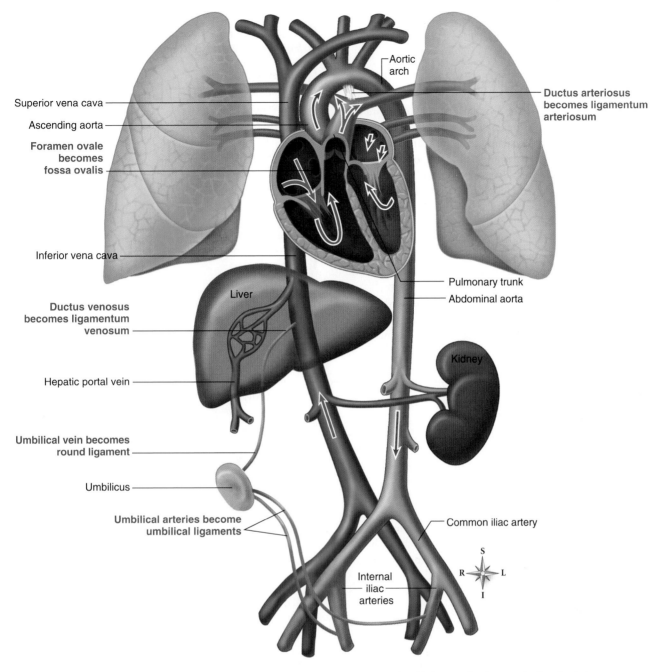

FIGURE 32-3 Changes in circulation after birth. Within the first year after birth, certain changes in the circulatory plan occur to adapt the body to life outside the womb. The placenta and portions of the umbilical vessels outside the infant's body are removed or fall off at, or shortly after, the time of birth. The internal portion of the umbilical vein constricts and becomes fibrous, eventually forming the round ligament of the liver. Likewise, the internal umbilical arteries become umbilical ligaments, the ductus venosus becomes the ligamentum venosum, and the ductus arteriosus becomes the ligamentum arteriosum. The fetal foramen ovale closes, forming a thin region of the atrial wall called the *fossa ovalis.* (From Patton KT, Thibodeau GA: *Anatomy & physiology,* ed 8, 2013, Mosby/Elsevier, Figure 21-37.)

- The *ductus arteriosus* contracts as soon as respirations are established and the PO_2 increases. The newborn's PO_2 must increase to >45 to 50 torr in order for the ductus arteriosus to close. Under normal conditions, the ductus arteriosus atrophies and becomes the **ligamentum arteriosum.** If this PO_2 is not reached, the ductus arteriosus will remain open. This condition results in **PPHN** (previously known as persistent fetal circulation).

- Finally, it should be noted that when the neonate's PO_2 increases sufficiently to close the ductus arteriosus, but then decreases within the first 24 to 48 hours after birth (e.g., because of meconium aspiration, respiratory distress syndrome, or a congenital heart defect), the ductus arteriosus will again reopen, and PPHN may again ensue. See the complete discussion of PPHN below.

Persistent Pulmonary Hypertension of the Newborn

Normally, shortly after birth there is a progressive decrease in the **pulmonary vascular resistance (PVR)** accompanied by a gradual increase in the **systemic vascular resistance (SVR)**. During this transitional period, the baby's pulmonary and systemic circulatory systems combine features of both fetal and adult circulatory patterns. The normal transitional period is a function of several factors, including the increased SVR that develops by the removal of the placenta, the normal catecholamine surge that occurs at birth, and the relatively cold extrauterine environment. On the other hand, factors that decrease the PVR include the infant's respirations—e.g., the mechanical expansion of the lungs, clearance of fetal lung fluid, and adequate alveolar ventilation and oxygenation (oxygen is a potent pulmonary arterial vascular dilator).

Persistent pulmonary hypertension of the newborn is described as a condition in which there is an abnormally high **PVR** after birth. As a result, the elevated PVR causes an increased right atrial pressure, which causes the foramen ovale to remain open. Because of these pathophysiologic changes, deoxygenated systemic venous blood, returning to the right heart, moves through the following fetal heart structures—and in this order: the *foramen ovale, left atrium, ductus arteriosus,* and into the *aorta.* Thus, as just outlined, the secondary pathophysiologic consequences of PPHN are as follows: (1) the venous blood (deoxygenated blood) moves from the right atrium through the foramen ovale to the left atrium—a *right-to-left shunt*—and mixes with the oxygenated blood returning to the left atrium from the lungs (venous admixture), (2) a large portion of the blood in the left atrium takes the path of least resistance and moves through the ductus arteriosus and empties into the aorta (another venous admixture), and (3) the newly mixed blood in the aorta—with a decreased PaO_2 and oxygen content—moves through the systemic circulation.

Etiology and Epidemiology

PPHN occurs primarily in term or late preterm infants (≥34 weeks' gestation). The prevalence of PPHN is estimated at 1.9 per 1000 births in the United States. Box 32-1 lists factors commonly associated with PPHN.

Conditions that disrupt the normal decline in the **pulmonary/systemic vascular resistance ratio (PVR/SVR ratio)**—which, in turn, prolong the transitional circulation of the newborn and result in PPHN—can generally be classified as one of three abnormalities: *maladaptation, underdevelopment,* and *maldevelopment.*

- **Maladaptation Abnormalities** (also known as acute pulmonary vasoconstriction conditions)—are the most commonly encountered clinical scenarios of PPHN. Although the lungs are fully developed, the pulmonary system can be affected by a variety of perinatal conditions that cause acute pulmonary arterial vasoconstriction. As a result of the acute pulmonary vasoconstriction, the normal postnatal decrease in PVR is delayed and PPHN ensues. Acute pulmonary vasoconstriction is also commonly caused by:

- **Alveolar hypoxia** secondary to parenchymal lung disease (such as meconium aspiration syndrome
- Respiratory distress syndrome
- Pneumonia
- Bacterial infections—especially those caused by group B *Streptococcus*
- Hypoventilation and alveolar hypoxia may also be caused by neurologic conditions or use of maternal depressants
- Hypothermia and hypoglycemia can also lead to acute pulmonary vasoconstriction and PPHN
- **Underdevelopment Abnormalities** (also known as hypoplasia of the pulmonary vascular bed conditions)—involve situations that reduce the cross-sectional area of the pulmonary vascular bed, resulting in a fixed elevation of the PVR. Causes of underdevelopment abnormalities and subsequent PPHN include congenital diaphragmatic

---

BOX 32-1 Factors Associated with Persistent Pulmonary Hypertension of the Newborn (PPHN)

Maternal Factors
- Diabetes
- Cesarean section
- Hypoxia

Cardiovascular Factors
- Systemic hypotension
- Congenital heart disease
- Shock

Fetal Factors
- Intrauterine stress
- Hypoxia
- Decreased pH
- Placental vascular abnormalities

Hematologic Factors
- Increased hematocrit
- Septicemia
- Maternal-fetal blood loss
- Placental abruption
- Placenta previa
- Acute blood loss

Respiratory Factors
- Meconium aspiration syndrome
- Respiratory distress syndrome
- Pneumonia

Other Factors
- Central nervous system disorders
- Hypoglycemia
- Hypocalcemia
- Neuromuscular disorders

hernia, cystic adenomatoid malformation of the lung, oligohydramnios with accompanying obstructive uropathy, and intrauterine growth restriction.

- **Maldevelopment Abnormalities** (also known as idiopathic pulmonary hypertension conditions)—include thickening of the muscle layer of the pulmonary arterioles and the extension of this muscle layer into small vessels that usually have thin walls and no muscle cells. In addition, the extracellular tissue that surrounds the pulmonary vessels may be thicker than normal. In newborns with PPHN caused by a maldevelopment abnormality, there is remodeling of the pulmonary vascular bed that usually occurs during the first 7 to 14 days after birth, with an accompanying fall in PVR.

Causes of maldevelopment abnormalities are uncertain, but vascular mediators are thought to play a role. For example, infants with PPHN are thought to have a higher plasma concentration of the vasoconstrictor **endothelin-1** and a lower concentration of cyclic guanosine monophosphate, a vasodilator. In addition, a genetic predisposition may influence the availability of the precursors for nitric oxide (NO), a vasodilator, which further impedes cardiopulmonary vascular adaptation at birth. Conditions associated with vascular maldevelopment and PPHN include postterm delivery, **meconium staining**, and meconium aspiration. In these disorders, the pulmonary vasculature usually responds poorly to therapies that normally decrease PVR, such as increased arterial oxygen tension and effective alveolar ventilation.

In addition, conditions that cause an excessive perfusion of the fetal lung are believed to predispose the pulmonary vasculature to maldevelopment. Such fetal conditions include premature closure of the ductus arteriosus (e.g., caused by maternal use of nonsteroidal antiinflammatory drugs such as ibuprofen), premature closure of the foramen ovale (e.g., caused by high placental vascular resistance), and total anomalous pulmonary venous drainage.

Diagnosis

The diagnosis of PPHN should always be suspected in any infant with nonresponsive or ongoing hypoxemia and cyanosis that are out of proportion to the degree of pulmonary disease, oxygen requirement, and mean airway pressure support. The diagnosis of PPHN is confirmed by **echocardiography**. When PPHN is present, echocardiography demonstrates normal structural cardiac anatomy with evidence of pulmonary hypertension (e.g., flattened or displaced ventricular septum). Doppler studies show *right-to-left* shunting through the patent ductus arteriosus and/or foramen ovale.

Clinical Manifestations

The newborn with PPHN generally presents with cyanosis and tachypnea. PPHN should be strongly considered in any neonate with severe cyanosis. PPHN should also be suspected when certain prenatal risk factors (such as heart abnormalities and **meconium-stained amniotic fluid**) or specific respiratory disorders (such as **meconium aspiration syndrome**, pneumonia, respiratory distress, diaphragmatic hernia, and pulmonary hypoplasia) are present.

The pulse oximeter often demonstrates a significant difference between the **preductal** and **postductal oxygen saturation**.[1] A >10% difference between the pre- and postductal oxygen saturation indicates right-to-left shunting. The chest radiograph is usually normal when no other pulmonary condition is present.

The diagnosis of PPHN is confirmed by echocardiography. The echocardiogram typically demonstrates normal cardiac structure and evidence of pulmonary hypertension (e.g., flattened or displaced ventricular septum or an estimated increase in the pulmonary arterial pressure). The differential diagnosis of PPHN includes cyanotic congenital heart disease, other pulmonary disorders, and sepsis.

Management

The **oxygenation index (OI)** is often used to assess the severity of hypoxemia in PPHN and other critical conditions to help determine the need for more aggressive therapies, such as **high frequency ventilation (HFV), inhaled nitric oxide (iNO)** administration, or **extracorporeal membrane oxygenation (ECMO)** support. The OI is calculated as follows:

$$OI = [(\text{mean airway pressure} \times FIO_2) \div PaO_2] \times 100.$$

In most cases of PPHN, the OI criteria are used while the infant is already receiving an FIO_2 of 1.0 and is being mechanically ventilated. Thus, the OI can be easily calculated from the mean airway pressure shown on the ventilator and the PaO_2. For example, if a newborn infant with PPHN is receiving ventilatory support with a mean airway pressure of 15 cm H_2O, an FIO_2 of 1.0, and a PaO_2 of 60, the OI would be calculated as follows:

$$OI = \frac{15 \times 1.0}{60} \times 100$$
$$= 25$$

Note: Because of the awkwardness of the mathematic notation associated with the result of the OI calculation—i.e., cm H_2O/mm Hg—the units are typically not included as part of the OI answer (in this case, 25). It should also be noted here that the OI discussed above is different from the oxygen desaturation index (ODI) discussed in Chapter 31 (Sleep Apnea).

Table 32-1 provides the OI ranges for mild, moderate, severe, and very severe hypoxemia. Infants with a severe OI (25 to 40) should receive care in a center where high-frequency ventilation, iNO, and ECMO are readily available in addition to general supportive care. In the infant with an OI <25 and an echocardiography that shows PPHN, a trial period of iNO may be administered to determine its effectiveness in (1) reversing the PPHN and (2) reducing the required mean airway pressure support.

---

[1]See discussion of pre- and postductal oxygenation saturation under Arterial Blood Gases in Newborns and Infants, page 448.

TABLE 32-1 Oxygenation Index Range

Clinical Severity of Hypoxemia	Range
Mild	5–15
Moderate	16–25
Severe	26–40
Very severe	>40

Oxygen—is a pulmonary vasodilator and should be administered in a concentration of 100% in an effort to reverse pulmonary vasoconstriction. However, because high concentrations of oxygen may eventually cause lung injury (**pulmonary oxygen toxicity**), the FIO_2 should be adjusted downward as soon as possible.[2] Efforts should be made to maintain the PaO_2 in the 50 to 90 mm Hg range (oxygenation saturation >90%). If adequate oxygenation cannot be achieved, more aggressive and invasive measures are required—e.g., high-frequency ventilatory support, iNO or ECMO.

Ventilatory Support—is used to prevent or reverse hypercarbia and acidosis, which both increase PVR. In newborns that require high peak inspiratory pressures (e.g., >30 cm H_2O) or high mean airway pressure (e.g., >15 cm H_2O), the use of **HFV** should be considered to reduce barotrauma and associated air leak syndrome. HFV in newborns may be accomplished with **high frequency oscillatory ventilation (HFOV)** or **high frequency jet ventilation (HFJV)**. During ventilatory support, attempts to achieve and maintain the $PaCO_2$ at 40 to 45 mm Hg and the pH between 7.35 and 7.45 are recommended. However, permissive hypercapnia may be utilized to prevent lung damage in patients with significant disease. The ultimate strategy of ventilator support is based on the presence or absence of pulmonary parenchymal disease and the infant's response to treatment. Sedation and analgesia with opioids are often required to achieve and maintain adequate mechanical ventilation in infants with PPHN.

Inhaled Nitric Oxide—provides a rapid relaxation of the smooth muscles of the pulmonary vascular system and reduces PVR. The administration of iNO is recommended in infants with an OI ≥25 or documented pulmonary hypertension as noted on the echocardiogram. It is a gas easily administered through the ventilator's inspiratory limb with an injector that assures an accurate "parts per million" (ppm) dose per breath. The initial recommended concentration of iNO is 20 ppm. In infants who respond to iNO, oxygenation is usually improved within a few minutes. Once the patient is stabilized, iNO should be gradually weaned to prevent rebound pulmonary vasoconstriction.

Extracorporeal Membrane Oxygenation—is needed in approximately 40% of infants with severe PPHN who remain hypoxemic despite full ventilatory support and the administration of iNO. One criterion for the institution of ECMO is an elevated OI (consistently ≥40) in a patient resistant to iNO. However, when the baby is receiving HFV, the mean airway pressures are typically higher than those seen with conventional ventilation. In these cases, the criterion to start ECMO is usually an OI ≥60. Common pulmonary disorders associated with the need for ECMO are meconium aspiration and congenital diaphragmatic hernia. The goal of ECMO is to maintain adequate tissue oxygenation and to avoid irreversible lung injury from mechanical ventilation while the infant's PVR decreases and the PPHN resolves. Infants with severe PPHN requiring ECMO therapy are at increased risk of developmental delay, motor disability, and hearing deficits. ECMO may also be used as a bridge therapy until lung transplantation is possible, in certain cases.

Circulatory Support—is often required to reduce right-to-left shunting and to augment tissue oxygenation. As discussed earlier, right-to-left shunting increases in PPHN because of the increased PVR. When the SVR is low or the cardiac output is poor, the right-to-left shunting will be even greater. Because the pulmonary arterial BP in infants with PPHN is at, or near, normal systemic BP, the systemic BP targets are typically set at the following upper limits of normal: mean BP between 45 and 55 mm Hg and systolic BP between 50 and 70 mm Hg. This is accomplished by (1) ensuring adequate vascular volume via intravenous fluids and transfusion of packed red blood cells and (2) providing vasopressor support, such as dopamine (most common), dobutamine, epinephrine, or norepinephrine.

Clinical Manifestations Common in Newborn and Early Childhood Cardiopulmonary Disorders

Respiratory disorders are the leading cause of admission to the neonatal intensive care unit (NICU). Essential to the understanding of neonatal respiratory distress is the axiom "Oxygen is the primary nutrient of the human body." The clinical manifestations presented by a baby in *early* respiratory distress include lethargy, cyanosis, increased respiratory rate, **nasal flaring**, **head bobbing**, **expiratory grunting, intercostal retractions,** substernal retraction, tachycardia, increased BP, and acute alveolar hyperventilation with hypoxemia. The *late*, ominous manifestations include a decreased respiratory rate, gasping respirations, apnea, bradycardia, decreased systemic BP, and acute ventilatory failure with both CO_2 retention and hypoxemia.

Although many of the pathophysiologic mechanisms and clinical manifestations presented by the newborn with a respiratory disorder are identical to those seen in the older child or adult, some are unique.

The more important clinical manifestations associated with neonatal respiratory disorders and the primary pathophysiologic mechanisms responsible for these clinical manifestations are discussed below.

---

[2]See more on this topic in Chapter 35, Respiratory Distress Syndrome.

Clinical Manifestations Associated with Increased Negative Intrapleural Pressures during Inspiration

The *thorax* of the newborn infant is quite flexible—i.e., the compliance of the infant's thorax is high. This flexibility is a result of the large amount of cartilage (compared with bone in the adult) found in the skeletal structure of newborns. Because of the structural alterations associated with many newborn respiratory disorders, however, the compliance of the infant's lungs is low. In an effort to offset the decreased lung compliance, the infant must generate more negative intrapleural pressures during inspiration. As shown in Figure 32-4, this condition causes the following:

- The soft tissues between the ribs retract during inspiration, causing **intercostal retractions**.
- The substernal area retracts and the abdominal area protrudes in a **seesaw** fashion during inspiration. The substernal retraction is caused by high negative intrapleural pressure, and the abdominal distention is caused by the contraction (depression) of the diaphragm during inspiration.
- The blood vessels in the more dependent portions of the thoracic and abdominal areas dilate and pool blood, causing these areas to appear mottled.

Flaring Nostrils (or Nasal Flaring)

Flaring nostrils (or nasal flaring) is frequently observed in infants in respiratory distress. This clinical manifestation is probably a facial reflex to facilitate the movement of gas into the tracheobronchial tree. The dilator naris, which originates from the maxilla and inserts into the ala of the nose, is the muscle responsible for this movement. When activated, the dilator naris pulls the alae laterally and widens the nasal aperture, providing a larger orifice for gas to enter during inspiration (Figure 32-5).

Expiratory Grunting

An audible **expiratory grunt** is frequently heard in infants with respiratory problems. Depending on the listener's auditory perception, the expiratory grunt may sound like an expiratory cry. It often is first detected on auscultation. The expiratory grunt is a natural physiologic mechanism that generates (high) positive pressures in the alveoli, which, at least in part, counteracts the alveolar collapse (atelectasis) and hypoventilation associated with the disorder (e.g., respiratory distress syndrome, discussed in detail in Chapter 35). In short, as the gas pressure in the alveoli increases, the infant's PAO_2 increases. During exhalation the infant's epiglottis covers the glottis, which causes the intrapulmonary air pressure to increase. When the epiglottis abruptly opens, gas rushes past the infant's vocal cords and produces an expiratory grunt or cry.

Head Bobbing

Head bobbing is a sign of respiratory distress in an infant. When in respiratory distress, the infant often uses the scalene and sternocleidomastoid accessory muscles of inspiration to assist in ventilation. When these muscles contract, the infant's head moves ("bobs") back and forth because the neck extensor muscles are not strong enough to stabilize the head.

Periodic Breathing

Periodic breathing is defined as 3 episodes of central apnea lasting at least 3 seconds, separated by no more than 20 seconds of normal breathing. It is considered benign in the newborn as long as there is no associated bradycardia or oxygen desaturation. It is most common during active sleep.

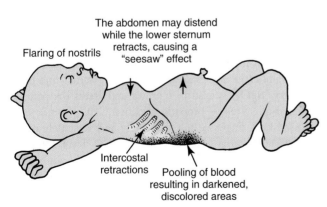

FIGURE 32-4 Clinical manifestations associated with increased negative intrapleural pressure during inspiration in infants. Common features include flaring of the nostrils, cyanosis of the dependent portions of the thoracic and abdominal areas, substernal and intercostal retractions, abdominal distention, and seesaw movement of the abdomen and chest.

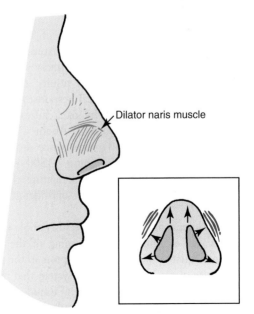

FIGURE 32-5 The dilator naris muscles cause the nostrils to dilate during a stressful inspiration.

BOX 32-2 Factors That Trigger Apnea in the Premature Infant

Control of Ventilation
- Rapid eye movement sleep
- Decreased hypoxic and hypercapnic response
- Congenital central hypoventilation syndrome (Ondine's curse, idiopathic alveolar hypoventilation)

Reflex Stimulation
- Suctioning of the nasopharynx and trachea
- Laryngeal stimulation
- Bowel movements (vagal response)
- Hiccups

Environmental Conditions
- Ambient temperature changes

Neurologic Disorders
- Seizures
- Intracranial hemorrhage
- Meningitis
- Drug-induced

Drug Depression
- Sedatives
- Analgesics
- Prostaglandins

Respiratory Disorders
- Respiratory distress syndrome
- Pneumonia

- Transient tachypnea of the newborn
- Meconium aspiration syndrome
- Bronchopulmonary dysplasia
- Diaphragmatic hernia

Cardiac Disorders
- Patent ductus arteriosus
- Congestive heart failure
- Right-to-left intracardiac shunting

Systemic Disease Processes
- Hypothermia
- Hypoglycemia
- Hyponatremia
- Hypocalcemia
- Sepsis (group B *Streptococcus*)

Body Position
- Head flexion

Anatomic Abnormalities
- Micrognathia
- Choanal atresia
- Macroglossia

Apnea of Prematurity

Apnea of prematurity is the cessation of breathing for >20 seconds or any apnea duration associated with cyanosis or bradycardia. It is due to the immaturity of the brainstem respiratory centers, which results in a reduced response to CO_2 and a paradoxical response to hypoxia that results in hypoxia—i.e., the hypoxia causes more episodes of apnea and hypoxia worsens. About 75% of premature babies weighing <1250 g experience severe apnea. More than 25% of infants weighing >1500 g manifest severe apnea. In general, the more premature the infant, the greater the number of apneic episodes that may occur.

Premature infants are believed to be susceptible to apneic episodes because of immature functioning of the chemoreceptors, inadequate functioning of receptors in the airways, and immaturity of the central nervous system that regulates oxygenation and carbon dioxide levels. Rapid eye movement sleep is also thought to play a role in the cause of central sleep apnea. Box 32-2 lists factors that trigger apneic episodes.

Arterial Blood Gases in Newborns and Infants

Because of the difficulty in obtaining an **arterial blood gas** (**ABG**)[3] sample in the newborn and pediatric patient (e.g., small vessels are difficult to palpate and puncture), a **capillary blood gas** (**CBG**) is usually performed to assess the pH, $PaCO_2$, and HCO_3^- values (the acid-base and ventilation status), and **pulse oximetry** (SpO_2) is used to monitor and assess the patient's oxygenation status. A properly obtained CBG, from a well-perfused heel, finger, or toe, can safely and accurately reflect the patient's arterial pH, $PaCO_2$, and HCO_3^- level. However, the PO_2 reading varies significantly—and, should not be used for clinical analysis! Typically, the PO_2 value in a CBG is much lower than the actual arterial PO_2 level.

[3]An ABG "stick" is generally reserved for the newborn or pediatric patient who is critically unstable or who has an unstable circulatory system. A poor circulatory system makes the peripheral CBG and SpO_2 measurements less likely to be accurate. In these infants, an in-line arterial catheter is typically inserted to minimize needle sticks and to allow for easy and rapid ABG monitoring.

Proper capillary sampling technique is needed to obtain a reliable, well-perfused sample. The lateral heel is the site of choice for infants 1 year of age. The lateral fingertip should be used for toddlers and older children. The puncture site is warmed for 3 to 5 minutes using an activated heel warmer or warmed washcloth wrap. The site is then cleaned with a povidone-iodine prep, and wiped dry with a 2 × 2 gauze. A puncture is made with a lancet or puncture device appropriate for infants (maximum puncture depth of 0.85 to 1.0 mm for newborns). The first drop of blood is wiped away with the gauze. The capillary tube is placed in the center of the drop of blood, keeping the capillary tube horizontal to avoid air entering the sample. If air enters, the tube should be tilted to release the air before proceeding. The capillary tube is filled to capacity. The foot or finger may require some gentle "milking" to increase blood flow; however, there should be no squeezing at the puncture site. Samples must be analyzed immediately to avoid clotting.

To obtain a reliable SpO_2, the oximeter probe is typically placed on the child's wrist, the medial surface of the palm, or the foot. Adequate cardiac output and skin blood perfusion are essential for accurate SpO_2 measurements. In addition, the pulse rate shown on the oximeter should correlate with the patient's actual pulse for accurate SpO_2 measurements. Common CBG and SpO_2 findings associated with newborn and early childhood respiratory disorders are (1) acute alveolar hyperventilation (acute respiratory alkalosis) with hypoxemia and (2) acute ventilatory failure (acute respiratory acidosis) with hypoxemia.

For the newborn in respiratory distress, pulse oximetry is often used to monitor both the **preductal SpO_2** and the **postductal SpO_2**. To measure the preductal SpO_2, the oximeter probe is placed on the right hand or wrist; to measure the postductal SpO_2, the probe is placed on either foot. A large difference between the two readings (>10%) indicates a *right-to-left shunt*, and **PPHN** is likely. Table 32-2 provides an overview of the SpO_2 and PaO_2 relationship for the newborn.

To summarize, the respiratory therapist must be careful in assessing the results of CBG measurements. The CBG provides a relatively accurate reading of the patient's pH, $PaCO_2$, and HCO_3^- status (the acid-base and ventilation status), but not the PO_2 or oxygenation status. Pulse oximetry (SpO_2) is used to monitor and evaluate the patient's oxygenation status.

Other Techniques

Other noninvasive techniques that may be used to monitor blood gases include (1) transcutaneous monitoring and (2) capnometry.

Transcutaneous gas monitoring requires the application of a miniaturized oxygen and carbon dioxide electrode to the infant's chest, abdomen or back. The electrode sensor is warmed to increase the capillary blood flow beneath, allowing for the measurement of the partial pressure of oxygen ($PtcO_2$) and carbon dioxide ($PtcCO_2$) through the skin's surface.

Capnometry uses infrared radiation to measure **end-tidal carbon dioxide ($ETco_2$)** in the exhaled gas. Mainstream devices direct an infrared beam through the exhaled gas; sidestream devices use a vacuum pump to pull exhaled gas into the measuring chamber. An airway adapter is placed on the endotracheal tube in the intubated patient for capnometry. A special cannula is used for the spontaneously breathing patient; this requires a sidestream device. Continuous $ETco_2$ monitoring is not routinely used in intubated newborns due to the dead space created by mainstream adapters and the dilution of exhaled gas with sidestream sampling. $ETco_2$ monitoring is routinely used in pediatric sleep studies.

Oxygen Toxicity

Hyperoxia should be avoided in newborns to prevent the resulting oxidative stress that can cause significant lung damage. The damage is caused by cytotoxic oxygen metabolites or oxygen radicals. Adult lungs have intact antioxidant enzymes, which can detoxify these radicals. However, premature infants lack these enzymes and can develop O_2 radical-induced chronic lung disease. Hyperoxia also contributes to another newborn complication, **retinopathy of prematurity**. Retinal vessels develop at 40 to 42 weeks' gestation. Very low-birth-weight infants born prematurely have the risk of developing retinal scarring, retraction, or detachment as oxygen promotes disorganized new vascularization and fibrovascular changes in the retina. The Vermont Oxford Network recently reported a 36% incidence of retinopathy of prematurity in such infants (500 to 1500 g).

Assessment of the Newborn

As discussed in Chapter 11, good assessment skills include (1) the systematic collection of clinical data, (2) the evaluation of the data, and (3) the formulation of an appropriate treatment plan. As with the older child or adult, the newborn with respiratory disease must be evaluated frequently. To enhance this process, Figure 32-6 illustrates objective data, assessments, and treatment plans commonly associated with newborn respiratory disorders.

Apgar Score

Another common assessment tool used at birth in the delivery room is the **Apgar score**. The Apgar score is a rating system for the rapid identification of newborn infants requiring immediate intervention or transfer to an NICU. The Apgar evaluation is performed 1 minute after birth and again 5 and 10 minutes later. It is based on a rating of five factors that reflect the infant's ability to adjust to extrauterine life. As shown in Figure 32-7, the infant's heart rate, respiratory effort, muscle tone, reflex irritability, and color are scored

TABLE 32-2 SpO_2 and PaO_2 Relationships in the Newborn

Oxygenation Status	SpO_2	PaO_2
Normal	91–96%	60–80
Mild hypoxemia	88–90%	55–60
Moderate hypoxemia	85–89%	50–59
Severe hypoxemia	<85%	<49

from a low value of 0 to a normal value of 2. Each of the five assessments are scored individually and then combined for a total score. A total score of 0 to 3 represents severe depression, a total score of 4 to 6 indicates moderate concern, and a total score of 7 to 10 represents normal adaptation to extra-uterine life. The totals are recorded at 1, 5, and 10 minutes. For example, an Apgar score of 7/9/10 is a score of 7 at 1 minute, 9 at 5 minutes, and 10 at 10 minutes.

The 5- and 10-minute scores are normally higher than the 1-minute score. A low 1-minute score requires immediate intervention, including oxygen administration and oral and nasal suctioning. A baby with a low score that remains low after 5 minutes requires expert care, which may include transfer to the NICU, continuous positive airway pressure, umbilical catheterization, and mechanical ventilation.

In the newborn who is lethargic, apneic, pale, cyanotic, and bradycardic at birth, and in whom resuscitation efforts are being done correctly and effectively, assessments typically follow this order: First, the heart rate returns to normal. This is followed by spontaneous respiratory movements and improved color. The last important response to be noted is improved tone and reflex irritability.

A   NEONATAL RESPIRATORY CARE POCKET CARD

HISTORY	OBJECTIVE DATA — Clinical manifestations that commonly develop in response to respiratory disease				ASSESSMENT	PLAN
	Inspection	Auscultation	ABGs/ Pulse Oximetry	Chest Radiograph	COMMON CAUSES OF CLINICAL INDICATORS	
Prematurity, maternal diabetes, C-section, multiple births, sibling with RDS	• Retractions • Nasal flaring • Paradoxical (see-saw) respirations • Cyanosis or pallor	• Expiratory grunting • Poor air entry • May have crackles	↓PO_2/SpO_2 while on ↑FIO_2 (Note: premature infants need PO_2 in 60-80 range) Avoid SpO_2 >95%	Reticulogranular, ground glass appearance with air bronchograms	RESPIRATORY DISTRESS SYNDROME (RDS) • Surfactant deficiency • Atelectasis	• Oxygen therapy • Hyperinflation therapy (CPAP/PEEP) • Mechanical ventilation • Surfactant administration
Prematurity, history of RDS, mechanical ventilation	• Decreased chest movement	• Diminished or distant breath sounds	Further ↓PO_2/SpO_2 while on ↑FIO_2	Small cystic areas with possibly flattened diaphragms	PULMONARY INTERSTITIAL EMPHYSEMA (PIE) • Air trapping	• Oxygen therapy • Decrease ventilator pressures • Permissive hypercapnia • Possibly high frequency ventilation and/or selective mainstem intubation • Monitor for barotrauma
Low birth weight, RDS, prolonged mechanical oxygen, slow growth	• Cyanosis if off O_2 • Barrel chest	• Wheezes • Crackles	↑PCO_2 with normal pH, ↓PO_2/SpO_2	Cystic pattern	BRONCHOPULMONARY DYSPLASIA (BPD) • Airtrapping • Bronchospasm	• Oxygen therapy • Bronchodilator therapy • Bronchial hygiene therapy • Permissive hypercapnia • Fluid management • Increased calorie intake
Usually full term, possibly C-section, perinatal complications	• Tachypnea • Retractions	• Crackles	↓PCO_2, ↓PO_2/SpO_2	Perihilar streaking with enlarged cardiac silhouette	TRANSIENT TACHYPNEA OF THE NEWBORN • Airway fluid	• Oxygen therapy • CPAP
Stress and/or asphyxia in utero, meconium noted in amniotic fluid, usually full term to post-term	• Dyspnea • Meconium-stained umbilical cord or fingernails	• Crackles	↓PCO_2 (May increase as patient fatigues), ↓PO_2/SpO_2	Hyperaeration	MECONIUM ASPIRATION SYNDROME (MAS) • Airway secretions • Air trapping	• Suction oropharynx and trachea before delivery • Oxygen therapy • Bronchial hygiene therapy • Possible hyperventilation (to further ↓PCO_2 and ↑pH) if hypertension likely • May need to consider ECMO, HFV, iNO • Monitor for barotrauma
Possible underlying problem with meconium aspiration, congenital heart disease, or perinatal asphyxia. Minimal ↑ PO_2 with 100% O_2 challenge	• Persistent cyanosis disproportionate to degree of pulmonary disease on CXR • Tachypnea	• Corresponds to underlying cardiopulmonary disorder	Fluctuations in PO_2/SpO_2	Normal to mild pulmonary parenchymal disease	PERSISTENT PULMONARY HYPERTENSION OF THE NEWBORN (PPHN) • Pulmonary vasoconstriction • Reopening of fetal circulation pathways	• Oxygen therapy • Mechanical ventilation • Treat underlying cause • May need to consider ECMO, HFV, iNO
May have normal pregnancy and delivery (full term), may have dusky, cyanotic episodes. Minimal ↑ PO_2 with 100% O_2 challenge.	• May be normal in appearance if Left → Right shunt present • Cyanotic if Right → Left shunt present	• Heart murmur may be present	PO_2 may vary widely depending on heart lesion: low with Right → Left shunt; more normal with Left → Right	May have irregular heart shape (e.g., boot or egg) depending on lesion	CONGENITAL HEART DISEASE • Pulmonary shunting	• Evaluation to identify problem • Cardiac catheterization • Surgery; pre- and post-op supportive care
Problems with breathing; difficulty with eating and breathing (e.g., dusky with feeding), noisy breathing	• Varies with lesion • Respiratory distress, drooling, gastric distension	• Varies with lesion	Usually ↓PCO_2 and ↓PO_2, extent of which varies with lesion	Normal to highly irregular, depending on lesion	CONGENITAL ANOMALIES of the respiratory system • Airway obstruction	• Evaluation to identify problem • Radiographic procedures/operative procedures to diagnose and treat • Pre- and post-op supportive care

FIGURE 32-6 (**A,B**) Common neonatal clinical manifestations (objective data), assessments, and treatment plans.

PEDIATRIC RESPIRATORY CARE POCKET CARD

HISTORY	OBJECTIVE DATA — Clinical manifestations that commonly develop in response to respiratory disease				ASSESSMENT	PLAN
	Inspection	Auscultation	ABGs/ Pulse Oximetry	Chest Radiograph	COMMON CAUSES OF CLINICAL INDICATORS	
Infant or young child (usually newborn–3 y.o.), upper respiratory infection, barking cough	• Tachypnea • Retractions • Nasal flaring • May have cyanosis	• Barking cough • Stridor	↓PCO$_2$ and ↓PO$_2$/SpO$_2$	Subglottic edema on neck radiograph– *steeple* sign	LARYNGOTRACHEO-BRONCHITIS (CROUP) (*typically parainfluenza viruses, occasionally bacterial in origin*) • Laryngeal edema	• Oxygen therapy • Cool mist • Racemic epinephrine • Steroids
Toddler or school age child (usually 2 y.o. or >), acute onset of fever and respiratory distress, non-immunized fever patient	• Stridor • Dyspnea • Drooling • May have cyanosis	• Stridor	↓PCO$_2$ and ↓PO$_2$/SpO$_2$	Epiglottis appears as large, round, soft tissue density on neck radiograph–*thumb* sign	EPIGLOTTITIS (*H. influenzae* Type B; vaccine available) • Edema	• Emergency attention • Oxygen therapy • Intubation in OR or tracheostomy in OR • Antibiotics
Upper respiratory infection, apnea (newborn–2 y.o. or older child with chronic cardiopulmonary condition)	• Tachypnea, re-tractions, nasal flaring, nasal secretions • Cyanosis if severe	• Wheezes	↓PO$_2$/SpO$_2$	May vary from normal to streaky infiltrates or hyperaeration	BRONCHIOLITIS (*typically RSV organism*) • Airway secretions • Bronchospasm possible • Airway inflammation/edema	• Supportive • Oxygen therapy • Suction • Trial of bronchodilator therapy if significant respiratory distress. • Mechanical ventilation; HFNC, CPAP
Upper respiratory infection, late onset of fever, may c/o earache	• Tachypnea, retrac-tions, nasal flaring, nasal secretions • Cyanosis if severe	• Crackles • Wheezes • Bronchial sounds	↓PO$_2$/SpO$_2$	Infiltrates and/or consolidation	PNEUMONIA • Consolidation • Airway secretions	• Supportive as above if viral • Antibiotics if bacterial with supportive care also provided
Wheezing, family history of asthma/allergies, frequent respiratory infections, or chronic unexplained cough	• Accessory muscle use • Decreased chest excursion • Pursed-lip breathing	• Wheezes, • Prolonged expiration • Crackles	↓PCO$_2$ (increasing PCO$_2$ is an ominous sign), ↓PO$_2$/SpO$_2$	May be normal or show hyperaeration	ASTHMA (*most common chronic disease in childhood; see Expert Guidelines ref. below*) • Inflammation • Reversible airway obstruction/bronchospasm	(*See Expert Guidelines ref. below*) • Plan varies with severity • Inhaled β$_2$ agonists, steroids, anticholinergics, mast cell stabilizers, leukotriene modifiers, PEF or FEV$_1$ assessments, oxygen therapy, possible mechanical ventilation • Discharge teaching of med use, peakflow self-monitoring, and school management plan
Meconium ileus at birth, excessive thick respiratory secretions, frequent respiratory infections, failure to thrive	• Accessory muscle use • Barrel chest • Clubbed fingertips	• Wheezes • Crackles	May have ↓PO$_2$/SpO$_2$	Hyperaeration, peribronchial thickening, bronchiectasis, increased AP diameter	CYSTIC FIBROSIS (*one of the most common hereditary disorders*) • Excessive secretions • Air trapping	• Bronchial hygiene therapy (postural drainage and percussion, PEP mask therapy, mucolytics) • Bronchodilators • Antibiotics if indicated • Oxygen therapy • Nutritional support • May need to consider lung transplant
Previously healthy, acute onset of choking, coughing. Occasionally chronic unexplained cough	• Drooling • Stridor • May have cyanosis	• Asymmetrical breath sounds • Wheezes	May be normal, May have ↓PO$_2$/SpO$_2$	Asymmetrical expansion of chest with forced expiratory film	FOREIGN BODY OBSTRUCTION • Airway obstruction	Rigid bronchoscopy with anesthesia, followed by bronchial hygiene therapy and bronchodilator therapy
Presence of underlying disorder such as shock, sepsis, near drowning, aspiration	• Dyspnea • Tachypnea progressing to cyanosis • Irritability	• Crackles • Bronchial sounds	↓PCO$_2$ (PCO$_2$ increases as disease progresses), ↓PO$_2$/SpO$_2$, which continues to worsen despite treatment	Normal early in course, progressively shows fluffy infiltrates and patchy, nodular densities	ADULT RESPIRATORY DISTRESS SYNDROME (ARDS) • Increased alveolar-capillary membrane • Atelectasis • Consolidation	• Oxygen therapy • Hyperinflation therapy (CPAP) • Mechanical ventilation • May need to consider HFV, ECMO • Monitor for barotrauma

Used with permission of author, Terry Des Jardins

FIGURE 32-6, cont'd

	0	1	2	1 minute	5 minutes	10 minutes
Heart rate	Absent	Slow, irregular	More than 100 beats per minute			
Respiratory effort	Apnea	Irregular, slow, shallow, gasping	Strong cry			
Muscle tone	Flaccid/limp	Some flexion of extremities	Well flexed			
Reflex irritability	None/no response to stimulus	Grimace (withdraws)	Crying			
Skin color	Pale blue (shock)	Blue hands and feet, body pink	Pink all over			

FIGURE 32-7 Apgar score interpretation (add the points in the 1-minute and 5-minute columns): 0 to 3 = severe distress; 4 to 6 = moderate distress; 7 to 10 = mild to no distress.

Newborn and Pediatric Treatment Protocols

Examples of respiratory protocols commonly used to treat the newborn and pediatric patient are provided below.*

*The authors would like to thank the Respiratory Care Department at Dayton Children's Hospital, Dayton, Ohio, for providing their newborn and pediatric treatment protocols.

Oxygen Therapy Protocol
For the Newborn and Pediatric Patient
PROTOCOL 32-1

Order for Oxygen Therapy Protocol

Evaluate for Indications

- Room air SpO$_2$ less than or equal to desired range
- Room air PaO$_2$ less than or equal to desired range
- Acute situation where hypoxemia is likely, as in significant respiratory distress
- Trauma with shock, hemorrhage
- Short-term postsedation
- Carbon monoxide poisoning

  Warning: Avoid high SpO$_2$ in LBW and VLBW infants who are prone to retinopathy of prematurity (ROP).

SpO$_2$ Goals: Generally Specific to Unit Policy or Respiratory Care Protocol

- VLBW newborn <1000 g: high risk for ROP, maintain at 85% to 95%. Avoid high SpO$_2$.
- LBW newborn >1000 g: moderate risk for ROP. Maintain at 85% to 95%.
- Term infant: 88% to 98%.
- PPHN: 90% to 95%.
- CHD: to be determined by managing physician based on patient history
- BPD: 88% to 98%; may need to keep toward the higher range to prevent BPD "fits" with transient hypoxia.
- Bronchiolitis: 91% to 94% or higher.
- Asthma 92% to 94% or higher.

- Pneumonia 92% to 94% or higher.
- Chronic CF: 88% to 92% or higher.
- Carbon monoxide poisoning: Ignore SpO$_2$ and deliver 100% oxygen until measured carboxyhemoglobin level drops to desired normal range (<5%).

Choose Device

Bag and Mask Blow-by or Assist

- Commonly used on a short-term basis for the newborn, infant, or child who is unstable and has the potential to deteriorate requiring either continuous positive airway pressure (CPAP) or assisted ventilation.
- Delivery gas may be 100% oxygen or blended.
- Anesthesia-type bags will deliver 100% of the source gas.
- Extended use in the delivery room to assist ventilation supports the use of a pressure-limited device.

Nasal Cannula

- Most common device used for the delivery of low to moderate concentrations of oxygen to newborns and children. Commercially available adhesive disks allow for the cannula to be gently taped to the newborn or infant's cheeks to prevent removal.
- Newborn oxygen therapy: An air-oxygen blender is commonly used with the nasal cannula. The blender is set to an FIO$_2$ to achieve the desired SpO$_2$ at a flow rate of 0.5 to 1.0 L/min Decrease FIO$_2$ to wean to room air. Home-going oxygen will require the newborn to be placed directly on oxygen. Oxygen flow rates may be adjusted in increments of 0.1 L/min for home with a special infant regulator.

Protocol 32-1 cont'd on page 453

- Bronchiolitis infants (generally <6 months of age) requiring oxygen by cannula should be set up on incrementally lower flow rates (i.e., 0.25 to 0.5 L/min, etc.) with oxygen flow titrated to desired SpO_2. Flows >1.5 to 2 L/min reflect significant FIO_2 in this age group, i.e., 1500 mL/min or 25 mL/s may provide the majority of the inspired flow and fill physiologic dead space, providing an FIO_2 of 0.60 or greater. Flow rates in excess of 1.5 or 2 L/min may reflect the need for increased flow rate to support positive pharyngeal pressure to reduce work of breathing. A high flow nasal cannula may be required.
- Older pediatric patients can be managed with cannular oxygen; higher flow rates, 4 to 6 L/min, may suggest a need to evaluate the patients actual FIO_2 with a venturi mask challenge. Using the venturi mask, adjust the FIO_2 and flow rate to get the desired SpO_2. Report this to the managing medical team to quantify the child's degree of hypoxemia.

High Flow Nasal Cannula

- High flow oxygen system applied via nasal cannula at 100% relative humidity at body temperature.
- An air-oxygen blender is commonly used to adjust FIO_2.
- High flow rates provide expiratory resistance and positive pharyngeal pressure to reduce work of breathing (flows of 4 to 8 L/min in newborns and infants, 15 to 40 L/min in children).
- Pharyngeal pressure varies with breathing cycle and leak through mouth.
- Unlikely to reverse atelectasis or increase FRC, but can be helpful in reducing work of breathing and preventing fatigue-related respiratory failure.

Simple Mask

Used primarily for short term, moderate oxygen use, possibly during a procedure or sedation. It may be used in the emergency department or in an emergency until a specific oxygen requirement is determined and a more comfortable device (nasal cannula, cool aerosol face mask, etc.) is set up.

Venturi Mask

Used for pediatric and adult-sized patients for short-term high flow oxygen delivery; precise FIO_2 delivery is helpful in quantifying the child's degree of $\dot{V}/\dot{Q}$ mismatch for the clinical team. Dry gas limits its long-term use.

Nonrebreather Mask

Used for quick pediatric application of high oxygen or specialty gas delivery in the ED or ICU. Flow should be set high enough to meet patient's inspiratory demand. Often used in trauma and carbon monoxide poisoning and can be used to deliver heliox. Dry gas prevents long-term use.

Cool Aerosol Face Mask or Face Tent

- Allows for delivery of continuous bland aerosol with accurate FIO_2 when total flow rate exceeds patient's inspiratory demand.
- Appropriate for cooperative pediatric patients.
- Face tent offers aerosol and FIO_2 control without direct contact to oronasal region, desirable with some trauma or surgical cases.

Oxygen Hood

- Used for short-term oxygen delivery in newborns or younger infants who are unable to roll over.
- Accurate FIO_2 when total flow rate exceeds infant's inspiratory flow rate, up to 100% oxygen.
- Hood limits access to face; FIO_2 fluctuates when hood is opened.
- May be used short term for oxygen challenge test.
- May be used postoperatively for infants with upper airway surgery, i.e., choanal atresia repair.

Mist Tent

- Rarely used in pediatric care for oxygen delivery since the introduction of adhesive disks that allow cannulas to be secured to an infant or child's cheeks.
- Difficult to maintain FIO_2 with tent opening to access patient.

Isolette

- Rarely used in newborn care for oxygen delivery
- Difficult to maintain FIO_2 with opening of side ports to access patient.

Assess Effectiveness of Oxygen Therapy

An oxygenation assessment should always include a respiratory assessment along with SpO_2; the frequency of assessments depends on the patient's acuity and stability: from continuous monitoring in critical care, intermittent Q2H for patient who has the potential to deteriorate or is labile, Q4h for acute respiratory admission, Q4h to Q6H for stable acute patient, Q6H when weaning, Q8H for chronic patient until stable. Continuous SpO_2 monitoring of general care patients often leads to nuisance alarms and has been shown to lengthen hospitalization.

Adjustment

Oxygen flow rate or FIO_2 should be adjusted to meet the SpO_2 goals or until a specific clinical goal is reached (i.e., carboxyhemoglobin level <5%). Generally, as the FIO_2 requirement drops, masks are transitioned to the nasal cannula for its ease of use during feeding, ambulation, etc.

Documentation and Communication

Document all respiratory assessments with SpO_2 in the medical record along with any adjustments in oxygen administration. Anytime oxygen is initiated, increased significantly, and/or FIO_2 exceeds 0.40 or the patient's SpO_2 does not reach the desired goal, the medical team should be notified to discuss additional treatment and/or diagnostics (chest x-ray, lab tests, etc.) to identify and treat the underlying condition.

BPD, Bronchopulmonary dysplasia; *CF*, cystic fibrosis; *CHD*, congenital heart disease; *LBW*, low birth weight (<2500 g); *PPHN*, persistent pulmonary hypertension of the newborn; *VLBW*, very low birth weight (<1500 g).

Bronchopulmonary Hygiene Therapy Protocol

For the Newborn and Pediatric Patient

PROTOCOL 32-2

Order for Bronchial Hygiene Protocol

Evaluate for Indications

- Difficulty with secretion clearance
- Evidence of retained bronchial secretions
- Chest x-ray (CXR) demonstrates atelectasis secondary to mucous plugging
- Cystic fibrosis (CF), primary ciliary dyskinesia
- Accumulation of purulent secretions in bronchopneumonia
- Residual secretions and debris after foreign body removal

Choose Applicable Techniques Based on Patient Age, Cooperation, Ability to Cough, and Disease Process

Suctioning

- Endotracheal suctioning is applicable to infants and children with an endotracheal tube or tracheostomy tube (PRN).
- Hypopharyngeal suction is applicable to infants or children with airway secretions who are unable to cough on demand due to age, muscle weakness or mental capacity (PRN).
- Noninvasive suction is often used to as an adjunct to gently remove secretions from the nares of small infants, the mouths of children with limited ability to cough, or the stoma area of chronic tracheostomy patients (PRN).

Cough Assist

- Applicable to a child with muscle weakness or lack of motor control to produce an effective cough (spinal muscular atrophy or muscular dystrophy). Device will deliver a pressurized breath then apply negative pressure to bring lower airway secretions into the upper airway for removal by hypopharyngeal or oral suction (QID + PRN).
- Contraindicated in patients with an effective cough.

Cough and Deep Breathing

- Indicated in all children who are able to cooperate and cough on demand with every encounter.
- Diaphragmatic breathing with pursed lip breathing is often utilized in relaxing an asthmatic child or a child with CF.
- **Huff cough** is used for effective coughing with CF patient's therapies.
- Adjuncts may be used to encourage deep breathing and mobilization of secretions, e.g., incentive spirometry, blowing bubbles, blowing pinwheels, laughing. Choose technique that matches the child's age and ability to perform.

Flutter Valve, PEP, and Oscillatory Positive Expiratory Pressure

- These techniques are used in cooperative children to encourage deep breathing and mobilization of secretions. Frequency depends on patient presentation. Any secretion-related atelectasis with hypoxemia requiring supplemental oxygen should increase treatment to Q4h or more frequently. Routine care at QID.
- Effective in patients with secretion-related atelectasis, bronchopneumonia, and/or chronic obstructive pulmonary disease.
- These therapies can be used for home therapy as well.
- These techniques encourage active participation in patients who may be passive with other therapies.

Chest Physical Therapy, Postural Drainage, and Percussion

Indications

- Secretion-related atelectasis, bronchitis, CF, and other childhood conditions where lower airway secretions are retained. Q4h for acute presentation, QID for chronic.
- May be used for localized removal of secretions or debris following foreign body removal.
- Choice of chest physical therapy or postural drainage as the method of bronchial hygiene is dependent on history of effectiveness, patient preference, ability to actively cough with each position, risk vs benefit of positioning (i.e., risk of extubation while on ventilator).
- Medicated aerosol therapy may be helpful before or after this procedure.

Contraindications

- Manual or mechanical percussion technique with positioning is currently contraindicated in newborns and young infants with highly compliant chest walls.
- A metaanalysis of chest physical therapy in bronchiolitis showed that it is not effective.
- Reflux and the risk of intraventricular hemorrhage in newborns and young infants make positioning in a head-down position contraindicated.
- Generally not performed when active hemoptysis is present.

Percussive Vest Therapy

- Alternative to chest physical therapy and postural drainage in secretion-related atelectasis (Q4h to QID).
- Size of vest may limit use in younger patients
- Alternate "wrap" vest may allow for easy application in ventilated patients
- Common method for airway clearance in chronic patients while hospitalized and at home.
- Patient may be able to take aerosol treatment during vest therapy.

IPV or MetaNeb

- These intrapulmonary percussive or high frequency oscillatory ventilation techniques are generally used with older cooperative pediatric patients. The patient uses a mouthpiece to inspire from a self-activated manifold. These devices deliver aerosolized medication while pulsating to mobilize secretions and stimulate cough (Q4h in acute care, QID in chronic care).
- For younger or less cooperative patients, use a positive pressure mask.
- Patient preference and history of effectiveness determine use. *Protocol 32-2 cont'd on page 455*

Cont'd Protocol 32-2

- Both devices can also be placed inline with a ventilator to mobilize secretions.
- Contraindications: This device delivers a pressure that could be dangerous in patients with a pneumothorax or at risk for air leak.

Medications to Facilitate Airway Clearance

- In the newborn with meconium aspiration syndrome, surfactant is indicated to help mobilize debris.
- Bronchodilators are used to improve aeration in patients with reactive airways disease and to promote an effective cough (Q4h or QID).
- Hypertonic saline (3%) has been recommended in the treatment of copious secretions in bronchiolitis (TID)
- Hypertonic saline 3% to 7% has been recommended for the mobilization of secretions in CF and primary ciliary dyskinesia (QID).
- DNAse Pulmozyme (dornase alfa) is a mucolytic, which breaks down the DNA of white blood cells to thin secretions in CF (QD or BID).
- Mucomyst (acetylcysteine), a mucolytic sometimes used in adults, is rarely used in pediatrics.

Bronchoscopy

- Assist with bronchoscopy in nonresolving atelectasis.

Assess Clinical Improvement Techniques after Each Treatment

Clinical Improvement Includes

- Breath sounds clear after treatment
- FIO_2 decreases, SpO_2 increases
- Subjective improvement
- Objective improvement: patient up and playing
- CXR improves
- On ventilator, airway resistance and lung compliance improve.

Weaning of Therapy

Reduce frequency of therapy to daytime hours (QID, TID, BID).

Discontinue in acute conditions if improvement is sustained over 24 hours.

Decrease treatment frequency to home regimen in chronic pulmonary conditions.

Consider lung expansion therapy if bronchial hygiene therapy is too painful for patient cooperation.

Lung Expansion Therapy Protocol
For the Newborn and Pediatric Patient
PROTOCOL 32-3

Newborn Applications

Goals

- To reduce work of breathing in respiratory distress syndrome (RDS) or transient tachypnea of the newborn (TTN)
- To improve functional residual capacity in restrictive lung disease
- To prevent or treat microatelectasis
- To stent airway tracheomalacia or bronchomalacia until airway matures or is surgically corrected

Common Newborn Treatment Modalities

High Flow Nasal Cannula

- High flow oxygen system applied via nasal cannula at 100% humidity at body temperature.
- An air-oxygen blender is generally used to adjust FIO_2.
- Provides expiratory resistance to reduce work of breathing and fatigue.
- Assists the infant in maintaining FRC.
- Good adjunct postextubation.

Bubble Nasal CPAP (B-NCPAP)

- Medical gas at desired FIO_2 is bubbled through water creating a vibratory, high frequency oscillatory CPAP; expiratory limb is immersed in water at the level of pressure desired (e.g., 4 cm H_2O).

- Applied via nasal prongs.
- Effective in the management of infants with mild respiratory distress postdelivery.

Nasal CPAP via ventilator (V-NCPAP)

- CPAP applied through nasal prongs via a conventional ventilator.
- Pressures of 6 to 9 cm H_2O are effective.
- Specific FIO_2 is controlled and weaned to desired SpO_2.

CPAP by Bag and Mask

- Often used in the delivery room or when an infant is unstable and may require assisted ventilation.
- Only for short-term use.
- Monitor CPAP pressure with a manometer.

Endotracheal CPAP

- CPAP through endotracheal tube via a conventional ventilator.
- Pressures of 5 to 6 cm H_2O are effective.
- Often combined with pressure support to overcome airway resistance of the endotracheal tube during spontaneous breathing.
- Specific FIO_2 is controlled and weaned to desired SpO_2.
- May be used postoperatively to prevent atelectasis or as an interim step between synchronized intermittent mechanical ventilation and extubation.

Frequency

- These are all continuous therapies and should be accompanied by continuous pulse oximetry and PRN suctioning of the airway to remove secretions and elicit cough.

Note: In premature infants with RDS, these therapies are applied in conjunction with surfactant administration.

Protocol 32-3 cont'd on page 456

Assessment

FIO$_2$, flow rate, and CPAP levels should be documented with a patient physical assessment Q2 to Q8H. Weaning the flow rate of a high-FLOW nasal cannula (HFNC) or CPAP pressure may begin once the patient's FIO$_2$ is <0.30 and chest x-ray (CXR) is improved. Use of CPAP for the treatment of airway malacia is often long term and may require continued home use.

Pediatric Applications

Goals

- To encourage cough and deep breathing
- To prevent postop atelectasis
- To reverse lung consolidation
- To treat obstructive sleep apnea (CPAP)

Is the patient cooperative and able to breathe without assistance? Yes or No?

If yes, consider these common pediatric treatment modalities:

Incentive Spirometry

- Primarily a technique for deep breathing and coughing.
- Can be a lung expansion technique in an older, cooperative child to prevent and treat atelectasis.
- Alternate deep-breathing therapies to substitute for younger children include blowing bubbles, blowing a pinwheel, laughing, etc. Emphasize the deep breathing prior to blowing.
- Encourage active coughing and expectoration.
- Frequency is usually (Q2 to Q4h) and supervised in the beginning, then tapered as the patient and family are able to assume care and the patient is not requiring oxygen.
- Reevaluate effectiveness Q24h.

Positive Expiratory Pressure or Oscillatory Positive Expiratory Pressure Therapy

- Indicated when there is evidence of lung consolidation with mild oxygen requirement.
- Positive expiratory pressure supports lower airway integrity and improves ventilation distribution.
- Effective in mobilizing secretions, particularly in cystic fibrosis.
- Encourages active coughing and expectoration.
- Frequency of Q2 to Q4h and supervised in beginning; wean to QID once oxygen is no longer required to maintain SpO$_2$.

Is the patient cooperative and able to deep breathe without assistance? Yes or No?

If no, consider these common treatment modalities:

IPPB Therapy

Caution: Active application of positive pressure is contraindicated when there is evidence of untreated air leak, i.e., pneumomediastinum, pneumothorax, subcutaneous air, etc.

- Intermittent application of positive airway pressure on inspiration; patient triggers breath with inspiratory effort for a 15-minute treatment.
- Pressure is adjusted to achieve good breath sounds and may be volume targeted to achieve one-third of predicted inspiratory capacity.
- May be applied by mask in patients unable to cooperate or by mouthpiece for cooperative patients.
- Generally used when there is CXR evidence of volume-related atelectasis.
- Patient may be positioned to elevate involved segment for better aeration.
- Frequency may be Q2 to Q4h at first, then tapered to Q4h to Q6h until CXR improves or oxygen requirement subsides.

CPAP Therapy

- Generally applied noninvasively via nasal mask, nasal-oral mask, or full face mask.
- Provides continuous positive airway pressure to build FRC and reverse atelectasis in the spontaneously breathing patient.
- Requires continuous pulse oximetry for acute use.
- CPAP pressure is adjusted to patient comfort, degree of atelectasis, and oxygen requirement, generally 5 to 10 cm H$_2$O pressure.
- May be applied during sleep for children with obstructive sleep apnea at the CPAP pressure prescribed following a CPAP titration sleep study.

Reevaluate the patient's progress toward specific goals with every intervention. Improvement is suggested by:

- Decreased respiratory rate
- Normal pulse rate
- Absence of fever
- Improved aeration over affected segment/lung field per breath sounds
- Resolution of atelectasis on CXR
- Improved muscle strength and effective cough
- Patient ambulation
- No supplemental oxygen required for SpO$_2$ goal

If goals are reached and patient's condition is improving: Reduce frequency and wean to most appropriate therapy for level of cooperation and participation. Consider family-directed care.

If patient does not improve: Advance care to IPPB or noninvasive CPAP or BiPAP. Consult with medical team for possible invasive support via mechanical ventilation with PEEP.

Document all assessments and communicate with medical team frequently if the patient does not progress as expected.

Recommend arterial blood gases when ineffective ventilation is a suspected cause of hypoxemia.

Aerosolized Medication
For the Hospitalized Newborn and Pediatric Patient
PROTOCOL 32-4

Indications

- To reverse bronchospasm and reduce work of breathing
- To determine response to bronchodilators or the presence of reversible airways disease (trial)
- To maximize ventilation prior to bronchial hygiene
- To reduce airway swelling in croup
- To liquefy and mobilize secretions
- To reduce airway inflammation and reactivity
- To provide topical antibiotics for treatment or prophylaxis

Methods of Delivery

Medicated Aerosol Via Hand-Held Nebulizer

- These aerosolized medications are commonly delivered by nebulizer: Tobi (tobramycin solution for inhalation), DNase, hypertonic saline, racemic epinephrine, Duo-Neb (albuterol/Ipratropium).
- The nebulizer used may be specific to the drug, as FDA approval of the drug includes the nebulizer used in the clinical trial. (E.g., Budesonide Respules, Tobi, and DNase are to be nebulized in the Pari LC nebulizer*).
- A mouthpiece is preferred over a mask for improved medication delivery; a mask may be used in a young, uncooperative child.
- Breath-activated nebulizers have been shown to improve drug delivery.

Metered Dose Inhaler with Valved Holding Chamber or Spacer

- Use of metered dose inhaler (MDI) with valved holding chamber (VHC) in the hospital allows the patient to practice proper technique for home use with each treatment.
- Infants can be treated effectively with MDI-VHC with mask.
- If policy is to provide asthma patients with individual MDI during hospital stay, this will ensure patient has an understanding of the MDI and the VHC at discharge for continued care.

Dry Powder Inhalers (DPIs)

- Several parasympatholytics, inhaled corticosteroids, and combination long-acting bronchodilators/inhaled corticosteroids come in a dry powder with a unique inhaler, which requires a coordinated breathing effort and a high peak inspiratory flow rate. These may not be suitable for young children under 6 years of age.

Continuous Albuterol Aerosol

- Children in status asthmaticus are often advanced to a continuous albuterol aerosol, which can run for hours until symptoms subside.
- Dosing can vary from 5 mg to 40 mg/h, using a syringe pump and a vibrating mesh nebulizer or a large volume medication nebulizer.
- Continuous electrocardographic monitoring is required and often this care is provided in an intensive care unit or emergency department (ED) (see Box 32-3).

Disease-Specific Drugs in Hospitalization

Disease	Type of medication	Drug	Method	Frequency
Asthma/Reactive airways disease	Rescue bronchodilator	Albuterol	Aerosol or MDI-VHC	Q20 minutes in ED, Q2 to Q6hours inpatient, Continuous in status. Up to 20 mg/h (Box 32-3). (some institutions use higher concentrations)
	Controller	Inhaled corticosteroids	MDI DPI aerosol	QD or BID
Bronchiolitis due to viral illness	Bronchodilator	Albuterol	Aerosol	Trial for moderate score or higher, continue if response (Q4h to Q6h)
	Decongestant	Racemic epinephrine	Aerosol	Trial for moderate score or higher and continue if improvement (Q4h to Q6h)
Croup	Decongestant	Racemic epinephrine	Aerosol	PRN for croup score in moderate range

*The Pari LC nebulizer is an effective jet nebulizer that is breath-enhanced and produces consistent particle size.

Protocol 32–4 cont'd on page 458

Disease	Type of medication	Drug	Method	Frequency
Cystic fibrosis	Bronchodilator	Albuterol	Aerosol	QID and PRN
	Mucolytic	Hypertonic saline	Aerosol or IPV delivery	QID
	Mucolytic	DNase	Aerosol	QD or BID
	Antibiotic	Variety of antibiotics specific to the patient's sensitivity: i.e., Tobi, colistin, Cayston (aztreonam), amphotericin	Aerosol	QD or BID
HIV positive/ immunosuppressed patient	Antibiotic prophylaxis	Pentamidine	Aerosol via filtered circuit and HEPA[†] system	Q30 days

[†]High efficiency particulate absorption (HEPA) refers to a filter used to protect the caregiver (e.g., HEPA hood) during treatment or clearing the room (room HEPA filter) after a treatment.

Assessment and Weaning

- Patients who are receiving aerosolized medications for acute relief are assessed at every encounter. Frequency of therapy is actively weaned using disease-specific scoring systems, e.g., asthma, bronchiolitis, or croup protocol.
- Any time patient does not progress as expected or needs to increase the frequency of aerosols to gain relief, the medical team must be notified to discuss need for additional treatment or diagnostics.
- Chronic patients are weaned to their home regimen.

Education

During assessments or treatments, particularly in the case of families with infants or children with chronic respiratory disease, the respiratory therapist should reinforce proper breathing technique, medication delivery, trigger avoidance, airway clearance, and when to seek medical help.

BOX 32-3 Procedure for Continuous Albuterol Aerosol Administration

Method 1

Using a large volume medication nebulizer, such as a Heart Nebulizer:

- Place 100 mL of normal saline into the Heart nebulizer.
- Add 16 mL of 0.5% albuterol (5 mg/mL × 16 mL = 80 mg of albuterol).
- Set flowmeter for the source gas at 10 L/min. At this flow rate, the nebulizer will nebulize over 4 hours, delivering approximately 20 mg of albuterol/h.

Method 2

Using a medication syringe pump with a small volume vibrating mesh nebulizer, such as the Aerogen:

- Determine desired albuterol dosing per hour.
- Using the chart below, mix specific albuterol volume with the normal saline volume and draw up the mixture in a 60-mL syringe.
- Attach the IV tubing to the syringe and the nebulizer.
- Prime the IV tubing, pushing the syringe until the solution reaches the nebulizer.
- Place the syringe in the pump and set the pump to 12 mL/h.

Drug Dose (mg/h)	IV Pump Rate (mL/h)	Albuterol (mL)	Saline (mL)	Total volume (mL)	Duration (h)
5	12	4	44	48	4
10	12	8	40	48	4
15	12	12	36	48	4
20	12	16	32	48	4

Newborns

Modes

- **Noninvasive positive pressure ventilation (NIPPV)** is preferred over invasive ventilation when it is effective in assisting ventilation in the spontaneously breathing infant. Special nasal interfaces/cannulas are available to support noninvasive bilevel ventilation with certain ventilators in newborn care.
- A volume-targeted mode for newborn ventilation is ideal to maintain consistent ventilation in the face of changing compliance. The actual mode chosen may be pressure controlled or pressure regulated as airway leaks may prevent the use of a volume-controlled mode. In the pressure-control mode, the therapist must ensure that pressure is adjusted to reach the desired weight-based V_T and to avoid overdistention and ventilator-associated lung injury.
- Pressure support is commonly used when available to counter the airway resistance associated with small endotracheal tubes, with spontaneous breathing.
- High frequency ventilation (HFV) should be considered when PIP rises above 30 cm H_2O pressure or when air leak is possible.
- Paralysis and sedation may be necessary in infants requiring significant control of mean airway pressure (MAP).

Settings

- **Delivered Tidal Volume (V_T):** 4 to 6 mL/kg, as set in a volume mode or as the targeted exhaled volume in pressure modes. Newer ventilators can be set to correct for compressible tubing volume to improve the accuracy of exhaled volume.
- **Inspiratory Time (IT)*:** 0.25 to 0.5 seconds, with higher inspiratory times used with obstructive conditions like meconium aspiration syndrome and lower with restrictive disease like RDS.
- **Respiratory Rate (RR)*:** Usually set to 20 to 40 breaths/ min, higher with restrictive disease, slower with obstructive disease. Higher rates may be necessary in cases where higher MAP is needed and raising PIP or PEEP is not desirable.
- **FIO$_2$:** Adjust to reach desired SpO$_2$ after setting appropriate ventilator parameters.
- **Peak Inspiratory Pressure (PIP):** Adjust initially to achieve an "easy breath" with good bilateral aeration and chest rise; when exhaled volume is measured, adjust to reach target of 4 to 6 mL/kg. Usually 18 to 25 cm H_2O pressure is adequate to begin; higher PIP may be necessary for

***Consider Time Constant:** This is the infant's airway resistance (Raw) × their lung compliance (V/P). Newborns with RDS have low Raw and low compliance requiring shorter inspiratory times and faster rates. Patients with high airway resistance and higher compliance, such as meconium aspiration syndrome, may need a longer inspiratory time and slower rates to ventilate.

NIPPV or with poor compliance as with significant pulmonary hypoplasia.

- **Positive End-Expiratory Pressure (PEEP):** Generally started at 4 to 5 cm H_2O for most newborn conditions. NOTE: this parameter has the most impact on MAP. Very low birth weight infants may require less (3 to 4 cm H_2O), especially after surfactant administration.

Monitoring

- Newborns with respiratory distress at birth will often have an **umbilical artery catheter** (UAC) placed for central monitoring of arterial blood gases. This line will remain in use until the patient improves, or generally up to 7 days.
- Infants who require ventilation, without the availability of a UAC, should be monitored with **capillary blood gases** and pulse oximetry, or a peripheral arterial line if critically unstable.
- Transcutaneous electrodes may be placed on the infant's chest or abdomen to monitor PtcCO$_2$ continuously.
- Newer ventilators for infants will give continuous feedback: exhaled volume with ventilator breaths, exhaled volume with spontaneous breaths, wave forms to demonstrate inspiratory effort, loops to show overdistention with prolonged inspiratory time, MAP trends, etc. This feedback should be used by the respiratory therapist to adjust ventilator settings.

Adjustments and Weaning in Patients Who Demonstrate Clinical Improvement

- Because surfactant quickly improves the infant's lung compliance, frequent monitoring and adjustments should be made to reduce PIP and, possibly, IT to reach the 4 to 6 mL/ kg V_T goal as soon possible after surfactant delivery. Weaning of the FIO$_2$ is usually needed to prevent overoxygenation.
- Chest x-ray (CXR) is helpful in determining the adequacy of ventilation. PIP and/or PEEP may need to be increased to achieve an adequate FRC or reduced to prevent overdistention. The diaphragm should generally be at the level of T8.
- Controlled or SIMV rate should be reduced incrementally to allow infants to assume more of their own minute ventilation. Pressure support prevents fatigue with spontaneous breaths.
- FIO$_2$ should be adjusted downward toward room air as soon as possible, following the SpO$_2$ goals for the newborn's gestational age and weight.
- Active weaning should occur with each assessment and blood gas with active communication with the medical management team. Goals should be updated daily at rounds.

Adjustments for Patients With Worsening Clinical Condition (Higher MAP, PIP, PEEP Required)

- Inline suction should be placed in the ventilator circuit to avoid drops in MAP during suctioning.
- As the required PIP approaches 30 cm H_2O pressure to achieve adequate V_T or FRC on CXR, HFV should be considered in restrictive lung diseases.

Protocol 32-5 cont'd on page 460

- The oxygenation index (OI) should be assessed using arterial blood gas PaO_2 and MAP and reported to the medical team.
- If HFOV is initiated, settings should begin with MAP set at 3 above the conventional setting, rate at 9 to 12 Hz (540 to 720 oscillations/min), IT at 33%, and amplitude set to produce the classic "**chest wiggle**" down to the umbilicus.
- Permissive hypercapnia may be permitted when appropriate.
- Sedation and paralysis may be necessary to manage the infant's ventilation and MAP.
- Persistent pulmonary hypertension of the newborn (PPHN) should be assessed by echocardiogram; a trial of iNO may determine effectiveness in reversing shunt-related hypoxemia.
- If underlying condition requires surgical repair, immediate surgery may be necessary.
- ECMO may be necessary for infants whose OIs are 40, or higher.

Pediatric Patients

Modes

- Modes will vary as significantly as in adult care, due to the wide range of conditions requiring ventilation—e.g., trauma, chronic and acute obstructive respiratory disease, neuromuscular weakness, respiratory depression, restrictive or parenchymal pulmonary disease, congenital disorders, infectious disease, acute respiratory distress syndrome (ARDS), etc. Follow Protocol 10-1 (see Chapter 10) for choice of ventilator mode.
- A ventilator with newborn, pediatric, and adult modes and capabilities is best suited to the pediatric intensive care unit. These ventilators must have the sensitivity to (1) sense the inspiratory effort of a small infant to an adult-sized teen, (2) deliver an accurate V_T across the newborn to adult spectrum, and (3) have a range of flow rates to meet the minimal inspiratory demands of a newborn as well as the largest, air-hungry teen. e.g., Servo i, Avea, PB 840, Drager V500, Hamilton G5.
- The choice of ventilator mode and method of triggering will depend on airway leaks, patient breathing effort, use of sedation or paralysis, and underlying disease state.
- NIPPV is preferred to invasive ventilation when it can assist the spontaneously breathing patient. Many critical care ventilators have noninvasive modes that are applicable through a variety of mask interfaces. Gaining a child's cooperation to wear a mask takes time and supervision to ensure continued use.
- Most pediatric intensive care units have both conventional and high frequency options for ventilating those children with severe hypoxemia requiring higher MAPs.
- Generally, infant ventilator circuits accommodate tidal volumes up to 120 mL; pediatric/adult circuits are used for tidal volumes above 80 to 100 mL.
- Acute ventilator patients are typically monitored continuously with pulse oximetry and capnography.

Settings

Delivered V_T[†]: 6 to 10 mL/kg. Generally, 6 to 8 mL is the common starting point, unless the patient has obstructive lung disease, in which case higher volume may be preferred due to increased physiologic dead space. Lower volumes are preferred when resulting PIP exceeds 35 cm H_2O pressure.

Inspiratory Time (IT): 0.5 to 1.2 seconds with the shorter IT for infants and longer IT for older patients or children with obstructive disease.

Respiratory Rate (RR): Age appropriate to produce a normal ventilation pattern, usually 12 to 30 breaths/min, with 30 for infants and as low as 12 for teens. Higher rates may be used when there is a need to increase MAP in patients who cannot tolerate increased PEEP or PIP.

Peak Inspiratory Pressure (PIP): In pressure cycled modes, adjust PIP to a pressure that produces an easy breath, bilateral aeration, and normal chest rise; when exhaled volume measurement is available, adjust PIP to achieve desired V_T of 6 to 10 mL/kg.

Positive End-Expiratory Pressure (PEEP): Generally, this should be set with the patient's lung condition in mind: 4 to 5 cm of H_2O is a common starting point for nearly all patients. In restrictive disease, the PEEP may need to be significantly increased, watching the patient's pressure-volume hysteresis curve and volume delivery to achieve optimal PEEP. In obstructive disease, the PEEP is typically set to 4 to 5 cm H_2O to provide airway stenting; inspiratory time and rate need to be adjusted to avoid "**auto-PEEP**" (air trapping), which can occur with insufficient expiratory time.

Pressure Support: Commonly used to overcome ET resistance with spontaneous breathing. Level is set to provide an easy, unlabored breath with spontaneous efforts.

Adjustment and Weaning of Patients with Clinical Improvement

- The child's clinical condition will impact the speed of weaning. Those ventilated for respiratory depression (i.e., postseizure, postop, postnarcotic overdose) will typically wean quickly as soon as the respiratory depression reverses.
- Those who have chronic pulmonary disease with an acute exacerbation or a condition such as ARDS, an immuno-suppressive disorder, a neuromuscular weakness, or congenital heart disease may require a longer weaning period, requiring a variety of modes to reach weaning goals.
- (Follow adult ventilator weaning protocol as in Protocol 10-2)

[†]**Note:** Newer ventilators can be set to correct for **compressible tubing volume**—i.e., the volume that expands the ventilator tubing that is not delivered to the patients. In older machines, compressible volume should be calculated, particularly in the younger patient. It is calculated as (PIP-PEEP) in cm H_2O pressure × tubing factor (i.e., 1 to 3 mL/cm H_2O pressure depending on the size of circuit used); subtract this volume from the displayed exhaled volume to determine the actual delivered tidal volume.

Protocol 32-5 cont'd on page 461

Adjustment and Weaning of Patients with Worsening Condition

- For patients who worsen due to ARDS or consolidation, lung recruitment strategies are needed. This typically involves higher PEEP to increase FRC and a raised MAP.
- Airway pressure-release ventilation (APRV) and high-frequency ventilation (HFV) are ventilator strategies that may be considered when the PIP exceeds 35 cm H_2O pressure (plateau pressure above 30 cm H_2O) or when OI exceeds 24 (see Protocol 10-1).
- Sedation and paralysis may be required in patients requiring a significantly high MAP.
- If high-frequency oscillatory ventilation (HFOV) is initiated, settings should begin with MAP at 5 above the conventional setting, rate at 5 to 6 Hz (300 to 360 oscillations/min), IT at 33%, and amplitude set to produce the classic "chest wiggle" down to the midthigh. Lower frequency Hz will increase bulk movement and help with CO_2 elimination. Children over 35 kg need an oscillator with increased flow capacity and power.
- Permissive hypercapnia becomes a physiologic goal when ventilation parameters increase and become more likely to induce ventilator-associated lung injury.
- Volumetric CO_2 Monitoring may be helpful in adjusting ventilator settings in patients who may be difficult to manage with increased physiologic dead space.
- Neurally activated ventilatory assistance (NAVA®) may be helpful in weaning patients who are weak or who have problems with asynchrony with spontaneous breathing efforts.

Surfactant Administration Protocol
PROTOCOL 32-6

Order

- Transport standing order for surfactant administration with specific drug and dosage.
- Order in electronic medical record for surfactant administration with specific drug and dosage.

Verify Indications

- Newborn exhibiting respiratory distress at birth
- Premature infants under 30 weeks' gestation
- Surfactant deficiency with presence of reticulogranular ground-glass appearance on chest x-ray (CXR)
- Meconium aspiration
- No contraindication present, e.g., significant air leak (tension pneumothorax requiring immediate treatment) or known nonviable condition

Procedure

1. Intubate infant with appropriate sized endotracheal tube (ET):
   - <1000 g   2.5 mm
   - 1000 to 2000 g   3.0 mm
   - 2000 to 3000 g   3.5 mm
   - >3000 g   3.5 mm to 4.0 mm

   If a large leak around the tube is present, the infant should be reintubated with the next larger size tube.
2. Assess ET position to ensure it is not in the esophagus or in the right or left mainstem bronchus.
   - Good symmetrical chest movement with each positive pressure breath
   - Equal breath sounds bilaterally
   - CXR shows tip of ET at T1 to T2
3. Place infant on mechanical ventilator and continuously monitor with pulse oximetry. Manual ventilation with pressure monitoring may also be used if a ventilator is not available.
4. Suction patient before surfactant administration.

5. Inspect the surfactant vial for discoloration; normal surfactant is off-white. Gently swirl the vial if drug has settled during storage. Do not shake. The drug should be at room temperature for 20 minutes or warmed by hand for at least 8 minutes.
6. Dosing is specific to the type of surfactant used. For example, initial Curosurf (poractant alfa) dose is 2.5 mL/kg per dose. Curosurf comes in 3-mL vials, so more than one vial is needed when the infant is over 1200 g. Slowly draw up the surfactant using an 18- to 19-gauge needle and a 5 mL-syringe.
7. Verify the infant's weight and the ordered dose with the infant's nurse before administration.
8. **Bolus dosing procedure (routine)**
   - Attach the feeding tube to the surfactant syringe.
   - Connect the multiaccess catheter adapter to the ET; re-attach the ventilator wye to continue ventilation.
   - Position the infant supine with the head midline.
   - Insert the feeding tube through the multiaccess port to the length required to just reach the end of the ET.
   - Quickly inject half of the dose. Remove the feeding tube.
   - Roll the infant laterally for 1 to 2 minutes.
   - Reposition the infant supine with the head and ET midline. Insert the feeding tube to the appropriate length.
   - Quickly inject the second half of the dose and remove the feeding tube.
   - Roll the patient to the other side for 1 to 2 minutes.
   - Replace the multiaccess adapter with the original ET 15 mm-adapter and attach to ventilator wye to continue ventilation.
9. **Drip dosing procedure:** This option may be considered when the infant is unstable and bolus delivery could add to instability. This is an older technique, using a 15-mm ET adapter with a Luer lock side port for the surfactant syringe attachment. The surfactant is instilled slowly with each mechanical inspiration, two half doses over 5

Protocol 32-6 cont'd on page 462

Cont'd Protocol 32-6

to 10 minutes each, with right and left side positioning after each half dose. If at any time the infant's SpO_2 drops significantly, dosing is paused and the PIP is increased (4–5 cm H_2O), and the FIO_2 is increased for several minutes until recovery.

10. **After dosing:**
    - Reevaluate the ET position to assure it was not dislodged during dosing.
    - As surfactant will quickly improve the infant's lung compliance, chest expansion, color, exhaled tidal volume, and SpO_2 must be monitored closely for 30 minutes after dosing. Frequently wean PIP and FIO_2 to avoid hyperventilation and hyperoxia. V_T goal is 4 to 6 mL/kg. Obtain blood gas at 30 minutes.
    - Infants should not be suctioned for at least 1 hour after surfactant administration unless clinically necessary.

11. **Documentation:** Document the indication for the surfactant administration, the method of administration, and the patient's tolerance and response. Relay any concerns to the medical team.

12. **Concerns**
    - If the infant continues to have a supplemental oxygen requirement (i.e., over 30% to 40%) or significant ventilator settings, a second dose of surfactant may be ordered based on the drug's specific recommended frequency. (Some surfactant preparations may recommend a repeat dose at 6 or 12 hours.) A second dose requires an additional order and dosage. E.g., Curosurf is dosed at half the initial dose at 1.25 mL/kg if given a second time
    - Watch for signs of pulmonary hemorrhage. This is a possible complication with surfactant administration, as the rapid improvement of lung compliance can result in pulmonary hyperperfusion. This occurs in the first few days of life.

SELF-ASSESSMENT QUESTIONS

Answers to questions can be found on Evolve. To access additional student assessment questions visit **http://evolve.elsevier.com/DesJardins/respiratory**.

1. Which of the following trigger(s) apneic episodes?
    1. Hypoglycemia
    2. Nasotracheal suctioning
    3. Head flexion
    4. MAS
        a. 4 only
        b. 2 and 3 only
        c. 2, 3, and 4 only
        d. 1, 2, 3, and 4

2. A newborn baby with PPHN is receiving ventilator support with a mean airway pressure of 10 cm H_2O, an FIO_2 of 1.00, a pH of 7.31, a $PaCO_2$ of 49, HCO_3^- 24, and a PaO_2 of 50. Based on this information, what is the patient's oxygenation index?
    a. 10
    b. 15
    c. 20
    d. 25

3. When resuscitation of the newborn is being done correctly, which of the following begins to improve first?
    a. Tone
    b. Heart rate
    c. Reflex irritability
    d. Respiratory movements

4. Which of the following is associated with PPHN?
    1. Hypoglycemia
    2. Decreased pH
    3. Hypercalcemia
    4. Systemic hypotension
        a. 1 only
        b. 3 only
        c. 2 and 4 only
        d. 1, 2, and 4 only

5. The Apgar evaluation is performed 1 minute after birth, 5 minutes after birth, and again:
    a. 5 minutes after birth
    b. 10 minutes after birth
    c. 15 minutes after birth
    d. 20 minutes after birth

33 Meconium Aspiration Syndrome

Chapter Objectives

After reading this chapter, you will be able to:

- List the anatomic alterations of the lungs associated with meconium aspiration.
- Describe the causes of meconium aspiration.
- List the cardiopulmonary clinical manifestations associated with meconium aspiration syndrome (MAS).
- Describe the general management of meconium aspiration.
- Describe the clinical strategies and rationales of the SOAPs presented in the case study.

Key Terms

"Ball-Valve" Effect
Chemical Pneumonitis
High-Frequency Oscillatory Ventilation
Inhaled Nitric Oxide (iNO)
Jet Ventilation
Meconium
Meconium Aspiration Syndrome (MAS)
Meconium Staining
Persistent Pulmonary Hypertension of the Neonate
Pneumomediastinum
Pneumothorax

Chapter Outline

Anatomic Alterations of the Lungs
Etiology and Epidemiology
Overview of the Cardiopulmonary Clinical Manifestations Associated with Meconium Aspiration Syndrome
General Management of Meconium Aspiration Syndrome
Case Study: Meconium Aspiration Syndrome (MAS)
Self-Assessment Questions

Anatomic Alterations of the Lungs

During normal intrauterine fetal development, the fetus periodically demonstrates normal rapid, shallow respiratory chest movements. This normal action moves pulmonary fetal fluid into and out of the oropharynx while the glottis remains closed. During periods of fetal hypoxemia, however, the fetus may demonstrate very deep, gasping inspiratory movements that may force the contents of the nasoooropharynx to pass through the glottis into the airways. The aspiration of minimal amounts of clear amniotic fluid is not usually associated with serious anatomic or functional problems of the lungs. During fetal hypoxemia, however, the aspirate may contain **meconium** and amniotic fluid—hence the phrase **meconium aspiration syndrome (MAS).**

MAS is a clinical entity seen primarily in full-term or postterm infants who have had some degree of fetal stress or hypoxemia either prenatally or during the birth process. When the fetus experiences in-utero hypoxia, the intestinal response is vasoconstriction, increased gastrointestinal peristalsis, anal sphincter relaxation, and passage of meconium into the amniotic fluid. Meconium is the material that collects in the intestine of the fetus and forms the first stools of the newborn. Meconium, an odorless, thick, sticky, blackish-green material, is a heterogeneous mixture of intestinal tract secretions, amniotic fluid, pulmonary fetal fluid, and intrauterine debris such as epithelial cells, mucus, lanugo, blood, and vernix. Aspiration of meconium leads to one or more of the following complications.

First, MAS causes a **chemical pneumonitis,** which is characterized by an acute inflammatory reaction and edema of the bronchial mucosa and alveolar epithelium. This reaction commonly leads to excessive bronchial secretions and alveolar consolidation. Meconium also promotes the growth of bacteria, which in turn augments the development of alveolar pneumonitis, infection, and consolidation. Meconium aspiration can also interfere with alveolar pulmonary surfactant production. When this occurs, respiratory distress syndrome also may complicate MAS.

Second, the physical presence of the meconium may result in an upper airway obstruction at birth because of the high viscosity of the meconium. In addition, if gasping inspirations are present, clumps of meconium can rapidly migrate past the glottis and penetrate the smaller airways (see Figure 33-1). In cases of severe intrauterine hypoxemia, meconium may already be present in the distal airways at birth. Although MAS primarily causes a restrictive lung pathophysiology, when thick particulate meconium is aspirated into the small airways, the meconium can partially or totally obstruct the airways. Airways that are partially obstructed are affected by a **"ball-valve" effect,** in which air can enter but cannot readily leave the distal airways and alveoli. This condition, in turn, may lead to air trapping and alveolar hyperinflation. Excessive hyperinflation may lead to alveolar rupture and air leak syndromes (see Chapter 36) such as **pneumomediastinum** or **pneumothorax.** Totally obstructed airways lead to alveolar shrinkage

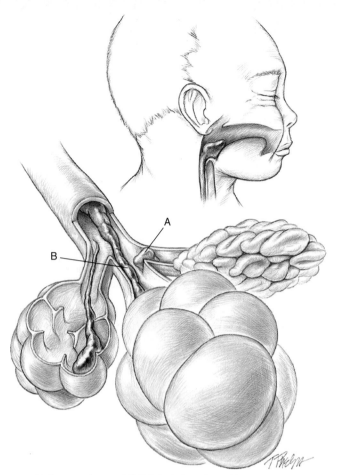

FIGURE 33-1 Meconium aspiration syndrome. (**A**) Total obstruction with meconium causing alveolar atelectasis. (**B**) Partial obstruction causing air trapping and alveolar hyperinflation.

and atelectasis. This combination of areas of overexpanded alveoli adjacent to areas of atelectasis creates both an increased functional residual capacity (FRC) and a decrease in airflow during exhalation.

Third, as a consequence of the hypoxemia associated with MAS, infants with the condition often develop hypoxia-induced pulmonary arterial vasoconstriction and vasospasm, which cause pulmonary hypertension. This results in blood shunting from *right-to-left* through the ductus arteriosus and the foramen ovale; intrapulmonary shunts are also occasionally seen. As a consequence, the blood flow is diverted away from the lungs (pulmonary hypoperfusion), which worsens the hypoxemia. Clinically, this condition is referred to as **persistent pulmonary hypertension of the neonate**, previously called *persistent fetal circulation*.

The major pathologic or structural changes associated with MAS are as follows:

- Physical presence of the meconium leading to:
  - Partially obstructed airways, air trapping, and alveolar hyperinflation
  - Pulmonary air leak syndromes (pneumomediastinum or pneumothorax)
  - Totally obstructed airways and absorption atelectasis
- Edema of the bronchial mucosa and alveolar epithelium

- Excessive bronchial secretions
- Alveolar consolidation (or secondary infection)
- Disrupted pulmonary surfactant production

Etiology and Epidemiology

About 10,000 to 15,000 infants are diagnosed with MAS annually. About 30% of them will require mechanical ventilation, and 10% to 15% will develop pneumothorax. The overall mortality rate is about 4%. As discussed earlier, the fetal passage of meconium is caused by fetal hypoxemia and stress. Fetal hypoxemia causes a vagal response that relaxes anal sphincter tone and allows meconium to move into the amniotic fluid.

MAS rarely is seen in infants born at less than 36 weeks' gestation because the release of meconium requires strong peristalsis and sphincter tone, which are not usually present in preterm infants. Thus, post-term infants (infants born after 42 weeks' gestation) are especially at risk for MAS, because both strong peristalsis and sphincter tone are present in babies of this age. Other infants who are at high risk for MAS are those who are small for gestational age, those who are delivered in the breech position, and those whose mothers are toxemic, hypertensive, or obese.

OVERVIEW of the Cardiopulmonary Clinical Manifestations Associated with Meconium Aspiration Syndrome

The following clinical manifestations result from the pathologic mechanisms caused (or activated) by atelectasis (see Figure 9-7), alveolar consolidation (see Figure 9-8), excessive bronchial secretions (see Figure 9-11), and airway obstruction—the major anatomic alterations of the lungs associated with MAS (Figure 33-1).

CLINICAL DATA OBTAINED AT THE PATIENT'S BEDSIDE

The Physical Examination

Vital Signs

Increased Respiratory Rate (Tachypnea)

Normally, a newborn infant's respiratory rate is about 40 to 60 breaths/min. In MAS the respiratory rate generally is well over 60 breaths/min. Several pathophysiologic mechanisms operating simultaneously may lead to an increased ventilatory rate:

- Stimulation of the peripheral chemoreceptors (hypoxemia)
- Decreased lung compliance–increased ventilatory rate relationship
- Stimulation of the central chemoreceptors
- Increased temperature

Increased Heart Rate (Pulse) and Blood Pressure

Apnea (see Box 32-3)

Clinical Manifestations Associated with More Negative Intrapleural Pressure during Inspiration

- Intercostal retractions
- Substernal retraction and abdominal distention (seesaw movement)
- Cyanosis of the dependent portion of the thoracic and abdominal areas
- Flaring nostrils

Chest Assessment Findings

- Wheezes
- Crackles

Expiratory Grunting

Cyanosis

Common General Appearance

- **Meconium staining** (brownish-yellow color) on:
  - Skin
  - Nails
  - Umbilical cord
  - Wrinkles and creases in the skin

Barrel chest (when airways are partially obstructed)

CLINICAL DATA OBTAINED FROM LABORATORY TESTS AND SPECIAL PROCEDURES

Pulmonary Function Test Findings
(Extrapolated Data for Instructional Purposes)
(Primarily Restrictive Lung Pathophysiology)

The anatomic alterations of the lungs associated with MAS primarily cause a restrictive lung pathophysiology. For example, in moderate to severe cases the following lung volumes and capacities will be lower than normal:

RV	IRV	VC	FRC	TLC
↓	↓	↓	↓	↓

When thick particulate meconium is aspirated into the small airways, the meconium may cause partial obstruction, air trapping, and alveolar hyperinflation. In these cases, an obstructive lung pathophysiology may develop—e.g., the following may be greater than normal:

RV	FRC
↑	↑

Arterial Blood Gases*

MILD TO MODERATE MECONIUM ASPIRATION SYNDROME

Acute Alveolar Hyperventilation with Hypoxemia[†]
(Acute Respiratory Alkalosis)

pH	$PaCO_2$	HCO_3^-	PaO_2	SaO_2 or SpO_2
↑	↓	↓ (but normal)	↓	↓

SEVERE MECONIUM ASPIRATION SYNDROME

Acute Ventilatory Failure with Hypoxemia[§]
(Acute Respiratory Acidosis)

pH[†]	$PaCO_2$	$HCO_3^{-[†]}$	PaO_2	SaO_2 or SpO_2
↓	↑	↑ (but normal)	↓	↓

---

*Note: Because of the difficulty of obtaining **arterial blood gas (ABG)** samples from newborn and pediatric patients, **capillary blood gas** samples may be used to determine the pH, $PaCO_2$, and HCO_3^- (i.e., the acid-base and ventilation status only). Capillary PO_2 values are unreliable and should not be used for clinical analysis. The standard way to evaluate the oxygenation status in these young patients is pulse oximetry (SpO_2) (see Chapter 32).

[†]See Figure 4-3 and related discussion for the acute pH, $PaCO_2$, and HCO_3^- changes associated with acute alveolar hyperventilation.

[§]See Figure 4-2 and related discussion for the acute pH, $PaCO_2$, and HCO_3^- changes associated with acute ventilatory failure.

[†]When tissue hypoxia is severe enough to produce lactic acid, the pH and HCO_3^- values will be lower than expected for a particular $PaCO_2$ level.

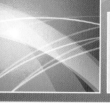
Oxygenation Indices*					
$\dot{Q}_S/\dot{Q}_T$	$DO_2{}^\dagger$	$\dot{V}O_2$	$C(a\text{-}\bar{v})O_2$	O_2ER	$S\bar{v}O_2$
↑	↓	N	N	↑	↓

RADIOLOGIC FINDINGS

Chest Radiograph

When alveolar atelectasis and consolidation are present, the chest radiograph shows irregular densities throughout the lungs. Although the chest radiograph is clearly different from that seen in respiratory distress syndrome, it is difficult to differentiate the radiograph appearance of MAS from that of pneumonia (Figure 33-2).

The chest radiograph may show local or generalized problem areas. When significant partial airway obstruction, air trapping, and alveolar hyperinflation are present, the chest radiograph appears hyperlucent and the diaphragm may be depressed. The respiratory therapist should be alert for the sudden development of a pneumothorax or pneumomediastinum in infants with MAS (Figure 33-3).

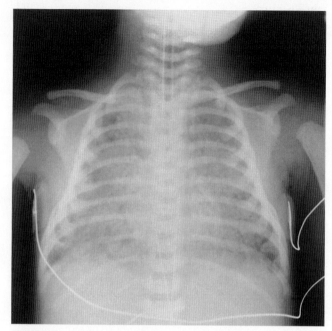

FIGURE 33-2 Chest radiograph of an infant with meconium aspiration syndrome. Patchy areas of increased density are observed in both lungs. (From Taussig LM, Landau LI: *Pediatric respiratory medicine*, ed 2, St Louis, 2008, Elsevier.)

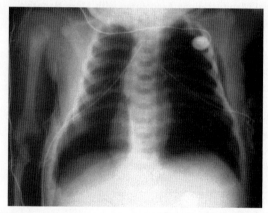

FIGURE 33-3 Meconium aspiration with bilateral pneumothorax.

*$C(a\text{-}\bar{v})O_2$, Arterial-venous oxygen difference; DO_2, total oxygen delivery; O_2ER, oxygen extraction ratio; $\dot{Q}_S/\dot{Q}_T$, pulmonary shunt fraction; $S\bar{v}O_2$, mixed venous oxygen saturation; $\dot{V}O_2$, oxygen consumption.
†Because the newborn normally has a higher hemoglobin level at birth (16.8 to 18.9 g/dL%), the DO_2 may actually be better than indicated by PaO_2 or SpO_2 (see Chapter 5, Total Oxygen Delivery).

General Management of Meconium Aspiration Syndrome

The respiratory therapist should be proactive whenever an infant is at risk for meconium aspiration. In other words, when the amniotic fluid is found to be stained with meconium—and when the infant is not actively breathing or crying immediately after delivery—the oropharynx should be emergently suctioned, even before drying and warming. With use of a laryngoscope for visualization, the infant's trachea

should be intubated and the trachea suctioned using a meconium aspirator attached to the endotracheal tube (ET). The ET acts as the suction catheter as it is withdrawn slowly while suction is applied until *all* the visible meconium has been cleared. This measure should be routine for all infants born through particulate meconium, even if meconium is not visualized in the oropharynx.

Positive-pressure ventilation should not be administered to a nonvigorous infant until a thorough suctioning of the upper airways has been completed, because any particulate meconium remaining in the upper airways likely will be forced into the lower airways in response to positive-pressure ventilation. Also, staff should not stimulate a meconium-stained infant to cry until **after** suctioning.

After the infant has been stabilized and transported to the neonatal intensive care unit, vigorous **bronchial hygiene** and PRN **suctioning** of the airways should be performed (see **Bronchopulmonary Hygiene Therapy Protocol**, Protocol 32-2). Although postural drainage and percussion may seem an appropriate therapy for the removal of thick meconium in the airway, the marginal effectiveness of this technique on a newborn's compliant chest wall is not worth the risk of over-stimulation in these very ill infants.

Appropriate **oxygen therapy** should be administered per protocol (see **Oxygen Therapy Protocol,** Protocol 32-1); in severe cases, continuous positive airway pressure (**CPAP;** see **Lung Expansion Protocol**, Protocol 32-3) or **mechanical ventilation** (see **Mechanical Ventilation Protocol**, Protocol 32-5) may be necessary. As already mentioned, however, mechanical ventilation should be avoided or applied cautiously to prevent the possibility of dislodging unseen particulate meconium and pushing it further down the infant's airways. In addition, a high incidence of pneumothorax is associated with MAS. If mechanical ventilation is necessary, an inspiration/expiration ratio that permits a long exhalation time (to allow expired gas enough time to flow past partially obstructed airways) should be used. Finally, the infant should be monitored closely for possible superimposed infection. Antibiotics may be indicated and steroids may be required to offset the inflammatory response in chemical pneumonitis. Because meconium aspiration disrupts normal surfactant production, exogenous pulmonary surfactant is often administered to infants with MAS (see **Surfactant Administration Protocol**, Protocol 32-6). Exogenous surfactant is also helpful as its low surface tension helps to wash out meconium particles while replacing surfactant stores. Current evidence shows that the use of surfactant with MAS within 6 hours of delivery reduces the need for extracorporeal membrane oxygenation.

In the event that the infant develops persistent pulmonary hypertension of the newborn, **inhaled nitric oxide (iNO)** is administered via mechanical ventilation. iNO is an inhaled gas and a potent pulmonary vasodilator. It is effective in dilating the pulmonary capillaries, which, in turn, decreases the pulmonary vascular resistance adjacent to effectively ventilated alveoli. This effect can greatly improve oxygenation by improving the ventilation/perfusion match in the ventilated regions of the damaged lung. iNO is administered in 1 to 20 parts/million (ppm) and titrated to the infant's oxygenation. When iNO fails to improve oxygenation in infants with MAS, ECMO may be required.

CASE STUDY Meconium Aspiration Syndrome

Admitting History and Physical Examination

A 38-week-gestation newborn male infant was delivered by emergency cesarean section because of sudden maternal vaginal hemorrhage. The mother, a primigravida, white 19-year-old, had no prenatal care. She was a heavy smoker and had an uncertain history of recreational psychopharmaceutical drug use during pregnancy. Rupture of membranes was believed to have occurred about 18 hours before delivery.

At delivery, the infant's umbilical cord was wrapped once around his neck. He was covered with meconium. He was limp and blue and did not show any spontaneous movement or respiratory effort when he was handed to the neonatologist, who was heading the resuscitation team, which also included a registered nurse and a registered respiratory therapist. With the aid of a laryngoscope, several clumps of meconium were suctioned from the infant's oral and pharyngeal areas. On one pass below the vocal cords, no meconium was visualized or suctioned.

Despite these efforts, the infant demonstrated no spontaneous respirations, and his heart rate was less than 60 beats/min. Because of this, manual ventilation could no longer be avoided. At this time, the respiratory therapist started to ventilate the infant with a bag-valve-mask resuscitation bag, at an FIO$_2$ of 1.0 and a respiratory rate of 50 breaths/min.

The nurse started chest compressions at about 90/min, with a rhythm of three compressions to one breath. Bilateral crackles were auscultated.

At 1 minute, the Apgar score was 1 for the heart rate. By the third minute, the heart rate was 80 beats/min. The infant was gasping occasionally and demonstrated improved color. Although compressions were stopped, bagging continued at 50 breaths/min. At 5 minutes, the Apgar score was 6 (heart rate 2, respirations 1, tone 1, reflex irritability 0, and color 2). At 10 minutes, the Apgar score was still 6. The neonatologist decided to intubate the baby with a 3.5-mm ET. The respiratory therapist confirmed the correct position of the ET by means of (1) careful auscultation and (2) the appearance of a "yellow" color on the CO$_2$ detector (i.e., a yellow color confirms CO$_2$ and a purple color indicates no CO$_2$). The respiratory therapist then taped the tube at the 9.0-cm mark at the infant's lips. The baby was transferred to the neonatal intensive care unit and placed on a ventilator. Initial ventilator settings were respiratory rate (RR) 26, inspiratory time (T$_1$) 0.5 second, FIO$_2$ 1.0, positive inspiratory pressure (PIP) +25, and positive end-expiratory pressure (PEEP) +5. The infant's SpO$_2$ was 94%. At that time the respiratory therapist documented the following in the infant's chart:

Respiratory Assessment and Plan

S N/A

O Apneic at birth, hypoactive, cyanotic, covered with meconium. Apgar score at 1 minute = 1, at 5 minute = 6. Bilateral crackles. Meconium suctioned from oral and pharyngeal areas. SpO_2: 94%.

A • Possible MAS (meconium in airway)
  • Airway secretions (meconium?) (crackles)
  • Probable asphyxic episode; likely combined respiratory and metabolic acidosis (history, cyanosis)
  • Adequate oxygenation and ventilation (SpO_2, auscultation, CO_2 detector)

P **Mechanical Ventilation Protocol** in combination with **Oxygen Therapy** and **Hyperinflation Therapy Protocol** (RR 26, FIO_2 100%, PIP +25, and PEEP 5). **Bronchopulmonary Hygiene Protocol** (suction). Surfactant protocol: administer surfactant per physician order. Monitor closely, weaning PIP to maintain exhaled V_T of 6 mL/kg, oximetry, vital signs, watch for signs of acute air leak, pulmonary hemorrhage).

Over the next hour, an umbilical artery catheter (UAC) was inserted; it showed a pH of 7.19, $PaCO_2$ 37 mm Hg, HCO_3^- 14 mEq/L, PaO_2 87 mm Hg, and SpO_2 94%. Although the infant's skin was now completely pink, bilateral crackles were still present. The chest radiograph revealed hyperinflation in both the right and left lungs. There was whiteout of the right upper and middle lobes, most likely caused by atelectasis. Clumps of white patches of atelectasis (resembling small popcorn balls) were seen throughout the remainder of the lungs. The ET tip was at the clavicle level, and the UAC tip was appropriately positioned at T-8.

The following SOAP note was recorded:

Respiratory Assessment and Plan

S N/A

O Pink skin. Bilateral crackles. CXR Atelectasis in the right upper and middle lobes. Air trapping right and left lower lobes. ABGs: pH 7.19, $PaCO_2$ 37, HCO_3^- 14, PaO_2 87, and SpO_2 94% (on FIO_2 1.0).

A • Airway secretions (crackles)
  • Atelectasis (CXR)
  • Uncompensated metabolic acidosis (ABG)

P Continue **Mechanical Ventilation Protocol** in combination with **Oxygen Therapy** and **Lung Expansion Therapy Protocols** (RR 26, TI 0.5, FIO_2 1.0, PIP +22 cm H_2O, and PEEP +5 cm H_2O). Continue **Bronchopulmonary Hygiene Protocol** (suction PRN). Discuss with the neonatologist possible ways to correct the uncompensated metabolic acidosis. (For example, in this sequence, bolus the infant with fluids, which may help to correct the metabolic acidosis. If this does not help, administer 2 mEq/kg HCO_3^- until the the pH is 7.25, or slightly higher). Monitor closely (vital signs, watch for signs of acute air leak, pulmonary hemorrhage).

Because the infant's mechanical ventilation was more than adequate (confirmed by a normal $PaCO_2$ of 37), the PIP was weaned to 22. The baby progressively improved over the next 4 days. On the fifth day, he was off the ventilator; on the seventh, he was discharged from the hospital. The mother was scheduled to see Social Services on a weekly basis.

Discussion

Inspection—the first step in the assessment process—was of the utmost importance in this case. The umbilical cord wrapped around the infant's neck, the presence of meconium, the blue skin, and the absence of spontaneous respirations were all important clinical indicators demonstrating the severity of the baby's condition. The fact that the baby was not manually ventilated—even though he had no spontaneous respirations—until after several clumps of meconium were suctioned from his oral and laryngeal areas is paramount. Great care must be taken not to drive any meconium, blood, or amniotic fluid deeper down the tracheobronchial tree. The neonatal team must always be alert for the presence of a ball-valve meconium obstruction and the possibility of a pneumothorax. A ball-valve obstruction was verified in this case by the identification of alveolar hyperinflation on the chest radiograph. Fortunately, a pneumothorax did not develop. The early administration of surfactant to infants with MAS should be part of routine care.

As with adult subjects, several of the clinical manifestations in this case can be traced back through the "clinical scenarios" associated with **atelectasis** (see Figure 9-7) and **excessive bronchial secretions** (see Figure 9-11). For example, the increased lung density caused by the atelectasis was revealed on the chest radiograph, and the crackles were produced by the excessive airway secretions recorded in the second SOAP.

Although it was not used here, **high-frequency oscillatory ventilation** or **jet ventilation** is often used in such cases. Either ventilator management approach appears to benefit the patient equally. Therapeutically, these techniques ventilate by air streams that flow down the center of the airways while gas leaving the lungs moves along the peripheral walls of the airways, thus moving meconium and secretions out of the lungs. However, both can have a negative effect in some cases where there is significant airway obstruction, causing more gas trapping.

These babies are very sensitive to external stimuli. Great caution should be taken not to overstimulate them. They should be suctioned only as needed. Chest physical therapy is contraindicated. When suctioning is necessary, the respiratory therapist should not prolong the suctioning process. Often, these babies are given eye patches and earplugs to decrease external sensory stimulation. Occasionally, they will be paralyzed to minimize their reactions to stimuli and resistance to ventilation. Inhaled nitric oxide is used in severe cases, when persistent pulmonary hypertension of the newborn is verified.

SELF-ASSESSMENT QUESTIONS

1. **When the fetus experiences in-utero hypoxia, which of the following occur(s)?**
   1. Vasoconstriction
   2. Inspiratory gasping
   3. Sphincter constriction
   4. Increased intestinal peristalsis
      a. 1 only
      b. 2 only
      c. 1, 2, and 4 only
      d. 2, 3, and 4 only
      e. 1, 2, 3, and 4

2. **Aspiration of meconium may lead to which of the following?**
   1. Ball-valve effect
   2. Atelectasis
   3. Total airway obstruction
   4. Alveolar hyperinflation
   5. Chemical pneumonitis
      a. 2 only
      b. 1, 2, and 4 only
      c. 2, 3, and 4 only
      d. 1, 2, 3, 4, and 5

3. **Which of the following is associated with MAS when a ball-valve effect is present?**
   a. Decreased RV
   b. Increased IRV
   c. Increased FRC
   d. All the lung volumes and capacities are decreased

4. **Which of the following clinical manifestations are associated with meconium aspiration syndrome?**
   1. Apnea
   2. Intercostal retractions
   3. Barrel chest
   4. Expiratory grunting
      a. 2 only
      b. 1, 2, and 4 only
      c. 2, 3, and 4 only
      d. 1, 2, 3, and 4

5. **What percentage of the infants with MAS who require mechanical ventilation will likely develop a pneumothorax?**
   a. 1% to 5%
   b. 5% to 10%
   c. 10% to 15%
   d. 15% to 20%

Transient Tachypnea
of the Newborn

Chapter Objectives

After reading this chapter, you will be able to:

- List the anatomic alterations of the lungs associated with transient tachypnea of the newborn.
- Describe the causes of transient tachypnea of the newborn.
- List the cardiopulmonary clinical manifestations associated with transient tachypnea of the newborn.
- Describe the general management of transient tachypnea of the newborn.
- Describe the clinical strategies and rationales of the SOAP presented in the case study.

Key Terms

Apgar Score
Grunting
Intercostal Retractions
Substernal Retractions
Interstitial Edema
Macrosomia
Nasal flaring
Perihilar Streaking (Starbursts or Sunbursts)
Pulmonary Capillary Congestion
Rapid and Shallow Breathing Pattern (Hallmark Clinical Manifestation)
Type II Respiratory Distress Syndrome
Wet Lung Syndrome

Chapter Outline

Anatomic Alterations of the Lungs
Etiology and Epidemiology
Overview of the Cardiopulmonary Clinical Manifestations Associated with Transient Tachypnea of the Newborn
General Management of Transient Tachypnea of the Newborn
Respiratory Care Treatment Protocols
Case Study: Transient Tachypnea of the Newborn
Self-Assessment Questions

Anatomic Alterations of the Lungs

Transient tachypnea of the newborn (TTN) (also called **type II respiratory distress syndrome** and **"wet lung" syndrome**) was first described in the literature in 1965. Within the first 4 to 6 hours after birth, TTN produces clinical signs very similar to those associated with the early stages of respiratory distress syndrome (see Chapter 35). However, the anatomic alterations of the lungs associated with TTN are very different from the pulmonary pathology seen in respiratory distress syndrome.

As shown in Figure 34-1, the infant with TTN has a delay in the pulmonary fluid absorption by the lymphatic system and pulmonary capillaries. It is thought that this condition results, in part, from the infant's hypoxemia and inadequate inspiratory effort, producing a delay in clearance of pulmonary fluid. As this condition worsens, the infant develops **pulmonary capillary congestion, interstitial edema**, decreased lung compliance, decreased tidal volume, and increased dead space. Because the swallowing and cough efforts of infants with TTN are commonly depressed, the clearance of bronchial secretions is compromised. Although TTN is primarily a restrictive lung disorder, excessive airway secretions may lead to air trapping and alveolar hyperinflation.

In severe cases, the excessive fluid accumulation throughout the alveolar-capillary interstitial tissue may also compress the bronchial airways. As a general rule, however, the abnormal anatomic alterations of the lungs associated with TTN usually begin to resolve about 48 to 72 hours after birth.

The major pathologic or structural changes associated with TTN are as follows:

- Decreased removal of fluid by pulmonary lymphatics
- Pulmonary capillary congestion
- Interstitial edema
- Excessive bronchial secretions and incomplete absorption of pulmonary fetal fluid
- Air trapping and alveolar hyperinflation
- Compressed bronchial airways (from excessive alveolar-capillary interstitial fluid)

Etiology and Epidemiology

TTN affects 1% to 2% of all newborns. Classically, TNN is most often seen in full-term infants. Risk factors include elective cesarean section, excessive administration of fluids to the mother during labor, male gender, and **macrosomia** (a newborn with excessive birth weight). The infant's history often includes maternal analgesia or anesthesia during labor and delivery or episodes of intrauterine hypoxia. TTN is also commonly associated with maternal bleeding, maternal diabetes, and prolapsed cord. TTN is occasionally seen in very small infants.

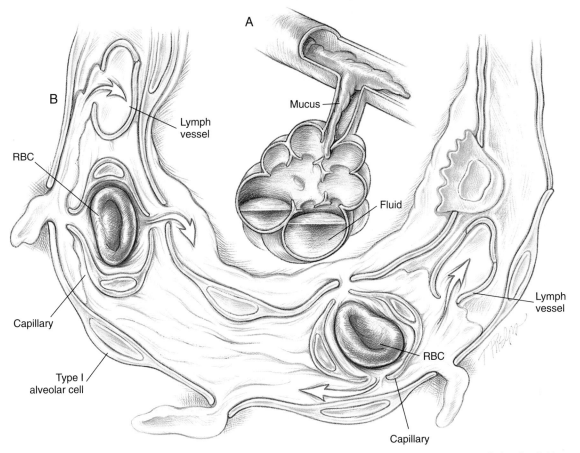

FIGURE 34-1 Transient tachypnea of the newborn. **A,** Excessive bronchial secretions and increased alveolar fluid. **B,** Cross-section of alveolus with interstitial edema, and pulmonary capillary congestion.

Although the precise mechanism is not known, it is believed that TTN results from a delayed absorption of fetal lung fluid. The delayed absorption of lung fluid is thought to be caused by any condition that increases the central venous pressure, which in turn slows the clearance of lung fluid by the lymphatic system. Infants with TTN are often lethargic at birth, resulting in a depressed cough effort and accumulation of airway secretions and mucus. The typical baby with TTN usually has good **Apgar scores** at birth. During the next few hours, however, signs of respiratory distress develop. Early clinical manifestations include tachypnea, chest retractions, **nasal flaring**, **grunting**, and cyanosis. It is common to see respiratory rates of 80 to 120 breaths/minute. In fact, the rapid and shallow breathing pattern is often considered a hallmark clinical manifestation of TTN. In addition, the infant may demonstrate a barrel chest and coarse crackles. Within 24 to 48 hours, the clinical manifestations of respiratory distress usually disappear.

General Management of Transient Tachypnea of the Newborn

Because of the relatively short course of TTN, the treatment consists mostly of proper stabilization, close monitoring, and frequent and thorough evaluations to rule out other, more serious conditions that may develop. Oxygen therapy is provided to maintain adequate oxygenation, and suctioning (bronchopulmonary hygiene therapy) may be performed to keep the airways clear of bronchial secretions. Lung expansion therapy (CPAP) is often used as a preventative measure, but mechanical ventilation is usually not required. Fluid restriction is usually ordered until the signs associated with TTN resolve. Oral feedings are usually started as soon as the infant is able to tolerate them (usually at a respiratory rate below 80). Diuretics do not affect the clinical course of the TTN. In cases in which pneumonia is suspected, the use of antibiotics is indicated.

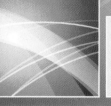

OVERVIEW of the Cardiopulmonary Clinical Manifestations Associated with Transient Tachypnea of the Newborn*

The following clinical manifestations result from the pathologic mechanisms caused (or activated) by Increased Alveolar-Capillary Membrane Thickness (see Figure 9-9), Excessive Bronchial Secretions (see Figure 9-11), and Airway Obstruction—the major anatomic alterations of the lungs associated with transient tachypnea of the newborn (TTN) (see Figure 34-1).

CLINICAL DATA OBTAINED AT THE PATIENT'S BEDSIDE

The Physical Examination

Vital Signs

Increased Respiratory Rate (Tachypnea)

Infants with TTN frequently breathe rapidly and shallowly. In fact, this rapid and shallow breathing pattern often is considered a hallmark clinical manifestation of TTN. Normally, a newborn infant's respiratory rate is about 40 to 60 breaths per minute. During the early stages of TTN, the respiratory rate is often 60 to 100 breaths per minute. Several pathophysiologic mechanisms operating simultaneously may lead to an increased ventilatory rate:

- Stimulation of the peripheral chemoreceptors (hypoxemia)
- Decreased lung compliance–increased ventilatory rate relationship
- Stimulation of the central chemoreceptors

Increased Heart Rate (Pulse) and Blood Pressure

Clinical Manifestations Associated with More Negative Intrapleural Pressure during Inspiration

- Intercostal retractions
- **Substernal retraction** and abdominal distention (seesaw movement)
- Cyanosis of the dependent portions of the thoracic and abdominal areas
- Flaring nostrils

Chest Assessment Findings

- Wheezes
- Crackles

Expiratory Grunting

Cyanosis

Barrel chest (when airways are partially obstructed)

CLINICAL DATA OBTAINED FROM LABORATORY TESTS AND SPECIAL PROCEDURES

Pulmonary Function Test Findings
(Extrapolated Data for Instructional Purposes)
(Primarily Restrictive Lung Pathophysiology)

The anatomic alterations of the lungs associated with TTN primarily cause a restrictive lung pathophysiology. For example, in moderate to severe cases, the following lung volumes and capacities will be lower than normal:

RV	IRV	VC	FRC	TLC
↓	↓	↓	↓	↓

When excessive airway secretions are present, air trapping and alveolar hyperinflation may develop. In these cases, an obstructive lung pathophysiology may develop—e.g., the following may be greater than normal:

RV	FRC
↑	↑

Arterial Blood Gases*

MILD TO MODERATE TRANSIENT TACHYPNEA OF THE NEWBORN

Acute Alveolar Hyperventilation with Hypoxemia[†]
(Acute Respiratory Alkalosis)

pH	$PaCO_2$	HCO_3^-	PaO_2	SaO_2 or SpO_2
↑	↓	↓	↓	↓
		(but normal)		

SEVERE TRANSIENT TACHYPNEA OF THE NEWBORN

Acute Ventilatory Failure with Hypoxemia[§]
(Acute Respiratory Acidosis)

pH[†]	$PaCO_2$	HCO_3^-[†]	PaO_2	SaO_2 or SpO_2
↓	↑	↑	↓	↓
		(but normal)		

---

*Note: Because of the difficulty of obtaining **arterial blood gas** (**ABG**) samples from newborn and pediatric patients, **capillary blood gas** (**CBG**) samples may be used to determine the pH, $PaCO_2$, and HCO_3^- (i.e., the acid-base and ventilation status only). Capillary PO_2 values are unreliable and should not be used for clinical analysis. The standard way to evaluate the oxygenation status in these young patients is pulse oximetry (SpO_2) (see Chapter 32).

[†]See Figure 4-3 and related discussion for the acute pH, $PaCO_2$, and HCO_3^- changes associated with acute alveolar hyperventilation.

[§]See Figure 4-2 and related discussion for the acute pH, $PaCO_2$, and HCO_3^- changes associated with acute ventilatory failure.

[†]When tissue hypoxia is severe enough to produce lactic acid, the pH and HCO_3^- values will be lower than expected for a particular $PaCO_2$ level.

---

*The clinical manifestations of TTN usually disappear in the first 24 to 48 hours. Severe TTN is rare.

Oxygenation Indices*

$\dot{Q}_S/\dot{Q}_T$	$DO_2^{\dagger}$	$\dot{V}O_2$	$C(a\text{-}\bar{v})O_2$	O_2ER	$S\bar{v}O_2$
↑	↓	N	N	↑	↓

*$C(a\text{-}\bar{v})O_2$, Arterial–venous oxygen difference; DO_2, total oxygen delivery; O_2ER, oxygen extraction ratio; $\dot{Q}_S/\dot{Q}_T$, pulmonary shunt fraction; $S\bar{v}O_2$, mixed venous oxygen saturation; $\dot{V}O_2$, oxygen consumption.

†It should be noted that because the newborn normally has a higher hemoglobin (Hb) level at birth (16.8 g to 18.9 g% Hb), the DO_2 may actually be better than the PaO_2 or SpO_2 indicates (see Chapter 5).

Radiologic Findings
Chest Radiograph

Initially, the chest radiograph appears normal. Over the next 4 to 6 hours, however, signs of pulmonary vascular congestion develop. These are revealed on the chest radiograph as prominent **perihilar streaking (commonly called *starbursts* or *sunbursts*)**, air bronchograms, and fluid in the interlobular fissures. Air trapping and hyperinflation may occur and are manifested by peripheral hyperlucency, flattened diaphragms, and bulging intercostal spaces. Patches of infiltrates may be seen in some infants. Mild cardiomegaly and pleural effusions also may be seen (see Figure 34-2).

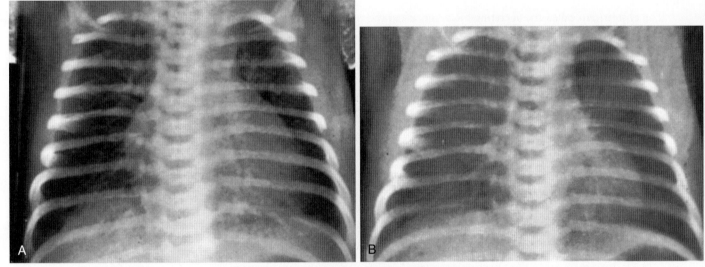

FIGURE 34-2 The large cardiovascular silhouette, air bronchogram, and streaky lung fields were seen at 2 hours of age (**A**) but had cleared by 24 hours of age (**B**), typical of transient tachypnea of the newborn or delayed clearance of lung liquid. (From Taeusch WH, Ballard RA, Gleason CA: *Avery's diseases of the newborn*, ed 8, Philadelphia, 2005, Saunders.)

Respiratory Care Treatment Protocols

Oxygen Therapy Protocol

Oxygen therapy is used to treat hypoxemia, decrease the work of breathing, and decrease myocardial work. Because of the hypoxemia that often develops in TTN, supplemental oxygen may be required (see **Oxygen Therapy Protocol**, Protocol 32-1).

Bronchopulmonary Hygiene Therapy Protocol

Because of the excessive airway secretions and accumulation associated with TTN, a number of bronchial hygiene treatment modalities may be used to enhance the mobilization of bronchial secretions (see **Bronchopulmonary Hygiene Therapy Protocol**, Protocol 32-2).

Lung Expansion Therapy Protocol

Lung expansion measures commonly are performed to offset the pulmonary capillary congestion and interstitial edema associated with TTN (see **Lung Expansion Therapy Protocol**, Protocol 32-3).

Mechanical Ventilation Protocol

Mechanical ventilation may occasionally be necessary to provide and support alveolar gas exchange and eventually return the patient to spontaneous breathing. Patients with TTN rarely require mechanical ventilation (see **Mechanical Ventilation** Protocol 32-5)

Admitting History and Physical Examination

A 27-year-old woman in the thirty-fifth week of her second pregnancy awakened at 2 AM with sudden lower abdominal pain and some bleeding. She had no contractions at the time. She woke her husband, who in turn called the obstetrician. The doctor instructed him to bring his wife to the hospital. On arrival at the hospital, she was immediately taken to the labor and delivery room. The nurse on duty placed an oxygen mask on the patient's face and started an intravenous (IV) line. The patient's vital signs were monitored closely. An ultrasound Doppler belt also was placed around the mother's lower abdominal area to monitor the baby's heart rate. Over the next 20 minutes, the mother continued to bleed, her blood pressure fell, and her heart rate increased. The baby's heart rate had increased from 155 beats/min to 170 beats/min.

The obstetrician called the operating room and asked the staff to prepare for an emergency cesarean section. The doctor also called for the neonatal resuscitation team (which consisted of a neonatologist, nurse, and respiratory therapist) and asked that they be on standby. The cesarean section was uneventful. The baby was a 3-kg girl. The neonatologist assessed the baby and gave a 1-minute Apgar score of 8 (2 heart rate, 2 respiratory rate, 1 tone, 1 reflex irritability, and 2 skin color). Within 30 minutes of delivery, the baby was tachypneic with a respiratory rate of 80 beats/min. Auscultation revealed bilateral mild crackles and occasional coarse crackles. The baby was transferred to the neonatal intensive care unit (NICU).

In the NICU, the baby was placed in a warmed Isolette with continuous pulse oximetry; SpO_2 was noted to be 82% to 84%. An IV line and nasogastric tube were also placed. Warm, humidified oxygen was started via a high-flow nasal cannula (HFNC)* at 4 L/min and an FIO_2 of 0.40. Ten minutes later the infant's vital signs were as follows: heart rate 155 beats/min, blood pressure 75/40, and respiratory rate 75 breaths/min. The infant's ventilatory pattern was described by the neonatologist as fast and shallow, however, she did not appear to be working hard to breathe. She had no intercostal retractions or nasal flaring at this time. Capillary blood gas values were as follows: pH 7.33, $PaCO_2$ 31 mm Hg, and HCO_3^- 21 mEq/L. The baby's SpO_2 was 88%. The FIO_2 was increased to 0.60 to achieve an SpO_2 of 93%.

About 2 hours later, however, the baby started to show signs of worsening. Her vital signs were as follows: heart rate 170 beats/min, blood pressure 75/45, and respiratory rate 100 breaths/min. She demonstrated abdominal respiratory efforts and nasal flaring. Her skin appeared pale and blue. Auscultation revealed moderate to severe bilateral crackles. On the same HFNC settings (4 L/min and an FIO_2 of 0.60),

*Also called high-humidity nasal cannula (HHNC).

her SpO_2 had dropped to 84%. Capillary blood gas values revealed the following acid-base and ventilation status: pH 7.52, $PaCO_2$ 28 mm Hg, and HCO_3^- 22 mEq/L.

A chest radiograph showed areas of infiltrates and microatelectasis throughout both lung fields, as well as prominent white-lined lung fissures (indicating fluid in the fissures). A starburst pattern was seen at the hilum of the lungs (indicating increased lymphatic fluid). The chest radiograph also showed air trapping and hyperinflation in the lower lobes (indicating fluid in the airways). The infant's diaphragm was flattened. The neonatologist charted a diagnosis of TTN in the baby's progress notes. The doctor also stated that he did not want to mechanically ventilate the baby at this time. The respiratory therapist entered the following assessment in the baby's chart.

Respiratory Assessment and Plan

S N/A

O Vital signs: HR 170/min, BP 75/45, and RR 100/min. Chest retractions, nasal flaring. Skin pale and blue. Moderate to severe bilateral crackles. CXR: Infiltrates and microatelectasis over both lungs, generalized hyperinflation. CBG on HFNC at 4 L/min and FIO_2 0.60: pH 7.52, $PaCO_2$ 28, HCO_3^- 22, SpO_2 84%.

A • TTN (neonatologist, CXR, history)
   • Infiltrates and atelectasis (CXR)
   • Air trapping (CXR)
   • Excessive bronchial secretions (rhonchi and crackles)
   • Acute alveolar hyperventilation with severe hypoxemia (capillary blood gas)

P **Lung Expansion Therapy Protocol** (nasal CPAP at +4 cm H_2O). Increase **Oxygen Therapy Protocol** (FIO_2 0.60 via CPAP at +4 cm H_2O setup adjusting to achieve desired SpO_2). **Bronchopulmonary Hygiene Therapy Protocol** (suction PRN). Continue to monitor closely.

Over the next 48 hours, the baby's condition progressively improved. She no longer required oxygen therapy, and her breath sounds were normal. Her last room air capillary blood gas values showed a pH of 7.38, $PaCO_2$ 39 mm Hg, and HCO_3^- 24 mEq/L. Her SpO_2 was 94%. Her chest radiograph was normal. The baby was discharged the next day.

Discussion

This case reinforces the importance of observation and inspection in the assessment process. The respiratory therapist must continuously inspect and analyze infants with TTN. This baby, for example, born at 35 weeks, may have had respiratory distress syndrome (RDS; see Chapter 35), but the clinical symptoms ruled out the diagnosis. For example, babies with RDS have alveolar collapse and consolidation; whereas babies with TTN have airway trapping and alveolar hyperinflation. In addition, the respiratory pattern of babies with RDS is commonly described as hard, fast, and deep breathing; whereas infants with TTN usually breathe rapidly and shallowly. In fact, this rapid and shallow breathing pattern often is considered a hallmark of TTN. Certainly, the rapid shallow breathing seen in this baby was caused, in part, by the **Increased Alveolar-Capillary Membrane Thickness** (see Figure 9-9)—and decreased lung compliance—associated with TTN.

Although apnea may occur in these babies, it is not common. Therapeutically, most do quite well with just oxygen via an HFNC. Occasionally, nasal continuous positive airway pressure (CPAP) may be used. Caution, however, must be taken not to give the baby too high of an inspiratory pressure or prolonged exposure to CPAP. The lungs of these babies are usually already hyperinflated. Too high of a CPAP pressure setting may expand the baby's lungs even more and may cause a tension pneumothorax. CPAP at +3 to +4 cm H_2O is usually safe. Mechanical ventilation rarely is needed for babies with TTN.

SELF-ASSESSMENT QUESTIONS

Answers to questions can be found on Evolve. To access additional student assessment questions visit **http://evolve.elsevier.com/DesJardins/respiratory**.

1. **Which of the following is/are associated with TTN?**
   1. Rapid and shallow breathing pattern
   2. PPHN
   3. Clinical signs similar to those of infant respiratory distress syndrome
   4. Reduced DO_2
      a. 1 only
      b. 2 and 4 only
      c. 2, 3, and 4 only
      d. 1, 2, 3, and 4

2. **The clinical manifestations associated with TTN usually disappear within:**
   a. 10 to 24 hours after birth
   b. 24 to 48 hours after birth
   c. 48 to 72 hours after birth
   d. 2 weeks after birth

3. **Which of the following is the hallmark clinical manifestation of TTN?**
   a. PPHN
   b. Rapid and shallow breathing pattern
   c. Substernal retraction and abdominal distention (seesaw movement)
   d. Expiratory grunting

4. **Radiologic findings associated with TTN include:**
   1. Flattened diaphragms
   2. Starbursts
   3. Air bronchograms
   4. Deviated trachea
      a. 1 and 3 only
      b. 2 and 4 only
      c. 1, 2, and 3 only
      d. 1, 2, 3, and 4

5. **Which of the following are the major anatomic alterations of the lungs associated with TTN?**
   1. Consolidation
   2. Bronchospasm
   3. Increased alveolar-capillary membrane thickness
   4. Atelectasis
   5. Excessive bronchial secretions
      a. 3 and 5 only
      b. 2 and 4 only
      c. 3, 4, and 5 only
      d. 1, 3, 4, and 5 only

Chapter Objectives

After reading this chapter, you will be able to:

- List the anatomic alterations of the lungs associated with respiratory distress syndrome.
- Describe the causes of respiratory distress syndrome.
- List the cardiopulmonary clinical manifestations associated with respiratory distress syndrome.
- Describe the general management of respiratory distress syndrome.
- Describe the clinical strategies and rationales of the SOAP presented in the case study.

Key Terms

Alveolar Type II Cells (Granular Pneumocytes)
Hyaline Membrane Disease
Infant Respiratory Distress Syndrome
Lecithin/Sphingomyelin Ratio (L:S Ratio)
Phosphatidylglycerol (PG)
Poractant Alfa (Curosurf)
Pulmonary Hyperperfusion
Pulmonary Hypoperfusion
Respiratory Distress Syndrome of the Newborn
Surfactant/Albumin Ratio (S:A Ratio)
Transient Pulmonary Hypertension
Volutrauma

Chapter Outline

Anatomic Alterations of the Lungs
Etiology and Epidemiology
Diagnosis
Overview of the Cardiopulmonary Clinical Manifestations Associated with Respiratory Distress Syndrome
General Management of Respiratory Distress Syndrome
Respiratory Care Treatment Protocols
Case Study: Respiratory Distress Syndrome
Self-Assessment Questions

Introduction

Respiratory distress syndrome (RDS) is the most common cause of respiratory failure in the preterm infant. Over the past several decades, a number of names have been used to identify infants with RDS (Box 35-1). A common thread running through most of the names is the term "respiratory distress," which characterizes an immature lung disorder in a preterm infant caused by inadequate pulmonary surfactant. RDS is a major cause of morbidity and mortality in the premature infant born at fewer than 37 weeks' gestation. The introduction of exogenous surfactant therapy has greatly improved the clinical course of this disorder and reduced the morbidity and mortality rates.

Anatomic Alterations of the Lungs

On gross examination, the lungs of an infant with RDS are dark red and liver-like. Under the microscope the lungs appear solid because of countless areas of alveolar collapse. The pulmonary capillaries are congested, and the lymphatic vessels are distended. Extensive interstitial and intraalveolar edema and hemorrhage are evident.

In what appears to be an effort to offset alveolar collapse, the respiratory bronchioles, alveolar ducts, and some alveoli dilate. As the disease intensifies, the alveolar walls become lined with a dense, rippled **hyaline membrane** identical to the hyaline membrane that develops in acute respiratory

---

BOX 35-1 Names Used to Identify Respiratory Distress Syndrome

- Infant respiratory distress syndrome
- Idiopathic respiratory distress syndrome
- Neonatal respiratory distress syndrome
- Respiratory distress syndrome of the newborn
- Hyaline membrane disease

---

distress syndrome (ARDS) (see Chapter 28). The membrane contains fibrin and cellular debris.

During the later stages of the disease, leukocytes are present, and the hyaline membrane is often fragmented and partially ingested by macrophages. Type II cells begin to proliferate, and secretions begin to accumulate in the tracheobronchial tree. The anatomic alterations in RDS produce a restrictive type of lung disorder (Figure 35-1).

As a consequence of the anatomic alterations associated with RDS, babies with this disorder often develop hypoxia-induced pulmonary arterial vasoconstriction and vasospasm, causing a state of **transient pulmonary hypertension.** This results in blood shunting from right to left through the ductus arteriosus and foramen ovale. Occasionally, intrapulmonary shunting may also occur. As a consequence, the blood flow is diverted away from the lungs (**pulmonary hypoperfusion**), which worsens the hypoxemia. It should be noted that if this condition does not resolve within 24 hours or so, shunting will begin to flow from left to right through the patent ductus arteriosus. This condition can lead to excessive lung fluid, **pulmonary hyperperfusion**, and pulmonary edema.

The major pathologic or structural changes associated with RDS are as follows:

- Interstitial and alveolar edema and hemorrhage
- Alveolar consolidation
- Intraalveolar hyaline membrane
- Pulmonary surfactant deficiency or qualitative abnormality
- Atelectasis
- Hyperperfusion (leads to excessive lung fluid and pulmonary edema in cases lasting longer than 24 hours)
- Pulmonary arterial hypoxia-induced vasoconstriction and vasospasm

Etiology and Epidemiology

Although the exact cause of RDS is controversial, the most popular theory suggests that the early stages develop as a result of (1) a pulmonary surfactant abnormality or deficiency, and (2) pulmonary hypoperfusion evoked by hypoxia, although (2) is probably a secondary response to the surfactant abnormality. The probable sequence of steps in the development of RDS is as follows:

1. Because of the pulmonary surfactant abnormality, alveolar compliance decreases, resulting in alveolar collapse.
2. The pulmonary atelectasis causes the infant's work of breathing to increase.
3. Alveolar ventilation decreases in response to the decreased lung compliance and infant fatigue, causing the alveolar oxygen tension (P_AO_2) to decrease.
4. The decreased P_AO_2 (alveolar hypoxia) stimulates a reflex pulmonary vasoconstriction.
5. Because of the pulmonary vasoconstriction, blood bypasses the infant's lungs through fetal pathways—the patent ductus arteriosus and the foramen ovale.
6. The lung hypoperfusion in turn causes lung ischemia and decreased lung metabolism.
7. Because of the decreased lung metabolism, the production of pulmonary surfactant is reduced even further, and a vicious circle develops (Figure 35-2).

It is estimated that approximately 30,000 cases of RDS occur annually in the United States. RDS is the leading cause of death in preterm infants. About 50% of the neonates born at 26 to 28 weeks' gestation develop RDS. About 25% of the babies born at 30 to 31 weeks' gestation develop

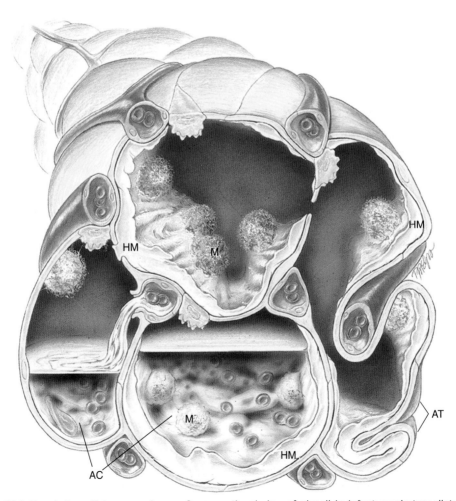

FIGURE 35-1 Respiratory distress syndrome. Cross-sectional view of alveoli in infant respiratory distress syndrome. *AC*, alveolar consolidation; *AT*, atelectasis; *HM*, hyaline membrane; *M*, macrophage.

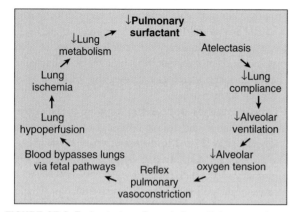

FIGURE 35-2 Early stages of respiratory distress syndrome.

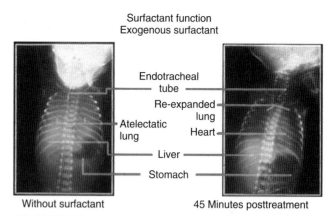

FIGURE 35-4 Chest x-ray films of an infant with respiratory distress syndrome before and after exogenous surfactant treatments.

RDS. The condition occurs more often in male babies and is usually more severe than in female babies. The higher incidence and severity of RDS in male infants is explained by the increased circulating androgens in males—which, in turn, slow the maturation of the infant's lung. The delayed lung maturation results in immature **alveolar type II cells (granular pneumocytes)** and decreased pulmonary surfactant production.

RDS is also more commonly seen in infants of diabetic mothers (the high fetal insulin levels decrease lung surfactant and structural maturation), white preterm babies compared with black preterm infants, and infants delivered by caesarean. RDS is also associated with low birth weight (1000 g to 1500 g), multiple births, prenatal asphyxia, prolonged labor, maternal bleeding, and second-born twins.

Diagnosis

There are three primary tests that can be performed on amniotic fluid to determine the lung maturity of the fetus:
1. The lecithin/sphingomyelin ratio.
2. The presence of phosphatidylglycerol.
3. The surfactant/albumin ratio.

Lecithin/sphingomyelin ratio (L:S ratio) is commonly used to test lung maturity. Lecithin, also called *dipalmitoyl phosphatidylcholine* (DPPC), is the most abundant phospholipid found in surfactant. When the concentration of lecithin is two times greater than sphingomyelin—an L:S ratio of 2:1—the infant's lung maturity is likely to be great enough that the lungs will produce adequate pulmonary surfactant at birth. Most infants with an L:S ratio less than 1:1 develop RDS. The L:S ratio is not reliable in pregnancies associated with diabetes and Rhesus (Rh) isoimmunization.

Phosphatidylglycerol (PG) is the second most abundant phospholipid found in surfactant. Because the PG level normally increases toward term, the presence of PG in the amniotic fluid indicates a low risk for RDS. When the amniotic fluid reveals an L:S ratio less than 2:1 and a lack of PG, the infant has a more than 80% risk of developing RDS. However, when the amniotic fluid shows an L:S ratio greater than 2:1 and when PG is present, the risk drops to almost zero.

Surfactant/albumin ratio (S:A ratio) is a more recently used indicator. It is reported as milligrams of surfactant per gram of protein. An S:A ratio of less than 35 indicates immature lungs. An S:A ratio of 35 to 55 indicates uncertain lung maturity. When the S:A ratio is greater than 55, adequate lung maturity is present.

General Management of Respiratory Distress Syndrome

Because of the decreased pulmonary surfactant associated with RDS, the administration of exogenous surfactant preparations, such as **beractant (Survanta), calfactant (Infasurf), or poractant alfa (Curosurf)** is helpful. Surfactant is generally administered as soon as possible (after birth) via an oral–tracheal tube and positive pressure ventilation (bagging) to distribute the surfactant throughout the airways. The term *exogenous*, used to describe these artificial surfactant agents, indicates that these preparations are from outside the patient's body. Exogenous surfactant preparations originate from other humans, from animals, or from laboratory synthesis. These agents replace the missing pulmonary surfactant of the premature or immature lungs of the baby with RDS until the lungs are mature enough to produce adequate pulmonary surfactant themselves (see Surfactant Procedure Protocol, Protocol 32-6).

Figure 35-4 provides comparison chest radiographs of an infant without exogenous surfactant and the same infant 45 minutes after treatment. The use of exogenous surfactant at birth in premature infants has significantly reduced mortality, as well as the incidence of pneumothorax and pulmonary interstitial emphysema previously associated with RDS. A surfactant administration protocol is often used to promote effective surfactant replacement therapy for prophylaxis and treatment (see Protocol 32-6).

During the early stages of RDS, **continuous positive airway pressure (CPAP)** is the treatment of choice (see Lung Expansion Therapy Protocol, Protocol 32-3). Mechanical ventilation is usually avoided as long as possible. CPAP generally works well with these patients because it (1) increases the functional residual capacity, (2) decreases the work of breathing, and (3) works to increase the PaO_2 through alveolar recruitment while the infant is receiving a lower inspired concentration of oxygen. **A PaO_2 of 40 mm to 70 mm Hg is normal for newborn infants.** No effort should be made to

The following clinical manifestations result from the pathologic mechanisms caused (or activated) by Atelectasis (see Figure 9-7), Alveolar Consolidation (see Figure 9-8), and Increased Alveolar-Capillary Membrane Thickness (see Figure 9-9)—the major anatomic alterations of the lungs associated with respiratory distress syndrome (RDS) (Figure 35-1).

CLINICAL DATA OBTAINED AT THE PATIENT'S BEDSIDE

The Physical Examination

Vital Signs

Increased Respiratory Rate (Tachypnea)

Normally, a newborn infant's respiratory rate is about 40 to 60 breaths per minute. During the early stages of RDS, the respiratory rate is generally well over 60 breaths per minute. The respiratory pattern of a baby with RDS is commonly described as "hard, fast, and deep breathing." Several pathophysiologic mechanisms operating simultaneously may lead to an increased ventilatory rate:

- Stimulation of peripheral chemoreceptors (hypoxemia)
- Decreased lung compliance–increased ventilatory rate relationship
- Stimulation of central chemoreceptors

Increased Heart Rate (Pulse) and Blood Pressure

Apnea (see Box 32-3)

Clinical Manifestations Associated with More Negative Intrapleural Pressures during Inspiration

- Intercostal retractions
- Substernal retraction and abdominal distention (seesaw movement)
- Acrocyanosis (mottling and cyanosis of the dependent portions of the thoracic and abdominal areas)
- Flaring nostrils

Chest Assessment Findings

- Bronchial (or harsh) breath sounds
- Fine crackles

Expiratory grunting

Cyanosis

CLINICAL DATA OBTAINED FROM LABORATORY TESTS AND SPECIAL PROCEDURES

Pulmonary Function Test Findings
(Extrapolated Data for Instructional Purposes)
(Primarily Restrictive Lung Pathophysiology)

The anatomic alterations of the lungs associated with RDS primarily cause a restrictive lung pathophysiology. For example, in moderate to severe cases, the following lung volumes and capacities will be lower than normal:

RV	IRV	VC	FRC	TLC
↓	↓	↓	↓	↓

Arterial Blood Gases*

MILD TO MODERATE RESPIRATORY DISTRESS SYNDROME
Acute Alveolar Hyperventilation with Hypoxemia[†]
(Acute Respiratory Alkalosis)

pH	$PaCO_2$	HCO_3^-	PaO_2	SaO_2 or SpO_2
↑	↓	↓	↓	↓
		(but normal)		

SEVERE RESPIRATORY DISTRESS SYNDROME
Acute Ventilatory Failure with Hypoxemia[§]
(Acute Respiratory Acidosis)

pH*	$PaCO_2$	HCO_3^- [†]	PaO_2	SaO_2 or SpO_2
↓	↑	↑	↓	↓
		(but normal)		

Oxygenation Indices[||]

$\dot{Q}_S/\dot{Q}_T$	DO_2[¶]	$\dot{V}O_2$	$C(a-\bar{v})O_2$	O_2ER	$S\bar{v}O_2$
↑	↓	N	N	↑	↓

*Note: Because of the difficulty of obtaining **arterial blood gas (ABG)** samples from newborn and pediatric patients, **capillary blood gas (CBG)** samples may be used to determine the pH, $PaCO_2$, and HCO_3^- (i.e., the acid-base and ventilation status only). Capillary PO_2 values are unreliable and should not be used for clinical analysis. The standard way to evaluate the oxygenation status in these young patients is pulse oximetry (SpO_2) (see Chapter 32)

[†]See Figure 4-3 and related discussion for the acute pH, $PaCO_2$, and HCO_3^- changes associated with acute alveolar hyperventilation.

[§]See Figure 4-2 and related discussion for the acute pH, $PaCO_2$, and HCO_3^- changes associated with acute ventilatory failure.

[†]When tissue hypoxia is severe enough to produce lactic acid, the pH and values will be lower than expected for a particular $PaCO_2$ level.

[||] $C(a-\bar{v})O_2$, Arterial–venous oxygen difference; DO_2, total oxygen delivery; O_2ER, oxygen extraction ratio; $\dot{Q}_S/\dot{Q}_T$, pulmonary shunt fraction; $S\bar{v}O_2$ mixed venous oxygen saturation; $\dot{V}O_2$, oxygen consumption.

[¶]It should be noted that because the newborn normally has a higher hemoglobin (Hb) level at birth (16.8 g% to 18.9 g% Hb), the DO_2 may actually be better than the PaO_2 or SpO_2 indicates (see Chapter 5).

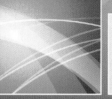
RADIOLOGIC FINDINGS

Chest Radiograph

• Increased opacity (ground-glass appearance)

On chest radiograph of infants with RDS, the air-filled tracheobronchial tree typically stands out against a dense opaque (or white) lung. This white density is often described as having a fine ground-glass appearance throughout the lung fields. Because of the pathologic processes, the density of the lungs is increased. Increased lung density resists x-ray penetration and is revealed on the radiograph as increased opacity. Therefore the more severe the RDS, the whiter the radiographic image (Figure 35-3).

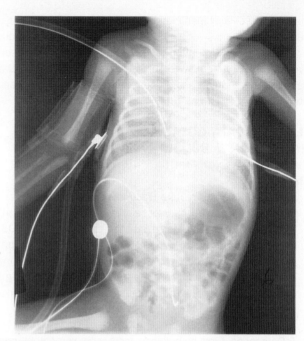

FIGURE 35-3 Whole body x-ray film of an infant with respiratory distress syndrome. Note the "whiteout," particularly of the left lower lobe and right upper lobe.

get an infant's PaO_2 within the normal adult range (80 mm to 100 mm Hg). Special attention should be given to the thermal environment of the infant with RDS because the infant's oxygenation can be further compromised if the body temperature is above or below normal.

Respiratory Care Treatment Protocols

Oxygen Therapy Protocol

Oxygen therapy is used to treat hypoxemia, decrease the work of breathing, and decrease myocardial work. Because of the hypoxemia that often develops in RDS, supplemental oxygen is usually required (see Oxygen Therapy Protocol, Protocol 32-1).

Surfactant Administration Protocol

Surfactant replacement is essential to replace the missing pulmonary surfactant in the premature or immature lungs of infants with RDS. Surfactant therapy should continue until the infant's lungs are mature enough to produce adequate surfactant. This protocol includes prophylaxis—as soon as possible after birth—and subsequent treatment dosing, which is based on established clinical criteria (such as oxygen requirement at a given age, i.e., 12 hours). In addition, the protocol includes safeguards, such as confirming endotracheal tube position before surfactant administration, the method of administration, and dosing specifics for the type of surfactant used required (see Surfactant Administration Protocol, Protocol 32-6).

Lung Expansion Therapy Protocol

Lung expansion therapies are commonly used to offset the pulmonary capillary congestion, interstitial edema, and atelectasis associated with RDS. CPAP is commonly used (see Lung Expansion Therapy Protocol, 32-3).

Mechanical Ventilation Protocol

Mechanical ventilation may be necessary to provide and support alveolar gas exchange and eventually return the patient to spontaneous breathing (see Mechanical Ventilation Protocol 32-5).

Admitting History and Physical Examination

A premature male infant was delivered after 28 weeks' gestation. The mother was a 19-year-old, unmarried primigravida patient who claimed to be in good health during the entire pregnancy until 6 hours before admission. At that time, she noticed the onset of painless vaginal bleeding. She called her obstetrician, who told her he would meet her in the emergency department of the medical center.

On examination she was found to be a healthy young woman, approximately 28 weeks pregnant, in early labor, and bleeding slightly from the vagina. Her vital signs were stable and within normal limits. A diagnosis of premature separation of the placenta was made. Because bleeding was minimal and both mother and fetus seemed to be doing well, it was decided to deliver the baby vaginally. She was monitored very closely, and labor progressed satisfactorily for about 8 hours, at which time she delivered the infant under epidural anesthesia without any obstetric complications. The baby weighed 1600 g. The Apgar scores were 7 after 1 minute and 9 after 5 minutes. Physical examination findings were entirely normal for an infant of this size.

On admission to the newborn nursery 30 minutes after delivery, the infant was noted to have some moderate respiratory distress. His respiratory rate was 56 breaths/min with nasal flaring. A chest radiograph obtained at this time was read by the radiologist as "having a reticulogranular appearance."

Within the next 30 minutes, the infant's respiratory distress became more marked with tachypnea, retractions, and grunting. The respiratory therapist was called to the nursery to evaluate this infant for possible surfactant administration. Upon arrival, the infant's respiratory rate was 64 breaths/min, heart rate 165 beats/min, and auscultation of the infant's chest revealed bilateral fine crackles. The infant was grunting on $\frac{1}{2}$ L/min oxygen per nasal cannula; nasal flaring was noted. A capillary blood gas showed: pH 7.14, $PaCO_2$ 68 mm Hg, HCO_3^- 22 mEq/L. The infant's SpO_2 was 85%.

Respiratory Assessment and Plan

S N/A (newborn)

O Increased work of breathing with worsening hypoxemia. Retracting and using accessory muscles. Flaring of nostrils. Vital signs: RR 64 with "grunting." HR 165. Bilateral fine crackles. CXR: Bilateral "ground-glass" haziness. CBGs on $\frac{1}{2}$ L/min oxygen: pH 7.14, $PaCO_2$ 68, HCO_3^- 22. SpO_2 85%.

A • **Infant respiratory distress syndrome** (history)
- Alveolar hyaline membrane, atelectasis (CXR)
- Acute ventilatory failure with severe hypoxemia (ABGs)
- Lactic acidosis likely (pH and HCO_3^- lower than expected for $PaCO_2$ of 68)
- (pH and HCO_3^- lower than expected for $PaCO_2$ of 68)

P **Surfactant Administration Protocol:** Apply CPAP by mask until intubation. Intubate, provide manual then mechanical ventilation; obtain chest radiograph to verify endotracheal tube placement. Draw up liquid surfactant using drug-specific mL per kg of infant's weight dose. Once tube is in the correct position (T2-T3), administer surfactant in small doses to avoid "drowning" the airway while providing mechanical ventilation.
- **Mechanical Ventilation Protocol:** Ventilate using positive end-expiratory pressure (PEEP) per neonatal intensive care unit (NICU) ventilator protocol. Focus effort on weaning PIP to maintain 4 mL/kg to 6 mL/kg tidal volume as the infant's lung compliance improves.
- **Oxygen Therapy Protocol:** Continuous Pulse Oximetry.

At this time, the baby was transferred to NICU, intubated, and put on a ventilator. The initial ventilator settings were respiratory rate (RR) 40/min, inspiratory time (TI) 0.35, FIO_2 0.40, positive inspiratory pressure (PIP) +25 cm H_2O, and positive end-expiratory pressure (PEEP) +5 cm H_2O. Artificial surfactant was administered without complication. Fluid and electrolyte balance was maintained within normal levels. While maintaining the exhaled V_T at 4 to 6 mL per kilogram, the PIP was progressively decreased. At 22 hours, the infant was weaned from mechanical ventilation to CPAP. He was weaned off the nasal CPAP and extubated at 30 hours. Chest x-ray examination on the fifth day was unremarkable. The baby was discharged on the tenth day and has been healthy ever since.

Discussion

RDS is a fascinating disorder in which meticulous respiratory care of the infant is crucial. Most respiratory therapy students greatly look forward to and enjoy their NICU rotation. In these units the expertise of the respiratory therapist is crucial to the functioning of the unit because the majority of patients there have respiratory disorders. Indeed, many of the first reports of therapist-driven protocols came from this setting.

Many of the clinical manifestations seen in this case are associated with **Atelectasis** (see Figure 9-7) and **Increased Alveolar-Capillary Membrane Thickness** (see Figure 9-9). For example, the use of accessory muscles of inspiration was likely to be a compensatory mechanism activated to offset the increased stiffness of the lungs (decreased lung compliance) caused by the atelectasis and alveolar hyaline membrane. The atelectasis and alveolar hyaline membrane were objectively verified by the chest radiograph. In addition, the severity level of the anatomic alterations and clinical manifestations seen in this case was very high. This was objectively confirmed by the capillary blood gas analysis that identified the acute ventilatory failure with hypoxemia (SpO_2: 85%).

Thus the aggressive implementation of mechanical ventilation and use of artificial surfactant were certainly justified.

Artificial surfactant has markedly improved the outlook for these infants. However, the respiratory therapist should be on the alert for sudden changes in lung compliance that often occur shortly after the administration of artificial surfactant. If the infant is on a pressure-cycled mode ventilator, this is especially important to avoid **volutrauma.*** As in adults with

ARDS, in which the pathology is very similar, constant attention must be given to the possibility of nosocomial infection, fluid overload, and cardiovascular instability. In addition, lung protection strategies such as PEEP, permissive hypercapnia, and use of small ventilator tidal volumes are commonly used in RDS cases.

---

*Volutrauma is defined as damage to the lung caused by over-distention by a mechanical ventilator set for an excessively high tidal volume.

SELF-ASSESSMENT QUESTIONS

ⓔ Answers to questions can be found on Evolve. To access additional student assessment questions visit **http://evolve.elsevier.com/DesJardins/respiratory.**

1. When transient pulmonary hypertension exists in respiratory distress syndrome, blood bypasses the infant's lungs through which of the following structures?
   1. Ductus venosus
   2. Umbilical vein
   3. Ductus arteriosus
   4. Foramen ovale
      a. 1 and 2 only
      b. 1 and 3 only
      c. 2 and 3 only
      d. 3 and 4 only

2. It is suggested that respiratory distress syndrome is a result of which of the following?
   1. Vernix membrane
   2. Decreased perfusion of the lungs
   3. Pulmonary surfactant abnormality
   4. Congenital alveolar dysplasia
      a. 1 and 3 only
      b. 2 and 3 only
      c. 1 and 4 only
      d. 2, 3, and 4 only

3. When an infant with respiratory distress syndrome creates more negative intrapleural pressure during inspiration, which of the following occurs?
   a. The soft tissue between the ribs bulges outward.
   b. The dependent blood vessels dilate and pool blood.
   c. The substernal area protrudes.
   d. The abdominal area retracts.

4. Infants with severe respiratory distress syndrome often have which of the following?
   1. Diminished breath sounds
   2. Bronchial breath sounds
   3. Hyperresonant percussion notes
   4. Fine crackles
      a. 1 and 4 only
      b. 3 and 4 only
      c. 2 and 3 only
      d. 2 and 4 only

5. Continuous positive airway pressure (CPAP) is often administered to infants with respiratory distress syndrome in an effort to do which of the following?
   1. Increase the infant's FRC
   2. Decrease the infant's work of breathing
   3. Increase the infant's PaO_2
   4. Decrease the FIO_2 necessary to oxygenate the infant
      a. 1 and 3 only
      b. 2 and 4 only
      c. 2, 3, and 4 only
      d. 1, 2, 3, and 4

36 Pulmonary Air Leak Syndromes

Chapter Objectives

After reading this chapter, you will be able to:

- List the anatomic alterations of the lungs associated with pulmonary air leak syndromes.
- Describe the causes of pulmonary air leak syndromes.
- List the cardiopulmonary clinical manifestations associated with pulmonary air leak syndromes.
- Describe the general management of pulmonary air leak syndromes.
- Describe the clinical strategies and rationales of the SOAP presented in the case study.

Key Terms

Air Embolism
Blebs (Emphysema-Like)
Bronchopulmonary Dysplasia
Cardiac Tamponade
Exogenous Surfactant
High Levels of Positive End-Expiratory Pressure (PEEP)
High-Frequency Ventilation
Iatrogenic Tension Pneumothorax
Iatrogenic Pneumothorax
Intravascular Air Embolism
Needle Thoracentesis
Peak Inspiratory Pressure (PIP)

Permissive Hypercapnia
Pneumomediastinum
Pneumopericardium
Pneumoperitoneum
Prolonged Inspiratory Time (T_I)
Pulmonary Air Leak Syndromes
Pulmonary Barotrauma
Pulmonary Interstitial Emphysema (PIE)
Pulmonary Volutrauma
Subcutaneous Emphysema
Syndrome of Inappropriate Antidiuretic Hormone (SIADH)
Transillumination of the Chest
Ventilator-Induced Lung Injury (VILI)

Chapter Outline

Anatomic Alterations of the Lungs
    Pulmonary Interstitial Emphysema
    Etiology and Epidemiology
Overview of the Cardiopulmonary Clinical Manifestations Associated with Pulmonary Air Leak Syndromes
General Management of Pulmonary Air Leak Syndromes
    Respiratory Care Treatment Protocols
Case Study: Pulmonary Air Leak Syndromes
Self-Assessment Questions

Introduction

Pulmonary air leak syndromes (also called *air block syndromes*) in the infant comprise a large spectrum of clinical entities, including **pulmonary interstitial emphysema (PIE)**, followed by, in severe cases, **pneumomediastinum, pneumothorax, pneumopericardium, pneumoperitoneum,** and, in rare cases, **intravascular air embolism.** Pulmonary air leak syndromes were common complications of mechanical ventilation in premature infants with respiratory distress syndrome before the introduction of **exogenous surfactant**.

It has long been known that mechanical ventilation can produce a variety of lung injuries referred to as **ventilator-induced lung injury (VILI), pulmonary volutrauma,** or **pulmonary barotrauma.** *VILI* is defined as stress fractures of the pulmonary capillary endothelium, epithelium, and basement membrane and, in severe cases, lung rupture. Lung ruptures can lead to leakage of fluid, protein, and blood into tissue and air spaces or leakage of air into tissue spaces. This condition can be followed by an inflammatory response and possibly a reduced defense against infection. *Pulmonary*

volutrauma is defined as damage to the lung caused by overdistention by a mechanical ventilator set for an excessively high tidal volume. *Pulmonary barotrauma* is defined as damage to the lungs caused by rapid or extreme pressures generated by mechanical ventilation.

Predisposing factors for VILI, pulmonary volutrauma, or pulmonary barotrauma include (1) mechanical ventilation with high peak inspiratory volumes and pressures, (2) mechanical ventilation with a high mean airway pressure, (3) structural immaturity of lung and chest wall, (4) surfactant insufficiency or inactivation, and (5) preexisting lung disease. Fortunately, newborn mechanical ventilator strategies today minimize lung injuries by keeping exhaled volumes low, accepting higher PCO_2 levels, or switching to high frequency ventilation when positive inspiratory pressures (PIPs) exceed safe limits. Pulmonary air leak syndrome, however, can still occur in certain clinical scenarios—especially when very high ventilator pressures are used or in the delivery room with aggressive ventilation during resuscitation (see Chapter 35).

Anatomic Alterations of the Lungs

Pulmonary Interstitial Emphysema

Virtually all pulmonary air leak syndromes begin with some degree of PIE. When high airway pressures are applied to an infant's lungs (e.g., during mechanical ventilation or excessive PEEP), the distal airways and alveoli often become overdistended—that is, they develop **blebs or emphysema-like** areas—and rupture (Figure 36-1). In addition, gas trapping from an insufficient expiratory time or auto-PEEP can also cause alveolar overdistention and rupture. Once the gas escapes, it is forced into (1) the loose connective tissue sheaths that surround the airways and pulmonary capillaries, and (2) the interlobular septa containing pulmonary veins. In severe cases, the gas continues to spread peripherally by dissecting along the peribronchial and perivascular spaces to the hilum of the lung, producing the classic radiographic appearance of PIE that shows bubbles of air in the interstitial cuffs (Figure 36-2 and Figure 36-3).

The overdistention associated with PIE forces the lungs into a full inflation position—which, in turn, decreases lung compliance (static lung compliance is reduced at *both* very low and very high lung volumes). Moreover, air trapped within the interstitial cuffs compresses the airways and increases airway resistance. In addition, the trapped air in the interstitial spaces impairs lymphatic function, resulting in fluid accumulation in the interstitial cuffs and alveoli, further decreasing lung compliance. Once the interstitial gas reaches the hilum of the lung, it either (1) coalesces to form large hilar blebs, or (2) tracks beneath the visceral pleura to form large subpleural pockets of air. In either case, the accumulation of gas can be large enough to significantly compress the lung or mediastinal structures.

A pneumomediastinum may occur when the excessive air associated with a PIE continues to track—and accumulate—through the perivascular and peribronchial cuffs and causes the gas in the hilar area to rupture into the mediastinum. In addition, the high gas pressures associated with a pneumomediastinum may also dissect into the pleural space and the fascial planes of the neck and skin, resulting in the condition known as **subcutaneous emphysema.**

A pneumothorax may occur because of the alveolar overdistention and subsequent rupture commonly associated with a PIE (Figure 36-4). A pneumopericardium can develop from direct tracking of interstitial air along the great vessels into the pericardial sac (Figure 36-5). Gas pressure in the pericardium restricts atrial and ventricular filling, resulting in a decreased stroke volume and, ultimately, a reduced cardiac

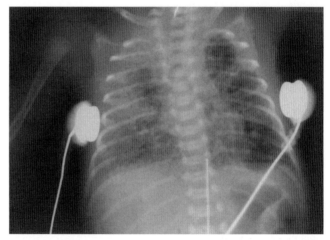

FIGURE 36-2 Pulmonary interstitial emphysema (PIE). Fine, bubbly appearance of the lungs in an infant with severe respiratory distress syndrome (RDS). (From Taussig LM, Landau LI: *Pediatric respiratory medicine*, ed 2, St Louis, 2008, Elsevier.)

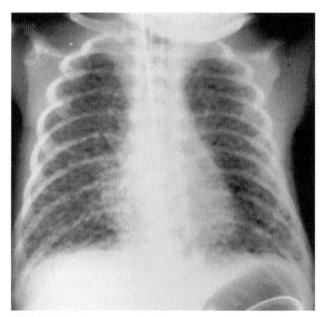

FIGURE 36-3 Pulmonary interstitial emphysema. The lung is grossly hyperinflated, with coarse radiolucencies extending from the pleura to the hilum. These radiolucencies represent bubbles of air in the perivascular and peribronchial interstitial cuffs. (From Taeusch WH, Ballard RA, Gleason CA: *Avery's diseases of the newborn*, ed 8, Philadelphia, 2005, Saunders.)

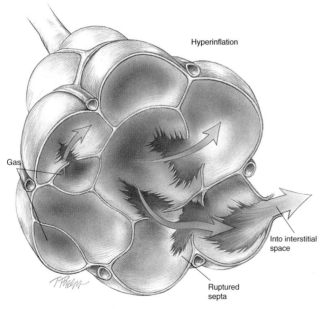

FIGURE 36-1 Pulmonary air leak syndromes.

output (**cardiac tamponade**) and systemic hypotension. During the late stages, inflammatory changes of the airways lead to increased capillary leakage and excessive bronchial secretions.

A **pneumoperitoneum** may develop from the tracking of gas along the sheaths of the aorta and vena cava which eventually may burst into the peritoneal cavity. Clinically, an infant with a pneumoperitoneum manifests a sudden onset

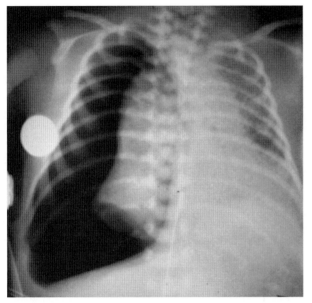

FIGURE 36-4 Tension pneumothorax. The lung on the involved (right) side is collapsed, and the mediastinum is shifted to the opposite side. Pleura can be seen bulging into the intercostal spaces. (From Taeusch WH, Ballard RA, Gleason CA: *Avery's diseases of the newborn*, ed 8, Philadelphia, 2005, Saunders.)

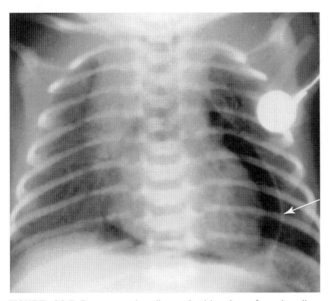

FIGURE 36-5 Pneumopericardium. A thin rim of pericardium (arrow) is visible and clearly separated from the heart by air within the pericardial sac. (From Taeusch WH, Ballard RA, Gleason CA: *Avery's diseases of the newborn*, ed 8, Philadelphia, 2005, Saunders.)

of abdominal distention. The pneumoperitoneum may be large enough to block the descent of the diaphragm and may require drainage. Finally, the excessive gas accumulation associated with a pneumoperitoneum may end up in the scrotum in male babies or the labia in females.

In very rare cases, an **intravascular air embolism** may occur. It is hypothesized that the air is actually pumped under high pressure through the pulmonary lymphatics into the systemic venous circulation. Intravascular air causes an abrupt cardiovascular collapse and is frequently diagnosed when air is observed in vessels on chest radiographs taken to establish the cause of cardiovascular collapse.

The major pathologic changes associated with pulmonary air leak syndromes are as follows:

- Atelectasis, caused by the following:
  - Collapsed alveoli adjacent to overdistended alveoli (e.g., blebs or emphysema-like area)
  - Pneumothorax
  - Pneumomediastinum
  - Pneumoperitoneum
- Airway compression (caused by interstitial air accumulation)
- Excessive bronchial secretions (late stages)

Etiology and Epidemiology

Preterm infants who weigh less than 1000 g at birth have an increased risk for the early occurrence of pulmonary air leak syndromes (often within the first 24 to 48 hours of life), especially because of the weak noncartilaginous structures of their distal airways. The most frequent causative factor resulting in pulmonary air leak syndromes in preterm infants is the use of mechanical ventilation. Pulmonary air leak syndromes commonly result from the use of **high levels of positive end-expiratory pressure (PEEP), high peak inspiratory pressures (PIPs),** and **prolonged inspiratory times (TIs).** The early use of surfactant and ventilator strategies, such as permissive hypercapnia*, to minimize peak pressures has resulted in a significant decrease in the incidence of air leak syndromes in premature infants. Occasionally, full-term babies will develop a spontaneous tension pneumothorax.

Permissive hypercapnia defined: Mechanical ventilation was traditionally applied with the goal of normalizing arterial blood gas values, particularly the arterial carbon dioxide tension ($PaCO_2$). However, this is no longer the primary objective of mechanical ventilation. Today, the emphasis is on maintaining adequate gas exchange while—and, importantly—minimizing the risks of mechanical ventilation. Common strategies used to reduce the risk of mechanical ventilation include (1) low tidal volume ventilation—to protect the lung from ventilator-associated lung injury in patients with acute lung injury (e.g., ARDS)—and (2) reduction of the tidal volume, respiratory rate, or both—to minimize intrinsic positive end-expiratory pressure (i.e., auto-PEEP) in patients with obstructive lung disease (e.g., COPD).

Although these mechanical ventilation strategies may result in an increased $PaCO_2$ level (hypercapnia), they do help to protect the lung from barotrauma (i.e., physical damage to lung tissues caused by excessive gas pressures). The lenient acceptance of the hypercapnia is called **permissive hypercapnia.** In most cases, the patient's $PaCO_2$ is adequately maintained by an increased ventilatory rate that offsets the decreased tidal volume. The $PaCO_2$, however, should not be permitted to increase to the point of severe respiratory acidosis. The most current consensus suggests it is safe to allow the pH to fall to at least 7.20 (www.ARDSNet.org).

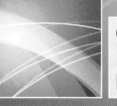

OVERVIEW of the Cardiopulmonary Clinical Manifestations Associated with Pulmonary Air Leak Syndromes

The following clinical manifestations result from the pathologic mechanisms caused (or activated) by Atelectasis (see Figure 9-7) and decreased lung compliance—the major anatomic alteration of the lungs associated with pulmonary air leak syndromes (see Figure 36-1).

CLINICAL DATA OBTAINED AT THE PATIENT'S BEDSIDE

The Physical Examination

Vital Signs

Increased Respiratory Rate (Tachypnea)

Normally, a newborn's respiratory rate is about 40 to 60 breaths per minute. During the early stages of pulmonary air leak syndromes, the respiratory rate is generally well over 60 breaths per minute. Several pathophysiologic mechanisms operating simultaneously may lead to an increased ventilatory rate:

- Stimulation of peripheral chemoreceptors (hypoxemia)
- Decreased lung compliance–increased ventilatory rate relationship
- Stimulation of central chemoreceptors

Increased Heart Rate (Pulse) and Blood Pressure
Apnea (see Box 32-3)

Clinical Manifestations Associated with More Negative Intrapleural Pressures during Inspiration

- Intercostal retractions
- Substernal retraction and abdominal distention (seesaw movement)
- Cyanosis of the dependent portions of the thoracic and abdominal areas
- Flaring nostrils

Chest Assessment Findings

- Diminished breath sounds (decreased air exchange)
- Crackles

Expiratory Grunting
Cyanosis
Increased Transillumination

Transillumination of the chest is performed by placing a high-intensity fiberoptic light source against the infant's chest in a darkened room. When free air is present in the chest cavity (that is a pneumothorax is present), an increased illumination is seen on the affected side.

CLINICAL DATA OBTAINED FROM LABORATORY TESTS AND SPECIAL PROCEDURES

Pulmonary Function Test Findings
(Extrapolated Data for Instructional Purposes)
(Primarily Restrictive Lung Pathophysiology)

The anatomic alterations of the lungs associated with pulmonary air leak syndromes primarily cause a restrictive lung pathophysiology. For example, in moderate to severe cases, the following lung volumes and capacities will be lower than normal:

RV	IRV	VC	FRC	TLC
↓	↓	↓	↓	↓

Arterial Blood Gases*

MILD TO MODERATE PULMONARY AIR LEAK SYNDROMES

Acute Alveolar Hyperventilation with Hypoxemia[†]
(Acute Respiratory Alkalosis)

pH	$PaCO_2$	HCO_3^-	PaO_2	SaO_2 or SpO_2
↑	↓	↓ (but normal)	↓	↓

SEVERE PULMONARY AIR LEAK SYNDROMES

Acute Ventilatory Failure with Hypoxemia[§]
(Acute Respiratory Acidosis)

pH*	$PaCO_2$	HCO_3^- [†]	PaO_2	SaO_2 or SpO_2
↓	↑	↑ (but normal)	↓	↓

*Note: Because of the difficulty of obtaining **arterial blood gas (ABG)** samples from newborn and pediatric patients, **capillary blood gas (CBG)** samples may be used to determine the pH, $PaCO_2$, and HCO_3^- (i.e., the acid-base and ventilation status only). Capillary PO_2 values are unreliable and should not be used for clinical analysis. The standard way to evaluate the oxygenation status in these young patients is pulse oximetry (SpO_2) (see Chapter 32).
[†]See Figure 4-3 and related discussion for the acute pH, $PaCO_2$, and HCO_3^- changes associated with acute alveolar hyperventilation.
[§]See Figure 4-2 and related discussion for the acute pH, $PaCO_2$, and HCO_3^- changes associated with acute ventilatory failure.
[†]When tissue hypoxia is severe enough to produce lactic acid, the pH and values will be lower than expected for a particular $PaCO_2$ level.

Oxygenation Indices*

$\dot{Q}_S/\dot{Q}_T$	DO_2†	$\dot{V}O_2$	$C(a\text{-}\bar{v})O_2$	O_2ER	$S\bar{v}O_2$
↑	↓	N	N	↑	↓

RADIOLOGIC FINDINGS
Chest Radiograph

The chest radiograph may show focal or generalized problem areas. When significant partial airway obstruction, air trapping, and alveolar hyperinflation are present, the chest radiograph appears hyperlucent and the diaphragms may be depressed.

---

*$C(a\text{-}\bar{v})O_2$, Arterial–venous oxygen difference; DO_2, total oxygen delivery; O_2ER, oxygen extraction ratio; $\dot{Q}_S/\dot{Q}_T$, pulmonary shunt fraction; $S\bar{v}O_2$ mixed venous oxygen saturation; $\dot{V}O_2$, oxygen consumption.

†It should be noted that because the newborn normally has a higher hemoglobin (Hb) level at birth (16.8 g% to 18.9 g% Hb), the DO_2 may actually be better than the PaO_2 or SpO_2 indicates (see Chapter 5).

The diagnosis of pulmonary interstitial emphysema (PIE) is commonly confirmed when the radiograph reveals lung hyperinflation and a fine, bubbly appearance (emphysema-like blebs) extending from the hilum to the pleura (see Figures 36-2 and 36-3). PIE may affect both lungs or may be present in one lung or one lobe.

The respiratory therapist should always be alert for the sudden development of a pneumomediastinum or pneumothorax in infants with pulmonary air leak syndromes. When the excessive air associated with a PIE continues to track—and accumulate—through the perivascular and peribronchial cuffs, it may cause the gas in the hilum area to rupture into the mediastinum, resulting in a pneumomediastinum. A pneumothorax may occur because of the alveolar overdistention and subsequent rupture commonly associated with PIE (see Figure 36-4). Figure 36-5 shows an infant with a pneumopericardium, which developed from the direct tracking of interstitial gas along the great vessels of the pericardial sac.

General Management of Pulmonary Air Leak Syndromes

Prevention is the best treatment for pulmonary air leak syndromes. These syndromes may be prevented by (1) using a manometer or pressure limited resuscitation device for manual ventilation, (2) using the lowest mechanical ventilator pressures (PIP, PEEP) to reach patient-appropriate exhaled tidal volumes, (3) adopting a strategy of permissive hypercapnia, (4) securing radiologic confirmation of the adequacy of PEEP and lung volume, and (5) implementing high frequency ventilation when required PIPs exceeds 30 cm H_2O.

Selective intubation of the unaffected or less affected lung may allow the injured lung time to heal. **High-frequency ventilation** has been successful in treating infants with pulmonary air leak syndromes. Survivors of pulmonary air leak syndromes often develop **bronchopulmonary dysplasia** (or chronic lung disease of infancy) (see Chapter 38) as a result of overly vigorous mechanical ventilation. Finally, the respiratory therapist must always be alert for signs and symptoms of subcutaneous emphysema, pneumothorax, pneumopericardium, pneumoperitoneum, pneumomediastinum, and intravascular air embolism.

Mechanical removal of free air from the intrathoracic cavity is necessary if the air accumulation is significant and prevents effective ventilation. **Needle thoracentesis** is a technique used to emergently relieve a significant or tension pneumothorax in these infants. Chest tube placement is the preferred method when a surgeon is present. Tapping and removing air from the pericardium or mediastinum may sometime be necessary, when vascular collapse or cardiac tamponade is present.

Respiratory Care Treatment Protocols
Oxygen Therapy Protocol

Oxygen therapy is used to treat hypoxemia, decrease the work of breathing, and decrease myocardial work. Because of the hypoxemia that often develops in pulmonary air leak syndromes, supplemental oxygen is required (see Oxygen Therapy Protocol, Protocol 32-1). Although 100% oxygen can be used in the acute treatment of an adult or child with a pneumothorax to speed the reabsorption of inert nitrogen, it is not considered for this purpose in the management of newborns with pulmonary air leak.

Bronchopulmonary Hygiene Therapy Protocol

Because of the excessive airway secretions and mucous accumulation associated with pulmonary air leak syndromes, suctioning may be used to enhance the mobilization of bronchial secretions (see Bronchopulmonary Hygiene Therapy Protocol, Protocol 32-2).

Lung Expansion Therapy Protocol

Cautious use of lung expansion measures commonly are administered to offset the pulmonary capillary congestion and interstitial edema and atelectasis associated with pulmonary air leak syndromes (see Lung Expansion Therapy Protocol, Protocol 32-3). Optimal PEEP is needed to improve lung compliance and reduce the need for higher PIP.

Mechanical Ventilation Protocol

Mechanical ventilation may be necessary to provide and support alveolar gas exchange and eventually return the patient to spontaneous breathing. Prevention is the best treatment for pulmonary air leak syndromes. Selective intubation of the unaffected or less affected lung may allow the injured lung time to heal. High-frequency ventilation has been successful in treating infants with pulmonary air leak syndromes (see Mechanical Ventilation Protocol, Protocol 32-5)

Needle Thoracentesis

This technique is used to emergently relieve the life-threatening pressure caused by a significant pneumothorax or tension pneumothorax that is impeding effective ventilation. Once the presence of free air is determined by chest radiograph, transillumination, or absence of breath sounds in a rapidly deteriorating infant, who is difficult to manually ventilate, a sheathed or catheter needle is inserted above the third intercostal space of the affected side at the mid-clavicular line or the mid-axillary line. The needle is advanced until it enters the pleural cavity, at which time a "pop" or release of air is heard. The needle is removed and the catheter is taped in placed and attached to a three-way stopcock for intermittent air removal by syringe. This technique allows for pressure relief until a chest tube is placed.

CASE STUDY Pulmonary Air Leak Syndromes

Admitting History and Physical Examination

A 32-week-gestation, preterm female infant was delivered by emergency caesarean section to a healthy 25-year-old mother. The infant weighed 2750 g. The mother's admitting history showed her to be a **primigravida** with normal prenatal care and no history of illness during her pregnancy. The cesarean section was performed because of repeated and prolonged fetal heart rate decelerations that did not improve with maternal positioning or oxygen administration. At delivery, the infant was found to have the umbilical cord twice wrapped tightly around her neck. She was limp, appeared pale and cyanotic, and was apneic. She showed no response to tactile stimuli, and her heart rate was 65 beats/min. Her 1-minute Apgar score was 1 (color 0, pulse 1, grimace 0, reflex irritability 0, muscle tone 0, respiratory 0).

Immediately the neonatologist, nurse, and respiratory therapist started compressions with manual ventilation with a bag-valve-mask at an FIO_2 of 1.0 and vigorous chest compressions. The 5-minute Apgar was 5 (color 1, pulse 2, grimace 0, reflex irritability 0, muscle tone 1, respiratory 1). Despite the fact that the baby's condition had started to improve, she suddenly took a turn for the worse. Her heart rate started to drop; she again appeared cyanotic, and her muscle tone decreased.

At this time, the respiratory therapist noted that the baby's breath sounds were absent over the right lung and severely decreased over the left upper and lower lobes. Her heart sounds were muffled and faint. Transillumination showed a large right pneumothorax. This was later confirmed by chest radiographic examination as a right tension pneumothorax. The neonatologist inserted a chest tube, and the baby was placed on a mechanical ventilator with the following settings: intermittent mandatory ventilation (IMV) 30, FIO_2 1.0, positive inspiratory pressure (PIP) +25 cm H_2O, positive end-expiratory pressure (PEEP) +5 cm H_2O, and inspiratory time (T_I) 0.35 seconds.

Moments later, an umbilical artery catheter (UAC) was inserted; it showed the following values: pH 7.19, $PaCO_2$ 77 mm Hg, HCO_3^- 19 mEq/L, PaO_2 31 mm Hg, and SaO_2 47%. The ventilator rate was increased immediately to 40 breaths/min. ABG values 20 minutes later were as follows: pH 7.33, $PaCO_2$ 43 mm Hg, HCO_3^- 22 mEq/L, PaO_2 47 mm Hg, and SaO_2 83%.

A second chest radiographic examination an hour later showed that the right lung had re-expanded, with scattered areas of segmental atelectasis throughout. At this time, the infant appeared pink and her vital signs were stable, with a heart rate of 155 beats/min and blood pressure of 68/35. Breath sounds revealed bilateral crackles. ABG values were as follows: pH 7.34, $PaCO_2$ 42 mm Hg, HCO_3^- 22 mEq/L, PaO_2 53 mm Hg and $SaO2$ 89%. The respiratory therapist recorded the following in the baby's chart:

Respiratory Assessment and Plan

S N/A

O Skin: Pink. HR 155 bpm, BP 68/35. Crackles throughout. ABGs: pH 7.34, $PaCO_2$ 42, HCO_3^- 22, PaO_2 53, and SaO_2 89%. CXR: Re-expanded right lung with scattered areas of segmental atelectasis throughout.

A • Preterm infant in respiratory distress at birth
   • Right tension pneumothorax, treated
   • Atelectasis—right lung (CXR)
   • Adequate ventilation and oxygenation on present ventilator settings (ABGs)
   • Excessive airway secretions (crackles and rhonchi)

P Continue **Mechanical Ventilation Protocol**. Attempt to reduce FIO$_2$ per **Oxygen Therapy Protocol**. Continue **Lung Expansion Therapy Protocol** (PEEP +5 cm H$_2$O). Start **Bronchopulmonary Hygiene Therapy Protocol** (Suction PRN). Monitor closely (vital signs, color, ABGs, transillumination).

Discussion

An **iatrogenic tension pneumothorax** caused by a resuscitation effort is not uncommon during resuscitation of the newborn. This is especially true when staff is inexperienced or perform resuscitation too aggressively because of the anxiety and urgency of the situation. Respiratory therapists must be prepared to attend deliveries, manage the airways, and provide ventilatory support as requested by the other members of the health-care team. In fact, most departments expect staff to have one or more of the following credentials: Neonatal Advance Life Support (NALS), Pediatric Advanced Life Support (PALS), or Registered Respiratory Therapist-Neonatal/Pediatric Specialist (RRT-NPS). With the simulation-baby and other computerized training manikins available, many respiratory therapists are trained and ready to participate on the rapid response teams.

Since the advent of surfactant therapy, pneumothoraces in mechanically ventilated infants in neonatal intensive care units (NICUs) have decreased. Tension pneumothorax is a potentially life-threatening emergency, and the respiratory therapist should always be alert for any signs or symptoms associated with this condition.

In this case the clinical manifestations associated with **Atelectasis** (see Figure 9-7) were quickly identified when the respiratory therapist noted the possibility of a pneumothorax by pointing out that the baby's breath sounds were absent over the right lung and severely decreased over the left upper and middle lobes. Transillumination further supported the presence of a pneumothorax. The chest radiograph confirmed a right lung pneumothorax. Caution should be used when evacuating air from a large pneumothorax as rapid re-expansion of a collapsed lung can cause a severe vasovagal reaction* and may also result in transient pulmonary edema.

Finally, it is not uncommon for infants with pulmonary air leak syndromes to develop fluid in their lungs shortly after a pneumothorax has resolved (i.e., the chest tube is no longer sucking any air out of the baby's chest). When this occurs, these infants retain fluid evidenced by rapid weight gain, demonstrate crackles, and require a higher FIO$_2$ to maintain their desired PaO$_2$ levels. The reason for this is that babies who have iatrogenic tension pneumothoraces often develop what is called a transient **syndrome of inappropriate antidiuretic hormone (SIADH)**. In other words, the pneumothorax causes the release of antidiuretic hormone, which inhibits urination. Some of the retained fluid accumulates in the baby's lungs. Often, a diuretic (such as furosemide), a little more airway pressure, an increased FIO$_2$, or an increased ventilator rate may be administered to offset this transient problem. The condition usually lasts only about 24 hours. The respiratory therapist should expect this condition and should not be overly concerned.

---

*Vasovagal reaction is defined as a reflex of the involuntary nervous system that causes the heart to slow down (bradycardia) and that, at the same time, affects the nerves to the blood vessels in the legs permitting those vessels to dilate (widen).

As a result the heart puts out less blood, the blood pressure drops, and what blood is circulating tends to go into the legs rather than to the head. The brain is deprived of oxygen and the fainting episode occurs. The vasovagal reaction is also called a vasovagal attack.

SELF-ASSESSMENT QUESTIONS

Answers to questions can be found on Evolve. To access additional student assessment questions visit **http://evolve.elsevier.com/DesJardins/respiratory**.

1. **The most frequent etiologic factor causing air leak syndromes in preterm infants is:**
   a. Infants who weigh less than 1000 g
   b. Mechanical ventilation
   c. Excessive bronchial secretions
   d. Increased expiratory grunting

2. **During the advanced stages of pulmonary air leak syndromes, the infant demonstrates a(n):**
   1. Increased $PaCO_2$
   2. Decreased HCO_3^-
   3. Increased pH
   4. Decreased PaO_2
      a. 1 and 4 only
      b. 2 and 3 only
      c. 1, 3, and 4 only
      d. 1, 2, 3, and 4

3. **Infants with pulmonary air leak syndromes often have:**
   1. Reduced urine output
   2. Increased transillumination
   3. Hypoxia-induced pulmonary arterial vasoconstriction
   4. Ventilator-induced lung injury
      a. 1 and 3 only
      b. 2 and 4 only
      c. 2, 3, and 4 only
      d. 1, 2, 3, and 4

4. **Which of the following are the major pathologic changes associated with pulmonary air leak syndromes?**
   1. Airway obstruction
   2. Consolidation
   3. Atelectasis
   4. Excessive bronchial secretions
      a. 3 and 4 only
      b. 1, 3, and 4 only
      c. 2, 3, and 4 only
      d. 1, 2, 3, and 4

5. **In pulmonary air leak syndromes, if the high interstitial lung pressure persists, the gas may:**
   1. Continue to spread peripherally
   2. Remain localized and restrict the airway lumen
   3. Cause a pneumomediastinum or pneumopericardium
   4. Rupture the visceral pleura
      a. 1 and 3 only
      b. 2 and 4 only
      c. 2, 3, and 4 only
      d. 1, 2, 3, and 4

Respiratory Syncytial Virus Infection (Bronchiolitis or Pneumonitis)

Chapter Objectives

After reading this chapter, you will be able to:

- List the anatomic alterations of the lungs associated with respiratory syncytial virus (RSV) infection.
- Describe the causes of RSV.
- List the cardiopulmonary clinical manifestations associated with RSV infection.
- Describe the general management of RSV.
- Describe the clinical strategies and rationales of the SOAPs presented in the case study.
- Define key terms and complete self-assessment questions at the end of the chapter.

Key Terms

"Ball-valve" Mechanism
Bronchiolitis
Enzyme Immuno Assay (EIA)
Palivizumab (Synagis)
Pneumonitis
Polymerase Chain Reaction (PCR)

Respiratory Infectious Disease Panel (RIDP)
Small Particle Aerosol Generator (SPAG)
Syncytium

Chapter Outline

Anatomic Alterations of the Lungs
Etiology and Epidemiology
    Laboratory Testing for Respiratory Syncytial Virus
Overview of the Cardiopulmonary Clinical Manifestations Associated with Respiratory Syncytial Virus Infection
General Management of Respiratory Syncytial Virus Infection (Bronchiolitis, Pneumonitis)
    Monitoring
    Oxygen Therapy Protocol
    Bronchopulmonary Hygiene Therapy Protocol
    Aerosolized Medication Protocol
    Antiviral Agents
    Corticosteroids
Case Study: Respiratory Syncytial Virus Infection
Self-Assessment Questions

Anatomic Alterations of the Lungs

The inhaled respiratory syncytial virus (RSV) moves down the respiratory tract by means of cell-to-cell transfer, causing **bronchiolitis** and, in severe cases, atelectasis and pneumonia in the child. The **syncytium** is defined as a "multinucleate mass of protoplasm produced by the merging of cells." At the level of the bronchioles the virus causes neighboring cells to fuse to form a syncytium, hence the name *respiratory syncytial virus*. The lower airways may also become infected when secretions from RSV-infected upper airways are aspirated.

RSV infection causes peribronchiolar mononuclear infiltration and necrosis of the epithelium of large and small airways. This condition leads to edema of the small airways and increased production of mucus. As the condition worsens, the epithelium of the small airways becomes necrotic and desquamates into the airway lumen. The combination of sloughing necrotic tissue, airway edema, and accumulation of mucus leads to (1) a decreased airway lumen and (2) either a partially or a completely obstructed airway. Partial airway obstruction leads to alveolar hyperinflation as a result of a **"ball-valve" mechanism** (see Figure 37-1).

Although RSV is primarily associated with obstructive lung pathophysiology, complete airway obstruction may lead to alveolar collapse or atelectasis. In these cases, pneumonic consolidation is common. RSV is also referred to as *bronchiolitis* or **pneumonitis**, although bacterial superinfection is uncommon.

The following major pathologic or structural changes are associated with RSV infection:

- Inflammation and swelling of the peripheral airways
- Excessive airway secretions
- Sloughing of necrotic airway epithelium
- Partial airway obstruction and alveolar hyperinflation
- Complete airway obstruction and atelectasis
- Consolidation

Etiology and Epidemiology

RSV is the most common viral respiratory pathogen seen in infancy and early childhood. Although RSV infection can occur at any age, it is the small infant who presents with the most severe symptoms requiring medical attention. RSV is commonly seen in premature infants, infants younger than 6 months of age, and infants with congenital heart disease,

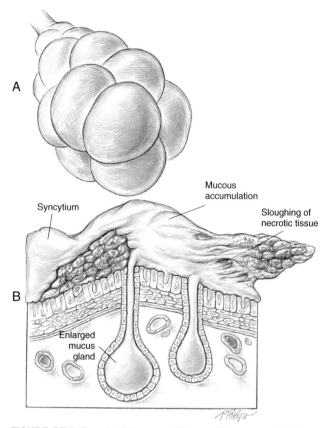

FIGURE 37-1 Bronchiolitis caused by respiratory syncytial virus. (**A**) Partial airway obstruction and alveolar hyperinflation. (**B**) Cross-section of inflamed airway.

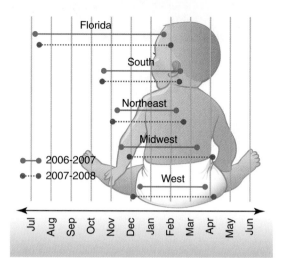

FIGURE 37-2 Respiratory syncytial virus season in the United States by region and in Florida. (Image and data modified from Centers for Disease Control and Prevention: www.cdc.gov/Features/dsRSV/.)

cystic fibrosis, weakened immune systems, or neuromuscular disease. Adults with compromised immune systems and those older than 65 years of age are also at risk.

RSV is commonly transmitted by young children who are infected with RSV and demonstrate the signs and symptoms of a mild upper respiratory tract infection or a "cold"—for example, coughing, sneezing, runny nose, decreased appetite, irritability, decreased activity, and respiratory distress. RSV is easily transmitted when droplets containing the virus are coughed or sneezed into the air. The lower respiratory tract is infected as the viral-laden nasopharyngeal secretions are aspirated. Infection occurs when the particles touch the nose, mouth, or eyes of uninfected individuals in the immediate area. RSV can also spread from direct or indirect contact with nasal or oral secretions from an infected person. For example, RSV can be contracted by kissing the face or hands of a child infected with RSV who has a runny nose. Indirect contact may occur when touching the hard surface of a table, crib rail, or doorknob that has been touched by a person infected with RSV. RSV can survive several hours on a hard surface. Common areas of RSV transmission include elementary schools and day care centers. Frequent hand washing and wiping hard surfaces with a disinfectant may help stop the spread of RSV.

Infants and children infected with RSV usually develop symptoms within 4 to 6 days of infection (range: 2 to 8 days). Most patients will recover in 1 to 2 weeks, but about 25% will have symptoms after 21 days. Infected individuals are usually contagious for up to 8 days. Some patients with a weakened immune system may be contagious for as long as 4 weeks.

Most otherwise healthy children with RSV do not require hospitalization. However, according to the Centers for Disease Control and Prevention, 75,000 to 125,000 children under the age of 1 year are hospitalized each year in the United States because of RSV infection. Of this group, most are under 6 months old.

Although the outbreak of RSV cases varies by location each year, the number of RSV cases typically increases during the fall, winter, and early spring months. It is not fully known why RSV outbreaks occur in certain regions more than in others, but temperature, climate, and humidity appear to play a role. Figure 37-2 shows the typical RSV season in the United States by region and in Florida according to the Centers for Disease Control and Prevention.

Laboratory Testing for Respiratory Syncytial Virus

RSV infection should be suspected when the clinical manifestations correlate to the time of year, the presence of a local outbreak, the age of the patient, and the history of the illness. RSV is most commonly diagnosed with commercially available **antigenassay tests**, typically ordered as an **RSV enzyme immuno assay (RSV-EIA)**. This test requires a nasopharyngeal aspirate or lavage sample, often obtained in the physician's office or emergency department (ED). It is a rapid and usually reliable screen—but a negative RSV-EIA does not rule out RSV. A more definitive test is the **respiratory infectious disease panel (RIDP)** by **polymerase chain reaction (PCR)**. This test identifies RSV plus other respiratory viruses such as rhinovirus, influenza, parainfluenza, adenovirus, and human metapneumovirus. The EIA test is less sensitive in older children and adults, making the RIDP by PCR the more frequently used test in adults.

OVERVIEW of the Cardiopulmonary Clinical Manifestations Associated with Respiratory Syncytial Virus Infection

The following clinical manifestations result from the pathologic mechanisms caused (or activated) by atelectasis (see Figure 9-7), alveolar consolidation (see Figure 9-8), and excessive bronchial secretions (see Figure 9-11)—the major anatomic alterations of the lungs associated with RSV infection (see Figure 37-1).

CLINICAL DATA OBTAINED AT THE PATIENT'S BEDSIDE

The Physical Examination

Vital Signs

Increased Respiratory Rate (Tachypnea)

During the early stages of RSV infection, the respiratory rate is generally higher than normal. Several pathophysiologic mechanisms operating simultaneously may lead to an increased respiratory rate:

- Stimulation of peripheral chemoreceptors (hypoxemia)
- Decreased lung compliance–increased ventilatory rate relationship
- Significant increased dead space to tidal volume ratio
- Stimulation of central chemoreceptors
- Fever (Increased temperature secondary to infection)

Increased Heart Rate (Pulse) and Blood Pressure

Apnea (see Box 32-3)

Clinical Manifestations Associated with More Negative Intrapleural Pressures during Inspiration

- Intercostal retractions
- Substernal retraction and abdominal distention (seesaw movement or paradoxical chest motion)
- Flaring nostrils

Chest Assessment Findings

- Wheezes
- Crackles
- Increased resonance to percussion (in severe cases when airways are partially obstructed)

Bronchial Secretions (Copious)

Expiratory Grunting

Cyanosis

CLINICAL DATA OBTAINED FROM LABORATORY TESTS AND SPECIAL PROCEDURES

Pulmonary Function Test Findings
(Extrapolated Data for Instructional Purposes)
(Primarily an Obstructive Lung Pathophysiology)

The anatomic or structural changes of the lungs associated with RSV primarily cause an obstructive lung pathophysiology. For example, in moderate to severe cases, the following will be higher than normal:

RV	FRC	RV/TLC ratio
↑	↑	↑

When alveolar consolidation and atelectasis are present, a primary restrictive lung pathophysiology may be present. In these cases, the following may be less than normal:

RV	IRV	VC	FRC	TLC
↓	↓	↓	↓	↓

Arterial Blood Gases*

MILD TO MODERATE RESPIRATORY SYNCYTIAL VIRUS INFECTION

Acute Alveolar Hyperventilation with Hypoxemia[†]
(Acute Respiratory Alkalosis)

pH	$PaCO_2$	HCO_3^-	PaO_2	SaO_2 or SpO_2
↑	↓	↓ (but normal)	↓	↓

SEVERE RESPIRATORY SYNCYTIAL VIRUS INFECTION

Acute Ventilatory Failure with Hypoxemia[§]
(Acute Respiratory Acidosis)

pH[†]	$PaCO_2$	HCO_3^-[†]	PaO_2	SaO_2 or SpO_2
↓	↑	↑ (but normal)	↓	↓

*Note: Because of the difficulty of obtaining **arterial blood gas** samples from newborn and pediatric patients, **capillary blood gas** (**CBG**) samples may be used to determine the pH, $PaCO_2$, and HCO_3^- (i.e., the acid-base and ventilation status only). Capillary PO_2 values are unreliable and should not be used for clinical analysis. The standard way to evaluate the oxygenation status of these young patients is pulse oximetry (SpO_2) (see Chapter 32).
[†]See Figure 4-3 and related discussion for the acute pH, $PaCO_2$, and HCO_3^- changes associated with acute alveolar hyperventilation.
[§]See Figure 4-2 and related discussion for the acute pH, $PaCO_2$, and HCO_3^- changes associated with acute ventilatory failure.
[†]When tissue hypoxia is severe enough to produce lactic acid, the pH and HCO_3^- values will be lower than expected for a particular $PaCO_2$ level.

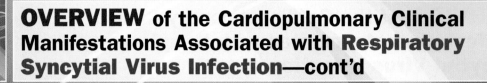

Oxygenation Indices*					
$\dot{Q}s/\dot{Q}\tau$	DO_2	$\dot{V}O_2$	$C(a-\bar{v})O_2$	O_2ER	$S\bar{v}O_2$
↑	↓	N	N	↑	↓

RADIOLOGIC FINDINGS
Chest Radiograph

RSV infection appears as both bronchiolitis and bronchopneumonia in infants and young children. The chest radiograph commonly shows streaky peribronchial opacities associated with air trapping and hyperinflation. Lobar atelectasis frequently is seen—particularly the right upper lobe—and alveolar and lobar pneumonic consolidation occasionally may be seen also (see Figure 37-3). Changes on chest radiographs may persist for up to 12 months after severe RSV infection.

*$C(a-\bar{v})O_2$, Arterial-venous oxygen difference; DO_2, total oxygen delivery; O_2ER, oxygen extraction ratio; $S\bar{v}O_2$, mixed venous oxygen saturation; $\dot{V}O_2$ oxygen consumption; $\dot{Q}s/\dot{Q}\tau$, pulmonary shunt fraction.

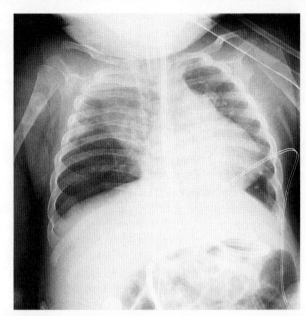

FIGURE 37-3 Chest x-ray film of a 6-month-old child with respiratory syncytial virus infection.

General Management of Respiratory Syncytial Virus Infection (Bronchiolitis, Pneumonitis)

The management of RSV bronchiolitis is largely supportive. Therapy includes carefully monitoring clinical status, providing adequate oxygenation, maintaining upper airway patency through secretion clearance, delivering adequate hydration, and providing parental education on home management. Table 37-1 shows an RSV bronchiolitis-scoring system commonly used to objectively evaluate the patient's condition and, importantly, to up-regulate or down-regulate therapy accordingly. Table 37-2 provides a helpful overview of an RSV bronchiolitis management protocol based on (1) the patient's response to aerosolized bronchodilators and (2) the patient's bronchiolitis score (see Table 37-1).

Monitoring

Close cardiopulmonary monitoring of the patient with RSV bronchiolitis is important in the detection of worsening clinical respiratory status, apnea, or bradycardia. CBGs to assess the patient's acid-base status and ventilation and pulse oximetry (SpO₂) to evaluate oxygenation should be routinely performed in all patients who are in significant respiratory distress, require high FIO₂ levels, demonstrate apneic or bradycardic episodes, or are slow to improve with aggressive care.

Oxygen Therapy Protocol

Oxygen therapy is used to treat hypoxemia, decrease the work of breathing, and decrease myocardial work. (See **Oxygen Therapy Protocol**, Protocol 32-1).

The oxygen therapy protocol for infants with RSV bronchiolitis includes the benefits provided by the high gas flow delivered with **high flow nasal cannula** (**HFNC**) therapy. HFNC therapy provides a constant flow that washes out the infant's upper airway dead space, decreases inspiratory resistance, provides increased humidity to help thin retained secretions, and can provide positive pressure during the respiratory cycle—which can decrease air trapping by stenting swollen airways and provides increased humidity to help thin retained secretions. Recent studies suggest:

- HFNC application is effective in reducing respiratory distress in RSV.
- The benefits of HFNC are seen within 60 to 90 minutes of application.
- HFNC with a flow rate ≥2 L/kg/min generates a clinically relevant pharyngeal pressure. Clinically, 5 to 8 L/min is commonly used for these small infants (3 to 4 kg).

Bronchopulmonary Hygiene Therapy Protocol

Airway Clearance with Suctioning

After oxygen therapy, airway clearance and suctioning are essential core therapy for RSV bronchiolitis. One third of an

TABLE 37-1 Bronchiolitis Scoring System*

	0—Normal	1—Mild	2—Moderate	3—Severe
Resp rate	<40	40–50	50–60	>60
Color	Normal	Normal	Normal	Dusky, mottled
SpO$_2$ on room air	>97%	94–96%	90–93%	<90%
Capillary refill	<2 s	<2 s	<2 s Normal color on O$_2$ ≤1 L/min	≥3 s Normal color on O$_2$ >1 L/min
Retractions/work of breathing	None	Subcostal	Intercostal and subcostal when quiet	Supraclavicular sternal paradoxical respiration
Breath sounds	Clear/good	Good entry End-expiratory wheeze ± crackles	Fair air entry Inspiratory and expiratory wheeze ± crackles	Poor/grunting Inspiratory and expiratory wheeze ± crackles
Level of consciousness	Normal/alert	Mild irritability	Restless when disturbed, agitated	Lethargic, hard to arouse

*Other factors used in evaluation of infants with suspected bronchiolitis:
  Signs of dehydration/difficulty feeding
  Parental ability to provide necessary care for child during acute infection
  Preexisting condition contributing to increased possibility of respiratory failure
Modified from Dayton Children's Hospital, Dayton, Ohio.

TABLE 37-2 General Overview: Management Protocol for Respiratory Syncytial Virus Bronchiolitis

Score	Aerosolized Bronchodilators*	Other Therapy
Normal 0–4	Assess Q6h	• Normal saline nose drops • Bulb syringe suction for home
Mild 5–7	Racemic epinephrine trial × 1. If the patient responds, give aerosols Q6h for scores ≥5. If no response, continue to assess the patient Q6h for airway clearance.	• Oxygen per protocol • Suction PRN
Moderate 8–10	Racemic epinephrine trial × 1. If the patient responds, continue aerosols Q4h. For scores ≥8, but no response to first medication, consider trial of alternate medicated aerosol. Continue to assess the patient Q4h	• Consider chest x-ray • Capillary blood gas • Normal saline nose drops • Suction PRN • IV fluids if patient exhibits dehydration or failure to feed • Oxygen per protocol
Severe 11–15	Racemic epinephrine trial. Evaluate response. If no response, consider a trial of alternate aerosol medication. If severity persists, consider PICU transfer and therapy with HFNC.	• Chest x-ray • IV fluids • Blood gas • If excessive PCO$_2$, acidosis, or hypoxia, transfer to ICU • Oxygen per protocol

*Aerosol bronchodilator trial: Patients will be suctioned if necessary, scored, given aerosol, and scored again. A positive response is defined as a decrease of the patient's postaerosol bronchiolitis score by 2 or more (decreased wheezing, WOB, RR, increased aeration). If the patient received an aerosol trial in the emergency department (ED), it is not necessary to repeat the trial when the patient is hospitalized.

Racemic epinephrine (0.5 mL) is generally the recommended aerosol medication for trial in hospitalized patients, unless patient responded to albuterol in the ED.
HFNC, High-flow nasal cannula; ICU, intensive care unit; IV, intravenous; PICU, pediatric intensive care unit.
Modified from Dayton Children's Hospital, Dayton, Ohio.

infant's total airway resistance derives from the nose. Bulb suctioning the infant's nares alone can significantly improve airflow. Nasal suctioning is typically performed before feeding and PRN. When nasal secretions obstruct the infant's nasal passages, nasopharyngeal suctioning with a lubricated, size-appropriate suction catheter is typically used to clear the nasal passages. In addition, the nasal catheter often stimulates a cough above the vocal cords, which helps to remove secretions.

In addition, **nebulized hypertonic saline (3%)** may be considered for those infants with documented copious secretions. The mechanism of hypertonic saline benefit includes:

- Inducing an osmotic flow of water into the mucus layer
- Rehydrating the airway surface liquid and improving mucus clearance
- Breaking ionic bonds within the mucus gel, lowering viscosity and elasticity
- Stimulating ciliary beats
- Absorbing water from the mucosa and submucosa, reducing edema of the airway.

Infants with RSV bronchiolitis do not benefit from chest percussion and drainage—in fact, its use is discouraged. Patient agitation associated with percussion therapy may exacerbate small airway obstruction (see **Bronchopulmonary Hygiene Therapy Protocol**, Protocol 32-2).

Aerosolized Medication Protocol

Bronchodilators

Serial use of bronchodilators are not beneficial in treating the airway edema associated with RSV bronchiolitis. The 2014 American Academy of Pediatrics (AAP) guidelines* suggest that bronchodilators may be more harmful than beneficial. Infants who swallow aerosolized bronchodilators often have an increase in their cardiac output while getting very little improvement in ventilation, resulting in $\dot{V}/\dot{Q}$ mismatch and transient hypoxemia. Multiple aerosols increase the infant's hypoxemia. Bronchodilator trials should be reserved for the moderate to severe RSV patient. A trial typically entails a single aerosol of racemic epinephrine or albuterol—to determine airway improvement, or lack of improvement. For the patient that does not demonstrate airway improvement, no further aerosolized bronchodilator therapy is given. However, for the occasional patient (usually with a family history of asthma or atopy), who does demonstrate a positive airway improvement after the aerosol bronchodilator trial, the serial use of bronchodilator therapy is provided (see Table 37-2 and, **Aerosolized Medication Protocol,** Protocol 32-4).

Antiviral Agents

Palivizumab (Synagis). This monoclonal antibody (directed against the fusion protein of RSV) is used as a preventive measure against RSV infection in high-risk infants. The American Academy of Pediatrics guidelines recommend that premature infants (less than 35 weeks' gestation), premature infants under 2 years of age with chronic lung disease, and infants with congenital heart disease receive a monthly injection of **palivizumab**—an immune globulin prophylaxis—once a month for at least 5 months starting 2 months before the RSV season is likely to occur. Research has shown that the use of palivizumab has significantly reduced the number of hospitalizations and the duration of hospitalization in high-risk infants.

Ribavirin (Virazole). Although ribavirin was widely used when it was first introduced, the routine use of nebulized **ribavirin** in infants and children with RSV is no longer recommended. The efficacy of ribavirin in this population has not been proven. In addition, ribavirin is expensive, requires special equipment, adds technical risk to ventilator care when used in line, and is associated with occupational exposure concerns. The **small particle aerosol generator (SPAG)** was used to deliver continuous ribavirin.

Corticosteroids

Steroid therapy given by inhalation or intravenous (IV), intramuscular (IM), or oral administration is not recommended for RSV bronchiolitis because of a lack of efficacy in numerous clinical trials.

---

*http://www.aap.org

CASE STUDY Respiratory Syncytial Virus Bronchiolitis

A 6-week-old male infant presented to the ED in respiratory distress. His mother noted that her son was unable to breast-feed because of his increasing congestion and that his symptoms began 3 days earlier. She also reported that her nephew whom they visited last weekend was diagnosed with something called "RSV."

Upon examination, this 4.5-kg infant had an heart rate of 168 beats/min, respiratory rate 64 breaths/min, and SpO$_2$ of 94% on room air. He exhibited moderate subcostal and intercostal retractions, nasal flaring, and white frothy secretions visible in his nares. His breath sounds upon auscultation showed good bilateral aeration with noisy, congested upper airways transmitted throughout, making it difficult to assess lower airway sounds. The infant appeared a little dry—the mother noted that he had been nursing poorly and had not had a wet diaper for 6 hours. The ED physician requested a fluid bolus to improve the infant's hydration. The physician directed the nurse caring for this infant to suction his nasopharynx prior to the IV insertion. The suctioning removed a moderate amount of tenacious white secretions. The physician explained to the mother that the infant would be observed for a few hours in the ED to see if the secretions reaccumulated and to assess his oxygen level during feeding and sleeping. During a nap in the ED, the infant's SpO$_2$ dropped into the high 80s. He was unable to breast-feed without difficulty because of secretions in his upper airway. An RIDP was ordered to determine the etiology of his viral bronchiolitis, as both RSV and influenza A were present in the community.

The infant was then admitted for supportive care, fluids, and ¼ L/min oxygen by nasal cannula. Respiratory therapy was called to assess and make recommendations for care. On admission to the general pediatric floor, the patient had heart rate of 142 beats/min, respiratory rate 48 breaths/min, and SpO_2 of 90%. on ¼ L/min oxygen per nasal cannula. Breath sounds revealed noisy upper airway sounds as a result of congestion, with bilateral wheezing and grunting on expiration. Moderate subcostal and intercostal retractions persisted with nasal flaring noted. The RIDP was positive for RSV only. The respiratory therapist wrote this SOAP note:

S N/A

O 6-week-old infant with viral bronchiolitis. RSV+ per RIDP. Vital signs: HR 142, RR 48, SpO_2 90% on ¼ L/min oxygen per nasal cannula. Moderate amount of tenacious white secretions. Persistent respiratory distress with subcostal and intercostal retractions, nasal flaring. Breath sounds: bilateral wheezing with grunting noted on expiration.

A • Wheezing—most likely because of mucosal edema
  • Hypoxemia (SpO_2: 90%)
  • Excessive secretions (noisy upper airway sound resulting from congestion, tenacious white secretions)
  • Possible atelectasis or $\dot{V}/\dot{Q}$ mismatch (history, positive for RSV, low SpO_2 during nap)
  • Potential for fatigue with persistent increased work of breathing

P **Aerosolized Medication Protocol Trial:** Bronchodilator (racemic epinephrine) trial to determine response
  • **Bronchopulmonary Hygiene Protocol:** Effective suction to remove upper airway secretions
  • Consider request for chest radiograph if oxygen requirement continues to increase
  • Recommend blood gas (capillary) to identify impending respiratory failure.
  • Oxygen therapy protocol: 1 L/min nasal cannula
    • May need to implement HFNC or continuous positive airway pressure (CPAP) to stent airways to prevent respiratory fatigue/failure.

A bronchodilator trial with racemic epinephrine was given after the patient was suctioned. The infant did not appear to respond to the aerosol by pre- and post-scores. The postaerosol SpO_2 was 91%. He did seem to improve after suctioning. The respiratory therapist told the mother that he would return in 4 hours to assess the infant again. Two hours later, the infant's nurse called to report that the infant's SpO_2 had dropped to 84% after a brief feeding and he was now on 1 L/min by oxygen nasal cannula. An NPO order was initiated and maintenance fluids were started.

One hour later, the infant demonstrated more significant respiratory distress, this time demonstrating subcostal, intercostal retractions with nasal head bobbing. The therapist arrived and suctioned a moderate amount of thin secretions from the infant's nasopharynx. The infant's heart rate was 176 beats/min and the respiratory rate was 62 breaths/min. Bilateral crackles and wheezing were heard on auscultation. The therapist called the physician and requested a CBG and chest radiograph. The CBG and pulse oximetry showed pH 7.33, $PaCO_2$ 57 mm Hg, HCO_3^- 29 mEq/L, and SpO_2 89%

on 1 L/min oxygen per nasal cannula. The chest radiograph showed patchy atelectasis in the right upper and lower lobes and the left lower lobe. A second bronchodilator trial with albuterol was given with no apparent response.

At this time, the respiratory therapist documented the following SOAP:

S N/A

O Infant in severe distress. HR 176, RR 62, subcostal, intercostal retractions with nasal flaring, head bobbing. Breath sounds, diminished in bases, crackles and wheezing present. CBG: pH 7.33, $PaCO_2$ 57, HCO_3^- 29. SpO_2: 89% on 1 L/min nasal cannula.

A • Excessive secretions (crackles, suctioned thin secretions)
  • Significant atelectasis (CXR: right upper and lower lobes and left lower lobe)
  • Hypercarbia despite increased minute volume effort (CBG)
  • Hypoxemia (SpO_2: 89%)
  • Impending respiratory failure (CBG and SpO_2)

P • Discontinue medicated aerosol trial: not effective in relieving symptoms
  • Bronchial hygiene: suctioned as needed
  • Oxygen therapy: need to advance to HFNC (5 to 8 L/min on FIO_2 0.50)
  • Place CPAP/mechanical ventilation on standby, if HFNC unable to reverse impending respiratory failure.

With the approval of the attending physician, the therapist started the infant on HFNC at 5 L/min of 50% oxygen in his room with central monitoring (see Figure 37-4). Despite this level of support, the infant's respiratory rate did not improve, continuing to track in the 60s. A repeat CBG after 60 minutes showed pH 7.31, $PaCO_2$ 60 mm Hg, and HCO_3^- 29 mEq/L. The SpO_2 was 91%. Because of the infant's general lack of improvement, he was transferred to the pediatric intensive care unit (PICU) and received a CPAP of

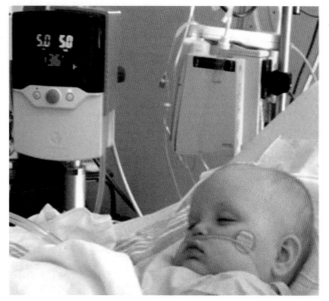

FIGURE 37-4 Infant on a high-flow nasal cannula (HFNC). Courtesy of Dayton Children's Hospital, Dayton, Ohio.

10 cm H_2O with an FIO_2 0.60 oxygen by nasal prongs. This support was initiated to reduce the infant's work of breathing by stenting his swollen airways open with continuous positive pressure. This also reduces physiologic dead space, improves alveolar ventilation, and effectively reduces hypercarbia during the acute phase of the illness. Suctioning and fluids continued in the PICU for supportive care. After 4 days, respiratory support was weaned to CPAP on room air and then to ambient room air.

Discussion

This case involves a 6-week-old infant who was exposed to the RSV virus by contact with another infant in the family. Family members could have easily transmitted RSV through hand contact. Strict attention to good hand hygiene is important for family members and medical personnel. Washing hands and using gloves, gowns, and masks are indicated when caring for an RSV-infected infant. The fact that several viruses were active in the community supported ordering the RIDP as both viruses can cause similar symptoms.

Most infants present with the inability to feed because of secretions. Nasopharyngeal suctioning with an IV fluid bolus to counter dehydration may be sufficient care in the ED, and the infant can be sent home after observation. The infant in this case was demonstrating hypoxemia requiring oxygen therapy along with fluids. Signs of increased respiratory distress (grunting, nasal flaring with wheezing, and tachypnea) warranted a bronchodilator trial (Aerosolized Medication Therapy Protocol). However, the effectiveness of bronchodilators in bronchiolitis has been shown to be marginal in many of these infants. The trial of bronchodilators in this case did not show clinical improvement from preassessment to postassessment scores.

The implementation of the **Bronchopulmonary Hygiene Therapy Protocol** (suctioning) was necessary to offset the **excessive bronchial secretions** (see Figure 9-11) (see **Bronchopulmonary Hygiene Therapy Protocol**, Protocol 32-2). However, postural drainage and percussion are not recommended in these infants. The goal of suctioning is to reduce airway resistance, reduce the work of breathing, and prevent fatigue.

The **Oxygen Therapy Protocol** is usually required in the RSV bronchiolitis patient and is often the reason for hospitalization (see **Oxygen Therapy Protocol**, Protocol 32-1). The goal is to maintain the SpO_2 at 91% to 94%. The use of HFNC—which delivers fully humidified and warmed gas mixtures—has had a dramatic positive effect on the treatment of infants with RSV bronchiolitis. HFNC is generally considered in RSV infants who (1) require higher oxygen cannula flow rates, (2) demonstrate a rising $PaCO_2$ despite increased minute ventilation, and (3) demonstrate increased atelectasis and consolidation on the CXR. In addition, HFNC provides expiratory resistance and flow to the upper airway, thus washing out dead space and possibly increasing pharyngeal pressure to help stent the airways. This can markedly decrease the work of breathing and improve air exchange in most infants. HFNC requires close monitoring and may be provided in special care or critical care units where central monitoring is available. Infants with RSV bronchiolitis typically recover faster with early use of HFNC; the goal is to prevent fatigue and respiratory failure. CPAP by nasal prongs can be used to give consistent positive end-expiratory pressure as a second noninvasive mode to prevent the need for intubation (see **Lung Expansion Protocol**, Protocol 32-3).

Mechanical ventilation may be necessary in the bronchiolitic infant who presents with persistent apnea or if fatigue with hypercapnia ensues despite HFNC or CPAP intervention. Ventilation of the infant with RSV bronchiolitis often requires sedation and paralysis and is generally given for several days.

Although palivizumab—an immune globulin prophylaxis—can be given once a month to high-risk infants to build their immunity against RSV and reduce the severity of symptoms, there is no vaccine available for all newborns. The development of a safe and effective vaccine to prevent RSV has been pursued for the last 50 years without great success. At present, there are vaccines for RSV under development and in clinical trials. Unfortunately, none of these potential vaccines will be effective in preventing RSV infection in infants under 6 months of age.

SELF-ASSESSMENT QUESTIONS

Answers to questions can be found on Evolve. To access additional student assessment questions visit **http://evolve.elsevier.com/DesJardins/respiratory**.

1. Which of the following are associated with RSV infection?
   1. Alveolar hyperinflation
   2. Atelectasis
   3. Excessive bronchial secretions
   4. Pneumonic consolidation
      a. 2 and 4 only
      b. 3 and 4 only
      c. 2, 3, and 4 only
      d. 1, 2, 3, and 4

2. Although the outbreak timing of RSV cases varies, the number of patients with RSV typically increases during:
   1. Summer
   2. Fall
   3. Winter
   4. Early spring
      a. 1 only
      b. 3 only
      c. 2, 3, and 4 only
      d. 1, 2, 3, and 4

3. How long is the typical patient with RSV typically contagious?
   a. 1 to 2 days
   b. 8 days
   c. 2 weeks
   d. 1 month

4. Although RSV infection can occur at any age, children younger than what age tend to be more severely affected?
   a. Less than 1 year old
   b. Less than 2 years old
   c. Less than 3 years old
   d. Less than 4 years old

5. Which of the following agents is/are are used to prevent RSV infection in high-risk babies?
   1. Virazole
   2. Synagis
   3. Streptomycin
   4. Ribavirin
      a. 1 only
      b. 2 only
      c. 3 only
      d. 1 and 4 only

Chapter Objectives

After reading this chapter, you will be able to:

- List the anatomic alterations of the lungs associated with bronchopulmonary dysplasia (BPD)
- Differentiate between the classic and "new" description of bronchopulmonary dysplasia.
- Describe the causes of BPD.
- List the cardiopulmonary clinical manifestations associated with BPD.
- Describe the general management of BPD.
- Describe the clinical strategies and rationales of the SOAP presented in the case study.

Key Terms

Alveolar Hypoplasia
Bronchopulmonary Dysplasia (BPD)
Canalicular Stage
Chronic Lung Disease of Prematurity
Exogenous Surfactant
Gentle Ventilation
Hyaline Membrane Disease
Hyperplasia

Metaplasia
"New" BPD
Permissive Hypercapnia
Pulmonary Barotrauma
Pulmonary Volutrauma
Stage I BPD
Stage II BPD
Stage III BPD
Stage IV BPD
Ventilator-Induced Lung Injury (VILI)

Chapter Outline

Anatomic Alterations of the Lungs
　The "New" Bronchopulmonary Dysplasia—Anatomic
　　Alterations of the Lungs
　Etiology and Epidemiology
Overview of the Cardiopulmonary Clinical Manifestations
　Associated with Bronchopulmonary Dysplasia
General Management of Bronchopulmonary Dysplasia
　Respiratory Care Treatment Protocols
Case Study: Bronchopulmonary Dysplasia
Self-Assessment Questions

Anatomic Alterations of the Lungs

Bronchopulmonary dysplasia (BPD), also referred to as **chronic lung disease of prematurity of infancy,** is the most common chronic lung disease of premature infants. BPD was first described by Northway and colleagues in 1967 as a severe chronic lung injury in premature infants who survived **hyaline membrane disease** (i.e., respiratory distress syndrome [RDS]) after being treated with high levels of mechanical ventilation and oxygen exposure for prolonged periods of time. Northway and colleagues described the following four pathologic stages of BPD:

Stage I BPD was said to occur during the first 2 to 3 days of life. This stage is often indistinguishable from RDS. During this period, alveolar hyaline membranes, patches of atelectasis, and lymphatic dilation were seen. In addition, early signs of bronchial mucosal necrosis appeared (see Figure 38-1, A). The chest radiographic findings revealed ground glass-like granular patterns and small lung volumes (Figure 38-2, A).

Stage II BPD was said to occur 4 to 10 days after birth. Atelectasis was more extensive during this period. In addition, metaplasia of the normal lung tissue cells caused bronchial necrosis, cellular debris, partial airway obstruction, air trapping, and alveolar hyperinflation. The patho-

logic findings during stage II were commonly described as alternating areas of atelectasis and emphysema (see Figure 38-1, B). These changes appeared on chest radiograph as patchy opaque areas of atelectasis next to areas of dark translucency (areas of hyperinflation) (see Figure 38-2, B).

Stage III BPD was said to occur at 11 to 30 days of age. Pathologic findings included extensive bronchial and bronchiolar **metaplasia** and **hyperplasia** (an increased number of cells), interstitial fibrosis, and excessive bronchial airway secretions. In addition, the alveolar hyperinflation continued to form circular groups of emphysematous bullae that were surrounded by patches of atelectasis (see Figure 38-1, C). On the chest radiograph, the lungs began to show circular or cystic areas surrounded by patches of irregular density (see Figure 38-2, C).

Stage IV BPD was said to occur after 30 days of life. During this stage, massive fibrosis of the lung and destruction of the bronchial airways, alveoli, and pulmonary capillaries occurred. Areas of emphysematous, or cystlike, regions continued to increase in size and number. Thin strands of atelectasis and normal alveoli were interspersed around emphysematous areas. In addition, pulmonary hypertension often developed, lymphatic and bronchial mucous gland deformation occurred, and excessive bronchial secretions

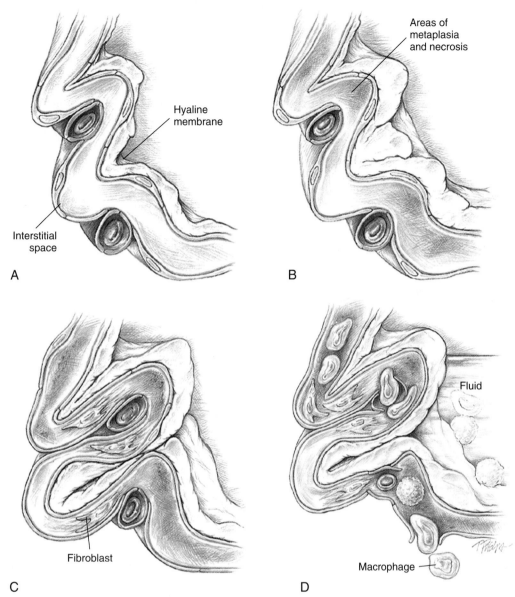

FIGURE 38-1 Alveolar changes during the four stages of bronchopulmonary dysplasia. (**A**) Stage I, the formation of hyaline membrane. (**B**) Stage II, the development areas of metaplasia and necrosis. (**C**) Stage III, extensive metaplasia, hyperplasia, and interstitial fibrosis. (**D**) Stage IV, progressive destruction of alveoli and airways.

continued (see Figure 38-1, D). The chest radiographs revealed fibrosis and edema with areas of consolidation adjacent to areas of overinflation (see Figure 38-2, D). Table 38-1 summarizes the original BPD stages, with pathologic and radiologic correlates.

The major pathologic or structural changes of the lungs associated with earlier descriptions of BPD are:

- Hyaline membrane formation
- Atelectasis
- Bronchial mucosal necrosis
- Excessive bronchial secretions
- Chronic alveolar fibrosis and bronchial smooth muscle hypertrophy
- Bronchial mucosal metaplasia and hyperplasia
- Alveolar hyperinflation
- Emphysematous areas surrounded by areas of atelectasis and normal alveoli

The "New" Bronchopulmonary Dysplasia—Anatomic Alterations of the Lungs

Much has been learned about BPD since it was first described in 1967. During the late 1960s, BPD occurred predominantly in larger preterm infants born at 30 to 34 weeks gestation, with a history of severe respiratory distress necessitating aggressive ventilatory support and high oxygen concentrations for prolonged periods of time. Today, BPD as it was originally described in 1967, has virtually disappeared. Infants who more commonly develop BPD today have very low birth weights (< 1500 g) and are born at less than 26 weeks gestation. They are now usually managed with several new and improved therapeutic techniques—including prenatal maternal steroids, postnatal **exogenous surfactant**, gentle ventilation techniques, controlled low oxygen concentrations,

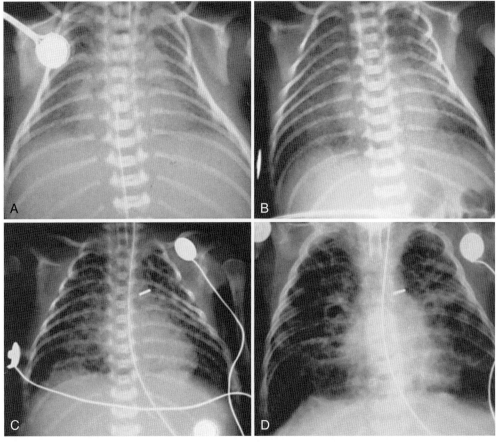

FIGURE 38-2 (**A**) Stage I; occurs during the first 2 to 3 days of life. The chest radiographic findings show ground glass-like granular patterns and small lung volumes. (**B**) Stage II; occurs 4 to 10 days after birth. The chest x-ray film shows patchy opaque areas with bronchograms (areas of atelectasis) next to areas of dark translucency (areas of hyperinflation). (**C**) Stage III; occurs at 11 to 30 days of age. The chest radiograph shows circular or cystic areas surrounded by patches of irregular density. (**D**) Stage IV; occurs after 30 days of life. The chest radiographs shows fibrosis and edema with areas of consolidation adjacent to areas of overinflation. (From Taeusch WH, Ballard RA, Gleason CA: *Avery's diseases of the newborn*, ed 8, Philadelphia, 2005, Saunders.)

nasal CPAP, fluid restriction, vitamin A, diuretics, bronchodilator therapy, bronchial hygiene therapy, postnatal corticosteroids, and inhaled nitric oxide.

In what is referred to as the **"new" bronchopulmonary dysplasia (new BPD)**, the pathologic findings of the lungs are described as "more uniformly inflated with minimal airway injury or fibrosis." The major anatomic pathology is a decrease in alveolar number, called **alveolar hypoplasia**. In the very preterm infant with the new BPD, the lung is just completing the **canalicular stage** of development at the time of birth. Interruption of the canalicular stage is thought to significantly disrupt the progress of alveolar growth and likely contributes to the development of the new BPD.

In response to awareness of new BPD, the National Institutes of Child Health and Human Development in 2001 sponsored a workshop on BPD and a new definition of BPD resulted. The new definition outlines specific diagnostic criteria, including the need for oxygen, positive pressure ventilation, and/or CPAP. It also includes the postnatal age to better assess the severity of BPD. Table 38-2 provides an overview of the diagnostic criteria for the new BPD.

Etiology and Epidemiology

BPD is the most common form of chronic lung disease in children. It is estimated that 10,000 to 12,000 infants are diagnosed with BPD in the United States annually. The current understanding is that multiple causative factors are associated with BPD. Table 38-3 provides an overview of the primary causes of BPD.

General Management of Bronchopulmonary Dysplasia

Several preventive methods are used today to avert or treat BPD. Mothers in preterm labor are often given steroids to hasten the lung maturity of the infant in an attempt to avoid mechanical ventilation. The most significant treatment for the prevention of BPD in the newborn is the administration of **exogenous surfactant**. This drug alone has significantly reduced the incidence of BPD; studies have shown a reduction in the incidence of BPD from 55% to 26% with use of surfactant. Dosing the infant with surfactant soon after birth

TABLE 38-1 Bronchopulmonary Dysplasia Staging (Northway)

Stage	Days after Birth	Radiologic Findings	Pathologic Findings
I	2–3	Ground-glass granular pattern; small lung volume	Atelectasis Hyaline membranes Lymphatic dilation
II	4–10	Patchy opaque areas with bronchograms (areas of atelectasis) adjacent to areas of dark translucency (areas of hyperinflation)	Widespread necrosis of alveolar epithelium Persistent alveolar hyaline membranes and atelectasis Metaplasia of bronchiolar smooth muscles Bronchial necrosis Emphysematous coalescence of alveoli
III	11–20	Circular or cystlike areas of hyperlucency, surrounded by patches of irregular density caused by atelectasis	Persisting injury to alveoli Interstitial edema and septal thickening Bronchial mucosal metaplasia and hyperplasia Emphysematous areas surrounded by atelectasis Excessive airway secretions
IV	>30	Increased size and numbers of cystlike areas of hyperlucency, surrounded by thinner stands of radiodensity	Increased size and numbers of emphysematous areas, next to collapsed alveoli and normal alveoli Septal fibrosis Pulmonary hypertension, lymphatic and bronchial mucous gland deformation Excessive airway secretions

From Northway WH Jr, Rosan RC, Porter DY: Pulmonary disease following respiratory therapy of hyaline-membrane disease: bronchopulmonary dysplasia. *N Engl J Med* 276:357–368, 1967.

TABLE 38-2 Diagnostic Criteria for the New Bronchopulmonary Dysplasia

Gestational Age	<32 Weeks	≥32 weeks
Time point of assessment	36 weeks' PMA or discharge to home, whichever comes first Treatment with >21% oxygen for at least 28 days, PLUS	>28 days but <56 days' postnatal age or discharge to home, whichever comes first
Mild BPD	Breathing room air at 36 weeks' PMA or discharge, whichever comes first	Breathing room air by 56 days' postnatal age or discharge, whichever comes first
Moderate BPD	Need* for <30% oxygen at 36 weeks' PMA or discharge, whichever comes first	Need* for <30% oxygen at 56 days' postnatal age or discharge, whichever comes first
Severe BPD	Need* for ≥30% oxygen and/or PPV or NCPAP at 36 weeks' PMA or discharge, whichever comes first	Need* for ≥30% oxygen and/or PPV or NCPAP at 56 postnatal age or discharge, whichever comes first

Modified from Jobe AH, Bancalari E: Bronchopulmonary dysplasia. *Am J Respir Crit Care Med* 163:1723–1729, 2001.
*A physiologic test confirming that oxygen supplementation is required at the time point of assessment has not yet been defined. This assessment may include a pulse oximetry saturation range.
BPD, Bronchopulmonary dysplasia; *NCPAP*, nasal continuous positive airway pressure; *PMA*, postmenstrual age; *PPV*, positive-pressure ventilation.

allows for effective ventilation at lower pressures with improved lung compliance (see **Surfactant Administration Protocol**, Protocol 32-6). Keeping the newborn's exhaled tidal volume at 4 to 6 mL/kg of body weight avoids volutrauma; it requires weaning the peak inspiratory pressure (PIP) as the infant's lung compliance improves.

Infants who may have coinfections or comorbidities that require higher ventilating pressures should be transitioned to high frequency ventilation to avoid high PIPs while maintaining mean airway pressure (MAP) necessary for oxygenation. **Permissive hypercapnia*** (allowing the PCO_2 to

primary objective of mechanical ventilation. Today, the emphasis is on maintaining adequate gas exchange while—and, importantly—minimizing the risks of mechanical ventilation. Common strategies used to reduce the risk of mechanical ventilation include (1) low tidal volume ventilation—to protect the lung from ventilator-associated lung injury in patients with acute lung injury (e.g., ARDS)—and (2) reduction of the tidal volume, respiratory rate, or both—to minimize intrinsic positive end-expiratory pressure (i.e., auto-PEEP) in patients with obstructive lung disease (e.g., COPD).

Although these mechanical ventilation strategies may result in an increased $PaCO_2$ level (hypercapnia), they do help to protect the lung from barotrauma (i.e., physical damage to lung tissues caused by excessive gas pressures). The lenient acceptance of the hypercapnia is called **permissive hypercapnia**. In most cases, the patient's $PaCO_2$ is adequately maintained by an increased ventilatory rate that offsets the decreased tidal volume. The $PaCO_2$, however, should not be permitted to increase to the point of severe acidosis. The most current consensus suggests it is safe to allow pH to fall to at least 7.20 (www.ARDSNet.org).

*****Permissive hypercapnia defined**: Mechanical ventilation was traditionally applied with the goal of normalizing arterial blood gas values, particularly the arterial carbon dioxide tension ($PaCO_2$). However, this is no longer the

TABLE 38-3 Causative Factors of Bronchopulmonary Dysplasia (BPD)

Host susceptibility and genetic predisposition	The single most important causative factor associated with the development of BPD is prematurity. In addition, the retardation or restriction of intrauterine growth and a family history of respiratory distress syndrome and asthma put the infant at a higher risk for BPD.
Oxygen toxicity	Even in the first cases of BPD reported by Northway and colleagues in 1967, it was clear that exposure to high concentrations of oxygen was a factor in causing BPD. Subsequent reports continue to show that prolonged exposure to high levels of supplemental oxygen puts infants at risk for BPD.
Inflammation	A severe inflammatory response also plays a major role in the development of BPD.
Neonatal infection	The development of postnatal bacterial sepsis puts the infant at risk for BPD. Even airway microbial colonization without frank sepsis may increase the risk of BPD.
Mechanical ventilation	The development of BPD is strongly associated with mechanical ventilation. The major causative factors linked to mechanical ventilation are (1) high peak inspiratory pressures, (2) high mean airway pressures, and (3) overdistention of the lungs. Overinflation of the lungs causes stress fractures of the capillary endothelium, epithelium, and basement membranes. This mechanical injury in turn causes leakage of fluid into the alveolar spaces, with additional inflammation.
Pulmonary edema and patent ductus arteriosus	Abnormalities of lung fluid volume are associated with BPD. Several reports have shown that patency of the ductus arteriosus has a high correlation with the incidence of BPD.
Poor nutrition	All of the above causative factors are intensified by a poor nutritional status.

rise above normal while keeping the pH around 7.3) is another method of avoiding lung injury. Continuous pulse oximetry allows the respiratory therapist to adjust oxygen settings to the infant's desired SpO_2 of 92% to 94%.

In general, the management of infants who are at high risk for development of BPD or who have evolving BPD is directed at (1) minimizing the administration of high concentrations of oxygen, (2) supporting and maintaining bronchial hygiene, (3) minimizing the need for ventilatory support, (4) using low inspiratory pressures, (5) managing the MAPs, and (6) supporting and maintaining an adequate FRC with PEEP or CPAP.

Respiratory Care Treatment Protocols

Oxygen Therapy Protocol

Oxygen therapy is used to treat hypoxemia, decrease the work of breathing, and decrease myocardial work. Because of the hypoxemia that often develops in BPD, supplemental oxygen may be required (see **Oxygen Therapy Protocol**, Protocol 32-1). It should be noted that prolonged exposure to supplemental oxygen should be minimized to reduce complications of BPD. Some physicians prefer allowing lower than normal SaO_2 values in the low birth weight infants.

Bronchopulmonary Hygiene Therapy Protocol

Because of the excessive airway secretions and accumulation associated with BPD, a number of bronchial hygiene treatment modalities may be used to enhance the mobilization of bronchial secretions (see **Bronchopulmonary Hygiene Therapy Protocol**, Protocol 32-2).

Mechanical Ventilation Protocol

Mechanical ventilation may be necessary to provide and support alveolar gas exchange and eventually return the patient to spontaneous breathing (see **Mechanical Ventilation Protocol**, Protocol 32-5).*

Table 38-4 provides an overview of the therapeutic measures used to prevent or manage infants with BPD.

---

*It has long been known that mechanical ventilation can produce a variety of lung injuries referred to as **ventilator-induced lung injury (VILI)**, **pulmonary volutrauma**, or **pulmonary barotrauma**. *VILI* is defined as stress fractures of the pulmonary capillary endothelium, epithelium, and basement membrane and, in severe cases, lung rupture. Lung ruptures can lead to leakage of fluid, protein, and blood into tissue and air spaces or leakage of air into tissue spaces. This condition can be followed by an inflammatory response and possibly a reduced defense against infection. *Pulmonary volutrauma* is defined as damage to the lung caused by over-distention by a mechanical ventilator set for an excessively high tidal volume. *Pulmonary barotrauma* is defined as damage to the lungs caused by rapid or extreme pressures generated by mechanical ventilation.

Predisposing factors for VILI, pulmonary volutrauma, or pulmonary barotrauma include (1) mechanical ventilation with high peak inspiratory volumes and pressures, (2) mechanical ventilation with a high mean airway pressure, (3) structural immaturity of lung and chest wall, (4) surfactant insufficiency or inactivation, and (5) preexisting lung disease. Fortunately, newborn mechanical ventilator strategies today minimize lung injuries by keeping exhaled volumes low, accepting higher PCO_2 levels, or switching to high frequency ventilation when positive inspiratory pressures (PIPs) exceed safe limits. Pulmonary air leak syndrome (see Chapter 36), however, can still occur in certain clinical scenarios—especially when very high ventilator pressures are used or in the delivery room with aggressive ventilation during resuscitation.

OVERVIEW of the Cardiopulmonary Clinical Manifestations Associated with Bronchopulmonary Dysplasia

The following clinical manifestations result from the pathologic mechanisms caused (or activated) by atelectasis (see Figure 9-7), increased alveolar-capillary membrane thickness (see Figure 9-9), and excessive bronchial secretions (see Figure 9-11)—the major anatomic alterations of the lungs associated with BPD (see Figure 38-1).

CLINICAL DATA OBTAINED AT THE PATIENT'S BEDSIDE

The Physical Examination

Vital Signs

Increased Respiratory Rate (Tachypnea)

Normally, a newborn's respiratory rate is about 40 to 60 breaths/min. During the early stages of BPD, the respiratory rate is generally well over 60 breaths/min. Several pathophysiologic mechanisms operating simultaneously may lead to an increased ventilatory rate:

- Increased stimulation of peripheral chemoreceptors (hypoxemia)
- Decreased lung compliance–increased ventilatory rate relationship
- Stimulation of central chemoreceptors
- Increased temperature (secondary to infection)

Increased Heart Rate (Pulse) and Blood Pressure

Clinical Manifestations Associated with More Negative Intrapleural Pressures during Inspiration

- Intercostal retractions
- Substernal retraction and abdominal distention (seesaw movement)
- Cyanosis of the dependent portions of the thoracic and abdominal areas
- Flaring nostrils

Chest Assessment Findings

- Wheezes
- Crackles

Expiratory Grunting

Cyanosis

CLINICAL DATA OBTAINED FROM LABORATORY TESTS AND SPECIAL PROCEDURES

Pulmonary Function Test Findings
(Extrapolated Data for Instructional Purposes)
(Primarily Restrictive Lung Pathophysiology)

The anatomic alterations of the lungs associated with BPD primarily cause a restrictive lung pathophysiology. For example, in moderate to severe cases, the following lung volumes and capacities will be lower than normal:

RV	IRV	VC	FRC	TLC
↓	↓	↓	↓	↓

However, when the airways are partially obstructed, and/or bullae, and/or emphysematous changes are present (e.g., in stage IV BPD), obstructive lung findings may be seen. In these cases, the following will be greater than normal:

RV	FRC	RV/TLC ratio
↑	↑	↑

Arterial Blood Gases*

MILD TO MODERATE BRONCHOPULMONARY DYSPLASIA

Acute Alveolar Hyperventilation with Hypoxemia[†]
(Acute Respiratory Alkalosis)

pH	$PaCO_2$	HCO_3^-	PaO_2	SaO_2 or SpO_2
↑	↓	↓	↓	↓
		(but normal)		

SEVERE BRONCHOPULMONARY DYSPLASIA

Chronic Ventilatory Failure with Hypoxemia[†]
(Compensated Respiratory Acidosis)

pH	$PaCO_2$	HCO_3^-	PaO_2	SaO_2 or SpO_2
N	↑	↑	↓	↓
		(significantly)		

ACUTE VENTILATORY CHANGES SUPERIMPOSED ON CHRONIC VENTILATORY FAILURE[§]

Because acute ventilatory changes are frequently seen in patients with chronic ventilatory failure, the respiratory therapist must be familiar with—and alert for—the following dangerous arterial blood gas (ABG) findings[§]:

- Acute alveolar hyperventilation superimposed on chronic ventilatory failure—which should further alert the respiratory therapist to record the following important ABG assessment: possible *impending acute ventilatory failure*.
- Acute ventilatory failure (acute hypoventilation) superimposed on chronic ventilatory failure.

---

*Note: Because of the difficulty of obtaining **ABG** samples from newborn and pediatric patients, **capillary blood gas** samples may be used to determine the pH, $PaCO_2$, and HCO_3^- (i.e., the acid-base and ventilation status only). Capillary PO_2 values are unreliable and should not be used for clinical analysis. The standard way to evaluate the oxygenation status of these young patients is pulse oximetry (SpO_2) (see Chapter 32).
[†]See Figure 4-3 and related discussion for the acute pH, $PaCO_2$, and HCO_3^- changes associated with acute alveolar hyperventilation.
[†]See Figure 4-2 and related discussion for the pH, $PaCO_2$, and HCO_3^- changes associated with chronic ventilatory failure.
[§]See TABLE 4-7 and related discussion for the pH, $PaCO_2$, and HCO_3^- changes associated with Acute Ventilatory Changes Superimposed on Chronic Ventilatory Failure.

		Oxygenation Indices*			
$\dot{Q}s/\dot{Q}T$	DO_2†	$\dot{V}O_2$	$C(a\text{-}\bar{v})O_2$	O_2ER	$S\bar{v}O_2$
↑	↓	N	N	↑	↓

RADIOLOGIC FINDINGS

Chest Radiograph

Using the classic description of BPD, Figure 38-2 provides a radiographic overview of the four stages of BPD. During stage I, the radiologic findings are analogous to those of severe respiratory distress syndrome (RDS), showing a ground-glass granular pattern and small lung volume (Figure 38-2, A). During stage II, patchy opaque areas with bronchograms (atelectasis) adjacent to areas of dark translucency (hyperinflation) appear. Identifying the precise cause of the haziness, whether pulmonary edema, alveolar consolidation, or atelectasis, is usually difficult (Figure 38-2, B).

The radiologic findings during stage III are more specific to BPD. Circular or cystlike areas of hyperlucency begin to appear and are surrounded by patches of irregular density areas caused by atelectasis. This condition generates a spongelike appearance of the lungs on the chest radiograph (Figure 38-2, C). Stage IV shows an increase in the size and number of cystlike areas of hyperlucency (emphysematous bullae), surrounded by thin strands of radiodensity (atelectasis and interstitial fibrosis). The emphysematous bullae and interstitial fibrosis around the bullae create a honeycomb appearance on the chest radiograph. Cor pulmonale may be seen during the advanced stages of BPD (Figure 38-2, D).

*$C(a\text{-}\bar{v})O_2$, arterial-venous oxygen difference; DO_2, total oxygen delivery; O_2ER, oxygen extraction ratio; $\dot{Q}s/\dot{Q}T$, pulmonary shunt fraction; $S\bar{v}O_2$, mixed venous oxygen saturation; $\dot{V}O_2$, oxygen consumption.
†Because the newborn normally has a higher hemoglobin level at birth (16.8 to 18.9 g/dL%), the DO_2 may actually be better than indicated by PaO_2 or SpO_2 (see Chapter 5, Total Oxygen Delivery).

TABLE 38-4 Therapeutic Measures Used to Prevent or Manage Infants with Bronchopulmonary Dysplasia (BPD)

Prenatal steroids	A single course of prenatal glucocorticoids administered to women who are at high risk for premature delivery results in a significant decrease in the mortality rate and in the morbidity associated with prematurity.
Gentle ventilation	Despite development of numerous sophisticated ventilators for the newborn, there is still no clear advantage to any one approach. The general approach is a ventilatory mode that prevents atelectasis, sustains or maintains FRC, uses a minimal tidal volume, and permits the infant to trigger his or her own ventilation as much as possible. Every effort should be made to minimize high peak inspiratory pressures, high mean airway pressures, and overdistention of the lungs. For example, high-frequency ventilation, low tidal volumes, and permissive hypercapnia are commonly used.
Low inspired oxygen concentrations	Every effort should be made to administer only the lowest concentration of oxygen that is necessary.
Nasal continuous positive airway pressure (CPAP)	Early application of nasal CPAP in high-risk respiratory distress syndrome and BPD infants is highly recommended during postnatal care.
Fluid restriction	Because fluid overload is a causative factor associated with BPD, fluid limitation may be helpful. However, care should be taken to avoid being overly aggressive when limiting fluids, because undernutrition is also associated with the development of BPD.
Vitamin A	Vitamin A is an essential nutrient for maintaining the epithelial cells of the tracheobronchial tree.
Diuretics	In infants with severe BPD, pulmonary edema is a major component. There is clear evidence that either daily or alternate-day therapy with furosemide improves lung mechanics and gas exchange in infants with established BPD.
Bronchodilator therapy	Increased airway resistance is highly associated with BPD. Short-term therapy with inhaled or parenteral beta$_2$-adrenergic agonists is frequently administered to infants with BPD. Inhaled albuterol has been the most widely used agent.
Bronchial hygiene therapy	Because of the high incidence of mucous plugging of the airways and endotracheal tubes, adequate humidification of the inspired gas is important. Routine suctioning is beneficial.
Postnatal corticosteroids	The administration of postnatal corticosteroids to preterm infants has been shown to reduce lung inflammation and the incidence of BPD. Postnatal corticosteroids are also believed to increase surfactant synthesis, enhance beta-adrenergic activity, increase antioxidant production, stabilize cell and lysosomal membranes, and inhibit prostaglandin and leukotriene synthesis.

CASE STUDY Bronchopulmonary Dysplasia

Admitting History and Physical Examination

An 1100-g baby boy was born at 28 weeks gestation to a mother who received no prenatal care. The mother had used cocaine and marijuana and may have had a vaginal infection during her pregnancy. Because of the baby's clinical presentation, mechanical ventilation was started moments after birth. Pulmonary surfactant was given to improve lung compliance and to avoid a prolonged ventilator course.

The infant worsened over 24 hours. He was diagnosed with RDS and group B streptococci pneumonia. An intravenous line and umbilical artery catheter were placed. Antibiotics were started. He required higher concentrations of oxygen (nasal cannula increased from 2 to 5 L/min), PIPs greater than 30 cm H_2O, and higher levels of PEEP to maintain oxygenation and adequate tidal volume.

He was placed on high frequency oscillatory ventilation for 4 days and was eventually transitioned back to conventional ventilation. He was placed on high flow nasal cannula oxygen at day 9. However, at day 14 he became tachypneic, with grunting and retractions, requiring an increase in FIO_2. A respiratory viral panel showed he was positive for influenza A, a virus contracted from his maternal grandmother who had been visiting the nursery. He developed pneumonia requiring another intubation and ventilator support. At this time the clinical team was concerned that this baby could have BPD.

At 3 weeks, the baby was still on a pressure-cycled mechanical ventilator with the following settings: PIP +25 cm H_2O, respiratory rate (RR) 35 breaths/min, inspiratory time (TI) 0.5 s, FIO_2 0.60, and PEEP +7 cm H_2O. His pulmonary mechanics showed increased airway resistance and decreased lung compliance. He demonstrated coarse bilateral crackles and some wheezes. Thick, clear mucus was suctioned. The chest radiograph showed patchy atelectasis and areas of pulmonary fibrosis. His arterial line ABG on an FIO_2 of 0.40 were pH 7.36, $PaCO_2$ 55 mm Hg, HCO_3^- 30 mEq/L, PaO_2 50 mm Hg, and SaO_2 of 84%. The doctor wrote the following order in the baby's chart: "Respiratory therapy to assess patient and begin to wean from ventilator."

The respiratory therapist charted the following assessment.

Respiratory Assessment and Plan

S N/A
O Marginal pulmonary mechanics—decreased compliance and increased airway resistance. Coarse crackles and wheezes. CXR: BPD with scattered areas of atelectasis and hyperinflation. ABGs on ventilator and FIO_2 0.40: pH 7.36, $PaCO_2$ 55, HCO_3^- 30, PaO_2 50, and SaO_2 84%.
A • Stiff lung with airway obstruction (pulmonary mechanics)
  • Chronic ventilatory failure with moderate hypoxemia (ABGs)

• Excessive bronchial secretions (crackles and suctioning results)
• Possible bronchospasm (wheezes—maybe caused by bronchial secretions)
• Appears ready for slow weaning trial

P Wean slowly per **Mechanical Ventilation Protocol** (decrease mandatory respiratory rate slowly; decrease need for pressure and rate; transition to pressure support ventilation). Continue **Oxygen Therapy Protocol** (FIO_2 to meet SpO_2 goals). Continue aggressive bronchopulmonary hygiene therapy per **Bronchopulmonary Hygiene Therapy Protocol** (suction PRN). Continue **Bronchodilator Therapy Protocol** (in-line neb with 0.25 mL of albuterol in 2.0 mL normal saline Q4H). Continue to monitor closely and assess frequently.

Over the next 10 weeks, the baby slowly improved. Five days before discharge, the mother was trained on respiratory and nursing procedures for home care. Over the following 4 years, the child's lungs continued to improve even though he had recurrent pneumonia and was seen monthly in the ED during the first 6 months. On one occasion, he was readmitted to the hospital for a week; he recovered and is now doing well. He is of normal weight and height for his age, runs and plays well with other children, and is about to enter preschool.

Discussion

Several comments should be made regarding this challenging pulmonary disorder of the newborn. First, infants with BPD have limited pulmonary reserves. Their lungs are seriously damaged, scarred, and fibrotic. They have increased airway resistance and decreased lung compliance. Because their lung tissues are constantly being bombarded by inflammatory stimuli, their hearts and lungs have a limited ability to recover from stress. *These infants may be slow to recover from procedures such as tracheal or nasopharyngeal suctioning.* Therefore health-care personnel should perform all therapeutic procedures as quickly and efficiently as possible.

Second, every attempt should be made to wean the baby off the ventilator—since ventilator pressures, rates, and high oxygen concentrations are the main factors causing the pulmonary damage. The longer the baby is on the ventilator, the more the lungs are being damaged. Also, because chronic ventilatory failure with hypoxemia commonly occurs in infants with chronic BPD, the respiratory therapist should not hurry to decrease the infant's $PaCO_2$ to the "normal" range of 35 to 45 mm Hg. Infants in the acute and chronic stages of BPD often have a high $PaCO_2$ and normal pH (compensated). A $PaCO_2$ of 50 to 60 mm Hg is often tolerated well. Therefore the therapist must be prepared to accept chronically high $PaCO_2$ levels. As the baby's lungs deteriorate, moreover, the ability of blood to flow easily through the lungs progressively declines. As the condition worsens, the work of the right side of the heart increases. If the BPD does not resolve, cor pulmonale may develop.

BPD is a disorder that requires a great deal of parental education and support at the time of the baby's discharge from the hospital. The respiratory therapist can be instrumental in working with the family both in the hospital and in the home to ensure that the parents are prepared to support the infant's respiratory care needs. For example, the parents must understand the procedures of oral and nasal suctioning, and aerosolized medication administration at home. Infants with BPD who have been discharged from the hospital commonly return to the hospital once or twice a year in acute respiratory distress. The majority of infants with severe BPD will develop some degree of airway hyperresponsiveness or reactivity. Therefore the importance of aggressive, long-term respiratory care in the home must be stressed to the family. For example, the value of good pulmonary hygiene therapy at home to offset the clinical manifestations associated with the accumulation of **Excessive Bronchial Secretions** (see Figure 9-11) cannot be overemphasized.

SELF-ASSESSMENT QUESTIONS

Answers to questions can be found on Evolve. To access additional student assessment questions visit **http://evolve.elsevier.com/DesJardins/respiratory**.

1. Which of the following is/are associated with the cause of bronchopulmonary dysplasia?
   1. History of RDS
   2. Low positive pressure mechanical ventilation
   3. High concentrations of oxygen
   4. Infant's weight greater than 2000 g
      a. 2 only
      b. 1 and 3 only
      c. 2, 3, and 4 only
      d. 1, 3, and 4 only

2. The anatomic alterations of the lungs associated with bronchopulmonary dysplasia are:
   1. Increased alveolar-capillary membrane thickness
   2. Atelectasis
   3. Excessive bronchial secretions
   4. Consolidation
      a. 2 and 4 only
      b. 3 and 4 only
      c. 1, 2, and 3 only
      d. 1, 2, 3, and 4

3. In what is referred to as the "new" bronchopulmonary dysplasia (new BPD), the major anatomic pathology is a decrease in alveolar number, called:
   a. Patches of atelectasis
   b. State IV BPD
   c. Alveolar hypoplasia
   d. Canalicular period of fetal development

4. Which of the following arterial blood gas values are associated with severe bronchopulmonary dysplasia?
   1. Decreased pH
   2. Increased $PaCO_2$
   3. Normal pH
   4. Decreased HCO_3^-
      a. 2 and 3 only
      b. 1 and 4 only
      c. 2, 3, and 4 only
      d. 1, 2, and 4 only

5. Which of the following clinical manifestations are associated with bronchopulmonary dysplasia?
   1. Crackles
   2. Intercostal retractions
   3. Normal or decreased FEV_T
   4. Increased $C(a-\bar{v})O_2$
      a. 1 and 4 only
      b. 2 and 3 only
      c. 1, 2, and 3 only
      d. 1, 2, 3, and 4

39 Congenital Diaphragmatic Hernia

Chapter Objectives

After reading this chapter, you will be able to:

- List the anatomic alterations of the lungs associated with congenital diaphragmatic hernia (CDH).
- Describe the causes of CDH.
- List the cardiopulmonary clinical manifestations associated with CDH.
- Describe the general management of CDH.
- Describe the clinical strategies and rationales of the SOAP presented in the case study.

Key Terms

Atelectasis
Bochdalek's Foramen
Bochdalek's Hernia
Congenital Diaphragmatic Eventration
Congenital Diaphragmatic Hernia (CDH)
Dextrocardia
Extracorporeal Membrane Oxygenation (ECMO)
Hemothorax
Inhaled Nitric Oxide (iNO)
Morgagni's Hernia
Pneumothorax
Posterior-Lateral Diaphragmatic Hernia
Pulmonary Hypertension
Pulmonary Hypoplasia
Scaphoid Abdomen

Chapter Outline

Anatomic Alterations of the Lungs
Etiology and Epidemiology
Overview of Cardiopulmonary Clinical Manifestations
   Associated with Congenital Diaphragmatic Hernia
General Management of a Congenital Diaphragmatic Hernia
Case Study: Diaphragmatic Hernia
Self-Assessment Questions

Anatomic Alterations of the Lungs

During normal fetal development, the diaphragm first appears anteriorly between the heart and liver and then progressively grows posteriorly. Between the eighth and tenth week of gestation, the diaphragm normally completely closes at the left **Bochdalek's foramen,** which is located posteriorly and laterally on the left diaphragm. At about the tenth week of gestation (close to the same time the Bochdalek's foramen is closing), the intestines and stomach normally migrate from the yolk sac. If, however, the bowels reach this area before Bochdalek's foramen closes, a hernia results—a **congenital diaphragmatic hernia (CDH)** (also called **Bochdalek's hernia** or **posterior-lateral diaphragmatic hernia**). In other words, Bochdalek's hernia is an abnormal hole in the posterolateral corner of the left diaphragm that allows the intestines—and in some cases the stomach—to move directly into the chest cavity and compress the developing lungs.*

---

*About 95% of CDHs are Bochdalek's hernias. Rare CDHs include **Morgagni's hernia** and **congenital diaphragmatic eventration** of the diaphragm. A **Morgagni's hernia** is characterized by herniation through the foramina of Morgagni, which are located immediately adjacent to the xyphoid process of the sternum. Most Morgagni's hernias occur on the right side of the body and are asymptomatic. A congenital diaphragmatic eventration is abnormal elevation of part or all of an otherwise intact diaphragm into the chest cavity. This rare form of CDH occurs when a region of the diaphragm is thinner (commonly caused by an incomplete muscularization of the diaphragm), which in turn allows the abdominal viscera to protrude upward.

As shown in Figure 39-1, the effects of a diaphragmatic hernia are similar to the effects of a **pneumothorax** or **hemothorax**—the lungs are compressed. As the condition becomes more severe, **atelectasis** and complete lung collapse may occur. When this happens, the heart and mediastinum are pushed to the right side of the chest—called **dextrocardia.** In addition, long-term lung compression in utero causes **pulmonary hypoplasia**, which is most severe on the affected (ipsilateral) side but also occurs on the unaffected (contralateral) side.

This pathologic process causes a marked reduction in the number of bronchial generations and alveoli per acinus. The concomitant increased muscularity of the small pulmonary arteries may contribute to the increased pulmonary vascular resistance and **pulmonary hypertension** commonly seen in these patients. Respiratory distress usually develops soon after birth. As the infant struggles to inhale, the increased negative intrathoracic pressure generated during each inspiration causes more of the intestines to be sucked into the thorax. Further compression of the lungs and heart occurs as the infant cries and swallows air, causing the intestine and stomach to distend further.

Finally, as a consequence of the hypoxemia associated with a diaphragmatic hernia, these babies often develop hypoxia-induced pulmonary arterial vasoconstriction and vasospasm, which produce a state of pulmonary hypertension. As a general rule, however, these babies only have a transient state of pulmonary hypertension until the diaphragmatic hernia is

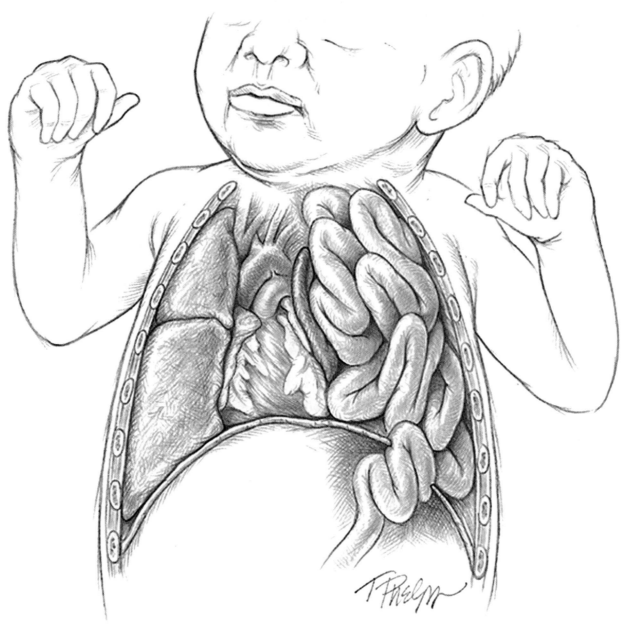

FIGURE 39-1 Diaphragmatic hernia.

repaired. This is different from persistent pulmonary hypertension of the newborn (see Chapter 32).

The major pathologic or structural changes associated with diaphragmatic hernia may include the following:

- Failure of the Bochdalek's foramen of the diaphragm to close
- Migration of intestines and stomach into the thorax
  - Atelectasis
  - Complete lung collapse
  - Mediastinal shift to the unaffected side of the thorax
  - Reduction in the number of bronchial generations and alveoli per acinus
  - Pulmonary hypoplasia
  - Transient pulmonary hypertension

Etiology and Epidemiology

The overall incidence of CDH ranges from 1 in 2000 to 4000 live births. The baby is usually mature, and two-thirds are male. About 95% of CDHs occur on the left side through Bochdalek's foramen. The mortality rate is about 40%. The prognosis depends on (1) the size of the defect, (2) the degree of hypoplasia, (3) the condition of the lung on the unaffected side, and (4) the success of the surgical diaphragmatic closure. Most cases of CDH are now diagnosed by prenatal ultrasound, allowing the infant to be delivered at a hospital where surgical repair of the diaphragmatic hernia can occur very shortly after birth. A few pediatric centers are performing high-risk prenatal surgery to repair the diaphragm.

The following clinical manifestations result from the pathologic mechanisms caused (or activated) by atelectasis (see Figure 9-7)—a common anatomic alteration of the lungs associated with diaphragmatic hernia (see Figure 39-1).

CLINICAL DATA OBTAINED AT THE PATIENT'S BEDSIDE

The Physical Examination

Vital Signs

Increased Respiratory Rate (Tachypnea)

Normally, a newborn's respiratory rate is about 40 to 60 breaths/min. When a diaphragmatic hernia is present, the respiratory rate is generally well over 60 breaths/min. Several pathophysiologic mechanisms operating simultaneously may lead to an increased ventilatory rate:

- Stimulation of peripheral chemoreceptors (hypoxemia)
- Decreased lung compliance–increased ventilatory rate relationship
- Stimulation of central chemoreceptors

Increased Heart Rate (Pulse) and Blood Pressure

Clinical Manifestations Associated with More Negative Intrapleural Pressures during Inspiration

- Intercostal retraction
- Substernal retraction
- Cyanosis of the dependent portions of the thoracic and abdominal areas
- Flaring nostrils

Chest Assessment Findings

- Diminished or absent breath sounds over the affected side
- Bowel sounds over the affected side
- Apical heartbeat heard over the unaffected side (usually right)

Expiratory Grunting

Cyanosis

Barrel Chest

When the intestines are in the chest and distended with gas, the baby often demonstrates a barrel chest.

Scaphoid Abdomen

Depending on the degree of intestinal displacement into the thorax, the infant's abdomen often appears flat or concave.

CLINICAL DATA OBTAINED FROM LABORATORY TESTS AND SPECIAL PROCEDURES

Pulmonary Function Test Findings
(Extrapolated Data for Instructional Purposes)
(Primarily Restrictive Lung Pathophysiology)

The anatomic alterations of the lungs associated with CDH primarily cause a restrictive lung pathophysiology. For example, in moderate to severe cases, the following lung volumes and capacities will be lower than normal:

RV	IRV	VC	FRC	TLC
↓	↓	↓	↓	↓

Arterial Blood Gases*

MILD TO MODERATE DIAPHRAGMATIC HERNIA

Acute Alveolar Hyperventilation with Hypoxemia[†]
(Acute Respiratory Alkalosis)

pH	$PaCO_2$	HCO_3^-	PaO_2	SaO_2 or SpO_2
↑	↓	↓ (but normal)	↓	↓

SEVERE DIAPHRAGMATIC HERNIA

Acute Ventilatory Failure with Hypoxemia[§]
(Acute Respiratory Acidosis)

pH[†]	$PaCO_2$	HCO_3^-[†]	PaO_2	SaO_2 or SpO_2
↓	↑	↑ (but normal)	↓	↓

Oxygenation Indices[||]

$\dot{Q}_S/\dot{Q}_T$	DO_2[¶]	$\dot{V}O_2$	$C(a-\bar{v})O_2$	O_2ER	$S\bar{v}O_2$
↑	↓	N	N	↑	↓

*Note: Because of the difficulty of obtaining **arterial blood gas (ABG)** samples from newborn and pediatric patients, **capillary blood gas** samples may be used to determine the pH, $PaCO_2$, and HCO_3^- (i.e., the acid-base and ventilation status only). Capillary PO_2 values are unreliable and should not be used for clinical analysis. The standard way to evaluate the oxygenation status of these young patients is pulse oximetry (SpO_2) (see Chapter 32).

[†]See Figure 4-3 and related discussion for the acute pH, $PaCO_2$, and HCO_3^- changes associated with acute alveolar hyperventilation.

[§]See Figure 4-2 and related discussion for the acute pH, $PaCO_2$, and HCO_3^- changes associated with acute ventilatory failure.

[†]When tissue hypoxia is severe enough to produce lactic acid, the pH and HCO_3^- values will be lower than expected for a particular $PaCO_2$ level.

[||] $C(a-\bar{v})O_2$, Arterial-venous oxygen difference; DO_2, total oxygen delivery; O_2ER, oxygen extraction ratio; $\dot{Q}_S/\dot{Q}_T$, pulmonary shunt fraction; $S\bar{v}O_2$, mixed venous oxygen saturation; $\dot{V}O_2$, oxygen consumption.

[¶]Because the newborn normally has a higher hemoglobin level at birth (16.8 to 18.9 g/dL%), the DO_2 may actually be better than indicated by PaO_2 or SpO_2 (see Chapter 5, Total Oxygen Delivery).

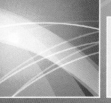

RADIOLOGIC FINDINGS
Chest Radiograph
Increased Opacity (Ground-Glass Appearance of Compressed Lung)

A typical radiograph shows fluid- and air-filled loops of intestine in the chest and a shift of the heart and mediastinum to the unaffected side. Atelectasis and complete lung collapse may be present. The lungs may appear hypoplastic and may not expand to meet the chest wall. A nasogastric tube (in the patient's stomach, it is hoped) may be seen on the chest radiograph. It is used to decompress the abdominal viscera. The presence of a diaphragmatic hernia on a chest radiograph usually confirms the need for surgery (see Figure 39-2).

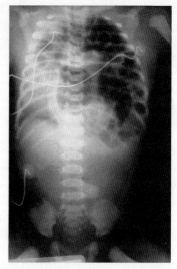

FIGURE 39-2 Chest radiograph of left diaphragmatic hernia.

General Management of a Congenital Diaphragmatic Hernia

Severe diaphragmatic hernia is one of the most urgent neonatal surgical emergencies. Although prompt surgical repair is imperative, a number of therapeutic measures may be instituted until the baby is stabilized for surgery, which may take several days.

As soon as the diagnosis of a diaphragmatic hernia is made, a double-lumen oral gastric tube should be inserted with intermittent or low continuous suction. This reduces the amount of gas in the stomach and bowels and thereby reduces lung compression. Oxygen therapy should be started immediately (see **Oxygen Therapy Protocol**, Protocol 32-1). The infant also may be placed in the semi-Fowler's position, which reduces the intrathoracic pressure and facilitates the downward positioning of the abdominal viscera. Placing the infant on the affected side aids expansion of the good lung. *The infant must not be manually ventilated with a bag and mask, because of the danger of air swallowing.*

The infant must, however, be intubated and ventilated. Mechanical ventilation should be applied with low peak airway pressures (<30 cm H$_2$O) and rapid respiratory rates. A typical set of ventilator parameters would be peak inspiratory pressure (PIP) +18 to +20 cm H$_2$O, respiratory rate (RR) 40, FIO$_2$ 1.0, positive end-expiratory pressure (PEEP) +2 to +3 cm H$_2$O, and inspiratory time (T$_I$) 0.4. High-frequency oscillatory ventilation and jet ventilation are sometimes successful (see **Mechanical Ventilation Protocol**, Protocol 32-5).

Because the infant's lungs are fragile and rupture easily, the incidence of pneumothorax is high. Therefore the physician may need to insert one or more chest tubes during mechanical ventilation. Paralysis with muscle relaxants and sedation are helpful at times. Paralysis eliminates air swallowing, which helps to keep the gastrointestinal contents compressed. Bronchial hygiene may be necessary to maintain the infant's airways (see **Bronchopulmonary Hygiene Therapy Protocol**, Protocol 32-2).

Occasionally, certain pharmacologic agents may be administered to offset the infant's pulmonary hypertension. Such drugs include digitalis, diuretics, nitroglycerin, and **inhaled nitric oxide (iNO)**. The physiologic action of iNO is believed to be similar to that of the vasoactive substance, endothelium-derived relaxing factor. The use of iNO has significantly reduced the need for **extracorporeal membrane oxygenation (ECMO)** therapy.

The surgical procedure entails repositioning the abdominal contents into the abdomen and closing the diaphragmatic defect. In some infants the peritoneal cavity may be too small to contain the abdominal contents. In these cases the surgeon leaves the fascia open and closes only the skin. This results in a ventral hernia that is repaired several months after the initial surgery. After surgery, the baby is placed back on the ventilator and weaned per ventilator protocol. Mechanical ventilation with PEEP and continuous positive airway pressure (CPAP) are commonly required to offset the atelectasis and hypoplasia associated with the disorder. Often, the lung on the affected side is hypoplastic, and days or weeks of therapy may be required for full expansion to occur (see **Lung Expansion Therapy Protocol**, Protocol 32-3).

ECMO may be indicated to treat circulatory and respiratory complications after surgery for infants who do not respond favorably to conventional medical therapy. While on ECMO, the infant is usually ventilated only three or four times per minute to keep the lungs inflated.

CASE STUDY Diaphragmatic Hernia

Admitting History and Physical Examination

A full-term baby boy was delivered at 2:25 AM with no remarkable problems to a mother who had received no prenatal care. After delivery, however, the baby made one cry and quickly became blue and limp, started to have bradycardia, and became apneic. The baby's 1-minute Apgar score was 3 (heart rate 1, respiration 0, tone 1, reflex irritability 1, color 0). The nurse handed the baby to a student intern, who immediately began manual ventilation. Both the respiratory therapist and the nurse noted that the baby's abdomen was scaphoid; the therapist stated that the baby might have a diaphragmatic hernia and that bagging should be stopped immediately. Moments later, the neonatologist entered the room, confirmed the **scaphoid abdomen**, noted that the lungs were very stiff in response to the bagging, and ordered a stat intubation with a 3.5-mm tube and a chest radiograph.

The infant was then transferred to the neonatal intensive care unit. The chest radiograph confirmed a left diaphragmatic hernia and hypoplastic left lung. At this time, a nasogastric tube was inserted, and suction was begun. The baby was sedated and placed on a pressure-limited mechanical ventilator. An intravenous line and umbilical artery catheter were then secured. The initial ventilator settings were respiratory rate 30 breaths/min, T_I 0.5, PEEP +4, PIP + 25, and FIO_2 1.0. Initial ABGs were pH 7.19, $PaCO_2$ 63 mm Hg, HCO_3^- 23 mEq/L, PaO_2 37 mm Hg, and SaO_2 56%. No breath sounds could be heard over the infant's left lung. The neonatologist diagnosed pulmonary hypertension of the neonate by cardiac echocardiogram. The respiratory therapist then adjusted the ventilator settings as follows: respiratory rate 35 breaths/min, T_I 0.4 second, PEEP +5, PIP +28 cm H_2O, and FIO_2 1.0. A second set of ABGs taken 15 minutes later showed pH 7.29, $PaCO_2$ 49 mm Hg, HCO_3^- 23 mEq/L, PaO_2 44 mm Hg, and SaO_2 74%.

The baby was started on iNO with little improvement in oxygenation. The team assumed this poor response was due to the severe pulmonary hypoplasia. He was then placed on ECMO, with the ventilator set to minimal settings. Even though the ECMO was doing all the oxygenation, the baby's lungs were expanded by the ventilator about four times a minute. Four days later, his pulmonary artery pressure was determined to be low enough for surgery. The diaphragmatic hernia was repaired, and the baby was returned to the unit with a chest tube in the left side of his chest. He was continued on a ventilator and ECMO.

The ventilator settings 3 days later were RR 8/min, T_I 0.6, PIP +20, PEEP and CPAP +4, and FIO_2 0.45. His vital signs were heart rate 145 beats/min, blood pressure 70/45, respiratory rate 65 (between ventilator breaths), and temperature 37°C (96.8°F). His skin was pink and normal. Good breath sounds were auscultated over the right lung, and coarse crackles could be heard over the left lung.

His ABGs at this time were pH 7.36, $PaCO_2$ 44 mm Hg, HCO_3^- 24 mEq/L, PaO_2 73 mm Hg, and SaO_2 94%. The baby's chest radiograph showed good lung expansion on the right side. Although the upper half of the left lung was well expanded, atelectasis and hypoplasia were still seen over the lower half of the left lung. Bubbles were no longer coming from the left-sided chest tube. A small amount of thin, clear secretions was suctioned from the baby's endotracheal tube three or four times an hour.

At that time the respiratory therapist wrote the following assessment in the infant's chart.

Respiratory Assessment and Plan

S N/A

O Vital signs: On ECMO HR 145, BP 70/45, RR 65 (8 mechanical breaths), T 37°C (96.8°F). Skin: pink and normal. Breath sounds: right lung—normal; left lung—coarse crackles. No chest tube bubbles. ABGs: pH 7.36, $PaCO_2$ 44, HCO_3^- 24, PaO_2 73, SaO_2 94%. CXR: Right lung normal; atelectasis and hypoplasia in left lower lung.

A • ECMO dependent on ventilator at minimal settings but improving (vital signs, skin color, ABGs)
  • Mild amount of large and small airway secretions (coarse crackles)
  • Atelectasis and hypoplasia of the left lower lobe (CXR)
  • May be ready to wean from ECMO—check with physician

P Mechanical Ventilation Protocol (continue to wean per protocol—wean pressures first, then FIO_2). **Lung expansion therapy protocol** (continue PEEP or CPAP per **mechanical ventilator protocol**). **Bronchopulmonary hygiene therapy protocol** (continue suction and CPT PRN). **Oxygen therapy protocol** (keep SpO_2 at 97% as the FIO_2 is decreased. Do not decrease FIO_2 more than 0.10 per hour).

ECMO was discontinued. The baby continued to improve over the next 5 days. On day 6, he was off the ventilator and discharged from the hospital 1 week later. The baby continued to develop normally over the next 4 years; at the time of this writing, he was about to enter kindergarten.

Discussion

This case nicely illustrates the importance of good assessment skills. Most diaphragmatic hernias are identified before the baby is born by high-resolution ultrasound of the maternal abdomen, visualizing the fetus in utero during routine prenatal care. Unfortunately, this mother had no prenatal care, and as a result, the baby's diaphragmatic hernia was a surprise. Fortunately, the respiratory therapist and nurse in this case quickly and correctly identified the possibility of the diaphragmatic hernia by noting the scaphoid abdomen. Had the student intern continued to bag the baby manually, more gas would have entered the stomach and intestines, compressing and compromising the infant's lungs even more. The atelectasis (see Figure 9-7) caused by the enlarged intestines was objectively confirmed on the chest radiograph. The **lung expansion therapy protocol** was clearly justified to offset the atelectasis after the diaphragmatic hernia was repaired (see **Lung Expansion Therapy Protocol**, Protocol 32-3).

This case further illustrates that the first objective in the management of the infant born with a diaphragmatic hernia is correction of the transient pulmonary hypertension. Often, as in this case, treatment requires that the infant be given ECMO for 3 or 4 days before surgery. After the pulmonary hypertension is controlled, the second objective is surgical repair of the hernia. Mechanical ventilation with PEEP is usually required after surgery to correct the atelectasis and hypoplasia associated with the disorder. Typically, weaning involves decreasing the FIO_2 while monitoring the baby's pulse oximetry. Ideally, the ventilator pressures are decreased first, followed by the ventilatory rates A target $PaCO_2$ of ≤40 mm Hg is commonly used. An infant on a ventilatory rate of 12 beats/min, a peak inspiratory pressure of +15 cm H_2O or less, and a PEEP of +3 cm H_2O or less is usually ready for a weaning trial. Infants who survive CDH require follow-up pulmonary care for the first years of life because they handle pulmonary infections poorly owing to their smaller than normal lungs as a result of the prenatal lung hypoplasia.

SELF-ASSESSMENT QUESTIONS

Answers to questions can be found on Evolve. To access additional student assessment questions visit **http://evolve.elsevier.com/DesJardins/respiratory**.

1. **The Bochdalek's foramen closes at the:**
   a. Fourth to sixth week of gestation
   b. Sixth to eighth week of gestation
   c. Eighth to tenth week of gestation
   d. Tenth to twelfth week of gestation

2. **Which of the following are associated with a congenital diaphragmatic hernia?**
   1. Females are affected more than males
   2. Left side (90%)
   3. A scaphoid abdomen at birth
   4. Bowel sounds on the affected side of chest
      a. 1 and 3 only
      b. 2 and 4 only
      c. 2, 3, and 4 only
      d. 1, 2, 3, and 4

3. **Which of the following arterial blood gas values is/are associated with mild to moderate congenital diaphragmatic hernia?**
   1. Increased pH
   2. Increased $PaCO_2$
   3. Increased PaO_2
   4. Increased HCO_3^-
      a. 1 only
      b. 1 and 4 only
      c. 2, 3, and 4 only
      d. 1, 2, and 4 only

4. **Which of the following clinical manifestations is or are associated with a congenital diaphragmatic hernia?**
   1. Diminished or absent breath sounds
   2. Intercostal retractions
   3. Normal or decreased FEV_T
   4. Increased $C(a-\bar{v})O_2$
      a. 3 and 4 only
      b. 1 and 2 only
      c. 1, 2, and 3 only
      d. 1, 2, 3, and 4

5. **Which of the following is/are associated with a congenital diaphragmatic hernia?**
   1. Increased alveolar-capillary membrane thickness
   2. Atelectasis
   3. Excessive bronchial secretions
   4. Pulmonary consolidation
      a. 2 only
      b. 3 only
      c. 1, 2, and 3 only
      d. 1, 2, 3, and 4

Chapter Objectives

After reading this chapter, you will be able to:

- List the anatomic alterations associated with common congenital heart defects.
- Describe the etiology and epidemiology of common congenital heart defects.
- List the cardiopulmonary clinical manifestations associated with common congenital heart defects.
- Describe the general management of the common congenital heart defects.
- Describe the clinical strategies and rationales of the SOAPs presented in the case study.

Key Terms

Aortic Ejection Click
Atrial Septal Defect (ASD)
Balloon Atrial Septostomy (BAS)
Coeur-en-sabot
Complex Transposition of the Great Arteries (complex TGA)
Congenital Heart Disease (CHD)
Conoventricular Ventricular Septal Defect
Dextrotransposition of the Great Arteries (d-TGA)
Differential Cyanosis
Foramen Ovale
Fossa Ovalis
"Hypercyanotic Spells"
Hyperoxia Test
Infundibular Stenosis
Inlet Ventricular Septal Defect
Ligamentum Arteriosum
Muscular Ventricular Septal Defect
Ostium Secundum ASD
Pansystolic Murmur
Patent Ductus Arteriosus (PDA)
Perimembranous Ventricular Septal Defect
Primum ASD
Prostaglandin E1
Pulmonary Flow to Systemic Flow ($\dot{Q}p/\dot{Q}s$) ratio
Simple Transposition of the Great Arteries (simple TGA)
Stenosis of the Pulmonary Artery
Subclavicular thrill

Systolic Thrill
Tetralogy of Fallot (TOF)
"Tet Spells"
Transposition of the Great Arteries
Valvular Stenosis
Ventricular Septal Defect

Chapter Outline

Patent Ductus Arteriosus
  Anatomic Alterations of the Heart
  Etiology and Epidemiology
  Diagnosis
  Clinical Manifestations
  Treatment
Atrial Septal Defect
  Anatomic Alterations of the Heart
  Etiology and Epidemiology
  Diagnosis
  Clinical Manifestations
  Treatment
Ventricular Septal Defect
  Anatomic Alterations of the Heart
  Etiology and Epidemiology
  Diagnosis
  Clinical Manifestations
  Treatment
Tetralogy of Fallot
  Anatomic Alterations of the Heart
  Etiology and Epidemiology
  Diagnosis
  Clinical Manifestations
  Treatment
Transposition of the Great Arteries
  Anatomic Alterations of the Heart
  Etiology and Epidemiology
  Diagnosis
  Clinical Manifestations
  Treatment
Case Study: Transposition of the Great Arteries
Self-Assessment Questions

Congenital heart diseases (CHDs) (also known as congenital heart defects) are anatomic abnormalities of the heart that are present at birth. CHDs can involve the (1) interior walls of the heart, (2) valves inside the heart, or (3) arteries and veins that carry blood to the heart or body. According to the National Heart, Lung, and Blood Institute, CHDs are the most common type of birth defect, affecting 8 of every 1000

newborns. According to the Centers for Disease Control and Prevention (CDC), nearly 40,000 infants are born with a heart defect each year in the United States, and more than 1 million adults are living with CHD here.

There are several types of CHDs ranging from simple defects with no symptoms to complex defects with severe, life-threatening symptoms. Many of the simple defects require no treatment or are relatively easy to repair. The complex defects require medical care and surgical repair soon after birth. The ability to diagnose and treat CHDs has greatly improved over the past few decades. Today, nearly all children born with complex CHDs survive to adulthood and lead active, productive lives.

CHDs commonly encountered by the respiratory therapist include **patent ductus arteriosus (PDA), atrial septal defect (ASD), ventricular septal defect (VSD), tetralogy of Fallot (TOF), and transposition of the great arteries (TGA).** These CHDs can be further classified as either a **noncyanotic** defect (a left-to-right shunting heart defect)—e.g., PDA, ASD, and VSD—or a **cyanotic defect** (a right-to-left shunting heart defect)—e.g., TOF and TGA.

In addition to the newborn's history, signs, symptoms, and physical examination findings, the **hyperoxia test** is used to help determine whether the infant's cyanosis is caused by lung disease or a CHD (e.g., TOF or TGA). The general procedure required for the hyperoxia test is as follows:

- First, obtain an arterial blood gas (ABG) while the patient is on room air. Review the results to confirm hypoxemia.
- If hypoxemia is present, the infant is then placed on an FIO_2 of 1.0 (e.g., head hood) for 10 minutes, followed by a second ABG.

If the infant's cyanosis is due to a lung disorder, the FIO_2 1.0 will increase the PaO_2—usually above 150 mm Hg. However, if the hypoxemia is caused by a CHD that produces a right-to-left pulmonary shunt, the increased oxygen will have little effect and the PaO_2 will remain below 100 mm Hg,

Patent Ductus Arteriosus

Anatomic Alterations of the Heart

Patent ductus arteriosus is a congenital heart defect in which the ductus arteriosus, which is normally open during fetal life, fails to close shortly after birth. As a result, a portion of the oxygenated blood from the aorta (which has a higher blood pressure) flows through the open ductus back to the pulmonary artery (Figure 40-1). The pathophysiologic effect of a PDA is a *left-to-right* shunt (noncyanotic disorder).[1] In other words, it allows blood from the systemic circulation to flow into the pulmonary circulation. Box 40-1 provides a brief review of the normal development and function of the ductus arteriosus.

A PDA results in excessive blood flow through the pulmonary circulation and hypoperfusion of the systemic circulation. Pulmonary engorgement results in decreased lung compliance—stiff lungs. Pulmonary blood flow can be up to three times greater than that of the systemic blood flow. The pathophysiologic consequences of the "ductal steal" depend on the size of the shunt and the response of the heart, lungs, and other organs impacted by the shunt. In preterm infants, a clinically significant PDA is associated with an increased

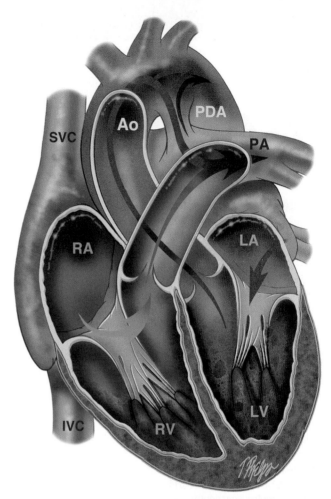

FIGURE 40-1 Patent ductus arteriosus (PDA) is a congenital heart defect in which the ductus arteriosus fails to close shortly after birth. The pathophysiologic effect of a PDA is a *left-to-right* shunt (noncyanotic disorder). When the infant has persistent hypertension of the newborn, a *right-to-left* shunt will develop (cyanotic disorder), resulting in a decreased PaO_2 and oxygen content. This figure illustrates both a left-to-right shunt and a right-to-left shunt. *Ao,* Aorta; *IVC,* inferior vena cava; *LA,* left atrium; *LV,* left ventricle; *PA,* pulmonary artery; *RA,* right atrium; *RV,* right ventricle; *SVC,* superior vena cava.

risk of pulmonary edema, pulmonary hemorrhage, bronchopulmonary dysplasia, and a decrease in pulmonary function.

Etiology and Epidemiology

PDA is associated with prematurity, low birth weight, high altitude and low atmospheric oxygen tension, hypoxia, and a variety of chromosomal abnormalities. It is more common in premature than in full-term infants, occurring in about eight of every 1000 premature babies, compared with two of every 1000 full-term babies. PDA is twice as common in girls as in boys. The prognosis is generally considered excellent in the newborn whose only problem is a PDA.

Diagnosis

The diagnosis of PDA is usually based upon its characteristic clinical findings—e.g., a loud systolic/diastolic heart murmur at the upper left sternal border—and confirmed by echocardiography. The combination of two-dimensional

---

[1]When persistent pulmonary hypertension of the newborn is present, a right-to-left shunt will develop (cyanotic disorder), causing decreased PaO_2 and oxygen content (see Box 40-1, and Chapter 32, page 404).

with a moderate or large ductal PDA usually develops signs and symptoms during the first 2 to 3 days after birth—as the pulmonary vascular resistance decreases—which, in turn, increases the *left-to-right* shunting through the lungs. When PDA is complicated by *persistent pulmonary hypertension of the newborn*, the clinical manifestations include tachycardia, dyspnea, **differential cyanosis** (i.e., cyanosis of the lower extremities but not the upper body), low PaO_2 and SpO_2, increased $PaCO_2$, loud systolic/diastolic murmur at the upper left sternal border (the S_2 is often obscured by murmur), cardiomegaly, left **subclavicular thrill**, prominent left ventricular impulse, bounding pulse (related to the high left ventricular stroke volume, which may cause systolic hypertension), and widened pulse pressure. Suprasternal or carotid pulsations may be prominent. Complications of PDA in the newborn include pulmonary edema, congestive heart failure, intraventricular hemorrhage, necrotizing enterocolitis, and bronchopulmonary dysplasia due to prolonged ventilator and/or oxygen support. A PDA in a newborn with any of these resulting conditions will likely require an extended hospitalization.

PDA patients who are 3 to 6 weeks old commonly present with tachypnea, diaphoresis, inability or difficulty with feeding, and weight loss or no weight gain. The patient with a moderate or large PDA may demonstrate a hoarse cry, cough, lower respiratory tract infection, atelectasis, or pneumonia. In the adult whose PDA has gone undiagnosed, the signs and symptoms include congestive heart failure, atrial arrhythmia, and differential cyanosis (i.e., cyanosis limited to the lower extremities).[2] The patient often reports decreased exercise tolerance.

Treatment

Treatment includes medication (e.g., indomethacin), catheter-based procedures, and/or surgery to permanently close the ductus. For the newborn, the standard respiratory care protocols—i.e., oxygen therapy protocol, bronchopulmonary hygiene therapy protocol, lung expansion therapy protocol, aerosolized medication therapy protocol, and ventilator support protocols—are all administered as needed (see Newborn Respiratory Therapy Protocols, Chapter 32)

Atrial Septal Defect

Anatomic Alterations of the Heart

Atrial septal defect is a congenital heart defect in which there is a hole in the septal wall between the right and left

---

echocardiographic imaging and Doppler color flow mapping is both sensitive and specific for the identification of PDA.

Clinical Manifestations

The patient with a PDA can present at any age. Typically, the newborn with a PDA is asymptomatic. The newborn

[2]Differential cyanosis occurs when cyanosis is more evident in the lower extremities than the upper extremities and the head. Differential cyanosis is seen in patients with a patent ductus arteriosus (PDA). These patients commonly develop progressive pulmonary vascular disease, and pressure overload of the right ventricle occurs. When pulmonary pressure exceeds aortic pressure, a shunt reversal occurs—i.e., a left-to-right shunt changes to a right-to-left shunt. The upper extremity remains pink because the brachiocephalic trunk, left common carotid trunk, and left subclavian trunk are given off proximal to the PDA.

During fetal development, the **ostium secundum** (also called foramen secundum or the "second opening") is an atrial orifice that develops in the **septum primum** during normal development. At birth, this orifice is partially covered and sealed by the *septum secundum*. The oval orifice that remains in the atrial wall—the **foramen ovale**—is covered, but not sealed, on the left atrium side by a flexible flap that is part of the *septum primum*. The increased blood pressure that develops in the left atrium shortly after birth causes the flexible flap to functionally close. It will eventually form part of the **fossa ovalis**. Complete structural closure usually takes about 9 months or more.

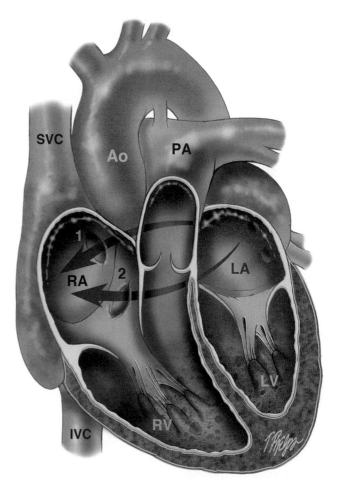

FIGURE 40-2 Atrial septal defect (ASD) is a congenital heart defect in which there is a hole in the septal wall between the right and left atrium. The two most common types of ASD are the **ostium secundum ASD** *(1)* and the **primum ASD** *(2)*. *Ao*, Aorta; *IVC*, inferior vena cava; *LA*, left atrium; *LV*, left ventricle; *PA*, pulmonary artery; *RA*, right atrium; *RV*, right ventricle; *SVC*, superior vena cava.

atrium (Figure 40-2). The two most common types of ASD are the **ostium secundum ASD** and the **primum ASD**.

The *ostium secundum ASD* is caused by arrested growth of the secundum septum or excessive absorption of the primum septum, resulting in an atrial septal wall defect. The secundum ASD presents as an isolated cardiac defect in the *fossa ovalis*. Box 40-2 provides a brief review of the normal development of the ostium secundum.

The *primum ASD* is caused by arrested growth of the apical portion of the atrial septum. It is associated with an anterior mitral valve cleft, which is often accompanied by mitral valve regurgitation. Box 40-3 provides a brief review of the normal development of the septum primum.

The degree of pathophysiology associated with an ASD depends on (1) the pulmonary and systemic vascular resistances, (2) the compliance of the left and right ventricles, and (3) the size of the ASD. At birth, the left atrial pressure becomes greater than right atrial pressure—resulting in a *left-to-right* shunt (noncyanotic disorder). Initially, the volume of blood shunted from left to right is small. This is because the right ventricle is still relatively thick and noncompliant. As the right ventricle remodels in response to the decreased pulmonary vascular resistance, its compliance increases—which, in turn, lowers the mean right atrial pressure. As a result, the left-to-right shunting increases in volume. In a large ASD, the **pulmonary flow to systemic flow ($\dot{Q}p/\dot{Q}s$) ratio** can be over 3:1. In other words, 75% of the blood returning to the left atrium from the lungs flows directly into the right atrium—via the ASD—and returns to the lungs; while 25% of the blood in the left atrium flows into the left ventricle and out to the systemic system.

The increased pulmonary blood flow is usually well tolerated for years. Heart failure is unusual before age 30. Beyond this age, the prevalence of heart failure increases substantially. Other complications include atrial arrhythmias such as flutter and fibrillation.

Etiology and Epidemiology

ASDs are common and account for approximately 13% of all patients with CHD. According to the CDC, over 1900 infants in the United States are born each year with an ASD.

During fetal development, the cavity of the primitive atrium is subdivided into right and left chambers by a structure called the **septum primum**, which grows downward between the two atrial cavities. As the septum primum grows downward, the progressively smaller gap below it—before it fuses with the endocardial cushion—is called the **ostium primum** ("the first opening"). Eventually, the septum primum fuses with the endocardial cushion and closes the ostium primum off completely.

Although the precise causes of ASDs are not known, abnormal genes in combination with certain maternal risk factors (e.g., environment, foods, and medicines) are believed to play a role.

Diagnosis

The diagnosis of ASD is usually based upon its characteristic clinical manifestations and confirmed by echocardiography. The combination of 2-dimensional echocardiographic

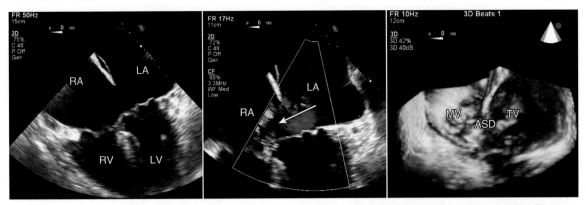

FIGURE 40-3 Echocardiograph of an ostium primum atrial septal defect (ASD) in a 64-year-old man. The Transesophageal echocardiogram (TEE) 4-chamber view (left) shows an ostium primum ASD, with color Doppler (center) showing left-to-right flow across the large defect. Three-dimensional imaging (right) shows the relationship between the ASD and the mitral valve (MV) and tricuspid (TV) valve. (From Otto CM: *Textbook of Clinical Echocardiography*, ed 5, 2013, Elsevier/Saunders.) *LA*, Left atrium; *LV*, left ventricle; *RA*, right atrium; *RV*, right ventricle.

imaging and Doppler color flow mapping is both sensitive and specific for the identification of ASD. Figure 40-3 shows an echocardiograph of an ostium primum ASD in a 64-year-old man.

Clinical Manifestations

The patient with an ASD can present at any age. In a small ASD, the baby may not have any remarkable signs or symptoms. The clinical manifestations are dependent on the size of the defect and the degree of shunting between the atria. In some infants with a moderate to large ASD, the clinical manifestations include heart failure, tachypnea, respiratory distress, substernal and intercostal retractions, crackles, failure to thrive, recurrent respiratory infection, and hepatomegaly.

In the older patient, common signs and symptoms include exercise intolerance, dyspnea, fatigue, heart arrhythmias (e.g., atrial flutter and fibrillation), heart failure, and swollen feet and hands. In all ages, a moderate to large ASD may produce a systolic murmur and a fixed split second heart sound (S_2), a QRS pattern suggestive of incomplete right bundle branch block, and a chest radiograph that shows cardiac enlargement and increased pulmonary vascularity. The heart murmur may be faint, and the diagnosis is easily overlooked, particularly in adults.

Treatment

Treatment is based on the seriousness of the signs and symptoms and the size of the ASD. Catheter-based procedures or surgery is required to repair the defect. Surgical risk and mortality is lowest when the ASD repair is performed under age 25 and before development of significant pulmonary hypertension.

For the newborn, the standard respiratory care protocols—i.e., oxygen therapy protocol, bronchopulmonary hygiene therapy protocol, lung expansion therapy protocol, aerosolized medication therapy protocol, and ventilator support protocols—are all administered as needed (see Newborn Respiratory Therapy Protocols, Chapter 32)

Ventricular Septal Defect

Anatomic Alterations of the Heart

A **ventricular septal defect** is a congenital heart defect in which there is an opening in the ventricular septum of the heart. There may be one or more openings in different locations of the ventricular septum. Common locations include:

- **Conoventricular Ventricular Septal Defect**—located where portions of the ventricular septum normally form below the pulmonary and aortic valves (see Figure 40-4-1)
- **Inlet Ventricular Septal Defect**—located near where blood enters the ventricles through the tricuspid and mitral valves. This congenital heart defect may be part of another heart defect called *atrioventricular septal defect (AVSD)* (see Figure 40-4-2).
- **Perimembranous Ventricular Septal Defect**—located in the upper portion of the ventricular septum (see Figure 40-4-3).
- **Muscular Ventricular Septal Defect**—located in the lower, muscular part of the ventricular septum. It is the most common type of VSD (see Figure 40-4-4).

The pathophysiology of a VSD depends upon the size of the defect and the pulmonary vascular resistance. At birth, the following physiologic events normally occur: (1) an immediate fall in pulmonary vascular resistance, (2) the removal of the low resistance placenta from circulation, and (3) the closure of the ductus arteriosus. In response to these normal physiologic changes, the left ventricle must contract against a higher systemic vascular resistance while, at the same time, the right ventricle contracts against a lower pulmonary vascular resistance. As a result of these vascular resistance changes, the pressure in the left ventricle quickly becomes greater (~80 to 90 mm Hg) than the pressure in the right ventricle (~20 mm Hg)—which, in turn, causes blood flow from the left to the right ventricle during each contraction. In short, a *left-to-right* shunt develops (noncyanotic disorder) (see Figure 40-4).

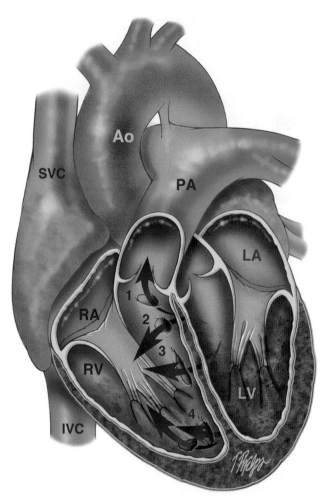

FIGURE 40-4 A ventricular septal defect (VSD) is a congenital heart defect in which there is an opening in the ventricular septum of the heart. Common VSDs are conoventricular ventricular septal defect *(1)*, inlet ventricular septal defect *(2)*, perimembranous ventricular septal defect *(3)*, and muscular ventricular septal defect *(4)*. *Ao*, Aorta; *IVC*, inferior vena cava; *LA*, left atrium; *LV*, left ventricle; *PA*, pulmonary artery; *RA*, right atrium; *RV*, right ventricle; *SVC*, superior vena cava.

A VSD has the following two net effects: First, the influx of blood into the right ventricle from the left ventricle increases the right ventricular pressure and volume; in turn, this can lead to pulmonary hypertension, arrhythmias, and heart failure. Second, the circuitous route of blood through the lungs and back to the heart causes a volume overload and elevated pressure in the left ventricle as well.

Etiology and Epidemiology

VSD is the most common congenital heart disorder. It occurs in almost 50% of all patients with CHD. According to the CDC, the prevalence of VSD is about 42 of 10,000 babies each year. Although the precise causes of VSDs are not known, abnormal genes in combination with certain maternal risk factors (e.g., environment, foods, and medicines) are believed to play a role. VSDs are frequently associated with certain congenital conditions, such as Down's syndrome.

Diagnosis

The diagnosis of VSD is usually based upon its characteristic clinical findings and confirmed by echocardiography. The combination of 2-dimensional echocardiographic imaging and Doppler color flow mapping is both sensitive and specific for the identification of VSD. Figure 40-5 shows an echocardiograph of a large VSD in a 26-year-old woman.

Clinical Manifestations

The patient with a VSD can present at any age. The size of the VSD influences what signs and symptoms, if any, are present. Often, if the opening is small, it closes on its own and the baby will never show any signs of a VSD. When the VSD is moderate or large, the early clinical manifestations include tachycardia, tachypnea, increased work of breathing, poor weight gain, failure to thrive, and diaphoresis. At 3 to 4 weeks of age, the baby usually manifests signs of heart failure, which include continued tachycardia and tachypnea, poor feeding (appears hungry, but tires easily and sweats with feeding), poor weight gain, hepatomegaly, pulmonary

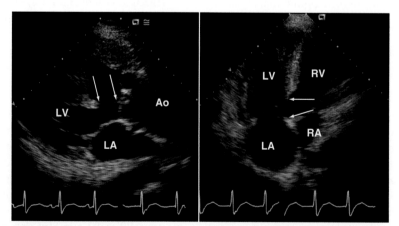

FIGURE 40-5 Echocardiograph of a large ventricular septal defect (VSD) in a 26-year-old woman. A large VSD (between arrows) is seen in a parasternal long-axis view (left) and an apical 4-chamber view (right). Severe RV hypertrophy is present. Doppler examination will show low-velocity bidirectional flow across the defect due to equalization of RV and LV pressures. (From Otto CM: *Textbook of Clinical Echocardiography*, ed 5, 2013, Elsevier/Saunders.) *Ao*, aorta; *LA*, left atrium; *LV*, left ventricle; *RA*, right atrium; *RV*, right ventricle.

crackles, grunting, intercostal retractions, and pallor (from peripheral vasoconstriction).

Cardiac clinical manifestations include systolic murmurs at the mid-to-lower left sternal border, an increased second heart sound (S_2), diastolic murmurs at the apex (indicates a Qp/Qs of 2:1 or greater), and diastolic murmurs at the mid-to-lower sternal border (indicating aortic or pulmonary regurgitation and left-to-right shunting). In addition, infants with a moderate to large VSD may develop a right ventricular heave as the pulmonary vascular pressure falls and the left-to-right shunt increases. Also, the dilated pulmonary trunk and pulmonary valve closure may be palpable, the cardiac apex may be displaced outside the midclavicular line as the heart enlarges, and vigorous precordial activity and a dynamic left ventricular impulse may be present.

In patients with VSD and aortic regurgitation, the left ventricle is especially overloaded because of both the regurgitated volume from the aorta and the increased volume of blood returning to the left atrium from the pulmonary circulation. Clinical features include neck pulsations, bounding pulse, wide pulse pressure, early diastolic murmur, diaphoresis, and vigorous precordial movement (particularly in the left lateral recumbent position). The electrocardiographic findings may indicate increased volume and pressure loads on the left and right ventricles. The chest radiograph may show increased pulmonary vascular markings, and enlargement of the left atrium, left ventricle and pulmonary artery. Magnetic resonance imaging may be helpful in showing how much blood is flowing to the lungs. Echocardiography is usually performed to confirm the diagnosis of a suspected VSD (see Figure 40-5).

Treatment

Smaller congenital VSDs often close within the first year of life as the heart grows. Moderate or large VSDs, however, usually require surgical intervention to close the defect. Continuing care may involve medications to support the heart (e.g., digitalis and diuretics) as well as close monitoring for early signs or symptoms of congestive heart failure. For the newborn, the standard respiratory care protocols—i.e., oxygen therapy protocol, bronchopulmonary hygiene therapy protocol, lung expansion therapy protocol, aerosolized medication therapy protocol, and ventilator support protocols—are all administered as needed (see Newborn Respiratory Therapy Protocols, Chapter 32)

Tetralogy of Fallot

Anatomic Alterations of the Heart

Tetralogy of Fallot (TOF) is a congenital heart defect with the following four major anatomic alterations:

- **Stenosis of the pulmonary artery**—This defect is commonly described as a narrowing of the right ventricular outflow tract. The obstruction can occur at the pulmonary valve—called a **valvular stenosis** or just below the pulmonary valve—called an **infundibular stenosis**. The infundibular stenosis is primarily caused by an overgrowth of the heart muscle wall. Note: *The degree of stenosis varies*

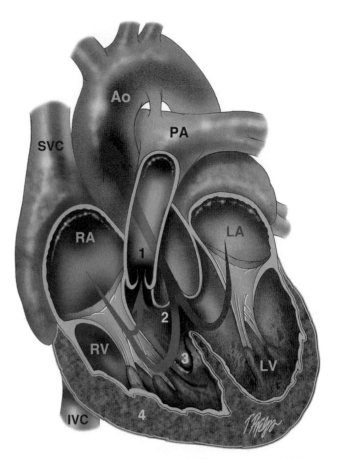

FIGURE 40-6 **Tetralogy of Fallot (TOF)** is a congenital heart defect that includes (**A**) stenosis of the pulmonary artery *(1)*, (**B**) deviation of the aorta to the right *(2)*, (**C**) ventricular septal defect *(3)*, and (**D**) right ventricular hypertrophy *(4)*. *Ao,* Aorta; *IVC,* inferior vena cava; *LA,* left atrium; *LV,* left ventricle; *PA,* pulmonary artery; *RA,* right atrium; *RV,* right ventricle; *SVC,* superior vena cava.

and is the primary determinant of symptoms and severity (see Figure 40-6, 1).

- **Deviation of the aorta to the right** (also known as a dextroposition of the aorta)—The aortic valve is situated directly over the ventricular septal defect, and connected to both the right and left ventricles. The degree to which the aorta is attached to the right ventricle is referred to as its degree of "override." The degree of aortic override is quite variable; between 5% and 95% of the aortic valve may be connected to the right ventricle (see Figure 40-6, 2).

- **Ventricular septal defect**—The defect is centered near the most superior portion of the ventricular septum, and is usually a single, large hole (see Figure 40-6, 3).

- **Right ventricular hypertrophy**—The right ventricle is more muscular than normal and causes a characteristic boot-shaped (**coeur-en-sabot**) appearance on the chest radiograph (Figure 40-7). Because of the pulmonic stenosis and increased obstruction to the right outflow tract, the right ventricular wall increases in size. Right ventricular hypertrophy is generally considered to be a secondary anomaly (see Figure 40-6, 4).

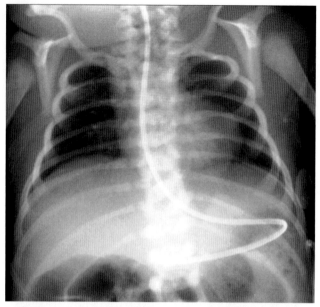

FIGURE 40-7 Tetralogy of Fallot (TOF). In TOF, **coeur-en-sabot** (French for "boot-shaped heart") is used to describe a radiologic silhouette of a heart that resembles that of a wooden shoe commonly see in patients with Tetralogy of Fallot. The "boot's toe" corresponds to an elevated cardiac apex, while the broad "foot" portion corresponds to an increased prominence of the left cardiac border caused by right cardiac hypertrophy. Coeur en sabot is the typical radiologic appearance of well-developed Tetralogy of Fallot—i.e., infundibular pulmonary valve stenosis, ventricular septal defect, right ventricular hypertrophy, and dextroposition of the aorta. (Image provided courtesy of Dayton Children's Hospital, Dayton, Ohio).

The pathophysiologic effects—and clinical symptoms—of TOF are largely dependent upon the degree of right ventricular outflow tract obstruction. The direction of blood flow across the VSD is determined by the path of least resistance, not the size of the VSD. For example, if the pulmonary vascular resistance is lower than the systemic vascular resistance, then there will be a predominant left-to-right shunt—and, in this case, the patient will not likely be cyanotic (noncyanotic disorder). However, when there is a significant right ventricular outflow tract obstruction—i.e., a significant pulmonary stenosis—there will be a *right-to-left* shunt across the VSD and cyanosis will ensue (cyanotic disorder).

One of the unique physiologic features of TOF is that the right ventricular outflow tract obstruction often fluctuates in response to transient increases and decreases in the resistance caused by obstruction. The precise mechanism for this obstruction variation is unclear, although several mechanisms, such as increased infundibular contractility, peripheral vasodilation, hyperventilation, and stimulation of the right ventricular mechanoreceptors, have been proposed. During the most dramatic fluctuation events, there can be a near complete occlusion of the right ventricular outflow tract, resulting in a very high resistance and a significant right-to-left shunting with profound cyanosis. These episodes are referred to as "**tet spells**" or "**hypercyanotic spells**." A typical tet spell is characterized by a sudden, marked increase in cyanosis, followed by syncope. Older children will often squat during a tet spell in an effort to increase systemic vascular resistance to help generate a temporary reversal of the right-to-left shunt.

Etiology and Epidemiology

The prevalence of TOF in the United States is about 4 per 10,000 live births, and it accounts for about 7% to 10% of the CHDs. According to the CDC, about 1600 infants are born each year with TOF. TOF is the most common congenital heart disorder to require intervention in the first year of life and occurs equally in males and females. Although the precise causes of TOF are not known, abnormal genes in combination with certain maternal risk factors (e.g., environment, foods, and medicines) are believed to play a role.

Diagnosis

TOF is generally confirmed by echocardiography. Additional tests include electrocardiogram and chest radiography. However, findings from these studies are often suggestive but not conclusive for the diagnosis of TOF. Cardiac catheterization may be needed to further delineate the anatomic alterations and to quantify the resulting hemodynamic pathology.

Clinical Manifestations

The clinical presentation of TOF depends on the degree of right ventricular outflow tract obstruction. Early signs and symptoms include episodes of pronounced cyanosis—i.e., "hypercyanotic "or "tet" spells—especially during crying or feeding. Oxygen saturation during hypercyanotic spells is low, although in between spells it is often normal. Feeding is usually difficult and the infant typically fails to thrive. Most infants are smaller than expected for their age.

On palpation, there may be a prominent right ventricular impulse and **systolic thrill** (i.e., a vibration felt by the examiner on palpation). Cardiac auscultation may reveal a single second heart sound (S_2) since the pulmonic component is rarely audible. An early systolic click (called an **aortic ejection click**) along the left sternal border may be heard, which is thought to be due to flow into the dilated ascending aorta. Symptoms of heart failure may be present. Although the chest radiograph often appears normal, the classic "boot-shaped" heart (coeur en sabot) is the hallmark of the disorder (see Figure 40-7).

A heart murmur is commonly heard primarily because of the right ventricular outflow tract obstruction—not the VSD. The murmur is described as a crescendo and decrescendo sound with a harsh systolic ejection quality. It is best heard along the left mid- to upper-sternal border. The murmur can have a more regurgitant quality that can be mistaken for a VSD. The murmur is caused by both the degree of obstruction and the amount of flow through the obstruction. Unlike an isolated pulmonary stenosis, in a TOF the amount of blood flow that can be pumped across the right ventricular outflow tract obstruction often varies—i.e., the blood flow decreases as the obstruction increases, and there is a right-to-left shunt. Thus, during periods of increased obstruction, the heart murmur will become softer. During severe hypercyanotic spells, the murmur may actually disappear as a result of the markedly diminished flow across the obstruction.

Treatment

The management of TOF entails initial medical care, surgical palliative care and intracardiac repair, and long-term postoperative care. The need for medical intervention is dependent on the degree of the right ventricular outflow tract obstruction. Severe cases may require intravenous prostaglandin therapy (alprostadil) to maintain ductal patency pending surgical repair. The step-wise management for patients who experience hypercyanotic ("tet") spells includes knee-chest positioning to increase systemic vascular resistance, oxygen therapy, intravenous morphine and fluid bolus, and, if these measures fail, intravenous beta-blockers. Patients with symptoms of heart failure may require diuretic therapy (e.g., furosemide) and digoxin.

Intracardiac repair can be performed by 3 months of age. The surgery consists of a patch closure of the ventricular septal defect and enlargement of the right ventricular outflow tract. Chronic postoperative complications include pulmonary regurgitation with associated right ventricular enlargement, residual right ventricular outflow tract obstruction, right ventricular dysfunction, aortic root dilation and aortic valve insufficiency, and arrhythmias including atrial and ventricular tachycardia. Long-term follow-up care includes routine health-care visits and cardiac testing (e.g., electrocardiogram, echocardiogram, Holter monitoring, exercise testing, and occasionally repeat cardiac magnetic resonance imaging or computed tomography).

The prognosis is poor for patients with uncorrected TOF. Surgical correction has shown excellent long-term survival. Patients who have surgery at a young age have a reported survival rate >90% at 25 years after the surgical repair. Arrhythmias and heart failure are the most common causes of death following surgical repair.

For the newborn, the standard respiratory care protocols—i.e., oxygen therapy protocol, bronchopulmonary hygiene therapy protocol, lung expansion therapy protocol, aerosolized medication therapy protocol, and ventilator support protocols—are all administered as needed (see Newborn Respiratory Therapy Protocols, Chapter 32).

Transposition of the Great Arteries

Anatomic Alterations of the Heart

Transposition of the Great Arteries (also known as transposition of the great vessels) is the most common cyanotic congenital heart lesion that presents in neonates. TGA is a congenital heart defect in which the pulmonary artery and the aorta are switched in position, or transposed. In short, the aorta arises from the right ventricle and the pulmonary artery arises from the left ventricle. The most common form of TGA is the **dextrotransposition of the great arteries (d-TGA),** in which the origin of the aorta is anterior and to the right of the pulmonary artery (see Figure 40-8).

TGA results in a pulmonary and systemic circulation that functions in "parallel," rather than "series." In other words, the deoxygenated venous blood returning to the right atrium and right ventricle is pumped directly back into the systemic

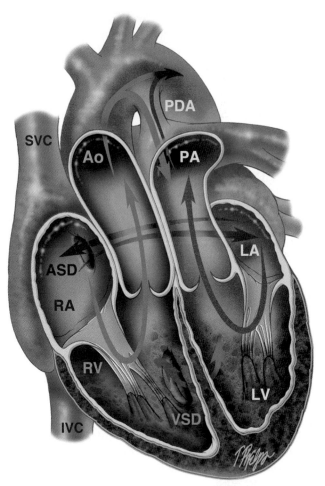

FIGURE 40-8 Transposition of the great arteries is a congenital heart defect in which the pulmonary artery and the aorta are switched in position, or transposed. TGA is commonly associated with an atrial septal defect, a ventricular septal defect, or a patent ductus arteriosus. *Ao,* Aorta; *ASD,* atrial septal defect; *IVC,* inferior vena cava; *LA,* left atrium; *LV,* left ventricle; *PA,* pulmonary artery; *PDA,* patent ductus arteriosus; *RA,* right atrium; *RV,* right ventricle; *SVC,* superior vena cava; *VSD,* ventricular septal defect.

circulation via the aorta, which is connected to the right ventricle—completely bypassing the lungs. This heart defect produces a *right-to-left shunt*—a cyanotic disorder. The oxygenated blood returning to the left atrium and ventricle from the lungs is pumped directly back into the pulmonary circulation via the pulmonary artery, which is connected to the left ventricle—completely bypassing the systemic circulation.

The severity of the symptoms associated with a TGA depends on whether there are additional heart defects that allow the two separate blood circulations to mingle—and, as a result, provide an alternative pathway for oxygenated blood to enter the systemic circulation. Fortunately (relatively speaking), a TGA is usually accompanied by one or more additional heart defects that provide a direct connection between these two circulations. The most common heart defects are the following:

- **Atrial septal defect**—is the most common. Depending on pressure differences between the right and left atrium at any given moment, blood may move in either direction through the ASD—i.e., either a left-to-right or right-to-left shunt. When oxygenated blood from the left atrium moves into the right atrium (a left-to-right shunt) and mixes with the nonoxygenated blood, the newly mixed blood can move into the right ventricle—and then on to the aorta and systemic circulation. However, when nonoxygenated blood moves from the right atrium into the left atrium (a right-to-left shunt) and mixes, some of this blood will move into the left ventricle and be pumped to the lungs via the pulmonary artery (see Figure 40-8).

- **Ventricular septal defect**—occurs in about 50% of TGA cases. Depending on pressure differences between the right and left ventricles at any given moment, blood may move in either direction through the VSD—i.e., either a left-to-right or right-to-left shunt. When oxygenated blood from the left ventricle moves into the right ventricle (a left-to-right shunt) and mixes with the nonoxygenated blood, some of this blood will be pumped through the aorta and out to the body. However, when nonoxygenated blood moves from the right ventricle into the left ventricle (a right-to-left shunt) and mixes, some of this blood will be pumped to the lungs via the pulmonary artery (see Figure 40-8).
- **Patent ductus arteriosus**—is often seen in patients with TGA. Again, depending on the pressure differences between the ductus arteriosus and the aorta at any given moment, blood may flow in either direction. When additional heart defects exist that allow oxygenated blood to enter the left ventricle, some of this blood may enter the systemic circulation when a right-to-left shunt is present (see Figure 40-8).

Other heart defects associated with TGA include a patent foramen ovale, left ventricular outflow tract obstruction, aortic arch obstruction, mitral and tricuspid valve abnormalities, and coronary artery anatomic variations. When no other heart defects are present, it is called **Simple Transposition of the Great Arteries (simple TGA)**. When other defects are present, it is a **Complex Transposition of the Great Arteries (complex TGA)**. The magnitude of these defects may impact cardiac function, mixing, and surgical approach.

Etiology and Epidemiology

The prevalence of TGA ranges from 2.3 to 4.7 per 10,000 live births in the United States. According to the CDC, approximately 1900 babies are born with TGA each year here. Although the precise cause of TGA is not known, it is associated with poor nutrition during pregnancy, rubella, or other viral illness during pregnancy, alcoholism, maternal age over 40 years, and Down's syndrome.

Diagnosis

The diagnosis of TGA is based on clinical suspicion of an underlying cyanotic CHD and is confirmed by echocardiography.

Clinical Manifestations

Infants with TGA commonly demonstrate cyanosis, tachypnea (respiratory rates >60 breaths/min), poor feeding, and clubbing of fingers and toes. When there is a VSD, a **pansystolic murmur** (a murmur occupying the entire systolic interval, from first to second hear sound) is usually present within a few days after birth at the lower left sternal borders. The intensity of the murmur is dependent on the turbulence of blood flow through the septal defect. In the patient with left ventricular outflow obstruction, there may be a systolic ejection murmur[3] along the upper left sternal border. The intensity of the murmur is a function of both the degree of obstruction and the amount of blood flow across the obstruction.

Treatment

The initial postnatal management of TGA is directed at stabilizing the patient's cardiac and pulmonary function and ensuring adequate systemic oxygenation. Therapy is focused on providing adequate mixing between the two circulatory systems. This can be accomplished by **prostaglandin E1** (alprostadil) therapy (to maintain patency of the ductus arteriosus), **balloon atrial septostomy (BAS)**,[4] and, ultimately, surgical repair. Surgical correction (e.g., arterial switch operation or atrial switch procedure) is necessary for survival in patients with TGA.

Complications of surgery include pulmonary artery stenosis, coronary artery insufficiency, neoaortic root dilation, neoaortic regurgitation, artery stenosis, coronary artery insufficiency, neoaortic root dilation, atrial arrhythmias, and progressive heart failure. Long-term follow-up care is required because of the potential complications. It entails a focused history, physical examinations, various tests such as echocardiography, electrocardiography, and angiography, and monitoring for atherosclerotic disease. Long-term survival is excellent with >90% survival after 20 years. Although patients may have reduced exercise tolerance, their typical daily level of activity is usually not restricted.

For the newborn, the standard respiratory care protocols—i.e., oxygen therapy protocol, bronchopulmonary hygiene therapy protocol, lung expansion therapy protocol, aerosolized medication therapy protocol, and ventilator support protocols—are all administered as needed (see Newborn Respiratory Therapy Protocols, Chapter 32).

---

[3]**Systolic ejection** or midsystolic **murmurs** are due to turbulent forward flow across the right and left ventricular outflow tract, aortic or pulmonary valve, or through the aorta or pulmonary artery.

[4]**Balloon atrial septostomy (BAS)** (also known as the Rashkind procedure) is a life-saving technique used to enlarge a hole between the right atrium and the left atrium. It is often used to manage patients with transposition of the great arteries. The larger hole improves oxygenation of the blood. This is normally a palliative procedure used to prepare patients for, or sustain them until, corrective surgery.

A 3.41-kg boy was delivered by vaginal delivery at 40 weeks to a 32-year-old mother. The mother had good prenatal care; her pregnancy was unremarkable, and her fetal ultrasound was read as normal. After being warmed and examined, the infant was taken to the regular nursery.

Upon arrival to the nursery, vital signs showed heart rate 150 beats/min, respiratory rate 50 breaths/min, blood pressure 70/35. The baby appeared to be comfortable, mildly tachypneic, and mildly cyanotic. Breath sounds were clear. No heart murmur was heard. A pulse oximeter was placed on the infant's right hand and the SpO_2 was 70%.

The nurse called for the respiratory team leader to assess the infant. She began blow-by oxygen with a resuscitation bag. When the respiratory team leader arrived, he noted that the infant was breathing comfortably; there was no nasal flaring, no grunting, no stridor, and good aeration with all lung fields clear. He checked the blow-by oxygen set-up to make sure that it was hooked up correctly to oxygen via the flowmeter in the nursery. It was set up correctly. The blow-by oxygen had raised the SpO_2 to 73%. The therapist also noted that, while placing his stethoscope on the infant's chest, the patient cried and his color appeared cyanotic. At this time, the respiratory therapist charted the following SOAP:

S N/A

O Term infant, HR 150, RR 50, B/P 70/35, SpO_2 73% and cyanotic on blow-by 100% oxygen. No apparent respiratory distress; no nasal flaring, grunting, or stridor. Mild tachypnea. Clear breath sounds in all fields. Crying appears to make the infant more cyanotic.

A Newborn condition that appears to be refractory to oxygen. Stable at the moment. Does not appear to be respiratory or neurologic in nature with good bilateral aeration and tachypnea. Need to rule out cardiac cause.

P Recommend hyperoxia challenge to rule out CHD.

The team leader removed the infant from the oxygen blow-by and obtained an ABG from the infant's right radial artery on room air. The results were pH 7.25, $PaCO_2$ 31 mm Hg, HCO_3^- 13 mEq/L, PaO_2 32 mm Hg, and SaO_2 54%. The respiratory therapist made a note of metabolic acidosis with hypoxemia. Next, the infant was placed in an oxygen head hood with 100% oxygen (an FIO_2 1.0) and sufficient flow to meet his inspiratory demand. A second ABG was drawn from the left radial 10 minutes later. The results were as follows: pH 7.23, $PaCO_2$ 30 mm Hg, HCO_3^- 12 mEq/L, PaO_2 44 mm Hg, and SaO_2 67%. The hyperoxia challenge strongly suggested that the infant had a congenital heart lesion with significant right-to-left shunting.

At this time, the nurse and team leader contacted the attending pediatrician with the hyperoxia test results. The doctor requested a stat cardiology consult, chest radiograph, electrocardiogram, and echocardiogram. Luckily, a cardiologist was available to assess the infant. He ordered prostaglandin infusion until a more definitive diagnosis could be made. While the prostaglandins were being sent up by pharmacy, the chest radiograph showed an "egg-shaped heart on a string," indicative of transposition of the great vessels. The cardiologist instructed the nursery charge nurse to arrange for transport of the infant to a tertiary pediatric center for cardiovascular surgery evaluation.

Discussion

When a respiratory therapist is faced with a cyanotic infant, he/she should first try to determine if the cause is respiratory, cardiac, or neurologic in origin. If an infant demonstrates respiratory distress with cyanosis, a respiratory cause should be expected. Oxygen and possibly surfactant with lung inflation/ventilation will be effective in treating this type of hypoxemia. If a cyanotic infant is born to a mother who is addicted to narcotics or overly sedated during delivery, the hypoxemia is likely the result of respiratory depression; the infant may present with apnea or ineffective respiratory effort. Manual ventilation or medications to reverse the narcotic effect can be used to improve oxygenation and ventilation until the infant recovers. The latter, however, may precipitate acute withdrawal symptoms in an infant born to an addicted mother.

An infant with CHD, who is cyanotic beyond the normal postdelivery period, generally presents with unlabored breathing and often tachypnea to compensate for a mild growing metabolic acidosis. This infant will not respond to oxygen, because the blood is being shunted away from the pulmonary vascular bed. If the hyperoxia test demonstrates a lack of response to 100% oxygen, the infant has a right-to-left shunt as a part of the cardiac defect. Defects of this magnitude warrant rapid evaluation by echocardiograph, and possibly medical treatment with prostaglandins or balloon septostomy to maintain mixing between the arterial and venous circulation.

In the case presented, the infant was cyanotic and failed to respond to supplemental oxygen administration; in addition, the hyperoxia test demonstrated a large right-to-left shunt. These findings are all consistent with the presentation of severe CHD in the newborn. The chest radiograph was suggestive of transposition of the great vessels. The cardiologist initiated a prostaglandin infusion to prevent the ductus arteriosus from closing, which would markedly worsen the infant's oxygenation and metabolic acidosis. Transferring the infant to a center with a pediatric cardiologist and eventually cardiothoracic surgery will be key to a successful outcome.

Today most severe CHD lesions are identified by prenatal ultrasound. Ideally these babies should be delivered at hospitals where pediatric cardiac services are available to diagnose and treat the newborn with CHD. It is important to remember that the pregnant mother is still the best transport incubator ever devised!

Note: Technical accuracy in the delivery of oxygen is also important when treating infants with oxygen or using oxygen to help diagnose a shunt. This was why it was important for the respiratory team leader to make sure that the delivery gas was actually oxygen. It is possible in a nursery (where medical air is available) for staff to connect their oxygen equipment to a medical air flowmeter. A mask attached to medical air would likely not improve the infant's SpO_2 and confuse the clinical team.

SELF-ASSESSMENT QUESTIONS

See Evolve Resources for answers. To access additional student assessment questions visit **http://evolve.elsevier.com/DesJardins/respiratory**.

1. **Which of the following congenital heart defects is associated with an infundibular stenosis?**
   a. Transposition of the great arteries
   b. Patent ductus arteriosus
   c. Tetralogy of Fallot
   d. Ventricular septal defect

2. **In a ventricular septal defect (VSD), all the following are correct EXCEPT:**
   a. The defect may be a muscular ventricular septal defect
   b. A right-to-left shunt develops
   c. The diagnosis is confirmed by echocardiography
   d. The patient with a VSD can present at any age

3. **"Hypercyanotic" or "tet spells" are associated with which of the following disorders?**
   a. Tetralogy of Fallot
   b. Ventricular septal defect
   c. Transposition of the great arteries
   d. Patent ductus arteriosus

4. **During normal fetal development, the cavity of the primitive atrium is subdivided into right and left chambers by a structure called the:**
   a. Septum secundum
   b. Ostium primum
   c. Ostium secundum
   d. Septum primum

5. **In which of the following congenital disorders is a balloon atrial septostomy sometimes used as a palliative procedure until a corrective surgery can be performed?**
   a. Transposition of the great arteries
   b. Ventricular septal defect
   c. Tetralogy of Fallot
   d. Atrial septal defect

Croup Syndrome: Laryngotracheobronchitis and Acute Epiglottitis

Chapter Objectives

After reading this chapter, you will be able to:
- List the anatomic alterations of the lungs associated with inspiratory stridor (croup) syndrome.
- Describe the causes of inspiratory stridor (croup) syndrome.
- List the cardiopulmonary clinical manifestations associated with inspiratory stridor (croup) syndrome.
- Describe the general management of inspiratory stridor (croup) syndrome.
- Describe the clinical strategies and rationales of the SOAPs presented in the case studies.

Key Terms

Acute Epiglottitis
Cool Aerosol Mist
Croup
Haemophilus Influenzae Type B
Inspiratory Stridor
Laryngotracheobronchitis (LTB)
Parainfluenza Viruses
Racemic Epinephrine
Steeple Point or Pencil Point (Lateral Neck Radiograph—LTB)
Subglottic Airway Obstruction
Subglottic Croup

Supraglottic Airway Obstruction
Supraglottic Croup
"Thumb Sign" (Lateral Neck Radiograph—Epiglottis)

Chapter Outline

Introduction

The word **croup** is a general term used to describe the inspiratory, barking or brassy sound associated with a partial upper airway obstruction. In other words, croup is actually a clinical sign (objective data) or a clinical manifestation—that is, the "barking or brassy sound" associated with a partial upper airway obstruction. Clinically, the inspiratory barking sound heard in a patient with a partial upper airway obstruction is called **inspiratory stridor**.

Most experts use the term *croup* and **laryngotracheobron-chitis (LTB)**—which is a **subglottic airway obstruction**—interchangeably. **Acute epiglottitis**—which is a **supraglottic airway obstruction**—is regarded as an entirely separate disease entity (Figure 41-1). Historically, this is probably a result, in part, of the fact that the inspiratory stridor (i.e., the

croup sound) associated with a patient with LTB is usually a loud and high-pitched brassy sound, whereas the inspiratory stridor associated with a patient with acute epiglottis is often lower in pitch, muffled, or even absent.

In addition, some sources refer to LTB as a **subglottic croup** and to acute epiglottitis as a **supraglottic croup**. In essence, these phrases (*subglottic croup* versus *supraglottic croup*) simply mean that the inspiratory stridor sound originates from either the subglottic area (i.e., in LTB) or the supraglottic area (i.e., in acute epiglottitis).

Thus, in view of the confusing nature of the term *croup* and the two types of partial upper airway disorders—LTB and acute epiglottis—for clarity, the phrase *inspiratory stridor* will always be used in place of the term *croup* throughout this chapter.

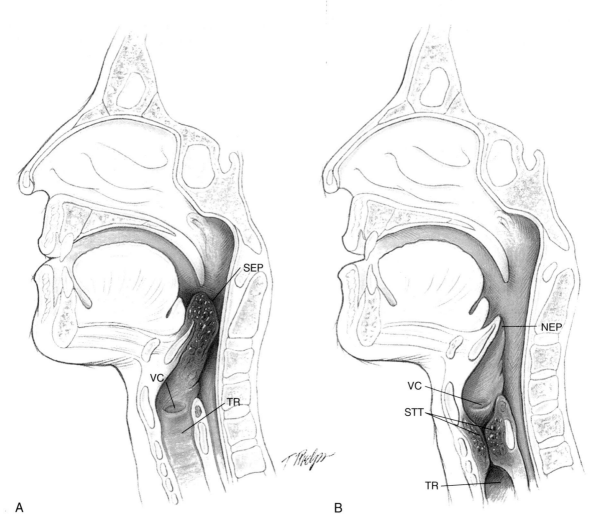

FIGURE 41-1 Laryngotracheobronchitis and acute epiglottitis. **A**, Acute epiglottitis. **B**, Laryngotracheobronchitis. *NEP*, Normal epiglottis; *SEP*, swollen epiglottis; *STT*, swollen tracheal tissue; *TR*, trachea. *VC*, vocal cords.

Anatomic Alterations of the Upper Airway

Laryngotracheobronchitis

Because laryngotracheobronchitis can affect the lower laryngeal area, trachea, and occasionally the bronchi, the term *laryngotracheobronchitis* is used as a synonym for "classic" subglottic obstruction (see Figure 41-1, B). Pathologically, LTB is an inflammatory process that causes edema and swelling of the mucous membranes. Although the laryngeal mucosa and submucosa are vascular, the distribution of the lymphatic capillaries is uneven or absent in this region. Consequently, when edema develops in the upper airway, fluid spreads and accumulates quickly throughout the connective tissues, which causes the mucosa to swell and the airway lumen to narrow. The inflammation also causes the mucous glands to increase their production of mucus and the cilia to lose their effectiveness as a mucociliary transport mechanism.

Because the subglottic area is the narrowest region of the larynx in an infant or small child, even a slight degree of edema can cause a significant reduction in cross-sectional area of the airway. The edema in this area is further aggravated by the rigid cricoid cartilage, which surrounds the subglottic trachea and prevents external swelling as fluid engorges the laryngeal tissues. The edema and swelling in the subglottic region decrease the ability of the vocal cords to abduct (move apart) during inspiration. This further reduces the cross-sectional area of airway in this region.

Acute Epiglottitis

Acute epiglottitis is a life-threatening emergency. In contrast to LTB, epiglottitis is an inflammation of the supraglottic region, which includes the epiglottis, aryepiglottic folds, and false vocal cords (see Figure 41-1, A). Epiglottitis does not involve the pharynx, trachea, or other subglottic structures. As the edema in the epiglottis increases, the lateral borders curl and the tip of the epiglottis protrudes posteriorly and inferiorly. During inspiration the swollen epiglottis is pulled (or sucked) over the laryngeal inlet. In severe cases, this may completely block the laryngeal opening. Clinically, the classic finding is a swollen, cherry-red epiglottis, severe respiratory distress and drooling.

The major pathologic or structural changes associated with *inspiratory stridor* are as follows:

- LTB—Airway obstruction caused by tissue swelling just *below* the vocal cords
- Epiglottitis—Airway obstruction caused by tissue swelling just *above* the vocal cords.

Etiology and Epidemiology

Laryngotracheobronchitis

The **parainfluenza viruses** cause most cases of LTB, with type 1 being the most common, type 3 less common, and type 2 infrequent. LTB also may be caused by influenza A and B, respiratory syncytial virus (RSV), herpes simplex virus, *Mycoplasma pneumoniae,* rhinovirus, and adenoviruses. LTB is primarily seen in children 6 months to 5 years of age, with peak prevalence in the second year of life. Boys are affected slightly more often than girls. The onset of LTB is slow (i.e., symptoms progressively increase over 24 to 48 hours), and it is most common during the fall and winter. A brassy or barking cough is commonly present. The child's voice is hoarse, and the inspiratory stridor is typically loud and high in pitch. The patient usually does not have a fever, drooling, swallowing difficulties, or a toxic appearance.

Acute Epiglottitis*

Acute epiglottitis is a bacterial infection that is almost always caused by **Haemophilus influenzae type B.** It is transmitted via aerosol droplets. Since 1985, when vaccinations with *H. influenzae* type B vaccine became widespread, the number of

reported cases of epiglottitis has decreased by over 95%. *H. influenzae* type B, however, is still responsible for 75% of the epiglottitis cases. Other causes of epiglottitis include aspiration of hot liquid and trauma from repeated intubation attempts.

Epiglottitis has no clear-cut geographic or seasonal incidence. Although acute epiglottitis may develop in all age groups (neonatal to adulthood), it most often occurs in children 2 to 6 years of age. Boys are affected more often than girls. The onset of epiglottitis is usually abrupt. Although the initial clinical manifestations are usually mild, they progress rapidly over a 2- to 4-hour period. A common scenario includes a sore throat or mild upper respiratory problems that quickly progresses to a high fever, lethargy, and difficulty in swallowing and handling secretions. The child usually appears pale and septic. As the supraglottic area becomes swollen, breathing becomes noisy, the tongue is often thrust forward during inspiration, and the child may drool. Compared with LTB, the inspiratory stridor is usually softer and lower in pitch. A cough is usually absent with acute epiglottitis. The voice and cry are usually muffled rather than hoarse. Older children commonly complain of a sore throat during swallowing. Acute epiglottitis in adults is typically seen in patients with neck trauma (e.g., blunt force neck injury or aspiration of hot liquid), in those who have been intubated repeatedly, and in drug abuse (crack cocaine) cases.

The general history and physical findings of LTB and epiglottitis are compared and contrasted in Table 41-1.

*It is of interest to note that George Washington, the first president of the United States, died in the winter of 1799 from acute epiglottitis during an epidemic of influenza. The details of the illness were fully recorded by his secretary, Tobias Lear, and this is the first published description in English of this condition. An account is given of the medical treatment and controversies that arose in criticism of the attendant doctors. (From Cohen B: The death of George Washington 1732–99: the history of cynanche. *J Med Biogr* 13:225–231, 2005.)

TABLE 41-1 General History and Physical Findings of Laryngotracheobronchitis (LTB) and Epiglottitis

	LTB	Epiglottitis
Age	6 months–5 years (with the peak prevalence in the second year)	2–6 years
Onset	Usually slow or gradual (24–48 hours)	Abrupt (2–4 hours)
Fever	Absent	Present
Drooling	Absent	Present
Radiograph findings	Haziness in subglottic area, "pencil point" or "steeple point"	Haziness in supraglottic area, "thumb sign"
Inspiratory stridor	High-pitched, brassy, loud sound	Low-pitched and muffled, or absent
Cough	Present (barking or brassy cough)	Absent
Hoarseness	Present	Absent
Swallowing difficulty	Absent	Present
White blood count	Normal (viral—parainfluenza viruses 1, 2, and 3; influenza A and B; respiratory syncytial virus)	Elevated (bacterial—*Haemophilus influenza* type B)

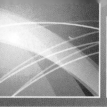
The following clinical manifestations result from the pathologic mechanisms caused (or activated) by an Upper Airway Obstruction—the major anatomic alteration of the lungs associated with laryngotracheobronchitis (LTB) and epiglottitis (see Figure 41-1). It should also be noted that an "upper airway" obstruction is *not* one of the major clinical scenarios discussed in Chapter 9.

CLINICAL DATA OBTAINED AT THE PATIENT'S BEDSIDE

The Physical Examination

Vital Signs

Increased Respiratory Rate (Tachypnea)

Several pathophysiologic mechanisms operating simultaneously may lead to an increased ventilatory rate:

- Increased stimulation of peripheral chemoreceptors
- Anxiety
- Increased temperature (seconday to infection)

Increased Heart Rate (Pulse) and Blood Pressure

Chest Assessment Findings

- Diminished breath sounds

Inspiratory Stridor

Under normal circumstances the slight narrowing of the upper (extrathoracic) airway that naturally occurs during inspiration is insignificant. Because the upper airway is relatively small in infants and children, however, even a slight degree of edema may become significant, particularly at the level of the cricoid cartilage. Thus when the cross-section of the upper airway is reduced because of the edema, the child will generate stridor during inspiration, when the upper airway naturally becomes smaller. It also should be noted that if the edema becomes severe, the patient may generate both inspiratory and expiratory stridor.

Cyanosis

Intermittent coughing spells may produce intermittent cyanosis as secretions obstruct an already limited airway.

Use of Accessory Muscles During Inspiration

Substernal and Intercostal Retractions

CLINICAL DATA OBTAINED FROM LABORATORY TESTS AND SPECIAL PROCEDURES

Arterial Blood Gases*
Mild to Moderate Laryngotracheobronchitis or Epiglottitis

Acute Alveolar Hyperventilation with Hypoxemia[†]
(Acute Respiratory Alkalosis)

pH	$PaCO_2$	HCO_3^-	PaO_2	SaO_2 or SpO_2
↑	↓	↓	↓	↓
		(but normal)		

SEVERE LARYNGOTRACHEOBRONCHITIS OR EPIGLOTTITIS

Acute Ventilatory Failure with Hypoxemia[§]
(This occurs in LTB with fatigue and epiglottitis with obstruction)
(Acute Respiratory Acidosis)

pH[†]	$PaCO_2$	HCO_3^- [†]	PaO_2	SaO_2 or SpO_2
↓	↑	↑	↓	↓
		(but normal)		

Oxygenation Indices[∥]

$\dot{Q}_S/\dot{Q}_T$	DO_2[¶]	$\dot{V}O_2$	$C(a-\bar{v})O_2$	O_2ER	$S\bar{v}O_2$
↑	↓	N	N	↑	↓

*Note: Because of the difficulty of obtaining **arterial blood gas** (ABG) samples from newborn and pediatric patients, **capillary blood gas** (CBG) samples are usually used to determine the pH, $PaCO_2$, and HCO_3^- (i.e., the acid-base and ventilation status only). Capillary PO_2 values are unreliable and should not be used for clinical analysis. The standard way to evaluate the oxygenation status in these young patients is pulse oximetry ($SpCO_2$) (see Chapter 32).

[†]See Figure 4-3 and related discussion for the acute pH, $PaCO_2$, and HCO_3^- changes associated with acute alveolar hyperventilation.

[§]See Figure 4-2 and related discussion for the acute pH, $PaCO_2$, and HCO_3^- changes associated with acute ventilatory failure.

[†]When tissue hypoxia is severe enough to produce lactic acid, the pH and values will be lower than expected for a particular $PaCO_2$ level.

[∥]$C(a-\bar{v})O_2$, Arterial-venous oxygen difference; DO_2, total oxygen delivery; O_2ER, oxygen extraction ratio; $\dot{Q}_S/\dot{Q}_T$, pulmonary shunt fraction; $S\bar{v}O_2$, mixed venous oxygen saturation; $\dot{V}O_2$, oxygen consumption.

[¶]It should be noted that because the newborn normally has a higher hemoglobin (Hb) level at birth (16.8 to 18.9 g% Hb), the DO_2 may be better than the PaO_2 or SpO_2 indicates (see Chapter 5).

OVERVIEW of the Cardiopulmonary Clinical Manifestations Associated with Laryngotracheobronchitis and Epiglottitis—cont'd

LATERAL NECK RADIOGRAPH

- Haziness in the subglottic area (LTB)
- Haziness in the supraglottic area (epiglottitis)
- Classic "thumb sign" (epiglottitis)

ANTERIO-POSTERIOR NECK RADIOGRAPH

- "Steeple point" or "pencil point" narrowing of the upper airway (LTB)

Although the diagnosis of epiglottitis or LTB can generally be made on the basis of the patient's clinical history, radiologic examinations are helpful. A lateral neck radiograph is usually done first to rule out the diagnosis of epiglottitis. Once this film is read as negative, an AP neck is ordered to define the degree of subglottic edema. When the patient has acute epiglottitis, a white haziness is evident in the supraglottic area. In addition, the epiglottitis often appears on a lateral neck radiograph as the classic "thumb sign." The epiglottis is swollen and rounded, giving it an appearance of the distal portion of a thumb (see Figure 41-2). Figure 41-3 shows an infant with new onset leukemia and epiglottitis.

When the patient has LTB, a white haziness is demonstrated in the subglottic area; the AP neck will show the classic "pencil point" or "steeple point" narrowing at the level of the cricoid cartilage (see Figure 41-4). It is also important to mention that a barky cough associated with partial airway obstruction can be caused by a foreign object in the airway—a not-so-infrequent cause in toddlers. Generally, the lateral and AP neck are helpful screens to suggest laryngoscopy in these cases.

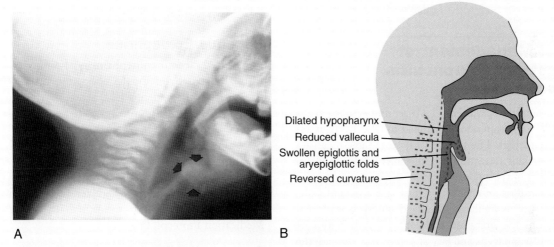

Dilated hypopharynx
Reduced vallecula
Swollen epiglottis and aryepiglottic folds
Reversed curvature

A   B

FIGURE 41-2 The classic "thumb sign" of an edematous epiglottis is evident in this lateral neck radiograph (see red arrows in **A**). The schematic illustrates the findings to look for in a lateral radiograph of a patient with suspected epiglottitis (**B**). Such radiographs are unnecessary in a child with the classic history, signs, and symptoms of epiglottitis; they can be of tremendous help, however, in diagnosing mild or questionable cases and explaining to parents the need for aggressive treatment. (From Ashcraft CK, Steele RW: Epiglottitis: A Pediatric Emergency, *J Respir Dis* 9:48, 1988.)

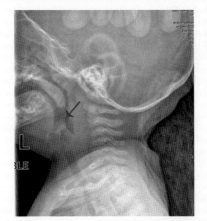

FIGURE 41-3 Young child with new onset leukemia and epiglottitis (see red arrow). (Image courtesy of Dayton Children's Hospital, Dayton, Ohio.)

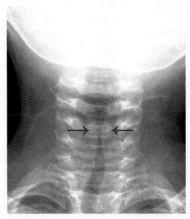

FIGURE 41-4 Classic "pencil point" or "steeple point" narrowing at the level of the cricoid cartilage (see red arrows). (Image courtesy of Dayton Children's Hospital, Dayton, Ohio.)

TABLE 41-2 LTB Scoring System

Score	0	1	2	3
Stridor	None	Mild	Moderate at rest	Severe with insp/exp or none with markedly decreased air entry
Retractions	None	Mild	Moderate	Severe marked use of accessory muscles
Air Entry	Normal	Mild decrease	Moderate decrease	Marked decrease
Color	Normal	Normal (0–Score)	Normal (0–Score)	Dusky or cyanotic
Level of Consciousness	Normal	Restless when disturbed	Anxious, agitated, restless when undisturbed	Lethargic, depressed
Scoring Guidelines				
Mild	0–2			
Moderate	3–5			
Severe	6–11			
Impending Ventilatory Failure:	>12			

General Management of Laryngotracheobronchitis and Epiglottitis*

There are a number of excellent LTB scoring systems available that allow the respiratory therapist to objectively assess and treat the patient. The typical LTB score table measures the patient's stridor, retractions, air movement, color and level of consciousness (Table 41-2).

Early recognition of epiglottitis may save a patient's life; it is a true airway emergency. Once the diagnosis is suspected or confirmed by the lateral neck radiograph, examination or inspection of the pharynx and larynx is *only* to be done in the operating room under general anesthesia with a fully trained team. *Under no circumstances should the mouth or throat be examined outside the operating room (even though depression of the tongue may reveal a bright red epiglottis and confirm the diagnosis) unless personnel and equipment are available to rapidly intubate or tracheostomize the patient. The patient usually maintains their limited airway by sitting up and leaning forward with their chin protruding—laying the patient down for examination will cause complete airway obstruction within minutes.* The patient with a confirmed diagnosis of acute epiglottitis should be intubated immediately!

After the diagnosis is established, the general management of LTB and acute epiglottitis is as follows:

Supplemental Oxygen

Because hypoxemia and significant work of breathing is associated with both LTB and epiglottitis, supplemental oxygen may be required. Oxygen therapy should be started when the patient's SpO_2 is under 92% (see Oxygen Therapy Protocol, Protocol 32-1).

*Although **cool aerosol mist** therapy was commonly used to treat patients with LTB in the past, it is rarely recommended today.

Racemic Epinephrine

Aerosolized **racemic epinephrine** is administered to children with LTB based on the LTB Scoring System (see Table 41-2). Using the patient's LTB score, the administration of racemic epinephrine protocol is as follows:

- 3–5: Consider racemic epinephrine
- >6: Administer racemic epinephrine 0.5 mL in 3 mL normal saline

This adrenergic agent is used for its vasoconstriction effect on mucosal edema and is recognized as an effective and safe aerosol decongestant for in-hospital use (see Aerosolized Medication Protocol, Protocol 32-4).

Corticosteroids

Corticosteroids, such as dexamethasone, have been shown to reduce the severity and duration of LTB, and are generally given when the patient presents with moderate to severe symptoms (see Appendix II).

Antibiotic Therapy

Because acute epiglottitis is almost always caused by *H. influenzae* type B, appropriate antibiotic therapy is part of the treatment plan. Ceftriaxone (Rocephin) and Ampicillin/sulbactam (Unasyn) often are prescribed to cover the most common organisms that cause acute epiglottitis.

Endotracheal Intubation or Tracheostomy

In the patient with a suspected acute epiglottitis, the examination or inspection of the pharyngeal and laryngeal areas is only to be performed in the operating room with a trained surgical team in attendance. This is because the epiglottis may obstruct completely in response to even the slightest touch or supine positioning during inspection. The physician, nurse, and respiratory therapist should not leave the patient's bedside until the endotracheal tube is secured. If the patient is anxious, restless, or uncooperative, restraints and sedation may be needed to prevent accidental extubation. After intubation, the patient should be transferred to the intensive care unit (ICU) and placed on continuous positive airway pressure (CPAP) or pressure support ventilation. Mechanical ventilation must be provided if paralysis is used to protect the airway in an uncooperative patient (see Mechanical Ventilation and Weaning Protocol, Protocol 32-5).

CASE STUDY 1 Laryngotracheobronchitis

Admitting History and Physical Examination

An 18-month-old boy had a mild viral upper respiratory infection and some hoarseness. At 10 PM on the third day of his illness, he rapidly developed a brassy cough and high-pitched inspiratory stridor. He became moderately dyspneic. The child was restless and appeared frightened. Rectal temperature was 37°C. The mother claimed that the child was "blue" on two occasions during a coughing episode. She was going to take the child to the emergency room, but the grandmother suggested that she try steam inhalation first. Accordingly, the child was taken to the bathroom, where the hot shower was turned on full force. The child was comforted by the grandmother and urged to breathe slowly and deeply. As the bathroom became filled with steam, the respiratory distress abated and within a few minutes the child was free of stridor, breathing essentially normally. The next day the same symptoms recurred, and the patient was taken to the emergency department.

Cough and inspiratory stridor were noted. Vital signs were: blood pressure 90/60, pulse 160 beats/min, respiratory rate 32 breaths/min. The room air SpO_2 was 94%. The patient's inspiratory stridor (croup) score was 7. The AP neck radiograph showed narrowing of the subglottic airway. The respiratory therapist documented the following assessment and plan.

Respiratory Assessment and Plan

S Mother reports patient had cough and inspiratory stridor.
O Confirms above. Lungs clear except for stridor and tracheal breath sounds throughout. Vital signs: BP: 90/60, P: 160/min, RR 32/min. Pallor noted. SpO_2 94% on room air. Inspiratory stridor (croup) score of 7. Soft tissue radiograph of neck suggests laryngotracheobronchitis.
A LTB, moderate (history and inspiratory stridor).
P Notify the physician. Start **Aerosolized Medication Protocol** (med. neb. treatment with racemic epinephrine per protocol).

Discussion

Home remedies sometimes do work. Any parent who has had a child with LTB will find this scenario familiar. What may not be as widely recognized is that sometimes inhalation of warm or cool mist may improve this syndrome. When this approach failed, the parents were wise to bring their son to the emergency department for prompt vasoconstrictive therapy and oral steroids. This resulted in prompt improvement.

CASE STUDY 2 Acute Epiglottitis

Admitting History and Physical Examination

A 2-year-old girl whose parents had an objection to routine infant and childhood immunizations appeared quite well in the evening and was put to bed at the usual time. She woke up 2 hours later, and her parents were immediately aware that she was in serious respiratory distress. She was feverish, sitting up in bed, drooling, unable to speak or cry, and breathing noisily. The parents wrapped the child in warm blankets and drove her to the emergency department of the nearest hospital.

On inspection, the child demonstrated a puffy face, drooling, inspiratory stridor, and cyanotic nail beds. At this time, she was placed on a 4 L/min nasal cannula. The emergency physician looked at the girl and listened to her chest but did not examine her mouth. Respiratory rate was 36 breaths/min, blood pressure was 80/50, and pulse was 140 beats/min. The rectal temperature was 103.6°F (39.8°C). The physician ordered a lateral soft-tissue radiograph of the neck, but while waiting for the radiograph, the child became increasingly dyspneic and more cyanotic. Her SpO_2 on 4 L/min nasal cannula was 88%. At this time, the following respiratory SOAP note was charted.

Respiratory Assessment and Plan

S Mother states that patient is in severe respiratory distress.

O RR 36/min, BP 80/50, P 140 regular. T 103.6° F (39.8° C). Child's face puffy, drooling. Inspiratory stridor (worsening). Nail beds cyanotic. On a 4 L/min nasal cannula: SpO$_2$ 88%. Soft tissue x-ray exam of neck pending.

A • Probable acute epiglottitis. No history of foreign body aspiration (general history).
  • Impending acute ventilatory failure (SpO$_2$ history, drooling, inspiratory stridor, and cyanosis)

P STAT page for anesthesiologist and ENT surgeon. Up-regulate the **Oxygen Therapy Protocol** (a nonrebreather with 100% oxygen [FIO$_2$ 1.0] if tolerated).

While the emergency page for the anesthesiologist and the ENT surgeon went out, a nonrebreathing oxygen mask was immediately "lightly" held to the child's face by the respiratory therapist. As soon as the physicians arrived (after about 10 minutes), the child was taken to the operating room. The surgeon stood by to perform an emergency tracheostomy while the anesthesiologist attempted to intubate the child.

Fortunately, the anesthesiologist was successful in spite of an enlarged, cherry-red epiglottis partially obstructing the larynx. As soon as the endotracheal tube was in place, the child relaxed and soon went to sleep. She was admitted to the intensive care unit (ICU), sedated, and placed on +5 cm H$_2$O continuous positive airway pressure (CPAP). IV ceftriaxone was administered. She was extubated the next day when she demonstrated a leak around her ET tube. She was discharged on the third hospital day. A throat culture taken in the OR was positive for *H. influenzae* (type B). She was discharged on a 7-day course of oral cefdinir (Omnicef).

Discussion

Acute epiglottitis is a life-threatening condition. The key point to remember is to refrain from examining the throat until a staff member qualified in pediatric intubation is nearby. Such manipulation is often unsuccessful, and unless qualified assistance is at hand, the child may asphyxiate. The treatment suitably selected here was placement of a nonrebreathing oxygen mask while the appropriate team was assembled. Typical of this disease is its abrupt onset, and once the airway is secured and antibiotics given, the symptoms and danger subside. Maintaining the intubated airway until a leak is heard is key to survival. In cases of acute epiglottitis, *H. influenzae* type B will grow from blood cultures, whereas airway or respiratory tract cultures will grow non-typeable *H. influenza*.

SELF-ASSESSMENT QUESTIONS

Ⓔ Answers to questions can be found on Evolve. To access additional student assessment questions visit **http://evolve.elsevier.com/DesJardins/respiratory**.

1. The onset of LTB is usually:
  a. 2 to 4 hours
  b. 5 to 10 hours
  c. 12 to 24 hours
  d. 24 to 48 hours

2. Which of the following is/are associated with epiglottitis?
  1. Parainfluenza viruses
  2. *Haemophilus influenza* type B
  3. RSV
  4. Influenza A and B
    a. 1 only
    b. 2 only
    c. 3 and 4 only
    d. 1, 3, and 4 only

3. Which of the following is/are clinical manifestations associated with LTB?
  1. Haziness in supraglottic area on x-ray film
  2. High-pitched and loud inspiratory stridor
  3. Swallowing difficulty
  4. Drooling
    a. 2 only
    b. 3 only
    c. 1 and 3 only
    d. 1, 3, and 4 only

4. The signs and symptoms associated with acute epiglottitis usually develop within:
  a. 1 to 2 hours
  b. 2 to 4 hours
  c. 8 to 10 hours
  d. 12 to 24 hours

5. Which of the following arterial blood gas values is/are associated with mild to moderate LTB or epiglottitis?
  1. Decreased pH
  2. Decreased PaCO$_2$
  3. Increased HCO$_3^-$
  4. Increased pH
    a. 1 only
    b. 4 only
    c. 2 and 4 only
    d. 1 and 3 only

CHAPTER

42 | Near Drowning/Wet Drowning

Chapter Objectives

After reading this chapter, you will be able to:
- List the anatomic alterations of the lungs associated with near drowning.
- Describe the causes of near drowning.
- List the cardiopulmonary clinical manifestations associated with near drowning.
- Describe the general management of near drowning.
- Describe the clinical strategies and rationales of the SOAPs presented in the case study.

Key Terms

Dry Drowning
First Responder
Hypothermia
Laryngospasm
Near Drowning
Noncardiogenic Pulmonary Edema

Permissive Hypercapnia[†]
Pulmonary Barotrauma
Pulmonary Volutrauma
Ventilatory-Induced Lung Injury (VILI)
Warming techniques
Wet Drowning

Chapter Outline

Anatomic Alterations of the Lungs
Etiology and Epidemiology
Overview of Cardiopulmonary Clinical Manifestations
    Associated with Near Wet Drowning
General Management
    The First Responder
    Management at the Hospital
Case Study: Near Drowning
Self-Assessment Questions

Anatomic Alterations of the Lungs

Drowning is defined as suffocation and death as a result of submersion in liquid. Drowning may be classified further as **near drowning, dry drowning,** and **wet drowning.** *Near drowning* refers to the situation in which a victim survives a liquid submersion, at least temporarily. In dry drowning the glottis spasms and prevents water from passing into the lungs. The lungs of dry drowning victims are usually normal.

In wet drowning the glottis relaxes and allows water to flood the tracheobronchial tree and alveoli. When fluid initially is inhaled, the bronchi constrict in response to a parasympathetic-mediated reflex. As fluid enters the alveoli, the pathophysiologic processes responsible for **noncardiogenic pulmonary edema** begin—that is, fluid from the pulmonary capillaries moves into the perivascular spaces, peribronchial spaces, alveoli, bronchioles, and bronchi. As a consequence of this fluid movement, the alveolar walls and interstitial spaces swell, pulmonary surfactant concentration decreases, and the alveolar surface tension increases.

As this condition intensifies, the alveoli shrink and **atelectasis** develops. Excess fluid in the interstitial spaces causes the lymphatic vessels to dilate and the lymph flow

to increase. In severe cases the fluid that accumulates in the tracheobronchial tree is churned into a frothy, white (sometimes blood-tinged) sputum as a result of air moving into and out of the lungs (generally by means of mechanical ventilation).

Finally, if the victim was submerged in unclean water (e.g., swamp, pond, sewage, or mud), a number of pathogens (e.g., *Pseudomonas*) and solid material may be aspirated. When this happens, pneumonia may occur, and in severe cases, acute respiratory distress syndrome (ARDS) may develop. Although the theory has been controversial in the past, it is now believed that the major pathologic changes of the lungs are essentially the same in fresh water and sea water wet drownings; both result in a reduction in pulmonary surfactant, alveolar injury, atelectasis, and pulmonary edema (see Figure 42-1).

The major pulmonary pathologic and structural changes associated with wet drowning are as follows:
- **Laryngospasm**
- Interstitial edema, including engorgement of the perivascular and peribronchial spaces, alveolar walls, and interstitial spaces
- Decreased pulmonary surfactant with increased surface tension of alveolar fluid

535

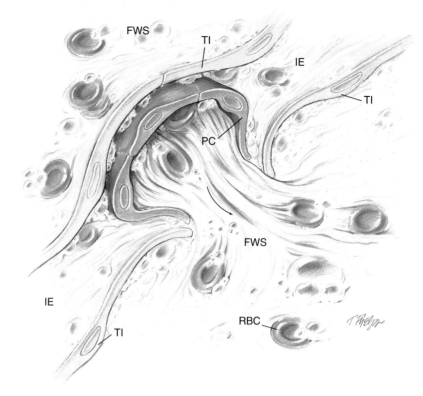

FIGURE 42-1 Near wet drowning. Cross-sectional, microscopic view of the alveolar-capillary unit. Illustration shows fluid moving from a pulmonary capillary to an alveolus. *FWS*, frothy white secretions; *IE*, interstitial edema; *PC*, pulmonary capillary; *RBC*, red blood cell; *TI*, type I alveolar cell.

- Frothy, white and pink secretions with stable bubbles throughout the tracheobronchial tree
- Alveolar shrinkage and atelectasis
- Alveolar consolidation
- Bronchospasm

Etiology and Epidemiology

According to the Center for Disease Control and Prevention's most recent data, about 1500 people drown every year in the United States. Drowning is the second leading cause of injury-related deaths in children aged one month to 14 years of age in the United States. The incidence of drowning in African–American children between the ages of 5 and 14 is almost three times that of white children in the same age range. For every child who dies from drowning, another five receive emergency department care for nonfatal submersion injuries. Most young children drown in swimming pools and bathtubs, while teens drown in natural bodies of water. Teen drowning is often associated with boating accidents, alcohol consumption, and illicit drug use. Nearly 80% of drowning victims are male. According to the World Health Organization (WHO), drowning is the third leading cause of death by unintentional injury worldwide. WHO estimates that each year there are more than 375,000 drowning deaths worldwide.

Box 42-1 summarizes the general sequence of events that occurs in drowning or near drowning. Victims submerged in cold water generally demonstrate a much higher survival rate than victims submerged in warm water. Table 42-1 lists favorable prognostic factors in cold-water near drowning.

BOX 42-1 Drowning or Near Drowning Sequence

1. Panic and violent struggle to return to the surface
2. Period of calmness and apnea
3. Swallowing of large amounts of fluid, followed by vomiting
4. Gasping inspirations and aspiration
5. Convulsions
6. Coma
7. Death

TABLE 42-1 Favorable Prognostic Factors in Cold-Water Near Drowning

Age	The younger, the better
Submersion time	The shorter, the better (60 minutes appears to be the upper limit in cold-water submersions)
Water temperature	The colder, the better (range, 27°F to 70°F)
Water quality	The cleaner, the better
Other injuries	None serious
Amount of struggle	The less struggle, the better
Cardiopulmonary resuscitation (CPR) quality	Good CPR technique increases the survival rate
Suicidal intent	Lower survival rate among victims who attempted suicide than among victims of accidental submersion

The following clinical manifestations result from the pathologic mechanisms caused (or activated) by Atelectasis (see Figure 9-7), Alveolar Consolidation (see Figure 9-8), Increased Alveolar-Capillary Membrane Thickness (see Figure 9-9), Bronchospasm (see Figure 9-10), and Excessive Bronchial Secretions (see Figure 9-11)—the major anatomic alterations of the lungs associated with near wet drowning (see Figure 42-1).

CLINICAL DATA OBTAINED AT THE PATIENT'S BEDSIDE

The Physical Examination

Apnea

Apnea is directly related to the length of time the victim is submerged and the temperature of the water. Cold water temperatures cause increased apnea. The longer the submersion, the more likely it is that the victim will not have spontaneous respiration. When spontaneous breathing is present, the respiratory rate is usually increased.

Vital Signs

Increased Respiratory Rate (Tachypnea)

Several pathophysiologic mechanisms operating simultaneously may lead to an increased ventilatory rate:

- Stimulation of peripheral chemoreceptors (hypoxemia)
- Decreased lung compliance–increased ventilatory rate relationship
- Stimulation of J receptors
- Anxiety (conscious patient)

Increased Heart Rate (Pulse) and Blood Pressure

Cyanosis

Cough and Sputum Production (Frothy, White or Pink, Stable Bubbles)

Pallor (extreme paleness)—particularly in cold water episodes

Chest Assessment Findings

- Crackles

CLINICAL DATA OBTAINED FROM LABORATORY TESTS AND SPECIAL PROCEDURES

Pulmonary Function Test Findings
(Extrapolated Data for Instructional Purposes)
(Primary Restrictive Lung Pathophysiology)

FORCED EXPIRATORY VOLUME AND FLOW RATE FINDINGS

FVC	FEV_T	FEV_1/FVC ratio	$FEF_{25\%-75\%}$
↓	N or ↓	N or ↑	N or ↓

$FEF_{50\%}$	$FEF_{200-1200}$	PEFR	MVV
N or ↓	N or ↓	N or ↓	N or ↓

LUNG VOLUME AND CAPACITY FINDINGS

V_T	IRV	ERV	RV
N or ↓	↓	↓	↓

VC	IC	FRC	TLC	RV/TLC ratio
↓	↓	↓	↓	N

DECREASED DIFFUSION CAPACITY (DL_{CO})

Arterial Blood Gases

MODERATE AND ADVANCED STAGES OF WET DROWNING

Acute Ventilatory Failure with Hypoxemia[†]
(Acute Respiratory Acidosis)

pH*	$PaCO_2$	HCO_3^-*	PaO_2	SaO_2 or SpO_2
↓	↑	↑ (but normal)	↓	↓

Oxygenation Indices[†]

$\dot{Q}_S/\dot{Q}_T$	DO_2	$\dot{V}O_2$[§]	$C(a-\bar{v})O_2$[§]	O_2ER	$S\bar{v}O_2$
↑	↓	N	N	↑	↓

[†]See Figure 4-2 and related discussion for the acute pH, $PaCO_2$, and HCO_3^- changes associated with acute ventilatory failure.

*When tissue hypoxia is severe enough to produce lactic acid (metabolic acidosis), the pH and values will be lower than expected for a particular $PaCO_2$ level.

[†] $C(a-\bar{v})O_2$, Arterial-venous oxygen difference; DO_2, total oxygen delivery; O_2ER, oxygen extraction ratio; $\dot{Q}_S/\dot{Q}_T$, pulmonary shunt fraction; $S\bar{v}O_2$, mixed venous oxygen saturation; $\dot{V}O_2$, oxygen consumption.

[§]The $\dot{V}O_2$ and $C(a-\bar{v})O_2$ may be decreased in cold water drowning.

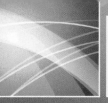

RADIOLOGIC FINDINGS
Chest Radiograph
· Fluffy infiltrates

The initial appearance of the radiograph may vary from being completely normal to showing varying degrees of pulmonary edema and atelectasis (Figure 42-2). It should be emphasized, however, that an initially normal chest radiograph still may be associated with significant hypoxemia, hypercapnia, and acidosis. In any case, radiographic deterioration may occur in the first 48 to 72 hours.

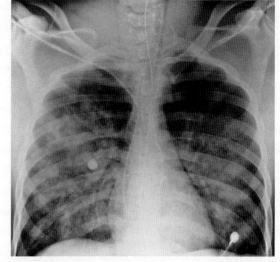

FIGURE 42-2 This radiograph of a young man, taken just after an episode of near drowning, shows a pulmonary edema pattern. Note the air bronchograms in both lungs reflecting atelectasis. (From Hansell DM, Armstrong P, Lynch DA, McAdams HP, eds: *Imaging of diseases of the chest,* ed 4, Philadelphia, 2005, Elsevier.)

General Management

The First Responder

For the **first responder,** the first objectives in treating a drowning victim are to remove the person from the water and, if the patient has no spontaneous ventilation and pulse, to call for help and immediately initiate cardiopulmonary resuscitation (CPR) with FIO_2 1.0. When the patient has been submerged for less than 60 minutes in cold water, fixed and dilated pupils do not necessarily indicate a poor prognosis. Because water is an excellent conductor of body heat (cold water can cool the body 25 times faster than air at the same temperature) and because evaporation further reduces an individual's body heat and produces **hypothermia**, the victim's wet clothing should immediately be removed and replaced with warm, dry coverings. High heat-loss areas of the body include the head and neck, axillae, and inguinal areas. The victim's vital signs, including rectal temperature, should be monitored closely during travel to the hospital. The victim's body temperature frequently falls during transport, and therefore measures to conserve the patient's body heat are extremely important. Victims with spontaneous ventilation should be monitored with pulse oximetry during transport, if at all possible.

Management at the Hospital

Treatment at the hospital is an extension of prehospital management. Virtually every near drowning victim suffers from hypoxemia, hypercapnia, and acidosis (acute ventilatory failure). Hypoxemia generally persists after aspiration of fluids in the airway (wet drowning) because of alveolar-capillary damage and continued intrapulmonary shunting. The degree of hypoxemia is directly related to the amount of alveolar-capillary damage. A chest radiograph should be obtained to help evaluate the magnitude of the alveolar-capillary injury. However, a normal initial chest radiograph does not rule out the possibility of alveolar-capillary deterioration during the first 24 hours.

Intubation and mechanical ventilation should be performed immediately for any victim with no spontaneous ventilations and for victims who are breathing spontaneously, but are unable to maintain a PaO_2 of 60 mm Hg with an FIO_2 of 0.50 or lower. Because of the nature of the alveolar-capillary injury seen in most wet drowning victims, mechanical ventilation with positive end-expiratory pressure (PEEP) or continuous positive airway pressure (CPAP) should be administered. It should be noted, however, that **pulmonary barotrauma, pulmonary volutrauma***, and **ventilatory-induced**

---

*It has long been known that mechanical ventilation can produce a variety of lung injuries referred to as **ventilator-induced lung injury (VILI), pulmonary volutrauma**, or **pulmonary barotrauma**. VILI is defined as stress fractures of the pulmonary capillary endothelium, epithelium, and basement membrane and, in severe cases, lung rupture. Lung ruptures can lead to leakage of fluid, protein, and blood into tissue and air spaces or leakage of air into tissue spaces. This condition can be followed by an inflammatory response and possibly a reduced defense against infection. Pulmonary volutrauma is defined as damage to the lung caused by over-distention by a

lung injury (VILI) are common complications of ventilatory therapy in these patients. Low tidal volume ventilation and **permissive hypercapnia**[†] are ventilator management techniques to consider when appropriate. The patient also may benefit from inotropic agents and diuretics.

Finally, warming the victim should progress concomitantly with all the other treatment modalities. Nearly all near drowning victims are hypothermic to some degree. Depending on the severity of the hypothermia and on the available resources, a number of **warming techniques** may be employed. For example, the body temperature can be increased by the intravenous administration of heated solutions; by heated lavage of the gastric, intrathoracic, pericardial, and peritoneal spaces; or by the administration of heated lavage to the bladder and rectum. Additional external heating techniques include warming of the patient's inspired air or gas mixtures, heating blankets, warm baths, and immersion in a heated Hubbard tank. In rare cases, extracorporeal circulation, with complete cardiopulmonary bypass and blood warming, has been successful. Resuscitation should not end even if the patient does not respond until a close approximation of normal body temperature is reached.

---

mechanical ventilator set for an excessively high tidal volume. Pulmonary barotrauma is defined as damage to the lungs caused by rapid or extreme pressures generated by mechanical ventilation

Predisposing factors for VILI, pulmonary volutrauma, or pulmonary barotrauma include (1) mechanical ventilation with high peak inspiratory volumes and pressures, (2) mechanical ventilation with a high mean airway pressure, (3) structural immaturity of lung and chest wall, (4) surfactant insufficiency or inactivation, and (5) preexisting lung disease.

[†]**Permissive Hypercapnia defined**: Mechanical ventilation was traditionally applied with the goal of normalizing arterial blood gas values, particularly the arterial carbon dioxide tension ($PaCO_2$). However, this is no longer the primary objective of mechanical ventilation. Today, the emphasis is on maintaining adequate gas exchange while—and, importantly—minimizing the risks of mechanical ventilation. Common strategies used to reduce the risk of mechanical ventilation include (1) low tidal volume ventilation—to protect the lung from ventilator-associated lung injury in patients with acute lung injury (e.g., ARDS)—and (2) reduction of the tidal volume, respiratory rate, or both—to minimize intrinsic positive end-expiratory pressure (i.e., auto-PEEP) in patients with obstructive lung disease (e.g., COPD).

Although these mechanical ventilation strategies may result in an increased $PaCO_2$ level (hypercapnia), they do help to protect the lung from barotrauma (i.e., physical damage to lung tissues caused by excessive gas pressures). The lenient acceptance of the hypercapnia is called **permissive hypercapnia**. In most cases, the patient's $PaCO_2$ is adequately maintained by an increased ventilatory rate that offsets the decreased tidal volume. The $PaCO_2$, however, should not be permitted to increase to the point of severe acidosis. The most current consensus suggests it is safe to allow pH to fall to at least 7.20 (www.ARDSNet).

CASE STUDY Near Wet Drowning

Admitting History and Physical Examination

A 12-year-old boy had a prior history of a seizure disorder but had not taken his medication for almost a year. On the morning of admission, he participated in a regular swimming class in the junior high school pool. According to the coach on duty, there had been a "pool check" 30 seconds before the patient's partner reported that the patient seemed to stay under water "too long."

When taken from the water, he was unconscious and "blue." He was given mouth-to-mouth resuscitation, and by the time the emergency medical technician (EMT) squad arrived about 20 minutes later, he was comatose, but he was breathing at a rate of 10 breaths/min, although his lips and fingers were still cyanotic. He was placed on 5 L/min oxygen and taken to the nearest hospital.

On admission the patient's blood pressure was 100/60 and his pulse was 140 beats/min. Rectal temperature was 98°F (36.1°C). Auscultation of his chest revealed fine crackles bilaterally. Clear secretions were suctioned from his oral airway. A chest radiograph showed bilateral diffuse increase in density, which suggested pulmonary edema or possible hemorrhage. His SpO_2 was 72%. Plans were made to transfer him to a nearby tertiary care medical center.

The respiratory therapist in the emergency department entered the following assessment moments before the patient transfer.

Respiratory Assessment and Plan

S N/A (patient comatose). History of near drowning.

O Comatose. Spontaneous breathing at 10/min, BP 100/60, P 140. Core temp 98°F (36.1°C) (normal). Crackles bilaterally. Nasotracheal suctioning yields clear fluid. Cyanotic. SpO_2 on 5 L/min O_2 per nasal cannula: 72%.

A • Near drowning. R/O seizure disorder (history)
• Increased airway secretions (suctioning of clear fluid)
• Poor oxygenation (cyanosis, SpO_2)
• Pulmonary edema (CXR)

P Stat ABG on FIO_2 1.0, then titrate per **Oxygen Therapy Protocol.** Have equipment to intubate on standby. Bag-mask ventilate, and PRN. Provide continuous pulse oximetry. Will accompany on transfer.

After transfer to the tertiary care medical center, the patient was described as a well-developed, slightly obese adolescent in obvious respiratory distress. He was now alert, oriented, but extremely apprehensive. His vital signs were: temperature (rectal) 100.8°F (38.2°C), blood pressure 112/70, pulse 140 beats/min, and respirations 60 breaths/min. The lips and fingertips were still cyanotic. The chest wall motion was paradoxical. There was marked substernal retraction. Breath sounds were diminished bilaterally, and loud crackles were heard over both lungs anteriorly.

Laboratory examination revealed a leukocytosis of $21,000/mm^3$ and 2+ albumin in the urine, but findings were otherwise within normal limits. There was no evidence of hemolysis. On bag-mask ventilation with an FIO_2 of 1.0, the arterial blood gas (ABG) values were pH 7.29, $PaCO_2$ 52 mm Hg, HCO_3^- 25 mEq/L, PaO_2 38 mm Hg, and SaO_2 67%. The patient's condition was rapidly deteriorating, and he developed even more severe crackles. He now had a spontaneous cough with frothy sputum production. The chest radiograph revealed pulmonary edema and nearly complete opacification of both lungs. The following was entered in the patient's chart.

Respiratory Assessment and Plan

S Anxious, dyspneic, crying. "I can't get my breath. Where am I? Am I going to die?"

O Afebrile. BP 112/70, P 140/min, RR 60/min. Cyanotic. Paradoxic chest/abdomen movements, sternal retraction. Crackles in both lungs anteriorly. Spontaneous cough with frothy sputum production, WBC $21,000/mm^3$. On FIO_2 1.0: pH 7.29, $PaCO_2$ 52, HCO_3^- 25, PaO_2 38, SaO_2 67%. CXR: "White-out."

A • Pulmonary edema secondary to near wet drowning (frothy sputum).
 • Acute ventilatory failure with severe hypoxemia (ABGs).

P Continue on FIO_2 1.0 and bag-mask ventilate. Page physician stat. Obtain intubation equipment and prepare to place patient on ventilator. Follow oximetry. Prepare to assist in placement of Swan-Ganz catheter.

The patient was intubated and paralyzed with succinylcholine. As soon as he was intubated, copious pink foam was aspirated from the endotracheal tube. He was alternately suctioned and ventilated with an Ambu bag. He was given 7 mg of morphine for sedation and was mechanically ventilated in continuous mechanical ventilation (CMV) mode at a rate of 10 breaths/min. On an FIO_2 of 1.0 and PEEP of 10 cm H_2O, his blood gases were pH 7.44, $PaCO_2$ 43 mm Hg, HCO_3^- 22 mEq/L, PaO_2 109 mm Hg, SaO_2 98%. At this time, the respiratory therapist started to slowly decrease the patient's FIO_2. Because he was still fighting the ventilator, he was paralyzed with pancuronium.

After several hours, the lungs were clear, the secretions were no longer present, and his blood gas values returned to normal on an FIO_2 of 0.50 and PEEP of 10 cm H_2O (pH 7.38, $PaCO_2$ 42 mm Hg, HCO_3^- 24 mEq/L, PaO_2 98 mm Hg, SaO_2 97%). His hemodynamic status was normal. The chest radiograph revealed considerable clearing of the earlier noted bilateral pulmonary infiltrates. A pulmonary artery catheter was not placed, as clinical improvement was clearly occurring. The respiratory therapist entered the following assessment and plan.

Respiratory Assessment and Plan

S N/A (patient sedated, paralyzed).

O Lungs clear. No secretions. On FIO_2 0.50 and +10 PEEP: pH 7.38, $PaCO_2$ 42, HCO_3^- 24, PaO_2 98, SaO_2 97%. CXR: Considerable improvement in bilateral infiltrates. Swan-Ganz catheter not inserted, as patient is improving.

A • Considerable improvement on CMV and PEEP (general improvement of clinical indicators)
 • Acceptable ventilation and oxygenation status on present ventilator settings (ABG)
 • Frothy airway secretions no longer present (clear lungs and no secretions)

P Contact physician to wean from muscle relaxant. Wean from mechanically ventilated breaths, FIO_2, and PEEP per **Mechanical Ventilation Protocol**. Change ventilator mode to synchronized intermittent mandatory ventilation (SIMV).

The patient was weaned from the ventilator over a period of 6 hours, after which he was extubated. The following morning, arterial blood gases on an FIO_2 0.28 venturi oxygen mask were as follows: pH 7.42, $PaCO_2$ 35 mm Hg, HCO_3^- 22 mEq/L, PaO_2 158 mm Hg, and SaO_2 98%. His chest radiograph was normal. An oxygen titration protocol was performed. He was discharged 2 days later.

Discussion

This case demonstrates initial worsening of the near wet drowning victim despite intensive respiratory care. The initial ABG values showed severe hypoxemia as a result of **Increased Alveolar-Capillary Membrane Thickness** and alveolar flooding (see Figure 42-1), as well as acute ventilatory failure and metabolic (probably lactic) acidosis. Bronchospasm never developed, and aggressive respiratory care prohibited the development of atelectasis and aspiration pneumonia.

When suctioning, supplemental oxygen and bag ventilation were no longer successful, the patient was intubated and mechanical ventilation with PEEP was begun. Even on these modalities, the patient remained anxious and was ultimately paralyzed to allow better respiratory synchrony and diminish the chance of ventilatory-associated lung injury (barotrauma or volutrauma). Morphine was used for its sedative qualities and as a vascular afterload reducer. The fact that the patient was fighting the ventilator some time after succinylcholine had been administered reflects the fact that it is a very short-acting paralyzing agent. Pancuronium has a much longer half-life, and its use is standard in settings where longer effectiveness is required. Once the abnormal pathology of the lungs associated with this case improved, the patient's cardiopulmonary status quickly returned to normal and the respiratory therapist was able wean the patient from the ventilation in a relatively short period of time.

This case demonstrates the necessity for frequent reassessment of the patient and therapeutic adjustments to follow the findings so observed. Note that the therapist appropriately documented the reason that one of his suggestions (the Swan-Ganz catheter) was not placed. In the protocol-rich environment, such documentation is vital, if only for medical legal reasons.

SELF-ASSESSMENT QUESTIONS

1. **In the United States, drowning is the:**
   a. leading cause of accidental death
   b. second leading cause of accidental death
   c. third leading cause of accidental death
   d. fourth leading cause of accidental death

2. **According to the Center for Disease Control and Prevention, about how many people drown each year in the United States?**
   a. 500
   b. 1000
   c. 1250
   d. 1500

3. **Which of the following are the major anatomic alterations of the lungs associated with near drowning victims?**
   1. Consolidation
   2. Bronchospasm
   3. Increased alveolar-capillary membrane thickness
   4. Atelectasis
   5. Excessive bronchial secretions
      a. 3 and 5 only
      b. 2 and 4 only
      c. 3, 4, and 5 only
      d. 1, 2, 3, 4, and 5

4. **Which of the following clinical manifestations are associated with near drowning victims?**
   1. Frothy, pink sputum
   2. Crackles
   3. Increased pH
   4. Increased $S\bar{v}O_2$
      a. 1 and 2 only
      b. 3 and 4 only
      c. 2, 3, and 4 only
      d. 1, 2, 3, and 4 only

5. **Which of the following pulmonary function testing values are associated with near drowning victims?**
   1. N or $\downarrow$ FEV_T
   2. $\downarrow$FVC
   3. $\downarrow$ RV
   4. N or $\uparrow FEV_1$/FVC ratio
      a. 1 and 2 only
      b. 3 and 4 only
      c. 2, 3, and 4 only
      d. 1, 2, 3, and 4

Smoke Inhalation, Thermal Injuries, and Carbon Monoxide Intoxication

Chapter Objectives

After reading this chapter, you will be able to:

- List the anatomic alterations of the lungs associated with smoke inhalation and thermal injuries.
- Describe the causes of smoke inhalation, thermal injuries, and carbon monoxide intoxication.
- List the cardiopulmonary clinical manifestations associated with smoke inhalation, thermal injuries, and carbon monoxide intoxication.
- Describe the general management of smoke inhalation and thermal injuries.
- Describe the clinical strategies and rationales of the SOAPs presented in the case study.

Key Terms

Body Surface Burns
Bronchiolitis Obliterans Organizing Pneumonia (BOOP)
Bronchospasm
Carbon Monoxide Poisoning
Carbonaceous Sputum
Carboxyhemoglobin
COHB Half-Life
CO-Oximetry
Cyanide Blood Level
Cyanide Poisoning
Cryptogenic Organizing Pneumonia (COP)
Eschar
Facial Burns
First-Degree Burn

Hyperbaric Oxygenation (HBO) Therapy
Multi-Organ Dysfunction Syndrome (MODS)
Noncardiogenic Pulmonary Edema
Parkland Formula (Fluid Resuscitation)
Pyrolysis
Second-Degree Burn
Smoke Inhalation Injury
Steam Inhalation
Thermal Injury
Third-Degree Burn

Chapter Outline

Anatomic Alterations of the Lungs

The inhalation of smoke, hot gases, and **body surface burns**—in any combination—continue to be a major cause of morbidity and mortality among fire victims and firefighters. In general, fire-related pulmonary injuries can be divided into thermal and smoke (toxic gases) injuries.

Thermal Injury

Thermal injury refers to injury caused by the inhalation of hot gases. Thermal injuries are usually confined to the upper airway—the nasal cavity, oral cavity, nasopharynx, oropharynx, and larynx. The distal airways and the alveoli are usually spared serious injury because of (1) the remarkable ability of the upper airways to cool hot gases, (2) reflex laryngospasm, and (3) glottic closure. The upper airway is an extremely efficient "heat sink." In fact, in 1945, Moritz and associates demonstrated that the inhalation of hot gases alone did not

produce significant damage to the lung. Anesthetized dogs were forced to breathe air heated to 500°C through an insulated endotracheal tube. The air temperature dropped to 50°C by the time it reached the level of the carina. No histologic damage was noticed in the lower trachea or lungs.

Even though thermal injury may occur with or without surface burns, the presence of **facial burns** is a classic predictor of thermal injury. Thermal injury to the upper airway results in blistering, mucosal edema, vascular congestion, epithelial sloughing, and accumulation of thick secretions. Acute upper airway obstruction (UAO) occurs in about 20% to 30% of hospitalized patients with thermal injury and is usually most marked in the supraglottic structures (see Figure 43-1).

Inhalation of steam at 100°C or greater usually results in severe damage at all levels of the respiratory tract. This damage occurs because steam has about 500 times the heat energy content of dry gas at the same temperature. Thermal injury to

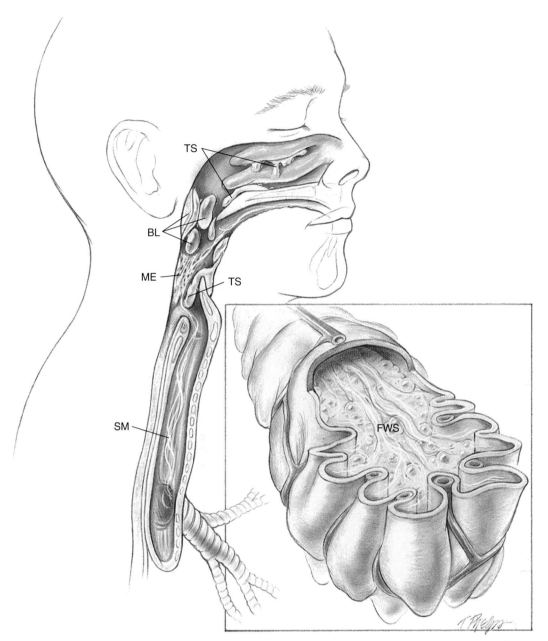

FIGURE 43-1 Smoke inhalation and thermal injuries. *BL*, Airway blister; *FWS*, frothy white secretions (pulmonary edema); *ME*, mucosal edema; *SM*, smoke (toxic gas); *TS*, thick secretions.

the distal airways results in mucosal edema, vascular congestion, epithelial sloughing, **cryptogenic organizing pneumonia (COP)**—also known as **bronchiolitis obliterans organizing pneumonia (BOOP)**—atelectasis, and pulmonary edema.

Therefore, direct thermal injuries usually do not occur below the level of the larynx, except in the rare instance of **steam inhalation**. Damage to the distal airways is mostly caused by a variety of harmful products found in smoke.

Smoke Inhalation Injury

The pathologic changes in the distal airways and alveoli are mainly caused by the irritating and toxic gases, suspended soot particles, and vapors associated with incomplete combustion and smoke. Many of the substances found in smoke are extremely caustic to the tracheobronchial tree and poisonous to the body. The progression of injuries that develop from

smoke inhalation and burns is described as the early stage, intermediate stage, and late stage.

Early Stage (0 to 24 Hours After Inhalation)

The injuries associated with smoke inhalation do not always appear right away, even when extensive body surface burns are evident. During the early stage (0 to 24 hours after smoke inhalation), however, the patient's pulmonary status often changes markedly. Initially, the tracheobronchial tree becomes more inflamed, resulting in **bronchospasm**. This process causes an overabundance of bronchial secretions to move into the airways, resulting in further airway obstruction. In addition, the toxic effects of smoke often slow the activity of the mucosal ciliary transport mechanism, causing further retention of mucus.

Smoke inhalation also may cause acute respiratory distress syndrome (ARDS), noncardiogenic high-permeability pulmonary edema—commonly referred to in smoke inhalation cases as "leaky alveoli." **Noncardiogenic pulmonary edema** also may be caused by overhydration resulting from overzealous fluid resuscitation (see insert panel in Figure 43-1). In severe cases, ARDS also may occur early in the course of the pathology.

Intermediate Stage (2 to 5 Days After Inhalation)

Whereas upper airway thermal injuries usually begin to improve during the intermediate stage (2 to 5 days after smoke inhalation), the pathologic changes deep in the lungs continue to be a problem. For example, production of mucus continues to increase, whereas mucosal ciliary transport activity continues to decrease. The mucosa of the tracheobronchial tree frequently becomes necrotic and sloughs (usually at 3 to 4 days). The necrotic debris, excessive production of mucus, and retention of mucus lead to mucous plugging and atelectasis. In addition, the mucous accumulation often leads to bacterial colonization, bronchitis, and pneumonia. Organisms commonly cultured include gram-positive *Staphylococcus aureus* and gram-negative *Klebsiella*, *Enterobacter*, *Escherichia coli*, and *Pseudomonas*. If not already present, ARDS may develop at any time during this period.

When chest wall (thorax) burns are present, the situation may be further aggravated by the patient's inability to breathe deeply and cough as a result of (1) pain, (2) the administration of narcotics, (3) immobility, (4) increased airway resistance, and (5) decreased lung and chest wall compliance.

Late Stage (≥5 Days After Inhalation)

Infections resulting from burn wounds on the body surface are the major concern during the late stage (≥5 days after smoke inhalation). These infections often lead to sepsis and **multi-organ dysfunction syndrome (MODS)**. Sepsis-induced MODS is the primary cause of death in seriously burned patients during this stage.

Pneumonia also continues to be a major problem during this period. In addition, pulmonary embolism also may develop within 2 weeks after serious body surface burns. Pulmonary embolism may develop from deep venous thrombosis secondary to a hypercoagulable state and prolonged immobility.

Finally, the long-term effects of smoke inhalation can result in restrictive and obstructive lung disorders. In general, a restrictive lung disorder develops from alveolar fibrosis and chronic atelectasis. An obstructive lung disorder is generally caused by increased and chronic bronchial secretions, bronchial stenosis, bronchial polyps, bronchiectasis, and bronchiolitis.

The major pathologic and structural changes of the respiratory system caused by thermal or smoke inhalation injuries are as follows:

Thermal injury (upper airway—nasal cavity, oral cavity, and pharynx):
- Blistering
- Mucosal edema
- Vascular congestion
- Epithelial sloughing
- Thick secretions
- Acute UAO

Smoke inhalation injury (tracheobronchial tree and alveoli):
- Inflammation of the tracheobronchial tree
- Bronchospasm
- Excessive bronchial secretions and mucous plugging
- Decreased mucosal ciliary transport
- Atelectasis
- Alveolar edema and frothy secretions (noncardiogenic pulmonary edema)
- ARDS (severe cases)
- COP (also called *bronchiolitis obliterans organizing pneumonia*)
- Alveolar fibrosis, bronchial stenosis, bronchial polyps, bronchiolitis, and bronchiectasis (severe cases)

Pneumonia (see Chapter 16) and pulmonary embolism (see Chapter 21) often complicate smoke inhalation injury.

Etiology and Epidemiology

According to the National Fire Protection Association (NFPA),[1] in 2012 there were 1,375,000 fires reported in the United States. These fires caused over 2800 deaths, 16,500 injuries, and $12.4 billion in property damage. The types of fires and subsequent deaths and property damage costs were as follows:

- 480,500 were structure fires, causing 2470 deaths, 14,700 injuries, and $9.8 billion in property damage;
- 172,500 were vehicle fires, causing 300 deaths, 800 injuries, and $1.1 billion in property damage;
- 692,000 were outside and other fires, causing 60 deaths, 825 injuries, and $813 million in property damage.

During 2012, US fire departments responded to a fire every 23 seconds. One structure fire was reported every 66 seconds. One home structure fire was reported every 85 seconds. One civilian fire injury was reported every 32 minutes. One fire death occurred every 3 hours. One outside fire was reported every 46 seconds. One vehicle fire was reported every 156 seconds.

The prognosis of fire victims is usually determined by the (1) extent and duration of smoke exposure, (2) chemical composition of the smoke, (3) size and depth of body surface burns (see Table 43-2), (4) temperature of gases inhaled, (5) age (the prognosis worsens in the very young or old), and (6) preexisting health status. When smoke inhalation injury is accompanied by a full-thickness or third-degree skin burn, the mortality rate almost doubles.

Smoke can result from either **pyrolysis** (smoldering in a low-oxygen environment) or combustion (burning, with visible flame, in an adequate-oxygen environment). Smoke is composed of a complex mixture of particulates, toxic gases, and vapors. The composition of smoke varies according to the chemical makeup of the material that is burning and the amount of oxygen being consumed by

---

[1]http://www.nfpa.org

TABLE 43-1 Toxic Substances and Sources Commonly Associated with Fire and Smoke

Substance	Source
Aldehydes (acrolein, acetaldehyde, formaldehyde)	Wood, cotton, paper
Organic acids (acetic and formic acids)	
Carbon monoxide, hydrogen chloride, phosgene	Polyvinylchloride
Hydrogen cyanide, isocyanate	Polyurethanes
Hydrogen fluoride, hydrogen bromide	Fluorinated resins
Ammonia	Melamine resins
Oxides of nitrogen	Nitrocellulose film, fabrics
Benzene	Petroleum products
Carbon monoxide, carbon dioxide	Organic material
Sulfur dioxide	Sulfur-containing compounds
Hydrogen chloride	Fertilizer, textiles, rubber manufacturing
Chlorine	Swimming pool water
Ozone	Welding fumes
Hydrogen sulfide	Metal works, chemical manufacturing

TABLE 43-2 The Approximate Percentage of Body Surface Area (BSA) for Various Body Regions of Adults and Infants

Anatomic Region	BSA in Adults (%)	BSA in Infants (%)
Entire head and neck	9	18
Each arm	9	9
Anterior trunk	18	18
Posterior trunk	18	18
Genitalia	1	1
Each leg	18	13.5

Note: *The* "rule of nines" is used to estimate percentage of injury; each of the areas listed here represents about 9% or 18% of the body surface area. This rule does not apply to infants' legs.

the fire. Table 43-1 lists some of the more common toxic substances produced by burning products that are frequently found in office, industrial, and residential buildings.

Although in some instances the toxic components of the smoke may be obvious, in most cases the precise identification of the inhaled toxins is not feasible. In general, the inhalation of smoke with toxic agents that have high water solubility (e.g., ammonia, sulfur dioxide, and hydrogen fluoride) affects the structures of the upper airway. In contrast, the inhalation of toxic agents that have low water solubility (e.g., hydrogen chloride, chlorine, phosgene, and oxides of nitrogen) affects the distal airways and alveoli. Many of the substances in smoke are caustic and can cause significant injury to the tracheobronchial tree (e.g., aldehydes [especially acrolein], hydrochloride, and oxides of sulfur).

Body Surface Burns

Because the amount and severity of body surface burns play a major role in the patient's risk of mortality and morbidity, an approximate estimate of the percentage of the body surface area burned is important. Table 43-2 lists the approximate percentage of surface area for various body regions of adults and infants. The severity and depth of burns are usually defined as follows:

First degree (minimal depth in skin): Superficial burn, damage limited to the outer layer of epidermis. This burn is characterized by reddened skin, tenderness, and pain. Blisters are not present. Healing time is about 6 to 10 days. The result of healing is normal skin.

Second degree (superficial to deep thickness of skin): Burns in which damage extends through the epidermis and into the dermis but is not of sufficient extent to interfere with regeneration of epidermis. If secondary infection results, the damage from a second-degree burn may be equivalent to that of a third-degree burn. Blisters are usually present. Healing time is 7 to 21 days. The result of healing ranges from normal to hairless and depigmented skin with a texture that is normal, pitted, flat, or shiny.

Third degree (full thickness of skin including tissue beneath skin): Burns in which both epidermis and dermis are destroyed, with damage extending into underlying tissues. Tissue may be charred or coagulated. Healing may occur after 21 days or may never occur without skin grafting if the burned area is large. The resultant damage heals with hypertrophic scars (keloids) and chronic granulation.

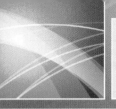

OVERVIEW of the Cardiopulmonary Clinical Manifestations Associated with Smoke Inhalation and Thermal Injuries

The following clinical manifestations result from the pathologic mechanisms caused (or activated) by atelectasis (see Figure 9-7), alveolar consolidation (see Figure 9-8), increased alveolar-capillary membrane thickness (see Figure 9-9), bronchospasm (see Figure 9-10), and excessive bronchial secretions (see Figure 9-11)—the major anatomic alterations of the lungs associated with smoke inhalation and thermal injuries (see Figure 43-1).

CLINICAL DATA OBTAINED AT THE PATIENT'S BEDSIDE

The Physical Examination

Vital Signs

Increased Respiratory Rate (Tachypnea)

Several pathophysiologic mechanisms operating simultaneously may lead to an increased ventilatory rate:

· Stimulation of peripheral chemoreceptors (hypoxemia)
· Decreased lung compliance–increased ventilatory rate relationship
· Stimulation of J receptors
· Pain, anxiety
· Fever (with infection)

Increased Heart Rate (Pulse) and Blood Pressure

Assessment of Acute Upper Airway Obstruction (Thermal Injury)

· Obvious pharyngeal edema and swelling
· Inspiratory stridor
· Hoarseness
· Altered voice
· Painful swallowing

Because the inhalation of hot gases often results in severe upper airway edema, the respiratory therapist always should be alert for any clinical manifestations of acute upper airway obstruction, even when the patient shows no remarkable upper airway problems or upper body or facial burns at admission.

Cyanosis

Cough and Sputum Production

When the patient experiences upper airway thermal injuries, abnormally thick and sometimes excessive secretions usually result. During the early stage of recovery from smoke inhalation, the patient generally expectorates a small amount of black, sooty sputum (**carbonaceous sputum**). During the intermediate stage the patient may produce moderate to large amounts of frothy secretions. During the late stage, purulent mucous production is common.

Chest Assessment Findings

· Normal breath sounds (early stage)
· Wheezing
· Crackles

CLINICAL DATA OBTAINED FROM LABORATORY TESTS AND SPECIAL PROCEDURES

Pulmonary Function Test Findings
(Extrapolated Data for Instructional Purposes)
(Primarily Restrictive Lung Pathophysiology)

FORCED EXPIRATORY VOLUME AND FLOW RATE FINDINGS

FVC	FEV_T	FEV_1/FVC ratio	$FEF_{25\%-75\%}$
↓	N or ↓	N or ↑	N or ↓

$FEF_{50\%}$	$FEF_{200-1200}$	PEFR	MVV
N or ↓	N or ↓	N or ↓	N or ↓

LUNG VOLUME AND CAPACITY FINDINGS

V_T	IRV	ERV	RV*
N or ↓	↓	↓	↓

VC	IC	FRC*	TLC	RV/TLC ratio
↓	↓	↓	↓	N

DECREASED DIFFUSION CAPACITY (DL_{CO})

Arterial Blood Gases

EARLY STAGES OF SMOKE INHALATION

Acute Alveolar Hyperventilation with Hypoxemia[§]
(Acute Respiratory Alkalosis)

pH	$PaCO_2$	HCO_3^-	PaO_2	SaO_2 or SpO_2
↑	↓	↓ (but normal)	↓ or Normal	↓ or Normal

SEVERE SMOKE INHALATION AND BURNS WITH METABOLIC ACIDOSIS

COHb	$pH^†$	$PaCO_2{}^†$	$HCO_3^-{}^†$	PaO_2	SaO_2 or SpO_2
↑	↓ (lactic acidemia)	↓	↓	↓ or Normal (but tissue hypoxemia is present)	↓ or Normal

COHb, Carboxyhemoglobin.

*↑when airways are partially obstructed.
[§]See Figure 4-3 and related discussion for the acute pH, $PaCO_2$, and HCO_3^- changes associated with acute alveolar hyperventilation.
[†]When tissue hypoxia is severe enough to produce lactic acid, the pH and HCO_3^- values will be lower than expected for a particular $PaCO_2$ level.
[‡]In severe burns with ARDS, the $PaCO_2$ may be elevated and combined respiratory and metabolic acidosis may be present.

When carbon monoxide (CO) or cyanide poisoning is present, the pH may be decreased during the early stages of smoke inhalation. This decrease in pH occurs because patients with severe CO or cyanide poisoning commonly have lactic acidemia as a result of tissue hypoxia—even in the presence of a normal PaO_2. Therefore when CO or cyanide poisoning is present, the patient may demonstrate the following arterial blood gas values.

SEVERE SMOKE INHALATION AND BURNS WITH RESPIRATORY AND METABOLIC ACIDOSIS

Acute Ventilatory Failure (Acute Respiratory Acidosis) and Metabolic Acidosis

COHb	pH*	$PaCO_2$†	HCO_3^-*	PaO_2	SaO_2 or SpO_2
↑	↓	↑	↓	↓	↓ or Normal

COHb, Carboxyhemoglobin.

Oxygenation Indices
Smoke Inhalation and Burns

	Early and Intermediate Stages	Late Stage
DO_2	↓	↓
$\dot{V}O_2$	↑	↓
$C(a-\bar{v})O_2$	↑	↓
O_2ER	↑	↓
$S\bar{v}O_2$	↓	↓

When CO or cyanide poisoning is present, the oxygenation indices are unreliable because the PaO_2 is often normal in the presence of **CO poisoning**, and when cyanide poisoning is present, the tissue cells are prevented from consuming oxygen. Both of these conditions cause falsely high pulse oximetry readings. For example, when CO is present, a normal DO_2 value may be calculated when, in reality, the patient's oxygen transport status is extremely low. When cyanide poisoning is present, the patient's $\dot{V}O_2$ may appear normal or increased, when in actuality the tissue cells are extremely hypoxic. Typically these problems are not present during the intermediate and late stages in the presence of appropriate treatment—i.e., once the carbon dioxide and/or cyanide has been removed.

Hemodynamic Indices
Cardiogenic Pulmonary Edema*

	Early Stage	Intermediate Stage	Late Stage
CVP	↓	Normal	↓
RAP	↓	Normal	↓
$\overline{PA}$	↓	Normal	↓
PCWP	↓	Normal	↓
CO	↓	Normal	↓
SV	↓	Normal	↓
SVI	↓	Normal	↓
CI†	↓	Normal	↓
RVSWI	↓	Normal	↓
LVSWI	↓	Normal	↓
PVR	Normal	Normal	↑
SVR	↑	Normal	↑

In general, the hemodynamic profile in patients with body surface burns relates to the amount of intravascular volume loss (hypovolemia) that occurs as a result of third-space fluid shifts. For example, during the early stage, the decreased values shown for the CVP, RAP, $\overline{PA}$, CWP, CO, SV, SVI, CI, RVSWI, and LVSWI reflect the reduction in pulmonary intravascular and cardiac filling volumes. Hypovolemia causes a generalized peripheral vasoconstriction, which is reflected in an elevated SVR. When appropriate fluid resuscitation is administered, the patient's hemodynamic indices are usually normal during the intermediate stage.

CARBON MONOXIDE POISONING

When a patient has been exposed to smoke, *CO poisoning must be assumed.* Although CO has no direct injurious effect on the lungs, it can greatly reduce the patient's oxygen transport because CO has an affinity for hemoglobin that is about 210 times greater than that of oxygen. CO attached to hemoglobin is called **carboxyhemoglobin (COHb)**. Breathing CO at a partial pressure of <2 mm Hg can result in a COHb of ≥40%. In other words, ≥40% of the hemoglobin oxygen transport system is then unavailable for oxygen transport.

In addition, high concentrations of COHb cause the oxyhemoglobin dissociation curve to move markedly to the left, which makes it more difficult for oxygen to leave the hemoglobin at the tissue sites. In essence, the tissue cells are better oxygenated

---

*When tissue hypoxia is severe enough to produce lactic acid, the pH and HCO_3^- values will be lower than expected for a particular $PaCO_2$ level.
†In severe burns with ARDS, the $PaCO_2$ may be elevated and combined respiratory and metabolic acidosis may be present.

---

*When ARDS is present, noncardiogenic pulmonary edema findings may be present (see Chapter 28, Acute Respiratory Distress Syndrome).
†*CI*, Cardiac index; *CO*, cardiac output; *CVP*, central venous pressure; *LVSWI*, left ventricular stroke work index; $\overline{PA}$, mean pulmonary artery pressure; *PCWP*, pulmonary capillary wedge pressure; *PVR*, pulmonary vascular resistance; *RAP*, right atrial pressure; *RVSWI*, right ventricular stroke work index; *SV*, stroke volume; *SVI*, stroke volume index; *SVR*, systemic vascular resistance.

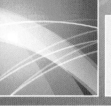
when 40% of the hemoglobin is absent (anemia) than when a COHb of 40% is present. Thus, it should be stressed that SpO_2 and pulse oximeter-based oxygen content measurements are misleading and unreliable in the presence of COHb. Arterial blood gas measurements (with **CO-oximetry**) provide important information regarding the presence of hypoxemia, widened alveolar-arterial oxygen gradient, acid-base status, and a correct measurement of both oxygen saturation (%) and COHb (%).

A COHb level in excess of 20% is usually considered CO poisoning, and a COHb level of ≥40% is considered severe. A COHb level in excess of 50% may cause irreversible damage to the central nervous system. If available, hyperbaric oxygen (HBO) therapy is usually used at a COHb >10%. Cigarette smokers may demonstrate COHb levels of ≥5% to 7%; in cigar smokers levels can be as high as 15%.

Table 43-3 lists the clinical manifestations associated with CO poisoning.

CYANIDE POISONING

When smoke contains cyanide, oxygen transport may be further impaired. Cyanide poisoning should be suspected in comatose patients who have inhaled fumes from burning plastic (polyurethane) or other synthetic materials. Inhaled cyanide is easily transported in the blood to the tissue cells, where it bonds to the cytochrome oxidase enzymes of the mitochondria. This inhibits the metabolism of oxygen and causes the tissue cells to shift to an inefficient (anaerobic) form of metabolism. The end-product of anaerobic metabolism is lactic acid. Cyanide poisoning may result in lactic acidemia, which is caused by an inadequate *tissue* oxygen level, even though the PaO_2 and SpO_2 are normal or above normal. Clinically, cyanide concentrations are easily measured with

commercially available kits. A **cyanide blood level** in excess of 1 mg/L usually is fatal.

RADIOLOGIC FINDINGS

Chest Radiograph

- Usually normal (early stage)
- Pulmonary edema, ARDS (May be present during early stage)
- Patchy or segmental infiltrates (late stage)

During the early stage, the radiograph is generally normal. Signs of pulmonary edema and ARDS may be seen during the intermediate and late stages. The chest radiograph reveals dense, fluffy opacities and patchy or segmental infiltrates (Figure 43-2).

TABLE 43-3 Blood Carboxyhemoglobin (COHb) Levels and Clinical Manifestations

COHb (%)	Clinical Manifestations
0–10	Usually no symptoms
10–20	Mild headache, dilation of cutaneous blood vessels
	Cherry red skin—but not always
20–30	Throbbing headache, nausea, vomiting, impaired judgment
30–50	Throbbing headache, possible syncope, increased respiratory and pulse rates
50–60	Syncope, increased respiratory and pulse rates, coma, convulsions, Cheyne-Stokes respiration
60–70	Coma, convulsions, cardiovascular and respiratory depression, and possible death
70–80	Cardiopulmonary failure and death

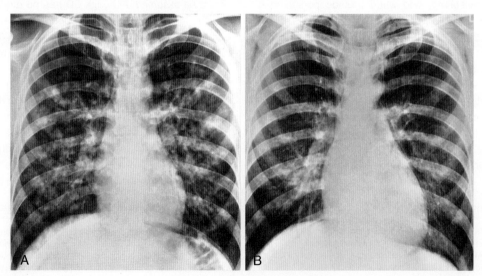

FIGURE 43-2 (**A**) Radiograph of a young man admitted after accidentally setting his kitchen on fire while intoxicated. (**B**) Prompt recovery after 72 hours. (From Hansell DM, Armstrong P, Lynch DA, McAdams HP, eds: *Imaging of diseases of the chest*, ed 4, Philadelphia, 2005, Elsevier.)

General Management of Smoke Inhalation and Thermal Injuries

General Emergency Care

The principal goals in the initial care of patients with smoke inhalation injury and burns include the immediate assessment of the patient's airway, respiratory status, cardiovascular status, percentage of body burned, and depth of burns. An intravenous line should be started immediately to administer medications and fluids. Easily separated clothing should be removed. Any remaining clothing should be soaked thoroughly before removing. When present, burn wounds should be covered to prevent shock, fluid loss, heat loss, and pain. Infection control includes isolation, room pressurization, air filtration, and wound coverings.

Fluid resuscitation with Ringer's lactate solution is usually initiated according to the **Parkland formula**—4 mL/kg of body weight for each percent of body surface area burned (see Table 43-2) over a 24-hour period. The patient's hemodynamic status will usually remain stable at this fluid replacement rate, with an average urine output target of 30 to 50 mL/h and a central venous pressure target of 2 to 6 mm Hg. Because this process may lead to overhydration and acute UAO and pulmonary edema, the patient's fluid and electrolyte status (weight, input and output, and laboratory values) must be monitored carefully.

Finally, knowledge of the exposure characteristics of the fire-related accident may be helpful in assessing the potential clinical complications. For example, did the accident involve a closed-space setting or entrapment? The amount and concentration of smoke are usually much greater under these conditions. What type of material was burning in the fire? Are the inhaled toxins known? Was CO or cyanide produced by the burning substances? Was the patient unconscious before entering the hospital? If the history warrants, tests for alcohol ingestion, poisoning, or drug overdose should be performed.

Airway Management

Early elective endotracheal intubation should be performed on the patient who has inhaled hot gases and demonstrates any signs of impending UAO (e.g., upper airway edema, blisters, inspiratory stridor, thick secretions). *This is a medical emergency.* Even though acute UAO is considered one of the most treatable complications of smoke inhalation, deaths still occur from UAO (hence the well-supported clinical guideline that states "When in doubt, intubate.").

Securing an endotracheal tube often is difficult in the presence of facial burns (typically wet wounds). Adhesive tape may cause further trauma to the burn wounds. Ingenuity and creativity may be required. Securing the endotracheal tube without traumatizing the patient has been successful with use of umbilical tape and a variety of helmets, halo traction devices, and Velcro straps.

Because of the infections associated with body surface burns and smoke inhalation, a tracheostomy should be reserved for patients in whom an airway cannot be established otherwise or who will require prolonged mechanical ventilation.

Bronchoscopy

Therapeutic bronchoscopy often is used to clear the airways of mucous plugs and eschar.[2] In addition, early bronchoscopy often is performed for inspection and evaluation of the upper airways. Mucosal changes distal to the larynx serve as good predictors of subsequent respiratory problems.

Hyperbaric Oxygen Therapy

Hyperbaric oxygenation (HBO) therapy is useful in the rapid elimination of CO and the enhancement of skin graft viability. Its clinical utility, however, is still a matter of debate in the medical literature. Although a PaO_2 >1500 mm Hg can be achieved with a hyperbaric chamber, it often is not possible or practical to institute this therapy. The chamber may not be immediately available. Can the patient be transported safely? Will the interruption of immediate therapy be detrimental?

Treatment for Cyanide Poisoning

The treatment for **cyanide poisoning** includes amyl nitrite inhalation and intravenous sodium thiosulfate.

Pharmacology

Antibiotic Agents

Antibiotics are used to treat burn wounds and pulmonary infections (see Appendix III).

Expectorants

Expectorants may be administered to facilitate expectoration (see Appendix V).

Analgesic Agents

Analgesics generally are ordered when surface burns are present.

Prophylactic Anticoagulants

Heparin and other anticoagulants often are administered to patients with severe, long-term fire-related injuries to reduce the risk of pulmonary embolism. Immobile patients also are treated with this therapy.

Respiratory Care Treatment Protocols

Oxygen Therapy Protocol

Oxygen therapy is used to treat hypoxemia, decrease the work of breathing, and decrease myocardial work. Because of the hypoxemia and **CO poisoning** associated with smoke inhalation, a high concentration of oxygen should always be administered immediately. The **COHb half-life** when a patient is breathing room air at 1 atmosphere is approximately 5 hours. In other words, a 40% COHb decreases

---

[2]An **eschar** is a slough or piece of dead tissue that is cast off from the surface of the skin or airway, particularly after a burn injury.

to about 20% in 5 hours and to about 10% in another 5 hours. Breathing 100% oxygen at 1 atmosphere reduces the COHb half-life to <1 hour. If available, HBO therapy is in order, especially in comatose smoke inhalation victims with COHb levels >10%. See Oxygen Therapy Protocol, Protocol 9-1.

Bronchopulmonary Hygiene Therapy Protocol

Because of the excessive mucous production and accumulation in the intermediate and late stages of smoke inhalation injuries, a number of respiratory therapy modalities may be used to enhance the mobilization of bronchial secretions. However, even though chest physical therapy is an excellent treatment modality to mobilize secretions, patients with severe chest burns or recent skin grafts do not tolerate chest percussion and vibration. Intermittent percussive ventilation may be a reasonable alternative (see Bronchopulmonary Hygiene Therapy Protocol, Protocol 9-2).

Lung Expansion Therapy Protocol

Lung expansion techniques are commonly used to offset the alveolar atelectasis and consolidation associated with smoke inhalation injuries. The administration of continuous positive airway pressure via an endotracheal tube or mask (when the patient has no facial or neck burns) may help minimize the development of pulmonary edema. Continuous positive airway pressure also supports the edematous airway and maintains or increases the patient's functional residual capacity (see Lung Expansion Therapy Protocol, Protocol 9-3).

Aerosolized Medication Protocol

Both sympathomimetic and parasympatholytic agents are used to produce vasoconstriction of the mucosa and to offset bronchial smooth muscle constriction. Inhaled gases must be humidified to aid in airway hydration and mobilization of secretions. Bland (saline) aerosols may be helpful. Mucolytics and antiinflammatory agents also may be administered as part of the Aerosolized Medication Protocol (see Protocol 9-4).

Mechanical Ventilation Protocol

Mechanical ventilation with positive end-expiratory pressure usually is required for patients who develop pulmonary edema, ARDS, and pneumonia. Mechanical ventilation should be implemented in the presence of acute or impending ventilatory failure (see Mechanical Ventilation Protocol, Protocol 10-1, and Mechanical Ventilation Weaning Protocol, Protocol 10-3).

CASE STUDY Smoke Inhalation and Thermal Injury

Admitting History and Physical Examination

A 21-year-old man, after smoking marijuana and falling asleep, suffered second- and third-degree burns on his face, chest, and abdomen after his bed caught fire. The extent of second- and third-degree burns was only 6% to 8% of his total body surface area. He had previously been in excellent health.

Shortly after admission, he developed respiratory distress and pulmonary edema. His blood pressure was 110/60, pulse 100 beats/min, and respiratory rate 30 breaths/min. His oral temperature was 98.8°F. Bilateral crackles and occasional wheezing were present. Spontaneous cough produced large amounts of thick, whitish-gray sputum. The chest radiograph revealed bilateral patchy infiltrates and consolidation. On 4 L/min oxygen, his arterial blood gas values were pH 7.51, $PaCO_2$ 28 mm Hg, HCO_3^- 21 mEq/L, PaO_2 45 mm Hg and SaO_2 86%. A COHb level was not obtained.

The patient was treated conservatively. He was placed on a oxygen mask, and the pulmonary edema progressively cleared over the next 48 hours. However, the respiratory distress and hypoxemia persisted, even on FIO_2 0.60 oxygen by venturi mask. Three days after admission, his condition was worsening. The patient was agitated and he complained of a productive cough, worsening shortness of breath, and substernal chest pain with deep breathing and coughing. Thick whitish-gray secretions were noted. Auscultation revealed bilateral crackles and expiratory wheezing. His vital signs were as follows: temperature 98.6°F (rectal), blood pressure 120/65, pulse 119 beats/min (regular sinus rhythm), respiratory rate 35 breaths/min. On an FIO_2 of 0.60, his arterial blood gas (ABG) values were as follows: pH 7.54, $PaCO_2$ 25 mm Hg, HCO_3^- 20 mEq/L, PaO_2 38 mm Hg and SaO_2 80%. His chest radiograph showed patchy infiltrates and some segmental consolidation. Fiberoptic bronchoscopy revealed extensive thermal damage and eschar in the trachea and large bronchi. A moderate amount of eschar and secretions was suctioned through the bronchoscope. At that time, the following respiratory assessment was documented.

Respiratory Assessment and Plan

S   Complains of productive cough, substernal chest pain when coughing, and dyspnea.
O   Afebrile. BP 120/65, P 119 and regular, RR 35. Bilateral crackles and expiratory wheezing. On FIO_2 0.60 O_2 by venturi mask: pH 7.54, $PaCO_2$ 25, HCO_3^- 20, PaO_2 38 and SaO_2 80%. CXR: Bilateral patchy infiltrates and consolidation. No cardiomegaly. Bronchoscopy—blackish eschar in oropharynx; reddened and inflamed larynx, trachea, and large airways. Thick, whitish-gray secretions noted.

A • Smoke inhalation with thermal burns of the oropharynx, larynx, and large airways (history and bronchoscopy)

• Alveolar infiltrates and consolidation (CXR)

• Acute alveolar hyperventilation with severe hypoxemia (ABGs)

• Impending ventilatory failure (general history and clinical trend)

• Excessive and thick airway secretions (sputum, bronchoscopy and expectorate)

P Confer with attending physician to intubate and initiate mechanical ventilation care per **Mechanical Ventilation Protocol. Oxygen Therapy Protocol:** FIO_2 at 1.0 via nonrebreather mask. **Aerosolized Medication Protocol** and **Bronchopulmonary Hygiene Protocol:** albuterol premix 2.0 mL via med. nebulizer. q2h (alternate with racemic epinephrine 6 drops in 2.0 mL normal saline). Gentle PRN nasotracheal and oral suctioning after med. neb. treatments. Check I&O status and daily weights.

The patient was intubated and started on intravenously administered steroids. He was ventilated with an FIO_2 of 0.60, rate of 12, and positive end-expiratory pressure of +10 cm H_2O. Because of the upper body burns, chest physical therapy and postural drainage were prohibited. The bronchial secretions, however, were loosened and mobilized adequately with an in-line ultrasonic nebulizer and frequent endotracheal suctioning. In-line aerosolized steroids also were administered at this time.

The patient's vital signs and blood gas values improved on this regimen. After 12 days of respiratory care, he was weaned to an FIO_2 of 0.40 and extubated. He continued to complain of exertional dyspnea with transfer activities but denied dyspnea at rest. Crackles were improved but still easily auscultated throughout all lung fields when the patient took deep breaths. Occasional expiratory wheezes also were heard.

Three days after extubation, on an FIO_2 of 0.35 via a venturi oxygen mask, his pH was 7.45, $PaCO_2$ 36 mm Hg, HCO_3^- 24 mEq/L, PaO_2 63 mm Hg and SaO_2 93%. On exercise, the SpO_2 fell to 85%. His peak expiratory flow rate (PEFR) was 40% of predicted. The infiltrates previously noted on chest radiograph were much improved. At that time, the respiratory therapist recorded the following assessment in the patient's chart.

Respiratory Assessment and Plan

S Complains of shortness of breath with any activity.

O Vital signs stable. Crackles heard over both lung bases. Some expiratory prolongation. ABGs (spontaneous breathing) (FIO_2 0.35 via venturi mask): pH 7.45, $PaCO_2$ 36, HCO_3^- 24, PaO_2 63 and SaO_2 93%. SpO_2 falls to 85% with exercise. PEFR 40% of predicted. CXR: Improvement in patchy lung infiltrates.

A • Mild to moderate hypoxemia secondary to thermal injury to lung (ABGs and history)

• Moderate obstructive pulmonary disease (PEFR)

P Complete pulmonary function tests ordered. Up-regulate **Oxygen Therapy Protocol** (increase FIO_2 to 0.40 via venturi mask). If patient is ambulatory, titrate oxygen therapy based on exercise SpO_2. If obstructive pulmonary disease is confirmed, restart **Bronchial Hygiene Protocol** and **Aerosolized Medication Protocol**.

Pulmonary function studies showed severely reduced expiratory flows and a sharply decreased diffusion capacity. Chest radiograph taken at regular intervals thereafter began to show emphysematous changes. The diaphragms were flattened, and bilateral coarse reticular infiltrates were evident. Despite vigorous therapy over the next 6 weeks, the patient's cardiopulmonary status continued to worsen. He died on day 59, 2 months after his original thermal and inhalational injury. The postmortem diagnosis at autopsy was cryptogenic organizing pneumonia (COP)—also known as *bronchiolitis obliterans organizing pneumonia* (BOOP).

Discussion

At the time of the first assessment, the patient demonstrated most of the pathophysiologic correlates of smoke inhalation and thermal injuries to the lung. His dyspnea reflected the increased work of breathing associated with **Bronchospasm** (see Figure 9-10), **Increased Alveolar-Capillary Membrane Thickness** (see Figure 9-9), and **Excessive Bronchial Secretions** (see Figure 9-11). The bronchospasm was treated with the vigorous use of both bronchodilator (albuterol) and decongestant (epinephrine) aerosols. The excessive bronchial secretions were treated with ultrasonic bland aerosols and airway suctioning. No specific treatment was available for the changes that occurred in the alveolar-capillary membrane.

This interesting case is instructive for these reasons. Primarily, all patients with burns of the upper chest, neck, or face should have a careful oropharyngeal examination to determine whether burns have indeed occurred in the upper airway. The presence of soot or eschar in the oropharynx is diagnostic of this problem; respiratory distress almost certainly will ensue if such findings are present, although this does not happen immediately. A 24- to 72-hour lag may occur between the burn and clinical obstruction of the airway. Second, a dreaded complication of smoke and heat inhalation is COP, which developed in this patient and ultimately was fatal. Lastly, failure to measure COHb on admission falls well below the standard of care.

This patient might have been considered a candidate for lung transplantation. This case study should remind the respiratory therapist that immediate intubation may be necessary over the diagnostic bronchoscope and that he or she should prepare accordingly.

SELF-ASSESSMENT QUESTIONS

Answers to questions can be found on Evolve. To access additional student assessment questions visit **http://evolve.elsevier.com/DesJardins/respiratory**.

1. About what percentage of hospitalized patients with thermal injury have an acute upper airway obstruction?
   a. 0% to 10%
   b. 10% to 20%
   c. 20% to 30%
   d. 30% to 40%

2. Except for the rare instance of steam inhalation, direct thermal injuries usually do not occur below the level of which of the following structures?
   a. Oral pharynx
   b. Larynx
   c. Carina
   d. Bronchi

3. When chest wall burns are present, the patient's pulmonary condition may be further aggravated by which of the following?
   1. Decreased lung and chest compliance
   2. Increased airway resistance
   3. Administration of narcotics
   4. Immobility
      a. 2 and 3 only
      b. 1 and 3 only
      c. 2 and 4 only
      d. 1, 2, 3, and 4

4. Which of the following is/are the pulmonary-related pathologic change(s) associated with smoke inhalation?
   1. Pneumomediastinum
   2. Bronchospasm
   3. Pulmonary edema
   4. Pulmonary embolism
      a. 1 only
      b. 2 only
      c. 3 and 4 only
      d. 2, 3, and 4 only

5. Which of the following produce carbon monoxide when burned?
   1. Polyurethanes
   2. Wood, cotton, paper
   3. Organic material
   4. Polyvinylchloride
      a. 1 only
      b. 2 only
      c. 3 and 4 only
      d. 1, 2, and 3 only

6. Which of the following oxygenation indices is or are associated with smoke inhalation and burns during the early and intermediate stages?
   1. Increased $\dot{V}O_2$
   2. Decreased $C(a\text{-}\bar{v})O_2$
   3. Increased DO_2
   4. Decreased $S\bar{v}O_2$
      a. 2 only
      b. 4 only
      c. 2 and 3 only
      d. 1 and 4 only

7. Which of the following hemodynamic indices is or are associated with body surface burns during the early stage?
   1. Decreased CO
   2. Increased SVR
   3. Decreased $\overline{PA}$
   4. Increased PCWP
      a. 1 only
      b. 3 only
      c. 2 and 4 only
      d. 1, 2, and 3 only

8. If an adult's entire right arm, right leg, and anterior trunk have been burned, approximately what percentage of the patient's body surface area is burned?
   a. 15%
   b. 25%
   c. 35%
   d. 45%

9. Healing time for a second-degree burn is:
   a. 1 to 7 days
   b. 7 to 21 days
   c. 21 to 31 days
   d. 1 to 2 months

10. Breathing 100% oxygen at 1 atmosphere reduces the COHb half-life to less than:
    a. 1 hour
    b. 2 hours
    c. 3 hours
    d. 4 hours

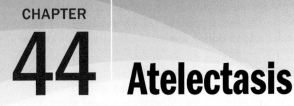
44 Atelectasis

Chapter Objectives

After reading this chapter, you will be able to:
- List the anatomic alterations of the lungs associated with atelectasis.
- Describe the specific causes of atelectasis.
- List the respiratory disorders associated with atelectasis.
- List the cardiopulmonary clinical manifestations associated with postoperative atelectasis.
- Describe the general management of atelectasis.
- Describe the clinical strategies and rationales of the SOAP presented in the case study.

Key Terms

Absorption Atelectasis
Air Bronchograms
Alveolar Degassing
Primary Atelectasis
Primary Lobule
Therapeutic Bronchoscopy

Chapter Outline

Anatomic Alterations of the Lungs
Etiology
Respiratory Disorders Associated with Atelectasis
Overview of the Cardiopulmonary Clinical Manifestations
    Associated with Postoperative Atelectasis
General Management of Postoperative Atelectasis
    General Considerations
    Respiratory Care Treatment Protocols
Case Study: Postoperative Atelectasis
Self-Assessment Questions

Anatomic Alterations of the Lungs

Atelectasis is an abnormal condition of the lungs characterized by the partial or total collapse of previously expanded alveoli—thus, resulting in (1) the prevention of respiratory exchange of carbon dioxide and oxygen in that part of the lung and, (2) reduced lung compliance. The failure of the lungs to expand at birth, most commonly seen in premature infants or those narcotized by maternal anesthesia, is known as **primary atelectasis**. Atelectasis may be limited to the smallest lung unit—i.e., alveolus or **primary lobule**[1]—or it may involve an entire lung or a segment or lobe of the lung (Figure 44-1).

The major pathologic and anatomic alterations associated with atelectasis include partial or total collapse of the following:
- Alveoli of primary lobules (microatelectasis or subsegmental atelectasis)—very common
- Lung segment—fairly common
- Lung lobe—less common
- Entire lung—rare

---

[1]A primary lobule is a cluster of alveoli that originates from a single terminal bronchiole. Each primary lobule is about 3.5 mm in diameter and contains about 2000 alveoli. Each lung contains about 150,000 primary lobules. A primary lobule also is called an *acinus, terminal respiratory unit,* or *functional lung unit.* The lung parenchyma consists of the terminal respiratory units.

Etiology

As shown in Box 44-1, there are many respiratory disorders associated with atelectasis. The etiologic factors linked to these disorders, and the subsequent atelectasis that ensues, can be further grouped into pulmonary conditions that (1) reduce alveolar ventilation (e.g., pulmonary edema, acute respiratory distress syndrome, smoke inhalation, thermal injuries), (2) enable alveolar "degassing" secondary to airway obstruction (e.g., cystic fibrosis, bronchiectasis, Guillain-Barré syndrome, myasthenia gravis), or (3) compress the lung tissue (e.g., flail chest, pneumothorax, pleural disease).

In this chapter, postoperative atelectasis is used as a prototype of the atelectasis process. Postoperative atelectasis is commonly seen after upper abdominal and thoracic surgical procedures. Lung expansion is often decreased after surgery because of postoperative alveolar hypoventilation (anesthesia), external compression, postoperative pain, or development of excessive airway secretions and mucous plugs—which, in turn, produce distal degassing of lung units (also called **absorption atelectasis**).[2]

In addition, good lung expansion depends on the patient's intact chest cage and the ability to generate an appropriate negative intrapleural pressure. Thoracic and upper abdominal procedures often result in a reduced ability to generate good

---

[2]In cases in which atelectasis is caused by excessive airway secretions, it is not uncommon to see this condition complicated by bronchospasm and wheezing.

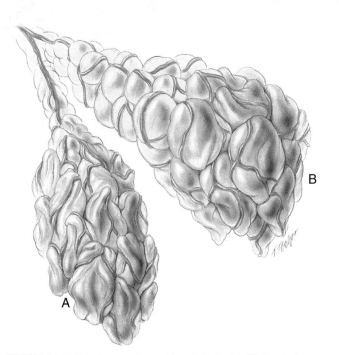

FIGURE 44-1 Alveoli in postoperative atelectasis. (**A**) Total alveolar collapse. (**B**) Partial alveolar collapse.

lung expansion and therefore are considered high-risk factors for subsequent development of postoperative atelectasis. Other precipitating factors of postoperative atelectasis include (1) obesity, (2) supine position, (3) advanced age, (4) inadequate tidal volume during mechanical ventilation, (5) malnutrition, (6) free fluid in the abdominal cavity (ascites), or (7) presence of a restrictive lung disorder (e.g., pleural effusion, pneumothorax, acute respiratory distress syndrome, pulmonary edema, interstitial lung disease, or pleural masses).

Finally, postoperative atelectasis is often associated with retained airway secretions and mucous plugs. Precipitating factors for retained secretions include (1) decreased mucociliary transport, (2) excessive secretions, (3) inadequate hydration, (4) weak or absent cough, (5) general anesthesia, (6) smoking history, (7) gastric aspiration, and (8) certain preexisting conditions (see Box 44-1). When total airway obstruction develops, alveolar oxygen is *absorbed* into the pulmonary circulation and **alveolar degassing** ensues. Breathing high oxygen concentrations favors this pathologic process.

BOX 44-1 Respiratory Disorders Associated With Atelectasis

- Bronchiectasis
- Cystic fibrosis
- Pulmonary edema
- Pulmonary embolism
- Flail chest
- Pneumothorax
- Pleural diseases
- Kyphoscoliosis
- Cancer of the lung
- Acute respiratory distress syndrome*

- Guillain-Barré syndrome*
- Myasthenia gravis*
- Meconium aspiration syndrome
- Respiratory distress syndrome
- Pulmonary air leak syndrome
- Respiratory syncytial virus
- Bronchopulmonary dysplasia
- Diaphragmatic hernia
- Near drowning
- Smoke inhalation and thermal injuries

*Common secondary anatomic alteration of the lungs associated with this disorder.

OVERVIEW of the Cardiopulmonary Clinical Manifestations Associated with Postoperative Atelectasis[3]

The following clinical manifestations result from the pathologic mechanisms caused (or activated) by atelectasis (see Figure 9-7)—the major anatomic alterations of the lungs associated with atelectasis (see Figure 44-1).

CLINICAL DATA OBTAINED AT THE PATIENT'S BEDSIDE

The Physical Examination

Vital Signs

Increased Respiratory Rate (Tachypnea)

Several pathophysiologic mechanisms operating simultaneously may lead to an increased ventilatory rate:

- Stimulation of peripheral chemoreceptors (hypoxemia)
- Decreased lung compliance–increased ventilatory rate relationship
- Stimulation of J receptors
- Pain, anxiety, fever

Increased Heart Rate (Pulse) and Blood Pressure
Cyanosis
Chest Assessment Findings

- Increased tactile and vocal fremitus
- Dull percussion note
- Bronchial breath sounds
- Diminished breath sounds (common when atelectasis in caused by mucous plugs)
- Crackles (usually heard initially in the dependent lung regions and during late inspiration)
- Whispered pectoriloquy

CLINICAL DATA OBTAINED FROM LABORATORY TESTS AND SPECIAL PROCEDURES

Pulmonary Function Test Findings
(Primarily Restrictive Lung Pathophysiology)

FORCED EXPIRATORY VOLUME AND FLOW RATE FINDINGS

FVC	FEV_T	FEV_1/FVC ratio	$FEF_{25\%-75\%}$
↓	N or ↓	N or ↑	N or ↓

$FEF_{50\%}$	$FEF_{200-1200}$	PEFR	MVV
N or ↓	N or ↓	N or ↓	N or ↓

LUNG VOLUME AND CAPACITY FINDINGS

V_T	IRV	ERV	RV
N or ↓	↓	↓	↓

VC	IC	FRC	TLC	RV/TLC ratio
↓	↓	↓	↓	N

DECREASED DIFFUSION CAPACITY (DL_{CO})

Arterial Blood Gases

SMALL OR LOCALIZED ATELECTASIS

Acute Alveolar Hyperventilation with Hypoxemia[†]
(Acute Respiratory Alkalosis)

pH	$PaCO_2$	HCO_3^-	PaO_2	SaO_2 or SpO_2
↑	↓	↓ (but normal)	↓	↓

WIDESPREAD ATELECTASIS

Acute Ventilatory Failure with Hypoxemia[†]
(Acute Respiratory Acidosis)

pH*	$PaCO_2$	HCO_3^-*	PaO_2	SaO_2 or SpO_2
↓	↑	↑ (but normal)	↓	↓

[†]See Figure 4-3 and related discussion for the acute pH, $PaCO_2$, and HCO_3^- changes associated with acute alveolar hyperventilation.
[†]See Figure 4-2 and related discussion for the acute pH, $PaCO_2$, and HCO_3^- changes associated with acute ventilatory failure.
*When tissue hypoxia is severe enough to produce lactic acid, the pH and HCO_3^- values will be lower than expected for a particular $PaCO_2$ level.

[3]The Overview of Cardiopulmonary Clinical Manifestations presented in this chapter apply to all cases of atelectasis—regardless of the etiology (see Box 44-1).

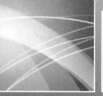

Oxygenation Indices*

$\dot{Q}_S/\dot{Q}_T$	$DO_2^\dagger$	$\dot{V}O_2$	$C(a\text{-}\bar{v})O_2$	O_2ER	$S\bar{v}O_2$
↑	↓	N	N	↑	↓

*$C(a\text{-}\bar{v})O_2$, Arterial-venous oxygen difference; DO_2, total oxygen delivery; O_2ER, oxygen extraction ratio; $\dot{Q}_S/\dot{Q}_T$, pulmonary shunt fraction; $S\bar{v}O_2$, mixed venous oxygen saturation; $\dot{V}O_2$, oxygen consumption.

$\dagger$The DO_2 may be normal in patients who have compensated to the decreased oxygenation status with (1) an increased cardiac output, (2) an increased hemoglobin level, or (3) a combination of both. When the DO_2 is normal, the O_2ER is usually normal.

RADIOLOGIC FINDINGS
Chest Radiograph
- Increased density in areas of atelectasis
- **Air bronchograms**
- Elevation of the hemidiaphragm on the affected side
- Mediastinal shift toward the affected side

Areas of increased density generally appear initially in dependent lung regions, such as the lower lobes, or posteriorly in patients who must recline in the supine position. Air bronchograms can be seen when large areas of atelectasis are present. An elevation of the hemidiaphragm or mediastinal shift toward the affected side is often seen when large areas of atelectasis exist. Figure 44-2, *A* shows left lung atelectasis caused by a misplaced endotracheal tube in the right main stem bronchus. Figure 44-2, *B* shows the same patient 20 minutes after the endotracheal tube was pulled back above the carina.

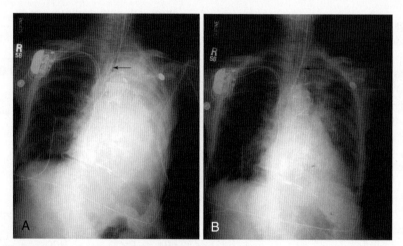

FIGURE 44-2 (A) Endotracheal tube tip misplaced in the right main stem bronchus (*arrow*). Note that the left lung has collapsed completely (i.e., white fluffy appearance in the left lung). **(B)** The same patient 20 minutes after the endotracheal tube was pulled back above the carina (*arrow*). Note that the left lung is better ventilated (i.e., appears darker). (Used, with permission, from author Terry Des Jardins.)

General Management of Postoperative Atelectasis

Precipitating factors for postoperative atelectasis should be identified during the pre- and postoperative assessments (see the previous section on etiology). High-risk patients should be monitored closely and are often treated with preventive measures. Bedside spirometry (vital capacity and inspiratory capacity) is useful in the early detection of atelectasis, and incentive spirometry is frequently prescribed to encourage good lung expansion. Preoperative patients with combined obstructive and restrictive pulmonary disease are generally considered extremely high risk for atelectasis. This is especially true if the patient has a condition associated with excessive airway secretions—e.g., chronic bronchitis. When postoperative atelectasis has been diagnosed, the following respiratory care procedures may be prescribed.

General Considerations
Whenever possible, treatment of the underlying cause of the postoperative atelectasis should be prescribed immediately (e.g., medication for pain, control/treatment of airway secretions, correction of inadequate tidal volumes during mechanical ventilation, repositioning of an endotracheal tube in the right main stem bronchus, or withdrawal of air or fluid from the pleural cavity).

Respiratory Care Treatment Protocols

Oxygen Therapy Protocol

Oxygen therapy is used to treat hypoxemia, decrease the work of breathing, and decrease myocardial work. Because of the hypoxemia that may develop in atelectasis, supplemental oxygen may be required. However, the hypoxemia that develops in postoperative atelectasis is caused by capillary shunting and therefore is often refractory to oxygen therapy (see Oxygen Therapy Protocol, Protocol 9-1).

Bronchopulmonary Hygiene Therapy Protocol

When atelectasis is caused by mucous accumulation and mucous plugs, a number of bronchial hygiene treatment modalities may be used to enhance the mobilization of airway secretions (see Bronchopulmonary Hygiene Therapy Protocol, Protocol 9-2).

Lung Expansion Therapy Protocol

Lung expansion therapy measures are routinely administered to offset atelectasis and reinflate collapsed lung areas (see Lung Expansion Therapy Protocol, Protocol 9-3).

Mechanical Ventilation Protocol

Short-term mechanical ventilation is often prescribed after major surgery, especially if the patient has one or more high-risk factors for postoperative atelectasis. For example, in patients undergoing cardiac surgery, mechanical ventilation generally is maintained until the cardiopulmonary parameters are stable (see Mechanical Ventilation Protocol, Protocol 10-1, and Mechanical Ventilation Weaning Protocol, Protocol 10-2).

CASE STUDY Postoperative Atelectasis

Admitting History and Physical Examination

A 62-year-old man with a 35-pack-year smoking history and long-standing productive cough had his left lower lobe resected because of small-cell lung carcinoma. Anesthesia had been given using a right-sided double-lumen endotracheal tube. At the end of the procedure, the patient was breathing well and the tube was removed.

In the recovery room 30 minutes after arrival, his respiratory rate increased from 22 breaths/min to 34 breaths/min. His pulse increased from 70 to 130 beats/min with regular rhythm, and his blood pressure decreased from 115/85 to 100/60 mm Hg. His SpO_2 dropped from 97% to 85% while he was on 2 L/min O_2 per cannula. Breath sounds were decreased in the left lower anterior chest. A chest radiograph showed atelectasis of the left lower lobe. Arterial blood gas (ABG) values (on 2 L/min O_2 per cannula) were pH 7.29, $PaCO_2$ 63 mm Hg, HCO_3^- 29 mEq/L, PaO_2 55 mm Hg, and SaO_2 84%.

At that time the respiratory therapist recorded the following SOAP note:

Respiratory Assessment and Plan

S N/A. Patient extubated, but still sedated from anesthesia.

O RR 34/min, P 130 and regular, BP 100/60. Breath sounds decreased in left lower chest anteriorly. CXR: Left lower lobe atelectasis. On 2 L/min O_2 per cannula: pH 7.29, $PaCO_2$ 63, HCO_3^- 29, SaO_2 84%.

A • Left lower lobe atelectasis; rule out mucous plugs (CXR and decreased breath sounds)
  • Acute ventilatory failure with moderate hypoxemia (ABGs)

P Stat: Contact physician regarding possible reintubation and **Mechanical Ventilation Protocol** (SIMV mode). **Oxygen Therapy Protocol** (FIO_2 0.50). **Bronchopulmonary Hygiene Therapy Protocol** (deep tracheal suction; discuss with physician the possibility of respiratory therapist assistance with therapeutic bronchoscopy). **Lung Expansion Therapy Protocol** after intubation (positive end-expiratory pressure based on titration study). Repeat ABGs in 30 minutes and reevaluate. Monitor SpO_2 for next 72 hours. When patient is alert, instruct in cough and deep breathing technique.

The patient was reintubated, ventilated, and oxygenated according to protocol. A mucolytic (acetylcysteine) was aerosolized and directly instilled into his endotracheal tube. Aggressive tracheobronchial suctioning was performed but produced small amounts of secretions with little or no benefit to the patient.

In view of this, a fiberoptic bronchoscope was inserted through the endotracheal tube, and a large mucous plug was identified in the orifice of the left lower lobe bronchus. The plug was removed under direct vision. After the bronchoscopy, the patient improved rapidly and could be extubated after about 60 minutes. A chest radiograph taken before that time showed full expansion of the left lower lobe. The patient was discharged on the sixth postoperative day.

Discussion

Care of a patient with postoperative **atelectasis** (see Figure 9-7) is one of the day-to-day responsibilities of the respiratory therapist and was well carried out in this case. Accordingly, the respiratory therapist must be extremely adept in the assessment and management of such patients. The development of immediate postoperative atelectasis is almost always related to **excessive bronchial secretions** (see Figure 9-11)—in this case caused by a large mucous plug obstructing the left lower lobe. Because such patients (in the immediate postoperative period) often cannot cough vigorously, particularly after thoracotomy, the decision to initiate **therapeutic bronchoscopy** immediately rather than to rely on physical therapy, suctioning and mucolytics was certainly in order.

In patients who have undergone abdominal surgery or those who develop atelectasis later, the simpler approaches should certainly be tried first. Atelectasis has a tendency to recur, and these patients need to be followed for at least 72 hours postoperatively to ensure that this has not happened. Therefore the therapist's suggestion to follow up with pulse oximetry and cough and deep breathing instruction was entirely appropriate.

As important as treatment is, prevention is better. In this regard, the **Bronchopulmonary Hygiene Protocol** and the **Lung Expansion Protocol** were very important. Indeed, the application of these simple protocols often prevents the late development of atelectasis in postoperative patients. Unfortunately, no preoperative aggressive respiratory care was recorded in this patient's care.

SELF-ASSESSMENT QUESTIONS

Answers to questions can be found on Evolve. To access additional student assessment questions visit **http://evolve.elsevier.com/DesJardins/respiratory**.

1. **Which of the following clinical manifestations are associated with postoperative atelectasis?**
   1. Frothy, pink sputum
   2. Crackles
   3. Air bronchograms
   4. Increased $S\bar{v}O_2$
      a. 1 and 2 only
      b. 2 and 3 only
      c. 3, and 4 only
      d. 2, 3, and 4 only

2. **Which of the following pulmonary function testing values are associated with postoperative atelectasis?**
   1. N or $\uparrow FEV_T$
   2. $\uparrow FVC$
   3. $\downarrow RV$
   4. N or $\uparrow FEV_1/FVC$ ratio
      a. 1 and 2 only
      b. 3 and 4 only
      c. 2, 3, and 4 only
      d. 1, 2, 3, and 4 only

3. **A primary lobule is a cluster of alveoli. About how many alveoli does a primary lobule contain?**
   a. 500 alveoli
   b. 1000 alveoli
   c. 1500 alveoli
   d. 2000 alveoli

4. **Which of the following are precipitating factors of postoperative atelectasis?**
   1. Obesity
   2. Anesthesia
   3. Postoperative pain
   4. Ascites
      a. 1 and 3 only
      b. 2 and 4 only
      c. 2, 3, and 4 only
      d. 1, 2, 3, and 4

5. **Which of the following arterial blood gas values are associated with small or localized postoperative atelectasis?**
   1. Increased PaO_2
   2. Decreased $PaCO_2$
   3. Increased pH
   4. Decreased HCO_3^- (but normal)
      a. 1 and 3 only
      b. 2 and 4 only
      c. 2, 3, and 4 only
      d. 1, 2, 3, and 4

Symbols and Abbreviations Commonly Used in Respiratory Physiology

Primary Symbols			
Gas Symbols		**Blood Symbols**	
P	Pressure	Q	Blood volume
V	Gas volume	$\dot{Q}$	Blood flow
$\dot{V}$	Gas volume per unit of time, or flow	C	Content in blood
F	Fractional concentration of gas	S	Saturation
Secondary Symbols			
Gas Symbols		**Blood Symbols**	
I	Inspired	a	Arterial
E	Expired	c	Capillary
A	Alveolar	v	Venous
T	Tidal	$\bar{v}$	Mixed venous
D	Dead space		
B	Barometric		

Abbreviations

Lung Volumes

VC	Vital capacity
IC	Inspiratory capacity
IRV	Inspiratory reserve volume
ERV	Expiratory reserve volume
FRC	Functional residual capacity
RV	Residual volume
TLC	Total lung capacity
RV/TLC (%)	Residual volume-to-total lung capacity ratio, expressed as a percentage
V_T	Tidal volume
V_A	Alveolar volume
V_D	Dead space volume
V_L	Actual lung volume

Respiratory Gas Flows and Rates

$\dot{V}_A$	Alveolar ventilation
$\dot{V}_D$	Dead space ventilation
f	Frequency (i.e., respiratory rate)

Spirometry

FVC	Forced vital capacity with maximally forced expiratory effort
FEV_T	Forced expiratory volume, timed
$FEF_{50\%}$	Forced expiratory flow at 50%

Continued

Lung Volumes

FEV_1	Forced expiratory volume in 1 second
FEV_2	Forced expiratory volume in 2 seconds
FEV_3	Forced expiratory volume in 3 seconds
FEV_1/FVC	Forced expiratory volume in 1 second/forced vital capacity ratio expressed as a percentage
$FEV_{1\%}$	Forced expiratory volume in 1 second (percentage)
$FEF_{200-1200}$	Average rate of air flow between 200 and 1200 mL of the FVC
$FEF_{25\%-75\%}$	Forced expiratory flow during the middle half of the FVC (*formerly called the maximal midexpiratory flow [MMF]*)
PEFR	Peak expiratory flow rate
$\dot{V}_{max}$	Forced expiratory flow related to the actual volume of the lungs as denoted by the subscript *x*, which refers to the amount of lung volume remaining when measurement is made (e.g., $\dot{V}_{50}$ = flow at 50% of FVC)

Mechanics

C_L	Lung compliance, volume change per unit of pressure change
CL_{dyn}	Dynamic lung compliance (lung compliance with flow)
CL_{stat}	Static lung compliance (lung compliance without flow)
R_{aw}	Airway resistance, pressure per unit of flow

Diffusion

D_{LCO}	Diffusing capacity of carbon monoxide

Other Symbols and Abbreviations

$C\bar{v}O_2$	Oxygen content of mixed venous blood
$\dot{V}/\dot{Q}$	Ventilation-perfusion ratio
$\dot{Q}_S/\dot{Q}_T$	Shunt fraction
$\dot{Q}_T$ or CO	Total cardiac output

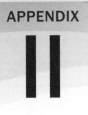
Agents Used to Treat Bronchospasm and Airway Inflammation

Medications Commonly Used in the Treatment of Chronic Obstructive Pulmonary Disease (COPD)*

Generic Name	Brand Name
Short-Acting Beta$_2$ Agents (SABAs)	
Albuterol	Proventil HFA, Ventolin HFA, ProAir HFA
Metaproterenol	Generic only
Levalbuterol	Xopenex, Xopenex HFA, Generic
Long-Acting Beta$_2$ Agents (LABAs)	
Salmeterol	Serevent Diskus
Formoterol	Perforomist, Foradil Aerolizer
Arformoterol	Brovana
Indacaterol	Arcapta Neohaler
Olodaterol	Striverdi Respimat
Anticholinergic Agents, Short-Acting	
Ipratropium	Atrovent HFA
Anticholinergic Agents, Long-Acting	
Tiotropium	Spiriva HandiHaler, Spiriva Respimat
Aclidinium	Tudorza Pressair
Umeclidinium	Incruse Ellipta
SABAs & Anticholinergic Agents (Combined)	
Ipratropium and Albuterol	DuoNeb, Combivent Respimat
LABAs & Anticholinergic Agents (Combined)	
Umeclidinium and Vilanterol	Anoro Ellipta
Inhaled Corticosteroids & Long-Acting Beta$_2$ Agents (Combined)	
Fluticasone and Salmeterol	Advair Diskus (250/50 mcg only)
Budesonide and Formoterol	Symbicort (60/4.5 mcg only)
Fluticasone and Vilanterol	Breo Ellipta
Systemic Corticosteroids	
Methylprednisolone	Medrol, Solu-Medrol
Hydrocortisone	Solu-Cortef
Xanthine Derivatives Used as Bronchodilators in COPD	
Theophylline	Theochron, Elxophyllin, Theo-24
Oxtriphylline	Oxtriphylline
Aminophylline	Generic
Dyphylline	Lufyllin
Phosphodiesterase-4 Inhibitor	
Roflumilast	Daliresp

*For the complete listing, doses, and administration of agents approved by the FDA, visit the Drugs@FDA website (www.accessdata.fda.gov/scripts/cder/drugsatfda/).

Controller Medications Used to Treat Asthma*

Generic Name	Brand Name
Long-Acting Beta$_2$ Agents (LABAs)	
Salmeterol	Serevent Diskus
Inhaled Corticosteroids (ICSs)	
Beclomethasone	QVAR
Flunisolide	Aerospan HFA
Fluticasone	Flovent HFA, Flovent Diskus, Arnuity Ellipta
Budesonide	Pulmicort Flexhaler, Pulmicort Respules
Mometasone	Asmanex Twisthaler, Asmanex HFA
Ciclesonide	Alvesco
Inhaled Corticosteroids & Long-Acting Beta$_2$ Agents (Combined)	
Fluticasone and Salmeterol	Advair Diskus, Advair HFA
Budesonide and Formoterol	Symbicort
Mometasone and Formoterol	Dulera
Leukotriene Inhibitors (Antileukotrienes)	
Zafirlukast	Accolate
Montelukast	Singulair
Zileuton	Zyflo, Zyflo CR
Monoclonal Antibody	
Omalizumab	Xolair
Xanthine Derivatives	
Theophylline	Theochron, Elxophyllin, Theo-24
Oxtriphylline	Chledyl SA
Aminophylline	Generic
Dyphylline	Lufyllin

*For the complete listing, doses, and administration of agents approved by the FDA, visit the Drugs@FDA website (www.accessdata.fda.gov/scripts/cder/drugsatfda/).

Reliever Medications (Rescue Medications) Used to Treat Asthma*

Generic Name	Brand Name
Ultra-short-Acting Bronchodilator Agents	
Epinephrine	Adrenalin
Racemic epinephrine	Generic
Short-Acting Beta$_2$ Agents (SABAs)	
Albuterol	Proventil HFA, Ventolin HFA, ProAir HFA, AccuNeb HFA, Generic
Metaproterenol	Generic
Levalbuterol	Xopenex, Xopenex HFA, Generic
Systemic Corticosteroids	
Methylprednisolone	Medrol, Solu-Medrol
Hydrocortisone	Solu-Cortef

*For the complete listing, doses, and administration of agents approved by the FDA, visit the Drugs@FDA website (www.accessdata.fda.gov/scripts/cder/drugsatfda/).

Antibiotics

Common Pathogens and Treatment of Respiratory Infections in Adults		
Respiratory Infection	**Pathogens**	**Treatment***
Sinusitis		
Acute (community acquired)	*Streptococcus pneumoniae, Haemophilus influenzae, Moraxella catarrhalis*	Amoxicillin-clavulanate or cefuroxime axetil or respiratory quinolone (levofloxacin or moxifloxacin or gemifloxacin) or macrolide/ketolide or TMP-SMX
Acute (hospital acquired)	*Pseudomonas aeruginosa, Acinetobacter* spp., *Staphylococcus aureus*	Ceftazidime or cefepime or aztreonam or a carbapenem and vancomycin
Chronic	*Bacteroides* spp., *Peptostreptococcus* spp., *Fusobacterium* spp.	Antibiotics are usually unsuccessful; sinus drainage may be required
Bronchitis		
Acute	*Mycoplasma pneumoniae, Chlamydia pneumoniae, Bordetella pertussis*	Antibiotics are usually not indicated; however, doxycycline or macrolide may be considered
Exacerbation of chronic bronchitis/COPD	*S. pneumoniae, H. influenzae, M. catarrhalis*	Value of antibiotics is controversial; doxycycline or macrolide may be considered
Pneumonia		
Community acquired	*S. pneumoniae, H. influenzae, M. catarrhalis, M. pneumoniae, C. pneumoniae, Legionella pneumophila*	Azithromycin, clarithromycin, telithromycin, or respiratory quinolone, or doxycycline or β-lactam (ceftriaxone, cefuroxime, amoxicillin-clavulanate) and a macrolide
Hospital acquired (nonneutropenic patient)	*S. pneumoniae, P. aeruginosa*	Cefepime, ceftazidime, or aztreonam or a carbapenem or piperacillin-tazobactam ± an aminoglycoside or ciprofloxacin ± vancomycin
Hospital acquired (neutropenic patient)	As listed for nonneutropenic patients and fungi such as *Aspergillus* spp., *Pneumocystis carinii* (especially if HIV positive)	Cefepime, a carbapenem, ceftazidime, or piperacillin-tazobactam + an aminoglycoside or ciprofloxacin ± vancomycin ± amphotericin B ± TMP-SMX
Aspiration suspected	*S. pneumoniae, Bacteroides fragilis, Peptostreptococcus* spp., *Fusobacterium* spp.	Amoxicillin-clavulanate, ampicillin-sulbactam, piperacillin-tazobactam, clindamycin ± quinolone
Patient with cystic fibrosis	*S. aureus, P. aeruginosa, Burkholderia cepacia*	Aminoglycoside + piperacillin-tazobactam or ceftazidime, cefepime ± TMP-SMX (*B. cepacia*)

HIV, Human immunodeficiency virus; *TMP-SMX*, trimethoprim-sulfamethoxazole.

*The potential treatments listed here are not listed in order of superiority. Choice of antimicrobials depends on the individual susceptibility pattern of the suspected organisms within the specific institution.

Modified from Gardenhire DS: *Rau's respiratory care pharmacology,* ed 8, St Louis, 2012, Elsevier/Mosby, Table 14-1.

Antifungal Class and Generic Name	Brand Name and Route	Common Uses (Microorganisms
Polyenes		
Amphotericin B	Fungizone IV, PO*	*Candida* spp., *Aspergillus* spp., *Cryptococcus neoformans*, *Histoplasma capsulatum*, *Blastomyces dermatitidis*, *Coccidioides immitis*
Amphotericin B colloidal dispersion (Amphotec)	Amphotec IV	*Candida* spp., *Aspergillus* spp., mucormycosis, *C. neoformans*
Amphotericin B lipid complex	Abelcet IV	*Candida* spp., *Aspergillus* spp., mucormycosis, *C. neoformans*
Liposomal amphotericin B	AmBisome IV	*Candida* spp., *Aspergillus* spp., mucormycosis, *C. neoformans*, *leishmaniasis*
Azoles		
Ketoconazole	Nizoral PO	*Candida* spp.[†], *C. neoformans*, *H. capsulatum*, *B. dermatitidis*
Fluconazole	Diflucan IV, PO	*Candida* spp.[†], *C. neoformans*
Itraconazole	Sporanox PO	*Candida* spp.[†], *Aspergillus* spp., *C. neoformans*, *H. capsulatum*, *B. dermatitidis*, *C. immitis*, *Sporothrix schenckii*
Voriconazole	Vfend IV, PO	*Candida* spp.[†], *Aspergillus* spp., *C. neoformans*, *C. immitis*, *H. capsulatum*, *B. dermatitidis*, *Fusarium* spp., *Scedosporium* spp.
Posaconazole	Noxafil PO	*Candida* spp.[†], *Aspergillus* spp., *C. neoformans*, *C. immitis*, *H. capsulatum*, *B. dermatitidis*, *Fusarium* spp., *Scedosporium* spp.
Echinocandins		
Caspofungin	Cancidas IV	*Aspergillus* spp., *Candida* spp.
Micafungin	Mycamine IV	*Aspergillus* spp., *Candida* spp.
Anidulafungin	Eraxis IV	*Aspergillus* spp., *Candida* spp.
Other Antifungals		
Flucytosine	Ancobon PO	*Aspergillus* spp., *Candida* spp., *C. neoformans*
Griseofulvin	Fulvicin PO	Tinea corporis, tinea cruris, tinea barbae, tinea capitis, and tinea unguium
Terbinafine	Lamisil PO, TOP	Tinea corporis, tinea pedis, tinea manuum, tinea cruris, tinea imbricata, tinea capitis, and tinea unguium

Modified from Gardenhire DS: *Rau's respiratory care pharmacology*, ed 8, St Louis, 2012, Elsevier/Mosby, Table 14-9.

IV, Intravenous; *PO*, oral; *TOP*, topical.

*The oral form of amphotericin B is not absorbed through the gastrointestinal tract.

[†]*Candida krusei* is intrinsically resistant to all azoles.

V | Mucolytic and Expectorant Agents

Mucolytics

Mucolytic agents are used to enhance the mobilization and thinning of thick bronchial secretions.

Agent	Trade Name	Adult Dosage
N-Acetylcysteine	Generic	Small volume nebulizer: 3–5 mL
Dornase alfa	Pulmozyme	Small volume nebulizer: 2.5 mg/ampule, one ampule daily
Aqueous aerosols: water, saline	N/A	Small volume nebulizer: 3–5 mL, as ordered, or 4 mL of a 3%–7% saline solution, twice a day
		Ultrasonic nebulizer: 3–5 mL, as ordered

Expectorants

Expectorants are agents used to increase bronchial submucous gland secretion, which in turn decreases viscosity of mucus. This facilitates the mobilization and expectoration of bronchial secretions.

Agents

Iodide-containing agents
Sodium bicarbonate (2%)
Guaifenesin (Robitussin, Naldecon Senior EX, Humibid LA)
Dissociating solvents (urea)
Oligosaccharides (dextran, mannitol, lactose)

Positive Inotropes and Vasopressors

Positive inotropes are drugs that increase the strength of the cardiac muscular contraction. Vasopressors are agents that cause contraction of the capillaries and arteries.

Agent	Alpha Stimulation (Capillary Constriction)	Beta$_1$ Stimulation (Heart and Rate Contractility)
Dopamine (Inotropin)	+ to +++*	+++*
Dobutamine (Dobutrex)	0 to +*	0 to +*
Epinephrine (Adrenalin)	+++*	+++
Isoproterenol (Isuprel)	0	+++
Norepinephrine (Levophed)	+++	++
Phenylephrine (Neo-Synephrine)	+++	0

Modified from Gardenhire DS: *Rau's respiratory care pharmacology*, ed 8, St Louis, 2012, Elsevier, Table 21-3.
*At higher doses: 0, effect; +, slight effect; ++, moderate effect; +++, pronounced effect.

VII Diuretic Agents

The primary purpose of diuretics is to lower the fluid volume in order to decrease blood pressure and/or clear the body of excess interstitial fluid.

Agents

Osmotic Diuretics

- Glycerin
- Isosorbide
- Mannitol
- Urea

Thiazide Diuretics

- Bendroflumethiazide
- Benzthiazide
- Chlorothiazide
- Chlorthalidone
- Hydrochlorothiazide
- Hydroflumethiazide
- Indapamide
- Methylclothiazide
- Metolazone
- Polythiazide
- Quinethazone
- Trichlormethiazide

Loop Diuretics

- Bumetanide
- Ethacrynic acid
- Furosemide
- Torsemide

Potassium-Sparing Diuretics

- Amiloride
- Spironolactone
- Triamterene

VIII The Ideal Alveolar Gas Equation

Clinically, the alveolar oxygen tension can be computed from the ideal alveolar gas equation. A useful clinical approximation of the ideal alveolar gas equation is as follows:

$$PAO_2 = FIO_2(PB - PH_2O) - PaCO_2 / RQ$$

where PB is the barometric pressure, PAO_2 is the partial pressure of oxygen within the alveoli, PH_2O is the partial pressure of water vapor in the alveoli (which is 47 mm Hg), FIO_2 is the fractional concentration of inspired oxygen, $PaCO_2$ is the partial pressure of arterial carbon dioxide, and RQ is the respiratory quotient. The RQ is the ratio of carbon dioxide production ($\dot{V}CO_2$) divided by oxygen consumption ($\dot{V}O_2$). Under normal circumstances, about 250 mL of oxygen/min is consumed by the tissue cells and about 200 mL of carbon dioxide is excreted into the lung. Thus, the RQ is normally about 0.8, but can range from 0.7 to 1.0. Clinically, 0.8 is generally used for the RQ.

Therefore, if a patient is receiving an FIO_2 of 0.40 on a day when the barometric pressure is 755 mm Hg and in whom the $PaCO_2$ is 55 mm Hg, the patient's alveolar oxygen tension (PaO_2) can be calculated as follows:

$$
\begin{aligned}
PAO_2 &= [PB - PH_2O] FIO_2 - PaCO_2/RQ \\
&= (755 - 47)\,0.40 - 55/0.8 \\
&= (708)\,0.40 - 68.75 \\
&= (283.2) - 68.75 \\
&= 214.45
\end{aligned}
$$

The ideal alveolar gas equation is part of the clinical information needed to calculate the degree of pulmonary shunting (see Chapter 4).

Physiologic Dead Space Calculation

The amount of physiologic dead space (V_D) in the tidal volume (V_T) can be estimated by using the dead space-to-tidal volume ratio (V_D/V_T) equation. The equation is arranged as follows:

$$V_D/V_T = \frac{PaCO_2 - P_{\bar{E}}CO_2}{PaCO_2}$$

For example, in a patient whose $PaCO_2$ is 40 mm Hg and whose $P_{\bar{E}}CO_2$ is 28 mm Hg:

$$V_D/V_T = \frac{40 - 28}{40}$$
$$= \frac{12}{40}$$
$$= 0.3$$

In this case, about 30% of the patient's ventilation is dead space ventilation. This is within the normal range.

Metric Weight

Grams	Centigrams	Milligrams	Micrograms	Nanograms
1	100	1000	1,000,000	1,000,000,000
0.01	1	10	10,000	10,000,000
0.001	0.1	1	1000	1,000,000
0.000001	0.0001	0.001	1	1000
0.000000001	0.0000001	0.000001	0.001	1

Weight

Metric	Approximate Apothecary Equivalents
Grams	**Grains**
0.0002	$\frac{1}{300}$
0.0003	$\frac{1}{200}$
0.0004	$\frac{1}{150}$
0.0005	$\frac{1}{120}$
0.0006	$\frac{1}{100}$
0.001	$\frac{1}{60}$
0.002	$\frac{1}{30}$
0.005	$\frac{1}{12}$
0.010	$\frac{1}{6}$
0.015	$\frac{1}{4}$
0.025	$\frac{3}{8}$
0.030	$\frac{1}{2}$
0.050	$\frac{3}{4}$
0.060	1
0.100	$1\frac{1}{2}$
0.120	2
0.200	3
0.300	5
0.500	$7\frac{1}{2}$
0.600	10
1	15
2	30
4	60

Liquid Measure

Metric	Approximate Apothecary Equivalents
Milliliters	
1000	1 quart
750	1½ pints
500	1 pint
250	8 fluid ounces
200	7 fluid ounces
100	3½ fluid ounces
50	1¾ fluid ounces
30	1 fluid ounce
15	4 fluid drams
10	2½ fluid drams
8	2 fluid drams
5	1¼ fluid drams
4	1 fluid dram
3	45 minims
2	30 minims
1	15 minims
0.75	12 minims
0.6	10 minims
0.5	8 minims
0.3	5 minims
0.25	4 minims
0.2	3 minims
0.1	1½ minims
0.06	1 minim
0.05	¾ minim
0.03	½ minim

Metric Liquid

Liter	Centiliter	Milliliter	Microliter	Nanoliter
1	100	1000	1,000,000	1,000,000,000
0.01	1	10	10,000	10,000,000
0.001	0.1	1	1000	1,000,000
0.000001	0.0001	0.001	1	1000
0.000000001	0.0000001	0.000001	0.001	1

Metric Length

Meter	Centimeter	Millimeter	Micrometer	Nanometer
1	100	1000	1,000,000	1,000,000,000
0.01	1	10	10,000	10,000,000
0.001	0.1	1	1000	1,000,000
0.000001	0.0001	0.001	1	1000
0.000000001	0.0000001	0.000001	0.001	1

Weight Conversions (Metric and Avoirdupois)

Grams	Kilograms	Ounces	Pounds
1	0.001	0.0353	0.0022
1000	1	35.3	2.2
28.35	0.02835	1	1/16
454.5	0.4545	16	1

Weight Conversions (Metric and Apothecary)

Grams	Milligrams	Grains	Drams	Ounces	Pounds
1	1000	15.4	0.2577	0.0322	0.00268
0.001	1	0.0154	0.00026	0.0000322	0.00000268
0.0648	64.8	1	$\frac{1}{60}$	$\frac{1}{480}$	$\frac{1}{5760}$
3.888	3888	60	1	$\frac{1}{8}$	$\frac{1}{96}$
31.1	31,104	480	8	1	$\frac{1}{12}$
363.25	373,248	5760	96	12	1

Approximate Household Measurement Equivalents (volume)

						1 tsp =	5 mL
					1 tbsp =	3 tsp =	15 mL
				1 fl oz =	2 tbsp =	6 tsp =	30 mL
			1 cup =	8 fl oz =			240 mL
		1 pt =	2 cups =	16 fl oz =			480 mL
	1 qt =	2 pt =	4 cups =	32 fl oz =			960 mL
1 gal =	4 qt =	8 pt =	16 cups =	128 fl oz =			3840 mL

Volume Conversions (Metric and Apothecary)

Milliliters	Minims	Fluid Drams	Fluid Ounces	Pints	Liters	Gallons	Fluid Quarts	Ounces	Pints
1	16.2	0.27	0.0333	0.0021	1	0.2642	1.057	33.824	2.114
0.0616	1	$\frac{1}{60}$	$\frac{1}{480}$	$\frac{1}{7680}$	3.785	1	4	128	8
3.697	60	1	$\frac{1}{8}$	$\frac{1}{128}$	0.946	$\frac{1}{4}$	1	32	2
29.58	480	8	1	$\frac{1}{16}$	0.473	$\frac{1}{8}$	$\frac{1}{2}$	16	1
473.2	7680	128	16	1	0.0296	$\frac{1}{128}$	$\frac{1}{32}$	1	$\frac{1}{16}$

Length Conversions (Metric and English System)

	Millimeters	Centimeters	Inches	Feet	Yards	Meters
1 Å =	$\frac{1}{10,000,000}$	$\frac{1}{100,000,000}$	$\frac{1}{254,000,000}$	$\frac{1}{3,050,000,000}$	$\frac{1}{9,140,000,000}$	$\frac{1}{10,000,000,000}$
1 nm =	$\frac{1}{1,000,000}$	$\frac{1}{10,000,000}$	$\frac{1}{25,400,000}$	$\frac{1}{305,000,000}$	$\frac{1}{914,000,000}$	$\frac{1}{1,000,000,000}$
1 μm =	$\frac{1}{1000}$	$\frac{1}{10,000}$	$\frac{1}{25,400}$	$\frac{1}{305,000}$	$\frac{1}{914,000}$	$\frac{1}{1,000,000}$
1 mm =	1	0.1	0.03937	0.00328	0.0011	0.001
1 cm =	10	1	0.3937	0.03281	0.0109	0.01
1 in =	25.4	2.54	1	0.0833	0.0278	0.0254
1 ft =	304.8	30.48	12	1	0.333	0.3048
1 yd =	914.40	91.44	36	3	1	0.9144
1 m =	1000	100	39.37	3.2808	1.0936	1

Poiseuille's Law

Poiseuille's Law for *Flow* Rearranged to a Simple Proportionality

$\dot{V} \simeq \Delta P r^4$, or rewritten as $\dfrac{\dot{V}}{r^4} \simeq \Delta P$

When ΔP remains constant, then

$$\frac{\dot{V}}{r_1^4} \simeq \frac{\dot{V}}{r_2^4}$$

Example 1—If the radius (r_1) is decreased to half its previous radius ($r_2 = \frac{1}{2} r_1$), then

$$\frac{\dot{V}}{r_1^4} \simeq \frac{\dot{V}}{(\frac{1}{2} r_1)^4}$$

$$\frac{\dot{V}_1}{r_1^4} \simeq \frac{\dot{V}_2}{(\frac{1}{16}) r_1^4}$$

$$(r_1^4) \frac{\dot{V}_1}{r_1^4} \simeq (r_1^4) \frac{\dot{V}_2}{(\frac{1}{16}) r_1^4}$$

$$\dot{V}_1 \simeq \frac{\dot{V}_2}{\frac{1}{16}}$$

$$(\tfrac{1}{16}) \dot{V}_1 \simeq (\tfrac{1}{16}) \frac{\dot{V}_2}{\frac{1}{16}}$$

$$(\tfrac{1}{16}) \dot{V}_1 \simeq \dot{V}_2$$

The gas flow ($\dot{V}_1$) reduces to $\frac{1}{16}$ its original flow rate [$\dot{V}_2 \simeq (\frac{1}{16}) \dot{V}_1$].

Example 2—If the radius (r_1) is decreased by 16% ($r_2 = r_1 - 0.16 r_1 = 0.84 r_1$), then

$$\frac{\dot{V}_1}{r_1^4} \simeq \frac{\dot{V}_2}{r_2^4}$$

$$\frac{\dot{V}}{r_1^4} \simeq \frac{\dot{V}}{(0.84 r_1)^4}$$

$$\dot{V}_2 \simeq \frac{(0.84 r_1)^4 \dot{V}_1}{r_1^4}$$

$$\dot{V}_2 \simeq \frac{0.4979 \, r_1^4 \dot{V}_1}{r_1^4}$$

$$\dot{V}_2 \simeq \tfrac{1}{2} \dot{V}_1$$

The flow rate ($\dot{V}_1$) decreases to half its original flow rate ($\dot{V}_2 \simeq \frac{1}{2} \dot{V}_1$).

Poiseuille's Law for *Pressure* Rearranged to a Simple Proportionality

$P \approx \dfrac{\dot{V}}{r^4}$ or rewritten as $P \cdot r^4 \approx \dot{V}$

When $\dot{V}$ remains constant, then

$$P_1 \cdot r_1^4 \approx P_2 \cdot r_2^4$$

Example 1—If the radius (r_1) is decreased to half its original radius [$r_2 = (\frac{1}{2})r_1$], then

$$P_1 \cdot r_1^4 \approx P_2 \cdot r_2^4$$

$$P_1 \cdot r_1^4 \approx P_2 [(\tfrac{1}{2})r_1]^4$$

$$P_1 \cdot r_1^4 \approx P_2 (\tfrac{1}{16}) r_1^4$$

$$\frac{P_1 \cdot \cancel{r_1^4}}{\cancel{r_1^4}} \approx \frac{P_2 (\tfrac{1}{16}) \cancel{r_1^4}}{\cancel{r_1^4}}$$

$$P_1 \approx P_2 \cdot (\tfrac{1}{16})$$

$$16 P_1 \approx 16 \cdot P_2 \cdot (\tfrac{1}{16})$$

$$16 P_1 \approx P_2$$

The pressure (P_1) increases to 16 times its original level ($P_2 = 16 \cdot P_1$).

Example 2—If the radius (r_1) is decreased by 16% ($r_2 = r_1 - 0.16r_1 = 0.84r_1$), then

$$P_1 \cdot r_1^4 \approx P_2 \cdot r_2^4$$

$$P_1 \cdot r_1^4 \approx P_2 (0.4979) \cdot r_1^4$$

$$\frac{P_1 \cdot \cancel{r_1^4}}{(0.4979 \, \cancel{r_1^4})} \approx P_2$$

$$2 \cdot P_1 \approx P_2$$

The pressure (P_1) increases to twice its original level ($P_2 = 2 \cdot P_1$).

PCO$_2$ /HCO$_3^-$ /pH Nomogram

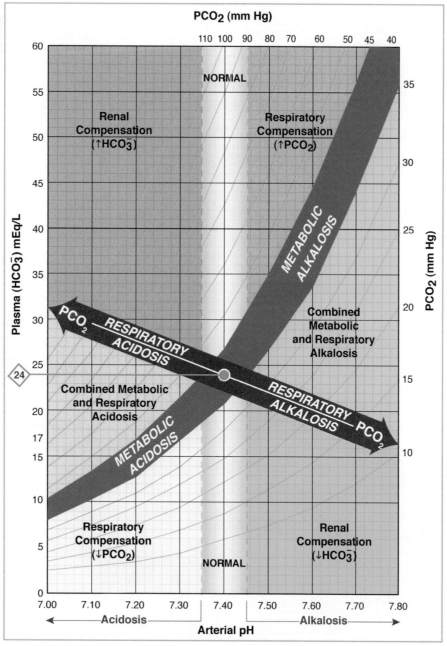

Nomogram of PCO$_2$/HCO$_3^-$/pH relationship. For explanation see text. The green box (with 24) and the green dot in the middle of the red arrow represent the normal pH, PCO$_2$, and HCO$_3^-$ relationship in the arterial blood. (Used, with permission, from author Terry Des Jardins.)

pH, PCO₂, HCO₃ RELATIONSHIP

PaCO₂		pH	HCO₃
100	≈	7.10	30
80	≈	7.20	28
60	≈	7.30	26
40	≈	7.40	24
30	≈	7.50	22
20	≈	7.60	20
10	≈	7.70	18

EX: ACUTE CHANGES ON CVF

AVF on CVF	CVF Baseline	AAH on CVF
	pH	
7.21 ⟵	7.39	⟶ 7.53
	PaCO₂	
110 ⟵	76	⟶ 51
	HCO₃	
43 ⟵	41	⟶ 37
	PaO₂	
34 ⟵	61	⟶ 46

CVF: Chronic ventilatory failure
ACF: Acute ventilatory failure
AAH: Acute alveolar hyperventilation

PaO₂ & SaO₂ RELATIONSHIP

	PaO₂	SaO₂
Normal	97	97
Range	> 80–100	> 95
Hypoxemia	< 80	< 95
Mild	60–80	90–95
Moderate	40–60	75–90
Severe	< 40	< 75

PaO₂, & SaO₂ RELATIONSHIP

PO₂ 30 ≈ 60% saturated

PO₂ 40 ≈ 75% saturated

PO₂ 50 ≈ 85% saturated

PO₂ 60 ≈ 90% saturated

FIO₂ & PaO₂ RELATIONSHIP

FIO₂		PaO₂
0.30	≈	150
0.40	≈	200
0.50	≈	250
0.80	≈	400
1.00	≈	500

O₂ TRANSPORT

		Normal Values
DO₂		1000 ml O₂/min
V̇O₂		250 ml O₂/min
C(a – v̄)O₂		5 vol%
O₂ER		25%
Sv̄O₂		75%

Cut out the above two-sided PCO₂/HCO₃⁻/pH nomogram and have it laminated for use as a handy, pocket-sized reference tool. See Chapter 4 for information about how to use the nomogram in the clinical setting.

XIII Calculated Hemodynamic Measurements

The following are the major hemodynamic values that can be calculated from the direct hemodynamic measurements listed in Table 6-1. The calculated hemodynamic values are easily obtained from a programmed calculator or by using the specific hemodynamic formula. Because the calculated hemodynamic measurements vary with the size of an individual, some hemodynamic values are "indexed" by body surface area (BSA). Clinically, the BSA is obtained from a height-weight nomogram (see Appendix XIV). In the normal adult, the BSA is 1.5 to 2 m^2.

Stroke Volume

The stroke volume (SV) is the volume of blood ejected by the ventricles with each contraction. The preload, afterload, and myocardial contractility are the major determinants of SV. SV is derived by dividing the cardiac output (CO) by the heart rate (HR):

$$SV = \frac{CO}{HR}$$

For example, if an individual has a cardiac output of 4 L/min (4000 mL/min) and a heart rate of 80 bpm, the SV is calculated as follows:

$$
\begin{aligned}
SV &= \frac{CO}{HR} \\
&= \frac{4000 \, mL/min}{80 \, beats/min} \\
&= 50 \, mL/beat
\end{aligned}
$$

Stroke Volume Index

The stroke volume index (SVI), also known as stroke index, is calculated by dividing the SV by the BSA:

$$SVI = \frac{SV}{BSA}$$

For example, if a patient has an SV of 50 mL/beat and a BSA of 2 m^2, the SVI is determined as follows:

$$
\begin{aligned}
SVI &= \frac{SV}{BSA} \\
&= \frac{50 \, mL/beat}{2 \, m^2} \\
&= 25 \, mL/beat/m^2
\end{aligned}
$$

Assuming that the HR remains the same, as the SVI increases or decreases, the cardiac index also increases or decreases. The SVI reflects the (1) contractility of the heart, (2) overall blood volume status, and (3) amount of venous return.

Cardiac Index

The cardiac index (CI) is calculated by dividing the cardiac output (CO) by the BSA:

$$CI = \frac{CO}{BSA}$$

For example, if a patient has a CO of 6 L/min and a BSA of 2 m^2, the CI is computed as follows:

$$CI = \frac{CO}{BSA}$$
$$= \frac{6\,L/min}{2\,m^2}$$
$$= 3\,L/min/m^2$$

Right Ventricular Stroke Work Index

The right ventricular stroke work index (RVSWI) measures the amount of work done by the right ventricle to pump blood. The RVSWI is a reflection of the contractility of the right ventricle. In the presence of normal right ventricular contractility, increases in afterload (such as those caused by pulmonary vascular constriction) cause the RVSWI to increase until a plateau is reached. When the contractility of the right ventricle is diminished by disease states, however, the RVSWI does not appropriately increase. The RVSWI is derived from the following formula:

$$RVSWI = SVI \times \left(\overline{PA} - CVP\right) \times 0.0136\,g/mL$$

where SVI is stroke volume index, $\overline{PA}$ is mean pulmonary artery pressure, and CVP is central venous pressure. The density of mercury factor 0.0136 g/mL is needed to convert the equation to the proper units of measurement—that is, gram/meters/m^2 (g/m/m^2).

For example, if a patient has an SVI of 40 mL, a $\overline{PA}$ of 20 mm Hg, and a CVP of 5 mm Hg, the RVSWI is calculated as follows:

$$RVSWI = SVI\left(\overline{PA} - CVP\right) \times 0.0136\,g/mL$$
$$= 40\,mL/beat/m^2 = (15\,mm\,Hg - 5\,mm\,Hg) \times 0.0136\,g/mL$$
$$= 40\,mL/beat/m^2 \times 10\,mm\,Hg \times 0.0136\,g/mL$$
$$= 5.44\,g/m/m^2$$

Left Ventricular Stroke Work Index

The left ventricular stroke work index (LVSWI) measures the amount of work done by the left ventricle to pump blood. The LVSWI is a reflection of the contractility of the left ventricle. In the presence of normal left ventricular contractility, increases in afterload (such as those caused by systemic vascular constriction) cause the LVSWI to increase until a plateau is reached. When the contractility of the left ventricle is diminished by disease states, however, the LVSWI does not increase appropriately. The following formula is used for determining this hemodynamic variable:

$$LVSWI = SVI \times (MAP - PCWP) \times 0.0136\,g/mL$$

where SVI is stroke volume index, MAP is mean arterial pressure, and PCWP is pulmonary capillary wedge pressure. The density of mercury factor 0.0136 g/mL is needed to convert the equation to the proper units of measurement—that is, gram/meters/m^2 (g/m/m^2).

For example, if a patient has an SVI of 40 mL, an MAP of 110 mm Hg, and a PCWP of 5 mm Hg, the patient's LVSWI is calculated as follows:

$$LVSWI = SVI \times (MAP - PCWP) \times 0.0136\,g/mL$$
$$= 40\,mL/beat/m^2 \times (110\,mm\,Hg - 5\,mm\,Hg) \times 0.0136\,g/mL$$
$$= 40\,mL/beat/m^2 \times (105\,mm\,Hg) \times 0.0136\,g/mL$$
$$= 59.84\,g/m/m^2$$

Vascular Resistance

As blood flows through the pulmonary and systemic vascular systems, resistance to flow occurs. The pulmonary vascular system is a low-resistance system. The systemic vascular system is a high-resistance system.

Pulmonary Vascular Resistance (PVR)

The PVR measurement reflects the afterload of the right ventricle. It is calculated by the following formula:

$$PVR = \overline{PA} - \frac{PCWP}{CO} \times 80$$

where $\overline{PA}$ is the mean pulmonary artery pressure, PCWP is the capillary wedge pressure, CO is the cardiac output, and 80 is a conversion factor for adjusting to the correct units of measurement (dyne × second × cm^{-5}).

For example, if a patient has a $\overline{PA}$ of 20 mm Hg, a PCWP of 5 mm Hg, and a CO of 6 L/min, the patient's PVR is calculated as follows:

$$
\begin{aligned}
PVR &= \overline{PA} - \frac{PCWP}{CO} \times 80 \\
&= \frac{20 \text{ mm Hg} - 5 \text{ mm Hg}}{6 \text{ L/min}} \times 80 \\
&= \frac{15 \text{ mm Hg}}{6 \text{ L/min}} \times 80 \\
&= 200 \text{ dynes} \times \sec \times cm^{-5}
\end{aligned}
$$

Systemic or Peripheral Vascular Resistance (SVR)

The SVR measurement reflects the afterload of the left ventricle. It is calculated by the following formula:

$$
SVR = \frac{MAP - CVP}{CO} \times 80
$$

where MAP is the mean arterial pressure, CVP is the central venous pressure, CO is the cardiac output, and 80 is a conversion factor for adjusting to the correct units of measurement (dyne × second × cm^{-5}). (*Note*: The right atrial pressure [RAP] can be used in place of the CVP value.)

For example, if a patient has an MAP of 90 mm Hg, a CVP of 5 mm Hg, and a CO of 4 L/min, the patient's SVR is calculated as follows:

$$
\begin{aligned}
SVR &= \frac{MAP - CVP}{CO} \times 80 \\
&= \frac{90 \text{ mm Hg} - 5 \text{ mm Hg}}{4 \text{ L/min}} \times 80 \\
&= \frac{85 \text{ mm Hg}}{4 \text{ L/min}} \times 80 \\
&= 1700 \text{ dynes} \times \sec \times cm^{-5}
\end{aligned}
$$

Note: For normal values of all these hemodynamic measurements, see Chapter 6 and Appendix XV.

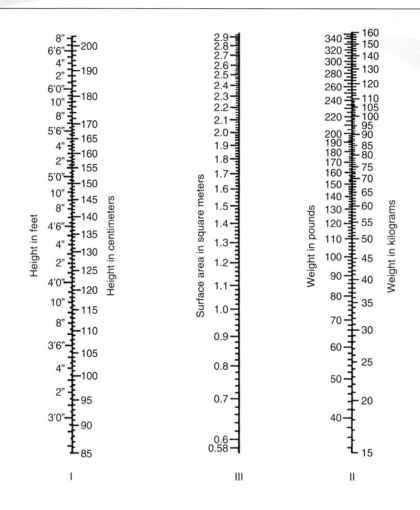

To find the body surface area of a patient, locate the height in inches (or centimeters) on Scale I and the weight in pounds (or kilograms) on Scale II, and place a straight edge (ruler) between these two points, which will intersect Scale III at the patient's surface area.

Representative examples of cardiopulmonary profile sheets used to monitor a critically ill patient.

Hemodynamic Status

| SVI mL-M^{-2} | CI L•min^{-1}•M^{-2} | RVSWI gm•M/M^2 | LVSWI gm•M/M^2 | PVR dyne•sec•cm^{-5} | SVR dyne•sec•cm^{-5} |

Stroke volume index | Cardiac index | Right ventricular stroke work index | Left ventricular stroke work index | Pulmonary vascular resistance | Systemic vascular resistance

Shaded areas represent normal range.

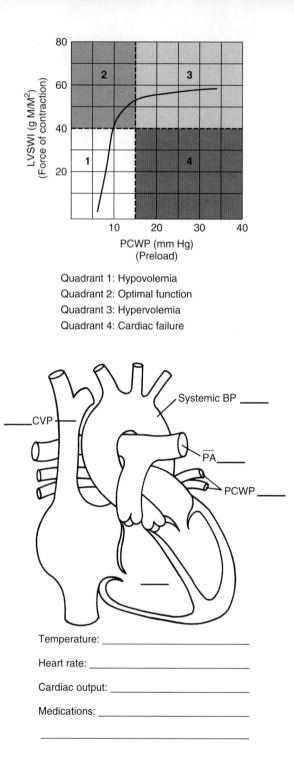

Quadrant 1: Hypovolemia
Quadrant 2: Optimal function
Quadrant 3: Hypervolemia
Quadrant 4: Cardiac failure

Temperature: _____

Heart rate: _____

Cardiac output: _____

Medications: _____

_____

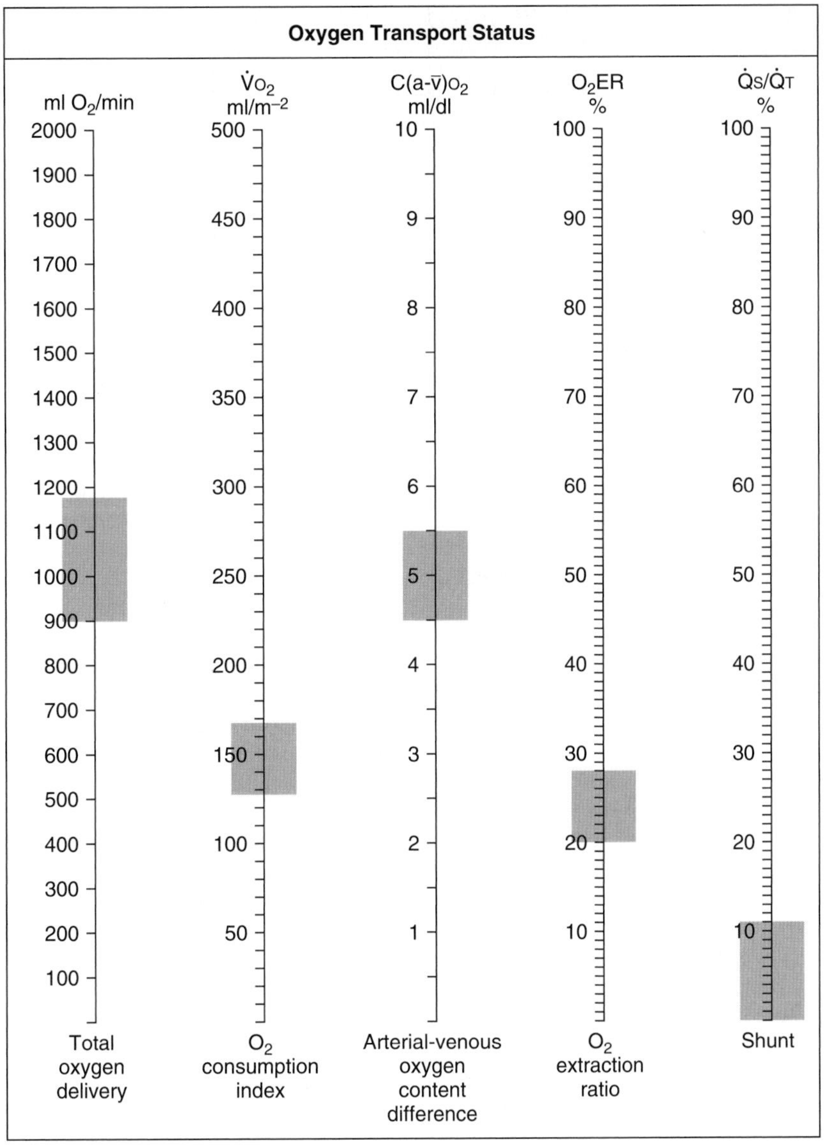

Oxygen Transport Status
ml O2/min
V̇O2 ml/m−2
C(a-v̄)O2 ml/dl
O2ER %
Q̇S/Q̇T %
2000 1900 1800 1700 1600 1500 1400 1300 1200 1100 1000 900 800 700 600 500 400 300 200 100
500 450 400 350 300 250 200 150 100 50
10 9 8 7 6 5 4 3 2 1
100 90 80 70 60 50 40 30 20 10
100 90 80 70 60 50 40 30 20 10
Total oxygen delivery
O2 consumption index
Arterial-venous oxygen content difference
O2 extraction ratio
Shunt

Shaded area represents normal range.

Blood Gas Values

pH ______________

$PaCO_2$ ______________

HCO_3^- ______________

PaO_2 ______________ **$P\bar{v}O_2$** __________

SaO_2 ___________% **$S\bar{v}O_2$** ________%

FIO_2 ______________ **Hb** __________

Mode(s) of Ventilatory

Support: ______________________

____

____

____

____

Patient's Name ______________________

Date ______________________

Time ______________________

Glossary

abscess Localized collection of pus that results from disintegration or displacement of tissue in any part of the body.

accessory muscles of expiration The accessory muscles of exhalation are often recruited when airway resistance becomes significantly elevated. When these muscles actively contract, intrapleural pressure increases and offsets the increased airway resistance. The major accessory muscles of exhalation are as follows: rectus abdominis, external oblique, internal oblique, transversus abdominis.

accessory muscles of inspiration During the advanced stages of chronic obstructive pulmonary disease, the accessory muscles of inspiration are activated when the diaphragm becomes significantly depressed by the increased residual volume and functional residual capacity. The accessory muscles assist or largely replace the diaphragm in creating subatmospheric pressure in the pleural space during inspiration. The major accessory muscles of inspiration are as follows: scalene, sternocleidomastoid, pectoralis major, trapezius.

acetylcholine (ACh) A direct-acting cholinergic neurotransmitter agent widely distributed in body tissues, with a primary function of mediating synaptic activity of the nervous system and skeletal muscles. Its half-life and duration of activity are short because it is rapidly destroyed by acetylcholinesterase. Its activity can also be blocked by atropine at junctions of nerve fibers with glands and smooth muscle tissue. It is a stimulant of the vagus and parasympathetic nervous system and functions as a vasodilator and cardiac depressant.

acidemia Decreased pH or an increased hydrogen ion concentration of the blood.

acidosis Pathologic condition resulting from accumulation of acid or loss of base from the body.

acinus Smallest division of a gland, a group of secretory cells surrounding a cavity; the functional part of an organ. (The respiratory acinus includes terminal [respiratory] bronchioles, alveolar ducts, alveoli, and all other structures therein.)

acquired bronchiectasis Destruction and widening of the large airways. If the condition is present at birth, it is called congenital bronchiectasis. If it develops later in life, it is called acquired bronchiectasis.

acute alveolar hyperventilation A condition marked by low levels of carbon dioxide and a high pH in the blood resulting from breathing excessively. Also called acute respiratory alkalosis.

acute alveolar hyperventilation with partial renal compensation A condition marked by low levels of carbon dioxide and a high pH in the blood resulting from hyperventilation, which is partly corrected by the excretion of HCO_3^- via the renal system.

acute epiglottitis A very rapidly progressive infection causing inflammation of the epiglottis (the flap that covers the trachea) and tissues around the epiglottis that may lead to abrupt blockage of the upper airway and death.

acute respiratory acidosis A condition marked by high levels of carbon dioxide and a low pH in the blood resulting from hypoventilation. Also called acute ventilatory failure.

acute respiratory alkalosis A condition marked by low levels of carbon dioxide and a high pH in the blood resulting from hyperventilation. Also called acute alveolar hyperventilation.

acute ventilatory failure A condition marked by high levels of carbon dioxide and a low pH in the blood resulting from hypoventilation. Also called acute ventilatory failure.

acute ventilatory failure with partial renal compensation A condition marked by high levels of carbon dioxide and a low pH in the blood resulting from hypoventilation, which is partly corrected by the retention of HCO_3^- via the renal system and/or the administration of HCO_3^-.—of rapid onset and characterized by severe symptoms and a short course; not chronic.

adenocarcinoma Any one of a large group of malignant epithelial cell tumors of the glandular tissue. Specific tumors are diagnosed and named by cytologic identification of the tissue affected; for example, an adenocarcinoma of the uterine cervix is characterized by tumor cells resembling the glandular epithelium of the cervix.—**adenocarcinomatous,** *adj.*

adenovirus Any one of the 49 medium-sized viruses of the Adenoviridae family, pathogenic to humans, that cause conjunctivitis, upper respiratory tract infection, cystitis, or gastrointestinal infection. After the acute and symptomatic period of illness, the virus may persist in a latent stage in the tonsils, adenoids, and other lymphoid tissue.

adhesion Fibrous band that holds together parts that are normally separated.

adolescent One in the state or process of adolescence; a teenager.

adrenergic Term applied to nerve fibers that, when stimulated, release epinephrine at their endings. Includes nearly all sympathetic postganglionic fibers except those innervating sweat glands.

adrenocorticotropic hormone (ACTH) A hormone secreted by the anterior pituitary. It is regulated by the corticotropin-releasing factor (CRF) from the hypothalamus and is essential to growth, development, and continued function of the adrenal cortex.

adventitious (abnormal) breath sounds Additional or different sounds that are not *normally* heard over a particular area of the thorax.

aerosol Gaseous suspension of fine solid or liquid particles.

afebrile Without fever.

afferent Carrying impulses toward a center, such as the central nervous system.

afferent nerves Nerves that transmit impulses from the peripheral to the central nervous system.

afterload The load, or resistance, against which the left ventricle must eject its volume of blood during contraction. The resistance is produced by the volume of blood already in the vascular system and by the constriction of the vessel walls.

air bronchogram When air can be visualized in the more peripheral intrapulmonary bronchi as a chest radiograph, this is known as the "air-bronchogram sign." This abnormality is usually caused by an infiltrate/consolidation that surrounds the bronchi.

air cyst Nonspecific term usually used to describe the presence in the lung of a thin-walled, well-defined, and well-circumscribed lesion, greater than 1 cm in diameter. Cysts may contain either air or fluid, but this term is usually used to refer to an air-containing lesion or air-filled cyst.

air trapping Trapping of alveolar gas.

airway resistance A measure of the impedance to air flow through the bronchopulmonary system. It is the reciprocal of airway conductance.

alkalemia Increased pH or decreased hydrogen ion concentration of the blood.

allergen Any substance that causes manifestations of allergy. It may or may not be a protein.

allergy Hypersensitivity to a substance (allergen) that normally does not cause a reaction. An allergic reaction is essentially an antibody-antigen reaction, but in some cases the antibody cannot be demonstrated. The reaction is caused by the release of histamine or histamine-like substances from injured cells.

α_1-antitrypsin Inhibitor of trypsin that may be deficient in persons with emphysema.

α-receptor Site in the autonomic nerve pathways where excitatory responses occur when adrenergic agents such as norepinephrine and epinephrine are released.

alpha waves One of the four brain waves, characterized by a relatively high voltage or amplitude and a frequency of 8 to 13 Hz. Alpha waves are known as the "relaxed waves" of the brain. They are commonly recorded when the individual is awake, but in a drowsy state and when the eyes are closed. Alpha waves are commonly seen during Stage N1 sleep. Bursts of alpha waves are also seen during brief awakenings from sleep-where they are called arousals. Alpha waves may also be seen during rapid eye movement (REM) sleep.

alpha$_1$-antitrypsin deficiency Blood test useful for individuals with a family history of emphysema, because a familial tendency to have a deficiency of alpha$_1$-antitrypsin antienzyme exists. A similar deficiency also exists in children with liver disease.

alteplase A tissue plasminogen activator.

alveolar hypoplasia Underdevelopment of the alveolar tissue.

anaerobic Metabolic pathway that does not require oxygen; such processes usually produce lactic acid.

anaerobic organisms Pertaining to the absence of air or oxygen.

anaphylaxis Allergic hypersensitivity reaction of the body to a foreign protein or drug.

anemia Condition in which there is a reduction in the number of circulating red blood cells per cubic millimeter, the amount of hemoglobin per 100 mL, or the volume of packed red cells per 100 mL of blood.

anemic hypoxia The PaO$_2$ is normal, but the oxygen-carrying capacity of the hemoglobin is inadequate.

aneurysm Localized dilation of a blood vessel, usually an artery.

angiogram Serial roentgenograms of a blood vessel taken in rapid sequence after injection of a radiopaque substance into the vessel.

angiography Roentgenography of blood vessels after injection of a radiopaque substance.

anion gap The balance between acids and bases in the blood plasma. Normally it results in a slightly alkaline state with an excess of hydroxyl ions in comparison to hydrogen. The balance is achieved by the offset of the ingestion and production of acidic and basic material by the amount of acidic and basic material metabolized and excreted by the body.

anoxia Absence of oxygen.

anterior axillary line An imaginary vertical line on the body wall continuing the line of the anterior axillary fold with the upper arm.

anterolateral In front and to one side.

anteroposterior radiograph Chest x-ray in which the x-ray beam travels from the front to the back of the body.

antibody Protein substance that develops in response to and interacts with an antigen. The antigen-antibody reaction forms the basis of immunity. Antibodies are produced by plasma cells in lymphoid tissue. Antibodies may be present because of previous infection, vaccination, or transfer from the mother to the fetus in utero, or may occur without known antigenic stimulus, usually as a result of unknown, accidental exposure.

antidysrhythmic agents Drugs used to treat irregularity or loss of normal heart rhythm.

antigen Substance that induces the formation of antibodies that interact specifically with it. An antigen may be introduced into the body or may be formed within the body.

antigen assay tests A laboratory assessment of the amounts of components in multimolecular antigen-antibody complexes. The assay is used in various diagnostic tests for collagen-vascular disorders, glomerulonephritis, vasculitis, hepatitis, and neoplastic diseases.

aortic valve Valve between the left ventricle and the ascending aorta that prevents regurgitation of blood into the left ventricle.

aperture Opening or orifice.

apex Top, end, or tip of a structure.

apical pulse The heartbeat as heard with a stethoscope placed on the chest wall or felt adjacent to the apex cordis.

apnea Complete absence of spontaneous ventilation.

apnea-hypopnea index (AHI) The diagnosis of obstructive sleep apnea is commonly based on the apnea-hypopnea index (AHI). *Apnea* is defined as the cessation of air flow—a complete obstruction for at least 10 seconds—with a simultaneous 2% to 4% decrease in the patient's SaO$_2$. *Hypopnea* is defined as a reduction of air flow of 30% to 50%, with a concomitant drop in the patient's SaO$_2$. The AHI is defined as the average number of apneas and hypopneas per hour of sleep. In adults, the normal AHI is <5/hr.

aponeurosis Flat, fibrous sheet of connective tissue that attaches muscle to bone or other tissues. May sometimes serve as a fascia.

arrhythmia Irregularity or loss of heart rhythm.

arterial catheter A tubular device that can be inserted into an artery either to draw blood or to measure blood pressure directly.

arteriole Very small artery that, at its distal end, leads into a capillary.

arthralgia Any pain that affects a joint.

ascending paralysis A condition in which there is successive flaccid paralysis of the legs, then the trunk and arms, and finally the muscles of respiration. Causes include poliomyelitis, Guillain-Barré syndrome, and exposure to toxic chemicals, for example, botulinum toxin.

asepsis The absence of germs; sterile.

asphyxia Condition caused by an insufficient uptake of oxygen.

aspiration Inhalation of gastric or pharyngeal contents into the pulmonary tree.

asymmetrical Unequal correspondence in shape, size, and relative position of parts on opposite sides of the midline.

asystole (cardiac standstill) Absence of contractions of the heart.

atelectasis Collapsed or airless lung. May be caused by obstruction of the airways by foreign bodies, mucus plugs, or excessive secretions or by compression from without, as by tumors, aneurysms, or enlarged lymph nodes.

atmospheric pressure Pressure of air on the earth at mean sea level—approximately 14.7 pounds per square inch (760 mm Hg).

atopic Of or pertaining to a hereditary tendency to develop immediate allergic reactions because of the presence of an antibody in the skin and sometimes the bloodstream.

atrial fibrillation Irregular and rapid randomized contractions of the atria working independently of the ventricles.

atrial flutter Extremely rapid (200 to 400/min) contractions of the atrium. In pure flutter a regular rhythm is maintained; in flutter with variable heart block the rhythm is irregular.

atrophy A wasting or decrease in size of an organ or a tissue.

atropine An alkaloid obtained from belladonna. It is a parasympatholytic agent.

auscultation The act of listening for sounds within the body to evaluate the condition of the heart, blood vessels, lungs, pleura, intestines, or other organs or to detect the fetal heart sound. Auscultation may be performed directly with the unaided ear, but most commonly a stethoscope is used to determine the frequency, intensity, duration, and quality of the sounds.

autoimmune disorders A condition in which a patient exhibits symptoms of a group of diseases, including Addison's disease, autoimmune thyroid disease, mucocutaneous candidiasis, hypoparathyroidism, and insulin-dependent diabetes.

autosomal recessive trait Pattern of inheritance in which the transmission of a recessive gene results in a carrier state if the person is heterozygous for the trait, and in an affected state if the person is homozygous for the trait. Males and females are affected with equal frequency.

bacillus Any rod-shaped bacterium.

bacteria Unicellular ovoid or rod-shaped organisms existing in free-living or parasitic forms. They display a wide range of biochemical and pathogenic properties.

Bacteroides fragilis A pleomorphic gram-negative bacillus and an obligate anaerobe of the gut.

Bacteroides melaninogenicus A member of the normal flora found in the upper respiratory tract.

Ball-valve effect (and/or mechanism) The intermittent opening and closing of an orifice by a buoyant, ball-shaped mass, which acts as a one-way valve. Some types of objects that may act in this manner are kidney stones, gallstones, and blood clots.

barotrauma Physical damage to body tissues caused by a difference in pressure between an air space inside or beside the body and the surrounding fluid.

basophils The least common of the granulocytes, representing about 0.01% to 0.3% of circulating white blood cells.

benign tumors Noncancerous and therefore not an immediate threat, even though treatment eventually may be required for health or cosmetic reasons.

beta waves Electroencephalogram (EEG) waves known as the "busy waves" of the brain. They are recorded when the patient is awake and alert with eyes open. They are also seen during Stage N1 sleep.

β-receptor Site in autonomic nerve pathways wherein inhibitory responses occur when adrenergic agents such as norepinephrine and epinephrine are released.

bicarbonate Any salt containing the HCO_3^- anion e.g., sodium bicarbonate.

bifurcation A separation into two branches; the point of forking.

Bilevel positive airway pressure (BiPAP) BiPAP is the brand name of a machine manufactured by Respironics (Pittsburgh, PA), which became popular in the 1980s as a home care device for treating sleep apnea. When BiPAP is administered, the patient receives both an inspiratory positive airway pressure (IPAP) and an expiratory positive airway pressure (EPAP). The IPAP is higher than EPAP when applied to patients. The term *BiPAP* has become so commonly used, it is often applied to any device that provides bilevel pressure control. Other names for BiPAP include the following: bilevel airway pressure, bilevel positive pressure, bilevel positive airway pressure, bilevel CPAP (continuous positive airway pressure), bilevel PEEP (positive end expiratory pressure), bilevel pressure assist, and bilevel pressure support.

biopsy Excision of a small piece of living tissue for microscopic examination; usually performed to establish a diagnosis.

Biot's respiration An abnormal respiratory pattern characterized by short episodes of rapid, uniformly deep inspirations followed by 10 to 30 seconds of apnea. Biot's respiration is symptomatic of meningitis or increased intracranial pressure.

bleb Blister or bulla. Blebs may vary in size from that of a bean to that of a goose egg and may contain serous, seropurulent, or bloody fluid.

blood pressure (BP) The pressure exerted by circulating blood on the walls of blood vessels, and is one of the principal vital signs. During each heartbeat, BP varies between a maximum (systolic) and a minimum (diastolic) pressure. The mean BP decreases as the circulating blood moves away from the heart through arteries, has its greatest decrease in the small arteries and arterioles, and continues to decrease as the blood moves through the capillaries and back to the heart through veins.

blood urea nitrogen (BUN) A measure of the amount of nitrogen in the blood in the form of urea and a measurement of renal function. *Urea* is a substance secreted by the liver and removed from the blood by the kidneys.

Bochdalek foramen A posterolateral opening in the fetal diaphragm. Its failure to close leaves a congenital posterolateral defect that may become a site for a congenital diaphragmatic hernia. Also called pleuroperitoneal hiatus hernia.

Body mass index (BMI) A key index for relating weight to height. BMI is a person's weight in kilograms (kg) divided by his or her height in meters squared. The National Institutes of Health (NIH) now defines normal weight, overweight, and obesity according to BMI rather than the traditional height/weight charts. Overweight is a BMI of 27.3 or more for women and 27.8 or more for men. Obesity is a BMI of 30 or more for either sex (about 30 pounds overweight). A very muscular person might have a high BMI without health risks.

body plethysmography A sensitive lung measurement used to detect lung pathology. This method of obtaining the absolute volume of air within one's lungs may also be used in situations where several repeated trials are required or where the patient is unable to perform the multi-breath tests. The technique requires moderately complex coaching and instruction for the subject.

body surface burns An assessment measure of burns of the skin. In adults, the "rule of nines" is used to determine the total percentage of area burned for each major section of the body. In some cases, the burns may cover more than one body part, or may not fully cover such a part—in these cases, burns are measured by using the casualty's palm as a reference point for 1% of the body.

body temperature Normal values upon the place in the body at which the measurement is made, and the time of day and level of activity of the body. Although the value 37.0° C (98.6° F) is the commonly accepted average core body temperature, the value of 36.8 ± 0.7° C, or 98.2 ± 1.3° F is an average oral (under the tongue) measurement. Rectal measurements, or measurements taken directly inside the body cavity, are typically slightly higher.

brachial pulse The pulse of the brachial artery is palpable on the anterior aspect of the elbow, medial to the tendon of the biceps, and, with the use of a stethoscope and sphygmomanometer (blood pressure cuff) often used to measure the blood pressure.

brachytherapy Radiation treatment given by placing radioactive material directly in or near the target, which is often a tumor.

bradycardia A slow heart rate, usually defined as less than 60 bpm. The word bradycardia is derived from two Greek roots: *bradys*, slow + *cardia*, heart = slow heart.

bradypnea Abnormally slow breathing. A respiratory rate that is too slow. The normal rate of respirations (breaths per minute) depends on a number of factors, including the age of the individual and the degree of exertion.

brady-tachy syndrome During periods of apnea the heart rate decreases, then increases after the termination of apnea.

bronchial Pertaining to the bronchi or bronchioles.

bronchial breath sounds A normal sound heard with a stethoscope over the main airways of the lungs, especially the trachea. An abnormal breath sound transmitted through consolidated lungs in pneumonia; they are similar to the sounds heard normally over the larger bronchi and are louder and harsher than vesicular breath sounds.

bronchiolitis Inflammation of the bronchioles, the airways that extend beyond the bronchi and terminate in the alveoli. Bronchiolitis is attributable to viral infections such as parainfluenza, influenza, adenovirus, and, especially, respiratory syncytial virus (RSV).

bronchoconstriction Constriction of the bronchial tubes.

bronchodilation Dilation of a bronchus.

bronchogenic carcinoma More than 90% of malignant lung tumors that originate in bronchi.

bronchography An x-ray examination of the bronchi after they have been coated with a radiopaque substance.

bronchopulmonary dysplasia (formerly *chronic lung disease of infancy*) A chronic lung disorder that is most common among children who were born prematurely, with low birth weights, and who received prolonged mechanical ventilation to treat respiratory distress syndrome.

bronchoscopy A visual examination of the tracheobronchial tree with the bronchoscope.

bronchospasm Involuntary contraction of the muscular layer of the bronchus, as in asthma.

bronchovesicular Breath sounds pertaining to the bronchi, bronchioles, and alveoli.

bulla Blister, cavity, or vesicle filled with air or fluid; a bleb.

calcification Process in which organic tissue becomes hardened by the deposition of calcium salts in tissue.

cannulation Placement of a tube or sheath enclosing a trocar to allow the escape of fluid after the trocar is withdrawn from the body.

capillary stasis Stagnation of the normal flow of blood in capillaries.

carbon dioxide (CO_2) Colorless, odorless, incombustible gas formed during respiration and combustion; normally constitutes only 0.03% of the atmosphere. Concentrations above 5% in inspired air stimulate respiration. CO_2 retention occurs in end-stage pulmonary disease.

carbon monoxide (CO) A product of incomplete combustion of fossil fuels. Also found in tobacco smoke, and highly toxic at high levels. Also used in pulmonary function testing to detect diffusion abnormalities.

carbon monoxide poisoning A toxic condition in which carbon monoxide gas has been inhaled and binds to hemoglobin molecules, thus displacing oxygen from the red blood cells and decreasing the capacity of the blood to carry oxygen to the cells of the body.

carcinoma Malignant tumor that occurs in epithelial tissue. These neoplasms tend to infiltrate and give rise to metastases.

cardiac diastole The period between contractions of the atria or the ventricles during which blood enters the relaxed chambers from the systemic circulation and the lungs. Ventricular diastole begins with the onset of the second heart sound and ends with the first heart sound.

cardiac output (CO) The volume of blood expelled by the ventricles of the heart with each beat (the stroke volume) multiplied by the heart rate. Cardiac output is commonly measured by the thermodilution technique. A normal, resting adult has a cardiac output of 4 to 8 L/min.

cardiac systole The contraction of the heart, driving blood into the aorta and pulmonary arteries. The occurrence of systole is indicated by the first heart sound heard on auscultation, by the palpable apex beat, and by the peripheral pulse.

cardiogenic Originating in the heart.

cardiotonic drugs Drugs that increase the tonicity (contraction strength) of the heart.

carotid pulse The pulse of the carotid artery, palpated by gently pressing a finger in the area between the larynx and the sternocleidomastoid muscle in the neck.

carotid sinus baroreceptors Sensory nerve endings located in the carotid sinus. Changes in pressure stimulate the nerve endings.

cartilage Dense, firm, compact connective tissue capable of withstanding considerable pressure and tension; located in all true joints, the outer ear, bronchi, and movable sections of the ribs.

caseous tubercles Cottage cheeselike mixture of fat and protein that appears in some body tissues undergoing necrosis. Also described as a nodule or a small eminence. For example, a small rounded nodule produced by infection with *Mycobacterium tuberculosis* is commonly described as a gray translucent mass of small spheric cells surrounded by connective cells.

catecholamines Biologically active amines that behave as epinephrine and norepinephrine. Catecholamines have marked effects on the nervous and cardiovascular systems, metabolic rate, temperature, and smooth muscle.

cavitation The formation of cavities or hollow spaces within the body such as those formed in the lung by tuberculosis.

cavity A hollow space within a larger structure, such as the peritoneal cavity or the oral cavity.

central sleep apnea (CSA) A form of sleep apnea resulting from decreased respiratory center output. It may involve primary brain stem medullary depression resulting from a tumor of the posterior fossa, poliomyelitis, or idiopathic central hypoventilation.

central venous pressure (CVP) Pressure within the superior vena cava. The pressure under which the blood is returned to the right atrium.

centrilobular emphysema One of the types of emphysema, characterized by enlargement of air spaces in the proximal part of the acinus, primarily at the level of the respiratory bronchioles. Also called *centriacinar emphysema*, *focal emphysema*.

cerebrospinal fluid (CSF) Liquid surrounding and protecting the brain and spinal cord.

chemoreceptor Sense organ or sensory nerve ending that is stimulated by and reacts to chemical stimuli and that is located outside the central nervous system. Chemoreceptors are found in the large arteries of the thorax and neck (carotid and aortic bodies), the taste buds, and the olfactory cells of the nose.

chemotherapy The treatment of cancer, infections, and other diseases with chemical agents. The term has been applied over the centuries to a variety of therapies, including malaria therapy with herbs and use of mercury for syphilis. In modern usage, chemotherapy usually entails the use of chemicals to destroy cancer cells on a selective basis.

Cheyne-Stokes respiration An abnormal pattern of respiration, characterized by alternating periods of apnea and deep, rapid breathing. The respiratory cycle begins with slow, shallow breaths that gradually become abnormally rapid and deep. Breathing gradually becomes slower and shallower and is followed by 10 to 20 seconds of apnea before the cycle is repeated. Each episode may last from 45 seconds to 3 minutes. A form of central sleep apnea (CSA).

Chlamydia Genus of viruslike microorganisms that causes disease in humans and birds. Some *Chlamydia* infections of birds can be transmitted to humans (e.g., ornithosis, parrot disease). The organisms resemble bacteria but are of similar size to viruses and are obligate parasites.

chronic Denoting a process that shows little change and slow progression and is of long duration.

chronotropic Agent that increases heart rate.

chylothorax A condition marked by the effusion of chyle from the thoracic duct into the pleural space. The cause is usually a traumatic injury to the neck or a tumor that invades the thoracic duct. Treatment is directed at repairing damage to the duct.

cilia Small, hairlike projections on the surface of epithelial cells. In the bronchi, they propel mucus and foreign particles in a whiplike movement toward the throat.

clinical manifestations Symptoms or signs demonstrated by a patient; may be subjective or objective.

coagulation Process of clotting. Coagulation requires the presence of several substances, the most important of which are prothrombin, thrombin, thromboplastin, calcium in ionic form, and fibrinogen.

coalesce To fuse, run, or grow together.

coccobacillus Short, thick bacterial rod in the shape of an oval or slightly elongated coccus.

coccus Bacterium with a spheric shape.

collagen Fibrous insoluble protein found in connective tissue, including skin, bone, ligaments, and cartilage. Collagen represents about 30% of the total body protein.

colloid Type of solution; a gluelike substance such as protein or starch whose particles (molecules or aggregates of molecules), when dispersed in a solvent to the greatest degree, remain uniformly distributed and fail to form a true solution.

compromise A blending of the qualities of two different things; an unfavorable change.

congenital Existing at and usually before birth; referring to conditions that are present at birth, regardless of their cause.

congestion Excessive amount of blood, tissue, or fluid in an organ or in tissue.

consolidation The process of becoming solid; a mass that has solidified.

continuous positive airway pressure (CPAP) The application of pressures above ambient to improve oxygenation in a spontaneously breathing patient.

contusion Injury in which the skin is not broken; a bruise. Symptoms are pain, swelling, and discoloration.

convex Having a rounded, somewhat elevated surface resembling a segment of the external surface of a sphere.

cor pulmonale Hypertrophy or failure of the right ventricle resulting from disorders of the lungs, pulmonary vessels, or chest wall.

core temperature The temperature of deep structures of the body, such as the liver, as compared to that of peripheral tissues.

corticosteroids Any of a number of hormonal steroid substances obtained from the cortex of the adrenal gland.

costophrenic angle The junction of the rib cage and the diaphragm.

cuirass A chest covering; breastplate, as in cuirass ventilator.

cyanide poisoning Poisoning resulting from the ingestion or inhalation of cyanide from such substances as bitter almond oil, wild cherry syrup, prussic acid, hydrocyanic acid, or potassium or sodium cyanide. Characterized by tachycardia, drowsiness, seizures, headache, apnea, and cardiac arrest, it may cause death within 1 to 15 minutes.

cyclic adenosine monophosphate (cAMP) Cyclic nucleotide participating in the activities of many hormones, including catecholamines, adrenocorticotropin, and vasopressin. It is synthesized from adenosine triphosphate and is stimulated by the enzyme adenylate cyclase.

cyst Closed pouch or sac with a definite wall that contains fluid, semifluid, or solid material.

cytoplasm Protoplasm of a cell exclusive of the nucleus.

D-dimer blood test A simple and confirmatory test for intravascular coagulation that can also indicate when a clot is lysed by thrombolytic therapy. The fragment D-dimer assesses both thrombin and plasmin activity.

deep venous thrombi (DVT) A disorder involving a thrombus in one of the deep veins of the body, most commonly the iliac or femoral vein. Symptoms include tenderness, pain, swelling, warmth, and discoloration of the skin. A deep vein thrombus is potentially life threatening. Treatment—including bed rest and use of thrombolytic and anticoagulant drugs—is directed to preventing movement of the thrombus toward the lungs.

delta waves Amplitude (>75 μV) broad waves. Although delta EEG activity is usually defined as <4 Hz, in human sleep scoring, the slow-wave activity used for staging is defined as EEG activity <2 Hz (>0.5 second duration) and a peak-to-peak amplitude of >75 μV. Delta waves are called the "deep-sleep waves." They are associated with a dreamless state from which an individual is not easily aroused. Delta waves are seen primarily during Stage N3.

demarcate To set or mark boundaries or limits.

demyelination The destruction or removal of the myelin sheath from a nerve or nerve fiber.

density Mass of a substance per unit of volume, the relative weight of a substance compared with a reference standard; e.g., gm/cc.

deoxyribonucleic acid (DNA) Type of nucleic acid containing deoxyribose as the sugar component and found principally in the nuclei of animal and vegetable cells, usually loosely bound to protein (hence termed *deoxyribonucleoprotein*).

depolarize To reduce to a nonpolarized condition. To reduce the amount of electrical charge between oppositely charged particles.

desensitization Prevention of anaphylaxis.

dextrocardia The location of the heart in the right hemithorax, either as a result of displacement by disease or as a congenital defect.

diabetes mellitus Chronic disease of pancreatic origin that is characterized by insulin deficiency or functional abnormality and a subsequent inability to process carbohydrates. This condition results in excess sugar in the blood and urine; excessive thirst, hunger, urination, weakness, and emaciation; and imperfect combustion of fats. If untreated, diabetes mellitus leads to acidosis, coma, and death.

diagnostic Pertaining to the use of scientific methods to establish the cause and nature of disease.

diastole Period in the heart cycle during which the muscle fibers relax and lengthen, the heart dilates, and the cavities fill with blood.

diastolic blood pressure The minimum level of blood pressure measured between contractions of the heart. It may vary with age, gender, body weight, emotional state, and other factors.

digitalis A cardiac glycoside.

dilation Expansion of an organ, orifice, or vessel.

dimorphism The quality of existing in two distinct forms.

diplopia Double vision caused by defective function of the extraocular muscles or a disorder of the nerves that innervate the muscles. It occurs when the object of fixation falls on the fovea in one eye and a nonfoveal point in the other eye or when the object of fixation falls on two noncorresponding points.

disseminate Scatter or distribute over a considerable area; when applied to disease organisms, scattered throughout an organ or the body.

distal Farthest from the center, from a medial line, or from the trunk.

double pneumonia Acute pneumonia affecting both lungs.

driving pressure Pressure difference between two areas.

ductus arteriosus Vessel between the pulmonary artery and the aorta. It bypasses the lungs in the fetus.

duplex ultrasonography A combination of real-time and Doppler ultrasonography.

dynamometer An instrument for measuring the force of muscular contractions. For example, a squeeze dynamometer is one by which the strength of the hand is measured.

Dynamic lung compliance Dynamic lung compliance is the **compliance** of the **lung** at any given time during actual movement of air.

dysphagia Difficulty in swallowing, commonly associated with obstructive or motor disorders of the esophagus. Patients with obstructive disorders such as esophageal tumor or a lower esophageal ring are unable to swallow solids but can tolerate liquids. Persons with motor disorders, such as achalasia, are unable to swallow solids or liquids. Diagnosis of the underlying condition is made through barium studies, the observed clinical signs, and evaluation of the patient's symptoms.

dysplasia Abnormal development of tissues or cells.

dyspnea Air hunger resulting in labored or difficult breathing, sometimes accompanied by pain. Symptoms include audible labored breathing, distressed anxious expression, dilated nostrils, protrusion of the abdomen with an expanded chest, and gasping.

edema A local or generalized condition in which the body tissues contain an excessive amount of fluid.

edrophonium chloride A cholinesterase inhibitor that acts as an antidote to curare and other nondepolarizing neuromuscular blockers and is an aid in the diagnosis of **myasthenia gravis**.

efferent Away from a central organ or section. Efferent nerves conduct impulses from the brain or spinal cord to the periphery.

efferent nerves Nerves that carry impulses having the following effects: motor, causing contraction of the muscles; secretory, causing glands to secrete; and inhibitory, causing some organs to become quiescent.

effusion Seeping or serous, purulent, or bloody fluid into a cavity, the result of such a seeping.

ejection fraction The proportion of the volume of blood in the ventricles at the end of diastole that is ejected during systole; it is the stroke volume divided by the end-diastolic volume, often expressed as a percentage. It is normally 65 ± 8 per cent; lower values indicate ventricular dysfunction.

elastase Enzyme that dissolves elastin.

electrocardiogram (ECG) Record of the electrical activity of the heart.

electrodiagnostic Use of electric and electronic devices for diagnostic purposes.

electroencephalogram (EEG) Record of the electrical activity of the brain.

electrolyte Substance that, in solution, conducts an electrical current which is decomposed by the passage of an electrical current. Acids, bases, and salts are electrolytes.

electromyogram (EMG) A graphic record of the contraction of a muscle as a result of electrical stimulation.

electrophoresis Movement of charged colloidal particles through the medium in which they are dispersed as a result of changes in electrical potential.

embolus Mass of undissolved matter present in blood or lymphatic vessels to which it has been brought by the blood or lymph current. Emboli may be solid, liquid, or gaseous.

empathy The ability to recognize and to some extent share the emotions and states of mind of another and to understand the meaning and significance of that person's behavior. It is an essential quality for effective psychotherapy.

empyema Pus in a body cavity, especially in the pleural cavity; usually the result of a primary infection in the lungs, or pleura.

encapsulated Enclosed in a fibrous or membranous sheath.

encephalitis Inflammation of the brain.

endemic A disease that occurs continuously in a particular population but has low mortality, such as measles.

endocarditis Inflammation of the endocardium. It may involve only the membrane covering the valves, or it may involve the lining of all the chambers of the heart.

endothelium The layer of epithelial cells that lines the cavities of the heart, blood and lymph vessels, and the serous cavities of the body; it originates from the mesoderm.

enuresis Involuntary discharge of urine, usually referring to involuntary discharge of urine during sleep at night or bedwetting beyond the age when bladder control should have been achieved.

enzyme Complex protein capable of inducing chemical changes in other substances without being changed itself. Enzymes speed chemical reactions.

eosinophil Cell or cellular structure that stains readily with the acid stain eosin. Specifically refers to a granular leukocyte.

epidemiology Scientific discipline concerned with defining and explaining the interrelationships of factors that determine disease frequency and distribution.

epinephrine Hormone secreted by the adrenal medulla in response to splanchnic stimulation.

epithelium Covering of the internal and external organs of the body, including the lining of vessels. It consists of cells bound together by connective material and varies in the number of layers and the types of cells.

epoch A period marked by distinctive character or reckoned from a fixed point or event.

erythema multiforme A hypersensitivity syndrome characterized by polymorphous eruptions of the skin and mucous membranes.

erythropoiesis Formation of red blood cells.

etiology Cause of disease.

exocrine gland Gland whose secretion reaches an epithelial surface either directly or through a duct.

expectoration To clear out the chest and lungs by coughing up and spitting out matter.

expiratory reserve volume (ERV) The maximum volume of gas that can be exhaled after a resting volume exhalation.

extracorporeal membrane oxygenator (ECMO) A device that oxygenates a patient's blood outside the body and returns the blood to the patient's circulatory system. The technique may be used to support an impaired respiratory gas exchange system.

extravascular Outside a vessel.

exudate Accumulation of fluid in a cavity; matter that penetrates through vessel walls into adjoining tissue.

facilitation The enhancement or reinforcement of any action or function so that it can be performed more easily.

fascia Fibrous membrane covering, supporting, and separating muscles.

Fatigue The overwhelming feeling of tiredness; a lack of energy or feeling of exhaustion; trouble initiating or completing voluntary efforts. Different from sleepiness, sadness, or weakness.

febrile Pertaining to a fever.

femoral pulse The pulse of the femoral artery, palpated in the groin.

fibrin Whitish, filamentous protein formed by the action of prothrombin on fibrinogen. The conversion of fibrinogen into fibrin is the basis for blood clotting. Fibrin is deposited as fine interlacing filaments in which are entangled red and white blood cells and platelets, the whole forming a coagulum or clot.

fibrinolytic Pertaining to the splitting (lysis) of fibrin.

fibroelastic Composed of fibrous and elastic tissue.

fibrosis Formation of scar tissue in the connective tissue framework of the lungs, or heart.

first responder The first emergency person to arrive at the scene of a traumatic or medical situation. This person is trained according to a national standard curriculum set up by the U.S. Department of Transportation.

fissure Cleft or groove on the surface of an organ, often marking the division of the organ into parts, as the lobes of the lung.

fistula Abnormal passage or communication, usually between two internal organs or leading from an internal organ to the surface of the body; designated according to the organs or parts with which it communicates.

flaccid paralysis Paralysis in which there is loss of muscle tone, loss or reduction of tendon reflexes, and atrophy and degeneration of muscles.

flare Flush or spreading area of redness that surrounds a line made by drawing a pointed instrument across the skin. It is the second reaction in the triple response of skin to injury and is caused by dilation of the arterioles.

flash burn A lesion caused by exposure to an extremely intense source of radiant energy or heat. Flash burn commonly occurs on the corneas of arc welders.

flow-volume loop A graph of the rate of air flow as a function of lung volume during a complete respiratory cycle consisting of a forced inspiration followed by a forced expiration. The plotted curve appears as a loop and is used in assessing pulmonary function.

fluorescent antibody microscopy Microscopic examination of antibodies tagged with fluorescent material for the diagnosis of infections.

fluoroscopy The examination of a part of the body or the function of an organ with a fluoroscope. The technique offers continuous imaging of the motion of internal structures and immediate serial images. It is invaluable in many clinical procedures, such as intrauterine fetal transfusion and cardiac catheterization.

focal emphysema Centriacinar emphysema associated with inhalation of environmental dusts, producing dilation of the terminal and respiratory bronchioles.

foramen ovale Opening between the atria of the heart in the fetus. This opening normally closes shortly after birth.

forced expiratory flow (FEF) The average volumetric flow rate during any stated volume interval while a forced expired vital capacity test is performed. It is usually expressed as a percentage of vital capacity.

forced expiratory flow$_{200-1200}$ (FEF$_{200-1200}$) The average flow rate between 200 and 1200 mL of a forced vital capacity measurement.

forced expiratory flow$_{25\%-75\%}$ (FEF$_{25\%-75\%}$) The average flow rate generated by the patient during the middle 50% of a forced vital capacity measurement.

forced expiratory flow$_{50\%}$ (FEF$_{50\%}$) The flow rate generated by the patient at the point in which 50% of a forced vital capacity has been exhaled.

forced expiratory volume in 1 second (FEV$_1$) The maximum volume of gas that can be exhaled in 1 second.

forced expiratory volume time (FEV$_T$) The maximum volume of gas that can be exhaled over a specific period.

forced expiratory volume in 1 second/forced vital capacity ratio (FEV$_1$/FVC ratio) Compares the amount of air exhaled in 1 second with the total amount exhaled during a forced vital capacity maneuver. Also called *forced expiratory volume 1 second percentage (FEV$_{1\%}$)*.

forced vital capacity (FVC) The maximum volume of gas that can be forcibly and rapidly exhaled after a full inspiration.

fossa Hollow or depression, especially on the surface of the end of a bone.

functional residual capacity (FRC) The volume of gas in the lungs at the end of a normal tidal volume exhalation. The functional residual capacity is equal to the residual volume plus the expiratory reserve volume.

fungal infection Any inflammatory condition caused by a fungus. Most fungal infections are superficial and mild, although persistent and difficult to eradicate. Some, particularly in older, debilitated, or immunosuppressed or immunodeficient people, may become systemic and life threatening.

gastric juice (or gastric secretions) Fluid produced by the gastric glands of the stomach. It contains pepsin, hydrochloric acid, mucin, small quantities of inorganic salts, and the intrinsic antianemic principle. Gastric juice is strongly acid, having a pH of 0.9 to 1.5.

gastroesophageal reflux disease (GERD) A backflow of contents of the stomach into the esophagus that is often the result of incompetence of the lower esophageal sphincter. Gastric juices are acidic and therefore produce burning pain in the esophagus. Repeated episodes of reflux may cause esophagitis, peptic esophageal stricture, or esophageal ulcer. In uncomplicated cases, treatment consists of elevation of the head of the bed, avoidance of acid-stimulating foods, and regular administration of antacids. In complicated cases, surgical repair may provide relief.

genus In natural history classification, the division between the family or tribe and the species; a group of species alike in the broad features of their organization but different in detail.

globulin Any of a group of simple proteins soluble in salt solutions and forming a large fraction of blood serum protein. The three principal subsets of globulin are alpha globulin, beta globulin, and gamma globulin, which are distinguished by their respective degrees of electrophoretic mobility.

glossopharyngeal nerve Ninth cranial nerve. Function: special sensory (taste), visceral sensory, and motor. Distribution: pharynx, ear, meninges, posterior third of the tongue, and parotid gland.

glycolysis Breakdown of sugar by enzymes in the body. This occurs without oxygen.

glycoprotein Any of a class of conjugated proteins consisting of a compound of protein with a carbohydrate group.

gram-negative organisms Having the pink color of the counterstain used in Gram's method of staining microorganisms. This property is a primary method of characterizing organisms in bacteriology. Some of the most common gram-negative pathogenic bacteria are *Bacteroides fragilis*, *Brucella abortus*, *Escherichia coli*, *Haemophilus influenzae*, *Klebsiella pneumoniae*, *Neisseria gonorrhoeae*, *Proteus vulgaris*, *Pseudomonas aeruginosa*, *Salmonella typhi*, *Shigella dysenteriae*, and *Yersinia pestis*.

gram-positive organisms Retaining the violet color of the stain used in Gram's method of staining microorganisms. This property is a primary method of characterizing organisms in microbiology. Some of the most common types of gram-positive pathogenic bacteria are *Bacillus anthracis*, *Clostridium* sp., *Mycobacterium leprae*, *Mycobacterium tuberculosis*, *Staphylococcus aureus*, *Streptococcus pneumoniae*, and *Streptococcus pyogenes*.

granuloma A chronic inflammatory lesion often caused by histoplasmosis, tubuculosis, and a fungal infection. It is characterized by an accumulation of macrophages; epithelioid macrophages, with or without lymphocytes; and giant cells into a discrete granule. Granulomas most often occur in the lungs. They may resolve spontaneously, remain static, become gangrenous, spread, or act as a focus of infection. Treatment depends on the cause and probable course of the particular granuloma.

Harrington rod One of the rigid, contoured metal rods inserted surgically, along with metal hooks, in the posterior elements of the spine to provide distraction and compression in treatment of scoliosis and other deformities.

hematocrit (Hct) Volume of erythrocytes packed by centrifugation in a given volume of blood. Hematocrit is expressed as a percentage of the total blood volume that consists of erythrocytes or as the volume in cubic centimeters of erythrocytes packed by centrifugation of the blood. The normal range is between 43% and 49% in men and between 37% and 43% in women.

hematology The scientific study of blood and blood-forming tissues.

hematopoietic Pertaining to the production and development of blood cells.

hemoglobin (Hb) A complex protein-iron compound in the blood that carries oxygen to the cells from the lungs and carbon dioxide away from the cells to the lungs. Each erythrocyte contains 200 to 300 molecules of hemoglobin; each molecule of hemoglobin contains four groups of heme; and each group of heme can carry one molecule of oxygen.

hemoptysis Expectoration of blood.

hemorrhage Abnormal internal or external discharge of blood; may be venous, arterial, or capillary.

hemothorax An accumulation of blood and fluid in the pleural cavity, between the parietal and visceral pleura, usually the result of trauma. Blood can also accumulate in the thoracic cavity as a result of erosion of pulmonary vessels, the rupture of blebs, or granulomas. Hemothorax may also be caused by the rupture of small blood vessels resulting from inflammation caused by pneumonia, tuberculosis, or tumors. Shock from hemorrhage, pain, and respiratory failure follow if emergency care is not available.

heparin Polysaccharide that has been isolated from the liver, lung, and other tissues. It is produced by the mast cells of the liver and by basophil leukocytes. It inhibits coagulation by preventing conversion of prothrombin to thrombin and blocking the liberation of thromboplastin from blood platelets.

hepatosplenomegaly Enlargement of both the liver and spleen.

Hering-Breuer reflex A neural mechanism that terminates inspiration and initiates expiration. The reflex is triggered by impulses that originate in stretch receptors of the bronchi and bronchioles in response to distension of the airway, increased intratracheal pressure, or pulmonary inflation. The impulses travel via afferent fibers of the vagus nerves to the medullary respiratory center. The Hering-Breuer reflex is well developed at birth and is hyperactive in conditions of restrictive ventilatory insufficiency.

heterozygote Individual with different alleles for a given characteristic.

high-frequency ventilation (HFV) A technique for providing ventilatory support to patients at a rate of at least 60 breaths/min with small tidal volumes. Types of HFV include high-frequency jet ventilation (HFJV) and high-frequency oscillation (HFO). HFJV uses a high-pressure gas source that can produce short, rapid jets of gas through a small-bore cannula into the airway above the carina at a rate of 100 to 400/min. HFO forces small impulses of gas into and out of the airway at a rate of 400 to 4000/min.

hilus Root of the lungs at the level of the fourth and fifth dorsal vertebrae.

histamine Substance normally present in the body; it exerts a pharmacologic action when released from injured cells. The red flush of a burn is caused by the local production of histamine. It is produced from the amino acid histidine.

homozygote Individual developing from gametes with similar alleles and thus possessing like pairs of genes for a given hereditary characteristic.

horizontal fissure A cleft that marks the separation of the upper and middle lobes of the right lung.

hormone Substance originating in an organ or gland that is conveyed through the blood to another part of the body where, by chemical action, it stimulates increased functional activity and increased secretion.

humoral Pertaining to body fluids or substances contained in them.

hyaline membrane A fibrous covering of the alveolar membranes in infants, caused by a lack of pulmonary surfactant associated with prematurity and low–birth-weight delivery.

hydralazine A vasodilator used in hypertension.

hydrostatic Pertaining to the pressure of liquids in equilibrium and to the pressure exerted on liquids by other forces.

hydrotherapy The use of water in the treatment of various disorders. Hydrotherapy may include continuous tub baths, wet sheet packs, or shower sprays.

hydrous Containing water, usually chemically combined.

hyperbaric oxygenation (HBO) The administration of oxygen at greater than normal atmospheric pressure. Also called *hyperbaric oxygen therapy*.

hypercarbia, hypercapnea Excess carbon dioxide in the blood; indicated by an elevated $PaCO_2$.

hypercoagulation Greater than normal clotting.

hyperinflation Distention of a part by air, gas, or liquid.

hyperplasia Excessive proliferation of normal cells in the normal tissue arrangement of an organ.

hyperpnea Increased depth (volume) of breathing with or without an increased frequency.

hyperpyrexia An extremely elevated temperature that sometimes occurs in acute infectious diseases, especially in young children.

hypersecretion Increased secretions from glands or cells.

hypersensitivity Abnormal increased sensitivity to a stimulus of any type.

hypertension Higher than normal blood pressure; greater than normal tension or tonus.

hyperthermia A much higher than normal body temperature.

hypertrophy Increase in size of an organ or structure that does not involve tumor formation.

hyperventilation Increased rate and/or depth of breathing, which in turn causes increased alveolar ventilation and a decreased $PaCO_2$.

hypochromic microcytic anemia A group of anemias characterized by a decreased concentration of hemoglobin in the red blood cells; a form of anemia in which the hemoglobin is deficient in proportion to the size of erythrocytes or the individual erythrocyte has the capacity to contain more hemoglobin, as in iron-deficiency anemia.

hypoperfusion Generalized or localized deficiency of blood coursing through the vessels of the circulatory system.

hypoproteinemia Decrease in the amount of protein in the blood.

hypotension An abnormal condition in which the blood pressure is not adequate for normal perfusion and oxygenation of the tissues. An expanded intravascular space, hypovolemia, or diminished cardiac output may be the cause.

hypoventilation Decreased rate and/or depth of breathing, which in turn causes decreased alveolar ventilation and an increased $PaCO_2$.

hypoxemia Refers to an abnormally low arterial oxygen tension (PaO_2) and is frequently associated with hypoxia, which is an inadequate level of tissue oxygenation.

hypoxia Refers to low or inadequate oxygen for aerobic cellular metabolism.

iatrogenic Any mental or physical condition induced in a patient by the effects of treatment by a physician or by the patient himself.

iatrogenic pneumothorax A condition in which air or gas is present in the pleural cavity as a result of mechanical ventilation, tracheostomy tube placement, or other therapeutic intervention.

idiopathic Disease or condition without a recognizable cause.

idiopathic pulmonary fibrosis A disorder of unknown cause characterized by fibrosis of the lungs. It may follow an earlier inflammation or disease, such as tuberculosis or pneumoconiosis.

immunoglobulin One of a family of closely related but not identical proteins that are capable of acting as antibodies. Five major types of immunoglobulins are normally present in the human adult: IgG, IgA, IgM, IgD, and IgE.

immunoglobulin E (IgE) An α-globulin produced by cells of the lining of the respiratory and intestinal tract. IgE is important in forming reagin antibodies; e.g., extrinsic asthma.

immunoglobulin G (IgG) antibodies An immunoglobulin produced by lymphocytes in response to bacteria, viruses, or other antigenic substances. An antibody is specific to an antigen. Each class of antibody is named for its action. Antibodies include **agglutinins, bacteriolysins, opsonins,** and **precipitin**.

immunoglobulin M (IgM) One of the five classes of antibodies produced by the body and the largest in molecular structure. It is found in circulating fluids and is the first immunoglobulin produced when the body is challenged by antigens. IgM triggers the increased production of IgG and the complement fixation required for effective immune response. It is the dominant antibody in ABO blood group incompatibilities. The normal concentration of IgM in serum is 40 to 120 mg/dL.

immunologic mechanism Reaction of the body to substances that are foreign or are interpreted as foreign.

immunotherapy Production or enhancement of immunity.

incubation period Development of an infection in a person from the time of entry into an organism up to the time of the first appearance of signs or symptoms.

infarction Necrosis of tissue after cessation of blood supply.

inferior vena cava (IVC) Venous trunk draining the lower extremities, the pelvis, and the abdominal viscera.

infiltrate v (verb)– To penetrate the interstices of a tissue or substance; *n*, the material or solution so deposited.

inflammation Localized heat, redness, swelling, and pain as a result of irritation, injury, or infection.

inotropic (positive) Increasing myocardial contractility.

insertion Manner or place of attachment of a muscle to the bone.

inspiratory capacity (IC) The maximum volume of gas that can be inhaled from the end of a resting exhalation. Equal to the sum of the tidal volume and the inspiratory reserve volume, it is measured with a spirometer.

inspiratory-to-expiratory ratio (I : E ratio) The ratio of the duration of inspiration to the duration of expiration. A range of 1 : 1.5 to 1 : 2 for an adult is considered acceptable for mechanical ventilation. Ratios of 1 : 1 or higher may cause hemodynamic complications, whereas ratios lower than 1 : 2 indicate lower mean airway pressure and fewer associated hazards.

inspiratory reserve volume (IRV) The maximum volume of gas that can be inhaled beyond a normal resting inspiration.

intercostal retraction Retraction of the chest. Sinking-in of the soft tissues of the chest is visible between and around the cartilaginous and bony ribs.

intermittent fever A fever that recurs in cycles of paroxysms and remissions, such as in malaria.

internal oblique One of a pair of anterolateral muscles of the abdomen, lying under the external oblique muscle in the lateral and ventral part of the abdominal wall. It is smaller and thinner than the external oblique muscle. It functions to compress the abdominal contents and assists in micturition, defecation, emesis, parturition, and forced expiration. Both muscles acting together serve to flex the vertebral column, drawing the costal cartilages toward the pubis. One side acting alone bends the vertebral column laterally and rotates it, drawing the shoulder of the opposite side downward.

interstitial Placed or lying between; pertaining to interstices or spaces within an organ or tissue.

interstitial edema An abnormal accumulation of fluid in interstitial spaces of tissues, such as in the pericardial sac, intrapleural space, peritoneal cavity, or joint capsules.

intrapleural pressure Pressure within the pleural cavity.

iodine Nonmetallic element belonging to the halogen group.

ion Atom, group of atoms, or molecule that has acquired a net electrical charge by gaining or losing electrons.

ischemia Deficiency of blood supply caused by obstruction of the circulation to a part.

isosorbide An antianginal agent.

isotope One of a series of chemical elements that have nearly identical chemical properties but differ in their atomic weights and electrical charges. Many isotopes are radioactive.

K complexes Are intermittent high-amplitude, biphasic Electroencephalogram (EEG) waves of at least 0.5 second duration that signals the start of Stage N2 sleep. A K complex consists of a sharp negative wave (upward deflection), followed immediately by a slower positive wave (downward deflection), that is, >0.5 second. K complexes are usually seen during Stage N2 sleep. They are sometimes seen in Stage N3. Sleep spindles are often superimposed on K complexes.

Kartagener's syndrome An inherited disorder characterized by bronchiectasis, chronic paranasal sinusitis, and transposed viscera, usually dextrocardia.

Kerley A and B lines Thickening of the interlobular septa as seen in chest roentgenography; may be caused by cellular infiltration or edema associated with pulmonary venous hypertension.

ketoconazole An antifungal agent.

kinetic Pertaining to or consisting of motion.

Klebsiella A genus of diplococcal bacteria that appear as small, plump rods with rounded ends. Several respiratory diseases, including bronchitis, sinusitis, and some forms of pneumonia, are caused by infection by species of *Klebsiella*.

Kulchitsky cell A cell containing serotonin-secreting granules that stain readily with silver and chromium; also known as an *argentaffin cell*.

Kussmaul breathing Abnormally deep, very rapid sighing respirations characteristic of diabetic ketoacidosis.

lactic acid Acid formed in muscles during activity by the anaerobic breakdown of sugar without oxygen.

lactic acidosis A disorder characterized by an accumulation of lactic acid in the blood, resulting in a lowered pH in tissue and serum. The condition occurs most commonly in tissue hypoxia but may also result from liver impairment, respiratory failure, burn trauma, neoplasms, and cardiovascular disease.

laryngospasm A spasmodic closure of the larynx.

latency State of being concealed, hidden, inactive, or inapparent, or delay.

lecithin-to-sphingomyelin ratio (L:S ratio) The ratio of two components of amniotic fluid, used for predicting fetal lung maturity. The normal L:S ratio in amniotic fluid is 2:1 or greater when fetal lungs are mature.

Legionella pneumophila A small gram-negative rod-shaped bacterium that is the causative agent in *Legionnaires' disease*.

lesion A wound, injury, or pathologic change in body tissue.

lethargy The state or quality of being indifferent, apathetic, or sluggish; stupor.

leukocytes White blood corpuscles, including cells both with and without granules within their cytoplasm.

leukopenia An abnormal decrease in the number of white blood cells to fewer than 5000 cells/mm^3.

linea alba Vertical white line of connective tissue in the middle of the abdomen from sternum to pubis.

lipids Any of numerous fats generally insoluble in water that constitute one of the principal structural materials of cells.

lobectomy The surgical excision of one or more lobes of a lung. It is performed to remove a malignant tumor or large benign tumor and to treat uncontrolled bronchiectasis, trauma with hemorrhage, congenital anomalies, or intractable tuberculosis.

longitudinal Parallel to the long axis of the body or part.

lubricant Agent, usually a liquid oil, that reduces friction between parts that brush against each other as they move. Joints are lubricated by synovial fluid.

lumen Inner open space of a tubular organ such as a blood vessel, intestine, or airway.

lung and chest topography The anatomic description of the lung and chest in terms of the region in which it is located.

lung biopsy Removal of a specimen of pulmonary tissue for histologic examination to diagnose pulmonary parenchymal disease, including carcinoma, granuloma, lung diseases caused by toxic exposure, sarcoidosis, and infection.

lung capacity A lung volume that is the sum of two or more of the four primary, nonoverlapping lung volumes. Lung capacities are **functional residual capacity**, **inspiratory capacity**, **total lung capacity**, and **vital capacity**.

lung compliance A measure of the ease of expansion of the lungs and thorax, determined by pulmonary volume and elasticity. A high degree of compliance indicates a loss of elastic recoil of the lungs, as in old age or emphysema. Decreased compliance means that a greater change in pressure is needed for a given change in volume, as in atelectasis, edema, fibrosis, pneumonia, or absence of surfactant. Dyspnea on exertion is the main symptom of diminished lung compliance.

lymph node Rounded body consisting of an accumulation of lymphatic tissue. Found at intervals in the course of lymphatic vessels.

lymphangitis carcinomatosa The condition of having widespread dissemination of carcinoma in lymphatic channels or vessels.

lymphatic vessels Thin-walled vessels conveying lymph from the tissues. Similar to veins, they possess valves ensuring one-way flow and eventually empty into the venous system at the junction of the internal jugular and subclavian veins.

macrocytic anemia A disorder of the blood characterized by impaired erythropoiesis and the presence of large red blood cells in the circulation. Macrocytic anemia is most often the result of a deficiency of folic acid or vitamin B$_{12}$.

macrophage Cell whose major function is phagocytosis of foreign matter.

malaise A vague feeling of body weakness, fatigue, or discomfort that often marks the onset of disease (see fatigue).

malignant tumor A neoplasm that characteristically invades surrounding tissue, metastasizes to distant sites, and contains anaplastic cells. A malignant tumor may cause death if treatment does not intervene.

malleolus The protuberance on both sides of the ankle joint, the lower extremity of the fibula being known as the *lateral malleolus* and the lower end of the tibia as the *medial malleolus*.

mannitol A poorly metabolized sugar used as an osmotic diuretic and in kidney function tests.

mast cell Connective tissue cells that contain heparin and histamine in their granules; important in cellular defense mechanisms, including blood coagulation; needed during injury or infection.

maximum voluntary ventilation (MVV) The maximum volume of gas that a person can inhale and exhale by voluntary effort per minute by breathing as quickly and deeply as possible. It is measured in pulmonary function tests.

mechanoreceptor Receptor that receives mechanical stimuli, such as pressure from sound or touch.

meconium A material that collects in the intestines of a fetus and forms the first stools of a newborn. It is thick and sticky, usually greenish to black, and composed of secretions of the intestinal glands, some amniotic fluid, and intrauterine debris, such as bile pigments, fatty acids, epithelial cells, mucus, lanugo, and blood. With ingestion of breast milk or formula and proper functioning of the gastrointestinal tract, the color, consistency, and frequency of the stools change by the 3rd or 4th day after the initiation of feedings. The presence of meconium in the amniotic fluid during labor may indicate fetal distress and may reflex a lack of oxygen and developmental delays.

meconium aspiration syndrome (MAS) The inhalation of meconium by a fetus or newborn. It can block the air passages and cause failure of the lungs to expand or cause other pulmonary dysfunction, such as pneumonia or emphysema.

meconium ileus Obstruction of the small intestine in the newborn by impaction of thick, dry, tenacious meconium, usually at or near the ileocecal valve. The condition results from a deficiency in pancreatic enzymes and is the earliest manifestation of cystic fibrosis.

mediastinoscopy An examination of the mediastinum through an incision in the suprasternal notch, by using an endoscope with light and lenses.

Mendelson's syndrome A respiratory condition caused by the aspiration of acidic gastric contents into the lungs. It usually occurs when a person vomits while inebriated, stuporous from anesthesia, or unconscious, as during a seizure. It is marked by bronchoconstriction and destruction of the tracheal mucosa, progressing to a syndrome resembling acute respiratory distress syndrome.

meningitis Any infection or inflammation of the membrane covering the brain and spinal cord.

mesothelioma A rare, malignant tumor of the mesothelium of the pleura or peritoneum; associated with early exposure to asbestos.

metabolic acidosis Acidosis in which excess acid is added to the body fluids or bicarbonate is lost from them. Acidosis is indicated by a pH of blood below 7.35. In starvation and in uncontrolled diabetes mellitus, glucose is not present or is not available for oxidation for cellular nutrition.

metabolic alkalosis An abnormal condition characterized by the significant loss of acid in the body or by increased levels of base bicarbonate. Alkalosis is indicated by a pH of blood above 7.45. Loss of acid may be caused by excessive vomiting, insufficient replacement of electrolytes, hyperadrenocorticism, or Cushing's disease.

metabolism Sum of all physical and chemical changes that take place within an organism; all energy and material transformations that occur within living cells.

metaplasia Conversion of one type of tissue into a form that is not normal for that tissue.

microvilli Minute cylindric processes on the free surface of a cell, especially cells of the proximal convoluted renal tubule and the intestinal epithelium; they increase the surface area of the cell.

mitosis A type of cell division of somatic cells in which each daughter cell contains the same number of chromosomes as the parent cell.

mitral valve Bicuspid valve between the left atrium and the left ventricle.

mixed sleep apnea A condition marked by signs and symptoms of both central sleep apnea and obstructive sleep apnea. It often begins as central sleep apnea and develops into the obstructive form. Mixed sleep apnea may also result from obstructive sleep apnea as hypoxia and hypercapnia induce signs and symptoms of the central form.

mononucleosis Presence of an abnormally high number of mononuclear leukocytes in the blood.

motile Having the power to move spontaneously.

mucous Pertaining to or resembling mucus; also glands secreting mucus.

mucus The free slime of the mucous membranes. It is composed of secretions of the glands along with various inorganic salts, desquamated cells, and leukocytes.

myelin Insulating material covering the axons of many neurons; increases the velocity of the nerve impulse along the axon.

myeloma Tumor originating in cells of the hematopoietic portion of bone marrow.

myocardial infarction Development of an area(s) of cellular death in the myocardium, the result of myocardial ischemia following occlusion of a coronary artery.

myocarditis Inflammation of the myocardium.

myocardium Middle layer of the walls of the heart, composed of cardiac muscle.

myopathy An abnormal condition of skeletal muscle characterized by muscle weakness, wasting, and histologic changes within muscle tissue.

necrosis Death of areas of tissue.

neoplasm New and abnormal formation of tissue, such as a tumor or growth. It serves no useful function but grows at the expense of the healthy organism.

nephritis Inflammation of the kidney. The glomeruli, tubules, and interstitial tissue may be affected.

nephrotic syndrome An abnormal condition of the kidney characterized by marked proteinuria, hypoalbuminemia, and edema.

neuroendocrine Pertaining to the nervous and endocrine systems as an integrated functioning mechanism.

neuromuscular junction The area of contact between the ends of a large myelinated nerve fiber and a fiber of skeletal muscle.

nitrogen oxides Automotive air pollutant. Depending on concentration, these gases cause respiratory irritation, bronchitis, and pneumonitis. Concentrations greater than 100 ppm usually cause pulmonary edema and result in death.

nocturnal Pertaining to or occurring in the night.

nodule A small aggregation of cells; a small node.

nomogram Graph consisting of three lines or curves (usually parallel) graduated for different variables in such a way that a straight line cutting the three lines gives the related values of the three variables. (For example, see Appendix XII).

non–small cell lung carcinoma (NSCLC) A general term comprising all lung carcinomas except small cell carcinoma, including adenocarcinoma of the lung, large cell carcinoma, and squamous cell carcinoma.

norepinephrine Hormone produced by the adrenal medulla, similar in chemical and pharmacologic properties to epinephrine.

normal flora Naturally occurring bacteria found in specific bodily areas. Normal flora has no detrimental effect.

oblique fissure The groove marking the division of the lower and the middle lobes in the right lung; the groove marking the division of the upper and the lower lobes in the left lung.

occlude To close, obstruct, or join together.

olfactory Pertaining to the sense of smell.

oncotic pressure Osmotic pressure resulting from the presence of colloids in a solution.

opacity Opaque spot or area; the condition of being opaque.

opaque Impervious to light rays or, by extension, to roentgen rays or other electromagnetic vibrations; neither transparent nor translucent.

open pneumothorax The presence of air or gas in the chest as a result of an open wound in the chest wall.

orbicularis oculi The muscular body of the eyelid; it is composed of the palpebral, orbital, and lacrimal parts.

orifice Mouth, entrance, or outlet to any aperture.

origin The more fixed attachment (usually proximal or central) part of a muscle.

orthopnea Respiratory complaint of discomfort in any but an erect sitting or standing position.

osmotic pressure Pressure that develops when two unequally osmolar solutions are separated by a semipermeable membrane.

osteoporosis Increased brittleness of bone seen most often in elderly persons.

ozone Formed by the action of sunlight on oxygen in which three atoms form the molecule O_3. It is an irritant to the respiratory tract.

P wave The component of the cardiac cycle shown on an electrocardiogram as an inverted U-shaped curve that follows the T wave and precedes the QRS complex. It represents atrial depolarization.

palatine arches Vault-shaped muscular structures forming the soft palate between the mouth and the nasopharynx.

palpation A technique used in physical examination in which the examiner feels the texture, size, consistency, and location of certain body parts with the hands.

panacinar emphysema One of the principal types of emphysema, characterized by relatively uniform enlargement of air spaces throughout the terminal bronchioles and alveoli. It is an inherited condition. Also called *panlobular emphysema*.

pancreas Fish-shaped, grayish pink gland that stretches transversely across the posterior abdominal wall in the epigastric region of the body. It secretes various substances, such as digestive enzymes, insulin, and glucagon.

pancreatic juice Clear alkaline pancreatic secretion that contains at least three different enzymes (trypsin, amylopsin, and lipase). It is poured into the duodenum, where, mixed with bile and intestinal juices, it furthers the digestion of food.

panlobular emphysema One of the principal types of emphysema, characterized by relatively uniform enlargement of air spaces throughout the terminal bronchioles and alveoli. It is an inherited condition. Also called *panacinar emphysema.*

paracentesis A procedure in which fluid is withdrawn from the abdominal cavity.

paradoxical Occurring at variance with the normal rule.

paramyxovirus Subgroup of viruses including parainfluenza, measles, mumps, German measles, and respiratory syncytial viruses.

parasite Any organism that grows, feeds, and is sheltered on or in a different organism while contributing nothing to the survival of the host.

parenchyma Essential parts of an organ that are concerned with its function.

paroxysmal Concerning the sudden, periodic attack or recurrence of symptoms of a disease.

paroxysmal nocturnal dyspnea (PND) A disorder characterized by sudden attacks of respiratory distress that awaken the person, usually after several hours of sleep in a reclining position. This occurs because of increased fluid central circulation with reclining position. It is most commonly caused by pulmonary edema resulting from congestive heart failure. The attacks are often accompanied by coughing, a feeling of suffocation, cold sweat, and tachycardia with a gallop rhythm. Sleeping with the head propped up on pillows may prevent PND, but treatment of the underlying cause is required to prevent fluid from accumulating in the lungs.

particulate Made up of particles.

patent ductus Open, narrow, tubular channel.

pathogen Any agent causing disease, especially a microorganism.

peak expiratory flow rate (PEFR) The greatest rate of air flow that can be achieved during forced expiration, beginning with the lungs fully inflated.

pectoralis major A large muscle of the upper chest wall that acts on the joint of the shoulder. Thick and fan-shaped, it arises from the clavicle, the sternum, the cartilages of the second to the sixth ribs, and the aponeurosis of the obliquus externus abdominis. It serves to flex, adduct, and medially rotate the arm in the shoulder joint.

pendelluft Shunting of air from one lung to another.

percussion A technique in physical examination of tapping the body with the fingertips to evaluate the size, borders, and consistency of some of the internal organs and to discover the presence of and evaluate the amount of fluid in a body cavity. **Immediate** or **direct percussion** is percussion performed by striking the fingers directly on the body surface. **Indirect, mediate,** or **finger percussion** involves striking a finger of one hand on a finger of the other hand (normally the second phalanx of the third digit) as it is placed over the organ.

perforation Hole made through a substance or part.

peribronchial Located around the bronchi.

peripheral airways Small bronchi on the outer portion of the lungs where most gas transfer takes place.

peritoneal dialysis Removal of toxic substances from the body by perfusing specific warm sterile chemical solutions through the peritoneal cavity.

perivascular Located around a vessel, especially a blood vessel.

permeability The quality of being permeable.

permeable Capable of allowing the passage of fluids or substances in solution.

permissive hypercapnia Ventilation that allows $PaCO_2$ to rise slowly over time as the pH becomes normalized. The goal is to reduce tidal volume and rate while preventing volutrauma during mechanical ventilation. Patients may need to be sedated during this.

pH Symbol for the logarithm of the reciprocal of the hydrogen ion concentration.

phagocytosis Envelopment and digestion of bacteria or other foreign bodies by cells.

phalanges Bones of the fingers or toes.

phenotype Physical makeup of an individual. Some phenotypes, such as the blood groups, are completely determined by heredity, whereas others, such as stature, are readily altered by environmental agents.

phenylketonuria Abnormal presence of phenylketone in the urine.

phlegmasia alba dolens Acute edema, especially of the leg, from lymphatic or venous obstruction, usually a thrombosis.

phosgene Carbonyl chloride ($COCl_2$), a poisonous gas causing nausea and suffocation.

phosphodiesterase Enzyme that catalyzes the breakdown of the second messenger (cyclic adenosine monophosphate) to adenosine monophosphate.

Pickwickian syndrome An abnormal condition characterized by obesity, alveolar hypoventilation, somnolence, and polycythemia.

plaque A flat, often raised patch on the skin, mucous surface or any other organ of the body. A patch of atherosclerosis. Example: *dental plaque,* usually a thin film on the teeth.

plasmapheresis The removal of plasma from previously withdrawn blood by centrifugation, reconstitution of the cellular elements in an isotonic solution, and reinfusion of this solution into the donor or another individual who needs red blood cells rather than whole blood.

platelets The smallest cells in the blood. They are formed in the red bone marrow and some are stored in the spleen. Platelets are disk-shaped, contain no hemoglobin, and are essential for the coagulation of blood and in maintenance of hemostasis. Normally between 200,000 and 300,000 platelets are found in 1 mL^3 of blood.

pleomorphic Multiform; occurring in more than one form.

pleural friction rub An abnormal coarse, grating sound heard on auscultation of the lungs during late inspiration and early expiration. It occurs when the visceral and parietal pleural surfaces rub against each other. The sound is not affected by coughing. A pleuropericardial rub indicates primary inflammatory, neoplastic, or traumatic pleural disease or inflammation secondary to infection or neoplasm.

pleurisy Symptoms of inflammation of the pleura.

pleuritis Inflammation of the pleura.

pneumomediastinum The presence of air or gas in the mediastinal tissues. In infants it may lead to pneumothorax or pneumopericardium, especially in those with respiratory distress syndrome or aspiration pneumonitis. In older children the condition may result from bronchitis, acute asthma, pertussis, cystic fibrosis, or bronchial rupture from cough or trauma.

pneumonectomy The surgical removal of all or part of a lung.

pneumonitis Inflammation of the lung. Pneumonitis may be caused by a virus or may be a hypersensitivity reaction to chemicals or organic dusts, such as bacteria, bird droppings, or molds. It is usually an interstitial, granulomatous, fibrosing inflammation of the lung, especially of the bronchioles and alveoli. Dry cough is a common symptom. Treatment depends on the cause but includes removal of any offending agents and administration of corticosteroids to reduce inflammation.

pneumopericardium The presence of air or gas in the pericardial sac.

pneumoperitoneum The presence of air or gas within the peritoneal cavity of the abdomen. It may be spontaneous, such as from rupture of a hollow, gas-containing organ, or induced for diagnostic or therapeutic purposes.

pneumothorax The presence of air or gas in the pleural space, causing a lung to collapse. Pneumothorax may be the result of an open chest wound that permits the entrance of air, the rupture of an emphysematous vesicle on the surface of the lung, or a severe bout of coughing. It may also occur spontaneously without apparent cause.

point of maximum impulse (PMI) The place where the apical pulse is palpated as strongest, often in the fifth intercostal space of the thorax, just medial to the left midclavicular line.

polyarteritis nodosa Necrosis and inflammation of small and medium-sized arteries and subsequent involvement of tissue supplied by these arteries.

polycythemia Excess of red blood cells.

polymorphonuclear leukocyte Subclass of white blood cells, including neutrophils, eosinophils, and basophils.

polyneuritis Inflammation of two or more nerves at once.

polyneuropathy Term applied to any disorder of peripheral nerves, but particularly used to describe those of a noninflammatory nature.

polyradiculitis Inflammation of nerve roots, especially those of spinal nerves as found in Guillain-Barré syndrome.

polyradiculoneuropathy Guillain-Barré syndrome.

popliteal pulse The pulsation of the popliteal artery, behind the knee, best palpated with the patient lying prone with the knee flexed.

positive inotropic agent A substance that influences the force of muscular contractions. An agent that increases the force of muscular contractions of the heart.

positron emission tomography (PET) A computerized radiographic technique that uses radioactive substances to examine the metabolic activity of various body structures. The patient either inhales or is injected with a metabolically important substance such as glucose, carrying a radioactive element that emits positively charged particles, or positrons. When the positrons combine with electrons normally found in the cells of the body, gamma rays are emitted. The electronic circuitry and computers of the PET device detect the gamma rays and construct color-coded images that indicate the intensity of metabolic activity throughout the organ involved. The radioactive isotopes used in PET are very short-lived, so that patients undergoing a PET scan are exposed to very small amounts of radiation. Researchers use PET to examine blood flow and the metabolism of the heart and blood vessels, to study and diagnose cancer, and to investigate the biochemical activity of the brain.

postpartum Occurring after childbirth.

postural drainage Drainage of secretions from the bronchi or a cavity in the lung by positioning the patient so that gravity will allow drainage of the particular lobe or lobes of the lung involved.

primigravida A woman pregnant for the first time.

prognostic Related to prediction of the outcome of a disease.

proliferation Increasing or spreading at a rapid rate; the process or results of rapid reproduction.

prophylactic Any agent or regimen that contributes to the prevention of infection and disease.

prostration A condition of extreme exhaustion.

proteolytic An enzyme producing proteolysis.

protocol(s) A standard sequential way of performing work. Usually consists of algorithms involving diagnostic and therapeutic components (e.g., Mechanical Ventilation Protocol).

proximal Nearest the point of attachment, center of the body, or point of reference.

Pseudomonas aeruginosa A species of gram-negative, non–spore-forming, motile bacteria that may cause various human diseases ranging from purulent meningitis to nosocomial infected wounds.

ptosis An abnormal condition of one or both upper eyelids in which the eyelid droops because of a congenital or acquired weakness of the levator muscle or paralysis of the third cranial nerve. The condition may be treated surgically by shortening the levator muscle.

pulmonary Concerning or involving the lungs.

pulmonary alveolar proteinosis A condition in which the air sacs of the lungs become filled with protein and lipids, progressing to respiratory failure. The cause is unknown.

pulmonary angiography The radiographic examination of the blood vessels of the lungs after the injection of radiopaque contrast medium into the pulmonary circulation. It is used to detect pulmonary emboli.

pulmonary artery catheter Any of various cardiac catheters for measuring pulmonary arterial pressures, introduced into the venous system through a large vein and guided by blood flow into the superior vena cava, the right atrium and ventricle, and the pulmonary artery.

pulmonary blood vessels Vessels that transport blood from the heart to the lungs and then back to the heart.

pulmonary circulation Passage of blood from the heart to the lungs and back again for gas exchange. The blood flows from the right ventricle to the lungs, where it is oxygenated and carbon dioxide is removed. The blood then flows back to the left atrium.

pulmonary embolectomy A surgical incision into a pulmonary artery for the removal of an embolus or clot, performed as emergency treatment for arterial embolism. The operation is done as soon as possible after a decrease in perfusion is detected. Before surgery, heparin may be administered, and an arteriogram may be used to identify the affected artery. A longitudinal incision is made in the artery and the embolus is removed. After surgery the blood pressure is maintained close to the level of the preoperative baseline, as a decrease might predispose to new clot formation.

pulse The regular, recurrent expansion and contraction of an artery, produced by waves of pressure caused by the ejection of blood from the left ventricle of the heart as it contracts. The pulse is easily detected on superficial arteries, such as the radial and carotid arteries, and corresponds to each beat of the heart.

pulse oximetry (SpO₂) A device that measures the amount of saturated hemoglobin in the tissue capillaries by transmitting a beam of light through the tissue to a receiver. This noninvasive method of measuring the saturated hemoglobin is a useful screening tool for determining basic respiratory function. This cliplike device may be used on either the earlobe or the fingertip. As the amount of saturated hemoglobin alters the wavelengths of the transmitted light, analysis of the received light is translated into a percentage of oxygen saturation (SO₂) of the blood. Also called (informally) *pulse ox.*

pulsus alternans A pulse characterized by a regular alternation of weak and strong beats without changes in the pulse rate.

pulsus paradoxus An exaggeration of the normal variation in the pulse volume with respiration. The pulse becomes weaker with inspiration and stronger with expiration. Pulsus paradoxus is characteristic of constrictive pericarditis and pericardial effusion. The changes are independent of changes in pulse rate.

purulent Containing or forming pus.

pyrexia An elevation of body temperature above the normal circadian range as a result of an increase in the body's core temperature.

radial pulse The pulse of the radial artery palpated at the wrist over the radius. The radial pulse is the one most often taken because of the ease with which it is palpated.

radiation therapy The treatment of neoplastic disease by using x-rays or gamma rays to deter the proliferation of malignant cells by decreasing the rate of mitosis or impairing DNA synthesis.

radiodensity The ability to stop or reduce the passage of x-rays. Bones have relative high radiopacity and therefore display as white areas on an exposed x-ray film. Lead has marked radiopacity and therefore is widely used to shield x-ray equipment and atomic power sources.

radiolucency The ability of materials of relatively low atomic number to allow most x-rays to pass through them, producing dark images on x-ray film, e.g. air.

radiopaque Impenetrable to x-radiation or other forms of radiation.

rapid eye movement (REM) sleep The stage of sleep that can be detected with an Electroencephalogram (EEG) and electrodes placed on the skin around the eyes so that tiny electric discharges from contractions of the eye muscles are transmitted to recording equipment. The REM sleep periods, lasting from a few minutes to half an hour, alternate with the non–rapid eye movement (NREM) periods. Dreaming occurs during REM time. Individual sleep patterns normally change throughout life because daily requirements for sleep gradually diminish from as much as 20 hours a day in infancy to as little as 6 hours a day in old age. Infants tend to begin a sleep period with REM sleep, whereas REM activity usually follows the four stages of NREM sleep in adults.

rectus abdominis One of a pair of anterolateral muscles of the abdomen, extending the whole length of the ventral aspect of the abdomen. The pair is separated by the linea alba. Each rectus arises in a lateral tendon from the crest of the pubis and is interlaced by a medial tendon with the muscle of the opposite side. The rectus abdominis inserts into the fifth, sixth, and seventh ribs. It functions to flex the vertebral column, tense the anterior abdominal wall, and assist in compressing the abdominal contents.

recumbent Lying down or leaning backward.

red blood cell (RBC) count A count of the number of erythrocytes in a specimen of whole blood, commonly made with an electronic counting device. The normal RBC count in the whole blood of males is between 4.6 to 6.2 million/mm^3. In females the count varies between 4.2 to 5.4 million/mm^3.

red blood cell indices A test routinely performed as part of a complete blood count to obtain information about the size, weight, and hemoglobin concentration of RBCs.

refractory Resistant to ordinary treatment; obstinate, stubborn.

remission Lessening of severity or abatement of symptoms; the period during which symptoms abate.

remittent fever Diurnal variations of an elevated temperature with exacerbations and remissions but never a return to normal.

residual volume (RV) The amount of air remaining in the lungs at the end of a maximum expiration.

residual volume/total lung capacity ratio The amount of air remaining in the lungs at the end of a maximum expiration/the volume of gas in the lungs at the end of a maximum inspiration. It equals the vital capacity plus the residual capacity.

respiration The molecular exchange of oxygen and carbon dioxide within the body's tissues.

resistance The property of being resistant (opposed) to a substance (e.g., antibiotic resistance) or therapy (e.g., CPAP resistant).

reteplase A recombinant form of tissue plasminogen activator used intravenously as a thrombolytic agent in treatment of myocardial infarction.

reticular formation Located in the brain stem, it acts as a filter from sense organs to the conscious brain. It analyzes incoming information for importance and influences alertness, waking, sleeping, and some reflexes.

rheumatoid arthritis A chronic, inflammatory, destructive, and sometimes deforming collagen disease that has an autoimmune component. It is characterized by symmetrical inflammation of synovial membranes and increased synovial exudate, leading to thickening of the membranes and swelling of the joints. Rheumatoid arthritis usually first appears when patients, most often women, are between 36 and 50 years of age. The course of the disease is variable but is most frequently marked by alternating periods of remission and exacerbation.

ribonucleic acid (RNA) Nucleic acid occurring in the nucleus and cytoplasm of cells that is involved in the synthesis of proteins. The RNA molecule is a single strand made up of nucleotides.

roentgenogram Film produced by roentgenography. Also referred to as an *x-ray*.

roentgenography Process of obtaining x-rays by the use of roentgen rays.

sawtooth waves Notched-jagged Electroencephalogram (EEG) waves of frequency in the theta range (3 to 7 Hz). They are commonly seen during REM sleep. Although sawtooth waves are not part of the criteria for REM sleep, their presence is a clue that REM sleep is present.

scalene Pertaining to one of the scalenus muscles or to lymph nodes near the scalene muscles.

scaphoid abdomen An abdomen with a sunken anterior wall.

scintillation camera Camera used to photograph the emissions that come from radioactive substances injected into the body.

segmentectomy Removal of a lung segment or segments of the lung.

semilunar valves Valves separating the left ventricle and aorta and right ventricle and pulmonary artery. Also referred to as the *aortic and pulmonary valves*.

semipermeable Permitting diffusion or flow of some liquids or particles but preventing the transmission of others, usually used in reference to a membrane.

septicemia Systemic disease caused by pathogenic organisms or toxins in the blood; may be a late development of any purulent infection.

septum Wall dividing two cavities.

serotonin Chemical present in platelets, gastrointestinal mucosa, mast cells, and carcinoid tumors; a potent vasoconstrictor.

serum (1) Clear, watery fluid, especially that moistening surfaces of serous membranes; (2) fluid exuded in inflammation of any of those membranes; (3) the fluid portion of the blood obtained after removal of the fibrin clot and blood cells; (4) sometimes used as a synonym for *antiserum*.

sibilant Hissing or whistling; applied to sounds heard in a certain crackle (or rhonchus).

sign Any objective evidence or manifestation of an illness or disordered function of the body. Signs are more or less definitive, obvious, and, apart from the patient's impressions, in contrast to symptoms, which are subjective.

silence Absence of noise or a state of producing no detectable signs or symptoms.

silica Silicon dioxide, an inorganic compound occurring in nature as agate, sand, amethyst, flint, quartz, and other stones. It is one of the major constituents of dental porcelain and a common filler in resin composites. In granular form it serves as a dental abrasive and polishing agent.

silicate Salt of silicic acid.

sinus arrhythmia An irregular cardiac rhythm in which the heart rate usually increases during inspiration and decreases during expiration. It is common in children and young adults and has no clinical significance except in elderly patients.

sinus bradycardia Beating of the sinus node at a rate below 60/min.

sinus tachycardia Uncomplicated tachycardia when sinus cardiac rhythm is faster than 100 bpm.

sleep spindles Are sudden bursts of EEG activity in the 12 to 14 Hz frequency (6 or more distinct waves) and duration of 0.5 to 1.5 seconds. Sleep spindles mark the onset of Stage N2. They may be seen in Stage N3, but usually do not occur in REM sleep.

small cell (or oat-cell carcinoma) A malignant, usually bronchogenic epithelial neoplasm consisting of small, tightly packed round, oval, or spindle-shaped epithelial cells that stain darkly and contain neurosecretory granules and little or no cytoplasm. Tumors produced by these cells do not form bulky masses but usually spread along submucosal lymphatics. Many malignant tumors of the lung are of this type. Usually surgical resection is not possible and chemotherapy and radiation therapy are not effective in treatment; thus the long-term prognosis is poor.

smooth muscle Muscle tissue that lacks cross-striations on its fibers; involuntary in action and found principally in visceral organs.

SOAP In a problem-oriented medical record, an abbreviation for *subjective*, *objective*, *assessment*, and *plan*, the four parts of a written account of the health problem. In taking and charting the patient history and physical examination, a SOAP statement is made for each syndrome, problem, symptom, or diagnosis. Charting by this method is said to be "soaped," and charts produced by using it are called "soap charts."

somatic nerve Nerve that innervates somatic structures (i.e., those constituting the body wall and extremities).

spasm Involuntary sudden movement or convulsive muscular contraction. Spasms may be clonic or tonic.

sphygmomanometer Instrument for determining arterial blood pressure non-invasive.

spinal fusion The fixation of an unstable segment of the spine, accomplished sometimes by skeletal traction or immobilization of the patient in a body cast but most frequently by a surgical procedure. Operative ankylosis may be performed in the treatment of spinal fractures or after diskectomy or laminectomy for the correction of a herniated vertebral disk. Surgical fusion involves the stabilization of a spinal section with a bone graft or synthetic device introduced through a posterior incision in the lumbar region; in the less frequently fused cervical region the incision may be anterior or posterior.

spontaneous pneumothorax The presence of air or gas in the pleural space as a result of a rupture of the lung parenchyma and visceral pleura with no demonstrable cause.

sputum Substance expelled by coughing or clearing the throat. It may contain cellular debris, mucus, blood, pus, caseous material, and microorganisms.

sputum culture A test for pathogenic bacteria in the sputum of patients with respiratory infections.

squamous cell carcinoma A slow-growing malignant tumor of squamous epithelium, frequently found in the lungs and skin, and occurring also in the anus, cervix, larynx, nose, and bladder. The neoplastic cells characteristically resemble prickle cells and form keratin pearls.

staging The classification of phases, quantity, or periods of a disease or other pathologic process, as in the TMN clinical method of assigning numerical values to various stages of tumor development.

stasis Stagnation of the normal flow of fluids, as of the blood, urine, or intestinal mechanism.

static lung compliance the change in volume for any given applied pressure during periods without gas flow, such an during an inspiratory pause (i.e., end-inspiration) (see dynamic lung compliance).

status asthmaticus Persistent and intractable asthma.

sternocleidomastoid A muscle of the neck that is attached to the mastoid process of the temporal bone and to the superior nuchal line and by separate heads to the sternum and clavicle. They function together to flex the head.

stridor An abnormal, high-pitched musical sound caused by an obstruction in the trachea or larynx. It is usually heard during inspiration. Stridor may indicate several neoplastic or inflammatory conditions, including glottic edema, asthma, diphtheria, laryngospasm, and papilloma.

stroke volume (SV) Amount of blood ejected by the ventricle at each beat.

subarachnoid space Space occupied by cerebrospinal fluid beneath the arachnoid membrane surrounding the brain and spinal cord.

subcutaneous Beneath the skin.

subcutaneous emphysema The presence of air or gas in the subcutaneous tissues. The air or gas may originate in the rupture of an airway or alveolus and migrate through the subpleural spaces to the mediastinum and neck. The face, neck, and chest may appear swollen. Skin tissues can be painful and may produce a crackling or popping sound as air moves under them. The patient may experience dyspnea and appear cyanotic if the air leak is severe. Treatment may require an incision to release the trapped air.

sulfur dioxide Common industrial air pollutant; causes bronchospasm and cell destruction.

superficial Confined to the surface.

superior vena cava Venous trunk draining blood from the head, neck, upper extremities, and chest. It begins by union of the two brachiocephalic veins, passes directly downward, and empties into the right atrium of the heart.

superior vena cava syndrome A condition of edema and engorgement of the veins of the upper body caused by obstruction of the superior vena cava by thrombi or primary pulmonary tumors. Signs and symptoms include a nonproductive cough, breathing difficulty, cyanosis, central nervous system disorders, and edema of the conjunctiva, trachea, and esophagus.

surface tension Condition at the surface of a liquid in contact with a gas or another liquid. It is the result of the mutual attraction of molecules to produce a cohesive state, which causes liquids to assume a shape presenting the smallest surface area to the surrounding medium. It accounts for the spheric shape assumed by fluids such as drops of oil or water.

surfactant Phospholipid substance important in controlling the surface tension of the air-liquid emulsion in the lungs; an agent that lowers the surface tension.

symmetrical Equal correspondence in shape, size, and relative position of parts on opposite sides of the body.

sympathomimetic Producing effects resembling those resulting from stimulation of the sympathetic nervous system, such as the effects following the injection of epinephrine.

symptom Any perceptible change in the body or its functions that indicates disease or the phases of a disease. Symptoms may be classified as objective, subjective, cardinal, and sometimes constitutional. However, another classification considers all symptoms as being subjective, with objective indications being called *signs*.

syncope Transient loss of consciousness resulting from inadequate blood flow to the brain.

syncytial Group of cells in which the protoplasm of one cell is continuous with that of adjoining cells.

syncytium A group of cells in which the cytoplasm of one cell is continuous with that of adjoining cells, resulting in a multinucleate unit.

systemic Pertaining to the whole body rather than to one of its parts.

systemic reaction Whole-body response to a stimulus.

systole Part of the heart cycle in which the heart is in contraction.

systolic blood pressure Maximum blood pressure; occurs during contraction of the ventricle.

T wave The component of the cardiac cycle shown on an electrocardiogram as a short, inverted, U-shaped curve after the S-T segment. It represents membrane repolarization phase 3 of the cardiac action potential.

tachycardia Abnormal rapidity of heart action, usually defined as a heart rate >100 bpm.

tachypnea A rapid breathing rate.

tactile fremitus A tremulous vibration of the chest wall during speaking that is palpable on physical examination. Tactile fremitus may be decreased or absent when vibrations from the larynx to the chest surface are impeded by chronic obstructive pulmonary disease, obstruction, pleural effusion, or pneumothorax. It is increased in pneumonia.

talc A native, hydrous magnesium silicate, sometimes containing a small proportion of aluminum silicate, used as a dusting powder and adsorbent in clarifying liquids.

temporal pulse The pulse points over the temporal artery in front of the ear.

tenacious Adhering to; adhesive; retentive.

tension of gas Gas pressure measured in millimeters of mercury (mm Hg).

tension pneumothorax Presence of air in the pleural space when pleural pressure exceeds alveolar pressure, caused by a rupture through the chest wall or lung parenchyma associated with the valvular opening. Air passes through the valve during coughing but cannot escape on exhalation. Unrelieved pneumothorax can lead to respiratory arrest.

theta waves Of the several types of electroencephalogram (EEG) waves, characterized by a relatively low frequency of 4 to 7 Hz and a low amplitude of 10 µV. Theta waves are the "drowsy waves" of the temporal lobes of the brain and appear in electroencephalograms when the individual is awake but relaxed and sleepy. Also called **theta rhythm**.

third degree burns In third-degree burns, the entire thickness of the epidermis and dermis is destroyed.

thoracentesis The surgical perforation of the chest wall and pleural space with a needle to aspirate fluid for diagnostic or therapeutic purposes or to remove a specimen for biopsy. The procedure is usually performed using local anesthesia, with the patient in an upright position. Thoracentesis may be used to aspirate fluid to treat pleural effusion or to collect fluid samples for culture or examination.

thrombocytopenia Abnormal decrease in the number of blood platelets.

thromboembolism Blood clot caused by an embolus obstructing a vessel.

thrombophlebitis Inflammation of a vein in conjunction with the formation of a thrombus; usually occurs in an extremity, most frequently a leg.

thrombus Blood clot that obstructs a blood vessel or a cavity of the heart.

thymectomy Surgical removal of the thymus gland.

thymoma A usually benign tumor of the thymus gland that may be associated with myasthenia gravis or an immune-deficiency disorder.

thymus Ductless gland situated in the anterior mediastinal cavity that reaches maximum development during early childhood and then undergoes involution. It usually has two longitudinal lobes. An endocrine gland, the thymus is now thought to be a lymphoid body. It is a site of lymphopoiesis and plays a role in immunologic competence.

tidal volume (V$_T$) The amount of air inhaled and exhaled per breath during normal ventilation. Inspiratory reserve volume, expiratory reserve volume, and tidal volume make up vital capacity.

titer A measurement of the concentration of a substance in a solution.

tone The state of a body or any of its organs or parts in which the functions are healthy and normal. In a more restricted sense, the resistance of muscles to passive elongation or stretch; normal tension or responsiveness to stimuli.

total lung capacity (TLC) The volume of gas in the lungs at the end of a maximum inspiration. It equals the vital capacity plus the residual capacity.

toxemia The condition resulting from the spread of bacterial products via the bloodstream; toxemic condition resulting from metabolic disturbances.

toxin Poisonous substance of animal or plant origin.

trachea Largest airway; a fibroelastic tube found at the level of the sixth cervical vertebra to the fifth thoracic vertebra; carries air to and from the lungs. At the carina it divides into two bronchi, one leading to each lung. The trachea is lined with mucous membrane, and its inner surface is lined with ciliated epithelium.

tracheobronchial clearance Mechanisms by which the airways are cleared of foreign substances; the act of clearing the airways by mucociliary action, coughing, or macrophages.

tracheostomy Operation entailing cutting into the trachea through the neck, usually for insertion of a tube to overcome upper airway obstruction.

tracheotomy Incision of the skin, muscles, and trachea.

transfusion Injection of blood or a blood component into the bloodstream; transfer of the blood of one person into the blood vessels of another.

transillumination The passage of light through body tissues for the purpose of examining a structure interposed between the observer and the light source. A diaphanoscope is an instrument introduced into a body cavity to transilluminate tissues.

translucent Transmitting light, but diffusing it so that objects beyond are not clearly distinguishable.

transmission Transference of disease or infection.

transpulmonary pressure The pressure difference between the mouth and intrapleural pressure.

transudate A fluid passed through a membrane or squeezed through a tissue or into the space between the cells of a tissue. It is thin and watery and contains few blood cells or other large proteins.

transverse Describing the state of something that is lying across or at right angles to something else; lying at right angles to the long axis of the body.

trauma Physical injury or wound caused by external forces.

tricuspid valve Right atrioventricular valve separating the right atrium from the right ventricle.

trypsin Proteolytic enzyme of the pancreas.

tuberculosis Infectious disease caused by the tubercle bacillus *Mycobacterium tuberculosis* and characterized by inflammatory infiltrations, formation of tubercles, caseation, necrosis, abscesses, fibrosis, and calcification. It most commonly affects the respiratory system.

ulcerate To produce or become affected with an open sore or lesion of the skin.

underventilation Reduced rate and depth of breathing.

uremia Toxic condition associated with renal insufficiency that is produced by retention in the blood of nitrogenous substances normally excreted by the kidney.

vaccinia A contagious disease of cattle that is produced in humans by inoculation with cowpox virus to confer immunity against smallpox.

vagus Pneumogastric or tenth cranial nerve. It is a mixed nerve, having motor and sensory functions and a wider distribution than any of the other cranial nerves.

varicella Chickenpox.

vasoactive Substances tending to cause vasodilation or vasoconstriction.

vasoconstriction Constriction of the blood vessels.

vasodilation An increase in the diameter of a blood vessel. It is caused by a relaxation of the smooth muscles in the vessel wall.

venous stasis Stagnation of the normal flow of blood caused by venous congestion.

ventilation Mechanical movement of air into and out of the lungs in a cyclic manner. The activity is autonomic and voluntary and has two components—an inward flow of air, called *inhalation* or *inspiration*, and an outward flow, called *exhalation* or *expiration*.

ventilatory rate The frequency of breathing per minute.

ventricle Either of the two lower chambers of the heart. The right ventricle forces blood into the pulmonary artery, the left into the aorta.

ventricular fibrillation A cardiac arrhythmia marked by rapid depolarizations of the ventricular myocardium. The condition is characterized by a complete lack of organized electric activity and of ventricular ejection. Blood pressure falls to zero, resulting in unconsciousness. Death may occur within 4 minutes. Cardiopulmonary resuscitation must be initiated immediately, with defibrillation and resuscitative medications given according to advanced cardiac life support protocol.

ventricular flutter A condition of very rapid contractions of the ventricles of the heart. Electrocardiograms show poorly defined QRS complexes occurring at a rate of 250 bpm or higher. Cardiac output is severely compromised or absent. The condition is fatal if untreated.

ventricular tachycardia Tachycardia with at least three consecutive ventricular complexes having a rate >100 bpm. It usually originates in a focus distal to the branching of the atrioventricular bundle.

verapamil A calcium channel blocker.

vernix Protective fatty deposit covering the fetus.

vertex waves Sharp negative (upward deflection) EEG waves, often in conjunction with high amplitude and short (2 to 7 Hz)

activity. The amplitude of many of the vertex sharp waves are greater than 20 µV and, occasionally, they may be as high as 200 µV. Vertex waves are usually seen at the end of Stage N1.

vesicular breath sound A normal sound of rustling or swishing heard with a stethoscope over the lung periphery. It characteristically has a higher pitch during inspiration and fades rapidly during expiration.

visceral pleura Pleura that invests the lungs and enters into and lines the interlobar fissures.

viscosity Stickiness or gumminess; resistance offered by a fluid to change of form or relative position of its particles caused by the attraction of molecules to one another.

viscous Sticky; gummy; gelatinous.

viscus Any internal organ enclosed within a cavity such as the thorax or abdomen.

vital capacity (VC) The maximum volume of air that can be expelled at the normal rate of exhalation after a maximum inspiration, representing the greatest possible breathing capacity.

vocal fremitus The vibration of the chest wall as a person speaks or sings that allows the person's voice to be heard by auscultation of the chest with a stethoscope.

volume percent (vol%) The number of cubic centimeters (milliliters) of a substance contained in 100 cc (or mL) of another substance.

walking pneumonia The phrase "walking pneumonia" has no clinical significance; it is often used to describe a mild case of pneumonia. For example, patients infected with *Mycoplasma pneumoniae*, who generally have mild symptoms and remain ambulatory, are sometimes told that they have walking pneumonia.

wedge resection The surgical excision of part of an organ, such as part of an ovary containing a cyst. The segment excised may be wedge-shaped.

wheal More or less round and evanescent elevation of the skin, white in the center, with a red periphery. It is accompanied by itching and is seen in urticaria, insect bites, anaphylaxis, and angioneurotic edema.

wheeze A form of rhonchus, characterized by a high-pitched or low-pitched musical quality. It is caused by a high-velocity flow of air through a narrowed airway and is heard during both inspiration and expiration. It may be caused by bronchospasm, inflammation, or obstruction of the airway by a tumor or foreign body. Wheezes are associated with asthma and chronic bronchitis. Unilateral wheezes are characteristic of bronchogenic carcinoma, foreign bodies, and inflammatory lesions. In asthma, expiratory wheezing is more common, although inspiratory and expiratory wheezes are heard.

whispering pectoriloquy The term used to describe the unusually clear transmission of the whispered voice of a patient as heard through the stethoscope.

white blood cell (WBC) count An examination and enumeration of the distribution of leukocytes in a stained blood smear. The different types of white cells are counted and reported as percentages of the total examined. Differential WBC count provides more specific information related to infections and diseases. Also called **differential leukocyte count**.

xenon-133 Radioactive isotope of xenon used in photo scanning studies of the lung.

Index

Modified British Medical Research Council (mMRC) Breathlessness Scale, 175
Modified Evan's blue dye test, unreliability, 258
Modified Medical Research Council Questionnaire, 175t
MODS. *See* Multi-organ dysfunction syndrome
Monocytes, 110
Morphine sulfate, 299
MRA. *See* Magnetic resonance angiography
MRI. *See* Magnetic resonance imaging
MRSA. *See* Methicillin-resistant *Staphylococcus aureus*
Mucociliary escalator, 41
Mucociliary transport, 41
Mucolytic agents, usage, 187
Mucous accumulation, 28f
  airway obstruction, combination, 412
  plug, 202f
Mucous blanket, 39–40
  production, 40–41
Multi-organ dysfunction syndrome (MODS), 544
Multiple drug-resistant *S. aureus* (MDRSA), 255
Multiple drug-resistant tuberculosis (MDRTB), 280
Muscle-specific receptor tyrosine kinase (MuSK), 412
Muscular ventricular septal defect, 519
Mutation analysis, 240
MVV. *See* Maximum voluntary ventilation
Myasthenia gravis
  acetylcholinesterase inhibitors, impact, 416
  admitting history, 417
  alveolar consolidation, 412
  anticholinesterase inhibitors, effectiveness, 416
  arterial blood gases, 415b
  atelectasis, 412
  bronchopulmonary hygiene therapy protocol, 416
  cardiopulmonary clinical manifestations, 415
  case study, 417–419
  chest assessment findings, 415
  chest radiograph, 415
  clinical classifications, 414b
  clinical presentation, 413
  conditions, evaluation, 414
  diagnosis, 413–414
  diagnostic tests (bedside diagnostic tests), 413
  differential diagnosis, 414
  discussion, 418–419
  edrophonium test (tensilon test), 413
  electrodiagnostic studies, 414
  electromyography, usage, 417
  etiology/epidemiology, 412–413
  gastric contents, aspiration, 418
  generalized myasthenia gravis, 411
  history, 413
  ice pack test, 413, 413f
  immunologic studies, 413–414
  immunotherapy, usage, 416
  impact, 412f
  intravenous immune globulin (IVIG), usage, 416
  laboratory tests/procedures, clinical data, 415
  lung expansion therapy protocol, 417
  lungs, anatomic alterations, 411–412
  management, 416–417
  maximum expiratory pressure (MEP), 416
  maximum inspiratory pressure (MIP), 416
  mechanical ventilation protocol, 417
  mucous accumulation, airway obstruction (combination), 412
  mycophenolate mofetil, usage, 416
  ocular myasthenia gravis, 411
  oxygenation indices, 415b
  oxygen therapy protocol, 416
  patient bedside, clinical data, 415
  physical examination, 415
  plasmapheresis (plasma exchange), 416
  pulmonary function test findings, 415b
  pulmonary function testing, 414
  pyridostigmine (Mestinon), selection, 416
  radiologic findings, 415
  rapid immunotherapies, 416
  repetitive nerve stimulation (RNS), 414
  respiratory assessment/pain, 417–418
  respiratory care treatment protocols, 416–417
  screening, 413–414
  seronegative myasthenia gravis, 412
  seropositive myasthenia gravis, 412
  signs/symptoms, 413
  thymectomy, 416

Myasthenic crisis, 412
Mycobacterium avium complex (MAC), 260
Mycobacterium tuberculosis, 105
  cultural appearance, 277f
  impact, 259
Mycophenolate mofetil, usage, 416
Mycoplasma organism, impact, 256
Mycoplasma pneumoniae
  cell wall, absence, 256f
  infection, 196, 254
Mycosis, 284
Mycotic disease, 284
Myocardial ischemia, 37
Myocoplasma organism, symptoms, 256
MZ phenotype, 173–174

N

N-3 polyunsaturated fatty acid, decrease, 206
N-6 polyunsaturated fatty acid, increase, 206
NAEPP. *See* National Asthma Education and Prevention
Narrative, assistance, 4–5
Nasal cannula
  high flow nasal cannula, 453
  usage, 452–453
Nasal flaring, 37, 446–447
Nasal polyps
  asthma, 215
  cystic fibrosis, 243
Nasal potential difference (NPD), 240
National Asthma Education and Prevention (NAEPP), 201, 211
  Expert Panel Report 3 (EPR-3), 201
National Heart, Lung, and Blood Institute (NHLBI), 201
National Institutes of Health (NIH), 201
Natural killer cells, 111
NCFB. *See* Noncystic fibrosis bronchiectasis
NCS. *See* Nerve conduction studies
Near drowning
  cold-water near drowning, prognostic factors, 536t
  etiology/epidemiology, 536
  lungs, anatomic alterations, 535–536
  sequence, 536b
Near wet drowning
  admitting history, 539
  apnea, 537
  cardiopulmonary clinical manifestations, 537–538
  case study, 539–540
  chest radiograph, 538
  diffusion capacity, decrease, 537b
  discussion, 540
  first responder, 538
  hospital management, 538–539
  laboratory tests/procedures, clinical data, 537
  management, 538–539
  oxygenation indices, 537b
  patient bedside, clinical data, 537
  physical examination, 537
  pulmonary function test findings, 537b
  radiograph, 538f
  radiologic findings, 538
  respiratory assessment/pain, 539–540
  respiratory rate (tachypnea), increase, 537
  vital signs, 537
  warming techniques, 539
Nebulized hypertonic saline, usage (consideration), 495–496
Necrotizing pneumonia, 254, 260
Needle thoracentesis, 488
Negative inspiratory force (NIF), 52
Negative intrapleural pressures
  clinical manifestations, 447
  increase, clinical manifestations, 447f
Neonatal intensive care unit (NICU), infant (placement), 474
Neonates
  clinical manifestations, 450f–451f
  persistent pulmonary hypertension, 464, 517
Neoplasm, 374
Nephrotic syndrome, 338
Nerve conduction studies (NCS), 405–406
Neuromuscular junction, 411
Neuromuscular scoliosis, 346
Neutrophils, 110
  band forms, 110

Newborn
  applicable techniques, 454
  applications, 455
  arterial blood gases, 448–449
  assessment, 449, 458
  bolus dosing procedure, 461
  bronchoscopy, 455
  bubble nasal CPAP (B-NCPAP), 455
  chest physical therapy, 454
  clinical condition
    adjustment/weaning, 460
    worsening, adjustments, 459–460
  clinical improvement
    adjustments/weaning, usage, 459
    techniques, assessment, 455
  clinical manifestations, 446
  conditions (worsening), adjustment/weaning, 461
  continuous albuterol aerosol, 457
  cough, 454
    assist, 454
  CPAP
    bag/mask, usage, 455
    therapy, 456
  deep breathing, 454
  drip dosing procedure, 461–462
  dry powder inhalers (DPIs), usage, 457
  endotracheal CPAP, 455
  expiratory grunting, 447
  flaring nostrils (nasal flaring), 447
  flutter valve, 454
  hand-held nebulizer, usage, 457
  head bobbing, 447
  high flow nasal cannula, 455
  high frequency ventilation (HFV), 459
  inspiratory time, 459
  IPPB therapy, 456
  IPV/MetaNeb, 454–455
  medicated aerosol, usage, 457
  metered dose inhaler, usage, 457
  modes, 459
  monitoring, 459
  nasal CPAP, 455
  negative intrapleural pressure, increase (clinical manifestations), 447f
  noninvasive positive pressure ventilation (NIPPV), 459
  oscillatory positive expiratory pressure, 444
  oxygen toxicity, 449
  partial pressure of oxygen, 18t
  peak inspiratory pressure (PIP), 459
  pediatric application, 456
  PEP, 454
  percussion, 454
  percussive vest therapy, 454
  periodic breathing, 447
  postural drainage, 454
  pressure support, 459
  pulse oximetry, 18t
  respiratory rate (RR), 459
  settings, 459
  SpO_2/PaO_2 relationships, 449t
  suctioning, 454
  therapy, weaning, 455
  thorax, flexibility, 447
  treatment protocols, 452–462
  valved holding chamber/spacer, 457
  ventilator nasal CPAP (V-NCPAP), 455
  volume-targeted mode, 459
  weaning, 458
New bronchopulmonary dysplasia
  diagnostic criteria, 503t
  lungs, anatomic alterations, 501–502
    alveolar hypoplasia, 502
NHLBI. *See* National Heart, Lung, and Blood Institute
Nicotine replacement products, 186
NICU. *See* Neonatal intensive care unit
NIH. *See* National Institutes of Health
NIPPV. *See* Noninvasive positive pressure ventilation
Nitrogen washout method, usage, 49f
Nitroglycerin (Nitro-Bid) (Minitra) (Nitrostat), 299
Nitroprusside (Nitropress), usage, 299
NIV. *See* Noninvasive ventilation
Nocardia, 260
Nocturnal asthma (sleep), 206
Nonallergic asthma, 204
Nonatopic asthma, 204

Wegener's granulomatosis, 364–365
  nodules, presence, 369f
Wells Clinical Prediction Rule, 304
Wells Scoring System, 304
Wet drowning
  etiology/epidemiology, 536
  lungs, anatomic alterations, 535–536
  near wet drowning, 537–538
  pulmonary pathologic/structural changes, 535–536
Wheezes, 25
  bibasilar wheezes, 193
  representation, 26f

Wheezing, development, 28f
Whirlpool therapy (hydrotherapy), 408
Whispered voice sounds, auscultation, 28f
Whispering pectoriloquy, 25
  representation, 28f
White blood cell (WBC)
  cell, increase (causes), 110t
  count, 108–111
    differential WBC count, 110b
Whiteout, presence, 480f
Why questions, usage, 6
Work efficiency, 63

Work of breathing, 28–30
World Health Organization (WHO), 201
  asthma estimates, 203

X

Xanthine derivatives, 187t
XDRTB. *See* Extensively drug-resistant TB

Z

Ziehl-Neelsen stain, 276–277
ZZ phenotype, 173–174